NUCLEAR CARDIOLOGY
STATE OF THE ART AND FUTURE DIRECTIONS
SECOND EDITION

NUCLEAR CARDIOLOGY
STATE OF THE ART AND FUTURE DIRECTIONS
SECOND EDITION

Barry L. Zaret, M.D.

Robert W. Berliner Professor of Medicine
Professor of Diagnostic Radiology
Chief, Section of Cardiovascular Medicine
Associate Chair for Clinical Affairs, Department of Internal Medicine
Yale University School of Medicine
New Haven, Connecticut

George A. Beller, M.D.

Ruth C. Heede Professor of Cardiology
Chief, Cardiovascular Division
Vice Chairman, Department of Medicine
University of Virginia Health Sciences Center
Charlottesville, Virginia

*with **643** illustrations including **30** four-color plates*

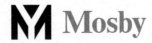

St. Louis Baltimore Boston Carlsbad Chicago Minneapolis New York Philadelphia Portland
London Milan Sydney Tokyo Toronto

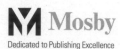

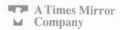

Editor: Elizabeth Corra
Associate Development Editor: Catherine Gray
Project Manager: Linda Clarke
Production Editor: Jennifer Harper
Composition Specialist: Fran D'Alessandro
Designer: Carolyn O'Brien
Cover Design: Maria Bellano
Manufacturing Manager: William A. Winneberger, Jr.
Publisher: Geoff Greenwood

Second Edition

Copyright © 1999 by Mosby, Inc.

Previous edition copyrighted 1993

Composition by Mosby Electronic Production, Philadelphia
Printing/binding by Maple-Vail Book Manufacturing Group

Mosby, Inc.
11830 Westline Industrial Drive
St. Louis, Missouri 63146

Library of Congress Cataloging-in-Publication Data
Nuclear cardiology : state of the art and future directions / [edited
   by] Barry L. Zaret, George A. Beller. — 2nd ed.
      p.   cm.
   Includes bibliographical references and index.
   ISBN 0-8151-1740-X
   1. Heart—Radionuclide imaging.   I. Zaret, Barry L.   II. Beller,
George A.
   [DNLM: 1. Heart—radionuclide imaging.   2. Coronary Disease—
radionuclide imaging.   WG 141.5.R3 N964 1999]
   RC683.5.R33N833   1999
   616.1'207575—dc21
   DNLM/DLC   98-33551
   for Library of Congress   CIP

99 00 01 02 03 / 9 8 7 6 5 4 3 2 1

Contributors

Aman M. Amanullah, M.D., Ph.D.
Assistant Professor of Medicine (Cardiology)
Allegheny University of Health Sciences
Director, Coronary Care Unit
Allegheny University Hospitals—Hahnemann
Philadelphia, Pennsylvania

Stephen L. Bacharach, Ph.D.
Head, Imaging Science Group
National Institutes of Health
Bethesda, Maryland

George A. Beller, M.D.
Ruth C. Heede Professor of Cardiology
Chief, Cardiovascular Division
Vice Chairman, Department of Medicine
University of Virginia Health Sciences Center
Charlottesville, Virginia

Daniel S. Berman, M.D.
Professor of Medicine
UCLA School of Medicine
Director, Nuclear Cardiology
Cedars-Sinai Medical Center
Los Angeles, California

Robert O. Bonow, M.D.
Professor of Medicine
Northwestern University Medical School
Chief, Division of Cardiology
Northwestern Memorial Hospital
Chicago, Illinois

Jeffrey S. Borer, M.D.
Gladys and Roland Harriman Professor of Cardiovascular
   Medicine
Professor of CV Medicine in Radiology
Cornell University Medical College
Attending Physician
The New York Hospital
New York, New York

Kenneth A. Brown, M.D.
Professor of Medicine
University of Vermont College of Medicine
Director, Nuclear Cardiology and Stress Laboratories
Medical Center Hospital of Vermont
Burlington, Vermont

Paul E. Christian, B.S.
Instructor, University of Utah School of Medicine
Director, Nuclear Medicine
University of Utah Health Sciences Center
Salt Lake City, Utah

Timothy F. Christian, M.D.
Associate Professor of Medicine
Mayo Clinic
Rochester, Minnesota

Mylan C. Cohen, M.D., M.P.H.
Cardiology Division, Maine Medical Center
Portland, Maine
University of Vermont College of Medicine
Burlington, Vermont

C. David Cooke, M.S.E.E.
Assistant Professor
Emory University School of Medicine
Division of Nuclear Medicine
Emory University Hospital
Atlanta, Georgia

Seth T. Dahlberg, M.D.
Assistant Professor
Department of Nuclear Medicine
University of Massachusetts Medical Center
Worcester, Massachusetts

Christophe Depre, M.D., Ph.D.
Research Fellow
University Louvain Medical School
Research Fellow
Institute of Cellular Pathology
Brussels, Belgium

E. Gordon DePuey, M.D.

Professor of Radiology
Columbia University College of Physicians and Surgeons
Director of Nuclear Medicine
St. Luke's—Roosevelt Hospital
New York, New York

Sanjay Dhar, M.D.

Senior Cardiology Fellow
Cedars-Sinai Medical Center
Los Angeles, California

Edward V. R. Di Bella, Ph.D.

Assistant Professor
University of Utah
Salt Lake City, Utah

Kim Allen Eagle, M.D.

Associate Professor of Internal Medicine
Associate Chief, Division of Cardiology
Director, Clinical Cardiology
Co-Director, Heart Care Program
University of Michigan Medical Center
Ann Arbor, Michigan

Tracy L. Faber, Ph.D.

Associate Professor of Radiology
Emory University School of Medicine
Atlanta, Georgia

Stefano Foresti, Ph.D.

Staff Scientist and Adjunct Professor
University of Utah
Center for High Performance Computing
Salt Lake City, Utah

Andrea T. Fossati, M.D.

Cardiology Fellow
University of Connecticut
Hartford Hospital
Hartford, Connecticut

John D. Friedman, M.D.

Assistant Clinical Professor of Medicine
University of California, Los Angeles
Associate Director, Nuclear Medicine
Cedars-Sinai Medical Center
Los Angeles, California

Ernest V. Garcia, Ph.D.

Professor of Radiology
Emory University School of Medicine
Director, Emory Center for PET
Emory University Hospital
Atlanta, Georgia

Bernhard L. Gerber, M.D.

University of Louvain—UCL
Assistant Professor of Cardiology
Hopital St. Luc
Brussels, Belgium

Guido Germano, Ph.D., M.B.A.

Associate Professor of Radiological Sciences
UCLA School of Medicine
Director, Nuclear Medicine Physics
Cedars-Sinai Medical Center
Los Angeles, California

Raymond J. Gibbons, M.D.

Professor of Medicine
Mayo Medical School
Consultant in Cardiovascular Diseases
Mayo Clinic
Rochester, Minnesota

David K. Glover, M.E.

Research Assistant Professor
University of Virginia
Charlottesville, Virginia

Robert J. Gropler, M.D.

Associate Professor of Radiology and Medicine
Washington University School of Medicine
Barnes-Jewish Hospital
St. Louis, Missouri

Grant T. Gullberg, Ph.D.

Professor of Radiology
University of Utah
Director of Medical Imaging Research Laboratory
Salt Lake City, Utah

Rory Hachamovitch, M.D.

Assistant Professor of Medicine
Cornell Medical College
Director, Nuclear Cardiology
New York Hospital
New York, New York

Sean Hayes, M.D.

Senior Cardiology Fellow
Cedars-Sinai Medical Center
Los Angeles, California

Gary V. Heller, M.D., Ph.D.

Associate Professor of Medicine and Nuclear Medicine
University of Connecticut School of Medicine
Director, Nuclear Cardiology
Hartford Hospital
Program Director, Cardiovascular Fellowship
UCONN Medical Health Center
Hartford and Farmington, Connecticut

Robert C. Hendel, M.D.

Assistant Professor of Medicine
Northwestern University Medical School
Co-Director, Nuclear Cardiology
Northwestern Memorial Hospital
Chicago, Illinois

Guy R. Heyndrickx, M.D.

Professor of Cardiovascular Physiology
University of Louvain Medical School
Brussels, Belgium
Associate Director
Cardiovascular Center
Aalst, Belgium

Ronald H. Huesman, Ph.D.

Senior Staff Scientist
E. O. Lawrence Berkeley National Laboratory
University of California
Berkeley, California

Ami E. Iskandrian, M.D.

William Penn Snyder III Professor of Medicine
Director, Cardiovascular Research Center
Director, Nuclear Cardiology
Medical College of Pennsylvania and Hahnemann University
Philadelphia, Pennsylvania

Diwakar Jain, M.D.

Assistant Professor of Medicine
Yale University School of Medicine
Attending Physician
Yale New Haven Hospital
New Haven, Connecticut

Robert L. Jesse, Ph.D., M.D.

Assistant Professor of Cardiology
Medical College of Virginia/Virginia Commonwealth University
Co-Director, Acute Cardiac Care Program & Coronary Intensive
    Care Units
Medical College of Virginia/Virginia Commonwealth University
McGuire VA Hospital
Richmond, Virginia

Xingping Kang, M.D.

Research Fellow
Cedars-Sinai Medical Center
Los Angeles, California

Sanjiv Kaul, M.D.

Professor of Medicine
Director, Cardiac Imaging Center
University of Virginia
Charlottesville, Virginia

Hosen Kiat, M.D.

Associate Cardiologist
Sydney Cardiology
Director, Sydney Nuclear Medicine
Westmead, Sydney, Australia

Michael A. King, Ph.D.

Professor of Nuclear Medicine
University of Massachusetts Medical Center
Worcester, Massachusetts

Takashi Kudoh, M.D.

Research Fellow
Department of Nuclear Medicine and Diagnostic Imaging
Kyoto University
Clinical Fellow
Kyoto University Hospital
Kyoto, Japan

Avijit Lahiri, M.B., B.S., M.Sc., M.R.C.P.

Consultant Cardiologist
Northwick Park Hospital
Harrow, Middlesex, United Kingdom

Jeffrey A. Leppo, M.D.

Professor of Medicine and Nuclear Medicine
University of Massachusetts Medical Center
Director of Nuclear Cardiology
Clinical Director of Nuclear Medicine
Worcester, Massachusetts

Howard C. Lewin, M.D.

Assistant Professor of Medicine
University of California, Los Angeles
Co-Director, Nuclear Cardiology Research
Cedars-Sinai Medical Center
Los Angeles, California

Karen E. Linder, M.S., Ph.D.

Research Fellow
Bracco Research USA
Princeton, New Jersey

Jonathan R. Lindner, M.D.

Assistant Professor of Medicine
Cardiovascular Division
University of Virginia
Charlottesville, Virginia

John J. Mahmarian, M.D.

Associate Professor of Medicine
Baylor College of Medicine
Associate Director
Nuclear Cardiology Laboratory, The Methodist Hospital
Co-Medical Director, HeartScan-Houston
Houston, Texas

Ichiro Matsunari, M.D.

Research Fellow
Der Technischen Universität München
Nuklearmedizinische Klinik und Poliklinik
Klinikum rechts der Isar
München, Germany

Jean C. Maublant, M.D., Ph.D.
Professor of Biophysics and Nuclear Medicine
Faculty of Medicine, University of Auvergne
Associate Director of the Division of Nuclear Medicine
Centre Jean Perrin
Clermont-Ferrand, France

Pascal Merlet, M.D.
Head of Clinical Section
Service Hospitalier Frédéric Joliot
Orsay, France

D. Douglas Miller, M.D.
Professor of Internal Medicine
Associate Chairman of Medicine
Saint Louis University School of Medicine
Director, Nuclear Cardiology
Director, SLUCare for Women
Saint Louis University Hospital
St. Louis, Missouri

Andreas J. Morguet, M.D.
Free University of Berlin
Department of Cardiology and Pulmology
Benjamin Franklin University Hospital
Teltow, Germany

Kenneth J. Nichols, Ph.D.
Associate Research Scientist
College of Physicians and Surgeons
Columbia University
Director of Nuclear Cardiology Physics
Division of Cardiology
St. Luke's/Roosevelt Hospital Center
New York, New York

Tsunehiko Nishimura, M.D., Ph.D.
Professor, Tracer Kinetics
Biomedical Research Center
Director, Nuclear Medicine
Osaka University Medical School
Osaka, Japan

Tinsu Pan, Ph.D.
Assistant Professor of Nuclear Medicine
University of Massachusetts Medical Center
Worcester, Massachusetts

Bryan W. Reutter, M.S.
Computer Scientist
Center for Functional Imaging
Lawrence Berkeley National Laboratory
Berkeley, California

Steven G. Ross, Ph.D.
Postdoctoral Fellow
University of Utah, Medical Imaging Research Laboratory
Salt Lake City, Utah

Heinrich R. Schelbert, M.D., Ph.D.
Professor of Pharmacology and Radiological Sciences
Vice Chair, Department of Molecular and Medical Pharmacology
Chief, Nuclear Medicine Service
UCLA School of Medicine
Los Angeles, California

Markus Schwaiger, M.D.
Professor of Nuclear Medicine
Technische Universitaet Muenchen
Nuklearmedizinische Klinik und Poliklinik
Klinikum R. D. Isar der tu Muenchen
Muenchen, Germany

Roxy Senior, M.D., M.R.C.P.
Consultant Cardiologist
Northwick Park Hospital
Harrow, Middlesex, United Kingdom

Albert J. Sinusas, M.D.
Associate Professor of Medicine and Diagnostic Radiology
Yale University School of Medicine
Associate Director, Cardiovascular Nuclear Imaging and Stress
  Laboratories
Yale—New Haven Hospital
New Haven, Connecticut

H. William Strauss, M.D.
Professor of Radiology
Stanford University School of Medicine
Chief, Division of Nuclear Medicine
Stanford University Hospital
Stanford, California

André Syrota, M.D., Ph.D.
Professor of Biophysics and Nuclear Medicine
Commissariat a L'Energie Atomique
Service Hospitalier Frédéric Joliot
Orsay, France

Eiji Tadamura, M.D., Ph.D.
Assistant Professor
Kyoto University Graduate School of Medicine
Kyoto University Hospital
Kyoto, Japan

Heinrich Taegtmeyer, M.D., D. Phil.
Professor of Medicine
University of Texas-Houston Medical School
Co-Director, Division of Cardiology
Hermann Hospital
Houston, Texas

Nagara Tamaki, M.D., Ph.D.
Professor and Chairman
Department of Nuclear Medicine
Hokkaido University School of Medicine
Sapporo, Japan

James L. Tatum, M.D.

Professor of Radiology and Medicine
Chairman, Division of Nuclear Medicine
Director, Nuclear Cardiology
Medical College of Virginia/Virginia Commonwealth University
Richmond, Virginia

Benjamin M. W. Tsui, Ph.D.

Professor of Biomedical Engineering and Radiology
University of North Carolina at Chapel Hill
Chapel Hill, North Carolina

James E. Udelson, M.D.

Associate Professor of Medicine
Tufts University School of Medicine
Director, Nuclear Cardiology
Co-Director, Heart Failure and Transplant Service
New England Medical Center Hospitals
Boston, Massachusetts

Kenneth F. Van Train, M.S.

Director, Computer Research and Development
Cedars-Sinai Medical Center
Los Angeles, California

Jean-Louis J. Vanoverschelde, M.D., Ph.D.

Professor of Cardiology
University of Louvain
Head, Division of Cardiology
Cliniques Universitaires St. Luc
Brussels, Belgium

Mario S. Verani, M.D.

Professor of Medicine
Baylor College of Medicine
Director, Nuclear Cardiology
The Methodist Hospital
Houston, Texas

Frans J. Th. Wackers, M.D.

Professor of Diagnostic Radiology and Medicine
Yale University School of Medicine
Director, Cardiovascular Nuclear Imaging Laboratories
Yale—New Haven Hospital
New Haven, Connecticut

Denny D. Watson, Ph.D.

Professor of Radiology
Director, Nuclear Cardiology
University of Virginia Health Sciences Center
Charlottesville, Virginia

Donald M. Wieland, Ph.D.

Professor of Internal Medicine
University of Michigan Medical Center
Director of Radiopharmaceutical Chemistry
Department of Internal Medicine
Division of Nuclear Medicine
Ann Arbor, Michigan

Barry L. Zaret, M.D.

Robert W. Berliner Professor of Medicine
Professor of Diagnostic Radiology
Chief, Section of Cardiovascular Medicine
Associate Chair for Clinical Affairs, Department of
    Internal Medicine
Yale University School of Medicine
New Haven, Connecticut

Gengsheng Lawrence Zeng, Ph.D.

Assistant Professor
University of Utah
Salt Lake City, Utah

***To our children and daughters-in-law**
Adam and Peggy, Elliot and Owen Zaret,
Michael and Mondy, Amy and Leslie Beller,
and our grandchildren: Jordan Zaret and Maxwell Beller.

Preface to the second edition

It has been 5 years since the publication of the first edition of *Nuclear Cardiology: State of the Art and Future Directions.* During this time, substantial advances have been made in the field of nuclear cardiology. Techniques that were in their infancy at the time of publication of the first edition have emerged as standard techniques: Gated single-photon emission computed tomography (SPECT) with technetium-labeled agents is just one example. Other techniques, such as planar perfusion imaging, have found lesser use. Finally, new approaches have been proposed and are in varying stages of development, validation and clinical application. The goal of the second edition is to address these developments in state-of-the-art reviews by acknowledged experts in the field and to consider the advances that will occupy the field in the next 5 years.

In the second edition, the total number of chapters has expanded from 31 to 37. Of the 37 chapters, 10 represent revisions of chapters published in the initial edition, whereas 27 represent entirely new contributions. Several of the authors who wrote chapters for the first edition have contributed entirely new chapters to the second edition, and many new authors have been recruited for the current edition. Chapters that have been revised have been modified and updated extensively.

The first edition of *Nuclear Cardiology: State of the Art and Future Directions* grew out of an international workshop held in Wintergreen, Virginia. This workshop has continued on a regular basis. However, the nature of this book transcends any one program, and, consequently, the format of the second edition is totally independent of the Wintergreen meetings.

The first section of this book deals with issues relating to radiopharmaceuticals and tracer kinetics. Watson and Glover provide an overview of kinetics and modeling. Maublant reviews issues relating to kinetics on a cellular level, and Dahlberg and Leppo review principles of tracer kinetics as studied in isolated heart models. Sinusas describes tracer kinetics in intact animal models. Gerber, Vanoverschelde, and Heyndrickx discuss animal models for studying positron emission tomography (PET) tracers. Two new chapters address newer radiopharmaceuticals. Nishimura discusses fatty acid analogs. Finally, Strauss and Lindner review current work with the nitroimidazoles, a new class of compounds for imaging hypoxic tissue.

The second section deals with instrumentation. Faber, Garcia, and Cooke review recent developments in SPECT quantification and display. Bacharach deals with new directions in PET

quantification. King, Tsui, and Pan address attentuation and scatter correction for SPECT, and Gullberg et al review principles and experimental data involving dynamic SPECT.

Three chapters address issues relating to measurement of ventricular function with nuclear techniques. Zaret and Jain review data on nonimaging probes. Borer discusses measurement of ventricular function and volume using predominately equilibrium techniques. DePuey and Nichols provide an overview of the newer area of regional and global ventricular functional analysis based on SPECT perfusion imaging.

Myocardial perfusion imaging remains the cornerstone of nuclear cardiology. Ten chapters are devoted to issues relating to myocardial perfusion imaging in patients with chronic stable coronary artery disease. Mahmarian addresses the state of the art for coronary disease detection using thallium-201(^{201}Tl), and Wackers reviews the state of the art for coronary artery disease detection with the newer technetium-99m(^{99m}Tc)– labeled perfusion agents. Berman et al review the general field of dual-isotope imaging, a technique developed and popularized by their laboratory. The issue of detecting coronary artery disease in women is discussed by Heller and Fossati. Iskrandrian discusses the state of the art of pharmacologic stress imaging. Of prime importance to the field are studies relating to outcomes and prognosis, an area reviewed by Brown. Cohen and Eagle discuss preoperative risk stratification, and Hendel reviews the assessment of coronary revascularization. Competing technology has challenged nuclear cardiology and its preeminent role in diagnosis of coronary artery disease. In this regard, Verani reviews issues involved in the comparison of stress echocardiography in nuclear imaging, and Lindner and Kaul discuss alternative nonnuclear myocardial perfusion imaging.

Four chapters are devoted to nuclear cardiology in the assessment of acute ischemic syndromes. Christian and Gibbons address the issue of perfusion studies at rest for assessment of the risk zone in acute myocardial infarction. Beller discusses risk stratification after acute myocardial infarction. Tatum and Jesse address emergency department triage using nuclear techniques. Miller discusses risk stratification in unstable angina pectoris.

Myocardial viability and metabolism has also been a fundamental of the nuclear cardiology armamentarium. Six chapters are devoted to this issue. Bonow discusses assessment of viability with thallium-201, and Udelson addresses assessment of viability using technetium-labeled perfusion agents. Metabolic assessment of viability is discussed and placed in a physiologic perspective by Depre and Taegtmeyer. The use of PET to assess viability using fluorodeoxy glucose is discussed by Morguet and Schelbert, and PET assessment of viability with acetate imaging is reviewed by Gropler. Tamaki and Tadamura address the general area of fatty acid imaging.

Finally, several newer approaches have been used in patient studies. Matsunari, Wieland, and Schwaiger discuss nuclear neurotransmitter imaging with PET or SPECT. Syrota and Merlet discuss receptor imaging. Lahiri and Senior present the general use of nuclear cardiology in the assessment of patients with congestive heart failure.

ACKNOWLEGMENTS

For this book to be published in a manner consistent with our current knowledge base, all authors have been asked to update their chapters with the most current references at the time of review of the copyedited manuscript. We thank all the contributors for responding to this and other requests.

The editorial and organizational assistance initially of Mia Cariño and, more recently, of Liz Corra and Cathy Gray at Mosby is appreciated. We acknowledge the outstanding secretarial support of Astrid Swanson in New Haven, Connecticut, and Jerry Curtis in Charlottesville, Virginia. Without such support, this second edition would not have been possible.

Barry L. Zaret, M.D.
George A. Beller, M.D.

Preface to the first edition

The strength and breadth of nuclear cardiology lie in its great potential for future creative growth. This growth involves the development of new biologically derived radiopharmaceuticals, advanced imaging technologies, and a broad-based set of research and clinical applications involving diagnosis, functional categorization, prognosis, evaluation of therapeutic interventions, and the ability to deal with many of the major investigative issues in contemporary cardiology such as myocardial hibernation, stunning, and viability. From a historical perspective, nuclear cardiology has grown enormously in the past 15 years. It is difficult to remember that the first nuclear cardiology studies were performed as early as 1927 by Blumgart and Weiss. These pioneers used modified Wilson cloud chambers to measure circulation times after intravenous injection of radon gas in humans. In 1965, Anger et al first demonstrated the ability to define cardiac transit with images from a prototype single-crystal scintillation camera. The early 1970s witnessed the onset of electrocardiographic gating of the equilibrium cardiac blood pool, stress perfusion imaging, and quantification of first-pass cardiovascular dynamics. In the mid-1970s, the imaging acute myocardial infarction was demonstrated, which introduced the era of the radionuclide study of the acutely ill patient. The late 1970s and 1980s heralded the onset of quantification of planar imaging and tomographic imaging with single-photon emission computed tomography (SPECT) and positron emission tomography (PET). In the 1980s, the prognostic applications of stress radionuclide imaging methods were defined and pharmacologic stress imaging approaches were validated. In the 1990s, the role of perfusion imaging in the assessment of myocardial viability is being established. In addition, new technetium-99m(^{99m}Tc)–labeled radiopharmaceuticals have been introduced and are currently undergoing experimental and clinical investigative study. At present, nuclear cardiology is an important cornerstone of cardiovascular evaluation and cardiovascular research. Its place within the spectrum of methods available for evaluating the cardiac patient seems to be assured.

The purpose of this book is to place the field of nuclear cardiology in appropriate perspective: that is, to assess the current state of the art and to speculate where future directions will take the discipline. This volume is not designed to be a comprehensive review of all that has or can be done in nuclear cardiology; rather, it is designed to focus on exciting areas of substantial investigative activity, to assess the scientific basis for many aspects of current clinical practice, and to help evaluate and forge the future of the discipline. This book should provide the reader with a sense of contemporary nuclear cardiology and give a perspective on its projected evolution over the next 5 years.

This book is an outcome of the International Nuclear Cardiology Workshop held in Wintergreen, Virginia, in July 1991. The researchers participating in that workshop each contributed a chapter to this volume based upon their presentations. The goal of the workshop and this text was to present state-of-the-art perspective of the field of nuclear cardiology. Current areas of active investigative and clinical interest were selected. In addition, several contributions were solicited from distinguished investigators who were not involved in nuclear cardiology but whose seminal contributions in the areas of cardiovascular physiology and metabolism have and will continue to contribute basic biologic information to the nuclear cardiologist's understanding of the field. These contributions involve assessment of the principles of tracer kinetics by Bassingthwaighte, specific physiologic issues relating to perfusion imaging and hibernation by Klocke, and assessment of the myocardial metabolism in ischemia and reperfusion by Liedtke. These chapters form conceptual cornerstones for many of the nuclear contributions.

The first section of this book deals with tissue tracer kinetics. Piwnica-Worms approaches this problem in myocyte cell culture. Leppo and Marshall discuss models involving isolated perfused hearts, and Gewirtz discusses data obtained in intact animal models.

The second section deals with specific aspects of imaging technology. Watson approaches this problem in the context of assessment of myocardial viability and ischemia using planar perfusion techniques. Germano et al discuss current concepts in SPECT. Bacharach deals with currently unanswered technical issues concerning cardiac PET. Garcia and Cooke provide an overview of computer approaches to nuclear cardiology.

The area of ventricular function, extremely active in the mid-1980s, has received less attention recently. Three chapters are devoted to this subject. Jones discusses his laboratory's experience with radionuclide angiography in patients with suspected or known coronary disease. Bonow discusses the role of equilibrium radionuclide angiocardiography for diagnostic and prognostic studies. Zaret and Jain discuss the newer method of continuous monitoring of left ventricular function using miniaturized nonimaging detectors.

Eight chapters are devoted to the assessment of myocardial perfusion in stable coronary disease. After an introductory chapter on physiology by Klocke, Brown deals with the role of thallium-201(^{201}Tl) perfusion imaging in the assessment of prognosis in patients with coronary disease. Iskandrian and Heo discuss the exciting and complex area of pharmacologic stress testing. Kaul compares aspects of perfusion imaging with exercise echocardiography for the evaluation of coronary disease. The next four chapters deal with aspects of the new ^{99m}Tc-labeled perfusion tracers. Maddahi et al review current experiences with sestamibi imaging. Wackers et al explore new approaches involving ^{99m}Tc sestamibi–gated echocardiographic imaging for the assessment of regional function. Johnson describes clinical experience with ^{99m}Tc teboroxime imaging. Verani contrasts the ^{99m}Tc perfusion agents with 201-Tl.

Seven chapters are devoted to imaging studies of myocardial infarction and viability, a topic that is particularly relevant in the era of reperfusion and thrombolysis. It is clear that this is one of the most exciting aspects of current nuclear cardiologic research. Beller reviews data on 201-Tl imaging for assessment of viability. Gibbons discusses the use of ^{99m}Tc sestamibi in the setting of acute infarction. Because of its unique properties, this particular agent can provide insight into areas at risk and directly assess the impact of reperfusion. Metabolic imaging may provide critical insights into issues of viability. After Liedtke's review of the fundamentals of myocardial metabolism in ischemia and reperfusion, Feinendegen discusses single-photon metabolic imaging. This is followed by chapters by Conversano and Bergmann, Wijns et al, and Schelbert and Czernin on PET studies in the setting of clinical and experimental myocardial infarction and reperfusion.

The concluding four chapters deal with new approaches to current cardiovascular problems. Hutchins and Schwaiger discuss the currently available alternatives for absolute quantification of myocardial blood flow with PET. Schwaiger et al review an exciting new area of neurocardiology in which neurotransmitter imaging within the left ventricular myocardium has become a reality. Dewhurst et al deal with the important area of imaging thrombosis. In this area of imaging, the direct applications to imaging of recent advances in the science of coagulation are readily evident. Lahiri et al summarize current experience with the use of antimyosin antibody imaging for detection of myocardial necrosis in acute infarction and other conditions.

Throughout this volume, we have attempted to emphasize not only where we are today but where the field is going. The dynamic aspect of nuclear cardiology has never been more apparent than in the present era. Indeed, the field has seemingly endless potential, limited only by our own creativity.

ACKNOWLEDGMENTS

This book grew out of an International Nuclear Cardiology Workshop held in Wintergreen, Virginia, on July 14–17, 1991. This workshop was sponsored by educational grants from E. I. DuPont de Vemours & Co.; Squibb Bristol-Myers; Mallinckrodt Medical, Inc.; McNeil Pharmaceutical; Capintec, Inc.; Marion-Merrell Dow, and Pfizer Laboratories. We gratefully acknowledge these contributions.

For this book to be published in a timely fashion, all contributors were required to submit their manuscripts promptly and to respond promptly to requested revisions. We thank all the contributors for their willingness to meet these specific and often demanding time constraints.

The editorial assistance of Anne S. Patterson and the staff at Mosby–Year Book is appreciated. We acknowledge the outstanding secretarial support of Joanne Mayfield and Astrid Swanson in New Haven, Connecticut, and Barbara Blum and Jane Bickers in Charlottesville, Virginia.

Barry L. Zaret
George A. Beller

Introduction

George A. Beller

The past decade has been characterized by major advances in nuclear cardiology that have greatly enhanced the clinical utility of the various radionuclide techniques used for the assessment of regional myocardial perfusion and regional and global left ventricular function under resting and stress conditions.[1,3,15,53,57,58,65] Despite the emergence of alternative noninvasive techniques for the diagnosis of coronary artery disease and the assessment of prognosis and viability, such as stress echocardiography, the use and application of nuclear cardiology techniques have continued to increase. The establishment of the American Society of Nuclear Cardiology (ASNC) and its educational programs has led to a greater diffusion of nuclear cardiology technology in the community hospital setting and has promoted the emergence and dissemination of imaging and procedural guidelines for nuclear cardiology methods.[21] The ASNC was also responsible for the introduction of a certification examination for competency in nuclear cardiology. The establishment of the *Journal of Nuclear Cardiology*, the official journal of the ASNC, allowed a greater number of manuscripts to be published in the field. The many superb reviews and editorials that appear in this journal highlight major advances and point out controversies for resolution. The *Journal of Nuclear Cardiology* has also begun to publish the abstracts of the biennial meeting of the International Congress of Nuclear Cardiology, again permitting the early dissemination of new discoveries and new clinical applications of nuclear cardiology techniques. The Wintergreen Conference, attended by leaders in nuclear cardiology from the United States and elsewhere every 2 years, was organized to identify areas of nuclear cardiology that required further emphasis and investigation, either in the basic laboratory or in clinical trials. Industry representatives also attend these conferences and actively participate in open discussions particularly on what was desired from them with respect to funding of bench research and clinical trials that could further enhance the field. A summary of the findings of the 1996 Wintergreen Conference was published in the *Journal of Nuclear Cardiology.*[52]

The postgraduate education of cardiologists, radiologists, and nuclear medicine physicians in nuclear cardiology has been markedly enhanced by the annual tutorials sponsored by the ASNC. These tutorials are highlighted by "read with the experts" sessions that demonstrate imaging systems and computer software. The goal of these sessions is for the audience participants to interpret unknown scans with an expert in the field. This should improve the skills in image interpretation for those who attend. Internet-based multimedia teaching programs and CD-ROMs are new additions to the continuing education of physicians responsible for the evaluation and interpretation of nuclear cardiology procedures.

Collectively, initiatives cited above have contributed enormously to the enhancement of the quality of nuclear cardiology laboratories and the expertise of physicians who are responsible for supervising and interpreting nuclear cardiology procedures.

In the sections to follow, three examples will be given in which advances in imaging technology or new knowledge from clinical research studies have contributed to enhanced decision making and the clinical care of patients.

EXAMPLE 1: GATED TECHNETIUM-99M SINGLE-PHOTON EMISSION COMPUTED TOMOGRAPHY FOR MORE ACCURATE DETECTION OF CORONARY ARTERY DISEASE

For many years, planar imaging and single-photon emission computed tomography (SPECT) with thallium-201 (^{201}Tl) imaging constituted the only scintigraphic techniques available for detecting coronary artery disease in patients undergoing stress testing. The major limitation of ^{201}Tl scintigraphy is the high false-positive rate observed in many laboratories, which is predominantly attributed to image attenuation artifacts and variants of normal that are interpreted as defects secondary to coronary artery disease.[18,39] Although quantitation of ^{201}Tl images improved specificity, the false-positive rate still remained problematic, particularly with imaging of obese persons and of women with defects that reflected breast attenuation artifacts. Such artifacts are sometimes difficult to distinguish from perfusion abnormalities secondary to inducible ischemia or myo-cardial scar.[39]

In the past decade, new ^{99m}Tc-labeled perfusion agents were introduced into clinical practice predominantly to enhance the specificity of SPECT (see Chapter 16). It was immediately apparent that the quality of images obtained with these new ^{99m}Tc-labeled radionuclides was superior to that of images obtained with ^{201}Tl because of the more favorable physical characteristics of ^{99m}Tc for imaging with a gamma camera. With

[99m]Tc, doses approximately 10 to 20 times higher than those that are feasible with ^{201}Tl can be administered, yielding images with higher count density. Technetium-99m demonstrates less scatter and attenuation than ^{201}Tl, which should be associated with fewer artifacts in patients who have no underlying coronary artery disease. Perhaps most important, ^{99m}Tc sestamibi or ^{99m}Tc tetrofosmin imaging allows easy gated acquisition, permitting the simultaneous evaluation of regional systolic thickening, global left ventricular function, and myocardial perfusion.[14,17,55]

The rationale for distinguishing attenuation artifacts from defects attributed to coronary artery disease on stress or resting SPECT images using gated ^{99m}Tc sestamibi or gated ^{99m}Tc tetrofosmin SPECT is that defects that reflect myocardial scar most often show decreased systolic thickening on gated tomograms, whereas defects secondary to artifact demonstrate normal systolic thickening.[17] The latter differentiation is most useful in patients with an intermediate-to-low pretest likelihood of coronary artery disease who have no history of infarction or electrocardiographic evidence of myocardial scar.

The patient population that benefits most from gated ^{99m}Tc SPECT imaging is women who present with chest pain and are referred for combined exercise or pharmacologic stress with radionuclide perfusion imaging. In a prospective study by Taillefer et al,[59] the diagnostic accuracy of ^{201}Tl SPECT and ^{99m}Tc sestamibi SPECT perfusion imaging for detection of coronary artery disease CAD in women was evaluated. Women in this study underwent both SPECT techniques; most also underwent coronary angiography. The overall sensitivities for detecting 50% or greater stenoses or 70% or greater stenoses were similar for ^{201}Tl SPECT and ^{99m}Tc sestamibi SPECT imaging. The specificity, however, was only 67% for ^{201}Tl SPECT when the definition of significant disease as stenosis of 70% or more was used. In the same patients, ^{99m}Tc sestamibi SPECT perfusion imaging alone increased specificity to 84.4%, and, when the gated images were analyzed, specificity further improved to 92.2% (Fig. I). Similar differences were observed when the definition of a significant stenosis was 50% or more in the women in this study. Thus, gated ^{99m}Tc sestamibi reduced the false-positive rate from 33% with ^{201}Tl to 8%.

A study performed in a heterogeneous population of patients with a low pretest likelihood of disease with those who had documented angiographic disease also demonstrated the value of gating of ^{99m}Tc sestamibi SPECT images.[55] This study showed that the addition of gating to standard perfusion ^{99m}Tc sestamibi SPECT reduced the number of borderline interpretations from 89 to 29 in the total group of 285 patients. In the 137 with a pretest likelihood of coronary artery disease of 10% or less, the addition of gated images added significantly to the percentage of interpretations that were designated as normal (74% to 93%) because of a reduction in borderline-normal and borderline-abnormal readings. Thus, the addition of electrographically-gated ^{99m}Tc sestamibi SPECT images to the reading of stress and rest perfusion images alone resulted in a significant shift in the final scan interpretations to a more normal designa-

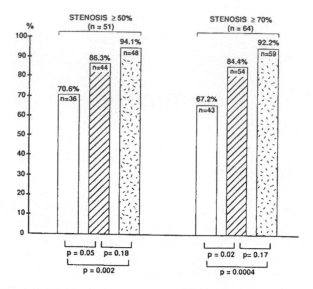

Fig. I. Specificity of thallium-201 (^{201}Tl) single-photoemission computed tomography (SPECT) (*open bars*), technetium-99m ^{99m}Tc-sestamibi SPECT (*striped bars*), and ^{99m}Tc sestamibi gated SPECT (*speckled bars*) for women with angiographically normal coronary arteries or with a less than 5% pretest likelihood of coronary artery disease. Note that the specificity of gated SPECT imaging is superior to the specificity of ^{201}Tl SPECT or ^{99m}Tc SPECT perfusion scintigraphy. (From Taillefer R, DePuey EG, Udelson JE, et al: Comparative diagnostic accuracy of Tl-201 and Tc-99m sestamibi SPECT imaging [perfusion and ECG-gated SPECT] in detecting coronary artery disease in women, *J Am Coll Cardiol* 29:69–77, 1997. Reprinted with permission from the American College of Cardiology.)

tion in patients with a low pretest likelihood of coronary artery disease and to more abnormal defects consistent with coronary artery disease in patients with known disease.

Another feature of electrocardiographic gating of ^{99m}Tc SPECT images is the elimination of a resting perfusion study in patients who undergo stress SPECT only imaging and have both normal myocardial perfusion and normal systolic thickening in all myocardial segments.[41] For example, women with a low-to-intermediate pretest likelihood of coronary artery disease who demonstrate anterior wall defects on stress tomograms that are associated with normal systolic thickening and no ischemic ST-segment depression do not require a resting study, because the defect surely represents a breast attenuation artifact. Inspection of the raw images should confirm this impression.

Finally, electrographically-gated SPECT yields important information about global left ventricular function that could previously only be obtained with a second test, such as radionuclide angiography, echocardiography, or contrast ventriculography.* The ability to accurately measure left ventricular ejection fraction with ^{99m}Tc sestamibi or ^{99m}Tc tetrofosmin adds supplementary value to the procedure with respect to prognostication. It has clearly been shown that patients with

*References 7,8,13,16,20,22,23,45,56,63,64.

left ventricular ejection fraction of 40% or less have a worse prognosis than patients with more normal global left ventricular function. In addition, the presence of systolic thickening in perfusion defects attributed to coronary artery disease provides an additional indication that such segments are viable. Viability is predicted when ^{99m}Tc sestamibi or ^{99m}Tc tetrofosmin counts exceed 50% or 60% of peak counts in irreversible defects.[61]

Thus, the introduction of gated ^{99m}Tc gated imaging has significantly enhanced the specificity of SPECT for the detection of coronary artery disease among patients presenting with chest pain, increased the detection rate of viable myocardium, and improved the ability to risk-stratify patients by providing information relevant to global left ventricular function. These features should be cost-effective for the diagnostic and prognostic evaluation of patients with suspected or known coronary artery disease. First, by enhancing specificity for detection of coronary artery disease and reducing the false-positive rate with gated ^{99m}Tc SPECT, fewer patients may be sent to unnecessary coronary angiography. By yielding less equivocal scan interpretation reports, the results of gated ^{99m}Tc SPECT reassure the clinician of the fact that when a scan is interpreted as normal or abnormal, the likelihood of an incorrect diagnosis is lower than that previously experienced with ^{201}Tl SPECT scintigraphy. Another cost-effective feature of gated ^{99m}Tc SPECT is the elimination of a resting study by performing a stress only ^{99m}Tc study in patients with a low pretest likelihood of coronary artery disease. With the demonstration of normal perfusion in all myocardial segments by quantitative criteria and normal systolic thickening, the probability that a resting study would provide further information on normalcy would be low. Finally, the measurement of left ventricular ejection fraction by ^{99m}Tc SPECT imaging could lead to the elimination of a second noninvasive test (such as echocardiography) in situations in which knowledge of both perfusion at rest and with stress and left ventricular function is required (for example, in the predischarge phase of acute myocardial infarction). New techniques[13,23,56] that permit automated determination of left ventricular ejection fraction by ^{99m}Tc gated tomography will only enhance the accuracy of the technique which already correlates well with that of other standard techniques for measurement of global left ventricular function.

EXAMPLE 2: STRESS RADIONUCLIDE IMAGING FOR PROGNOSTICATION AND DETERMINATION OF WHICH PATIENTS BENEFIT MOST FROM REVASCULARIZATION

The prognostic value of exercise and pharmacologic stress myocardial perfusion imaging has been established in thousands of patients in the past 20 years.* As discussed in Chapter 20, the major prognostic variables on stress perfusion imaging are a large defect that occupies more than 20% of the left ventricular myocardium, extensive reversible defects in one or

*References 6,9,10,11,24,26-29,30,31,33-36,40,50,57,60.

more coronary vascular regions, a multivessel disease scan pattern with inducible defects in the distribution of more than one of the three major coronary arteries, increased lung uptake of ^{201}Tl on the initial poststress anterior view image, and transient or persistent left ventricular cavity dilation seen on stress and rest images. A remarkable observation reported in one study after another, whether ^{201}Tl or ^{99m}Tc sestamibi was used as the imaging agent, is the extremely low cardiac event rate (death or myocardial infarction) in patients with a normal perfusion scan on symptom-limited exercise or pharmacologic stress testing.[9] The finding of a high negative predictive value of a normal scan for no subsequent events has greatly changed the manner in which patients with chest pain and suspected coronary artery disease are evaluated in terms of cost-effectiveness. This is because one major goal of noninvasive risk stratification is the identification of patients at low risk for future cardiac events based on scintigraphic findings; such patients can be spared unnecessary referral for invasive evaluation. Conversely, patients with high-risk scan findings are at increased risk for future ischemic events and therefore may benefit from revascularization. The underlying assumption of this noninvasive approach to risk stratification is that patients with important perfusion abnormalities during stress conditions have survival benefit with coronary revascularization compared with medical therapy because a substantial amount of jeopardized myocardium in the distribution of severely stenotic vessels is revascularized. Patients with minimal or no evidence of ischemia would not derive a survival benefit from revascularization; thus, a normal or low-risk perfusion study would often lead to the decision to continue with medical therapy; institute primary prevention measures; or search for a noncardiac cause of chest pain, such as gastroesophageal reflux.

Many published studies have shown that incremental prognostic information is obtained when assessment of variables from myocardial perfusion imaging is added to information acquired solely from the clinical history, physical examination, and exercise electrocardiography treadmill test results.[6,27,28,32,50] In fact, some reports have indicated that when clinical, exercise electrocardiographic, and scintigraphic variables are known, coronary angiographic variables yield little additional prognostic information. What has been most impressive is the low rate of cardiac catheterization in patients with a low-risk myocardial perfusion scan, even in the presence of a high likelihood of coronary artery disease on the basis of treadmill exercise test variables, such as the Duke treadmill score. Hachamovitch et al[28] showed that the catheterization rate was only 1% in 834 patients who had an "intermediate" Duke treadmill score after exercise testing (Fig. II). The combined death and infarction rate in the 834 patients with an intermediate Duke treadmill score and a normal scan was only 0.4% per year (Fig. II). Patients with normal scans were infrequently referred for catheterization in all Duke treadmill score categories. In a study by Iskandrian et al,[32] the treadmill score was not a significant predictor of prognosis, even by univariate analysis, in 121 patients with no coronary artery disease and 316 patients

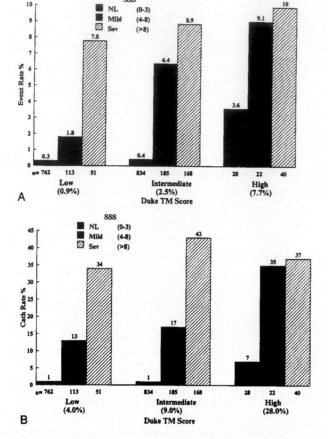

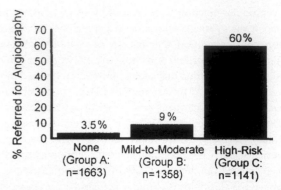

Fig. III. Relation between single-photoemission computed tomography (SPECT) reversibility on stress scintigraphy and subsequent referral for coronary angiography as determined from a retrospective analysis of 4162 patient studies. A study was categorized as high-risk if more than two of the following three criteria were met: reversibility of the left anterior descending territory, multivessel disease scan pattern, or abnormal lung uptake of thallium-201. All other scans showing reversible defects were categorized in the mild-to-moderate group (group B). (From Bateman TM, O'Keefe JHJ, Dong VM, et al: Coronary angiography rates after stress single-photon emission computed tomographic scintigraphy, *J Nucl Cardiol* 2:217-223, 1995. Reprinted with permission from the American Society of Cardiology.)

Fig. II. A, Cardiac event rate (death or nonfatal infarction) based on the presence of a normal summed stress score *(SSS)*, a mild SSS, and a severe SSS relative to the Duke treadmill score categorized as a low-risk score, an intermediate-risk score, and a high-risk score. **B**, The cardiac catheterization rate based on the SSS presented for patients with a low-risk, intermediate-risk, and high-risk Duke treadmill score. Note the low rate of referral for cardiac catheterization in patients with a normal scan *(first columns)*. (From Hachamovitch R, Berman DS, Kiat H, et al: Exercise myocardial perfusion SPECT in patients without known coronary artery disease. Incremental prognostic value and use in risk stratification, *Circulation* 93:905-914, 1996 by the American Heart Association, Inc.)

with angiographically determined coronary artery disease who underwent treadmill exercise ^{201}Tl SPECT.

The prognostic value of stress perfusion imaging has not only been demonstrated in centers of excellence but also has been shown to exist in a community population. Miller et al[43] evaluated the prognostic value of ^{201}Tl imaging in a community-based population of 446 residents of Olmstead County, Minnesota. Only five variables (age, history of myocardial infarction, number of abnormal ^{201}Tl segments on postexercise images, trauma, and increased lung uptake of ^{201}Tl) contained the most independent prognostic information.

Bateman et al[2] also reported that patients categorized as low risk by stress SPECT scintigraphy were rarely referred for coronary angiography. As shown in Fig. III, only 3.5% of 1663 patients with a normal perfusion scan had coronary angiogra-

phy soon after testing. Of interest, only 9% of patients with mild-to-moderate SPECT reversibility were referred for angiography after testing compared with 60% of patients referred for angiography with high-risk SPECT reversibility. In a subsequent report, this group gave follow-up data on the 91% of patients with non–high-risk SPECT reversibility who did not undergo early invasive management. With medical therapy, the unadjusted actuarial 3-year survival rate for cardiac death or nonfatal infarction was only 2% in this medically managed group with mild-to-moderate ischemia. Only 4% of the patients crossed over to subsequent coronary revascularization. This study suggests that the results of SPECT imaging can assist in deciding which patients will do well with medical therapy as reflected by low mortality and infarction rates.

The Cedars–Sinai group recently reported similar results.[29] They found that the annual cardiac death rate was only 0.8% in patients with a mildly abnormal stress perfusion scan who received medical treatment and an annual cardiac death rate of 0.9% in patients with a mildly abnormal scan who underwent revascularization. In contrast, patients with moderately abnormal and severely abnormal scans benefited from revascularization early after nuclear testing in this retrospective analysis.

Thus, stress myocardial perfusion imaging may function as a gatekeeper for referral for cardiac catheterization because it may identify low-risk groups who have an excellent prognosis treated with medical treatment and do not benefit from early revascularization.[5,38,44,46,62] This strategy, in which referral for cardiac catheterization is ischemia driven, could reduce healthcare costs, because coronary angiography could be avoided in patients with low-risk radionuclide studies regardless of clinical characteristics, treadmill exercise test results, and even

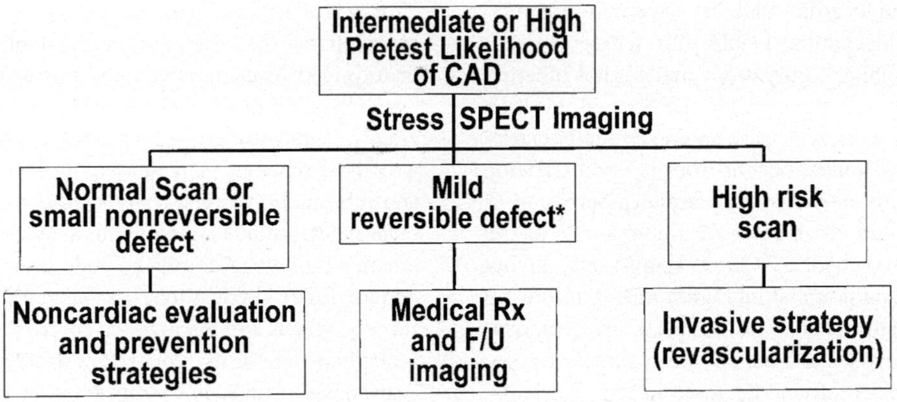

*A mild reversible defect is one that is confined to one coronary vascular region and does not include the entire risk zone of the left anterior descending coronary artery (apex, anterolateral wall, and septum).

Fig. IV. Proposed decision-making algorithm for stable patients with an intermediate or high pretest likelihood of coronary artery disease *(CAD)* who undergo stress single-photoemission computed tomography imaging.

Table 1. Comparison of two testing strategies in patients matched for age, sex, and clinical variables.

Variable	Strategy A	Strategy B
Cardiac death, %	2.8	3.3%
Normal coronary angiography result %	33.0	52.0*
Coronary revascularization, %	13.7	26.3*
Composite cost per patient, $	4882	8212*

From Miller D, Shaw LJ, Travin MI, Heller GV, et al: Downstream economic impact of failing to document myocardial ischemia before coronary angiography in stable angina patients, Circulation 94(suppl):I-60, 1996 (abstract).
*= p<0.01.

coronary angiographic findings. Brown et al[12] reported that patients with angiographically documented coronary artery disease have the same low risk for subsequent cardiac death and infarction with a normal scan as patients who have normal coronary arteries or a 5% or less pretest likelihood of coronary artery disease and normal scans.

Finally, Miller et al[42] reported the preliminary results of a multicenter study that compared the cost-efficiency of two testing strategies in patients who were matched for age, sex, and clinical variables. These patients were classified as having stable angina and were followed for 3 years. Strategy A (5826 patients) involved stress perfusion imaging as the first test, followed by coronary angiography in patients who had ischemia (1613). Strategy B was undertaken in 5423 patients and involved proceeding directly to coronary angiography as the first test for the evaluation of chest pain without previous stress perfusion imaging. The outcomes for the two strategies are shown in Table 1. Although both testing strategies achieved similar clinical outcomes, the 40% greater composite of cost accrued with direct referral to catheterization for patients with angina-type chest pain as a result of the increased downstream use of revascularization for strategy B and an increased normal coro-

nary angiographic rate in such patients who had no history of ischemia before angiography.

Thus, the data from the studies cited above clearly indicate that stress perfusion imaging provides important prognostic information that supplements clinical and exercise electrocardiographic stress test data and can be highly cost-effective in the identification of low-risk patients who can be treated medically and do not need to be referred for early angiography. The identification of high-risk patients who would probably benefit from early revascularization on the basis of an expected high cardiac event rate with medical treatment can also be accomplished. The former group comprises patients with normal myocardial perfusion scans or mild perfusion abnormalities, such as those that might be observed in the distribution of one coronary supply region. Patients in the latter group, who are at high risk for ischemic events when medically treated, most often have extensive areas of stress-induced hypoperfusion, particularly of the reversible type. Figure IV is a proposed decision-making algorithm for stable patients who present with chest pain and an intermediate or high pretest likelihood of coronary artery disease who then undergo stress SPECT.

Cost-effectiveness analysis has begun to be applied to nuclear cardiology, as evidenced by the recent instructive reviews on the subject.[48,49,54] As stated by Shaw et al,[54] "In the managed-care era, there is tremendous concern over the incremental or marginal cost of additional diagnostic and prognostic information." Combining stress perfusion imaging with exercise electrocardiography from the outset in patients with an intermediate or high pretest likelihood of coronary artery disease is highly cost-effective.

EXAMPLE 3: DETECTION OF MYOCARDIAL VIABILITY FOR PREDICTING OUTCOMES

Another area in which nuclear cardiology has made a major impact with respect to clinical decision making and that may have the potential for reduction in medical costs is the noninvasive assessment of myocardial viability. Accurate noninvasive determination of myocardial viability to distinguish irreversible myocardial cellular injury from myocardial hibernation is critically important with respect to the optimal selection of patients with coronary artery disease and resting left ventricular dysfunction who will most benefit from revascularization strategies.[4] Patients with extensive myocardial hibernation as assessed by ^{201}Tl scintigraphy or PET–[18]F-fluorodeoxyglucose imaging who are treated medically have significantly higher rates of cardiac death and nonfatal infarction during follow-up than do patients who are treated with coronary revascularization strategies.[4] It is proposed that patients with extensive coronary artery disease and a profound decrease in left ventricular ejection fraction will experience improvement in left ventricular function, alleviation of heart failure symptoms, and enhanced survival if revascularization results in improvement in segmental cardiac function in areas of viable but underperfused myocardium. Even in the absence of enhanced systolic function after revascularization, restoring blood flow to zones of chronic hypoperfusion or repetitive stunning could improve such outcomes as cardiac mortality and infarction. This is because some areas that are comprised of subendocardial scar may not demonstrate improved regional function after revascularization, but revascularization may still reduce the probability for future cardiac events. As reviewed in Chapters 29 and 32, the greater the extent of viability in patients with left ventricular dysfunction and coronary artery disease, the better the improvement in global left ventricular function and the better the outcome with coronary revascularization. Ragosta et al[51] showed that in a 15-segment model, the left ventricular ejection fraction increased after coronary artery bypass graft surgery from 0.29 to 0.41 when 7 or more asynergic segments were judged to be viable. The remaining group of patients with fewer than 7 viable asynergic segments had no statistically significant increase in left ventricular ejection fraction after CABG surgery.

It should also be pointed out that surgeons are often reluctant to perform CABG surgery in patients with coronary artery disease who have severely depressed left ventricular ejection fraction unless they can be assured that the operative mortality rate is reasonable and that the long-term outcome will be salutary. Thus, noninvasive radionuclide techniques that can accurately distinguish viable myocardium from myocardial scar would be of great benefit for optimal preoperative evaluation of ischemic cardiomyopathy patients who are being considered for revascularization.

Certain patients with severe congestive heart failure referred for heart transplantation may benefit from revascularization despite absence of anginal symptoms. Patients who will benefit most from revascularization rather than transplantation should demonstrate substantial preserved viability in asynergic myocardium. In one study,[19] 46 patients with an average left ventricular ejection fraction of 23% underwent CABG surgery instead of transplantation; in this group, the 2-year survival rate was 87%.

Revascularization strategies for patients with ischemic cardiomyopathy who demonstrate substantial viability could ultimately lead to cost reductions. For example, the subsequent hospitalization rate for exacerbations of heart failure would decrease, and hospitalizations for recurrent ischemic events would be reduced in patients with ischemic cardiomyopathy and substantial regions of myocardial viability who underwent revascularization. Patients with ischemic cardiomyopathy and hibernating myocardium who undergo revascularization should require fewer medications for heart failure and angina after surgery, which will also reduce costs.

Perhaps one of the important considerations with respect to cost considerations is the observation that patients with predominantly nonviable myocardium have a rather poor outcome after coronary revascularization.[47] Thus, rejecting patients with severe left ventricular dysfunction and predominantly scarred myocardium for revascularization could create a reduction in cost as a result of avoiding a surgical intervention that is not likely to be of long-term benefit and that is associated with an increased perioperative mortality.

The influence of viability testing on short-term outcome after CABG surgery is well reflected in the study by Haas et al[25] who compared 35 patients who were referred for revascularization with coronary artery disease and left ventricular dysfunction based only on clinical and angiographic criteria with 34 patients who were referred to surgery on the basis of clinical, angiographic and noninvasive viability information. The 30-day mortality rate for the group referred for revascularization without a viability study was 11.4% compared with 0% for the group referred for surgery with a preoperative viability study. The 12-month mortality rate was 14.3% compared with 2.9%, respectively, for the two groups ($p<0.05$). The left ventricular ejection fraction significantly increased only CABG surgery in the group referred to surgery with viability assessment. The event-free survival for the two groups are shown in Fig. V.

Thus, this example of using nuclear cardiology testing for distinguishing myocardial viability from irreversible myocardial injury shows that valuable information for decision making that can improve patient outcomes can be gained. In addition, the costs of managing patients with ischemic cardiomyopathy can be reduced. A proposed decision-making algorithm is presented (Fig. VI) that uses viability testing to determine which patients with ischemic cardiomyopathy will benefit most from revascularization.

SUMMARY

These three examples of the use of nuclear cardiology testing clearly show how nuclear cardiology techniques can assist in the decision-making process in selecting strategies that have been shown to be cost-effective. The predominant theme in this chapter, which recurs through many chapters, is that nuclear cardiology testing can serve as the gatekeeper for more costly and more riskier invasive strategies in the evaluation and treatment of patients with stable coronary artery disease, acute myo-cardial infarction, or significant left ventricular dysfunction. Throughout

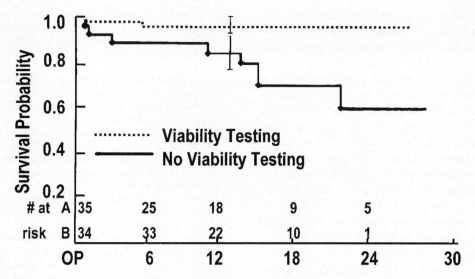

Fig. V. Probability of survival after coronary artery bypass graft surgery in patients with coronary artery disease and left ventricular function who were referred for revascularization on the basis of whether preoperative viability testing was performed with clinical and angiographic assessment. Note that the event-free survival rate was significantly better in patients who had viability testing before referral for coronary revascularization. (Adapted from Haas F, Haehnel CH, Picker W, et al: Preoperative positron emission tomographic viability assessment and perioperative and postoperative risk in patients with advanced ischemic heart disease, *J Am Coll Cardiol* 30:1693-1700,1997. Reprinted with permission from the American College of Cardiology.)

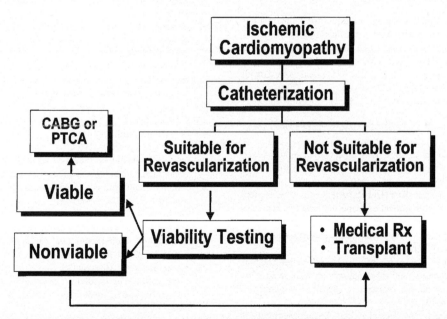

Fig. VI. Decision-making algorithm for referral of patients with ischemic cardiomyopathy for revascularization or medical management and possible subsequent cardiac transplantation. Patients with substantial myocardial viability reflecting myocardial hibernation seem to benefit most from coronary artery bypass graft surgery *(CABG)* or multivessel percutaneous transluminal coronary angioplasty *(PTCA)*.

this book, many examples are given in which stress or rest perfusion imaging or rest or stress radionuclide angiography provides diagnostic and prognostic information that supplements clinical, electrocardiographic, and treadmill test variables.

Coincident with the emergence of many clinical research studies validating the utility of nuclear cardiology techniques have come major improvements in instrumentation and in radiopharmaceuticals. The advent of ^{99m}Tc-labeled agents for use with gated SPECT is one of the most important advances in nuclear cardiology, and its value is highlighted in Example 1.

Finally, no matter how useful nuclear cardiology testing may seem from publications in the literature, the same accuracy will not be achieved throughout the United States and abroad in community hospital settings without proper attention to quality control, optimal instrumentation and computer software programs, and experienced interpreters who are trained to distinguish between artifacts or variants of normal from scar on SPECT images. The activities and contributions of the American Society of Nuclear Cardiology and other scientific and professional organizations have their predominant mission in this area. That is, the goal of these organizations is to enhance the quality of nuclear cardiology testing worldwide and to educate physicians about the value and limitations of the various nuclear imaging technologies and protocols. The information included in this book should contribute to enhancing the knowledge base of all physicians who actively engage in conducting and supervising nuclear cardiology procedures or who refer patients for such testing. The next decade should see even greater advances in the field, and such breakthroughs will be instrumental in further enhancing the information that can be derived from functional testing for the assessment of myocardial blood flow, cardiac function, and myocardial viability.

REFERENCES

1. Bairey Merz CN, Berman DS: Imaging techniques for coronary artery disease: current status and future directions, *Clin Cardiol* 20:526–532, 1997.

2. Bateman TM, O'Keefe JH Jr, Dong VM, et al: Coronary angiography rates after stress single-photon emission computed tomographic scintigraphy, *J Nucl Cardiol* 2:217–223, 1995.

3. Beller GA: *Clinical nuclear cardiology*, Philadelphia, 1995, W.B. Saunders.

4. Beller GA: Assessment of myocardial viability, *Curr Opin Cardiol* 12:459–467, 1997.

5. Berman DS, Kiat H. Friedman JD, et al: Clinical applications of exercise nuclear cardiology studies in the era of healthcare reform, *Am J Cardiol* 75:3D–13D, 1995.

6. Berman DS, Hachamovitch R, Kiat H, et al: Incremental value of prognostic testing in patients with known or suspected ischemic heart disease: a basis for optimal utilization of exercise technetium-99m sestamibi myocardial perfusion single-photon emission computed tomography, *J Am Coll Cardiol* 26:639–647, 1995.

7. Berman DS, Germano G: Evaluation of ventricular ejection fraction, wall motion, wall thickening, and other parameters with gated myocardial perfusion single-photon emission computed tomography, *J Nucl Cardiol* 4:S169–S171, 1997.

8. Boonyaprapa S, Ekmahachai M, Thanchaikkun N, et al: Measurement of left ventricular ejection fraction from gated technetium-99m sestamibi myocardial images, *Eur J Nucl Med* 22:528–531, 1995.

9. Brown KA: Prognostic value of myocardial perfusion imaging: state of the art and new developments, *J Nucl Cardiol* 3(6 Pt 1):516–537, 1996.

10. Brown KA, Boucher CA, Okada RD, et al: Prognostic value of exercise thallium-201 imaging in patients presenting for evaluation of chest pain, *J Am Coll Cardiol* 1:994–1001, 1983.

11. Brown KA, Altland E, Rowen M: Prognostic value of normal technetium-99m-sestamibi cardiac imaging, *J Nucl Med* 35:554–557, 1994.

12. Brown KA, Rowen M: Prognostic value of a normal exercise myocardial perfusion imaging study in patients with angiographically significant coronary artery disease, *Am J Cardiol* 71:865–867, 1993.

13. Calnon DA, Kastner RJ, Smith WH, et al: Validation of a new counts-based gated single photon emission computed tomography method for quantifying left ventricular systolic function: comparison with equilibrium radionuclide angiography, *J Nucl Cardiol* 4:464–471, 1997.

14. Chua T, Kiat H, Germano G, et al: Gated technetium-99m sestamibi for simultaneous assessment of stress myocardial perfusion, postexercise regional ventricular function and myocardial viability. Correlation with echocardiography and rest thallium-201 scintigraphy, *J Am Coll Cardiol* 23:1107–1114, 1994.

15. DePuey EG: The technical maturation of cardiovascular nuclear medicine: an art becoming a science, *J Nucl Med* 36:905–906, 1995.

16. DePuey EG, Nichols K, Dobrinsky C: Left ventricular ejection fraction assessed from gated technetium-99m-sestamibi SPECT, *J Nucl Med* 34:1871–1876, 1993.

17. DePuey EG, Rozanski A: Using gated technetium-99m-sestamibi SPECT to characterize fixed myocardial defects as infarct or artifact, *J Nucl Med* 36:952–955, 1995.

18. Desmarais RL, Kaul S, Watson DD, et al: Do false positive thallium-201 scans lead to unnecessary catheterization? Outcome of patients with perfusion defects on quantitative planar thallium-201 scintigraphy, *J Am Coll Cardiol* 21:1058–1063, 1993.

19. Dreyfus GD, Dubue D, Blasco A, et al: Myocardial viability assessment in ischemic cardiomyopathy: benefits of coronary revascularization, *Ann Thorac Surg* 57:1402–1407, 1994.

20. Everaert H, Franken PR, Flamen P, et al: Left ventricular ejection fraction from gated SPET myocardial perfusion studies: a method based on the radial distribution of count rate density across the myocardial wall, *Eur J Nucl Med* 23:1628–1633, 1996.

21. Garcia EV: Imaging guidelines for nuclear cardiology procedures. Part 1. American Society of Nuclear Cardiology, *J Nucl Cardiol* 3:G1–G46, 1996.

22. Germano G, Kiat H, Kavanagh PB, et al: Automatic quantification of ejection fraction from gated myocardial perfusion SPECT, *J Nucl Med* 36:2138–2147, 1995.

23. Germano G, Erel J, Lewin H, et al: Automatic quantitation of regional myocardial wall motion and thickening from gated technetium-99m sestamibi myocardial perfusion single-photon emission computed tomography, *J Am Coll Cardiol* 30:1360–1367, 1997.

24. Gibbons RJ: Role of nuclear cardiology for determining management of patients with stable coronary artery disease, *J Nucl Cardiol* 1(5 Pt 2):S118–S130, 1994.

25. Haas F, Haehnel CH, Picker W, et al: Preoperative positron emission tomographic viability assessment and perioperative and postoperative risk in patients with advanced ischemic heart disease, *J Am Coll Cardiol* 30:1693–1700, 1997.

26. Hachamovitch R: Prognostic characterization of patients with mild coronary artery disease with myocardial perfusion single photon emission computed tomography: validation of an outcomes-based strategy, *J Nucl Cardiol* 5:90–95, 1998.

27. Hachamovitch R, Berman DS, Kiat H, et al: Effective risk stratification using exercise myocardial perfusion SPECT in women: gender-related differences in prognostic nuclear testing, *J Am Coll Cardiol* 28:34–44, 1996.

28. Hachamovitch R, Berman DS, Kiat H, et al: Exercise myocardial perfusion SPECT in patients without known coronary artery disease: incremental prognostic value and use in risk stratification, *Circulation* 93:905–914, 1996.

29. Hachamovitch R, Berman DS, Shaw LJ, et al: Incremental prognostic value of myocardial perfusion single photon emission computed tomography for the prediction of cardiac death: differential stratification for risk of cardiac death and myocardial infarction, *Circulation* 97:535–543, 1998.

30. Hilton TC, Shaw LJ, Chaitman BR, et al: Prognostic significance of exercise thallium-201 testing in patients aged greater than or equal to 70 years with known or suspected coronary artery disease, *Am J Cardiol* 69:45–50, 1992.

31. Iskandrian AS, Haleki AH, Kane-Marsch S: Prognostic implications of exercise thallium-201 scintigraphy in patients with suspected or known coronary artery disease, *Am Heart J* 110(1 Pt 1):135–143, 1985.

32. Iskandrian AS, Johnson J, Lett, et al: Comparison of the treadmill exercise score and single-photon emission computed tomographic thallium imaging in risk assessment *J Nucl Cardiol* 1(2 Pt 1):144–149, 1994.

33. Kaul S, Lilly DR, Gascho JA, et al: Prognostic utility of the exercise thallium-201 test in ambulatory patients with chest pain: comparison with cardiac catheterization, *Circulation* 77:745–758, 1988.

34. Kaul S, Finkelstein DM, Homma S, et al: Superiority of quantitative exercise thallium-201 variables in determining long-term prognosis in ambulatory patients with chest pain: a comparison with cardiac catheterization, *J Am Coll Cardiol* 12:25–34, 1988.

35. Ladenheim ML, Pollock BH, Rozamski A, et al: Extent and severity of myocardial hypoperfusion as predictors of prognosis in patients with suspected coronary artery disease, *J Am Coll Cardiol* 7:464–471, 1986.

36. Machecourt J, Longere P, Fazret D, et al: Prognostic value of thallium-201 single-photon emission computed tomographic myocardial perfusion imaging according to extent of myocardial defect. Study in 1,926 patients with follow-up at 33 months, *J Am Coll Cardiol* 23:1096–1106, 1994.

37. Maddahi J, Rodrigues E, Berman DS, et al: State-of-the-art myocardial perfusion imaging, *Cardiol Clin* 12:199–222, 1994.

38. Maddahi J, Gambhir SS: Cost-effective selection of patients for coronary angiography, *J Nucl Cardiol* 4(2 Pt 2):S141–S151, 1997.

39. Mannting F, Morgan-Mannting MG: Gated SPECT with technetium-99m-sestamibi for assessment of myocardial perfusion abnormalities, *J Nucl Med* 34:601–608, 1993.

40. Marie P-Y, Damchin N, Durand JF, et al: Long-term prediction of major ischemic events by exercise thallium-201 single-photon emission computed tomography. Incremental prognostic value compared with clinical, exercise testing, catheterization and radionuclide angiographic data, *J Am Coll Cardiol* 26:879–886, 1995.

41. Milan E, Ginbbini R, Gioia G, et al: A cost-effective sestamibi protocol in the managed health care era, *J Nucl Cardiol* 4:509–514, 1997.

42. Miller D, Shaw LJ, Travin MI, Heller GV, et al: Downstream economic impact of failing to document myocardial ischemia before coronary angiography in stable angina patients, *Circulation* 94(suppl):I 60, 1996 (abstract).

43. Miller TD, Christian TF, Clements IP, et al: Prognostic value of exercise thallium-201 imaging in a community population, *Am Heart J* 135:663–670, 1998.

44. Nallamothu N, Pancholy SB, Leek R, et al: Impact on exercise single-photon emission computed tomographic thallium imaging on patient management and outcome, *J Nucl Cardiol* 2:334–338, 1995.

45. Nichols K, DePuey EG, Rozanski A: Automation of gated tomographic left ventricular ejection fraction, *J Nucl Cardiol* 3(6 Pt 1):475–482, 1996.

46. O'Keefe JH Jr, Bateman TM, Ligsn RW, et al: Outcome of medical versus invasive treatment strategies for non-high-risk ischemic heart disease, *J Nucl Cardiol* 5:28–33, 1998.

47. Pagley PR, Beller GA, Watson DA, et al: Improved outcome after coronary bypass surgery in patients with ischemic cardiomyopathy and residual myocardial viability, *Circulation* 96:793–800, 1997.

48. Patterson RE: Cost-effectiveness analysis in diagnosis of cardiac disease: overview of its rationale and method, *J Nucl Cardiol* 3:334–341, 1996.

49. Patterson RE, Eisner RL, Horowitz SF: Comparison of cost-effectiveness and utility of exercise ECG, single photon emission computed tomography, positron emission tomography, and coronary angiography for diagnosis of coronary artery disease, *Circulation* 91:54–65, 1995.

50. Pollock SG, Abbott RD, Buncher CA, et al: Independent and incremental prognostic value of tests performed in hierarchical order to evaluate patients with suspected coronary artery disease. Validation of models based on these tests, *Circulation* 85:237–248, 1992.

51. Ragosta M, Beller GA, Watson DD, et al: Quantitative planar rest-redistribution ^{201}Tl imaging in detection of myocardial viability and prediction of improvement in left ventricular function after coronary bypass surgery in patients with severely depressed left ventricular function, *Circulation* 87:1630–1641, 1993.

52. Proceedings of the 3rd Wintergreen Nuclear Cardiology Invitational Conference. July 14-16, 1996, *J Nucl Cardiol* 4(1 Pt 1):83–98, 1997.

53. Ritchie JL, Bateman TM, Bonow RO, et al: Guidelines for clinical use of cardiac radionuclide imaging. Report of the American College of Cardiology/American Heart Association Task Force on Assessment of Diagnostic and Therapeutic Cardiovascular Procedures (Committee on Radionuclide Imaging), developed in collaboration with the American Society of Nuclear Cardiology, *J Am Coll Cardiol* 25:521–547, 1995.

54. Shaw LJ, Hachamovitch R, Eisenstien EL, et al: A primer of biostatistic and economic methods for diagnostic and prognostic modeling in nuclear cardiology: Part I, *J Nucl Cardiol* 3(6 Pt 1):538–545, 1996.

55. Smanio PEP, Watson DD, Segalla DL, et al: Value of gating of technetium-99m sestamibi single-photon emission computed tomographic imaging, *J Am Coll Cardiol* 30:1687–1692, 1997.

56. Smith WH, Kastner RJ, Calnon DA, et al: Quantitative gated single photon emission computed tomography imaging: a counts-based method for display and measurement of regional and global ventricular systolic function, *J Nucl Cardiol* 4:451–463, 1997.

57. Stratmann HG, Williams GA, Wittry MD, et al: Exercise technetium-99m sestamibi tomography for cardiac risk stratification of patients with stable chest pain, *Circulation* 89:615–622, 1994.

58. Strauss HW: Myocardial perfusion imaging: perspectives from a turbulent twenty-five years, *Q J Nucl Med* 40:20–26, 1996.

59. Taillefer R, DePuey EG, Udelson JE, et al: Comparative diagnostic accuracy of Tl-201 and Tc-99m sestamibi SPECT imaging (perfusion and ECG-gated SPECT) in detecting coronary artery disease in women, *J Am Coll Cardiol* 29:69–77, 1997.

60. Travin MI, Boucher CA, Newell JB, et al: Variables associated with a poor prognosis in patients with an ischemic thallium-201 exercise test *Am Heart J* 125(2 Pt 1):335–344, 1993.

61. Udelson JE, Coleman PS, Metherall J, et al: Predicting recovery of severe regional ventricular dysfunction. Comparison of resting scintigraphy with ^{201}Tl and ^{99m}Tc-sestamibi, *Circulation* 89:2552–2561, 1994.

62. Wackers FJTh, Zaret BL: Radionuclide stress myocardial perfusion imaging: the future gatekeeper for coronary angiography, *J Nucl Cardiol* 2:358–359, 1995 (editorial).

63. Williams KA, Taillon LA: Gated planar technetium 99m-labeled sestamibi myocardial perfusion image inversion for quantitative scintigraphic assessment of left ventricular function, *J Nucl Cardiol* 2:285–295, 1995.

64. Yang KT, Chen HD: A semi-automated method for edge detection in the evaluation of left ventricular function using ECG-gated single-photon emission tomography, *Eur J Nucl Med* 21:1206–1211, 1994.

65. Zaret BL, Wackers FJ: Nuclear cardiology(1), *N Engl J Med* 329:775–783, 1993.

66. Zaret BL, Wackers FJ: Nuclear Cardiology(2), *N Engl J Med* 329:855–863, 1993.

Contents

NUCLEAR CARDIOLOGY
STATE OF THE ART AND FUTURE DIRECTIONS
SECOND EDITION

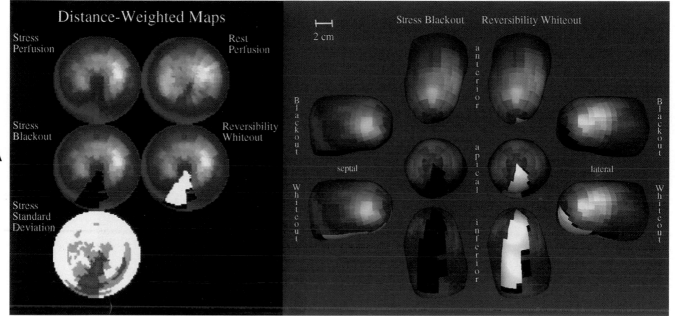

Color Plate 1. **A,** Polar maps displaying the results of perfusion quantification. The top row shows the quantitated stress and rest perfusion. The middle row shows the stress blackout map *(left)* and the whiteout reversibility map *(right)*. The bottom left map displays the number of standard deviations below normal of each myocardial sample of the stress perfusion. This patient had a completely reversible inferior perfusion defect. **B,** Three-dimensional displays of the stress blackout and reversibility whiteout information from the same patient. Clockwise from the top are shown an anterior, lateral, inferior, and septal views. An apical view is shown in the middle of the display. *(See also Fig. 8-2, A & B.)*

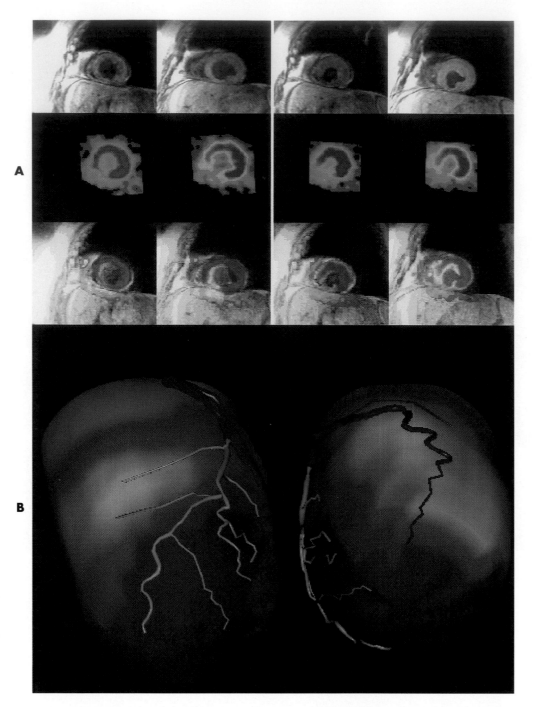

Color Plate 2. Multimodality registration. **A,** Cardiac metabolism information in positron emission tomograms (PET) created by using fluoro-deoxyglucose, registered with anatomic magnetic resonance (MR) images of the same patient. From top to bottom, MR images, registered PET, and unified MR images and PET. The first two columns show two short-axis slices at end diastole; the final two columns show the same short-axis slices at end systole. **B,** Demonstration of unifying three-dimensional coronary artery trees with single-photon emission computed tomography perfusion images. The left side is approximately a septal view; the right view is approximately lateral. Perfusion is color-coded onto the left ventricular epicardial surface; the blacked-out region indicates an anterior or apical perfusion defect. The green portion of the left anterior descending coronary artery indicates the segment of the artery distal to the stenosis. Note the overlap between the stenosed artery and the perfusion defect. (Courtesy of Dr. Shantanu Sinha, University of California, Los Angeles.) *(See also Fig. 8-5, A & B.)*

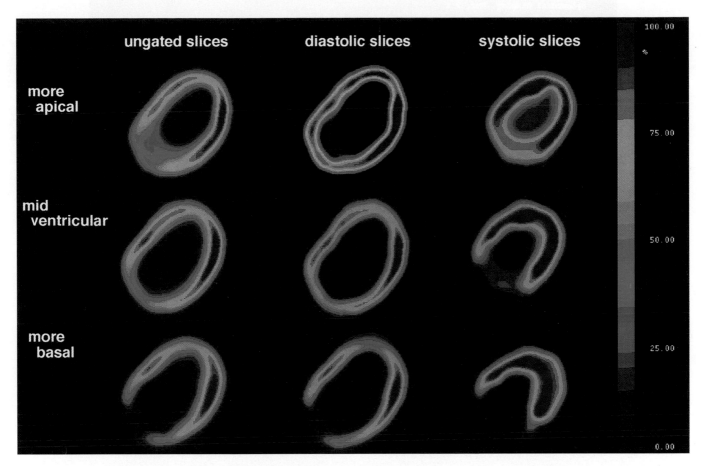

Color Plate 3. Positron emission tomographic images simulated from actual gated magnetic resonance images of a human subject by setting the myocardium uniformly to a value of 100 and blurring according to 7 mm in plane resolution and 12.5 mm in axial resolution. Each row shows images from a different level in the heart. The columns *(left to right)* show ungated images, gated end diastole images, and gated end systole images, respectively. The underlying activity distribution is perfectly homogeneous. The inhomogeneities are produced by imperfect resolution and motion blurring. *(See also Fig. 9-2.)*

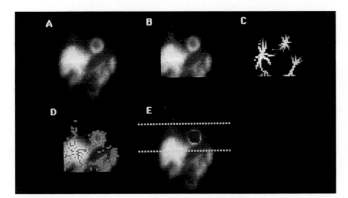

Color Plate 4. Cluster analysis before Gaussian myocardial wall detection is demonstrated. The left anterior oblique summed tomogram **(A)** is masked **(B)**, then convolved with a two-dimensional Gaussian function **(C)**. Circles identifying local clusters **(C)** are compared with clusters of local maxima **(D)** to identify the single region that most likely represents myocardium **(E)**. (From Germano G et al: Operatorless processing of myocardial perfusion SPECT studies, *J Nucl Med* 36:2127-2132, 1995. By permission of the Journal of Nuclear Medicine.) *(See also Fig. 14-5, A-E.)*

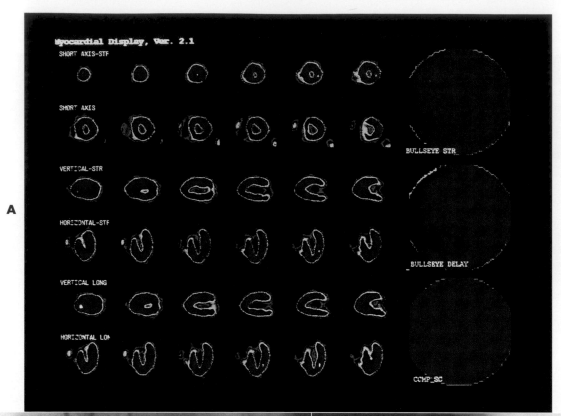

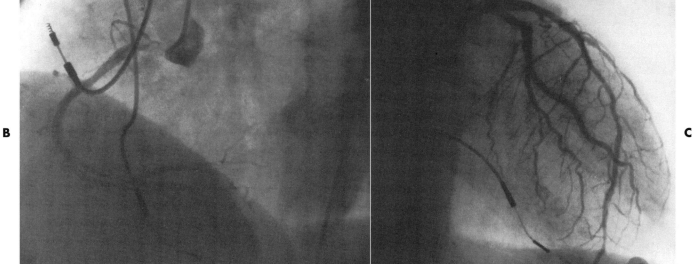

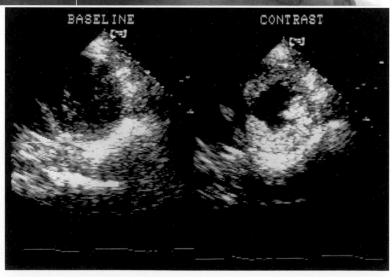

Color Plate 5. Stress single-photon emission computed tomography reoriented and polar plot images. **A,** right coronary artery anteriogram; **B,** left anterior descending coronary artery arteriogram; **C,** circumflex coronary arteriogram; and the short-axis two-dimensional echocardiographic images **D** at baseline *(left)* and after contrast injection down the LAD coronary artery *(right)*. Although this patient had a normal dobutamine thallium-201 SPECT with no discernible perfusion defect after defect after comparison to the normal databank (COMPSC) **A,** The right coronary artery is noted to have a subtotal ostial stenosis **B,** No collaterals are observed to the right coronary artery after left main contrast injection (**C**). However, on echocardiography (**D**), intense contrast enhancement is noted in the inferior wall after injection of sonicated microbubbles down the LAD, verifying the presence of coronary collaterals to the right coronary artery. Despite a severe right coronary artery stenosis, this patient did not develop a stress perfusion defect because of the well-developed collateral circulation, which was apparent on echocardiography but not arteriography. *(See also Fig. 15-14, A-D.)*

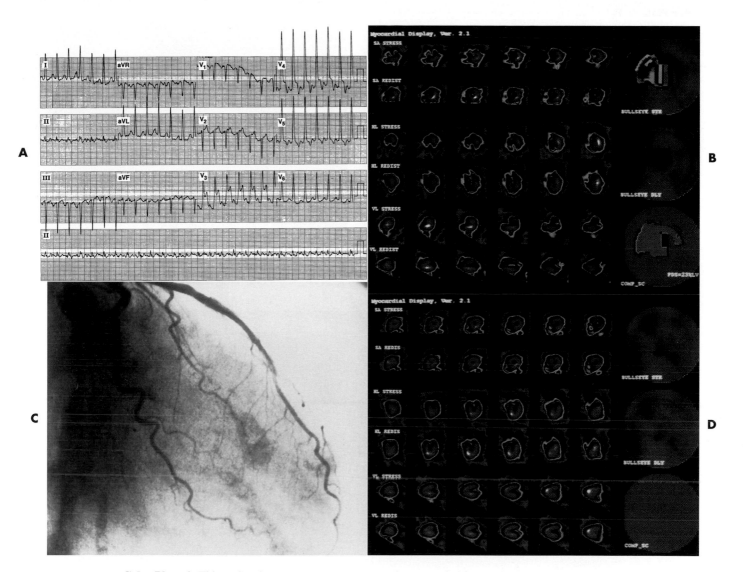

Color Plate 6. This patient has coronary artery spasm who responded favorably to calcium-channel antagonist therapy. During the initial exercise single-photon emission computed tomography (SPECT) study, the patient developed chest pain and significant ST-segment elevation on 12-lead electrocardiography (**A**). The corresponding SPECT images (**B**) show an anterior exercise (stress)-induced perfusion defect that normalizes on 4-hour redistribution (REDIST) imaging. The polar maps *(right)* show a 23% total perfusion defect after comparison with a normal databank (COMPSC). The patient underwent coronary angiography and was found to have normal coronary arteries (**C**). After starting antiischemic medical therapy, a repeat exercise SPECT was performed several weeks later (**D**) that was now entirely normal. Medical therapy eliminated exercise-induced ischemia in this patient as assessed by sequential SPECT imaging. Black = scar; Green = ischemia; DLY = delay; HL = horizontal long axis, PDS = perfusion defect size; SA = short axis; STR = stress; VL = vertical long axis. *(See also Fig. 15-24, A-D.)*

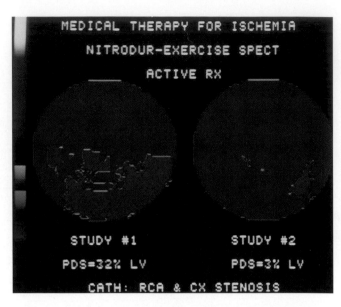

Color Plate 7. Polar maps in a patient with angiographic stenosis of the right (RCA) and circumflex (CX) coronary arteries before *(left)* and after *(right)* nitrate patch therapy. The polar map on the left demonstrates a 32% ischemic perfusion defect *(blue)* following symptom-limited treadmill exercise. The patient underwent a second exercise test 6 days after starting nitrate patch therapy. The polar map after therapy *(right)* showed almost complete resolution of scintigraphic ischemia. PDS = perfusion defect size. (Reproduced from Mahmarian JJ and Verani MS: Use of radionuclide imaging in assessing medical therapy. In Iskandrian AS [ed.], Myocardial Perfusion Imaging, Part II: Acute Coronary Syndromes and Interventions, *Am J Cardiol CME Series,* 19, 1993.) *(See also Fig. 15-26.)*

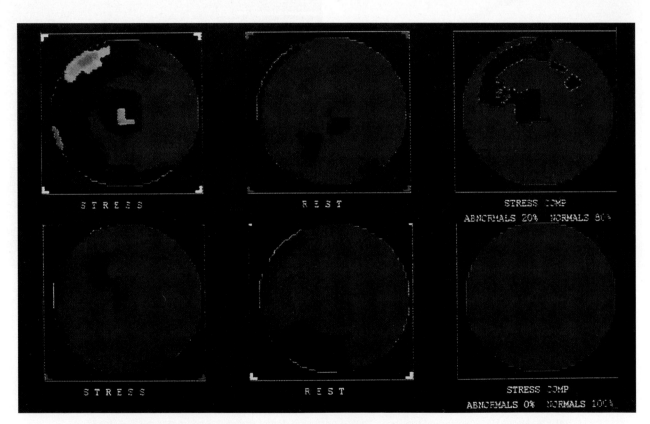

Color Plate 8. The raw data and statistical polar maps of a patient at baseline (study 1) *(upper panel)* and while receiving 21-mg nicotine patches (study 3) *(lower panel)* are displayed. The improvement in myocardial perfusion on the raw data stress polar map at study 3 compared with baseline is evident. The quantified 20% exercise-induced perfusion defect at baseline (STRESS COMP) *(green)* is virtually eliminated at study 3 despite severe stenosis of the proximal left anterior descending coronary artery. This patient stopped smoking while receiving nicotine patch therapy and had a dramatic reduction in exhaled carbon monoxide levels (from 13 ppm to 3 ppm). Plasma nicotine levels increased from 13.8 ng/ml at baseline to 39.6 ng/ml while the patients was receiving 21-mg patch therapy. *(See also Fig. 15-29.)*

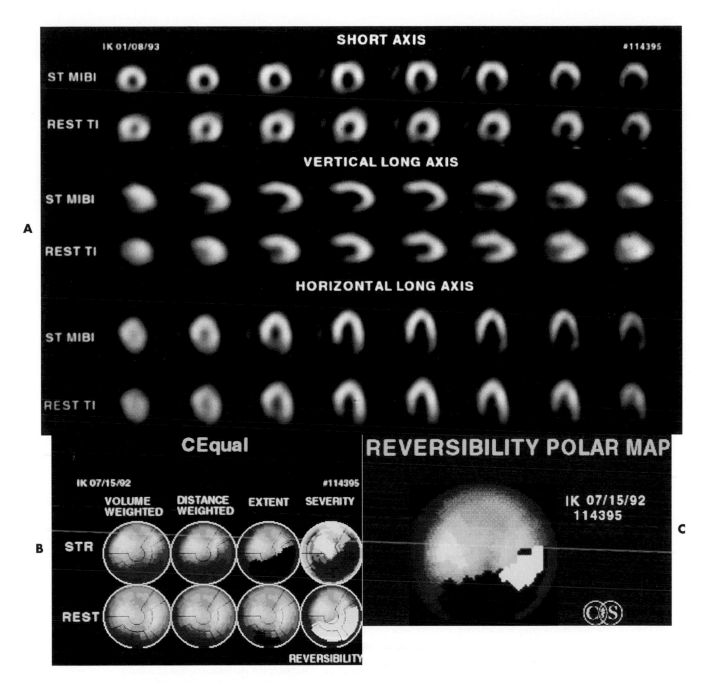

Color Plate 9. A, A case example of separate acquisition dual-isotope myocardial perfusion single-photon emission computed tomography demonstrating a small reversible defect in the inferolateral wall and a nonreversible defect in the inferior left ventricular wall. **B,** Cedars-Emory quantitative analysis (CEqual) quantitation using the standard normal limits of same-day rest-stress technetium-99m sestamibi demonstrates close correspondence to the visual abnormalities with respect to the extent of the stress defect but a lack of correspondence in defect reversibility. **C,** The reversibility in polar map using special dual-isotope normal limits is shown. This map shows the small reversible component and the larger nonreversible component, which accurately represents the visual findings in this patient. *(See also Fig. 17-12, A-C.)*

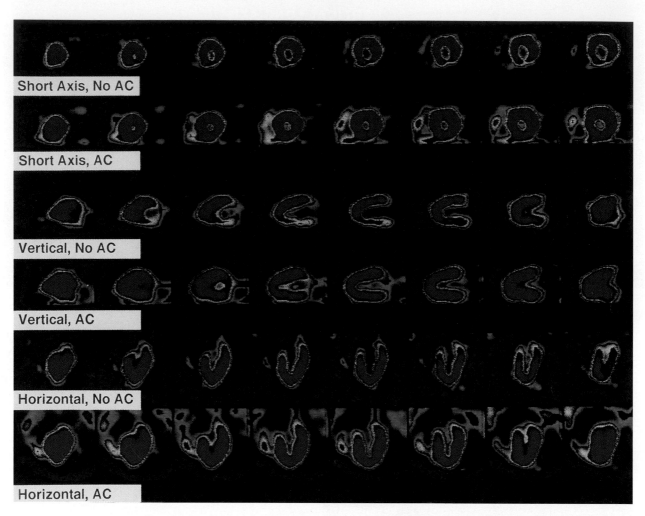

Color Plate 10. Inferoposterior photon attenuation causing an apparent perfusion defect in a short, obese male patient. The apparent defect disappears after photon attenuation correction using gadolinium-153 line sources and a dual-headed SPECT system. *(See also Fig. 22-1.)*

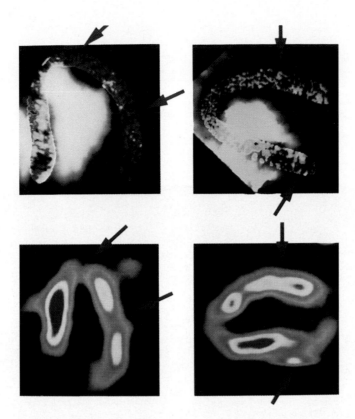

Color Plate 11. Perfusion defects in two patients with previous myocardial infarction. The top panels show images obtained with intermittent harmonic myocardial contrast echocardiography; the bottom panels show images obtained using technetium-99m sestamibi. The first patient (*left,* four-chamber view) has a large anterolateral defect. The second patient (*right,* two-chamber view) has defects in two vascular territories: the anteroapical and the upper posterior walls. The contrast echocardiographic image from the apical two-chamber view in this patient is placed on its side to correspond to the vertical two-chamber view obtained using technetium sestamibi. (From Kaul S, Senior R, Dittrich H, Raval U, Khattar R, Lahiri A: Detection of coronary artery disease with myocardial contrast echocardiography: comparison with 99mTc-sestamibi single-photon emission computed tomography, *Circulation* 96:785-792, 1997.) *(See also Fig. 23-13.)*

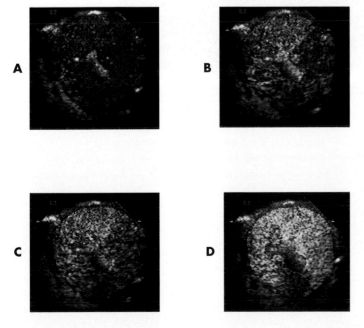

Color Plate 12. End-systolic images obtained at a constant left anterior descending artery flow at four pulsing intervals (316, 536, 1608, and 5360 ms, respectively, in **A** to **D**). Images were color coded so that the progression from red to yellow to orange to white denote increasing background-subtracted video intensity. (From Wei K, Jayaweera AR, Firoozan S, et al: Quantification of myocardial blood flow with ultrasound-induced destruction of microbubbles administered as a constant venous infusion, *Circulation* 97:473-483, 1998. With permission of the American Heart Association.) *(See also Fig. 23-22, A-D.)*

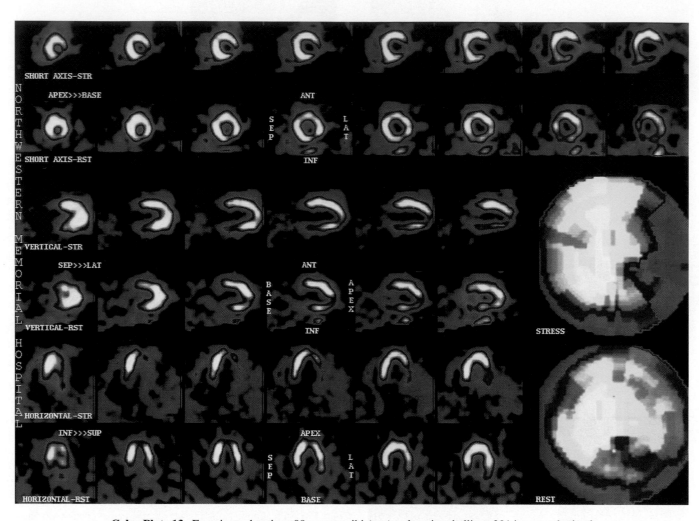

Color Plate 13. Exercise technetium-99m sestamibi *(top)* and resting thallium-201 images obtained as part of an exercise dual-isotope protocol in a man with recent-onset chest pain, demonstrating a moderate-sized region of severely decreased activity in the lateral wall. The patient was subsequently found to have 95% stenosis of the proximal left circumflex coronary artery. He underwent successful coronary angioplasty of this vessel. *(See also Fig. 24-7.)*

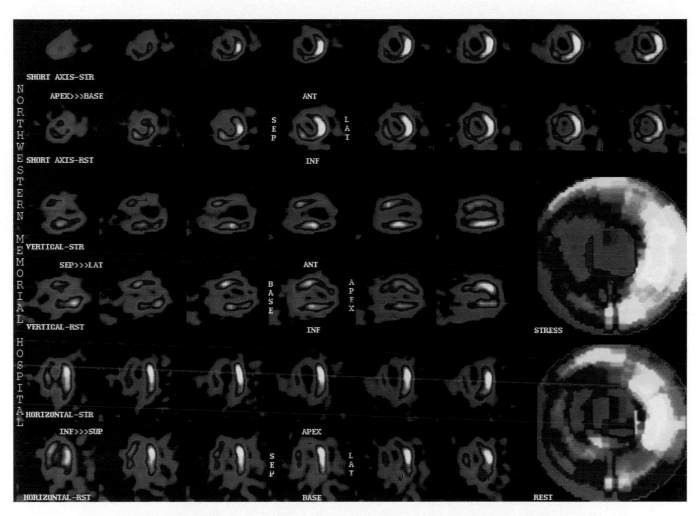

Color Plate 14. Dual-isotope images of a 47-year-old man who presented 5 days earlier with acute myocardial infarction and underwent successful percutaneous transluminal coronary angioplasty of the left anterior descending and first diagonal arteries. A moderately large defect of moderate severity is noted in the anterior, apical, and septal walls, with substantial (albeit not complete) reversibility. Because of recurrent symptoms 2 weeks later, he underwent repeated angiography, which revealed widely patent vessels. This study reveals the potential for a false-positive examination shortly after angioplasty. *(See also Fig. 24-10.)*

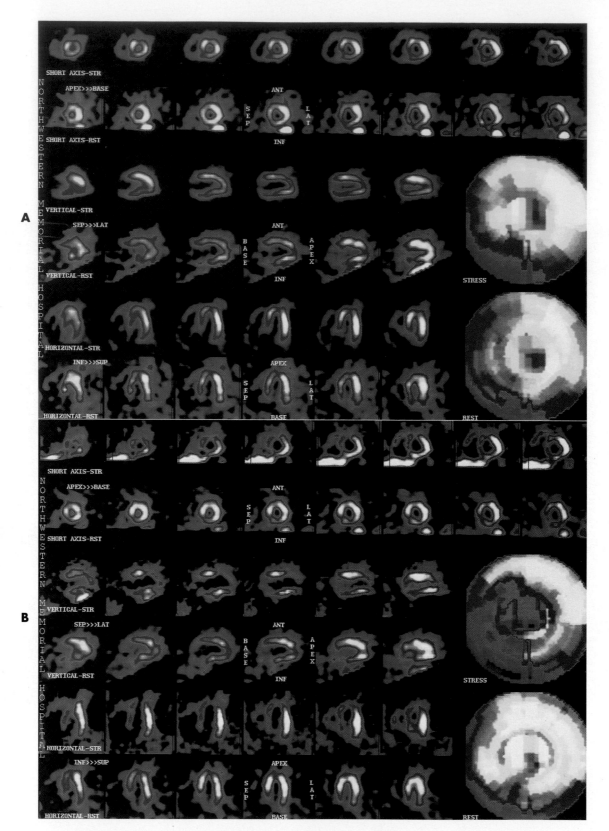

Color Plate 15. These images are of a 52-year-old man who sustained an anterior wall myocardial infarction, treated urgently with an angioplasty of the left anterior descending *(LAD)* coronary artery. **A,** The first dual-isotope perfusion study *(top)* was obtained approximately 3 weeks later and was thought to be normal except for diaphragmatic attenuation. His chest pain subsequently recurred, and at 3.5 months after the initial event, he underwent a second perfusion study. These images *(middle)* show a large, reversible perfusion defect in the anterior, septal, and apical walls. In addition, the ejection fraction measured by gated single-photon emission computed tomography decreased from 51% on the first study to 40% on the second. Repeated angiography demonstrated restenosis in the proximal LAD, for which a stent was most in place. **B,** Repeated perfusion imaging after percutaneous transluminal coronary angioplasty demonstrates resolution of ischemia. *(See also Fig. 24-14, A & B.)*

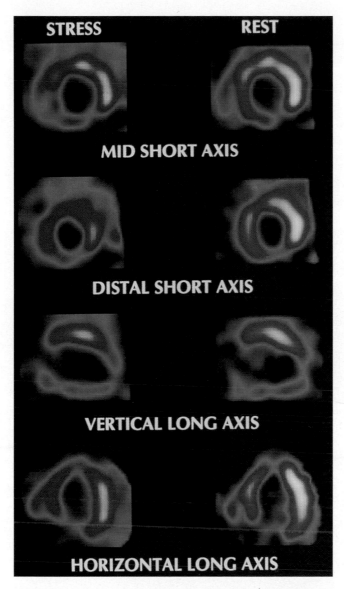

Color Plate 16. Stress *(left row)* and rest *(right row)* technetium-99m sestamibi SPECT images obtained in a patient who underwent submaximal exercise testing 1 week after an uncomplicated acute myo-cardial infarction. Note the nonreversible inferior defect consistent with the patient's inferior myocardial infarction. A defect in the anterior wall and intraventricular septum can be seen that demonstrates reversibility on the resting tomograms. This is consistent with remote ischemia in the supply region of the left anterior descending coronary artery. *(See also Fig. 26-6.)*

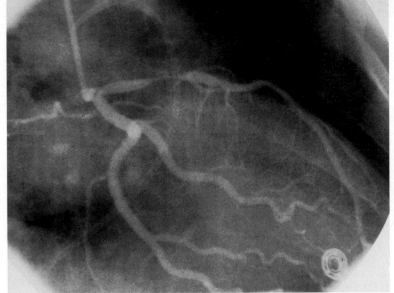

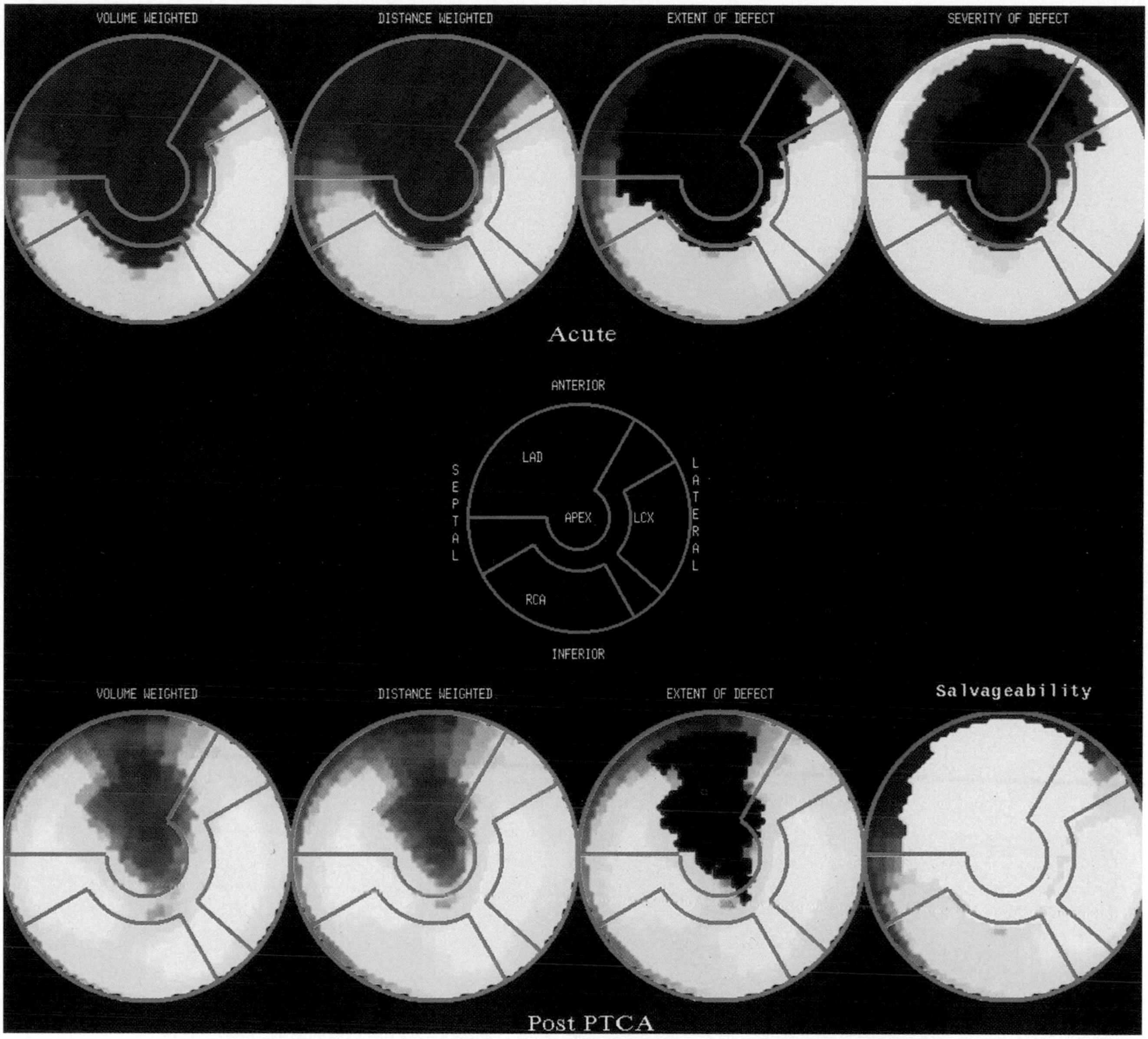

Color Plate 17. A 32-year-old women who experienced intermittent chest pain for 3 days. The presenting electrocardiogram **(A)** showed only T-wave changes that were considered suspicious but nonspecific. The patient was assigned to Acute Cardiac Team level 4. Acute technetium-99m sestamibi single-photon emission computed tomography (SPECT) **(B)** showed an extensive high-grade anteroseptal defect, and cardiac catheterization **(C)** demonstrated a high-grade proximal left anterior descending defect that led to immediate percutaneous transluminal coronary angioplasty (PTCA). Repeated resting sestamibi SPECT MIBI before hospital discharge (day 5) **(D)** demonstrates significant salvage of myocardium compared with the acute risk area. This is also seen his comparing the acute and post-PTCA polar maps with salvageability displayed in lower right corner **(E)**. *(See also Fig. 21-1, A- E.)*

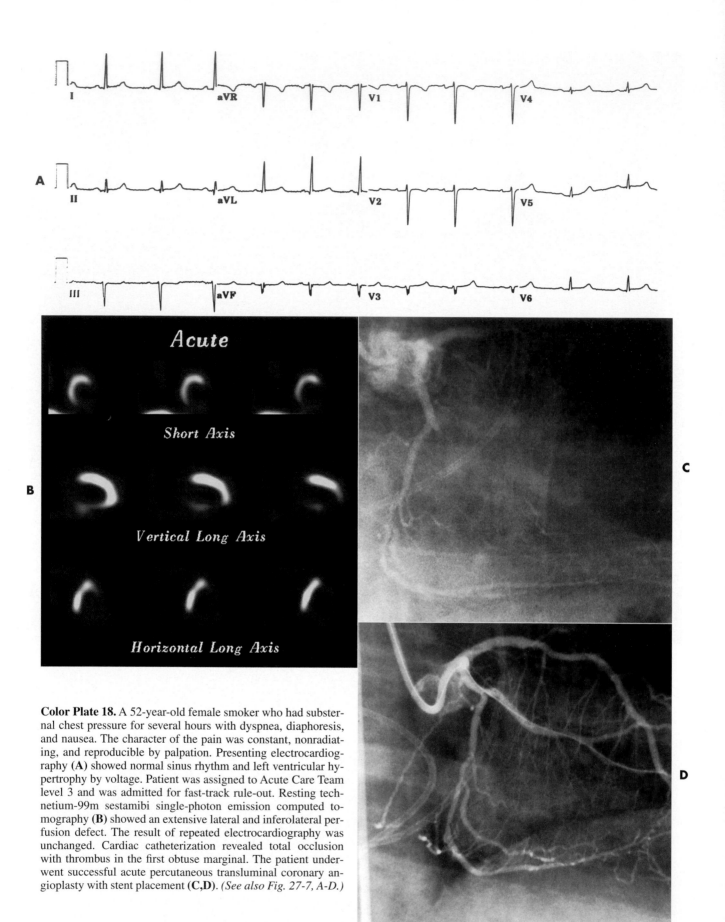

Color Plate 18. A 52-year-old female smoker who had substernal chest pressure for several hours with dyspnea, diaphoresis, and nausea. The character of the pain was constant, nonradiating, and reproducible by palpation. Presenting electrocardiography (**A**) showed normal sinus rhythm and left ventricular hypertrophy by voltage. Patient was assigned to Acute Care Team level 3 and was admitted for fast-track rule-out. Resting technetium-99m sestamibi single-photon emission computed tomography (**B**) showed an extensive lateral and inferolateral perfusion defect. The result of repeated electrocardiography was unchanged. Cardiac catheterization revealed total occlusion with thrombus in the first obtuse marginal. The patient underwent successful acute percutaneous transluminal coronary angioplasty with stent placement (**C,D**). *(See also Fig. 27-7, A-D.)*

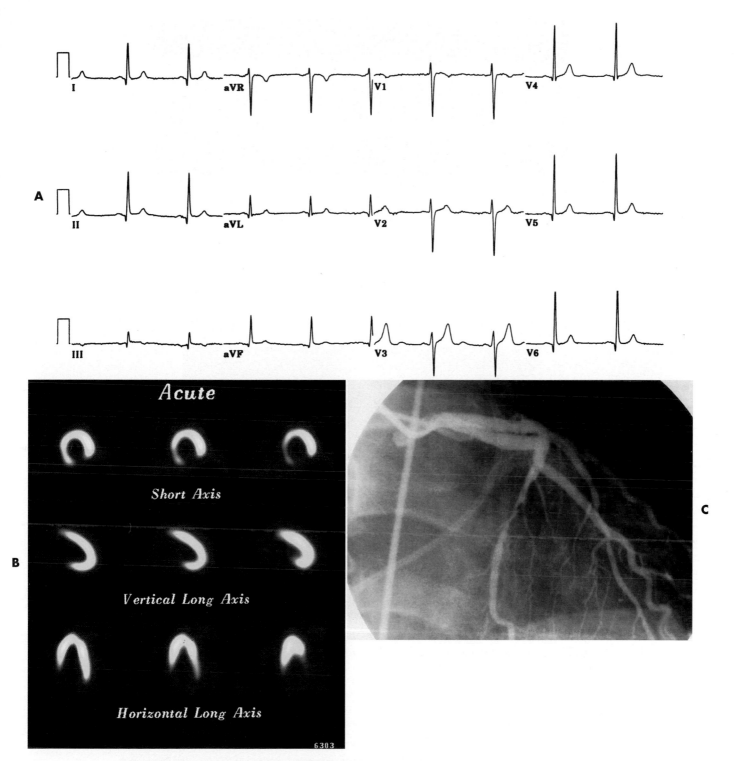

Color Plate 19. A 54-year-old man with known hypertension had had intermittent chest pain for 2 days. The burning character of the pain was attributed to eating spicy foods. Presenting electrocardiography (**A**) demonstrated normal sinus rhythm with left ventricular hypertrophy by voltage. The patient was assigned to Acute Cardiac Team level 4. Resting technetium-99m sestamibi single-photon emission computed tomography (**B**) showed an extensive high-grade inferior perfusion defect. The patient was admitted to the coronary intensive care unit. Two hours later, he developed ST elevation and received tissue plasminogen activator. Cardiac catheterization performed 24 hours later (**C**) revealed a long high-grade circumflex lesion. The patient underwent successful percutaneous transluminal coronary angioplasty an uneventful postintervention course. *(See also Fig. 27-8, A-C.)*

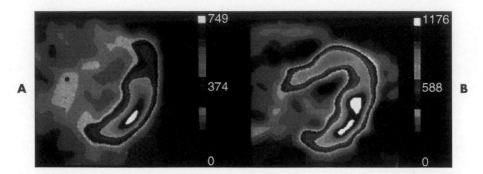

Color Plate 20. Transversal myocardial positron emission tomographic sections showing distribution of 2-[18F]fluoro-2-deoxy-glucose in a normal volunteer under fasting conditions **(A)** and after oral glucose loading **(B)**. The markedly diminished tracer accumulation in the septum under fasting conditions improves after glucose loading. (Reprinted by permission of the author and the Society of Nuclear Medicine from: Gropler RJ, Siegel BA, Lee KJ, et al. Nonuniformity in myocardial accumulation of fluorine-18-FDG in normal fasted humans, *J Nucl Med* 31:1749-1756, 1990.) *(See also Fig. 32-3, A & B.)*

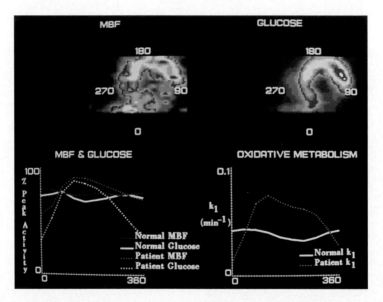

Color Plate 21. Flow and metabolism in irreversibly dysfunctional myocardium (no change in mechanical dysfunction on serial-wall motion studies) in the inferolateral wall. The midventricular images of flow *(upper left)* and glucose metabolism *(upper right)* are displayed in true short-axis orientation. The lateral wall is at 90? and the anterior wall is at 180 degrees. At the lower left are circumferential profiles of the relative values for regional perfusion (blue interrupted curve) and glucose metabolism *(yellow interrupted curve)*. Profiles representing the lower limits of normal (derived from 10 normal controls) for regional flow and glucose utilization are depicted by the solid red and white curves, respectively. At the lower right is the profile representing regional values for the myocardial turnover rate constant of acetate (k1) for this patient *(blue interrupted curve)* superimposed on the profile depicting the lower limits of normal *(white solid curve)*. Myocardial blood flow *(MBF)* and glucose metabolism are reduced concordantly in the inferolateral wall; the values are decreased to less than the lower limits of normal, a pattern consistent with irreversibly damaged tissue. Myocardial oxidative metabolism in the inferolateral wall is also decreased to less than the lower limits of normal for this region, consistent with irreversibly dysfunctional myocardium (Reproduced with permission: Rubin PJ, Lee DS, Davila-Roman VG, et al: Superiority of C-11 acetate compared with f-18 fluorodeoxyglucose in predicting myocardial functional recovery by positron emission tomography in patients with acute myocardial infarction, *Am J Cardiol* 78:1230-1235, 1996.) *(See also Fig. 33-3.)*

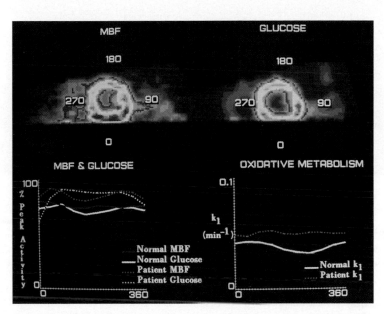

Color Plate 22. Flow and metabolism in the anterior wall with reversibly dysfunctional myocardium (akinesia present initially, with normal function on follow-up). In the anterior wall, both flow and glucose metabolism are within the normal range predictive of functional recovery. Myocardial oxidative metabolism in the anterior wall is within the normal range as well. (Reproduced with permission: Rubin PJ, Lee DS, Davila-Roman VG, et al: Superiority of C-11 acetate compared with F-18 fluorodeoooxyglucose in predicting myocardial functional recovery by positron emission tomography in patients with acute myocardial infarction, *Am J Cardiol* 78:1230–1235, 1996.) *(See also Fig. 33-4.)*

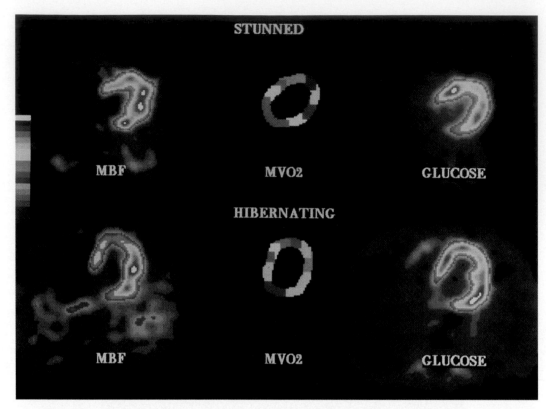

Color Plate 23. Images of myocardial perfusion and metabolism in patients with diverse perfusion and reversibly dysfunctional segments. The images to the left show relative perfusion with oxygen-15 water; the images in the middle are parametric displays of regional values of myocardial clearance of carbon-11 activity after the administration of 11C acetate and reflect regional oxidative metabolism; images on the right depict regional glucose metabolism with fluorine-18 fluorodeoxyglucose. The color bars are a linear representation of activity in all of the images. The septum is to the left and the anterior wall is on top. In the upper example, reversible dysfunction was present in the anterior wall, but myocardial blood flow was normal at 1.2 ml/g/min. Both oxidative metabolism and glucose metabolism were comparable to values in the normally functioning lateral wall. These findings are consistent with stunned myocardium. In the lower panel, reversible dysfunction is present in the anteroapical wall. Perfusion was reduced at 0.50 ml/g/min. Oxidative metabolism was reduced relative to that in the normally functioning posterolateral wall. Glucose metabolism was increased relative to flow. These findings probably reflect myocardial hibernation (Reproduced with permission: Conversano A, Walsh JF, Geltman FM, et al: Delineation of myocardial stunning and hibernation by positron emission tomography in advanced coronary artery disease, *Am Heart J* 131:440-450, 1996.) *(See also Fig. 33-5.)*

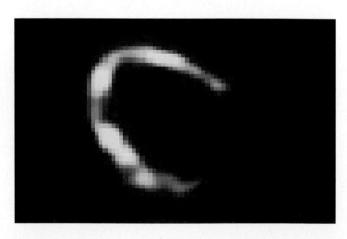

Color Plate 24. Representative midventricular tomogram acquired with positron emission tomography after intravenous administration of carbon-11 choline glycerophosphatide in a normal patient. This ligand binds with high affinity to the externalized βreceptors. The left ventricle is to the left. The lateral left ventricular wall is to the left, the septum is to the right, and the anterior wall is at the top. The regional distribution of the tracer is homogenous, and the heart to lung ratio of activity high. *(See also Fig. 36-1.)*

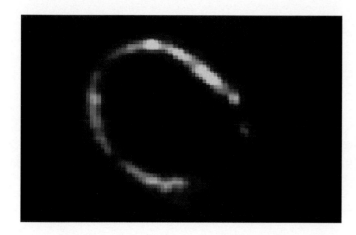

Color Plate 25. Midventricular tomogram acquired after intravenous administration of carbon-11 choline glycerophosphatide (CGP) in a patient with severe left ventricular dysfunction related to idiopathic dilated cardiomyopathy. Compared with the normal patient, the myocardial uptake of labeled CGP seems to be high. However, decreased concentration of available receptor sites was found when mathematical analysis was done, because the images are normalized. *(See also Fig. 36- 2.)*

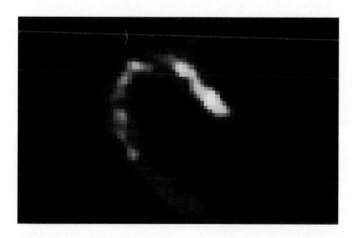

Color Plate 26. Midventricular tomogram acquired after intravenous administration in a normal subject of carbon-11 N-methyl 3-quinuclidinyl benzilate, an antagonist of the muscarinic acetylcholine receptors. The orientation is the same as that in Colorplate 24. A high activity is seen in the myocardium. Activity in the right ventricle is lower than that in the left ventricle. Lungs and blood activities are very low. *(See also Fig. 36-3.)*

Color Plate 27. Midventricular tomogram acquired after intravenous administration of carbon-11 N-methyl 3-quinuclidinyl benzilate in a patient with nonischemic dilated cardiomyopathy. In such patients, an increased number of muscarinic acetylcholine receptors was seen by using this positron emission tomographic approach. *(See also Fig. 36-4.)*

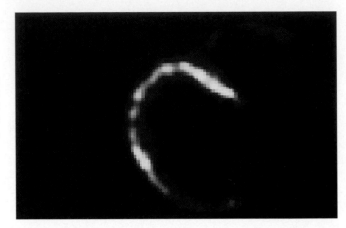

Color Plate 28. Midventricular tomogram acquired after administration of carbon-11 choline glyceropeptide in a patient with primary hypertrophic cardiomyopathy who had had an episode of decompensed heart failure. A significant decrease in breceptor sites has been found in such patients, similar to that found in patients with idiopathic dilated cardiomyopathy. *(See also Fig. 36-5.)*

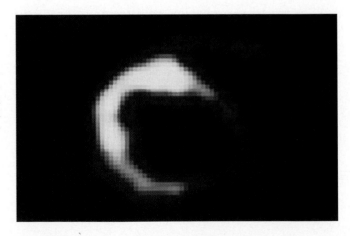

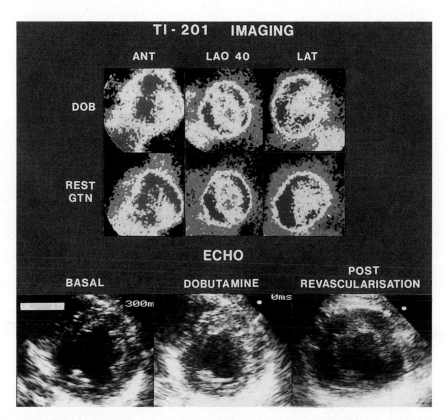

Color Plate 29. Composite image of a patient with a preoperative left ventricular ejection fraction of 17%, triple-vessel disease, and New York Heart Association class IV congestive heart failure. Top, dobutamine and rest-redistribution ^{201}Tl imaging at 1 hour after treatment with glyceryl trinitrate (GTN) shows retained viability in the anterior, septal, and lateral walls. Bottom, short-axis end-systolic echocardiographic images at rest (basal) *(left)* and low-dose dobutamine *(middle)* before surgery and at rest 3 months after revascularization *(right)*. The basal echocardiogram shows discordance caused by severe global hypokinesia (left ventricular ejection fraction, 17%). The dobutamine echocardiogram shows improved wall thickening in the anteroseptal, lateral, and inferior walls (left ventricular ejection fraction 30%) but not in the inferoposterolateral wall, which shows a matching perfusion defect in the same region with [201]Tl. Three months after revascularization, improved contractility was seen in the antero-septal and lateral walls (predicted by ^{201}Tl and dobutamine echocardiography). The postoperative left ventricular ejection fraction improved to 32%. Reduced anterolateral perfusion can be seen on ^{201}Tl imaging during dobutamine infusion despite increased contractility as demonstrated by echocardiography in the same region. (From Senior R, Glenville B, Basu S, et al: Dobutamine echocardiography and thallium-201 imaging predict functional improvement after revascularization in severe ischaemic left ventricular dysfunction, *Br Heart J* 74:358-364, 1995.) *(See also Fig. 37-4.)*

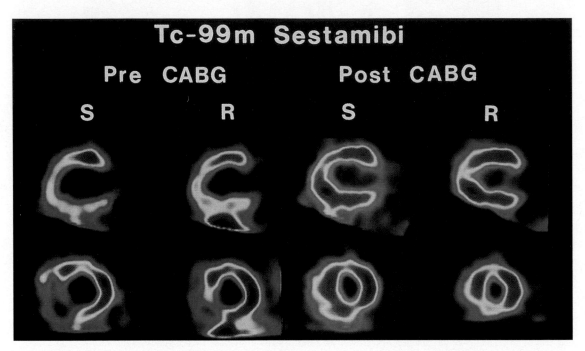

Color Plate 30. Technetium-99m sestamibi (MIBI) single-photon emission computed tomography in a 42-year-old man with New York Heart Association class IV heart failure (CHF) who was awaiting heart transplantation. The rest *(R)* nitrate-enhanced MIBI image shows extensive myocardial viability despite left ventricular ejection fraction of 17%. Extensive ischemia was noted by stress *(S)* MIBI after, 2 minutes of a modified Bruce protocol. Three months after triple-vessel revascularization, exercise tolerance increased to 10 minutes of Bruce protocol, with a normal MIBI, improvement in left ventricular ejection fraction to 48%, and no evidence of CHF. *(See also Fig. 37-7.)*

RADIO-PHARMACEUTICALS/ TRACER KINETICS

Chapter 1

Overview of kinetics and modeling

Denny D. Watson and **David K. Glover**

Over the past two decades of myocardial perfusion imaging, many observations have been made from laboratory data and human studies that relate to tracer kinetics. These observations highlight several clinically important questions, including the sensitivity of various tracers in showing a substantial reduction of coronary flow reserve, the use and limitations of redistribution and reinjection, and how various tracers can be used to differentiate viable from nonviable myocardium

Although many studies have been performed, they do not lead easily to a coherent overall pattern from which we can understand the kinetic behavior of tracers. The sum total of the literature forms a tapestry that can be as confounding as the astronomical data when the motion of planets was being described by earth-centered Ptolemaic epicycles. Kepler's model of planets orbiting the sun under the captivating force of gravity is an example of how a simple model can enable our understanding. Although this model did not illuminate deeper scientific questions, such as the cause of gravitational attraction, it gave us a simple way to understand such practical matters as day and night, summer and winter, the tides, and daylight savings time.

In this chapter, we use a solute absorption model to foster an understanding of the relation of tracer extraction to capillary perfusion and also a simplified compartmental exchange model to help understand tracer redistribution. These models are not concerned with the biochemical process of tracer transport and ignore much of the complexity of the physiologic system. We use them in the spirit of Kepler's model: to bring the mass of laboratory data into a coherent pattern and to help answer some of the practical questions encountered in clinical practice.

TRACER EXTRACTION

It is a common mis-statement that tracer extraction is proportional to blood flow. This would only be true for completely extracted tracers, such as microspheres. From a systemic injection, the number of tracer atoms that pass through a capillary bed will be proportional to the fraction of total cardiac output that passes through the capillary bed. If all of the tracer atoms are extracted, the number per unit volume of tissue will be proportional to the fraction of cardiac output per unit volume of perfused tissue.

The tracers used for clinical imaging of myocardial blood flow are not completely extracted. For these tracers, the fraction of tracer extracted when passing through a capillary bed depends on the blood flow through the capillary bed. A model of a diffusible tracer traveling through a cylindrical capillary based on the work of Gosselin and Stibitz[4] provides insight into this process. The tracer can diffuse outward from the blood across the capillary endothelium, but it can also diffuse back into the blood from outside the capillary endothelium. The outward and back-diffusion coefficients can be different. The extraction coefficient reflects the net loss in tracer concentration between the arterial and venous ends of the capillary. This leads to a tracer "extraction fraction" of the form:

$$1 - e^{-\frac{PS}{b}} \tag{1}$$

where PS is a product of capillary permeability and surface area and b is the capillary blood flow. The relation between blood flow and tracer extraction is shown in Fig. 1-1. The top curve with $PS = 4$ would represent a tracer with very high first-pass extraction; the lower curve with $PS = 1$ would represent a tracer with lower first-pass extraction.

The amount of tracer retained by the myocardium shortly after bolus injection is the product of extraction fraction and myocardial flow per unit of volume, which would be represented by the equation:

$$\text{Myocardial extraction} \propto b(1 - e^{-\frac{PS}{b}}) \qquad (2)$$

The curve with the functional form shown above has been ubiquitous in representing myocardial uptake as a function of myocardial blood flow. Although the equation was derived for solute exchange in a single capillary, the functional form remains unchanged for a generalized distribution of capillaries if the variables are taken to represent the averages over the entire capillary distribution.

A flaw in the basic model of Gosselin and Stibitz is that it does not account for the possibility that the capillary blood volume may depend on flow, which would be true if flow regulation involves the opening and closing of capillary channels or changes in the effective capillary diameter; such a phenomenon has been experimentally demonstrated.[6,12] To include the possible effect of variable capillary volumes, we would extend the model as follows: The first factor in Equation 2 is replaced by F, which represents flow per unit of myocardial volume. The term b in the exponential represents flow per unit of open capillary volume. We therefore introduce a new relation:

$$\frac{F}{b} = 1 - e^{-F} \qquad (3)$$

This term relates the flow in the open capillaries to the flow per unit of myocardial volume determined by the supply vessels. Equation 3 introduces the assumption that capillary blood volume decreases as flow is reduced because of capillary closure or constriction and increases to some maximal value when all of the capillary channels are fully used at high flow. Figure 1-2 shows the relative capillary volume assumed by equation 3, which qualitatively agrees with the observations of Wu et al.[12] The exact manner in which capillary volume changes in the

course of vasoregulation is unknown. Our purpose here is limited to showing what effect (if any) this change would have on tracer extraction. To this end, we can introduce the assumption shown as a hypothesis in Fig. 1-2 to demonstrate the effect of capillary closure, if it indeed follows a pattern similar to that shown in Fig. 1-2.

The effect of capillary closure can be seen in Fig. 1-3. The curves of first-pass extraction become less dependent on blood flow. The first-pass extraction fraction at low flow is much less than would be predicted by the basic model of Gosselin and Stibitz.[4] The corresponding curves of the myocardial flow–extraction product for tracers with high and low first-pass extraction are shown in Fig. 1-4.

Figure 1-5 shows extraction fraction curves generated by using the modified model for PS values of 3.1 and 1.6. These values for the PS coefficient are then used to predict myocardial uptake versus flow, and the curves with an overall normalization are plotted by using experimental data from Glover et al.[2] The predicted curves fit the experimental data quite well.

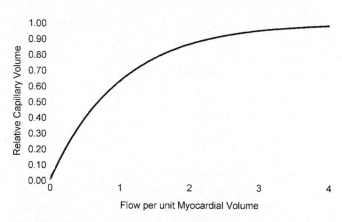

Fig. 1-2. Relation between the fraction of open capillary volume and myocardial blood flow per unit of myocardial volume.

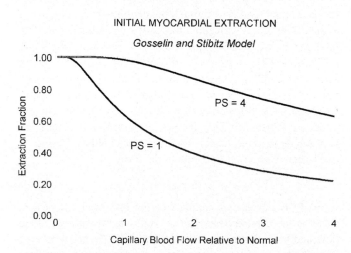

Fig. 1-1. Tracer extraction fraction as predicted by the Gosselin and Stibitz model. Curves are shown for $PS = 1$, representing a poorly extracted tracer, and $PS = 4$, representing a tracer with very high first-pass extraction.

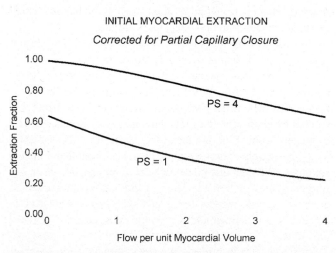

Fig. 1-3. Tracer extraction fraction for the same values of $PS = 1$ and $PS = 4$ as those shown in Fig. 1-1. These curves show the changes in first-pass extraction caused by the introduction of variable capillary volume as assumed in Figure 1-2.

The curves of Fig. 1-6 represent a transition from a low-flow state, where tracer extraction is flow limited and therefore proportional to flow, to high-flow states, where extraction is limited by membrane diffusion and is therefore not dependent on flow. Another way of thinking of this is that the tracer spends less time in the capillary at higher flows and consequently has a lower probability of being extracted in a single pass through the capillary. At sufficiently low flows, more of the tracer atoms can be extracted, and the tracer acts more like an ideal (that is, a microsphere) flow tracer. If the capillary pathways close substantially as flow decreases, the increased extraction at low flow is less marked and tracer extraction remains linear over a wider range of flow. The introduction of capillary closure was essential so the model could simultaneously predict the first-pass extraction fractions and fit the uptake-versus-flow data. Without the assumption of capillary closure, the basic model overesti-

mates extraction at low flow for values of PS that fit the myocardial uptake curves.

The nonlinearity of tracer uptake versus flow is striking and may seem to be at odds with many reports that tracer uptake is proportional to myocardial blood flow. Figures 1-7 and 1-8 illustrate how this may occur. Figure 1-7 shows some data from studies on dogs in our research laboratory. A linear curve fit has been performed for which the correlation coefficient is very high. The straight line intersects above the origin. On the basis of this data, it could be said that uptake is linearly proportional to flow and that tracer uptake overestimates flow at low flows.

Figure 1-8 shows exactly the same data as Fig. 1-7, except that the range has been extended to display tracer uptake at lower and higher levels of myocardial blood flow. The failure of the straight line to fit is now obvious. The curve shown in Fig. 1-8 is the prediction of the Gosselin and Stibitz model, which is

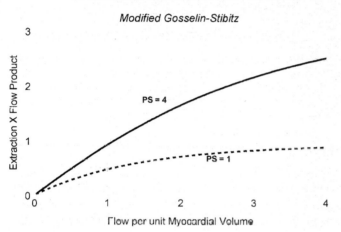

Fig. 1-4. Curves of myocardial uptake as a function of total flow per unit volume to the myocardium. These curves are based on the predicted extraction fraction with variable capillary volume.

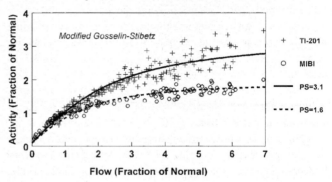

Fig. 1-6. Solid curves are the predicted values of tracer activity versus myocardial blood flow using the values for PS based on first-pass extraction coefficients and the modified model with variable capillary volume. Data were obtained from an animal model.

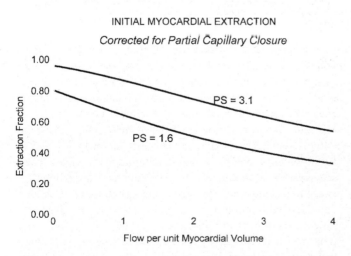

Fig. 1-5. Extraction fraction curves for specific values of $PS = 1.6$, representing the first-pass extraction fraction of technetium-99m sestamibi, and $PS = 3.1$, representing the first-pass extraction of thallium-201.

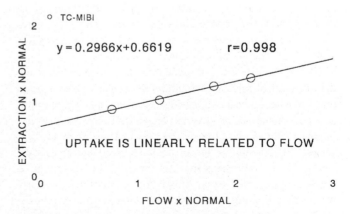

Fig. 1-7. Extraction of technetium-99m sestamibi from an animal model with data obtained over a limited range of flow. These data seem to fit a straight line that intersects above the origin.

EXTRACTION vs FLOW DURING ADENOSINE

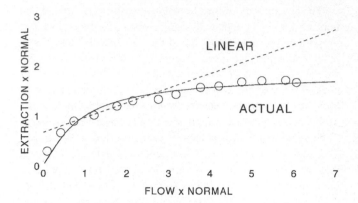

Fig. 1-8. These are the same data as those shown in Fig. 1-7, with the addition of more data over a wider range of myocardial flow values. Tracer uptake is now seen to be nonlinear.

clearly a better predictor than the linear model. Tracer uptake starts out being proportional to flow at very low flows, but it falls off rapidly and becomes flow independent at high flow.

In practical myocardial imaging, we do not observe absolute flow or tracer uptake but compare samples in presumably abnormal segments with those from a presumably normal segment. Figure 1-9 shows an actual tracer extraction curve that has progressively decreasing extraction as flow increases. However, the curve is normalized to indicate tracer uptake of 1.0 when myocardial flow is 1.0. Compared with a linear extraction with the same normalization, the actual curve seems to overestimate myocardial flow for values less than one and to underestimate for values greater than one. On a relative scale, in which all tracers are normalized to unity at normal resting blood flow, a tracer with a lower extraction will appear to overestimate low flows to a greater extent than a tracer with higher extraction. Both tracers underestimate flow compared with an ideal tracer, but the degree of underestimation is less for the tracer of higher extraction. On a relative scale, this underestimation makes it seem that tracers of lower extraction overestimate low flow. On an absolute scale, the tracer underestimates all flow values; on a relative scale, the tracer overestimates low flow values. Therefore, both statements are true.

The flow dependence of myocardial tracer uptake has more than theoretical relevance. It limits the sensitivity of a given tracer to detect coronary artery disease. It has significant implications for pharmacologic stress agents and may be the determining factor in choosing the best tracer for a given circumstance. The flattening of the curves of tracer uptake versus myocardial blood flow means that the defect in the tracer will be much less than the actual blood flow disparity, particularly when a flow-limiting lesion causes a reduction in the reserve capacity of a vessel so that a normal segment that has greatly increased flow is compared with an abnormal segment that has only slightly increased flow. The study by Glover et al showed that obstructions that only limit flow reserve can produce mini-

RELATIVE FLOW EXTRACTION PRODUCT

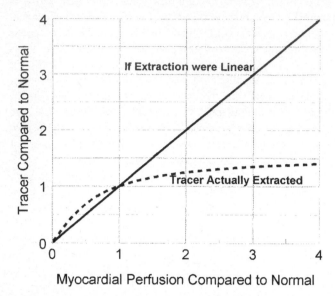

Fig. 1-9. Actual nonlinear tracer uptake compared with an ideal linear uptake (such as microspheres). If both curves are normalized to pass through the point (1,1), the nonlinear tracer will seem to overestimate low flow and underestimate high flow relative to the ideal.

mal tracer defect contrast despite maximum vasodilatation with adenosine.[2] Tracers with higher first-pass extraction will track blood flows over a wider range than will tracers with lower first-pass extraction. This does not apply to scar, because tracers with different extraction coefficients will indicate myocardial scar with equal contrast. As a result, comparison of the sensitivity of different tracers for the detection of coronary artery disease should separate patients who have infarcts from those who have only perfusion defects with viable muscle.

TRACER RETENTION

A highly diffusible tracer may be efficiently extracted, but it will diffuse back across the membrane into the blood as rapidly as it was extracted unless there is some mechanism to trap or bind the extracted molecule. Teboroxime belongs to a class of neutral molecules that are highly diffusible but unbound. Its initial extraction is fairly proportional to the fraction of cardiac output passing through the capillary bed, but the molecules diffuse back out of the myocardium within a few minutes. There seems to be no mechanism for maintaining a differential between intracellular and intravascular concentration. As a result, delayed equilibrium imaging does not reflect myocardial blood flow or viability. The initial washout rate of these diffusible molecules is modulated by regional blood flow. Dynamic measurements of regional washin and washout rates could potentially provide valid and quantitative information about regional blood flow. Such a class of tracers is not presently in widespread use, probably because available single-photon emission computed tomography (SPECT) units are too limited for use in rapid dynamic imaging.

Sestamibi is extracted with an intermediate first-pass extraction and bound within myocardial cells largely by the mitochondrial membrane potential.[10] Tetrofosmin and furifosmin have progressively lower first-pass extraction[3,7] and have similar binding. The process of redistribution (a term used for delayed imaging of thallium-201 (^{201}Tl) and reversibility (a term used for rest and stress imaging with technetium-99m [^{99m}Tc] agents) is related to the retention and exchange of these tracers.

REDISTRIBUTION

The mechanism

Most myocardial tracers are not fixed in the myocardium but have some intrinsic rate of washout. If the tracer were injected only in the myocardium, its washout rate would reflect myocardial blood flow (that is, higher blood flow would encourage more rapid tracer washout).[5] This intuitive statement is not useful when systemic injections are used. After a systemic tracer injection, no more than 3% to 5% of the tracer is delivered to the myocardium; the rest is distributed throughout the other body compartments. After the initial distribution, the tracer then starts to exchange between the various compartments. The amount of "washout" from the myocardium depends not only on how much tracer is leaving the myocardium, but also on how much continuously accumulates by exchange from other compartments. It is simplistic and incorrect to expect the net washout to simply reflect myocardial perfusion.

The process of redistribution is still a subject of investigation, and it has been a central issue in the detection of myocardial ischemia and viability. Use of a compartmental exchange model will foster a better understanding of the redistribution process. We tailored the model specifically for ^{201}Tl for two reasons: It is the most important example of using redistribution as part of clinical practice, and it is an unusually simple example of a multicompartmental model. It is simple because the extraction process is rapid, the membrane exchange process is of intermediate duration (about 1 hour), and the systemic excretion process is long (more than 10 hours). Under these circumstances, the differential equations describing the process can be uncoupled effectively, resulting in a very simple, closed analytic solution of multiple exponentials with coefficients that can be interpreted intuitively. In keeping with our desire not to get bogged down in mathematics, some illustrations are provided.

Figure 1-10 shows the myocardial uptake and washout of an exchangeable tracer that is injected intravenously. The curves of Figure 1-10 are based on parameters that reflect ^{201}Tl. Specifically, a blood clearance half-time of 1 to 5 minutes is assumed, a systemic excretion of about 10 hours is assumed, and the intrinsic myocardial membrane transport coefficient is taken as 0.01, representing a half-time of 69 minutes in accordance with experimental data.[5] The curves show rapid early myocardial uptake that is roughly proportional to myocardial perfusion. Blood levels of the tracer decrease rapidly as it is extracted by the heart and all of the other systemic compartments

TI-201 REDISTRIBUTION

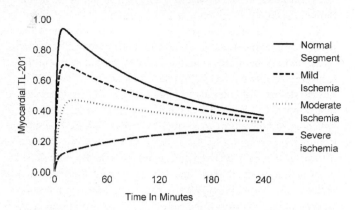

Fig. 1-10. Multicompartmental model of thallium-201 including extraction, redistribution, and systemic excretion. Myocardial tracer uptake is shown for normal flow and transiently reduced flows to 75%, 50%, and 25% of normal, respectively.

in relation to the distribution of cardiac output. After initial extraction, the tracer molecules are slowly released back into the blood, maintaining an almost constant low-level blood concentration of tracer. The subsequent exchange of tracer between blood and myocardial cells continues until an equilibrium is reached in which the myocardium loses one tracer molecule for each new molecule it picks up from the blood. This exchange equilibrium does not depend on blood flow. It depends only on the relative concentrations of intravascular and extravascular tracer molecules. The level of net tracer uptake at equilibrium is determined by the residual blood concentration of tracer and by the magnitude of the intracellular–extracellular concentration gradient supported by the membrane potentials or active membrane transport.

The clinically relevant parts of this process can be summarized as follows: (1) The initial myocardial extraction reflects the distribution of blood flow at the time of injection, and (2) the delayed uptake after equilibrium has been reached is flow independent, but it reflects an intact myocardial cell membrane and membrane potential and therefore is a marker of cell viability. This is the principle behind redistribution imaging. Because delayed uptake is flow independent, redistribution can still occur if a myocardial segment is chronically hypoperfused, even when injection is performed at rest. As shown in Fig. 1-11, rest redistribution has been demonstrated experimentally for both thallium and sestamibi.[11]

Redistribution versus persistent defect

Flow tracers that are trapped by membrane potentials are not retained by infarcted myocardium; therefore, the infarcted tissue will have a negligible tracer concentration. However, most perfusion defects are not samples of totally infarcted myocardium but consist of some infarcted myocardium mixed with normal or ischemic myocardium. In addition, the infarct borders are usually ragged and ill-defined. Because the resolution of imaging systems is too low to show the details of an infarct, infarcted tissue is usually sampled along with noninfarcted tissue.

Consider the example in Fig. 1-12, which compares one myocardial segment that is a half-and-half mixture of infarcted tissue and normal tissue with another myocardial segment that is entirely viable but has 50% reduced blood flow. The half-infarcted defect will continue to have half the uptake of the normal sample. The ischemic segment starts with an uptake that is half normal but returns to normal by redistribution. Examination of the curves in Fig. 1-12 shows that at any one time the difference between the fixed defect and the redistributing defect is surprisingly small. The signal (representing the difference between the two curves) is weak and comparable to the noise (representing the error of measurement) involved in real clinical imaging. Thus, under the best of circumstances, differentiation of partly infarcted from moderately ischemic myocardium will be subtle and subject to some uncertainty. We will return to this point when we discuss reinjection.

Reinjection

Redistribution of 201-Tl is used as a marker of myocardial viability, but it may significantly underestimate myocardial viability.[13] It has been reported that reinjection of ^{201}Tl at rest shows more redistribution than does delayed imaging alone, which enhances detection of viability.[1] We model this process in Fig. 1-13, which shows the same comparison of a myocardial segment that is half-normal and half infarcted, with a segment that is transiently ischemic with half-normal tracer uptake at stress. We assumed that blood flow returns to normal after stress and that reinjection of half of the initial dose takes place 150 minutes after stress injection. Figure 1-13 shows that tracer reinjection has two effects: It adds more tracer to both the normal and the abnormal segments. It adds more redistribution—the sudden equivalent of about 2 more hours of redistribution. Figure 1-14 shows data from an animal study in which a severe perfusion defect (resulting from mild subendocardial infarction and surrounding ischemia) was followed for 3 hours of redistribution and after reinjection. As indicated by the compartmental model, we see a severe defect with slow redistribution and the sudden addition of a bit more reversibility on reinjection. The change in response to reinjection is predictable—the equivalent of about 2 more hours of redistribution—but it is not dramatic.

Neither the model in Fig. 1-13 nor the animal data in Fig. 1-14 shows an absence of redistribution in a defect that reverses on reinjection. However, the juxtaposition of initial and delayed images with reinjection images sometimes creates the appearance of a patently fixed defect that suddenly reverses on reinjection. We have no physiologically logical model for that phenomenon, and no quantitative measurements confirm such behavior. Why, then, do scintiphotographs show visually persuasive examples of such behavior?

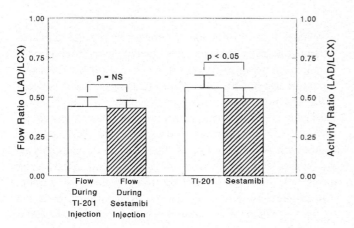

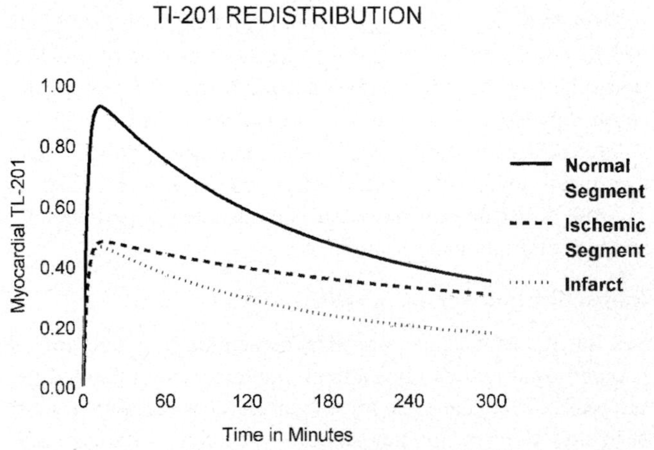

Fig. 1-11. Rest redistribution of thallium-201 and technetium-99m sestamibi in a canine model with 2 hours of sustained low flow. Note that although both tracers demonstrated rest redistribution, the amount was greater for thallium-201.

TI-201 REDISTRIBUTION

Fig. 1-12. Myocardial uptake and redistribution for a normal segment, a segment with half normal myocardium and half scar, and a viable segment with flow reduced to 50% of normal.

TI-201 REDISTRIBUTION
Post Mild Infarct

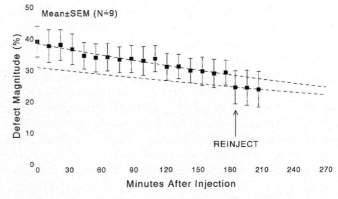

Fig. 1-13. Serial myocardial uptake measurements of defect to normal ratio after thallium-201 injection in a severely ischemic region. Reinjection was performed after 180 minutes.

Scintiphoto images give an amplified perception of reversibility after reinjection for two reasons. First, most images, particularly those of SPECT slices, have some background suppression. Severe defects that have some tracer uptake as well as some redistribution may have too little tracer to be visible above the background suppression level. The addition of more tracer activity by reinjection can lift the level of activity in these regions over the suppression level, resulting in the abrupt appearance of significant activity in regions that have previously seemed devoid of significant tracer uptake.

A second important factor has to do with sampling statistics. The amount of "tracer activity" in a sampled myocardial segment is not the ground truth; rather, it is an estimate based on a sample that is represented as an intensity level in an image. In SPECT images, the intensity level of a pixel representing myocardial tracer uptake is computed from a large number of statistically noisy samples. The presence of statistical noise means that if two images are acquired while the myocardial tracer uptake is identical, the uptake represented by the images will be different to the extent of the uncertainty of statistical sampling. In comparing images from only two samples, the amount of redistribution will be underestimated half of the time simply by virtue of sampling error. If we set aside all the image examples for which redistribution was shown (including the statistical overestimates) and select those examples for which redistribution was not demonstrated (including the statistical underestimates), a third sample will have a high probability (around 50%) of showing "reversibility" on re-sampling. If we had performed reinjection in the interim, we would have attributed the additional reversibility to reinjection. This is a classic example of a statistical phenomenon called "regression to the mean."

We have argued that additional reversibility on reinjection will inevitably be observed as a result of nonlinear count representation in images and also as a result of sampling statistics. However, these situations usually arise from underestimates of redistribution (either by imaging problems or sampling error); the second imaging procedure followed by reinjection will tend to correct the problem. Therefore, reinjection followed by additional imaging can identify more viable segments than are identified by delayed imaging alone. However, we argue that there are logical reasons for this phenomenon that do not require postulation that the ischemic muscle has some mysterious affinity for freshly reinjected tracer after refusing to extract previously injected tracer.

Ischemia versus viability

Ischemia is often confused with viability. This problem may have started in the early days of imaging when abnormal myocardial segments were seen as being either ischemic or infarcted. Redistribution indicated ischemia and its absence was taken to indicate scar. Various situations, including stunned and hibernating myocardium, are now recognized. We also recognize that stunned, hibernating, ischemic, infarcted, and normal myocardium can be interdigitated or mixed in the sampling volume. Significant residual tracer uptake, even without redistribution or reversibility, indicates significant residual myocardial viability. However, the definition of "significant viability" needs clarification. Usually, significant viability is assumed if reperfusion improves myocardial contractile function. If ischemia can be demonstrated, it is indicative that improved myocardial function will result from relief of ischemia. Significant residual tracer uptake may also be found without an overt indication of myocardial ischemia; this indicates the presence of functioning myocytes. If this is seen in an akinetic segment, it could indicate stunned myocardium or suggest an area that is prone to adverse remodeling if perfusion to this region is compromised. The findings of "significant viability" and "ischemia" should be distinguished and treated as having different clinical implications.

Tracers that do not redistribute

All tracers must redistribute to some extent; it is merely a question of degree. Technetium-labeled tracers that use a cationic, lipophilic molecule are more firmly trapped by membrane potentials after they diffuse out of the vascular bed. This means that the intrinsic transmembrane transport half-time is long and that the time to reach exchange equilibrium is correspondingly long. This time, for Tl-201, is on the order of 1 hour. That means that half of all of the remaining possible redistribution will take place each hour. As a result, redistribution times of 2 to 4 hours represent two to four half-times in the equilibration process and are adequate to see most of the significant redistribution. The lipophilic, cationic molecules represented by sestamibi and tetrofosmin seem to be sufficiently bound so that the exchange times are one order of magnitude longer. This puts the intrinsic transport half-time on the order of 10 hours and the corresponding time for redistribution from a systemic injection at about 20 to 40 hours. Because the technetium-99m decay half-time is 6 hours, there is a catch-22 for these isotopes: They decay before they redistribute. Again, we should expect to have some redistribution, but the amount is probably not sufficient to be clinically

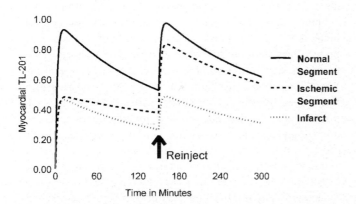

TI-201 REDISTRIBUTION

Fig. 1-14. Model of myocardial tracer activity that shows redistribution and the effect of reinjection at 150 minutes.

useful within the time frame when there is enough tracer for adequate imaging.

Reverse redistribution

A focal defect in a stress image is often seen that appears to be more severe on rest images. In addition a defect is sometimes seen on rest images that was not seen on stress images. This phenomenon has been called reverse redistribution. The cause or causes of this phenomenon should be examined before a conclusion is reached about its significance.

The kinetic transport models provide no logical explanation as to why a defect grows larger in delayed images. It is not logical for the myocardium to initially extract a normal amount of tracer (implying normal flow and extraction) and then lose tracer to the extent that a defect grows in the delayed images. There is no way to make the tracer uptake curves cross over, if we assume that the abnormal segment had normal uptake and extraction during the first-pass phase. This leaves us with a puzzle, to explain the frequent observations of reverse redistribution.

There are many ways to create the appearance of reverse redistribution, such as:

1. Motion artifact on the rest images.

2. Tissue attenuation artifact on the rest images caused by position shifts.

3. Misalignment on SPECT slices so that the rest image slice cuts through the edge of a fixed defect, but the stress slice misses the edge of the defect.

4. Changes in the image scale factor that make mild fixed defects appear more severe on rest images. This can happen because of tracer washout or because of higher visceral activity in rest images that can set the maximum image scale to a higher value and reduce the relative intensity of uptake in the defect region.

Because all these situations are common, the appearance of reverse redistribution must result in part from image artifact. Two physiologic situations are now recognized. One is the result of comparing an infarct to an ischemic segment in the mistaken assumption that there is a normal myocardial segment for reference. Suppose that we had an ischemic segment and a segment that was partly infarcted, as shown in Fig. 1-12. Suppose further that the normal segment was not visible, which could happen in cases of diffuse multiple vessel disease that was so extensive that there is no normal segment for reference. In such a case, tracer uptake is initially reduced in both the ischemic and infarct segments. The tracer then redistributes into the ischemic segment so that it ends up with more uptake than the partly infarcted segment, creating the appearance of a defect in the delayed or rest images that was not apparent in the stress images.

We have observed another appearance of reverse redistribution in segments with subendocardial scar that were supplied by vessels with restored patency. A logical theory for this is that during stress the epicardium surrounding the subendocardial

scar becomes more hyperemic compared with normal myocardium because of the increased wall stress. The hyperemic epicardium tends to obscure the subendocardial defect. In rest images, the amount of epicardial hyperemia is smaller, and the defect is thus more visible.

Therefore, two situations, one created by global severe multivessel disease and one created by a recanalized vessel feeding a subendocardial infarct, can logically explain the pattern of reverse redistribution. Multivessel disease is common, but a complete absence of any well-perfused myocardial reference sample is unusual. The occurrence of a recanalized vessel after a subendocardial infarct usually can be recognized from the clinical situation.

When neither of these physiologic explanations is available to account for the appearance of reverse redistribution, our experience has been that it is one of the several artifacts mentioned above. We can find no convincing evidence that a more mysterious explanation exists.

DETECTION OF CORONARY ARTERY DISEASE

We showed that highly extractable tracers are extracted in proportion to the fraction of total cardiac output passing through the capillary bed. Once the tracer leaves the capillary bed, it must be trapped by some mechanism, or it will rapidly diffuse back out of the myocardium. Thallium-201 is an example of a cationic, potassium-like tracer that is retained within the sarcolemmal membrane. At equilibrium, the tracer will be concentrated in the membrane relative to the blood pool; therefore, the intracellular concentration of tracer will be much greater than the blood pool concentration. There is a continuous exchange between intracellular and extracellular ions, giving rise to the process of redistribution. The cationic molecular tracers using technetium-99m behave in a similar manner, except that they are more firmly bound, probably within the mitochondrial membrane. These tracers are exchanged more slowly, and because they decay more rapidly than they exchange, redistribution is insignificant.

None of these tracers is completely extracted in a single capillary passage. The first-pass extraction coefficients vary from about 54% for tetrofosmin[3] to about 65% for sestamibi[9] and about 85% for [201]Tl.[8] Tracers with a lower extraction fraction are more blood flow–dependent, with lower extraction at higher blood flow. The blood flow dependence of tracer extraction imposes a limitation on the ability to detect coronary artery disease at the level where coronary reserve capacity is diminished. When comparing a myocardial segment with greatly enhanced flow caused by stress or vasodilator with another segment with less enhanced flow because of a flow-limiting stenosis, the tracers will greatly underestimate the flow disparity. Because this effect is related to the extraction coefficient, tracers with higher extraction coefficients will be more sensitive for the detection of mild flow-limiting stenoses. Detection of infarction or severe reduction of myocardial flow will be similar for tracers with different extraction fractions.

MYOCARDIAL VIABILITY

The cationic tracers retained by membrane potentials will be viability agents, in the sense that significant tracer uptake requires both delivery, implying perfusion, and retention, implying enough cellular integrity to generate membrane potentials. These tracers include ^{201}Tl, ^{99m}Tc sestamibi, tetrofosmin, and furifosmin. However, tracer uptake alone is not enough to answer the clinical question of whether improved perfusion can improve myocardial function. When myocardial function is depressed, the demonstration of resting ischemia leads to the logical conclusion that function will improve if adequate perfusion is restored. This can be shown by the redistribution of ^{201}Tl after injection at rest. It must be noted that reinjection will not be helpful after a rest injection, when any redistribution that had taken place would simply be obscured by a second rest injection. Sestamibi and similar compounds do not redistribute sufficiently to be of value.

However, thallium and sestamibi can both be used to demonstrate substantial residual tracer uptake by a myocardial segment. Substantial uptake of these tracers indicates viability. If a segment is deemed viable by evidence of tracer uptake but is not contracting, we may reasonably expect that the myocardium is stunned or hibernating and that improving perfusion to the myocardium may improve its function. As a result, we are led to another viability tool. If significant tracer uptake its obtained in a myocardial region that has discordantly poor contractile function, it suggests a favorable outcome from repair of the obstructed supply arteries.

SUMMARY

In this chapter, we examined a model of tracer extraction. It showed very nonlinear extraction of tracers that are not completely extracted, with higher extraction at low flow and with extraction that was almost independent of flow when myocardial blood flow was elevated. This was shown to be in good accord with experimental data. The model was extended to include the effects of capillary dilatation and recruitment with increasing blood flow. This had little effect on the general shape of the curve of myocardial tracer uptake versus flow in the region of high flow; however, it had a significant effect on tracer extraction at low flows. The addition of a term representing changes in capillary blood volume as a result of dilatation and recruitment brought the model into even better agreement with existing data. In particular, it allowed us to consistently predict both first-pass extraction and the flow dependence of myocardial uptake with the same *PS* coefficient.

The clinical implication is that most existing flow tracers significantly underestimate the actual amount of myocardial flow impairment. Tracers with higher extraction coefficients give a better representation of actual flow impairment. The extent to which capillary recruitment is involved in flow regulation is an important determinant of tracer extraction in regions of subnormal flow. This could have significant implications in regions that are supplied by stenotic vessels. It has been suggested that if there is a significant pressure gradient across a stenotic lesion, capillary recruitment or dilatation occurs to maintain normal flow until the reserve is exhausted. If this is true, further vasodilatation induced by vasodilators or perhaps by increasing oxygen demand would not further increase capillary blood volume, and the effect of capillary volume changes would be diminished. As of now, data are not sufficient to enable us to exploit this as a tool for probing the coronary reserve capacity.

Tracer retention and redistribution also play an important role in the use of myocardial blood flow tracers. The compartmental exchange model gives us a compact way to study temporal changes in myocardial tracer activity after initial extraction. Tracer retention should be long enough to allow imaging after stress; thallium-201 is a good example. If retention is too long, the amount of redistribution will become insignificant, which seems to be the case with sestamibi. Because sestamibi can give a good indication of regional wall thickening, the best viability marker for this tracer may be the indication of disparity between regional perfusion and function.

Redistribution is determined by membrane transport not by blood flow. This gives us a clinical tool to determine membrane viability in chronically underperfused myocardium. Redistribution is a gradual process, and the signal that indicates redistribution is very subtle if some scar mixed is in the myocardial region being sampled. As a result, redistribution can be difficult to detect. Reinjection can be helpful in enhancing the detection of reversibility; however, reinjection would diminish the detection of redistribution in chronically hypoperfused (hibernating) regions. Reverse redistribution can be modeled in cases of multivessel disease, in which a partly scarred region is being compared with an ischemic region. We can also model reverse redistribution in subendocardial scar if the scar causes stress-induced epicardial hyperemia. We have neither a model nor clear experimental evidence for reverse redistribution associated with simple transient ischemia.

The arsenal of myocardial perfusion tracers is growing, and tracers that reflect myocardial metabolism and ischemia may soon be available. All tracers show patterns of uptake, redistribution, and reversibility that seem complex but have the potential to yield more detailed clinical information. It seems unlikely that the full potential clinical value of these tracers is understood. Continued study and a deeper understanding of these tracers should be fruitful.

REFERENCES

1. Dilsizian V, Rocco TP, Nanette MD, et al: Enhanced detection of ischemic but viable myocardium by the reinjection of thallium after stress-redistribution imaging, *N Engl J Med* 323:141–146, 1990.
2. Glover DK, Ruiz M, Edwards NC, et al: Comparison between ^{201}Tl and ^{99m}Tc sestamibi uptake during adenosine-induced vasodilation as a function of coronary stenosis severity, *Circulation* 91:813–820, 1995.
3. Glover DK, Ruiz M, Yang JY, et al: Comparison between Tl-201 and Tc-99m tetrofosmin uptake during adenosine vasodilatation in a canine model of either critical or mild coronary stenosis, *Circulation* 92:I-789, 1995 (abstract).

4. Gosselin RE and Stibitz GR: Rates of solute absorption from tissue depots: theoretical considerations, *Pflugers Arch* 318:85–98, 1970.

5. Grunwald AM, Watson DD, Holszgrefe HH, et al: Myocardial thallium-201 kinetics in normal and ischemic myocardium, *Circulation* 64:610–618, 1981.

6. Lindner JR and Kaul S: Insights into the assessment of myocardial perfusion offered by different cardiac imaging modalities, *J Nuc Cardiol* 2:446–460, 1995.

7. McGoron AJ, Gerson MC, Biniakiewicz DS, et al: Effects of ouabain on technetium-99m-Q12 and thallium-201 extraction and retention by isolated rat heart, *J Nucl Med* 37:752–756, 1996.

8. Moore CA, Cannon J, Watson DD, et al: Thallium 201 kinetics in stunned myocardium characterized by severe postischemic systolic dysfunction, *Circulation* 81:1622–1632, 1990.

9. Mousa SA, Cooney JM, and Williams SJ: Relationship between regional myocardial blood flow and the distribution of ^{99m}Tc-sestamibi in the presence of total coronary artery occlusion, *Am Heart J* 119:842–847, 1990.

10. Piwnica-Worms D, Chiu ML, and Kronauge JF: Divergent kinetics of ^{201}Tl and ^{99m}Tc-SESTAMIBI in cultured chick ventricular myocytes during ATP depletion, *Circulation* 85:1531–1541, 1992.

11. Sansoy V, Glover DK, Watson DD, et al: Comparison of thallium-201 resting redistribution with technetium-99m-sestamibi uptake and functional response to dobutamine for assessment of myocardial viability, *Circulation* 92:994–1004, 1995.

12. Wu XS, Ewert DL, Liu YH, et al: In vivo relation of intramyocardial blood volume to myocardial perfusion. Evidence supporting microvascular site for autoregulation, *Circulation* 85:730–737, 1992.

13. Yang LD, Berman DS, Kiat H, et al: The frequency of late reversibility in SPECT thallium-201 stress-redistribution studies, *J Am Coll Cardiol* 15:334–344, 1990.

Chapter 2

Kinetics on a cellular level

Jean C. Maublant

When using myocardial blood flow (MBF) imaging agents, it is anticipated that their tissue uptake at the time of imaging will be proportional to the regional MBF. Ideally, a linear relationship should link the detected activity of the agents and the MBF. There are three ways to achieve this.

1. Identification of a mechanical blockage of labeled particles, such as microspheres, would be the most desirable approach, because MBF is by far the principal variable related to the number of trapped particles in a given territory.[6] However, peripherally injected microspheres are stopped at the pulmonary level, as in lung perfusion imaging. Reaching arterially perfused organs would mean administering an arterial injection. In addition, unless a selective arterial injection is performed, some vessels in all peripheral organs would be embolized by the microspheres, which is an unacceptable situation. Except in some research protocols in which microspheres are selectively injected into a coronary artery, such a method cannot be used in routine clinical practice.

2. In a second approach, the radiolabeled molecules may be bound to the cell membrane. Such receptor binding is a strong possibility, although it has not been developed in MBF imaging. Because the cell membrane is a lipid structure, highly lipophilic neutral molecules are naturally attracted to it. This mechanism does not require any cellular energy and seems to be an attractive replacement for the microsphere method. However, the plasma membranes of the myocytes are not the only lipophilic structures that a peripherally injected agent encounters during its vascular tour. Circulating proteins and cells are also attractive sites, and the obstacle presented by the capillary wall must be taken into account. The problem can become even more complicated if the molecule is structurally unstable, resulting in a superimposed release phenomenon. The multiple factors involved in the seemingly global kinetics of such an agent can make it very complex and difficult to understand if the effect of each factor cannot be assessed separately.

3. A third approach involves the use of agents that can cross the membrane of the myocytes either passively or actively. Passive crossing, or diffusion, does not require energy directly from the cell but does require that some imbalance be created that results in an inward movement of the tracer. Active crossing involves the consumption of energy, usually in the form of adenosine triphosphate (ATP). Whether active or passive, such mechanisms result in complex behaviors because they must combine with mechanisms involved in tracer movements in blood and at the capillary level. Moreover, different types of mechanisms can be combined to varying degrees, so a possible intracellular compartmentation of the agent must also be taken into account. Most of the commercially available radiopharmaceuticals belong to this third category.

Is a sound clinical use of MBF tracers required to understand the mechanisms involved in their uptake, especially at the cellular level, or is the observation of the in vivo or ex vivo tracer kinetics in various experimental or clinical situations enough? It is likely that both are necessary. The problem with clinical application is that there are always cases in which it is difficult to explain the observation. This occurs because complete knowledge of the biological behavior of available MBF imaging agents does not exist.

With experiments performed in animal models, it is also difficult to control all of the variables. Moreover, the complexity, cost, and difficulty of these experiments mean that only selected situations are explored. The reproducibility of the results is often questionable, and their variability can sometimes conceal an important phenomenon. Finally, the results of experiments in animals cannot always be extrapolated to human situations. It seems that looking specifically at the mechanisms involved at the cellular level can solve at least part of the problem; but that part can be very detrimental to the general objective of using a given MBF agent. For instance, demonstrating that an agent is taken up passively by the cell implies that it will be of no use in assessing myocardial viability, whereas if another agent is taken up through the consumption of ATP, it means that this agent has the potential to assess myocardial viability. Such differences can be difficult to identify from clinical data alone. Knowledge of the cellular mechanisms of accumulation also can promote the use of an agent in a particular clinical indication.

MODELS OF CARDIAC CELL CULTURES
Methods

In nuclear cardiology, most of the experimental work has been conducted with embryonic[7] or neonatal[15] cardiac cells because these cells, unlike adult cells, readily attach to the culture dish and develop as a monolayer. They are an ideal tool for measuring uptake with radiolabeled agents because all of the cells are in direct contact with the medium of incubation, from which they can be easily separated by removal of the medium. These cells also spontaneously contract, providing an easy way to check for their viability. Adult cells are more difficult to prepare and are prone to the "calcium paradox" phenomenon.

Embryonic cells are prepared from the hearts of 10-day-old chicks. The hearts are trimmed of connective tissue and atria, minced, and exposed to 0.024% (wt/vol) of trypsin in Ca^{++}- and Mg^{++}-free Earle salt solution for 7 minutes at 37° C. After isolation by 400 g-centrifugation for 10 minutes, the cells are resuspended to yield a suspension of 500,000 cells ml^{-1}. After 3 to 4 days in a humidified atmosphere of 5% carbon dioxide (CO_2) and 95% air, a confluent layer of spontaneously contracting myocytes is obtained in 25-mm diameter coverslips. The cell water space of these myocytes has been measured at 6.9 µl/mg of protein^{-1}.[37]

To prepare myocytes from a neonatal rat, a technique originally described by Harary and Farley is used.[15] After killing 2-day to 4-day-old Sprague–Dawley rats, the heart is removed, trimmed of connective tissue and atria, and finely minced and trypsinized in a 0.2% concentration for 10 minutes. After centrifugation at 900 g for 5 minutes, the pellet is resuspended in complemented Ham F-10 growth medium. The fibroblasts are separated using the differential attachment technique, and the final suspension is plated at a concentration of 300,000 cells/ml^{-1} in 35-mm diameter culture dishes (2 ml per dish). After 3 to 4 days of incubation in a humidified atmosphere of 5% CO_2 and 95% air at 37° C, a confluent layer of spontaneously contracting myocytes with a water space of 2 µl/mg^{-1} is obtained.[27,49]

Advantages and Limitations

The main advantage of using cultured cells is that the incubation medium is in direct contact with the plasma cell membrane. All uncertainties from the patency of the small vessels and capillaries to the diffusion through the capillary walls, are resolved. However, this can be seen as a disadvantage, because it makes extrapolation to the clinical situation difficult. However, it is the only way to clearly isolate the mechanism of cellular accumulation, which is the major mechanism responsible for overall tissue uptake.

Another advantage of using cultured cells is that the surrounding variables—temperature, pH, and extracellular volume—are easily controlled. Compared with whole hearts or freshly dissected preparations, cultured cells are in a stable condition and do not show signs of injury. Several groups have validated the use of cultured heart preparations as models of reversible and irreversible cell injury for assessing morphology, contractility, electrophysiology, ionic movements, and metabolic activity.[2,16,18,26,33] Although their use does not allow duplication of pathological situations, it permits the systematic examination of specific causes of irreversible injury.[53] However, cultures of embryonic or newborn myocytes are prone to the rapid growth of nonmuscular, fibroblast-like cells. They are more dependent than adult cells on glycolysis and lack neuronal connections. Because species differences are obvious, great care must be taken before extrapolating results to humans. Even if the mechanisms of membrane exchange are probably the same in vitro and in vivo, quantitative differences are likely to exist because the environment is more complex in vivo, with more barriers and surrounding factors that usually slow down the exchange process. In addition, the extracellular compartment is very different. At normal blood flow, the vascular space is equivalent to a large extracellular compartment, whereas in ischemic conditions, the stagnant blood is confined to small volume. At the opposite extreme, the extracellular compartment in cultured cells has the same volume in control and ischemic conditions. The viability of preparations can vary widely because of the many variables involved in the process of cell culturing, including those that are unknown or uncontrolled. The problem with viability is that it cannot be measured straightforwardly. The simplest approach is the trypan blue exclusion method, which is highly subjective.

BIOLOGICAL BASIS OF CELLULAR EXCHANGES
Mechanisms of transmembrane exchange

The exchange of molecules through the cell membrane involves a passive or an active mechanism. Passive exchange is always directed down the concentration gradient of the molecule. It can result from simple diffusion across the membrane, mainly from small neutral molecules, such as oxygen (O_2), CO_2, and urea, and from hydrophobic molecules, such as lipid vitamins and steroid hormones. Other molecules, such as glucose, can only efficiently cross the membrane by binding reversibly to a specialized membrane protein; this mechanism is called facilitated diffusion. In passive exchange by simple or by facilitated diffusion, the movement of the solute is governed only by the difference in concentration across the membrane. The molecules move down the concentration gradient until the internal and external concentrations equalize.

Active exchange always results in the movement of molecules across the membrane against the gradient of concentration, a process that requires energy and involves mostly charged solutes. Adenosine triphosphate is a common source of energy in the cells. Molecules using this active transport usually bind reversibly to a membrane protein that transforms the energy of ATP hydrolysis into a transport against the concentration gradient. A well-known example of such an active transporter is Na^+/K^+-ATPase; however, other sources of energy are possible. Established gradients of concentration or transmembrane electrical potentials represent various forms of stored energy that can be used to drive the transmembrane movement of an ionic solute against the concentration gradient. To separate active exchange that requires immediate ATP consumption from active exchange that uses other forms of energy, the former is called primary active transport and the latter is called secondary active transport or exchange.

The rate of diffusion of a solute across a membrane is limited by the permeability coefficient, which increases with the size of the molecule. This applies to passive diffusion and secondary active exchanges. Transport mechanisms involving membrane proteins, either by facilitated diffusion or by primary or secondary active transports, are primarily limited by the number of protein channels available. This is ususally not a problem in scintigraphy, because of the low concentration of radiotracer used in vivo ($\ll 1$ μM).

Kinetics of membrane exchange

The kinetics of exchange between the internal and external cellular volumes can be described in a first approximation, by using a two-compartment model. Washin and washout time-activity curves are single exponential functions that tend toward equilibrium. If passive exchanges are involved, equilibrium corresponds to the equalization of the internal and external concentrations. With active exchanges, the ratio between the internal and external concentrations at equilibrium, expressed as $(C_i/C_e)_{eq}$, is governed by the transmembrane potential, according to the Nernst equation. This ratio must be greater than 1 and as high as possible for suitable radiopharmaceuticals.

The exchange of a solute across a membrane is usually described quantitatively by using the exchange rate, a variable that is expressed as a molar concentration per unit of time (for example as fmol/min^{-1}). This concentration should be given per cell and per unit of membrane surface. When dealing with a culture of several hundreds of thousands of confluent cells in a culture dish, it is very difficult to estimate the total number of cells. However, for a given preparation of monolayer cells the total surface of cell membrane exposed to the medium and the total number of cells correlate highly with the amount of protein in the dish, a parameter that can be measured by routine biochemical methods. Consequently, the exchange rate is usu-

ally normalized to the mass of protein and expressed as fmol/min^{-1}(milligrams of protein)$^{-1}$. Because the exchange rate can be directed inward or outward, the rates are called *influx* and *efflux* rates, respectively.

At steady state, the total amount of radiotracer retained with the cellular fraction, either on the membrane or inside the cell, is called the *cellular accumulation* (in fmol [milligrams of protein]$^{-1}$), although it is more often (but improperly) termed the *cellular uptake* of the tracer. Steady state is not synonymous with the absence of exchange but with the presence of equilibrated exchanges. Before equilibrium, the rate of tracer accumulation is not constant; it can be called the *rate of uptake*. After equilibrium, if the extracellular medium has been replaced with a nonradioactive medium, the washout of tracer by the cells can be called the *rate of release*. This is easily demonstrated by derivation of the time function of the cellular concentration when, at the very beginning of the process (time zero), the rates of uptake and release are equal to the influx and efflux rates, respectively (Fig. 2-1).

Practical measurements

The extracellular compartment and the whole cells are the most easily accessible components for radioactivity measurements in a culture dish. The activity present in the extracellular compartment can be followed by direct sampling in the medium, which is an easy and nondestructive approach. Because the extracellular volume is controlled (added medium), the extracellular tracer concentration (C_e) can be easily calculated and followed over time. Measurement of the intracellular concentration with ($C_i/C_e)_{eq}$ is more difficult because it is dif-

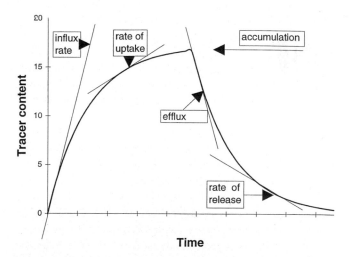

Fig. 2-1. This curve simulates the phases of cellular tracer accumulation and release, on the basis of a two-compartment model. Experimentally, the curve is not continuous but is made of a limited number of data points. The slope at the origin of each phase corresponds to the influx and efflux rates, which are constant for a given preparation. The slopes measured on the rest of the curve represent the rates of uptake or release, which vary with time. Accumulation, or "uptake," corresponds to the near-plateau of the uptake phase.

ficult to attempt to properly separate the plasma membranes from the intracellular compartment. Most of the time, the radioactivity of both is counted together. In addition, measurement of the intracellular volume is difficult.

It is possible to use indirect methods based on the diffusion of labeled neutral, nonmetabolizable molecules such as tritiated methylglucose,[23] but for a given technique of cell culture preparation, a regression equation is usually used to estimate this volume from the amount of protein. Unfortunately, knowing the intracellular concentration (C_I) is more important than knowing C_e, because C_e remains fairly stable as a result of the very large extracellular volume relative to the intracellular volume, whereas C_I varies widely (from 0 to its value at equilibrium). Eventually, the uptake at a given time can be expressed as C_i (in fmol/ml^{-1}), as C_i/C_e (a dimensionless variable); or as relative to its value at steady state, $(C_i)_{eq}$ and $(C_i/C_e)_{eq}$, respectively, leading to $C_i/(C_i)_{eq}$, and $(C_i/C_e)/(C_i/C_e)_{eq}$, which can be expressed as a percentage. These values can be followed during the accumulation phase, providing access to the rate of uptake at different times, and to the influx rate by extrapolating its value at time zero. It must be remembered that C_i is only the apparent intracellular concentration, because the agent can also be bound to the cell membrane or compartmentalized in the cell. The rates of release and efflux can be measured by measuring them after the extracellular medium has been replaced by an identical but not radioactive solution.

Examination of the subcellular distribution of the tracer requires cell fractionation. The sarcolemmal membranes are the easiest to isolate by disruption through osmotic lysis and washout of all medium. The separation of organelles, such as mitochondria, is more complex and requires ultracentrifugation. In any case, labeling with the tracer studied can be done either before or after separation, with specific limitations in each situation. Before separation, the relative distribution of the agent among the various cellular structures can be determined by assuming that the separation process has not modified the original distribution. After separation, subcellular variables such as O_2 consumption and tracer concentration can be measured by assuming that the separation process has not altered the isolated subcellular fraction.

What can be learned from these measurements? Some general observations arise when considering the distribution of radiotracers in cellular or subcellular structures.

1. For MBF imaging, the cellular uptake of the ideal agent should have a positive linear relation with MBF. Consequently, potent agents must be overconcentrated in the cells and can be expressed as $[(C_i/C_e)_{eq} >> 1]$. Because active transport is defined as any mechanism that produces a transmembrane concentration gradient of the free agent, all of the agents used for MBF scintigraphy that enter the cell undergo active transport. Some agents can seem to be overconcentrated, but this is the result of membrane binding and a passive mechanism of accumulation. In any case, when cells are placed in a medium that contains the radiotracer the activity of the cells or of the isolated subcellular fractions increases with time until equilibrium is reached.

2. The rate of tracer uptake depends greatly on the physical chemical properties of the tracer, the mechanisms of uptake involved in the process, and the cellular structure. Because several mechanisms and structures are usually present, it is very difficult to model the whole process. However, in vitro observations demonstrate that the uptake curves usually fit accurately with a single exponential. This strongly suggests that among all the compartments that may be involved in the global uptake process only one plays a major role. If this hypothesis is accepted, the influx rate can be calculated.

3. In every compartment model, the distribution of the tracer uptake tends toward equilibrium. This equilibrium is a function not only of the cell structure and metabolic state but also of the chemical, physical, and biological properties of the radiotracer. At equilibrium, the apparent exchanges between the extracellular and cellular compartments stop, or at least in seem to, because opposite but equal exchanges may still be occurring. It is difficult to determine experimentally the precise time equilibrium will be reached, whereas the level of equilibrium itself can be fairly well measured. A good way to proceed is to measure the half-time to equilibrium: that is, the time necessary to reach 50% of the plateau level. These two measurements allow a useful comparison of different agents.

How can the level at equilibrium be interpreted? If the tracer is transported only by passive diffusion and there was no driving potential other than the initial difference of concentration, equilibrium will be reached when the intracellular and extracellular concentrations become equal; therefore, it is useful to be able to measure C_i/C_e. In practice, with most of the available molecules, some degree of passive diffusion is present, but it is generally associated with another driving potential that is electrical or chemical in origin. Consequently, the level of equilibrium cannot be predicted precisely, even if the transmembrane electrical potential provides a good indication of the level that should be attained by positively charged molecules. The relation of this potential should always be viewed critically because adjunct mechanisms can play a role (such as compartmentation, ion channels, or exchange membrane proteins) and modify the final equilibrium of the molecule, despite a given transmembrane electrical potential.

THALLIUM-201

Thallium (Tl) uptake was initially measured in noncardiac cells, such as frog skeletal muscle,[32] erythrocytes,[12,50] cultured rabbit lenses,[22] squid axon,[24] and *Streptococcus lactis*.[20] The movements of Tl$^+$ were often assessed with ^{204}Tl as a marker, a 0.77 megaelectronvolts beta emitter with a 4-year half-life. There was already clear evidence that influx[32] and efflux[22] could be well approximated by a single exponential curve and that Na$^+$,K$^+$-ATPase has a greater affinity for Tl$^+$ than for K$^+$.[50] Even when cardiac cells were first used, the concentration range studied was usually between 10 μM and 10 millimolar, far higher than the concentration likely to be found during imaging in humans (<1 μM). For instance, Delano and associates[8] observed in cultured myocardial cells from newborn rats,

10 mM of Tl^+ competes with 10 mM of K^+, and that Tl^+ influx is inhibited by 0.15 mM and 10 mM of ouabain. Competition between K^+ and Tl^+ in the 3- to 7-mM concentration range was also documented in isolated mitochondria.[9]

The initial reference work dealing with the use of a model of cultured cardiac cells for the specific assessment of a MBF imaging agent with realistic tracer concentrations was a study by McCall and associates of ^{204}Tl.[25] Primary cultures of myocardial cells from 1-day-old to 2-day-old rats were prepared. After trypsinization of the ventricular tissue and 4 to 5 days of incubation, synchronously beating monolayers of 1 to 1.5 million cells per dish were obtained. The cellular content was measured after equilibration in a medium containing ^{42}K or ^{204}Tl and washing of the extracellular activity with a $0°$ C isotonic Na^+- and K^+-free calcium–sorbitol solution. Kinetics measurements confirmed that the washin and washout of Tl in the 10-nM to 10-µM range of concentrations can be described by a single exponential with a similar constant rate in both directions because the measured half-time of exchange was 4.95 ± 0.51 minutes at influx and 5.09 ± 0.46 minutes at efflux. Equilibrium was reached after 20 to 30 minutes, and the internal/external concentration ratio was approximately 50:1. Of note, the exchange rate of ^{47}K is longer, with a mean half-time of around 12 minutes.

Ouabain was observed to have an inhibitory effect on the influx rate of thallium at concentrations higher than 0.1 µM. Inhibition was half-maximal at 20 µM of ouabain, but it never exceeded 60% of thallium influx; this suggests that the remaining 40% was not mediated through the Na^+,K^+-ATPase. Both fractions were equally sensitive to the extracellular concentration of potassium, which acts as a competitive inhibitor. For example, the total and ouabain-insensitive thallium influx decreased from 13.56 ± 0.59 mol^{-14}/cm^{-2} and 2.86 ± 0.07 mol^{-14}/cm^{-2}, respectively, in a K-free medium, to 2.10 ± 0.15 and 0.84 ± 0.05 in K^+ 10 mM. However, Tl^+ was also found to act as a competitive inhibitor for K^+ influx, and at much lower concentrations. In effect, the inhibitor constant for K^+ was calculated at 1.2 mM, whereas it was 6 µM for Tl^+, suggesting that the affinity of the receptor for Tl^+ is 200 times greater than for K^+. Neither ouabain nor external potassium could modify the washout rate of Tl. The results of this study represent the major reference for in vitro assessment of Tl.

The role of Na^+,K^+-ATPase seems to vary with the type of cells in cultures. The presence of ouabain, 0.5 mM, induced only a small decrease of the total uptake of ^{204}Tl in calcium-tolerant cultured cardiac cells from the adult rat, whereas nearly 50% inhibition was observed in calcium-sensitive, damaged cells.[44] In the same work, a strong reduction in Tl uptake was induced by tetraethylammonium, 5 mM, suggesting that a passive influx by membrane channels that are sensitive to this chemical plays a major role in calcium-tolerant cardiac cells. These results are at variance with those of a study in which it was found that in calcium-resistant adult rat cardiac cells, as in neonatal cells, nearly half of the Tl^+ uptake occurs through Na^+,K^+-ATPase[17].

It was demonstrated that the effect of ouabain is more pronounced when the rate of sodium entrance is increased, probably as a result of stimulation of the Na^+,K^+-ATPase. This may explain the variability of the effect of ouabain in different reported experimental models. The latter work is also of interest because it is the only published study that explores the mechanism of uptake of the ouabain-insensitive fraction, which was found to remain constant when magnesium is removed by ethylenediamine tetraacetic acid and then restored, suggesting that it is independent of the Na^+/K^+ gradient. However, it was totally inhibited by the presence of rotenone and carbonyl cyanide p-trifluoromethoxyphenylhydrazone, agents that depleted the level of ATP by more than 95%. Therefore, the ouabain-independent Tl^+ uptake seems to be an ATP-dependent mechanism, but not much more is known about it.

In the ventricular myocytes of newborn rats, a period of 6 minutes for ^{201}Tl washout and of less than 5 minutes for washin[29] has been reported. Incubation with ouabain, 0.01 mM, did not change the level of the plateau, but a mixture of cyanide 5 mM, and iodoacetate, 0.1 mM, decreased Tl accumulation to 66% of its control level while the contractions of the myocytes were stopped.

The effect of true hypoxia on Tl washout has been studied by using a model of chick embryo myocardial cells infused with a normoxic or hypoxic (<12 mm Hg) medium.[11] The cellular exponential component of the washout curves was found to be moderately but significantly decreased during hypoxia, with respective rate constants of 0.26 ± 0.06 min^{-1} and 0.23 ± 0.05 min^{-1} ($p<0.01$). A 13% decrease in cellular Tl uptake during hypoxia was also noted. A dose-dependent decrease in thallium cellular content was observed with ouabain; the maximum decrease was 61% with 1 mM of ouabain. Use of such a model of actual hypoxia is certainly a better approach than the use of metabolic inhibitors to simulate in vivo ischemia. However, a drawback of this model is that it takes several minutes to attain low oxygen concentration in the circulating medium, and it is not known whether the other variables can be kept constant during equilibration.

Finally, the in vitro studies have all reported the important but partial role of ouabain in the mechanism of cellular uptake of ^{201}Tl, which explains why cellular accumulation is sensitive to any injury that alters the production of ATP. The period of transmembrane exchange was also found to be very short (in the 5-minute range) (Table 2-1).

TECHNETIUM-99M ISONITRILES

The first potential technetium-99m (^{99m}Tc)–labeled agent for MBF imaging, 1,2-bis(dimethylphosphino)-ethane (DMPE), was a member of the isonitrile family that was complexed with technetium(I). Its cellular accumulation in cultured myocytes from neonatal rats[8] and human erythrocytes[47] was shown to be unrelated to the presence of ouabain, Tl^+, or K^+ in the external medium, suggesting that unlike thallium-201, cellular uptake of DMPE does not involve the Na^+,K^+-ATPase. There was also evidence that it does not bind to the cell membrane, because no ac-

Table 2-1. Variables of Accumulation of Thallium-201 in Cultured Myocardial Cells

Thallium-201 Half-life	Intracellular Volume at Equilibrium*	Intracellular Volume/ Extracellular Volume at Equilibrium†	Reference
11.7 ± 2.9	240 ± 41‡	35/1	17
4.95 ± 0.51	–	50/1	25
4.33 ± 0.05	–	–	11
6	–	130/1	28
5	–	–	26
5	43.8 ± 7.2§	–	38

* $(C_i)_{eq}$.
† $(C_i/C_e)_{eq}$.
‡ pmol (milligrams of protein)$^{-1}$
§ fmol (milligrams of protein)$^{-1}$ $(nM_0)^{-1}$

tivity was counted with the cell debris resulting from the action of trichloroacetic acid. Unfortunately, DMPE was not effective for imaging in man. However, other Tc(I)-labeled members of the isonitrile family were synthesized. The kinetics of uptake of hexakis(t-butylisonitrile) (TBI) and hexakis-isopropylisonitrile were studied by using neonatal rat myocytes[48] according to the method described by Delano and associates.[8] A plateau was attained in about 20 minutes with TBI and in 2 hours with IPI; these plateaus were not modified by the presence of ouabain, 0.15 mM, nor KCl, 10 mM. Most of the activity was associated with the myocyte membranes. These experiments convincingly demonstrated that as in the case of DMPE, the mechanism of cellular complexion of this family of isonitrile complexes does not involve the Na$^+$,K$^+$-ATPase. A similar observation was reported with another derivative, hexakis(carbomethoxyiso-propylisonitrile).[37] At that point, the documented high lipophilicity of these compounds and their seeming membrane binding led to the hypothesis that no other mechanism was involved, although it could not explain the observed lack of nonspecific accumulation in blood cells and vessels. It has been stated that the uptake of ^{99m}Tc sestamibi "appears to be totally by a process of passive diffusion,"[31] a concept that still prevails, even if it can be challenged with the biochemical definitions of transport mechanisms and even if it should instead be called a secondary active transport.[28]

The fundamental explanation of the mechanism responsible for cellular accumulation of ^{99m}Tc sestamibi was provided by Piwnica-Worms, Kronauge, and Chiu in 1990.[41] By using a model of cultured embryonic chick ventricular myocytes, they demonstrated that the amount of accumulated cellular ^{99m}Tc sestamibi could be modified by various ionophores and inhibitors that are known to affect the electrical potentials of the plasma and mitochondrial membranes (E_m and $\Delta\Psi$, respectively). Conversely, during their less than 60-minute duration of action these agents did not modify the cellular ATP content, thereby excluding the possibility of any primary active transport. It is interesting to look in detail into the methodology of this work because a wide palette of the tools available to test the ionic transmembrane exchanges is described. At the sarcolemmal level, exchanging three internal Na$^+$ for two external K$^+$ at

the expense of ATP hydrolysis, Na$^+$,K$^+$-ATPase is the main electrogenic, primary active transporter at the origin of the internal hyperconcentration of K$^+$ and the hypoconcentration of Na$^+$ relative to the extracellular compartment. Ouabain, as mentioned, is a specific inhibitor. The resultant internal under-concentrated Na$^+$ can be exchanged through an Na$^+$/H$^+$ exchanger with external H$^+$, an example of secondary active exchange that is inhibited by amiloride. The overconcentrated internal K$^+$ can leave the cell through activation of an electroneutral K$^+$,H$^+$ exchange that is mediated by the ionophore nigericin. Valinomycin is a K$^+$ ionophore that allows a rapid equilibration of the external and internal concentrations of K$^+$, destroying the transmembrane electrical potential. Nigericin and valinomycin are also active at the level of the inner membrane of the mitochondria. Nigericin is known to equilibrate the pH gradient across that membrane, resulting in an increased transmembrane mitochondrial electrical potential.

Other agents can block specific sites of the respiratory chain in the mitochondria. Carbonyl cyanide-m-chlorophenylhydra-zone and 2,4-dinitrophenol are rapid-action protonophores that depolarize the mitochondrial membrane. Rotenone and azide block the electron-chain transport and have delayed effects on the membrane potential. Oligomycin blocks the synthesis of ATP at the end of the electron chain, resulting in hyperpolarization of the membrane. The measurements of the cellular uptake of ^{99m}Tc sestamibi must be interpreted in light of the effects of these ionophores and inhibitors on the transmembrane electrical potential.

Simple proof of the dependence of membranes' electrical potential on ^{99m}Tc-sestamibi uptake lies in fact that (1) incubation of the cells with an external concentration of 130-mM K$^+$ identical to their internal concentration, which nearly depolarizes the plasma membrane, lowers the cellular uptake to 17% of control levels; (2) the addition of 1 µg/ml^{-1} of valinomycin, which annihilates the mitochondrial potential, further decreases the cellular uptake to a background level (Fig. 2-2); and (3) Nigericin, 5 µg/ml^{-1} by hyperpolarizing the mitochondria, increases ^{99m}Tc sestamibi uptake (Fig. 2-3). This last effect was even more pronounced and was found to be partly the result of plasma membrane hyperpolarization in a model of cultured

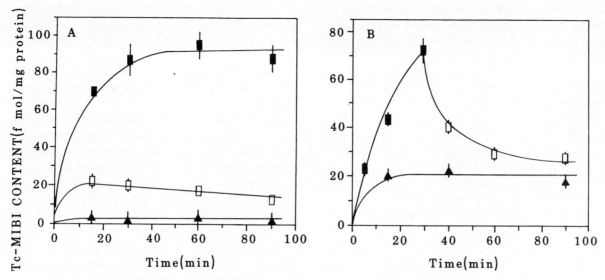

Fig. 2-2. Kinetics of uptake of technetium-99m sestamibi in embryonic chick myocardial cells. **A,** Compared with the control cells (*dark squares*), the level of cellular accumulation decreases when the extracellular medium contains potassium, 130 mM (*white squares*) and decreases even more when valinomycin is added (*dark triangles*). **B,** Accumulation suddenly decreases when the control medium (*dark squares*) is replaced by a medium containing potassium, 130 mM (*white squares*). Kinetics when the medium permanently contains 130 mM of potassium is also shown (*dark triangles*). (From Piwnica-Worms D, Kronauge JF, Chiu ML: *Circulation* 82:1826, 1990.)

fibroblasts that had a larger pH gradient at the inner mitochondrial membrane than did the chick embryo myocytes (Fig. 2-4).[5] Additional evidence lies in the lack of effect of metabolic inhibitors that directly block the electron chain and the production of ATP, such as rotenone, 10 µM, and azide, 10 mM, when their effect is evaluated during the first 20 minutes of incubation. This means that the lack of mitochondrial ATP production does not have an immediate effect on the membrane potential; this observation may now be explained by ATP compartmentation. Other results can only be interpreted through sometimes speculative cascades of interactions among ion concentrations, membrane potentials, and transporters. However, it must be emphasized that similar observations have been reported with other small, lipophilic cations, such as ^{3}H-tetraphenylphosphonium or fluorescent rhodamine-123, which are used as probes of membrane potentials in optically transparent preparations in biochemistry and histology that are not readily accessible to microelectrode techniques.[10] Further supporting evidence for this mechanism was provided by the enhancement of ^{99m}Tc sestamibi uptake in cultured chick-embryo cardiac cells in the presence of hydrophobic anions, such as tetraphenylborate.[42] Piwnica-Worms, Kronauge, and Chiu explained that because of the complex structure of the cell membrane the transmembrane potential profile consists of negative potential wells near the surface and broad positive energy barriers near the middle of the membrane, resulting in a serious obstacle for translocation of lipophilic cations. Incubation of the cells with hydrophobic anions results in a lowering of these internal barriers, thereby facilitating the translocation and the influx rate of ^{99m}Tc sestamibi. However, explanation of the increased accumulation

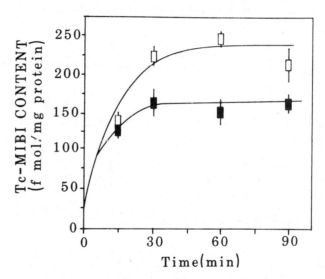

Fig. 2-3. Kinetics of uptake of technetium-99m sestamibi in embryonic chick myocardial cells. When the membrane is hyperpolarized by the K+/H+ ionophore nigericin (5 µg/mL[-1]) (*open squares*), the level of accumulation is significantly higher than that in the controls (*dark squares*). (From Piwnica-Worms D, Kronauge JF, Chiu ML: *Circulation* 82:1826, 1990.)

observed at equilibrium is more difficult, because it would imply that the adjuvant molecule can modify the plasma or more likely the mitochondrial transmembrane potential.

Although these experiments demonstrated the basic role of the transmembrane electrical potential in the cellular retention of ^{99m}Tc sestamibi, there was only indirect evidence of the involvement of mitochondria. This observation was strongly supported by the work of Crane and associates,[6] who isolated the mitochondrial fraction of myocardial samples in guinea pigs that were injected with [99mTc] sestamibi 10 minutes before they were sacrificed. Subcellular fractionation of cardiac homogenates revealed that [99mTc] sestamibi was specifically retained in the mitochondrial pellet, whereas in control animals, most of the thallium-201 was found in the supernatant. By using a variety of homogenization solutions, 80% to 90% of [99mTc] sestamibi was always recovered in the mitochondrial fraction. The same observations could be made with hepatic, pulmonary, and femoral skeletal muscle and renal tissue samples. However, direct evidence that [99mTc] sestamibi concentrates specifically and strongly in mitochondria was provided by Backus et al.[1] By using quantitative electron-probe x-ray microanalysis with a $\times 12{,}400$ times magnification of freeze-dried cryosections of cultured embryonic chick heart cells that were incubated for 60 minutes with [99mTc] sestamibi, they were able to observe a strong mitochondrial concentration of this agent. For example, at 36 μM of extracellular [99mTc] sestamibi, the intracellular concentration was 16 ± 1.3 mM, which means that the a C_i/C_e ratio was more than 400:1. They also showed that the mitochondrial transmembrane potential could be calculated from these values by using the Nernst equation.

A demonstration that the presence of a transmembrane electrical potential was sufficient to drive the accumulation of [99mTc] sestamibi was given later.[4] Negatively charged lipophilic membranes were created using artificial unilamellar vesicles of egg phosphatidylcholine, 114 nm in diameter, that were loaded with 160 m millimolar of K^+. By increasing the permeability of the membrane to K^+ with valinomycin, the diffusion membrane electrical potential could be clamped at the Nernst potassium equilibrium potential. Vesicular accumulation of [99mTc] sestamibi was determined with variable concentrations of extravesicular K^+. An excellent correlation was observed between the membrane potential estimated from the Nernst equation using [99mTc] sestamibi and the K^+ diffusion potential (Fig. 2-5).

Preliminary studies of the kinetics of uptake and release of [99mTc] sestamibi demonstrated that compared with thallium-201, exchanges of [99mTc] sestamibi are slower[29] and show a pattern that agrees with the two-compartment model, which closely approximates a single exponential curve. This is only an approximation, because modeling should be based on a three-compartment model involving the extracellular medium, the cytosol, and the intramitochondrial compartment. The main parameter for the influx rate is the plasma membrane potential, whereas the rate-limiting step for the efflux seems to

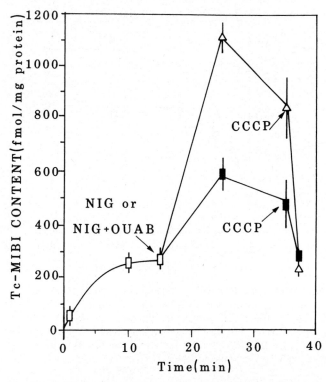

Fig. 2-4. Kinetics of uptake of technetium-99m sestamibi in mouse fibroblasts (BALB/c 3T3). The increased accumulation is induced by the addition of nigericin, 5 μg/ml⁻¹ (*open triangles*) and is diminished by the addition of oubabain, 0.1 mM (*dark squares*). In both situations, a sharp decrease is observed when the mitochondrial potential is collapsed by the addition of CCCP 5 μM. (From Chiu ML, Kronauge JF, Piwnica-Worms D: Effect of mitochondrial and plasma-membrane potential on accumulation of hexakis [2-methoxyisobutylisonitrile], *J Nucl Med* 31:1646, 1990. Reprinted by permission of the Society of Nuclear Medicine.)

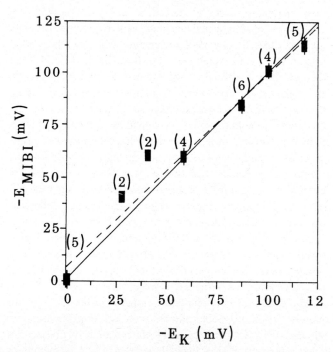

Fig. 2-5. Membrane electrical potential calculated by applying the Nernst equation to the technetium-99m sestamibi distribution into artificial unilamellar vesicles shows excellent correlation with their potassium diffusion potential ($r = 0.97$). (From Chernoff DM, Strichartz GR, Piwnica-Worms D: *Biochim Biophys Acta* 1147:262, 1993. With kind permission from Elsevier Science-NL, Sara Burgerhartstraat 25, 1055 KV Amsterdam, The Netherlands.)

be the mitochondrial membrane potential.[41] The half-time of accumulation was reported to be 9.3 ± 1.5 minutes in chick embryo[39] and about 30 minutes in newborn rats[24] (Fig. 2-6), with $(C_i/C_e)_{eq}$ values between 25 to 50 and 150, respectively, and a cellular concentration of 206.7 ± 14.0 fmol (milligrams of protein)$^{-1}$ (nanomolar extracellular ^{99m}Tc sestamibi)$^{-1}$ in chick embryo.[40] The period of release was 28 minutes (Fig. 2-7). Because endothelial and fibroblast-like cells constitute 5% to 10% of the mass of heart cells, Caldwell et al examined the uptake of ^{99m}Tc sestamibi by these cells.[3] Using cells isolated from adult rats, they observed greater uptake of ^{99m}Tc sestamibi compared with ^{201}Tl in endothelial cells but not as much as in the myocytes.

The consequences of simulated ischemia have also been assessed. It seemed that a moderate metabolic inhibition by a mixture of cyanide, 5 mM, and iodoacetate, 0.1 mM, did not affect ^{99m}Tc sestamibi uptake after 20 minutes of incubation, whereas uptake of ^{201}Tl decreased by 34%.[29] Interestingly, a low dose of ouabain (10 µM) did not affect ^{201}Tl uptake, but it increased ^{99m}Tc sestamibi uptake by 10%. The influx rates of these two agents have also been compared in cultured chick ventricular myocytes that were inhibited for up to 2 hours by iodoacetate, 1 mM, to inhibit glycolysis and rotenone, 10 µM, to inhibit mitochondrial respiration.[40] Despite a decrease in ATP level, these poisons had little effect on lactate dehydrogenase release, suggesting modest cell injury. The influx rate of ^{201}Tl rapidly decreased to 30% ± 13% of control levels during the first 20 minutes of incubation and then remained stable. This residual activity was insensitive to ouabain, a result that is consistent with the observation that about 60% of ^{201}Tl influx is

mediated by the Na$^+$/K$^+$-ATPase.[25] With ^{99m}Tc sestamibi, the influx rate showed a 44% increase at 10 minutes and then monotonously declined, crossing the control level after 1 hour (Fig. 2-8), suggesting hyperpolarization of the plasma membrane. When the effect of metabolic inhibition on the efflux of the two agents was assessed, a more rapid washout of ^{99m}Tc sestamibi than of ^{201}Tl was seen, suggesting depolarization of the mitochondrial membrane and the presence of a somewhat metabolically insensitive component of ^{201}Tl retention.

In the light of what is now known about the mechanisms of cellular accumulation of these agents, these results are consistent with the fact that only metabolic interventions severe enough to alter the transmembrane potentials can modify uptake of ^{99m}Tc sestamibi. It must be remembered that in the event of cellular injury, the ionic transmembrane gradients, especially potassium (and therefore its electrical diffusional potential), are the last abnormalities to appear. Their loss is associated with irreversible injury.

These various in vitro experiments provide consistent observations about the mechanisms of accumulation of ^{99m}TC sestamibi in myocardial cells. First, ^{99m}Tc sestamibi concentrates in the cells as a function of transmembrane electrical potentials. Second, because the membranes are more negatively charged at the mitochondrial level than the sarcolemmal level, the tracer concentrates preferentially in the mitochondria. Third, metabolic alterations that are capable of altering the myocardial uptake of ^{99m}TC sestamibi must also alter the transmembrane potentials, which can be induced only by a toxic chemical intervention or an intervention that correspond to a severe ischemic situation.

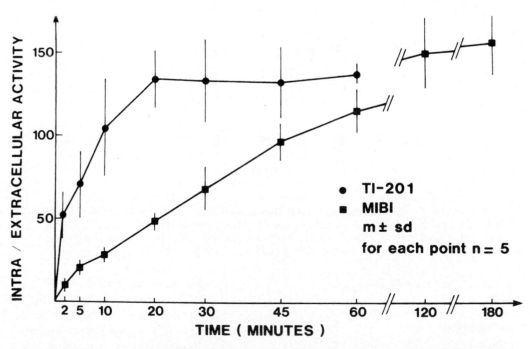

Fig. 2-6. Kinetics of accumulation of thallium-201 and techetium-99m sestamibi in cultured myocardial cells of newborn rats. (From Maublant J, Gachon P, Moins N: Hexakis [2-methoxy-isobutylisontrile] technetium-99m and thallium-201 chloride, *J Nucl Med* 29:48, 1988. Reprinted by permission of the Society of Nuclear Medicine.)

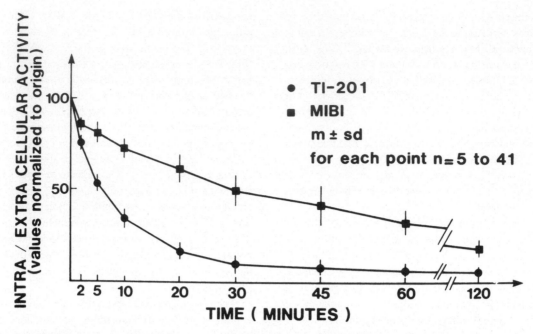

Fig. 2-7. Kinetics of release of thallium-201 and technetium-99m sestamibi in cultured myocardial cells of newborn rats. (From Maublant J, Gachon P, Moins N: Hexakis [2-methoxyisobutylisontrile] technetium-99m and thallium-201 chloride, *J Nucl Med* 29:48, 1988. Reprinted by permission of the Society of Nuclear Medicine.)

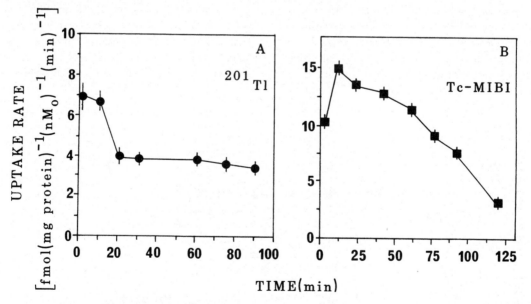

Fig. 2-8. Display of the uptake rate of thallium-201 and technetium-99m sestamibi, shown as a function of the duration of metabolic inhibition by a mixture of iodoacetate, 1 mM, and rotenone, 10 mM. Thallium-201 rapidly decreases and then plateaus at about 50% of its initial level, whereas the ^{99m}Tc sestamibi influx is initially stimulated and then monotonously decreases to a very low level. (From Piwnica-Worms D, Chiu ML, and Kronauge JF: *Circulation* 85:1531, 1992.)

OTHER MYOCARDIAL BLOOD FLOW IMAGING AGENTS

Technetium-99m teboroxime

In addition to charged molecules, neutral ^{99m}Tc-labeled agents have been tested for MBF imaging. A member of the family of the boron derivatives, (chloro(methylboron(1-)-tris

[1,1-cyclohexane-dionedixime(1-)]-N,N′,N″,N‴,N⁗,N⁗′)Tc, or SQ30217,[35] has been available on the U.S. market. This agent and another member of the same family, SQ32014, have been shown to very rapidly attain (<2 minutes) a plateau level in the cultured myocytes of newborn rats.[30] The value for $(C_i/C_e)_{eq}$ was 15 times greater with SQ30217 than with SQ32014 (585 ± 66 vs 34.7 ± 4.5). It was not affected by any

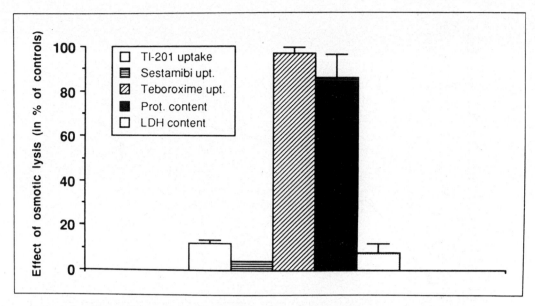

Fig. 2-9. Effect of osmotic lysis of cultured newborn rat myocytes on the accumulation of tracer, protein content, and release of lactate dehydrogenase. Only the accumulation of ^{99m}Tc teboroxime was not altered by disruption of the cell membrane. (From Maublant J et al: *J Nucl Med* 34:255, 1993.)

combination of cyanide, 1 mM; iodoacetate, 0.1 mM; and ouabain, 1mM, demonstrating its total independence relative to metabolism.[27] A dramatic difference with ^{201}Tl and ^{99m}Tc sestamibi was observed in free membranes obtained from cells subjected to osmotic lysis (Fig. 2-9). When incubated for 20 minutes, uptake of ^{201}Tl and ^{99m}Tc sestamibi was less than 15% of control values in whole cells, whereas SQ30217 uptake, which was normalized to the amount of protein remaining in the dishes, was not modified. All of these results strongly suggest that the mechanism of cellular uptake of SQ30217 is totally different than that of the two other agents, probably as a result of simple partitioning in the lipid phase of the cell membranes. However, the stability of the molecules also differs. When samples of the activity released by the cells during the washout experiments are used for uptake measurements in fresh preparations, ^{201}Tl and ^{99m}Tc sestamibi attain their usual $(C_i/C_e)_{eq}$ levels, but ^{99m}Tc teboroxime in that form of release is only minimally concentrated in or on the cells (Unpublished data). These results suggest that the structure of ^{201}Tl and ^{99m}Tc sestamibi is not modified by transit through the cell (which is obvious for the ion ^{201}Tl), whereas ^{99m}Tc teboroxime undergoes a conformational change, probably through enzymatic action, that makes it unsuitable for cellular reuptake. This could explain its in vivo apparent washout, which is nearly as fast as in vitro. By contrast, the in vivo washout of ^{201}Tl and ^{99m}Tc-sestamibi, which is much slower than the values observed in vitro, could result from reuptake of most of their released activity.

Technetium-99m tetrofosmin

Technetium-99m tetrofosmin is a recently introduced MBF imaging agent.[21] A lipophilic technetium-phosphino-dioxo

cation, it has been studied in vitro by using a model of adult rat ventricular myocytes[43] that were obtained by infusion of a collagenase solution into the perfused heart of male rats. Noncontracting rod-shaped cells were isolated and incubated with ^{99m}Tc tetrofosmin. At the end of the incubation phase, the cells were separated from the supernatant after 3 minutes of centrifugation. Subcellular fractionation was also performed. At uptake, a plateau was reached after approximately 60 minutes (Fig. 2-10). Washout was slow, with 65% of the initial activity being retained by the cells after 1 hour. Metabolic blockade by iodoacetate, 1 mM, and 2,4-dinitrophenol, 10 μM (an uncoupler of mitochondrial respiration) resulted in a 71% drop in tracer accumulation. Channel inhibitors, such as ouabain, amiloride, and bumetanide, had no effect. The kinetics of ^{99m}Tc tetrofosmin was found to be comparable to ^{99m}Tc sestamibi in a model of cultured smooth-muscle cells.[34]

Technetium-99m tetrofosmin was also assessed in isolated mitochondria.[54] This was a definite way to demonstrate the localization of this kind of agent in these organelles. Mitochondria were prepared from the hearts of adult rats. After mechanical homogenization in a protease-containing buffer, the mitochondria were isolated by differential centrifugation of the homogenate. Their volume, which was determined by a dual-isotope technique, was 1.16 ± 0.23 μl (milligrams of protein)$^{-1}$. The percentage of uptake was independent of tracer concentration but was closely proportional to the number of mitochondria. The addition of dinitrophenol induced a rapid and nearly complete release of the tracer (Fig. 2-11), whereas stimulation of oxygen consumption by Ca^{++}, 0.2 mM, caused a partial and reversible release and inhibition of ADP phosphorylation by Ca^{++}, 1 mM, produced an irreversible loss of ^{99m}Tc tetrofosmin (Fig. 2-12).

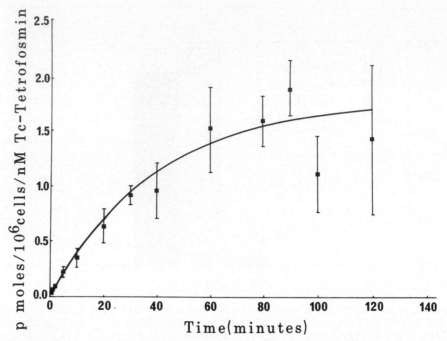

Fig. 2-10. Kinetics of accumulation of technetium-99m tetrofosmin in cultured adult rat myocytes. (From Platts EA et al: *J Nucl Cardiol* 2:317, 1995.)

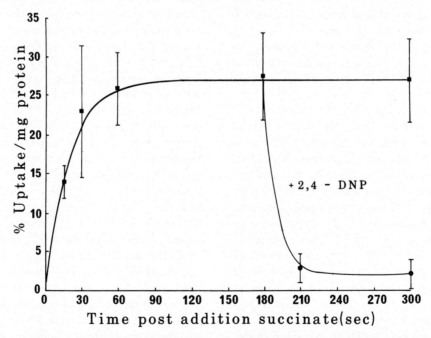

Fig. 2-11. Kinetics of uptake of technetium-99m tetrofosmin in isolated mitochondria from adult rat hearts. A plateau is attained after 60 seconds. Addition of the uncoupler 2,4-dinitrophenol (DNP) results in fast release of the tracer. (From Younès A et al: *J Nucl Cardiol* 2:327, 1995.)

Technetium-99m furifosmin

Technetium-99m furifosmin, a new lipophilic cation labeled with technetium(III) is currently under investigation.[45] Its kinetics of uptake and retention have been assessed in a model of cardiac myocytes and mitochondria from adult rats.[45] In terms of the concentration of the agent per milligram of protein, mitochondria were 5 to 10 times more active than intact cells. There was also evidence that mitochondrial retention was related to transmembrane potential, because it collapsed with the addition of FCCP, an uncoupler of the proton ionophore type. These results strongly suggest that ^{99m}Tc furifosmin behaves like the other ^{99m}Tc-labeled lipophilic cations.

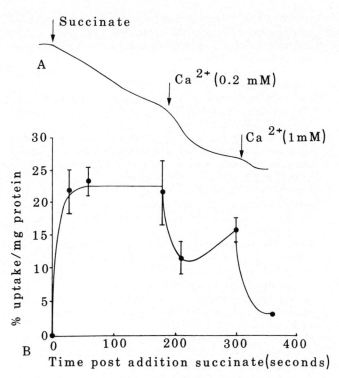

Fig. 2-12. Effect of added calcium on the mitochondrial respiration (**A**) and uptake of technetium-99m tetrofosmin (**B**). Respiration is represented by the negative slope of the curve in **A**. When a low concentration of calcium (0.2 mM) is added, respiration is temporarily stimulated and ^{99m}Tc tetrofosmin accumulation is temporarily depressed. When a higher concentration of calcium (1 mM) is added, respiration and tracer accumulation are irreversibly collapsed. (From Younès A et al: *J Nucl Cardiol* 2:327, 1995.)

Technetium-99m NOET

Bis(N-ethoxy,N-ethyl dithiocarbamato)nitrido ^{99m}Tc (V) (^{99m}Tc-NOET) is a neutral lipophilic myocardial perfusion imaging agent that is also being investigated.[36] Experiments in beating myocardial cells of newborn rats found a half-time of 11.5 ± 0.7 minutes to attainment of plateau during the accumulation phase but no appreciable release of activity during washout.[14] The metabolic or ion transport inhibitors rotenone, iodoacetic acid, amiloride, ouabain, and bumetamide did not modify ^{99m}Tc NOET accumulation; however it was reduced by the calcium channel blockers verapamil, 1 mM, and diltiazem, 10 mM, to $67\% \pm 11\%$ and $65\% \pm 14\%$ of control values, respectively ($p<0.01$ for both), whereas it was increased to $171\% \pm 12\%$ by the calcium channel activator BayK8644. Technetium-99m NOET shows high binding to myocardial cell membranes,[51] as well as to red blood cells,[19] which may explain its apparent redistribution, which has been documented in animals.[12] However, in vitro results suggest that the mechanism of this redistribution differs from that of ^{201}Tl.

CONCLUSIONS

Cultured cardiac cells are very useful in understanding the mechanism of tissue uptake of MBF imaging agents, which is a complex, multifactorial, and hard-to-predict phenomenon.[38] However, such cells cannot explain everything, because they only represent a part of the whole process of tissue accumulation of tracer. These cells enable isolation of the crucial part of transmembrane exchange.

Demonstration that the translocation of an agent is not at all related to a primary or secondary metabolic process is sufficient to claim that it will never be useful to assess myocardial viability in vivo but that the agent is a potential candidate for MBF imaging. This kind of finding can be obtained rapidly and at relatively low cost, and could avoid costly, lengthy, and useless clinical studies. The same is true for an agent to which accumulation seems to be related in vitro to cellular metabolism through a primary or secondary active exchange mechanism. This finding makes it worthwhile to suggest that it could be of interest in detecting myocardial viability and in justifying some clinical studies. In the future, it is hoped that new agents will become commercially available only after such basic data become available.

REFERENCES

1. Backus M, Piwnica-Worms D, Hackett D, et al: Microprobe analysis of Tc-MIBI in heart cells: calculation of mitochondrial membrane potential, *Am J Physiol* 265 (1 pt 1): C178–C187, 1993.
2. Buja LM, Hagler HK, Parsons D, et al: Alterations of ultrastructure and elemental composition in cultured neonatal rat cardiac myocytes after metabolic inhibition with iodoacetic acid, *Lab Invest* 53:397–412, 1985.
3. Caldwell JH, Mertens H, Linssen MC, et al: Uptake kinetics of technetium-99m-methoxyisobutylisonitrile and thallium-201 in adult rat heart endothelial and fibroblast-like cells in comparison to myocytes, *J Nucl Med* 33:102–107, 1992.
4. Chernoff DM, Strichartz GR, and Piwnica-Worms D: Membrane potential determination in large unilamellar vesicles with hexakis(2-methoxyisobutylisonitrile) technetium(I), *Biochim Biophys Acta* 1147:262–266, 1993.
5. Chiu ML, Kronauge JF, and Piwnica-Worms D: Effect of mitochondrial and plasma membrane potentials on accumulation of hexakis(2-methoxyisobutylisonitrile) technetium(I) in cultured mouse fibroblasts, *J Nucl Med* 31:1646–1653, 1990.
6. Crane P, Laliberte R, Heminway S, et al: Effect of mitochondrial viability and metabolism on technetium-99m-sestamibi myocardial retention, *Eur J Nucl Med* 20:20–25, 1993.
7. DeHaan RL and Gottlieb SH: The electrical activity of embryonic chick heart cells isolated in tissue culture singly or in interconnected cell sheets, *J Gen Physiol* 52:643–665, 1968.
8. Delano ML, Sands H, and Gallagher BM: Transport of ^{42}K$^+$, ^{201}Tl$^+$, and [^{99m}Tc(dmpe)$_2$.Cl$_2$]$^+$ by neonatal rat myocyte cultures, *Biochem Pharmacol* 34:3377–3380, 1985.
9. Diwan JJ and Lehrer PH: Inhibition of mitochondrial potassium ion flux by thallous ions, *Biochem Soc Trans* 5:203–205, 1977.
10. Emaus RK, Grunwald R, and Lemasters JJ: Rhodamine 123 as a probe of transmembrane potential in isolated rat-liver mitochondria: spectral and metabolic properties, *Biochim Biophys Acta* 850:436–448, 1986.
11. Friedman BJ, Beihn R, and Friedman JP: The effect of hypoxia on thallium kinetics in cultured chick myocardial cells, *J Nucl Med* 28:1453–1460, 1987.
12. Gehring PJ and Hammond PB: The uptake of thallium by rabbit erythrocytes, *J Pharmacol Exp Ther* 145:215–221, 1964.
13. Ghezzi C, Fagret D, Arvieux CC, et al: Myocardial kinetics of TcN-NOET: a neutral lipophilic complex tracer of regional myocardial blood flow, *J Nucl Med* 36:1069–1077, 1995.

14. Ghezzi C, Fagret D, Riou L, et al: In vitro uptake kinetics of bis (N-ethoxy N-ethyl dithiocarbamato) nitrido technetium-99m (V), a myocardial perfusion imaging agent: a study in cultured cardiac cells, *J Nucl Cardiol* 4:S20, 1997.

15. Harary I and Farley B: In vitro studies of single isolated beating heart cells, *Science* 132:1674–1675, 1960.

16. Hasin Y and Barry WH: Myocardial metabolic inhibition and membrane potential, contraction, and potassium uptake, *Am J Physiol* 247:H322–H329, 1984.

17. Hunter DR, Haworth RA, Goknur AB, et al: Control of thallium and sodium fluxes in isolated adult rat heart cells by anthopleurin-A, verapamil and magnesium, *J Mol Cell Cardiol* 18:1125–1132, 1986.

18. Ishida H, Kohmoto O, Bridge JH, et al: Alterations in cation homeostasis in cultured chick ventricular cells during and after recovery from adenosine triphosphate depletion, *J Clin Invest* 81:1173–1181, 1988.

19. Johnson G III, Nguyen KN, Pasqualini R, et al: Interaction of technetium-99m-N-NOET with blood elements: potential mechanism of myocardial redistribution, *J Nucl Med* 38:138–143, 1997.

20. Kashket ER: Active transport of thallous ions by *Streptococcus lactis, J Biol Chem* 254:8129–8131, 1979.

21. Kelly JD, Forster Am, Higley B, et al: Technetium-99m-tetrofosmin as a new radiopharmaceutical for myocardial perfusion imaging, *J Nucl Med* 34:222–227, 1993.

22. Kinsey VE, McLean IW, and Parker J: Studies on the crystalline lens/XVIII, Kinetics of thallium (Tl$^+$) transport in relation to that of the alkali metal cations, *Invest Ophthalmol* 10:932–942, 1971.

23. Kletzien RF, Pariza MW, Becker JE, et al: A method using 3-O-methyl-D-glucose and phloretin for the determination of intracellular water space of cells in monolayer culture, *Anal Biochem* 68:537–544, 1975.

24. Landowne D: A comparison of radioactive thallium and potassium fluxes in the giant axon of squid, *J Physiol (Lond)* 252:79–96, 1975.

25. McCall D, Zimmer LJ, and Katz AM: Kinetics of thallium exchange in cultured rat myocardial cells, *Circ Res* 56(3):370–376, 1985.

26. McCall D, Zimmer LJ, and Katz AM: Effect of ischemia-related metabolic factors on thallium exchange in cultured rat myocardial cells, *Can J Cardiol* 2:176–183, 1986.

27. Maublant J and Baggott J: Technetium-99m-sestamibi cellular uptake: passive or secondary active transport? *J Nucl Med* 38:1170, 1997.

28. Maublant J, Gachon P, and Moins N: Hexakis (2-methoxy isobutyl-isonitrile) technetium-99m and thallium-201 chloride: uptake and release in cultured myocardial cells, *J Nucl Med* 29:48–54, 1988.

29. Maublant J, Moins N, and Gachon P: Uptake and release of two new Tc-99m-labeled myocardial blood flow imaging agents in cultured cardiac cells, *Eur J Nucl Med* 15:180–182, 1989.

30. Maublant J, et al: Uptake of technetium-99m-teboroxime in cultured myocardial cells: comparison with thallium-201 and technetium-99m-sestamibi, *J Nucl Med* 34:255–259, 1993.

31. Mousa SA, Williams SJ, and Sands H: Characterization of in vivo chemistry of cations in the heart, *J Nucl Med* 28:1351–1357, 1987.

32. Mullins LJ and Moore RD: The movement of thallium ions in muscle, *J Gen Physiol* 43:759–773, 1960.

33. Murphy E, Le Furgey A, and Lieberman M: Biochemical and structural changes in cultured heart cells induced by metabolic inhibition, *Am J Physiol* 253:C700–C706, 1987.

34. Nakamura K, Sammiya T, Hashimoto J, et al: Comparison of cationic myocardial perfusion agents: characteristics of accumulation in cultured smooth muscle cells, *Ann Nucl Med* 10:375–381, 1996.

35. Narra RK, Nunn AD, Kuczynski BL, et al: A neutral technetium-99m complex for myocardial imaging, *J Nucl Med* 30:1830–1837, 1989.

36. Pasqualini R, Duatti A, Bellande E, et al: Bis(dithiocarbamato) nitrido

37. Piwnica-Worms D, Kronauge JF, Holman BL, et al: Hexakis (carboxymethoxyisopropylisonitrile) technetium(I), a new myocardial perfusion imaging agent: binding characteristics in cultured chick cells, *J Nucl Med* 29:55–61, 1988.

38. Piwnica-Worms D, Chiu ML, and Kronauge JF: Divergent kinetics of ^{201}Tl and 99mTc-SESTAMIBI in cultured chick ventricular myocytes during ATP depletion, *Circulation* 85:1531–1541, 1992.

39. Piwnica-Worms D, Kronauge JF, and Chiu ML: Uptake and retention of hexakis (2-methoxyisobutyl isonitrile) technetium(I) in cultured chick myocardial cells, Mitochondrial and plasma membrane potential dependence, *Circulation* 82:1826–1838, 1990.

40. Piwnica-Worms D, Kronauge JF, and Chiu ML: Enhancement by tetraphenylborate of technetium-99m-MIBI uptake kinetics and accumulation in cultured chick myocardial cells, *J Nucl Med* 32:1992–1999, 1991.

41. Piwnica-Worms D, Kronauge JF, Delmon L, et al: Effect of metabolic inhibition on technetium-99m kinetics in cultured chick myocardial cells, *J Nucl Med* 31:464–472, 1990.

42. Piwnica-Worms D, Kronauge JF, Holman BL, et al: Comparative myocardial uptake characteristics of hexakis (alkylisonitrile) technetium(I) complexes, Effect of lipophilicity, *Invest Radiol* 24:25–29, 1989.

43. Platts EA, North TL, Pickett RD, et al: Mechanism of uptake of technetium-tetrofosmin, I: Uptake into isolated adult rat ventricular myocytes and subcellular localization, *J Nucl Cardiol* 2:317–326, 1995.

44. Rauch B and Kübler W: Kinetics of cellular uptake of tracers used in myocardial scintigraphy, *Basic Res Cardiol* 80 Suppl 1:65–68, 1985.

45. Rossetti C, Paganelli G, Vanoli G, et al: Biodistribution in humans and preliminary clinical evaluation of a new tracer with optimized properties for myocardial perfusion imaging: [^{99m}Tc]Q12, *J Nucl Biol Med* 36:29–31, 1992.

46. Roszell NJ, McGoron AJ, Biniakiewicz DS, et al: ^{99m}Tc Q12 handling by isolated rat cardiac myocytes and mitochondria, *Circulation* 92:I-181, 1995.

47. Sands H, Delano ML, and Gallagher BM: Uptake of hexakis(t-butyl-isonitrile) technetium (I) and hexakis-(isopropylisonitrile) technetium (I) by neonatal rat myocytes and human erythrocytes, *J Nucl Med* 27;404–484, 1986.

48. Sands H, Delano ML, Camin LL, et al: Comparison of the transport of ^{42}K$^+$, ^{22}Na$^+$, ^{201}Tl$^+$, and [^{99m}Tc(dmpe)2 X Cl$_2$]$^+$ using human erythrocytes, *Biochim Biophys Acta* 812:665–670, 1985.

49. Simpson P, McGrath A, and Savion S: Myocyte hypertrophy in neonatal rat heart cultures and its regulation by serum and by catecholamines, *Circ Res* 51:787–801, 1982.

50. Skulskii IA, Manninen V, and Järnefelt J: Factors affecting the relative magnitudes of the ouabain-sensitive and the ouabain-insensitive fluxes of thallium ion in erythrocytes, *Biochim Biophys Acta* 506:233–241, 1978.

51. Uccelli L, Giganti M, Duatti A, et al: Subcellular distribution of technetium-99m-N-NOET in rat myocardium, *J Nucl Med* 36:2075–2079, 1995.

52. Wagner HN Jr, Rhodes BA, Sasaki Y, et al: Studies of the circulation with radioactive microspheres, *Invest Radiol* 4(6):374–386, 1969.

53. Watanabe A, Green FJ, and Farmer BB: *Preparation and use of cardiac myocytes in experimental cardiology,* In Fozzard HA, et al, eds, *The heart and cardiovascular system*, New York, 1986, Raven Press.

54. Younès A, Songadele JA, Maublant J, et al: Mechanism of uptake of technetium-tetrofosmin, II: Uptake into isolated adult rat heart mitochondria, *J Nucl Cardiol* 2:327–333, 1995.

Chapter 3

Tracer kinetics in the isolated heart model

Seth T. Dahlberg and Jeffrey A. Leppo

Over the past few decades, myocardial perfusion imaging with radiolabeled tracers has become a standard method for diagnosing and assessing coronary artery disease. Significant coronary artery disease can be diagnosed when impaired coronary flow reserve reduces regional tracer deposition during hyperemic stress. In addition, the severely reduced myocardial uptake of some tracers at rest can indicate irreversibly injured or infarcted myocardium.

The deposition of imaging tracers requires that they be extracted from myocardial capillaries and subsequently retained by cardiac myocytes.[4,6,9,48,55] Extraction from capillaries requires tracer diffusion or active transport across endothelial, interstitial, and sarcolemmal barriers. Tracer extraction across these barriers generally decreases as coronary flow increases. If cellular tracer retention requires active, energy-dependent processes, cell death may result in tissue loss or washout of intracellular tracer.[18–20,27,34,36,45,50,54,73] Therefore, regional deposition of perfusion tracers is affected by two factors: the level of coronary flow and cardiac myocyte viability.

The isolated heart model can be used to assess the separate effects of these factors on myocardial uptake of perfusion tracers. Tracer extraction across the endothelial and interstitial barriers of normal tissue can be measured while coronary flow is varied independent of myocardial metabolic needs. The effect of drugs, toxins, or ischemic injury on myocardial tracer retention can be determined while coronary flow is kept constant.

MYOCARDIAL PERFUSION TRACERS

Many cationic perfusion tracers, including thallium (Tl), rubidium (Rb), potassium (K), and cationic technetium (Tc) compounds, have been studied with the isolated heart model. The properties of several of these perfusion tracers are shown in Table 3-1.

Because of favorable physiologic properties for assessing blood flow and myocardial viability, ^{201}Tl is the most widely used single-photon tracer for myocardial perfusion imaging.[2,15,21,49,66,71] Thallium is a monovalent cation similar in size to K^+ and Rb^+.[62] Whereas the cellular uptake of Tl is in part caused by active transport by Na^+,K^+ adenosinetriphosphate Tl^+ has other mechanisms of cellular transport (including transport via Na channels[38]) that result in higher extraction and larger intracellular volume of distribution than K^+ or Rb^+.[10,28,29,57,59,60,62] However, despite favorable physiologic properties as a diffusible tracer, the suboptimal dosimetry and photon energy of ^{201}Tl have led to the development of ^{99m}Tc-labeled perfusion agents.

Several ^{99m}Tc-labeled compounds, including the isonitrile sestamibi and the phosphine compounds tetrofosmin, furifosmin (Q12), and Q3,[17,30,31,37,44] have been studied as myocardial perfusion tracers. Sestamibi and tetrofosmin, which are currently available for clinical use, share properties of moderate myocardial extraction, stable retention, and moderate liver uptake.

Two neutral ^{99m}Tc-labeled perfusion tracers have been studied with the isolated heart model. Technetium-99m teboroxime, a BATO (boronic acid adduct of technetium dioxime) compound with high myocardial extraction and rapid clearance, is a neutral, lipophilic perfusion agent currently approved for clinical use.[52,63] Technetium-99m-NOET (bis[N-ethoxy,N-ethyldithiocarbamato]), a neutral nitrido compound with moderate myo-cardial extraction and clearance, was recently developed for perfusion imaging.[32,39,65] The myocardial clearance kinetics of both of these neutral compounds are affected by binding to blood components.

ISOLATED HEART MODEL

The isolated perfused heart model can be used to assess tracer kinetics by measuring cardiac time–activity curves with an external scintillation detector, or coronary sinus blood can be collected for determination of venous outflow dilution curves. In either method, a heart is harvested from a small animal (such as a rat or rabbit)[51,72] or, less commonly, from a larger animal (such as a dog).[10] The heart is perfused in a retrograde manner with warmed perfusate through the aorta by using the Langendorff technique. Left ventricular chamber pressure and aortic perfusion pressure are continuously monitored. Although the retrograde perfusion can use either constant pressure or constant flow, the latter is preferred for the study of perfusion flow tracers.

Cardiac perfusate includes isotonic buffer, such as Krebs–Henseleit buffer, and metabolic substrate, such as glucose, lactate, pyruvate, or fatty acids. A membrane oxygenator is used to maintain physiologic perfusate pH and oxygen levels.

Although the heart can be perfused with oxygenated buffer alone, the very perfusate flow required for adequate oxygen delivery and the low oncotic perfusate pressure can result in poor ventricular function and nonphysiologic tracer kinetics. The addition of albumin and washed erythrocytes to the perfusate permits lower physiologic coronary flow, improved energy metabolism, higher left ventricular developed pressure, and higher dP/dT.[16,41] However, some perfusion tracers can bind to circulating blood components, which could affect measured tracer kinetics in this experimental model.

INDICATOR-DILUTION ANALYSIS OF TRACER KINETICS

In evaluating a diffusible perfusion tracer, it is important to understand general transport principles. As a bolus of tracer moves through the coronary arteries and arterioles, it is confined to the intravascular space. However, during passage through the myocardial capillaries, the tracer may diffuse through endothelial cells or intercellular gap junctions into the interstitial space. Tracer that remains in the capillaries will emerge in the venous blood earlier than extracted tracer that resides in the interstitial space before eventually diffusing back into the capillaries and emerging in the venous outflow. The delay in the appearance of the extracted tracer can be measured as a prolonged myocardial transit time. Tracer that is extracted and retained in cardiac myocytes will have longer myocardial transit time.[4,6]

To evaluate the kinetics of perfusion tracers with the multiple indicator-dilution technique, diffusible compounds, such as Tl or ^{99m}Tc-labeled compounds, are coinjected into the aorta along with an intravascular reference tracer, such as albumin labeled with indium-111–diethylenetriamine pentaacetic acid (DTPA) or iodine-125.[4,6,7,9,47] An interstitial reference tracer, such as carbon-14 sucrose or cobalt-58 ethylenediamine tetraacetic acid (EDTA), can also be included. After tracer injection, samples of venous flow are collected from the coronary sinus, and the measured isotope concentrations are used to plot indicator-dilution venous outflow curves for each tracer. For each injection, normalized coronary sinus indicator-dilution curves, referred to as $h(t)$ curves (equation 1), are calculated for each of the coinjected tracers, where F is coronary flow (in ml/min), $C(t)$ is isotope activity (in counts per minute [cpm]/ml) at time t (in seconds) after injection, and q_0 (cpm) is the dose of injected tracer.[4,5]

$$h(t) = \frac{C(t) \cdot F}{q_0} \qquad (1)$$

The unextracted intravascular reference tracer, $h_R(t)$, has the highest peak because all tracer is collected in the venous blood. Although the diffusible tracers, $h_D(t)$, have lower early $h(t)$ peaks because extracted tracer remains in the heart, the higher tails of the diffusible curves indicate delayed efflux of the initially extracted tracer. The $h(t)$ curves are used for all further calculations of tracer kinetics.

Each point on an $h(t)$ curve represents the fraction of injected tracer dose emerging from the coronary sinus per second. The $h(t)$ curves usually have a rapid rise to a relatively sharp peak, followed by a prolonged tail. This shape results from dispersion caused by heterogeneous flow in the cardiac vascula-

Table 3-1. Single-Photon Myocardial Perfusion Agents*

Variable	Thallium-201	Sestamibi	Teboroxime	Tetrofosmin†	Furifosmin	NOET
E_{max}	0.80	0.39	0.89	0.30	0.26	0.48
E_{net} at 5 minutes	0.60	0.41	0.71	0.30	0.12	0.24
P_{scap}, ml/min/g	2.95	0.44	3.7	0.66	0.48	1.02
Cell injury reduces tracer uptake	++++	++++	+/−	++++	++	++
Speed of myocardial clearance	Moderate	Slow	Rapid	Slow	Slow	Moderate
Redistribution	Yes	Minimal	Yes	No	No	Yes
Ability to measure hyperemic flow	Good	Adequate	Excellent	Adequate	Adequate	Adequate

*E_{max} = maximum tracer extraction; E_{net} = net tracer extraction; NOET = bis (n-ethoxy,N-ethyldithiocarbamato) nitrido. PS_{cap} = tracer permeability–surface area product. All compounds except thallium-201 are labeled with technetium-99m in isolated hearts.
† Tetrofosmin data from isolated rat hearts; all others from rabbit hearts.

ture as well as laminar flow within the system. Because albumin is assumed to be confined to the vascular space (an assumption that is appropriate for the time frame of the experimental period),[12] the shape of the albumin $h(t)$ curve (the solid lines in Figs. 3-1, A and 3-2, A) reveals this overall dispersive effect. However, the shapes of the $h(t)$ curves for the diffusible tracers result not only from this global dispersion but also from the escape of tracer from the vasculature into extravascular compartments (interstitium, membranes, and parenchymal cells).

Closer examination of the $h(t)$ curves reveals important differences among the tracers. When the early peak of the albumin curve is higher than the diffusible tracer $h(t)$ curve (Tl, solid circles; Tc, open circles; Figs. 3-1, A and 3-2, A), a net blood-to-tissue transport is indicated. The lowest peak of the venous $h(t)$ curve of the diffusible tracer indicates the highest maximal myocardial tracer extraction. Myocardial extraction of teboroxime is greater than that of Tl, and the extraction is greater than that of sestamibi. When the later tail of the albumin $h(t)$ curve is lower than the diffusible $h(t)$ curve (as shown on the semilog

$h(t)$ plots of Figs. 3-1, B and 3-2, B), a net efflux or clearance of diffusible tracer from the myocardium back to the intravascular space is indicated.[3] As for extraction, myocardial clearance of teboroxime is greater than that of Tl and clearance of Tl is greater than that of sestamibi.

Because the difference between the $h_R(t)$ of the albumin reference and the $h_D(t)$ of Tl or the Tc compounds indicates an escape or extraction of diffusible tracer from the perfusate as it passes through the heart, instantaneous extraction, $E(t)$, for each diffusible tracer can be calculated from the $h(t)$ curves as:

$$E(t) = \frac{h_R(t) - h_D(t)}{h_R(t)} \qquad (2)$$

where $h_D(t)$ is the venous outflow dilution curve of the diffusible tracer and $h_R(t)$ is the transport function of albumin, the intravascular reference. The variable E_{max} is the highest early value of $E(t)$ up to the peak of the albumin $h(t)$ curve and is the best estimate of fractional tissue extraction for each diffusible tracer. This instantaneous fractional extraction, $E(t)$, is plotted for teboroxime and Tl (Fig. 3-1, C) and for sestamibi and Tl (Fig. 3-2, C). In contrast to the Tl and teboroxime $E(t)$ curves,

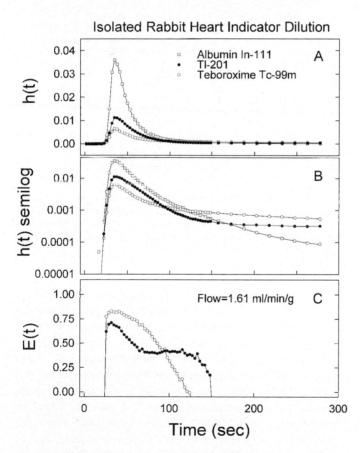

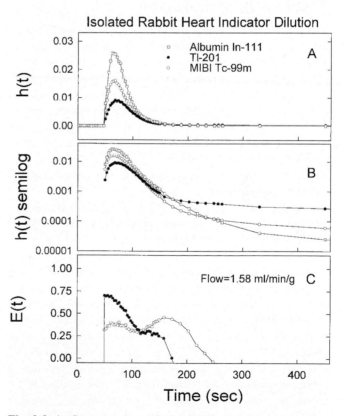

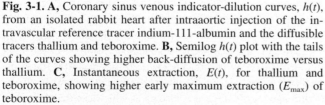

Fig. 3-1. A, Coronary sinus venous indicator-dilution curves, $h(t)$, from an isolated rabbit heart after intraaortic injection of the intravascular reference tracer indium-111-albumin and the diffusible tracers thallium and teboroxime. **B,** Semilog $h(t)$ plot with the tails of the curves showing higher back-diffusion of teboroxime versus thallium. **C,** Instantaneous extraction, $E(t)$, for thallium and teboroxime, showing higher early maximum extraction (E_{max}) of teboroxime.

Fig. 3-2. A, Coronary sinus venous indicator-dilution $h(t)$ curves from an isolated rabbit heart with indium-111-albumin intravascular reference and the diffusible tracers thallium and sestamibi. **B,** Semilog $h(t)$ plot with the tails of the curves showing lower back-diffusion of sestamibi versus thallium. **C,** Instantaneous extraction, $E(t)$, for thallium and sestamibi, showing more prolonged early extraction of sestamibi.

sestamibi shows a lower extraction with a relatively long and high plateau phase. This suggests that the extraction mechanism for sestamibi differs from that of Tl or teboroxime and that it seems to have a much slower exchange process.

The value for E_{max} can then be used in the calculation of the Crone–Renkin permeability–surface area product (PS_{cap}):

$$PS_{cap} = -F \cdot \ln(1 - E_{max}) \qquad (3)$$

where PS_{cap} is the permeability–surface area product for capillary–tissue diffusion (ml/min · g); F is coronary flow (ml/min · g); and E_{max} is maximum value of $E(t)$, as defined above.

The net tissue extraction, $E_{net}(t)$, of a diffusible compound can also be derived from the $h(t)$ curves. The value for E_{net} reflects the integral balance of extraction and clearance up to the time t and E_{net} is calculated as:

$$E_{net}(t) = \frac{\int_0^t [h_R(\tau) - h_D(\tau)]d\tau}{\int_0^t h_R(\tau)d\tau} \qquad (4)$$

where τ is a dummy variable for integration.[6]

MYOCARDIAL TRACER EXTRACTION AS A FUNCTION OF BLOOD FLOW

The E_{max} values versus blood flow for sestamibi, teboroxime, and Tl are shown in the upper panels of Figs. 3-3 and 3-4.[51,52] Maximal extraction of teboroxime is consistently higher than that of Tl determined simultaneously over a physiologic flow range (Fig. 3-3). There is an inverse linear relation of E_{max} versus flow, and the best-fit linear regression lines are shown. Figure 3-4 shows the individual values of E_{max} and coronary blood flow for Tl and sestamibi. There is also an inverse linear relationship between E_{max} and blood flow for each tracer, and sestamibi values are always less than corresponding thallium determinations.

The capillary flux values (PS_{cap}) for Tl, sestamibi, and teboroxime are seen in the lower panels of Figs. 3-3 and 3-4. The least-square, best-fit linear regression lines are shown for each isotope. The (PS_{cap}) (Fig. 3-3) for teboroxime is always higher than that of Tl determined simultaneously, whereas PS_{cap} for Tl is greater than that of sestamibi (Fig. 3-4). However, there is a positive linear relation between PS_{cap} and flow for all three flow tracers because the increase in flow is proportionally greater than the relatively smaller decrease in peak extraction. The higher PS_{cap} slope for teboroxime compared with that for Tl suggests that teboroxime has a more linear initial deposition of tracer than does Tl. This predicts better initial myocardial uptake properties for teboroxime compared with Tl, whereas the reverse is true for sestamibi. However, sestamibi has better imaging properties later (after 10 to 15 minutes) because of its relatively small amount of back-diffusion and high cellular retention. A similar relation between extraction and blood flow for sestamibi and thallium has been shown by Marshall et al,[56] who used a blood-perfused rabbit heart model.

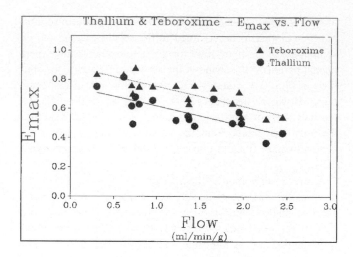

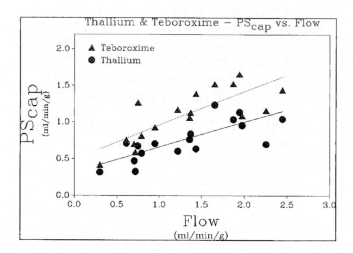

Fig. 3-3. Comparison of peak extraction E_{max} (*upper panel*) and capillary permeability PS_{cap} (*lower panel*) versus coronary flow for teboroxime (*triangles*) and thallium (*dots*) in isolated perfused rabbit hearts. (From Leppo JA and Meerdink DJ: *J Nucl Med* 31:67, 1990.)

Although a relatively high first-pass extraction and PS_{cap} value are regarded as important attributes of a perfusion tracer,[3,6] it is equally important that the initial extraction of the radionuclide remain stable in the tissue during imaging. Therefore, the values for E_{max} and PS_{cap} must be combined with calculations of E_{net} to account for the first-pass transcapillary extraction and the net tissue clearance (back-diffusion) of the initially extracted tracer. The E_{net} curves for several myocardial perfusion tracers are shown in Figs. 3-5 and 3-6. Thallium, teboroxime, and Tc NOET all show significant myocardial clearance of extracted tracer, which is associated with the clinical phenomenon of tracer redistribution. In contrast, sestamibi and tetrofosmin show high retention of extracted tracer and do not undergo substantial redistribution. Although the peak E_{net} value of Tl is initially higher than that of sestamibi or tetrofosmin, this disparity is reduced 15 to 20 minutes after tracer injection. On the basis of the observed myocyte retention of sestamibi and tetrofosmin, it is also clear why these tracers can be

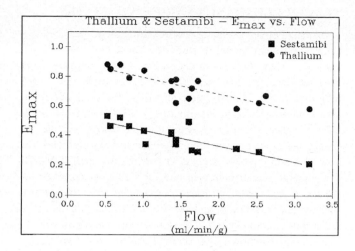

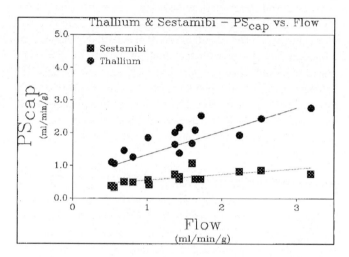

Fig. 3-4. The comparison shown in Fig. 3-3 except that sestamibi (*boxes*) replaces teboroxime. (From Leppo JA and Meerdink DJ: *Circ Res* 65:632, 1989.)

imaged longer after injection without substantial loss of initial regional tracer activity.

TRACER UPTAKE VERSUS FLOW

The myocardial tissue concentration, or initial uptake, of a diffusible tracer is a function of both the quantity of tracer delivered by coronary flow (the arterial input) and the extraction fraction of the tracer. Because extraction of perfusion agents decreases as coronary flow increases (Figs. 3-3 and 3-4), the myocardial deposition of these tracers is not linear compared with flow. Myocardial uptake of diffusible compounds can be calculated as

$$\text{Uptake} = E_{net}(t) \cdot F \qquad (5)$$

where $E_{net}(t)$ is net extraction and F is coronary flow. Therefore, uptake (expressed as ml/min · g) is a measure of tissue content of diffusible tracer.[22,26,33,48,56,67] Tracer uptake compared with coronary flow for teboroxime, thallium, and sestamibi are shown in Fig. 3-7 with a nonlinear regression for

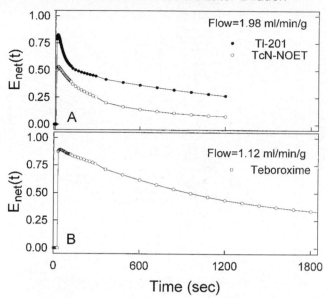

Fig. 3-5. A, Net extraction (E_{net}) for thallium, technetium-99m NOET, and **B,** teboroxime in isolated rabbit hearts showing moderate myo-cardial clearance of the three tracers.

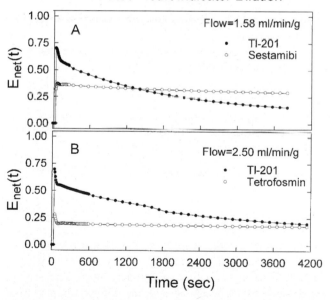

Fig. 3-6. A, Net extraction (E_{net}) for thallium and sestamibi in a rabbit heart, and **B,** tetrofosmin and thallium in a rat heart that contrasts the moderate myocardial washout of thallium with the stable retention of sestamibi and tetrofosmin.

each tracer. The E_{net} of tracer at 5 minutes after injection was used in the calculation of uptake. The variable levels of coronary flow were produced by using a peristaltic pump to vary the perfusate flow supplied to the hearts. During higher levels of coronary flow (>2.5 ml/min · g), intraaortic adenosine was in-

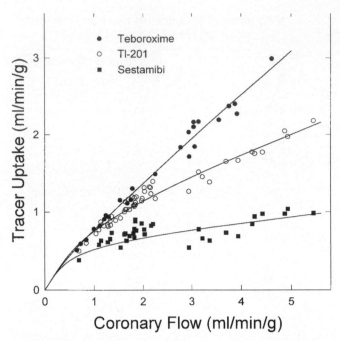

Fig. 3-7. Tracer uptake ($E_{net} \times$ flow) versus coronary flow for teboroxime, thallium, and sestamibi. The tracer data was fit with the nonlinear regression:
Uptake = F $[1 - e^{-(a + b \cdot flow)/F}]$ with $r = 0.99$ and $p < 0.001$ for each tracer. The higher coronary flows (> 2.5 ml/min/g) were produced during intraaortic adenosine infusion.

fused to permit high delivered flow without extreme increases in perfusion pressure.

Nonlinear regression for uptake versus flow was obtained by rearranging the terms in Equation 3[40] to derive

$$E = 1 - e^{-PS/F} \qquad (6)$$

The data in Figs. 3-3 and 3-4, as well as data from Caldwell et al[23] indicate that tracer permeability–surface area (*PS*) is linearly related to coronary flow as follows:

$$PS = b_1 \cdot flow + b_0 \qquad (7)$$

Tracer uptake ($E \times F$) can therefore be described as:

$$Uptake = F \cdot [1 - e^{-(b_1 \cdot F + b_0)/F}] \qquad (8)$$

The nonlinear regressions found by using this equation fit the data for each tracer in Fig. 3-7, with $r = 0.99$ and $p < 0.001$. At higher levels of coronary flow, a plateau in uptake versus flow occurs because the diffusion limitation of these tracers is such that tracer uptake underestimates flow. This plateau is most apparent for sestamibi uptake and least apparent for teboroxime uptake, which is nearly linear over a relatively wide range of coronary flows. Therefore, whereas uptake of all diffusible tracers underestimates hyperemic flow, uptake of teboroxime is closest to measured flow, followed by uptake of thallium and uptake of sestamibi. Although the available isolated heart data are more limited for tetrofosmin, this tracer seems to have uptake characteristics similar to those of sestamibi.

TRACER CLEARANCE VARIES WITH FLOW

Marshall et al[56] used a nonrecirculating blood-perfused isolated rabbit heart model to study the kinetics of thallium and sestamibi. Their data, illustrated in Fig. 3-8, show mean tracer washout data for five hearts perfused at high (2.8 ± 0.6 ml/g/min) and five hearts perfused at low (0.7 ± 0.2 ml/g/min) levels of coronary flow. Maximum E_{net} of Tl is initially significantly higher than that of sestamibi ($p < 0.001$), but the decrease in E_{net} of Tl over time is greater at both high and low flow. Perfusion tracers, such as Tl, teboroxime, and Tc NOET, that undergo redistribution in clinical studies generally show significant myocardial clearance of extracted tracer. In contrast, such tracers as sestamibi and tetrofosmin, which show minimal redistribution, are cleared very slowly from the myo-cardium. The E_{net} curves showing myocardial washout for these tracers are given in Figs. 3-5 and 3-6.

The neutral compound teboroxime shows transiently high myocardial uptake followed by rapid myocardial clearance and redistribution.[70] The rapid in vivo myocardial clearance of teboroxime contrasts with the moderate efflux of this compound observed in cell culture and isolated heart models.[52,58] Whereas cellular and isolated heart washout of teboroxime is faster than that of sestamibi, efflux of teboroxime in these models is similar to that of Tl. The rapid washout of teboroxime that occurs in vivo is probably caused by binding of the compound to blood components.

Rumsey, Rosenspire, and Nunn[69] observed that aliquots of teboroxime in blood withdrawn from the circulation of donor rats showed a progressive decrease in extraction by isolated rat hearts, whereas the extraction of Tl and sestamibi remained unchanged. We also observed reduced teboroxime extraction (but not reduced Tl or sestamibi extraction) in isolated rabbit hearts after incubation of teboroxime with erythrocytes.[25] Teboroxime incubated with erythrocytes or mixed even briefly with erythrocyte-enriched perfusate showed rapid myocardial clearance that contrasted with the slower myocardial clearance of teboroxime mixed only in saline before injection (Fig. 3-9). Therefore, the early rapid cardiac clearance of teboroxime seems to be due to erythrocyte binding, which reduces the amount of free tracer available for myocardial extraction.

A similar increased tracer clearance for the neutral compound Tc NOET has been observed by Johnson et al[43] who used isolated rat hearts perfused with blood as opposed to buffer. When Tc NOET was injected into rat hearts perfused with crystalloid buffer, the compound showed virtually no myocardial clearance, an effect similar to that with sestamibi. Efflux of Tc NOET from cultured myocytes has also been shown to be slow.[74] However, when injected into hearts perfused with erythrocyte-enriched and albumin-enriched perfusate, Tc NOET showed accelerated myocardial clearance. By using blood-perfused isolated rabbit hearts, we have observed moderate myocardial washout similar to that of Tl.[24] The moderate myocardial clearance of Tc NOET is much slower than that of teboroxime, and it is clear that the choice of perfusate components can

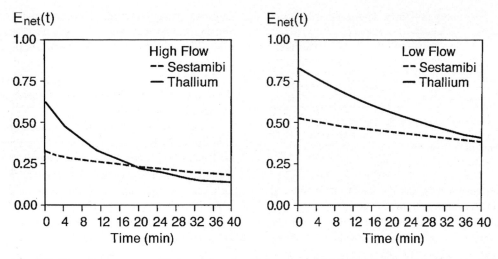

Fig. 3-8. Plot of mean myocardial retention $E_{net}(t)$ for sestamibi (*dashed lines*) and thallium (*solid lines*) from 5 high-flow (*left panel*) and 5 low-flow (*right panel*) rabbit hearts. (From Marshall RC, et al: *Circulation* 82:998, 1990.)

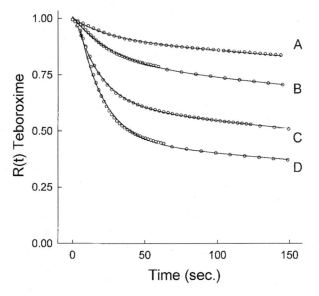

Fig. 3-9. Isolated rabbit heart residual cardiac tracer activity ($R(t)$) or fraction of injected dose) after intraaortic injection of teboroxime. Teboroxime is injected in saline (**A** and **B**), in erythrocyte-enriched perfusate (**C**), or human erythrocytes (**D**). Hearts were maintained with nonrecirculating (**A**) or recirculating (**B** through **D**) perfusate. Teboroxime in saline has the slowest myocardial clearance. Teboroxime in perfusate or human erythrocytes shows much faster clearance because of reduced extraction. Open circles represent teboroxime data and solid lines represent fitted biexponential curves. (From Dahlberg ST, Gilmore MP, Leppo JA: *J Nucl Cardiol* 1:270, 1994.)

have a marked effect on the measured kinetics of neutral perfusion tracers.

MODEL ESTIMATE ANALYSIS

For more rigorous analysis of indicator-dilution curves, the heart can be defined as an aggregate of capillary tissue units in parallel, an idea described elsewhere in more detail.[3,8,46]

Briefly, each unit is a three-region (capillary, interstitial fluid, and cell), two-barrier, axially distributed convection–diffusion model. This model is an extension of the one-barrier model of Bassingthwaighte[3] and is similar in concept to the two-barrier model of Rose, Goresky, and Bach.[68] The variables of the model for fitting the dilution curves are as follows:

1. F_s, average solvent flow (ml/g/min) = coronary blood flow × (1-hematocrit)

2. PS_c, capillary permeability–surface area product, ml/g/min

3. V'_I, volume of interstitial fluid distribution, mL/g (estimated from the interstitial tracer dilution curve for EDTA and held constant for the diffusible tracer fittings)

4. PS_{pc}, permeability–surface area product of parenchymal cell (sarcolemma of cardiac myocytes), ml/g/min

5. V'_{pc}, volume of tracer distribution within the parenchymal cells (cardiac myocytes), ml/g

An automated adjustment program is used to optimize the values of the variables to maximize the goodness-of-fit by using sensitivity functions described elsewhere.[53] The coefficient of variation is used as a measure of the overall goodness-of-fit and in the adjustment of variable stimates. The heterogeneity of flows (distribution of regional flows) is represented by five or seven regions as determined in rabbit heart experiments.[46] The greatest accuracy in estimation of the variables results from a reduction in the degrees of freedom given a physiologically appropriate model. Therefore, PS_c for albumin and PS_{pc} for EDTA are set at zero, which is appropriate for the relatively short observation times. Consequently, the large-vessel transport function can be defined by the albumin curve, the measured average flow, the distribution of regional flow, and an assumed capillary volume of 0.035 ml/g.[11]

For sestamibi and Tl, transport through endothelial capillary cells and consumption of tracer in the parenchymal cell are not included. The variables PS_c, PS_{pc}, and V'_{pc} are free for fitting

Table 3-2. Model Estimates of Tracer Tissue Distribution*

Model Estimates	Sestamibi	Thallium
PS_c, ml/g/min	0.6	2.9
PS_{pc}, ml/g/min	52	4.8
V'_{pc}, ml/g	13	7.5

*PS_c = permeability–surface area product at the capillary level; PS_{pc} = permeability–surface area product at the parenchymal cell level; V'_{pc} = parenchymal cell volume of distribution.

the diffusible tracer curves, whereas V'_I is set to the value estimated from the EDTA transport function.

As seen in Table 3-2, the mean PS_c values for sestamibi are substantially lower than the corresponding Tl values.[51,61] However, mean PS_{pc} and V'_{pc} values for sestamibi are both significantly greater than the corresponding Tl measurements. An estimate of myocardial tracer residence time can be made from the model variable estimates. Tracer retention is related to the reciprocal of the $[PS_c/(V'_{pc}+V'_I)]$ value (in minutes), which relates the capillary exchange rate to the apparent volume of distribution. When the mean estimates for PS_c, V'_{pc}, and V'_I were used, sestamibi retention was 20.6 minutes compared with 3.1 minutes for Tl. This should not be confused with a $t_{1/2}$ value; rather, it expresses a sixfold to sevenfold higher organ retention of tracer that has left the vascular space over this physiologic flow range for sestamibi compared with Tl. Marshall et al[56] also noted an accelerated washout of myocardial Tl activity related to increased flow that was almost fourfold higher than corresponding sestamibi measurements.

EFFECTS OF CELL INJURY ON TRACER RETENTION

In addition to their use in assessing regional coronary flow, myocardial perfusion tracers have more recently been studied as markers of myocardial viability. When used for this purpose, the retention of a perfusion tracer in an isolated heart independent of flow is compared at the control value and after irreversible myocardial injury caused by ischemia, metabolic poisoning, or membrane detergent. To remove the confounding effect of variable flow on tracer washout, flow must be maintained constant at the control value and during the experimental intervention. Tracer retention can then be assessed by measuring net myocardial tracer extraction by doing indicator-dilution analysis or by comparing rates of cardiac tracer clearance with an external sodium iodide detector. A summary of the effect of cellular injury on tracer uptake is included in Table 3-1.

Several indicator-dilution studies in which isolated rat or rabbit hearts were used have shown accelerated myocardial clearance of Tl after ischemic injury, resulting in decreased net tracer retention.[39,61,72] In a recent indicator-dilution study, ischemic injury was shown to reduce E_{net} for tetrofosmin in isolated rat hearts.[72] Beanlands et al[13] showed that metabolic injury with cyanide or membrane disruption with Triton X-100 deter-

gent caused severe myocyte injury manifested by release of creatine kinase and lactate dehydrogenase and confirmed by triphenyl tetrazolium staining and electron microscopy. This cell damage resulted in reduced accumulation and accelerated washout of infused sestamibi despite constant perfusate flow. Therefore, the myocardial uptake of these cationic tracers is a marker of myocardial viability.

A consistent effect of ischemic myocardial injury on the kinetics of infused teboroxime has not been observed in isolated rat hearts. One study showed accelerated cardiac teboroxime washout after global ischemia,[64] whereas another study found little effect of ischemia on teboroxime kinetics.[14] Because the effect of ischemia on teboroxime uptake has been inconsistent with in vivo models,[1,35] use of this compound in the assessment of myocardial viability requires further study.

In a preliminary indicator-dilution study of Tc NOET, 45 minutes of global ischemia caused a moderate reduction in tracer extraction, but this reduction was not as great as the effect of ischemia on Tl retention.[39] Johnson et al[42] found that ischemia had little effect on Tc NOET clearance, although membrane disruption caused rapid cardiac loss of infused tracer. Therefore, myocardial retention of Tc NOET may be affected by viability, but further studies of this tracer are warranted.

CONCLUSIONS AND FUTURE DIRECTIONS

Isolated heart models permit the accurate measurement of tracer kinetics with time–activity curves of high temporal resolution. Arterial input of tracer can be controlled without the confounding effect of tracer recirculation, and coronary blood flow can be controlled independent of myocardial metabolic demands.

Table 3-1 summarizes the properties of the myocardial perfusion tracers discussed in this chapter. Because extraction of diffusible tracers decreases with increasing coronary flow, the uptake of myocardial perfusion tracers is not linear versus flow. Although the uptakes of teboroxime and Tl are closest to measured flow, the low photon energy of Tl and rapid washout of teboroxime are disadvantages. The somewhat lower initial extractions of sestamibi and tetrofosmin are offset by stable myocardial retention of these tracers. In addition to their usefulness in noninvasively assessing coronary flow, retention of the cationic tracers Tl, sestamibi, and tetrofosmin can be used as a marker of myocardial viability. The effect of viability on the retention of neutral tracers, such as teboroxime and Tc NOET, is less clear and warrants further study. Knowledge of the differing properties of these perfusion tracers can aid in the optimal performance and interpretation of myocardial perfusion imaging studies.

ACKNOWLEDGMENTS
We are grateful for the secretarial assistance of Harriet Kay.

REFERENCES
1. Abraham SA, Mirecki FN, Levine D, et al: Myocardial technetium-99m-teboroxime activity in acute coronary artery occlusion and reperfusion: Relation to myocardial blood flow and viability, *J Nucl Med* 36: 1062-1068, 1995.

2. Atkins HL, Budinger TF, Lebowitz E, et al: Thallium-201 for medical use. Part 3: Human distribution and physical imaging properties, *J Nucl Med* 18:133-140, 1977.

3. Bassingthwaighte JB: A concurrent flow model for extraction during transcapillary passage, *Circ Res* 35:483-503, 1974.

4. Bassingthwaighte JB: Physiology and theory of tracer washout techniques for the estimation of myocardial blood flow: flow estimation from tracer washout, *Prog Cardiovasc Dis* 20:165-189, 1977.

5. Bassingthwaighte JB and Goresky CA: *Modeling in the analysis of solute and water exchange in the microvasculature.* In Renkin EM, Michel CC, eds: *Handbook of physiology. sect. 2, the cardiovascular system. vol. IV. The Microcirculation.* Bethesda, Md., American Physiological Society, 1984.

6. Bassingthwaighte JB and Holloway GA, Jr: Estimation of blood flow with radioactive tracers, *Semin Nucl Med* 6:141, 1976.

7. Bassingthwaighte JB, Raymond GM, and Chan JI: *Principles of tracer kinetics.* In Zaret BL and Beller GA eds: *Nuclear Cardiology: State of the Art and Future Directions.* St. Louis, Mosby, 1993.

8. Bassingthwaighte JB, Winkler B, and King RB: Potassium and thallium uptake in dog myocardium, *J Nucl Med* 38:264-274, 1997.

9. Bassingthwaighte JB, Yipintsoi T, and Harvey RB: Microvasculature of the dog left ventricular myocardium, *Microvasc Res* 7:229-249, 1974.

10. Bassingthwaighte JB, Chinard FP, Crone C, et al: Terminology for mass transport and exchange, *Am J Physiol* 250(4 Pt 2): H539-H545, 1986.

11. Bassingthwaighte JB, Krikke JT, Chan IS, et al: A comparison of ascorbate and glucose transport in the heart, *Am J Physiol* 249 (1 Pt 2): H141-H149, 1985.

12. Bean CP: *The physics of porous membranes—neutral pores.* In Eisenman G (ed): *Membranes, vol. I.* New York, Dekker, 1972.

13. Beanlands RSB, Dawood F, Wen WH, et al: Are the kinetics of technetium-99m methoxyisobutyl isonitrile affected by cell metabolism and viability? *Circulation* 82:1802-1814, 1990.

14. Beanlands RSB, DeKemp RA, Harmsen E, et al: Myocardial kinetics of technetium-99m teboroxime in the presence of postischemic injury, necrosis and low flow reperfusion, *J Am Coll Cardiol* 28:487-494, 1996.

15. Beller GA: *Myocardial perfusion imaging with thallium-201.* In Marcus ML, Skorton DS, Schelbert HR, et al, eds: *Cardiac imaging: a companion to* Braunwald's Heart Disease. Philadelphia, W.B. Saunders, 1991.

16. Bergmann SR, Clark RE, and Sobel BE: An improved isolated heart preparation for external assessment of myocardial metabolism, *Am J Physiol* 236:H644-H651, 1979.

17. Berman DS, Kiat H, Van Train K, et al: Technetium 99m sestamibi in the assessment of chronic coronary artery disease, *Semin Nucl Med* 21:190-212, 1991.

18. Bolli R: Mechanism of myocardial "stunning," *Circulation* 82:723-738, 1990.

19. Bolli R: Myocardial "stunning" in man, *Circulation* 86:1671-1691, 1992.

20. Bonow RO and Dilsizian V: Thallium 201 for assessment of myocardial viability, *Semin Nucl Med* 21:230-241, 1991.

21. Bradley-Moore PR, Lebowitz E, Greene MW, et al: Thallium-201 for medical use. II. Biologic behavior, *J Nucl Med* 16:156-160, 1975.

22. Caldwell JH, Martin GV, Link JM, et al: Iodophenylpentadecanoic acid–myocardial blood flow relationship during maximal exercise with coronary occlusion, *J Nucl Med* 30:99-105, 1990.

23. Caldwell JH, Martin GV, Raymond GM, et al: Regional myocardial flow and capillary permeability–surface area products are nearly proportional, *Am J Physiol* 267(2 Pt 2):H654-H666, 1994.

24. Dahlberg ST, Gilmore MP, and Leppo JA: Interaction of technetium 99m-labeled teboroxime with red blood cells reduces the compound's extraction and increases apparent cardiac washout, *J Nucl Cardiol* 1:270-279, 1994.

25. Dahlberg ST, Meerdink DJ, Gilmore MP, et al: Myocardial extraction of technetium-99m-[2-(1-methoxybutyl) isonitrile] in the isolated rabbit heart: a myocardial perfusion agent with high extraction and stable retention, *J Nucl Med* 34:927-931, 1993.

26. Dahlberg ST, Gilmore MP, Flood M, Leppo JL, et al: Extraction of technetium-99m-N-NOET in the isolated rabbit heart. *Circulation* 90:I-368(Abstract), 1994.

27. Dilsizian V and Bonow RO: Current diagnostic techniques of assessing myocardial viability in patients with hibernating and stunned myocardium, *Circulation* 87:1-20, 1993.

28. Gehring PJ and Hammond PB: The uptake of thallium by rabbit erythrocytes, *J Pharmacol Exp Ther* 145:215-221, 1964.

29. Gehring PJ and Hammond PB: The interrelationship between thallium and potassium in animals, *J Pharmacol Exp Ther* 155:187-201, 1967.

30. Gerson MC, Lukes J, Deutsch E, et al: Comparison of technetium-99 m-Q3 and thallium-201 for detection of coronary artery disease in humans, *J Nucl Med* 35:580-586, 1994.

31. Gerson MC, Millard RW, Roszell NJ, et al: Kinetic properties of ^{99m}Tc-Q12 in canine myocardium, *Circulation* 89:1291-1300, 1994.

32. Giganti M, Cittanti C, Colamussi P, et al: Biodistribution in man of bis [(N-ethyl, N-ethoxy) dithiocarbamate] nitrido technetium (V), a promising new tracer for myocardial perfusion imaging, *J Nucl Med* 35:155P(Abstract), 1994.

33. Goldstein RA, Mullani NA, Marani SK, et al: Myocardial perfusion with rubidium-82. II. Effects of metabolic and pharmacologic interventions, *J Nucl Med* 24:907-915, 1983.

34. Gropler RJ and Bergmann SR: Flow and metabolic determinants of myocardial viability by positron-emission tomography, *Coron Art Dis* 4:495-504, 1993.

35. Heller LI, Villegas BJ, Reinhardt CP, et al: Teboroxime is a marker of reperfusion after myocardial infarction, *J Nucl Cardiol* 3:2-8, 1996.

36. Hendel RC and Bonow RO: Disparity in coronary perfusion and regional wall motion: effect on clinical assessment of viability, *Coron Art Dis* 4:512-520, 1993.

37. Higley B, Smith FW, Smith T, et al: Technetium-99m-1,2-bis[bis(2-ethoxyethyl) phosphino]ethane: human biodistribution, dosimetry and safety of a new myocardial perfusion imaging agent, *J Nucl Med* 34:30-38, 1993.

38. Hille B: *Ionic channels of excitable membranes.* Sunderland, Mass, Sinauer Associates, 1984.

39. Holly TA, et al: Effect of ischemic injury on the cardiac transport of Tc-99m-NOET in the isolated rabbit heart, *Circulation* 95:I-789-I-790(Abstract), 1995.

40. Huang SC and Phelps ME: *Principles of tracer kinetic modeling in positron emission tomography and autoradiography.* In Phelps ME, Mazziotta JC, Schelbert HR, eds: *Positron emission tomography and autoradiography.* New York, Raven Press, 1986.

41. Isoyama S, Apstein CS, Wexler LF, et al: Acute decrease in left ventricular diastolic chamber distensibility during simulated angina in isolated hearts, *Circ Res* 61:925-933, 1987.

42. Johnson G III, Allton IL, Nguyen KN, et al: Clearance of technetium 99m N-NOET in normal, ischemic-reperfused, and membrane-disrupted myocardium, *J Nucl Cardiol* 3:42-54, 1996.

43. Johnson G III, Nguyen KN, Pasqualini R, et al: Interaction of technetium-99m-N-NOET with blood elements: potential mechanism of myocardial redistribution, *J Nucl Med* 38:138-143, 1997.

44. Kelly JD, Forster AM, Higley B, et al: Technetium-99m-tetrofosmin as a new radiopharmaceutical for myocardial perfusion imaging, *J Nucl Med* 34:222-227, 1993.

45. Kuijper AFM, van Eck-Smit BL, Bruschke AV, et al: Flow and cellular function: clinical assessment of myocardial viability by single-photon agents, *Coron Art Dis* 4:505-511, 1993.

46. Kuikka J, Levin M, and Bassingthwaighte JB: Multiple tracer dilution estimates of D- and 2-deoxy-D-glucose uptake by the heart, *Am J Physiol* 250(1 Pt 2):H29-H42, 1986.

47. Kuikka JT, Bassingthwaite JB, Henrich MM, et al: Mathematical modeling in nuclear medicine, *Eur J Nucl Med* 18:351-362, 1991.

48. Lassen NA, Perl W: *Tracer kinetic methods in medical physiology.* New York, Raven Press, 1979.

49. Lebowitz E, Greene MW, Fairchild R, et al: Thallium-201 for medical use. I, *J Nucl Med* 16:151-155, 1975.

50. Leppo JA: Overview: clinical assessment of myocardial viability, *Coron Art Dis* 4:481-485, 1993.

51. Leppo JA and Meerdink DJ: Comparison of the myocardial uptake of a technetium-labeled isonitrile analogue and thallium, *Circ Res* 65:632-639, 1989.

52. Leppo JA, and Meerdink DJ: Comparative myocardial extraction of two technetium-labeled BATO derivatives (SQ30217, SQ32014) and thallium, *J Nucl Med* 31:67-74, 1990.

53. Levin M, Kuikka J, and Bassingthwaighte JB: Sensitivity analysis in optimization of time-distributed parameters for a coronary circulation model, *Med Prog Technol* 7:119-124, 1980.

54. Lucas JR, Botvinick EH, and Dae MW: Myocardial viability: evidence provided by the analysis of left ventricular systolic function, *Coron Art Dis* 4:485-494, 1993.

55. Marcus ML, Harrison DG: *Physiologic basic for myocardial perfusion imaging.* In Marcus ML, Skorton DJ, Schelbert HR, et al, eds: *Cardiac imaging: a companion to* Braunwald's heart disease. Philadelphia, W.B. Saunders, 1991.

56. Marshall RC, Leidholdt EM Jr, Zhang DY, et al: Technetium-99m hexakis 2-methoxy-2-isobutyl isonitrile and thallium-201 extraction, washout, and retention at varying coronary flow rates in rabbit heart, *Circulation* 82:998-1007, 1990.

57. Marshall RC, Taylor SE, Powers-Risius P, et al: Kinetic analysis of rubidium and thallium as deposited myocardial blood flow tracers in isolated rabbit heart, *Am J Physiol* 272(3 Pt 2):H1480-H1490, 1997.

58. Maublant JC, Moins N, and Gachon P: Uptake and release of two new Tc-99m labeled myocardial blood flow imaging agents in cultured cardiac cells, *Eur J Nucl Med* 15:180-182, 1989.

59. McCall D: Cation exchange and glycoside binding in cultured rat heart cells, *Am J Physiol* 236:C87-C95, 1979.

60. McCall D, Zimmer LJ, and Katz AM: Kinetics of thallium exchange in cultured rat myocardial cells, *Circ Res* 56:370-376, 1985.

61. Meerdink DJ and Leppo JA: Myocardial transport of hexakis (2-methoxyisobutylisonitrile) and thallium before and after coronary reperfusion, *Circ Res* 66:1738-1746, 1990.

62. Mullins LJ and Moore RD: The movement of thallium ions in muscle, *J Gen Physiol* 43:759-773, 1960.

63. Narra RK, Nunn AD, Kuczynski BL, et al: A neutral technetium-99m complex for myocardial imaging, *J Nucl Med* 30:1830-1837, 1989.

64. Okada RD, Glover DK, Moffett JD, et al: Kinetics of technetium-99m-teboroxime in reperfused nonviable myocardium, *J Nucl Med* 38:274-279, 1997.

65. Pasqualini R, Duatti A, Bellande E, et al: Bis(dithiocarbamato) nitrido technetium-99m radiopharmaceuticals: a class of neutral myocardial imaging agents, *J Nucl Med* 35:334-341, 1994.

66. Pohost GM, Alpert NM, Ingwall JS, et al: Thallium redistribution: mechanisms and clinical utility, *Semin Nucl Med* 10:70-93, 1980.

67. Renkin EM: Transport of potassium-42 from blood to tissue in isolated mammalian skeletal muscles, *Am J Physiol* 197:1205-1210, 1959.

68. Rose CP, Goresky CA, and Bach GG: The capillary and sarcolemmal barriers in the heart. An exploration of labeled water permeability, *Circ Res* 41:515-533, 1977.

69. Rumsey WL, Rosenspire KC, and Nunn AD: Myocardial extraction of teboroxime: effects of teboroxime interaction with blood, *J Nucl Med* 33:94-101, 1992.

70. Stewart RE, Hutchins GD, Brown D, et al: Myocardial retention and clearance of the flow tracer Tc-99m SQ30217 in canine heart, *J Nucl Med* 30:860(Abstract), 1989.

71. Strauss HW, Harrison K, Langan J, et al: Thallium-201 for myocardial imaging. Relation of thallium-201 to regional myocardial perfusion, *Circulation* 51:641-645, 1975.

72. Takahashi N, Dahlberg ST, Gilmore MP, et al: Effects of acute ischemia and reperfusion on the myocardial kinetics of technetium 99m-labeled tetrofosmin and thallium-201, *J Nucl Cardiol* 4:524-531, 1997.

73. Tamaki N: Assessment of myocardial viability by use of multiple clinical parameters and effect on prognosis, *Coron Art Dis* 4:521-528, 1993.

74. Zhang Z, Maublant JC, Ollier M, et al: Cellular uptake of Tc-99m-NOET, a potent myocardial blood flow imaging agent: Comparison with Tl-201, Tc-99m sestamibi and Tc-99m teboroxime, *Circulation* 86:I-708, 1992.

Chapter 4

Role of intact biological models for evaluation of radiotracers

Albert J. Sinusas

The development of radiolabeled tracers for clinical application in humans has been critically dependent on evaluation and testing in biological models. Although in vitro models have been important in the evaluation of radiotracers, this chapter will focus only on the use of intact models. Initial evaluation of a radiotracer generally focuses on assessment of in vivo organ selectivity as determined by biodistribution and pharmacokinetics.[34] Often, radioloabeled compounds are evaluated in various species to assure that behavior of a compound does not demonstrate important species differences. More importantly, radiotracers must be evaluated for specific organ pharmacokinetics in different disease processes.[33]

This chapter will define the role of intact biological models in the evaluation of radiotracers for use in the diagnosis and management of cardiovascular disease. Important species differences will be defined as they relate to cardiovascular disease. The selection of short-term versus long-term animal models will be discussed, with particular attention to the need for conscious or sedated models. Approaches for determination of myocardial radiotracer kinetics will be reviewed, including dynamic imaging (planar imaging or single-photon emission computed tomography [SPECT]), miniature detectors, serial biopsies, and postmortem tissue well counting or autoradiography. Approaches for evaluation of radiotracer biodistribution and myocardial radiotracer uptake and clearance will be reviewed briefly, with emphasis on the effect of cellular viability, flow, metabolic inhibitors, and pharmacologic stress on radiotracer kinetics.

Animal models are often used to validate specific clinical applications of radiolabeled tracers. This chapter will also focus on the use of animal models for evaluation of radiotracers for detection of coronary artery disease, assessment of the extent of myocardial ischemia or infarction, and evaluation of congestive heart failure. For these clinical applications, radiotracers must provide measures or indices of myocardial flow and coronary flow reserve, myocardial metabolism, tissue oxygenation, and regional and global ventricular function. In the future, radiotracers may provide insight into the atherosclerotic process and ischemic injury. To understand the underlying physiology and evaluate potential future clinical applications, specific physiologic states must be modeled (such as ischemia, infarction, stunning, and hibernation).

SELECTION OF ANIMAL MODEL

Use of small mammals for definition of biodistribution

The first step in the evaluation of any radiopharmaceutical involves determination of the normal biodistribution of a radiotracer over time. These initial screening studies are usually performed in mice, rats, or rabbits, to minimize cost. A measured dose is injected intravenously, and the percentage of uptake per gram of tissue is determined for critical organs.[54,59] Uptake in the heart, the target organ, is compared with adjacent background structures at multiple time points after injection. Blood clearance can be easily derived by serial sampling of blood for gamma well counting. Tissue clearance curves can be derived by either sacrificing animals at different time points or by performing serial imaging. Segregation of tissue into cell fractions can provide information on tracer localization in specific cellular fractions.[43] This information may offer insight into the mechanism of uptake and retention. The smaller hearts in these animals lend themselves to microautoradiography.

Use of small mammals for evaluation of specific disease processes

A limited number of biological models are currently available in smaller mammals for evaluation of specific cardiovascular disease processes. The Syrian hamster model is an example of a small model for evaluation of radiotracer kinetics under cardiomyopathic conditions. Other researchers have developed rabbit models of congestive heart failure.[32,76] Investigators created a chronic volume-overloaded condition by mechanically disrupting the aortic valve, instigating aortic insufficiency.[37] It is more difficult to create a small-animal model of regional ischemia or infarction. However, this has been accomplished by placing a ligature or small clamp around a proximal coronary artery. In the rat, this occlusion can be done blindly with a small needle and suture. Unfortunately, this approach necessitates disruption of both venous drainage and arterial inflow. Recently, Reinhardt et al used a rabbit model of regional ischemia.[58] In the rabbit, it is possible to selectively isolate and occlude a proximal coronary artery. Production of graded ischemia in smaller animals is nearly impossible. The use of radiolabeled microspheres for independent assessment of regional myocardial blood flow is more difficult in these preparations. In addition, these preparations do not permit regional arterial–venous balance measurement for the independent assessment of regional metabolism.

We are at the beginning of a new era for radiopharmaceutical testing, with the development of transgenic models for many cardiovascular disease processes. However, the effect of testing radiopharmaceuticals in transgenic models remains undefined.

Use of large mammals for evaluation of specific disease processes

Dogs, pigs, and sheep are the large mammals most commonly used for the evaluation of cardiovascular physiology. These models have been used for many years, and the methodologies of their use are well established. The higher cost of large-animal models almost precludes their use for simple biodistribution studies; rather, they are usually used to evaluate radiotracer kinetics in specific disease processes. In the evaluation of radiotracers, dogs and pigs have been most commonly used. Important interspecies differences in radiotracer uptake have been observed over the years. The most notable example is the uptake of technetium-99m (^{99m}Tc) 1,2-bis(dimethylphosphino)ethane. This ^{99m}Tc-labeled perfusion tracer showed favorable uptake characteristic in rats, dogs, rabbits, and monkeys; however, in phase I trials, no appreciable uptake was noted in the hearts of pig or humans. Although there was transient uptake of this radiotracer by human heart, trapping was not observed because of a reductive mechanism that is prominent in human myocardium.[13]

Canine models have been used for many years in fundamental cardiac physiologic studies. All of the important physiologic conditions (ischemia, infarction, stunning, and even hibernation) have been modeled in dogs, and all of the currently approved radiotracers have been evaluated in canine models. Thus, the characteristics of new tracers can be easily compared with existing data on older tracers. However, it is becoming prohibitively expensive to use dogs in these types of studies.

The dog has a dominant left coronary system. In almost all cases, the left circumflex coronary leads to the posterior descending coronary artery; very rarely does the right coronary artery provide any of the blood supply to the left ventricle. The coronary vascular tree in the dog is also highly collateralized. Therefore, some investigators claim that the dog is the ideal model of chronic coronary artery disease in humans because patients with longstanding critical coronary disease frequently are highly collateralized. In addition, the dog is very tolerant of ischemic injury. In contrast, pigs and sheep have limited native collaterals and tolerate ischemic insults less reliably. When conducting radioisotope experiments in the dog, it may sometimes be necessary to tie off superficial epicardial collaterals to minimize the nearly instantaneous opening of epicardial collateral circuits. Dogs can also be trained to walk on a treadmill, providing an effective model for evaluation of pharmacologic stress agents.

The pig has a coronary circulation that is more similar than that of the dog to human coronary circulation in that both the right and left coronary artery supply the left ventricle with blood. Pig coronary circulation systems have less native coronary collaterals, a characteristic akin to normal coronaries in humans. Therefore, the pig may be a better model of acute coronary occlusion in humans because under conditions of acute occlusion, coronary collaterals may not have yet developed. In recent years, porcine models of ischemia, infarction, stunning, and hibernation have been established. However, sheep may provide the best model for studying chronic infarction and left ventricular remodeling.

In all of these large animal models, acute coronary occlusion may be created surgically[57] or with a balloon angioplasty catheter under fluoroscopic guidance.[6,12] In acute and chronic models, partial occlusions can be created with the aid of a hydraulic occluder or partially occluding ligature. A better way to achieve chronic partial or total occlusion may be placement of an ameroid occluder. An ameroid occluder is a small ring which is surgically placed around a vessel. This device slowly swells over 3 to 4 weeks. A complete or partial coronary occlusion is thus created very gradually, allowing for the development of coronary collaterals.

Large-animal models offer important advantages over studies in smaller animals. First, studies in larger animals allow for more complete instrumentation and regional interventions. Second, the distribution of a radiotracer can be easily evaluated with standard radionuclide imaging equipment. Finally, independent regional measures of flow, function, and metabolism are much easier to obtain in larger animals.

Many physiologic issues can be addressed by using acute animal models. However, to evaluate changes over an extended period of time, chronic models must be used. Chronic models also offer the ability to evaluate radiotracer behavior under conscious conditions. Animals are usually surgically instrumented and allowed to recover for at least 1 week after surgery. After full surgical recovery, an ischemic insult is implemented or stress is applied while the animal is conscious.

Selection of anesthesia

Selection of the method of anesthesia may have a greater effect on radiotracer uptake than many investigators realize. Uptake of perfusion and metabolic tracers can be substantially affected by heart rate, contractile state, systemic pressures, and loading conditions. All of these hemodynamic variables are altered by anesthesia.

The cardiovascular effects of anesthesia in experimental animals have been recently reviewed.[23] These effects vary with different species and with dosages. Opioids tend to decrease preload, contractility, afterload, and heart rate.[23] Benzodiazepines induce taming effects in animals, facilitating imaging of chronically instrumented animals. These drugs may affect the cardiovascular system as a result of their central nervous system effects. Narcotic analgesics tend to have less cardiovascular effects than do general anesthetics. However, these agents require additional use of neuromuscular blocking agents. Inhalant anesthetics tend to decrease contractility, aortic pressure,

and cardiac output and cause a compensatory increase in heart rate. Halothane is the most commonly used inhaled anesthetic for research purposes. Halothane at low end-tidal concentrations (1%) has little effect on the coronary circulation.

METHODS OF MEASUREMENT
Dynamic imaging

Pharmacodynamics can be evaluated noninvasively with serial planar imaging, SPECT, and dynamic positron emission tomography (PET) immediately after injection of a radiotracer. Dynamic imaging sequences allow determination of blood clearance and clearance of a radiotracer from the heart and other critical noncardiac structures. All of these imaging approaches can be easily applied to both open-chest and long-term models.

Planar imaging. Planar imaging offers some advantages for evaluation of radiotracer pharmodynamics, including high temporal and spatial resolution. Planar imaging of the heart is complicated by superimposition of activity in adjacent extracardiac structures. This can be obviated in open-chest models by isolation of the heart from other structures by using a flexible lead sheet.[10] It is critical that the shielding material is placed directly under the heart, thereby completely isolating the beating heart from extracardiac structures. Time–activity curves can be derived for determination of blood and regional myocardial pharmacodynamics. In this type of kinetic analysis, placement of the regions of interest is critical. We have found that moving the myocardial region of interest one pixel toward or away from the blood pool can greatly alter the myocardial clearance curves. To facilitate optimal placement of the myocardial region of interest, we generate a reference image by subtracting an early blood pool image from a later image (Fig. 4-1). An initial left-ventricular blood-pool image can be derived by reconstruction of the left ventricular phase of the first-pass list mode acquisition. A myocardial perfusion image can be derived by summing the last 1 minute of the dynamic image

Bloodpool	Perfusion	Subtraction
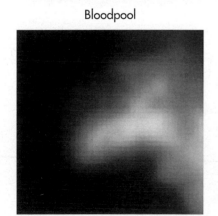	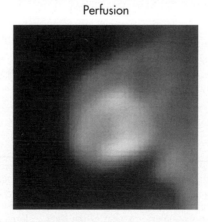	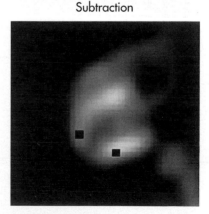

Fig. 4-1. Generation of myocardial uptake and clearance curve from serial planar images. An early blood-pool image (*left*) can be subtracted from the last perfusion image (*middle*) to define the myocardial regions within the image that were relatively devoid of blood-pool contamination. A typical subtraction image is shown (*right*). Regional myocardial uptake and clearance can be derived from regions of interest placed on the subtraction image.

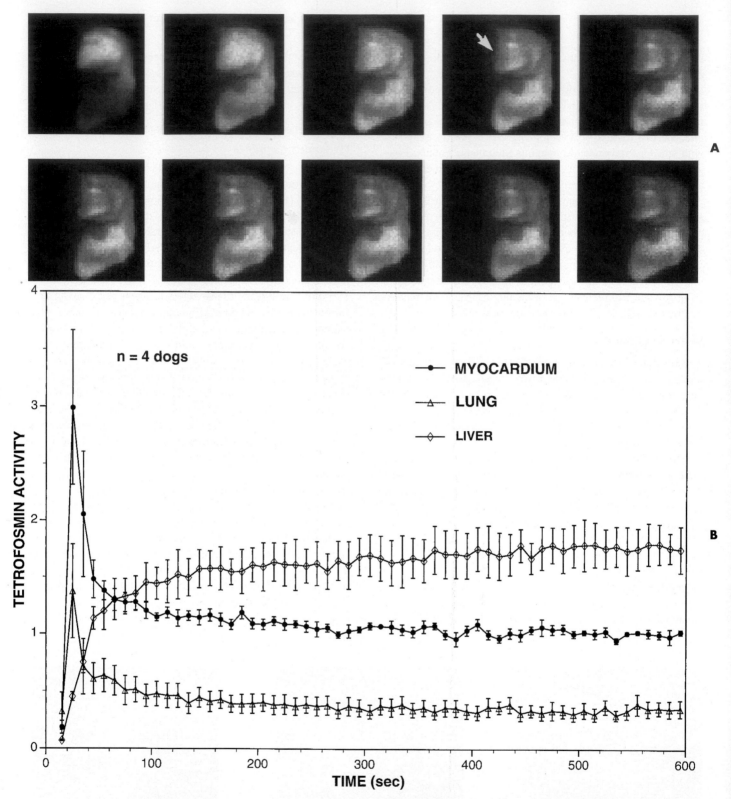

Fig. 4-2. A, Dynamic lateral technetium-99m tetrofosmin image sequence. One-minute images were acquired during the first 10 minutes after injection. The initial image (*upper left*) reflects right ventricular (superior) and left ventricular (inferior) blood-pool activity. The apex of the heart points toward the left lower corner of each image. The liver is seen below the heart. The rib spreader produces an attenuation defect in the superior aspect of the liver. A large dense anteroapical defect is seen (*arrow*). **B,** The tissue clearance curves for technetium-99m tetrofosmin (in 4 dogs) are shown. Activity of ^{99m}Tc tetrofosmin is expressed as a percentage of the nonischemic myocardial activity at the time of sacrifice. The clearance of ^{99m}Tc tetrofosmin in a nonischemic region is shown relative to hepatic and lung clearance. (From Sinusas AJ, Shi QX, Saltzberg MT, et al: *J Nucl Med* 35:664-671, 1994. Reprinted with permission of the Society of Nuclear Medicine.)

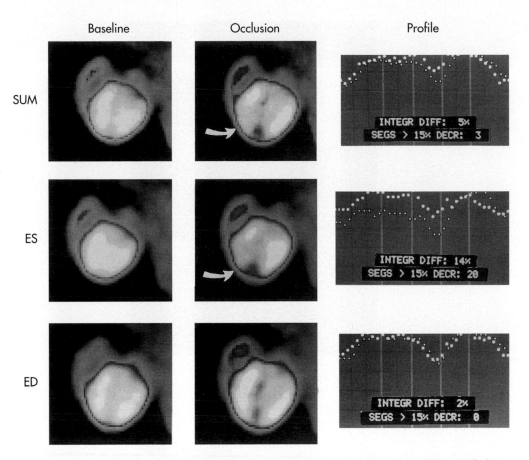

Fig. 4-3. Images showing that regional left ventricular dysfunction creates an artifactual perfusion defect. Technetium-99m sestamibi was injected during baseline conditions before coronary occlusion and reperfusion. Shown are lateral planar images obtained at baseline (*left*) and during coronary artery occlusion (*middle*). A large anteroapical defect (*arrow*) is seen both on summed (*SUM*) and end-systolic (*ES*) images during coronary artery occlusion. This artifact is less evident on the end-diastolic (*ED*) image. The corresponding baseline and occlusion quantitative profiles are superimposed on the right. White dots represent the circumferential profile derived from each baseline image. Black-and-white dots represent the corresponding occlusion profile. Changes in defect scores are also shown. (From Sinusas AJ, Shi QX, Vitols PJ, et al: *Circulation* 88:2224-2234, 1993. Reprinted with permission.)

sequence. The initial blood-pool image is then subtracted from the final perfusion image, providing an index myocardial image that is minimally contaminated by blood pool. The myocardial clearance curves generated by using this planar imaging approach can provide useful information on myocardial uptake and clearance of radiotracer in carefully controlled experimental models of regional ischemia or infarction. This model allows for selective arterial and venous sampling for simultaneous determination of regional metabolism or radiotracer extraction. Figure 4-2 shows a dynamic image series and corresponding clearance curves that can be derived from it.

In 1979, it was recognized that distortion of global and regional left ventricular geometry could cause artifact defects in perfusion images obtained with thallium-201 (^{201}Tl) or intracoronary administration of technetium-99m (^{99m}Tc)–labeled albumin microspheres.[20] More recently, we demonstrated that changes in regional function may confound analysis of planar ^{99m}Tc sestamibi images.[66] Thus, changes in regional myocar-

dial thickening may lead to misinterpretation of myocardial tracer uptake or clearance because of partial volume effects.[66] *Partial volume effects* refers to the underestimation of count density from a structure that is thinner than twice the resolution of the imaging system (usually 12 to 20 mm for a gamma camera). In models of regional ischemia, systolic thinning may occur in ischemic or postischemic stunned regions. Differences in wall thickness would be most prominent at end systole. The potential impact of these partial volume errors are illustrated in Fig. 4-3. We found that analysis of end-diastolic images may compensate somewhat for the partial volume effect associated with regional dyskinesis.

Dynamic planar imaging has been used by several investigators to establish the clearance kinetics of ^{201}Tl,[52] ^{99m}Tc sestamibi,[50] ^{99m}Tc tetrofosmin,[65] and ^{99m}Tc teboroxime.[72] Serial planar imaging permits nontraumatic serial assessment of changes in regional activity. However, dynamic planar imaging is limited by camera resolution, partial volume effects, and po-

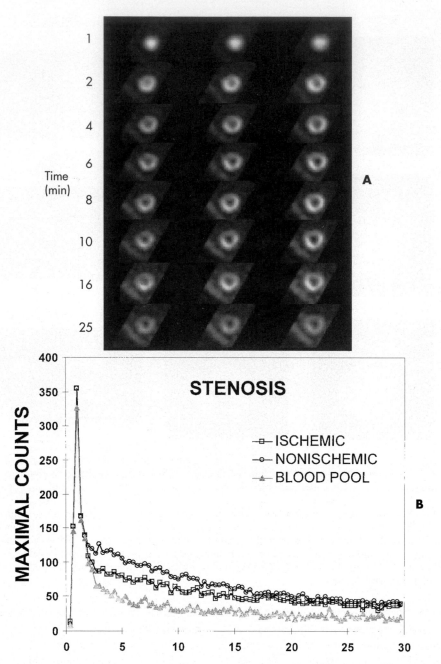

Fig. 4-4. Dynamic single-photon emission computed tomography technetium 99m (^{99m}Tc) teboroxime images were acquired (20 seconds per image) over 30 minutes in an open-chest dog after creation of a partial occlusion of the left anterior descending region. **A,** Short-axis ^{99m}Tc teboroxime images are shown from mid-ventricle over time. A perfusion defect is seen in the anteroapical region. Blood-pool and myocardial clearance curves were generated from this dynamic image set. **B,** Maximum counts from ischemic, nonischemic, and blood pool regions are plotted over time. Differences in regional ^{99m}Tc teboroxime clearance are evident.

tential motion artifacts and may be influenced by background scatter and tissue cross-talk.

Single-photon emission computed tomography. High-quality tomographic images can be acquired to evaluate the biodistribution of a radiotracer. Imaging by SPECT provides better separation of organs than does planar imaging. Dynamic SPECT imaging has only recently become feasible, with the de-velopment of multidetector cameras. Several investigators have used dynamic SPECT imaging for kinetic modeling.[44,69,73] Stewart et al performed dynamic tomographic imaging with ^{99m}Tc teboroxime in closed-chest dogs by using a single-photon ring tomographic system.[73] These investigators demonstrated monoexponential clearance of ^{99m}Tc teboroxime with this approach. By using a triple-detector SPECT system, Smith et al

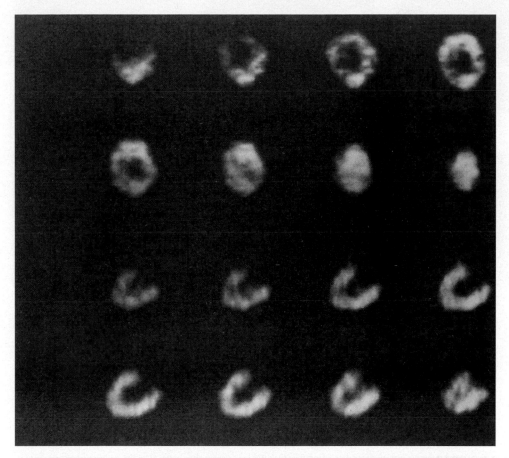

Fig. 4-5. Pinhole technetium-99m sestamibi single-photon emission computed tomography images of a rat heart. Shown are short-axis images (upper two rows) and long-axis images (lower two rows). (From Weber DA, Ivanovic M, Franceschi D, et al: *J Nucl Med* 35:342-348, 1994. Reprinted with permission of the Society of Nuclear Medicine.)

demonstrated the feasibility of acquiring dynamic 10-second tomographic data with a continuous acquisition protocol.[69] Analysis of washin of ^{99m}Tc teboroxime in myocardial tissue measured by using this dynamic SPECT approach in conjunction with compartmental modeling provided an index of regional myocardial blood flow. Smith et al also demonstrated that the use of attenuation correction in conjunction with dynamic SPECT was critical for compartmental analysis of ^{99m}Tc teboroxime. Figure 4-4 provides an example of a series of high-quality images and corresponding clearance curves derived from dynamic SPECT in a dog. The potential advantage of kinetic modeling with SPECT over PET is the greater availability of SPECT equipment and reduced cost. However, the accuracy of the dynamic SPECT approach is not established.

Pinhole SPECT systems have been developed to evaluate regional properties of radiopharmaceuticals in small animals.[28, 82] Unfortunately, the tenfold gains in resolution of these systems are at the expense of a 100-fold loss in sensitivity.[81] This limitation has been overcome by using multidetector SPECT systems.[28] Optimal reconstruction of the pinhole images will probably require more computer-intensive, three-dimensional maximum-likelihood-expectation-maximum algo-rithms.[81] Although these systems cannot compete with the high resolution of microautoradiography, they may provide an alternative to macroautoradiography or well counting. Recently, Hirai et al demonstrated the feasibility of serial SPECT with pinhole collimators for estimation of flow and metabolism in vivo in rat hearts (Fig. 4-5).[26]

Positron emission tomography. Dynamic positron emission tomography (PET) in large animal models plays an important role in evaluation of the kinetics of positron-emitting radiopharmaceuticals. However, this chapter will not review this topic. Technetium-94m, a positron emitter with a 53 minute half-life, can be used to evaluate the biodistribution and pharmacokinetics of Tc radiopharmaceuticals for SPECT.[47,74] Performing PET in animal models with Tc-labeled compounds allows in vivo evaluation of regional myocardial uptake and clearance kinetics. Figure 4-6 provides an example of [94m]Tc sestamibi PET images. Imaging with PET offers great advantages in the evaluation of SPECT tracers: It provides high temporal and spatial resolution and reliable attenuation correction. Labeling of SPECT tracers with [94m]Tc allows the direct comparison of SPECT radiotracers with PET compounds.

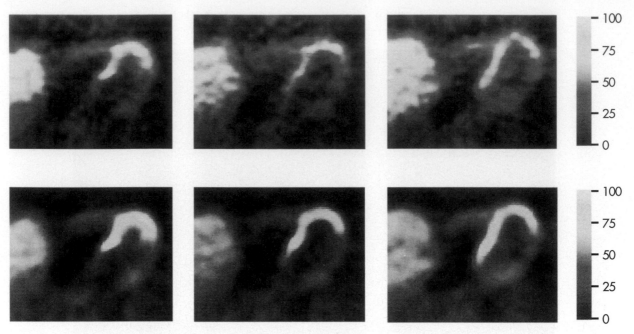

Fig. 4-6. Technetium-94m (^{94m}Tc) sestamibi and nitrogen-13 (^{13}N) ammonia positron emission tomography images in a 66-year-old woman with previous posterolateral wall myocardial infarction. Shown are transaxial ^{94m}Tc sestamibi images (*top row*) and ^{13}N ammonia images (*bottom row*). Greater hepatic uptake is seen on the ^{94m}Tc sestamibi images. (From Stone CK, Christian BT, Nickles RJ, et al: *J Nucl Cardiol* 5:425-433, 1994. Reprinted with permission of the American Society of Nuclear Cardiology.)

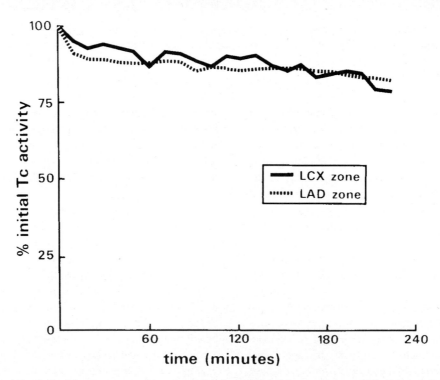

Fig. 4-7. Typical decay-corrected myocardial time–activity clearance curves derived from miniature cadmium telluride probes for an ischemic left circumflex (*LCX*) and control left anterior descending (*LAD*) region in a dog with a critical coronary stenosis. Both probes were positioned on the epicardial surface of the left ventricle. In this example, there was minimal and equal washout from the two regions. (From Okada RD, Glover D, Gaffney T, et al: *Circulation* 77:491-498, 1988. Reprinted with permission.)

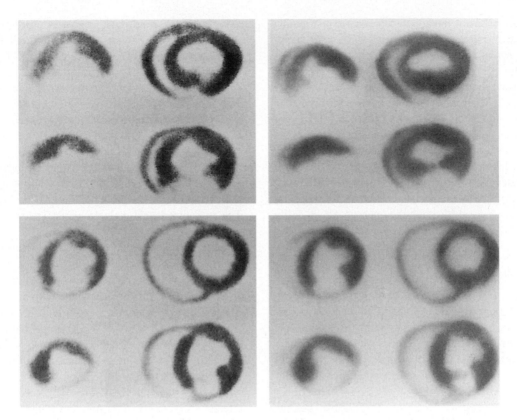

Fig. 4-8. Comparability of technetium-99m sestamibi gamma camera ex vivo slice images (*left*) and macroautoradiographs (*right*). Shown are images from two dogs that underwent 3 hours of left anterior descending coronary artery occlusion followed by 3 hours of reperfusion. Technetium-99m sestamibi was injected during coronary occlusion (*top*) in one dog and after 90 minutes of reperfusion in the second dog (*bottom*). (From Sinusas AJ, Trautman KA, Bergin JD, et al: *Circulation* 82:1424-1437, 1990. Reprinted with permission.)

Miniature detectors

Myocardial radiotracer kinetics can also be derived in large open-chest animal preparations with the use of miniature radiation detectors. In many studies by Okada et al, miniature cadmium telluride radiation detectors were used to evaluate myocardial uptake and clearance of several radiopharmaceuticals, including ^{201}Tl and ^{99m}Tc sestamibi.[49-51] These probes allow continuous monitoring and display of regional myocardial activity.[30] High-quality myocardial clearance curves derived by using a cadmium telluride detector are shown in Fig. 4-7. The use of these probes can be complicated by changes in myocardial thickness and underlying blood pool beneath the probe and the stability of the instrumentation. In some studies, probes have been placed on the myocardium in combination with a device to measure wall thickening. This system allows online correction of changes in counts associated with cyclic wall thickening. More recently, Stewart et al measured myocardial clearance of ^{99m}Tc teboroxime with a 1-inch collimated sodium–iodine (Tl) probe.[72] The first component of ^{99m}Tc teboroxime washout derived by using this probe was related to microsphere blood flow. This miniature probe approach allows continuous monitoring of regional myocardial activity under different isch-emic conditions or during pharmacologic stress.

Despite the potential limitations of these miniature probes, much insight into the in vivo behavior of ^{201}Tl and newer ^{99m}Tc-labeled compounds has been derived from probe studies.

Serial myocardial biopsy

Investigators have obtained serial myocardial biopsy specimens after injection of a radiotracer to evaluate changes in absolute myocardial activity over time.[19,22,36] This approach is the most accurate method to serially determine changes in absolute myocardial counts per gram. However, serial myocardial biopsy results in myocardial injury, necessitates the analysis of very small pieces of tissue, and has a potential sampling error.

Postmortem imaging

Imaging of excised organs or tissues can be very useful to establish the final distribution of a radiotracer that has been injected in vivo under a specific physiologic condition. Some investigators have acquired high-resolution, tomography-like images by placing slices of the heart on the surface of a gamma camera (Fig. 4-8).[67] Images acquired by using this method are similar to those obtained by using macroautoradiography. The gamma camera approach enables the simultaneous acquisition of high-resolution images by using multiple energy windows.

Investigators have used this method to compare the distribution of perfusion and metabolic tracers labeled with different radioisotopes. Effective application of this method necessitates sectioning the heart in slices of uniform thickness, which requires an automated slicing device. Alternatively, a complete 3-dimensional set of short-axis images of the intact heart can be acquired ex vivo with a SPECT camera (Fig. 4-9). This eliminates the need for precision slicing of the heart, and avoids the problems of attenuation and motion. To simulate the in vivo geometry of the heart, hearts are generally stuffed with gauze or frozen in a distended state. All methods of postmortem imaging eliminate partial volume errors associated with cardiac deformation. Images derived by using this method can be easily quantified and be readily compared with postmortem histochemical stains.

Autoradiography

Microautoradiology and macroautoradiography have been critical in the development and evaluation of radiopharmaceuticals.[37,67,83,84] One of the major limitations of this approach is that each animal provides data for only a single experimental time point, possibly two if dual-isotope autoradiographs are acquired. However, these approaches also offer several advantages.

Microautoradiography. Microautoradiography permits high-resolution assessment of the distribution of radioactivity within an organ. This approach allows several isotopes to be compared directly if they can be separated on the basis of differences in half-life. The appropriate use of this technique requires preparation of tissue standards for each isotope in exponentially increasing activity concentrations.[29,84] Tissue standards are necessary to convert autoradiographic intensity into tracer activity. Digitized autoradiographs can be quantitatively analyzed if the appropriate standards are used; the details of this approach have been reported elsewhere.[83] Figure 4-10 provides an example of digitized dual-isotope microautoradiographs and quantitative profiles comparing the myocardial distribution of ^{201}Tl and ^{99m}Tc teboroxime in a rabbit model of acute coronary occlusion.

The resolution of autoradiographs depends on the energy level of the tracers and the thickness of the sections.[77] Hearts are typically cut into sections that are 20 to 50 μm thick. For quantitative analysis, a high-precision cryotome is required and the thickness of the specimen must be uniform. Spatial resolution is improved if the specimen is firmly pressed onto the film. This technique is relatively economical because a gamma well-counter is not required.

Macroautoradiography. Lower-resolution macroautoradiographs can be more easily obtained in larger animal hearts.[67] This approach does not even require a cryotome. Thin slices (2 to 5 mm) can be obtained with an inexpensive meat slicer. These myocardial slices are laid flat on cardboard, are covered in plastic wrap, and inverted on x-ray film. Macroautoradiographs obtained in this manner can provide information on the spatial distribution of a radiotracer under experimental conditions of low-flow ischemia, myocardial stunning, or infarction. As shown in Fig. 4-11, macroautoradio-graphs can be directly compared with postmortem stains to relate radiotracer uptake to myocardial viability

Postmortem tissue well-counting

Postmortem tissue well-counting is the most widely applied approach for assessment of myocardial uptake and clearance of a radiotracer. This technique is applied in larger animal models in which specific physiologic states can be modeled. In general, the radiotracer under evaluation is injected during a specific

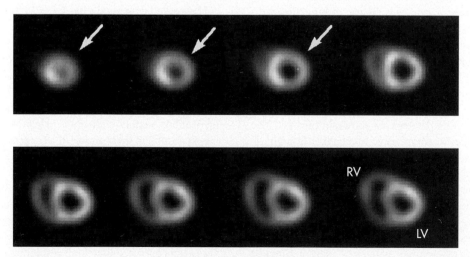

Fig. 4-9. Postmortem ex vivo technetium-99m sestamibi single-photon emission computed tomography images oriented in standard short-axis format. Technetium-99m sestamibi was injected during inotropic stress in the presence of a partial stenosis of the left anterior descending coronary artery. Short-axis images (5 mm thick) are shown from apex to base. The right ventricle (*RV*) is seen on left and left ventricle (*LV*) on right of each image. A mild perfusion defect is seen in the anteroapical region (*arrows*).

physiologic condition; the activity retained in the myocardium is determined by doing gamma well counting of the excised tissue. If hearts are excised within minutes of injection, the initial myocardial distribution of a radiotracer can be determined. Hearts excised hours after injection provide information about the relative late retention of a radiotracer.

The initial uptake of a tracer is dependent on flow or delivery of the radiotracer to the tissue and the extraction of the tracer by the tissue. Retention of a tracer may be influenced by perturbations in regional metabolism, cellular viability, or flow. Frequently, the distribution of a radiotracer under evaluation is compared with independent measures of regional myocardial blood flow determined using the radiolabeled microsphere technique.

Tissue is counted in a gamma well-counter, which has excellent energy discrimination and permits simultaneous evaluation of as many as six radiotracers if each one has gamma emissions at distinguishable energy ranges. Activity spillover from the energy window of one radiotracer to another can be corrected for with a matrix derived from counting pure specimens of each radiotracer. This approach has been described in detail by Heymann et al[24] and has been applied by many other investigators.[42] Identification of ^{201}Tl redistribution was accomplished using this approach (Fig. 4-12).[55]

Gamma well-counting in postmortem tissue has obvious advantages and disadvantages. A major disadvantage is that the myocardial distribution of a radiotracer can only be determined

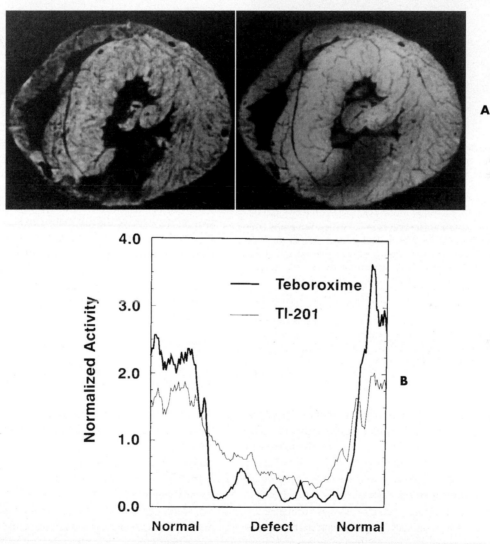

Fig. 4-10. **A,** Dual-isotope microautoradiographs showing technetium-99m (^{99m}Tc) teboroxime *(left)* and thallium-201 (^{201}Tl) *(right)*. Myocardial activity distributions in the same rabbit heart during coronary artery occlusion. Microautoradiographs were obtained from 30 μm thick short-axis slices. Note the increased contrast and clearer delineation of normal and low-flow zones produced by ^{99m}Tc teboroxime compared with ^{201}Tl simultaneously injected. **B,** A representative pair of dual-isotope ^{99m}Tc teboroxime and ^{201}Tl profiles across the defect. Normal-to-defect contrast was increased and normal-to-defect transition was sharper for ^{99m}Tc teboroxime compared with ^{201}Tl. (From Weinstein H, Reinhardt CP, Wironen JF, et al: *J Nucl Med* 34:1510-1517, 1993. Reprinted with permission of the Society of Nuclear Medicine.)

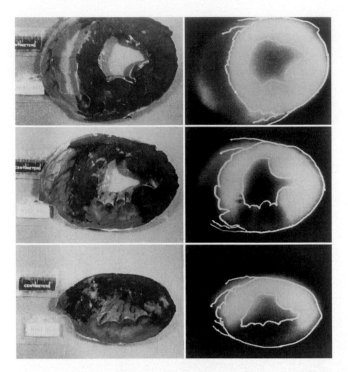

Fig. 4-11. Postmortem dual-perfusion maps (*left*) and technetium-99m (^{99m}Tc) sestamibi macroautoradiographs (*right*) from a dog undergoing 3 hours of left anterior descending coronary artery occlusion followed by 3 hours of reperfusion. Technetium-99m sestamibi was injected 90 minutes into the reperfusion period. Shown are three slices oriented with the right ventricle on the left and the anterior wall on the bottom. The risk area is stained brick-red with triphenyltetrazolium chloride (TTC). The infarct area is the pale unstained region within the risk area. Defects seen on the unenhanced macroautoradiographs with superimposed overlay (*right*) correlate closely with the area of infarction defined by TTC staining. No significant ^{99m}Tc sestamibi activity is seen in the central necrotic region, whereas some activity is seen in the perinecrotic area. This approach allows for direct comparison of macroautoradiographs with postmortem stains to evaluate radiotracer uptake to myocardial viability. (From Sinusas AJ, Trautman KA, Bergin JD, et al: *Circulation* 82:1424-1437, 1990. Reprinted with permission.)

at discrete time points. In addition, a given animal can be examined only once. Finally, the resolution of this approach is dependent on how finely the heart is sectioned, usually in 0.3-gm samples. On the other hand, this approach is very reproducible and avoids interference of background activity. To facilitate comparisons of results between animals, myocardial radiotracer activity is usually normalized. One way to normalize activity is to express activity in each segment as a percentage of a predefined normal region.[68] This method enables evaluation of the myocardial activity within an ischemic or infarcted region relative to a normal region in a manner analogous to the interpretation of clinical images. Alternatively, regional myocardial activity can be normalized by the computed average activity for each heart, as proposed by Yipintsoi et al.[86] A less desirable approach normalizes activity in each myocardial segment according to the segment with the highest activity.[18]

Evaluation of tracer kinetics and kinetic modeling

Regional myocardial uptake of a diffusible tracer is dependent on flow and myocardial extraction. The simplest approach to kinetic modeling assumes a monoexponential clearance. Under these conditions, dynamic image data are fitted to a monoexponential equation, $(A = A_0 e^{-kt})$, where A_0 represents initial activity, K the decay constant, in the elapsed time. Myocardial clearance half-time can be derived from the slope of the linear regression of the natural logarithmic transformation of the raw counts over time ($t_{1/2} = \ln 2/k$). To further simplify the analysis, the initial data from 0 to 2 minutes after injection may be excluded to avoid potential blood-pool contamination. More sophisticated compartmental modeling is often required. The dynamic data can be derived from both planar imaging and SPECT; this topic is covered in detail in other sections of the book.

PHYSIOLOGIC MODELS

To define the behavior of a new radiopharmaceutical under different clinical cardiovascular conditions, the myocardial kinetics of a radiotracer are evaluated in animal models. Clinical applicability can be evaluated by testing a radiotracer under specific physiologic states. Important ischemic conditions include acute and chronic low-flow ischemia (hibernation), postischemic dysfunction (stunning), and transmural or nontransmural myocardial infarction. A major goal of radionuclide imaging in the evaluation of patients with ischemic heart disease is noninvasive discrimination of stunned, hibernating, and infarcted myocardium. Important nonischemic conditions include myocardial hypertrophy and dilated cardiomyopathy.

The most frequently used short-term and long-term physiologic models are reviewed below. Most of these models are experimental, although some models of cardiovascular disease occur naturally.

Myocardial infarction

It has been well established in canine models of coronary occlusion that myocardial necrosis progresses from the subendocardium to the subepicardium in a wavefront manner.[56,57] Advancing myocardial necrosis can be halted by coronary reperfusion. In canine models, permanent cellular injury begins after approximately 40 minutes of occlusion. The extent of necrosis depends on the area at risk and the duration of occlusion. In dogs, the maximum degree of infarction occurs after about 6 hours of occlusion. However, the extent of infarction may be affected by heart rate and left ventricular loading conditions. Thus, in anesthetized models, the method of anesthesia may affect infarct size. Myocardial flow following reperfusion varies and is critically dependent on timing after reperfusion because a period of hyperemic flow is often seen following release of an occlusion.

Connelly et al reported that complete coronary occlusion in the rabbit produced an expanding necrotic wavefront from the subendocardium.[11] This effect is similar to the phenomenon first described by Reimer and Jennings in the canine model of

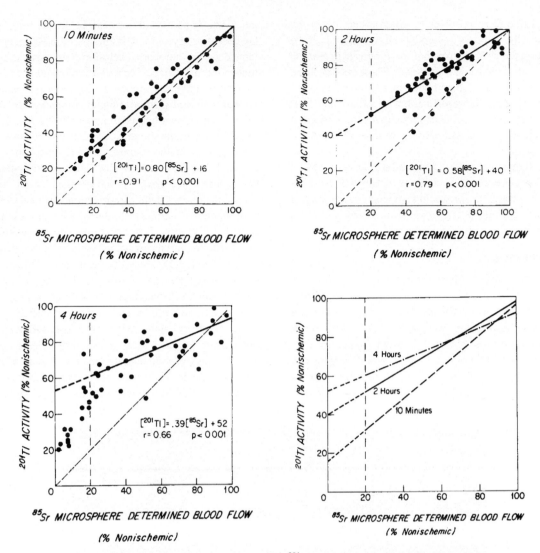

Fig. 4-12. Relationship of myocardial thallium-201 (^{201}Tl) activity and radiolabeled microsphere regional myocardial blood flow as determined by gamma well-counting. Thallium-201 was injected in the presence of a fixed coronary stenosis. The myocardial distribution of ^{201}Tl was compared with the strontium-85 microsphere–determined blood flow at the time of radiotracer injection in animals sacrificed at 10 minutes (*upper left*), 2 hours (*upper right*), and 4 hours (*lower left*) after radiotracer injection. The left ventricle was cut into 1-gm to 3-gm pieces for gamma well-counting. Regional myocardial ^{201}Tl activity and flow were expressed as a percentage of nonischemic region. The solid line represents the line of regression; the dashed line represents the line of identity. Linear regression analysis was performed only on the 20% to 100% flow range. The graph in the lower right shows the superimposed regression lines for each subset of animals. The regression lines become progressively lower between 10 minutes, 2 hours, and 4 hours, with a ^{201}Tl excess relative to the ischemic flow region. This is consistent with a relative increase in ^{201}Tl in the ischemic region relative to the nonischemic region and represents ^{201}Tl redistribution. (From Pohost GM, Okada RD, O'Keefe DD, et al: *Circ Res* 48:439-446, 1981. Reprinted with modification and permission.)

occlusion.[56] In the rabbit, mild subendocardial necrosis can be detected by nitroblue tetrazolium staining as early as 15 minutes after occlusion; 1 hour of coronary occlusion consistently produces completed transmural infarction.

Coronary occlusion can be produced by various noninvasive and invasive methods.[23] Noninvasive closed-chest approaches include sustained coronary occlusion with angioplasty catheters[6,12]; selective coronary embolization[75]; and deployment of intracoronary copper coils,[31] which promote thrombosis. Some

of these approaches permit subsequent reperfusion. More invasive surgical approaches involve acute occlusion with a surgical ligature[56,57] or more gradual occlusion after implantation of an ameroid occluder.[60]

Experimental models of coronary occlusion and reperfusion are frequently used to assess the behavior of radiolabeled perfusion tracers under conditions of reduced flow and in the presence of myocardial necrosis. The myocardial uptake and retention of a perfusion tracer is critically dependent on the timing of injection relative to reperfusion.[3,22] Appropriate use of experimental occlusion–reperfusion models allows analysis of the uptake and clearance characteristics of a radiotracer in relation to cellular viability independent of flow.[67] These models have also been used to evaluate sympathetic innervation of the heart after coronary occlusion and reperfusion with iodine-123 (^{123}I) metaiodobenzyl-guanidine[12] or to examine myocardial metabolism with radiolabeled tracers of aerobic or anaerobic metabolism.[6,7,41,48]

A model of chronic congestive heart failure can be produced by repeated coronary embolization[75,87] or by surgery.[1] Animals with extensive infarction producing extensive myocardial necrosis can be created by repetitive transmyocardial direct current shocks.[40]

Myocardial stunning

Myocardial stunning is characterized by a condition of postischemic mechanical dysfunction that persists after reperfusion despite the absence of irreversible injury. In the dog, a coronary occlusion lasting less than 20 minutes does not result in any myocardial necrosis; however, it produces regional dysfunction that may persist for hours.[5,25] Myocardial stunning can also be produced by repeated brief (5- or 10-minute) coronary occlusions.[46] In other species with less coronary collaterals,

much briefer periods of coronary occlusion result in myocellular necrosis. Myocardial stunning can also occur after a prolonged partial coronary occlusion,[39] in association with nontransmural infarction,[35] or with exercise-induced ischemia.[27]

We recently developed a long-term canine model of ameroid-induced gradual subtotal coronary occlusion resulting in regional myocardial dysfunction (Fig. 4-13). Although resting flow was normal in these animals on PET imaging with nitrogen-13 ammonia coronary flow reserve was markedly impaired in response to adenosine. This model matches the clinical scenario reported by Vanoverschelde et al, in which reversible left ventricular dysfunction was identified in patients with viable collateralized occluded coronary arteries with preserved resting flow.[79] In our canine model, dysfunctional regions with impaired coronary flow reserve also demonstrate increased fluorine-18 deoxyglucose uptake, similar to the clinical condition reported by Camici et al.[9] This supports the contention that the chronic regional dysfunction may be caused by repetitive stress–induced ischemia in the setting of normal resting flows and impaired flow reserve. This chronic model should prove useful in the evaluation of radiolabeled fatty acids, such as ^{123}I-B-methyl-iodophenyl-pentadecanoic acid, which are reportedly "memory" markers of reversible ischemic injury.[48]

All radiopharmaceuticals directed at evaluating myocardial

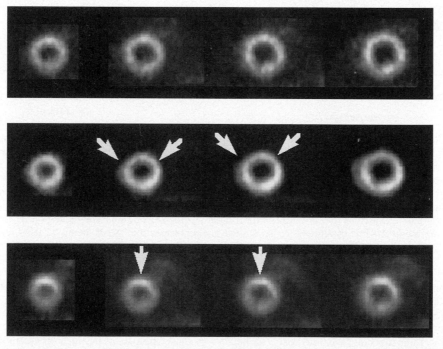

Fig. 4-13. Long-term canine model of ischemic dysfunction. Positron emission tomography (PET), perfusion, and metabolic imaging was performed in dogs 5 weeks after implantation of an ameroid occluder. Images from PET with nitrogen-13 ammonia (*top row*) demonstrate normal resting flow. Nitrogen-13 ammonia images during adenosine stress (*middle row*) demonstrate reduced flow in the anterior wall (*between arrows*). Increased accumulation of fluorine-18 deoxyglucose (*arrow*) is seen in the area of impaired flow reserve (*bottom row*). A coronary angiogram at 4 weeks showed 90% stenosis of the left anterior descending coronary artery at the site of the ameroid occluder. Magnetic resonance imaging and serial echocardiography showed profound regional dysfunction; however, postmortem examination revealed no significant necrosis in this region. This animal model seems to be analogous to the condition observed clinically in patients with collateralized viable myocardium subtended by a subtotal occlusion. Regional dysfunction can be attributed to repeated myocardial stunning.

metabolism should be evaluated in one of these pure experimental models of myocardial stunning. These models allow evaluation of a radiotracer under conditions of predominantly altered metabolism. As in infarct models of occlusion-reperfusion, the timing of radiotracer injection during conditions of postreperfusion stunning is critical because of a transient period of hyperemic flow. The reperfusion hyperemia observed following a brief period (<15 minutes) of ischemia tends to be more intense but shorter in duration.

Myocardial hibernation

The term *myocardial hibernation* has generally been applied to patients with coronary artery disease who have chronically depressed left ventricular function in the absence of myocardial infarction that improves after coronary revascularization. It is unclear whether chronic left ventricular dysfunction in humans represents an adaptive response to chronic reduction in coronary blood flow.[78] Impairment of left ventricular function under these conditions has been regarded as a protective mechanism by which the heart downregulates its energy requirements, thereby preventing irreversible myocardial injury.

This condition of chronic low-flow perfusion-contraction matching has been difficult to model experimentally. Short-term canine and porcine studies have successfully demonstrated sustained (1- to 5-hour) matching of reduced flow and function.[2,16,39] However, chronic models have been much more difficult to establish. Recently, investigators succeeded in producing regional dysfunction over extended periods in pigs and dogs.[15,17,62] In each of these studies, the severity of regional dysfunction was out of proportion to the reduction in regional myocardial blood flow. In a clinical study, Vanoverschelde et al suggested that chronic regional myocardial dysfunction in the presence of relatively preserved resting coronary flow may be attributed to repetitive stunning associated with intermittent stress–induced ischemia.[79] The presence of ^{201}Tl rest redistribution in patients with reversible left ventricular dysfunction supports the idea that true myocardial hibernation with chronic resting reduction in flow can and does occur.[4] Whereas a resting defect may be attributed to partial volume errors, the presence of ^{201}Tl redistribution suggests differential myocardial clearance that is most likely secondary to reduced resting myocardial flow. Animal models of chronic hibernation are needed to establish the pathophysiology of reversible ischemic dysfunction in the presence of coronary artery disease. The application and evaluation of new metabolic radiotracers in these models will be critical for advancing our understanding of this important clinical condition. These low-flow models also will be invaluable in assessing new radiolabeled perfusion tracers.

We developed a short-term canine model of sustained low-flow ischemia (Fig. 4-14).[14,63,68] A hydraulic occluder is placed around a proximal coronary artery, allowing for the creation of a variable stenosis. The distal coronary artery is cannulated with a non–flow-obstructing catheter, which permits accurate regulation of the stenosis severity on the basis of measurement of distal coronary artery pressure and transstenotic pressure gradient. The degree of ischemic dysfunction can be assessed by measuring regional myocardial thickening with epicardial Doppler thickening probes.

Changes in regional metabolism can also be assessed in this model by selective venous sampling for arterial–venous balance measurements. Additional application of atrial pacing or intravenous administration of inotropic agents can provide a model of stress–induced ischemia as it may occur in patients with critical coronary artery disease.[63] Many investigators have used this type of low-flow model to evaluate radiolabeled tracers of perfusion, myocardial metabolism, and tissue hypoxia.[21,55,63,68] Using this experimental model of sustained low flow, the perfusion tracer ^{99m}Tc NOET (bis[N-ethoxy, N-ethyl dithiocarbamato] nitrido) demonstrates susbstantial redistribution,[21] as was previously observed for ^{201}Tl[55] and ^{99m}Tc sestamibi.[64]

Dilated cardiomyopathy

Many canine species are known to have idiopathic dilated cardiomyopathies.[23] This is seen almost exclusively in the larger breeds of dogs, and is characterized by biventricular cardiac dilatation. Dilated cardiomyopathies have also been seen in domestic cats and there is a cardiomyopathic strain of Syrian hamsters.

Several investigators have developed experimental models of congestive heart failure associated with ventricular dilation. Chronic rapid atrial or right ventricular pacing in the dog or pig produces dilated cardiomyopathy.[53,70,71] Chronic mitral insufficiency also results in dilated cardiomyopathy. This can be accomplished surgically or noninvasively by cutting chordae tendineae of the mitral valve with a urologic forceps.[42,88] Other investigators have created a volume-overloaded state by creating aortic insufficiency.

Magid et al developed a rabbit model of chronic aortic insufficiency.[38] The regurgitant fraction and resulting left ventricular dilatation and hypertrophy produced by this rabbit model are similar to those reported in severe aortic insufficiency in human beings. Lu et al used this model to evaluate the value of indium-111 (^{111}In)–labeled antimyosin antibody Fab fragment imaging for identification of myocyte necrosis associated with chronic aortic insufficiency.[37] These types of experimental studies help to generate hypotheses about the potential role of radionuclide imaging in the evaluation and management of patients with acute or chronic aortic insufficiency.

Atherosclerosis

Animal models of atherosclerosis generally involve use of a high-fat diet in combination with endothelial injury. Vascular injury can be produced by direct physical injury, chemical injury, or immunologic injury. Some animals develop atherosclerosis as a naturally occurring disease: The Watanabe heritable hyperlipidemic rabbit, for example, provides a natural model for homozygous familial hypercholesterolemia.[80] The most commonly used animal model of atherosclerosis is the high-cholesterol-diet–fed rabbit.[23] The pig is also commonly used as a model of atherosclerosis. To reduce the problems associated with use of this large species, miniaturized breeds of swine have been developed. Nonhuman primates are considered to provide a model of

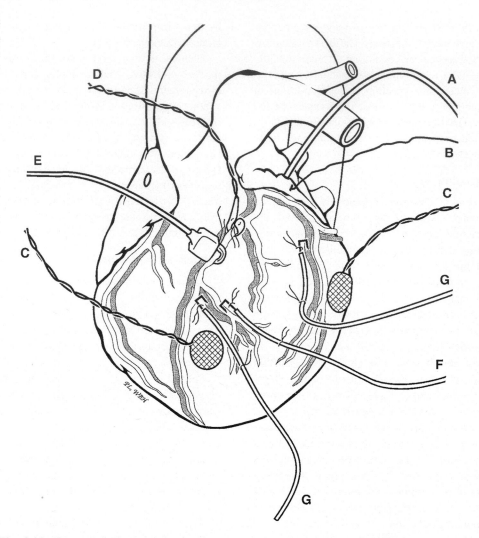

Fig. 4-14. Heart surgical preparation and instrumentation of a model of partial coronary occlusion and pacing-induced demand ischemia. **A,** Left atrial catheter; **B,** atrial pacing wire; **C,** Doppler thickening crystals; **D,** Doppler flow probes; **E,** hydraulic occluder; **F,** distal coronary artery catheter; and **G,** coronary venous catheters. (From Shi CQX, Sinusas AJ, Dione DP, et al: *J Nucl Med* 36:1078-1086, 1995. Reprinted with permission of the Society of Nuclear Medicine.)

atherosclerosis that is most similar to the atherosclerosis seen in humans. Limitations of the nonhuman primate include expense and the rapid development of atherosclerotic lesions.

Naturally or artificially created animal models of atherosclerosis have been used to study aspects of coronary restenosis with radiolabeled monoclonal antibodies.[45] Narula and associates suggested that ^{111}In-Z2D3 antibody imaging could be used for noninvasive assessment of the rate of smooth-muscle cell proliferation after coronary angioplasty.[45]

Short-term versus long-term models

Short-term and long-term models have important practical and physiologic differences, some of which are outlined above. Whereas long-term models are much more expensive and labor-intensive to maintain, they offer the important advantage of evaluating a physiologic state at multiple time points with multiple radiotracers. Long-term models also offer the option of

evaluating a radiotracer under conscious, unsedated conditions, which may be particularly important in the evaluation of metabolic tracers or pharmacologic stressors. Radiotracer kinetics even can be evaluated during treadmill exercise in permanently instrumented animals. To facilitate the injection of diffusible radiotracers and radiolabeled microspheres in conscious animals during different physiologic conditions, indwelling vascular access devices can be implanted. These devices are implanted under the skin between the scapula; the end of the device can be tunneled subcutaneously for insertion in the left atrium through a small thoracotomy. They can also be implanted in the neck for direct and repeated access to the carotid artery.

Evaluation of pharmacologic stressors

Radiotracers are often used in conjunction with pharmacologic stressors, particularly for the detection of coronary artery disease. Recent evidence suggests that radiotracer pharmacokinetics may be influenced by the type of pharmacologic stress applied.[8,61,85] Therefore, biological models have an important role in evaluation of pharmacologic stressors.

The effects of pharmacologic stress on radiotracer kinetics can be initially evaluated in short-term anesthetized models. However, the effects of inotropic agents, such as dobutamine and arbutamine, on global hemodynamics, regional myocardial flow, and function may be greatly influenced by the type of anesthesia. For example, the anesthetized dog is more sensitive to inotropic stimulation; in contrast, it requires much higher doses of adenosine to elicit the same effect on coronary flow. These differences must be taken into consideration when designing experimental protocol involving a pharmacologic stressor. Ultimately, pharmacologic stressors must be evaluated in long-term conscious experimental models to define their true effects on radiotracer kinetics.

CONCLUSIONS

Intact biological models play a critical role in the evaluation of radiotracers for application in the diagnosis and management of cardiovascular disease. The toxicity, biodistribution, and dosimetry of a radiotracer can be determined effectively with small animal models. Larger animal models permit evaluation of myocardial radiotracer kinetics under control and ischemic conditions. This kinetic analysis can be accomplished by using dynamic imaging (planar or SPECT), miniature detectors, serial biopy, postmortem tissue well-counting, or autoradiography.

Animal models are often used to validate specific clinical application of radiolabeled tracers. To understand the underlying physiology and evaluate these potential clinical applications, specific physiologic states must be modeled. I described short-term and long-term models of ischemia, infarction, stunning, hibernation, and congestive heart failure. The development of more advanced instrumentation and image reconstruction may permit kinetic analysis of new radiotracers in smaller animals. These advances may allow for application of transgenic models in our evaluations of radiotracers in specific diseases.

In the future, study of radiotracers by using intact animal models may provide fundamental insight into our understanding of the pathophysiology of the cardiovascular system. We may be better able to define such processes as atherosclerosis or ischemic injury. Radiotracer studies will certainly provide insight into membrane transport and receptor binding and regulation in the heart and vasculature. Study of intact biological models will be necessary for optimal development of diagnostic approaches that use radioisotopes. These diagnostic approaches can ultimately be used to assess the efficacy of new pharmacologic or mechanical therapies. Through application of radiotracers in physiologic models, we will learn more about metabolic regulation of the cardiovascular system and the interrelation of cardiovascular structure and function.

REFERENCES

1. Anversa P, Loud AV, Levicky V, et al: Left ventricular failure induced by myocardial infarction. I. Myocyte hypertrophy, *Am J Physiol* 248 (6 Pt 2):H876–H882, 1985.

2. Arai AE, Pantely GA, Anselone CG, et al: Active downregulation of myocardial energy requirements during moderate ischemia in swine, *Circ Res* 69:1458–1469, 1991.

3. Beller GA, Glover DK, Edwards NC, et al: ^{99m}Tc-sestamibi uptake and retention during myocardial ischemia and reperfusion, *Circulation* 87:2033–2042, 1993.

4. Berger BC, Watson DD, Burwell LR, et al: Redistribution of thallium at rest in patients with stable and unstable angina and the effect of coronary artery bypass surgery, *Circulation* 60:1114–1125, 1979.

5. Bolli R, Zhu WX, Thornby JI, et al: Time course and determinants of recovery of function after reversible ischemia in conscious dogs, *Am J Physiol* 254(1 Pt 2):H102–H114, 1988.

6. Buxton DB and Schelbert HR: Measurement of regional glucose metabolic rates in reperfused myocardium, *Am J Physiol* 261(6 Pt 2):H2058–H2068, 1991.

7. Buxton DB, Mody FV, Krivokapich J, et al: Quantitative assessment of prolonged metabolic abnormalities in reperfused canine myocardium, *Circulation* 85:1842–1856, 1992.

8. Calnon DA, Glover DK, Beller GA, et al: Effects of of dobutamine stress on myocardial blood flow, Tc99m-sestamibi uptake, and systolic wall thickening in the presence of coronary artery stenosis: Implications for dobutamine stress testing, *Circulation* 96:2353-2360, 1997.

9. Camici P, Araujo LI, Spinks T, et al: Increased uptake of ^{18}F-fluorodeoxyglucose in postischemic myocardium of patients with exercise-induced angina, *Circulation* 74:81–88, 1986.

10. Chang PI, Shi Q-X, Saltzberg MT, et al: Myocardial distribution and clearance of Tc99m-teboroxime during reperfusion after acute myocardial infarction, *Circulation* 86:I-707, 1992.

11. Connelly CM, Vogel WH, Hernandez YM, et al: Movement of necrotic wavefront after coronary occlusion in rabbit, *Am J Physiol* 243:H682–690, 1982.

12. Dae MW, O'Connell JW, Botvinick EH, et al: Acute and chronic effects of transient myocardial ischemia on sympathetic nerve activity, density, and norepinephrine content, *Cardiovasc Res* 30:270–280, 1995.

13. Deutsch E, Ketring AR, Libson K, et al: The Noah's Ark experiment: species dependent biodistributions of cationic ^{99m}Tc complexes, *Int J Nucl Med Biol*16:191–232, 1989.

14. Edwards NC, Sinusas AJ, Bergin JD, et al: Influence of subendocardial ischemia on transmural myocardial function, *Am J Physiol* 262 (2 Pt 2):H568–H576, 1992.

15. Fallavollita JA, Perry BJ, and Canty JM Jr: Transmural variation in ^{18}F-2-deoxyglucose (FDG) deposition in pigs with collateral-dependent myocardium and chronic hibernation, *Circulation* 92(suppl): I-386, 1995.

16. Fedele FA, Gewirtz H, Capone RJ, et al: Metabolic response to prolonged reduction of myocardial blood flow distal to a severe coronary artery stenosis, *Circulation* 78:729–735, 1988.

17. Gerber B, Laycock SK, Melin JA, et al: Perfusion-contraction matching, inotropic reserve and vasodilatory capacity in a canine model of dysfunctional collateral-dependent myocardium, *Circulation* 92(suppl): I-314, 1995.

18. Meleca MJ, McGoron AJ, Gerson MC, et al: Flow versus uptake comparisons of ^{201}Thallium with six ^{99m}technetium perfusion tracers in a canine model of myocardial ischemia, *J Nucl Med* 38:1847–1856, 1997.

19. Gerson MC, Millard RW, Roszell NJ, et al: Kinetic properties of ^{99m}Tc-Q12 in canine myocardium, *Circulation* 89:1291–1300, 1994.

20. Gewirtz H, Grote GJ, Strauss HW, et al: The influence of left ventricular volume and wall motion on myocardial images, *Circulation* 59:1172–1177, 1979.

21. Ghezzi C, Fagret D, Brichon P-Y, et al: Redistribution of bis (N-ethoxy, N-ethyl dithiocarbamato) nitrido technetium-99m-(V), a new myocardial perfusion imaging agent: Comparison with ^{201}thallium redistribution, *Circulation* 94:I-302, 1996.

22. Granato JE, Watson DD, Flanagan TL, et al: Myocardial thallium-201 kinetics during coronary occlusion and reperfusion: influence of

method of reflow and timing of thallium-201 administration, *Circulation* 73:150–160, 1986.

23. Gross DR: *Animal models in cardiovascular research.* In ed 2, Dordrecht, The Netherlands: Kluwer Academic Publishers, 1994.

24. Heymann MA, Payne BD, Hoffman JIE, et al: Blood flow measurements with radionuclide-labeled particles, *Prog Cardiovasc Dis* 20:55–79, 1977.

25. Heyndrickx GR, Millard RW, McRitchie RJ, et al: Regional myocardial functional and electrophysiological alterations after brief coronary artery occlusion in conscious dogs, *J Clin Invest* 56:978–985, 1975.

26. Hirai T, Nohara R, Hosokawa R, et al: Evaluation of flow and metabolism in rat heart using "pinhole" SPECT system, *J Nucl Cardiol* 4:S113(Abstract), 1997.

27. Homans DC, Sublett E, Dai XZ, et al: Persistence of regional left ventricular dysfunction after exercise-induced myocardial ischemia. *J Clin Invest* 77:66–73, 1986.

28. Ishizu K, Mukai T, Yonekura Y, et al: Ultra-high resolution SPECT system using four pinhole collimators for small animal studies, *J Nucl Med* 36:2282–2287, 1995.

29. Ito T and Brill AB: Validity of tissue paste standards for quantitative whole-body autoradiography using short-lived radionuclides, *Int J Rad Appl Instrum [A]* 41:661–667,1990.

30. Jacobs ML, Okada RD, Daggett WM, et al: Regional myocardial radiotracer kinetics in dogs using miniature radiation detectors, *Am J Physiol* 242:H849–H854, 1982.

31. Kordenat RK, Kezdi P, and Stanley EL: A new catheter technique for producing experimental coronary thrombosis and selective coronary visualization, *Am Heart J* 83:360–364, 1972.

32. Kubota K, Som P, Oster ZH, et al: Detection of cardiomyopathy in animal model using quantitative autoradiography, *J Nucl Med* 29:1697–1703, 1988.

33. Lambrecht RM: *Biological models in radiopharmaceutical development.* In: Dordrecht, The Netherlands: Kluwer Academic Publishers, 1996.

34. Lambrecht RM and Eckelman WC: *Animal models in radiotracer design.* In: New York: Springer-Verlag, 1983.

35. Lavallee M, Cox D, Patrick TA, et al: Salvage of myocardial function by coronary artery reperfusion 1, 2, and 3 hours after occlusion in conscious dogs, *Circ Res* 53:235–247, 1983.

36. Li QS, Solot G, Frank TL, et al: Myocardial redistribution of technetium-99m-methoxyisobutyl isonitrile (SESTAMIBI), *J Nucl Med* 31:1069–1076, 1990.

37. Lu P, Zanzonico P, Goldfine SM, et al: Antimyosin antibody imaging in experimental aortic regurgitation, *J Nucl Cardiol* 4(1 Pt 1):25–32, 1997.

38. Magid NM, Opio G, Wallerson DC, et al: Heart failure due to chronic experimental aortic regurgitation, *Am J Physiol* 267(2 Pt 2): H556–H562, 1994.

39. Matsuzaki M, Gallagher KP, Kemper WS, et al: Sustained regional dysfunction produced by prolonged coronary stenosis: gradual recovery after reperfusion, *Circulation* 68:170–182, 1983.

40. McDonald KM, Francis GS, Carlyle PF, et al: Hemodynamic, left ventricular structural and hormonal changes after discrete myocardial damage in the dog, *J Am Coll Cardiol* 19:460–467, 1992.

41. Miller DD, Gill JB, Livni E, et al: Fatty acid analogue accumulation: a marker of myocyte viability in ischemic-reperfused myocardium, *Circ Res* 63:681–692, 1988.

42. Morais DJ, Richart TS, Fritz AJ, et al: The production of chronic experimental mitral insufficiency, *Ann Surg* 145:500–508, 1957.

43. Morishita S, Kusuoka H, Yamamichi Y, et al: Kinetics of radioiodinated species in subcellular fractions from rat hearts following administration of iodine-123-labelled 15-(p-iodophenyl)-3-(R,S)-methylpentadecanoic acid (^{123}I-BMIPP), *Eur J Nucl Med* 23:383–389, 1996.

44. Nakajima K, Taki J, Bunko H, et al: Dynamic acqusition with a three-headed SPECT system: application to technetium-99m-SQ30217 myocardial imaging, *J Nucl Med* 32:1273–1277, 1991.

45. Narula J, Kolodgie F, Virmani R, et al: Should assessment of the rate of smooth muscle cell proliferation by In-111-Z2D3 antibody imaging allow for predicting post-angioplasty restenosis? *J Nucl Med* 38(suppl):3P(Abstract), 1997.

46. Nicklas JM, Becker LC, and Bulkley GH: Effects of repeated brief coronary occlusion on regional left ventricular function and dimension in dogs, *Am J Cardiol* 56:473–478, 1985.

47. Nickles RJ, Nunn AD, Stone CK, et al: Technetium-94m-teboroxime: synthesis, dosimetry and initial PET imaging studies, *J Nucl Med* 34:1058–1066, 1993.

48. Nishimura T, Sago M, Kihara K, et al: Fatty acid myocardial imaging using ^{123}I-β-methyl-iodophenyl pentadecanoic acid (BMIPP): comparison of myocardial perfusion and fatty acid utilization in canine myocardial infarction (occlusion and reperfusion model), *Eur J Nucl Med* 15:341–345, 1989.

49. Okada RD: Kinetics of thallium-201 in reperfused canine myocardium after coronary artery occlusion, *J Am Coll Cardiol* 3:1245–1251, 1984.

50. Okada RD, Glover D, Gaffney T, et al: Myocardial kinetics of technetium-99m-hexakis-2-methoxy-2-methylpropyl-isonitrile, *Circulation* 77:491–498, 1988.

51. Okada RD, Jacobs ML, Daggett WM, et al: Thallium-201 kinetics in nonischemic canine myocardium, *Circulation* 65:70–77, 1982.

52. Okada RD and Pohost GM: The use of preintervention and postintervention thallium imaging for assessing the early and late effects of experimental coronary arterial reperfusion in dogs, *Circulation* 69:1153–1160, 1984.

53. Packer DL, Bardy GH, Worley SJ, et al: Tachycardia-induced cardiomyopathy: a reversible form of left ventricular dysfunction, *Am J Cardiol* 57:563–570, 1986.

54. Pasqualini R, Duatti A, Bellande E, et al: Bis(dithiocarbamato) nitrido technetium-99m radiopharmaceuticals: a class of neutral myocardial imaging agents, *J Nucl Med* 35:334–341, 1994.

55. Pohost GM, Okada RD, O'Keefe DD, et al: Thallium redistribution in dogs with severe coronary stenosis of fixed caliber, *Circ Res* 48:439–446, 1981.

56. Reimer KA and Jennings RB: The "wavefront phenomenon" of myocardial ischemic cell death. II. Transmural progression of necrosis within the framework of ischemic bed size (myocardium at risk) and collateral flow, *Lab Invest* 40:633–644, 1979.

57. Reimer KA, Lowe JE, Rasmussen MM, et al: The wavefront phenomenon of ischemic cell death. 1. Myocardial infarct size vs duration of coronary occlusion in dogs, *Circulation* 56:786–794, 1977.

58. Reinhardt CP, Weinstein H, Marcel R, et al: Comparison of iodine-125-BMIPP and thallium-201 in myocardial hypoperfusion, *J Nucl Med* 36:1645–1653, 1995.

59. Reske SN, Sauer W, Machulla HJ, et al: Metabolism of 15(p ^{123}I iodophenyl-)pentadecanoic acid in heart muscle and noncardiac tissues, *Eur J Nucl Med* 10:228–234, 1985.

60. Roth DM, Maruoka Y, Rogers J, et al: Development of coronary collateral circulation in left circumflex Ameroid-occluded swine myocardium, *Am J Physiol* 253(5 Pt 2):H1279–H1288, 1987.

61. Ruiz M, Calnon DA, Desta H, et al: Tc99m-sestamibi (MIBI) defect magnitude during dobutamine stress underestimates the magnitude of ischemia in dogs with mild coronary stenoses, *J Am Coll Cardiol* 27:353A, 1996.

62. Shen YT and Vatner SF: Mechanism of impaired myocardial function during progressive coronary stenosis in conscious pigs: Hibernation versus stunning? *Circ Res* 76:479–488, 1995.

63. Shi CQX, Sinusas AJ, Dione DP, et al: Technetium-99m-nitroimidazole (BMS181321): a positive imaging agent for detecting myocardial ischemia, *J Nucl Med* 36:1078–1086, 1995.

64. Sinusas AJ, Bergin JD, Edwards NC, et al: Redistribution of ^{99m}Tc-sestamibi and ^{201}Tl in the presence of a severe coronary artery stenosis, *Circulation* 89:2332–2341, 1994.

65. Sinusas AJ, Shi Q, Saltzberg MT, et al: Technetium-99m-tetrofosmin

to assess myocardial blood flow: experimental validation in an intact canine model of ischemia, *J Nucl Med* 35:664–671, 1994.

66. Sinusas AJ, Shi Q, Vitols PJ, et al: Impact of regional ventricular function, geometry, and dobutamine stress on quantitative 99mTc-sestamibi defect size, *Circulation* 88(5 Pt 1):2224–2234, 1993.

67. Sinusas AJ, Trautman KA, Bergin JD, et al: Quantification of area at risk during coronary occlusion and degree of myocardial salvage after reperfusion with technetium-99m methoxyisobutyl isonitrile, *Circulation* 82:1424–1437, 1990.

68. Sinusas AJ, Watson DD, Cannon JM Jr, et al: Effect of ischemia and postischemic dysfunction on myocardial uptake of technetium-99m-labeled methoxyisobutyl isonitrile and thallium-201, *J Am Coll Cardiol* 14:1785–1793, 1989.

69. Smith AM, Gullberg GT, Christian PE, et al: Kinetic modeling of teboroxime using dynamic SPECT imaging of a canine model, *J Nucl Med* 35:484–495, 1994.

70. Spinale FG, Fulbright BM, Mukherjee R, et al: Relation between ventricular and myocyte function with tachycardia-induced cardiomyopathy, *Circ Res* 71:174–187, 1992.

71. Spinale FG, Zellner JL, Tomita M, et al: Tachycardia-induced cardiomyopathy: effects on blood flow and capillary structure, *Am J Physiol* 261(1 Pt 2):H140–H148, 1991.

72. Stewart RE, Heyl B, O'Rourke RA, et al: Demonstration of differential post-stenotic myocardial technetium-99m-teboroxime clearance kinetics after experimental ischemia and hyperemic stress, *J Nucl Med* 32:2000–2008, 1991.

73. Stewart RE, Schwaiger M, Hutchins GD, et al: Myocardial clearance kinetics of technetium-99m-SQ30217: a marker of regional myocardial blood flow, *J Nucl Med* 31:1183–1190, 1990.

74. Stone CK, Christian BT, Nickles RJ, et al: Technetium 94m-labeled methoxyisobutyl isonitrile: dosimetry and resting cardiac imaging with positron emission tomography, *J Nucl Cardiol* 1(5 Pt 1):425–433, 1994.

75. Stone HL, Bishop VS, and Guyton AC: Cardiac function after embolization of coronaries with microspheres, *Am J Physiol* 204:16–27, 1963.

76. Takatsu H, Uno Y, and Fujiwara H: Modulation of left ventricular iodine-125-MIBG accumulation in cardiomyopathic Syrian hamster using the renin-angiotensin system, *J Nucl Med* 36:1055–1061, 1995.

77. Tomoike H, Ogata I, Maruoka Y, et al: Differential registration of two types of radionuclides on macroautoradiograms for studying coronary circulation: concise communication, *J Nucl Med* 24:693–699, 1983.

78. Vanoverschelde JLJ, Wijns W, Borgers M, et al: Chronic myocardial hibernation in humans. From bedside to bench, *Circulation* 95:1961–1971, 1997.

79. Vanoverschelde JLJ, Wijns W, Depre C, et al: Mechanism of chronic regional postischemic dysfunction in humans. New insights from the study of noninfarcted collateral-dependent myocardium, *Circulation* 87:1513–1523, 1993.

80. Watanabe Y: Serial inbreeding of rabbits with hereditary hyperlipidemia (WHHL-rabbit), *Atherosclerosis* 36:261–268, 1980.

81. Weber DA and Ivanovic M: Pinhole SPECT: ultra-high resolution imaging in small animal studies (editorial), *J Nucl Med* 36:2287–2289, 1995.

82. Weber DA, Ivanovic M, Franceschi D, et al: Pinhole SPECT: an approach to in vivo high resolution SPECT imaging in small laboratory animals, *J Nucl Med* 35:342–348, 1994.

83. Weinstein H, Reinhardt CP, and Leppo JA: Teboroxime, sestamibi and thallium-201 as markers of myocardial hypoperfusion: comparison by quantitative dual-isotope autoradiography in rabbits, *J Nucl Med* 34:1510–1517, 1993.

84. Weinstein H, Reinhardt CP, Wironen JF, et al: Myocardial uptake of thallium-201 and technetium 99m-labeled sestamibi after ischemia and reperfusion: comparison by quantitative dual-tracer autoradiography in rabbits, *J Nucl Cardiol* 1:351–364, 1994.

85. Wu JC, Yun JJ, Heller EN, et al: Limitations of dobutamine for enhancing flow heterogeneity in the presence of single coronary stenosis: implications for technetium-99m sestamibi imaging, *J Nucl Med* 39:417–425, 1998.

86. Yipintsoi T, Dobbs WA Jr, Scanlon PD, et al: Regional distribution of diffusable tracers and carbonized microspheres in the left ventricle of isolated dog hearts, *Circ Res* 33:573–587, 1973.

87. Young DF, Cholvin NR, and Roth AC: Pressure drop across artificially induced stenoses in the femoral arteries in dogs, *Circ Res* 36:735–743, 1975.

88. Zile MR, Tomita M, Nakano K, Mirsky I, Usher B, Lindroth J, and Carabello BA: Effects of left ventricular volume overload produced by mitral regurgitation on diastolic function, *Am J Physiol* 261(5 Pt 2). H1471–H1480, 1991.

Chapter 5

Animal models for the study of positron emission tomography tracers

Bernhard L. Gerber, Jean-Louis J. Vanoverschelde, and **Guy R. Heyndrickx**

The major incentives for the use of animal models for imaging by positron emission tomography (PET) are:

1. To develop new PET tracers and to define and validate accurate tracer kinetics models that allow quantitative measurements to be made noninvasively.

2. To explore the physiopathology of such disease states as acute myocardial ischemia, stunning, and chronic contractile dysfunction to understand the underlying metabolic abnormalities.

The use of PET in intact animals models will likely increase in the near future. It is an ideal tool for noninvasive assessment of the efficacy of drugs or other therapeutic interventions aimed at improving myocardial blood flow and metabolism in various models of heart disease. By revealing the sites and mechanisms of interaction of radiolabeled drugs with cardiac receptors, PET may also provide valuable insights into cardiac pharmacology.

The first part of this chapter illustrates how PET tracers can be developed and validated in animal models and how kinetic tracer models can subsequently be applied to allow a quantitative exploration of myocardial metabolic pathways in vivo. The second part surveys different animal models in which PET has been used to unravel the underlying physiopathology.

DEVELOPMENT AND VALIDATION OF POSITRON EMISSION TOMOGRAPHY TRACERS IN ANIMAL MODELS

The feature of PET that makes it different from other noninvasive imaging techniques is its ability to measure tissue concentrations of radioisotope tracer in absolute terms (such as in counts per gram of cardiac tissue). Combined with the possibility of dynamic imaging and kinetic tracer modeling, PET offers the unique opportunity to trace biochemical pathways noninvasively in vivo and to assess quantitatively physiologic parameters, such as organ perfusion and tissue metabolism, directly in humans. The mathematical basis of modeling is outlined in detail elsewhere in this book. This chapter illustrates how kinetic tracer models in PET can be developed and validated in vitro and in vivo by using animal models.

Theoretical considerations concerning the development of positron emission tomography tracers

Most available PET tracers are derived from metabolic tracers already used in classic biochemistry or in isolated organ preparations. For example, the use of freely diffusible tracers, such as [^{3}H]$_2$O, to trace regional blood flow in vitro fostered the development of the myocardial PET blood flow tracer H$_2$[^{15}O]. Similarly, the use of [^{14}C]-6-desoxyglucose preceded that of [^{18}F]-6-desoxyglucose and the use of [^{3}H]-labeled receptor ligands led to the emergence of receptor tracers labeled with positron-emitting radionuclides. In many cases, myocardial PET tracers were initially not developed for use in cardiac physiology but rather to assess the function of other organs, such as the brain. Accordingly, the development of cardiac specific models has often relied on the knowledge acquired in these other organ systems. Only problems specific to myocardial imaging, such as partial volume or spillover effects, had to be taken into account. The successive steps involved in the development of a de novo PET tracer are illustrated schematically in Fig. 5-1.

Choice of the optimal tracer is the crucial step when exploring the possibility of probing a specific metabolic pathway. Before developing a new tracer, one must ascertain that the substance of interest does not participate in any other undesirable metabolic pathways or enter metabolic pools whose size might be unstable under pathophysiologic conditions and thereby might influence measurements. The biochemical behavior of the potential candidate for tracer should also have been thoroughly studied in isolated cellular or organ preparations. The next step is radiochemical synthesis of the substance by using positron-emitting isotopes. The following are prerequisites for successful radiosynthesis of a tracer:

1. Synthesis must be sufficiently rapid to permit incorporation of the short-lived positron-emitting radioisotope.

2. The radioisotope must have a sufficiently long physical half-life to permit complete exploration of the biochemical pathway of interest.

3. The process of incorporation of the radionuclide into the tracer must be automated as much as possible to limit exposure to radiation.

Once radiosynthesis has been achieved, autoradiographic studies in small animals (such as rats or hamsters) and in vivo PET in larger animals and humans are needed to test whether the tracer is suitable for imaging of the myocardium. To be clinically useful, the PET tracer must have a large myocardial extraction to permit satisfactory imaging of the heart. In addition, uptake of the tracer by the lung, liver, and spleen must be sufficiently low to minimize spillover due to cross-contamination from these organs.

Once the feasibility of PET has been demonstrated, the properties of the tracer must be better defined. To this end, the tracer is usually studied in vitro in isolated heart preparations. Because PET tracers have short half-lifes, such studies are often performed with tracers labeled with a beta- or gamma-emitting radioisotope, such as [^{14}C] or [^{3}H], rather than with a positron-emitting isotope. Myocardial retention is studied by repeated tissue sampling after bolus injections of the tracer. This allows one to determine the first-pass extraction, clearance, and accumulation rates. Isolated heart preparations are useful to follow the metabolic fate of the tracer, such as by freeze-clamping the heart at different intervals after tracer injection and biochemically analyzing radiolabeled compounds by using high-performance liquid chromatography (HPLC). From this knowledge and from the determination of the number of compartments in which the tracer is distributed, one can formulate a mathematical kinetic model that describes the accumulation and clearance of the tracer. This model then must be validated, and the rate constants of the individual variables must be fitted under different conditions by matching external detection measurements of the labeled tracer in the isolated heart.

The next step is analysis of the targeted process in vivo in dogs or pigs by using PET imaging. The extraction and clearance rates obtained under physiologic and pathologic conditions must corroborate those obtained in vitro. Because PET scanners have a limited spatial resolution compared with the thickness of the myocardium, corrections must be made for partial volume and spillover. This is best achieved by measuring radioactivity directly in tissue sampled from open-chest animals and comparing these data with radioactivity externally determined by using PET. Finally, one must validate the resulting kinetic model with conventional methods of assessing the biochemical or physiologic pathways in intact closed-chest animals.

Clearly, the development of a new myocardial tracer for PET is an elaborate and time-consuming procedure. Many tracers that seem promising on a conceptual basis turn out to be useless for PET, because of their poor imaging quality or their complex kinetic behavior. Examples of tracers that failed to become useful in clinical practice because of imaging problems are [^{11}C]-O-methyl-glucose, [^{15}O]-labeled oxygen, and [^{18}F]-fluoro-midazole.

Animal models used to develop and validate positron emission tomography

In vitro studies used to develop and validate PET tracers are frequently performed in the isolated, retrogradely perfused rat or rabbit heart model (Fig. 5-2). After excision from the animal, the heart is suspended and perfused retrogradely through the

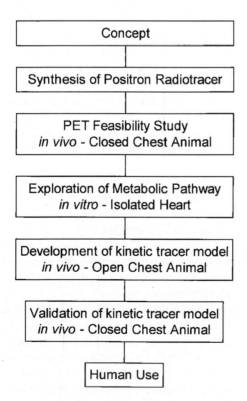

Fig. 5-1. Steps involved in the development and validation of a positron emission tomography tracer.

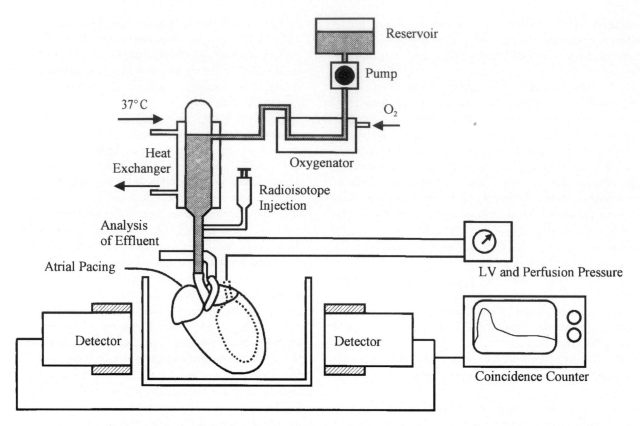

Fig. 5-2. Diagram of a Langendorff isolated perfused working heart model, which is used for in vitro development of positron emission tomography tracers. (Modified with permission from Bergmann SR, et al: The dependence of accumulation of 13-N-ammonia by myocardium on metabolic factors and its implications for quantitative assessment of perfusion, *Circulation* 61:34, 1980.)

aorta. The pulmonary artery is cannulated, and the cardiac effluent is sampled for continuous monitoring of oxygen consumption and tracer extraction by measuring the arteriovenous difference. Heart rate can be controlled by atrial pacing. A balloon can then be introduced through the left atrium through the mitral valve into the left ventricular cavity to measure left ventricular pressure and to modify the loading conditions. Perfusion and left ventricular pressure are recorded by using pressure transducers. The retrogradely perfused heart has the advantage of remaining stable over a prolonged period of time and allowing precise control of cardiac work, blood flow, oxygen tension, and substrate availability. Residue curves in the isolated heart model can be obtained by direct tissue sampling, recording of external radioactivity by using a coincidence counter or a simple gamma or beta detector placed directly over the heart, or both. These residue curves permit calculation of the extraction, clearance, and accumulation rates of the tracer in the heart (Fig. 5-3). Extraction and clearance rates must be studied under various metabolic and physiologic conditions. In vitro preparations are also useful in determining the metabolic fate of the tracer at different times after injection and indicating the number of metabolic compartments, an obligatory step for the development of appropriate kinetic models of a tracer. Therefore, the isolated heart is removed from the perfusion apparatus and rapidly freeze-clamped in liquid nitrogen at different times after tracer injection. The preparation is homogenized, and the la-

beled metabolites are studied by doing autoradiography and HPLC of the supernatant. The number of metabolically relevant compartments can be verified by fitting the residual curve to different numbers of exponential functions.

In vivo studies are performed later in the procedure, usually in open-chest dogs or pigs (Fig. 5-4). The animals are anesthetized and, after a left thoracotomy, the heart is exposed and suspended in a pericardial cradle. Catheters are introduced into the left atrium and the aorta for simultaneous coinjection of radioactive microspheres to measure blood flow. Another catheter is introduced into the coronary sinus for venous sampling to calculate extraction of tracer, oxygen, and substrate by the heart. The animal is then placed in a PET scanner, and radioactivity is recorded externally after injection of the PET tracer. The externally determined extraction, retention, and kinetic values are studied under various conditions, depending on the expected use of the tracer.

Tracers of myocardial blood flow must be studied over a wide range of coronary flow. In typical experiments, low coronary flow is obtained by placing a hydraulic or snare occluder around the left circumflex or left anterior descending coronary artery to partially or completely occlude them; hyperemia flows are obtained by intracoronary infusion of dipyridamole, adenosine, or papaverine. Similarly, tracers for the study of cardiac metabolism must be investigated under different loading conditions. Workload is modified by positive or negative inotropic

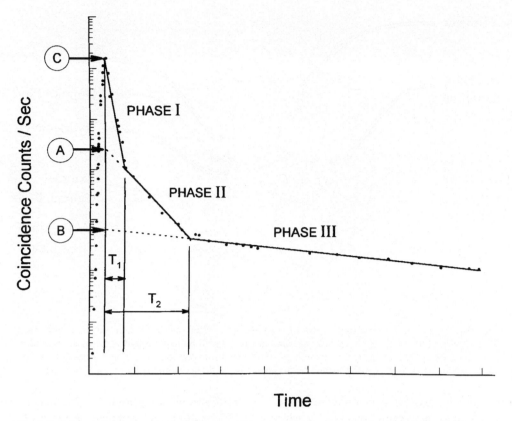

Fig. 5-3. Schematic time–activity curve describing the estimate of retention fraction and clearance rate using the washout phases of a radiotracer. For descriptive purposes, the curves have been considered in terms of three consistently observed prominent phases. Phase I represents a rapid decline in radioactivity associated with independently measured washout of the tracer in the vascular compartment. Phase II reflects redistribution of the tracer between interstitial and intracellular fluid and slow washout of tracer entering the right ventricular cavity. Phase III represents an apparent monoexponential decline of nitrogen-13 counts after sequestration in the myocardium. Back-extrapolation of phase III to the time of peak counts (B/C) defines a residual fraction. Clearance ($t_{1/2}$) is calculated as the half-time required for elimination of sequestered tracer from the best-line fit monoexponential conforming to phase III values. (Redrawn with permission from Bergmann SR, et al: The dependence of accumulation of 13-N-ammonia by myocardium on metabolic factors and its implications for quantitative assessment of perfusion, *Circulation* 61:34, 1980.)

drugs, such as norepinephrine or propranolol, or by atrial pacing. Tracer use by the myocardium can also be modified by varying the dietary state of the animals or by perfusing the animals with glucose and insulin. Acidosis can be induced by reducing external ventilation, and alkalosis can be produced by hyperventilation or by injection of bicarbonate.

Tracers that probe the sympathetic nervous system require specific procedures. Sympathetic fibers in discrete areas of the heart can be destroyed selectively in certain regions by applying a solution of 88% phenol in ethanol on the epicardial surface. Permanent denervation is obtained by superior cranial ganglionectomy. Reuptake of catecholamines from the axonal cytoplasm into storage vesicles can be blocked by an injection of desipramine or reserpine. The release of catecholamines by the nerve endings can be induced by tyramine, and ganglion blockade can be obtained by infusion of trimethaphan.

Because anesthesia and surgery alter the metabolic conditions under which animals are studied, the final validation of PET tracers requires the use of constantly instrumented, con-

scious animals and appropriate reference methods. Flow tracers must be compared with microsphere flow, and metabolic tracers need to be tested against Fick extraction methods under several physiopathologic situations.

The process of developing and validating PET tracers on animal models can be illustrated by examples of a metabolic tracer, [^{11}C]-acetate, and a flow tracer, [^{13}N]-ammonia.

Development of a metabolic positron emission tomography tracer: [^{11}C]-acetate

The metabolic tracer [^{11}C]-acetate is one of the few examples in which a PET tracer has been specifically developed for the heart.

Because all major myocardial oxidative fuels are oxidized by conversion to acetyl coenzyme A and proceed through the tricarboxylic acid cycle (TCA), [^{11}C]-acetate was developed to assess overall oxidative metabolism and oxygen consumption by PET. Because of the relative simplicity of its metabolic pathway, acetate is usually preferred over other fuels for shunting

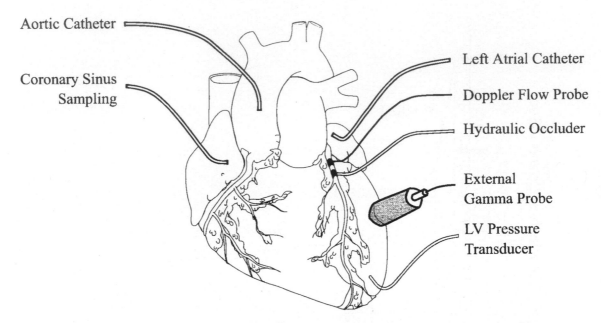

Fig. 5-4. Typical in vivo dog model used for validation of PET tracers in later stages. Myocardial blood flow in the left anterior descending coronary is reduced by using a hydraulic occluder and is monitored by a Doppler probe. Catheters are introduced into the left atrium and aorta for microsphere and radioisotope injection. Radiotracer uptake is recorded externally by using a gamma probe.

into the TCA cycle. Acetate is avidly taken up by myocardial cells[81] and rapidly converted into acetyl-coenzyme A, which becomes available for shunting into the TCA cycle[54] and oxidation to carbon dioxide (CO_2). In vitro studies of isolated heart models in which [^{14}C]-acetate was used indicated that acetate does not participate in metabolic pathways other than TCA flux and, in particular, does not enter the fatty acid synthesis pathway.[81] Initial studies with [^{11}C]-acetate[51] showed the feasibility of imaging the myocardium in vivo in dogs[2] and humans[51] and demonstrated that clearance of acetate from the myocardium was monoexponential and was reduced in ischemic tissue. The biochemical fate of the tracer was studied in detail in retrogradely perfused Langendorff preparations.[11,14]

Because of the short half-time of [^{11}C] (20 minutes), the initial studies were performed with [^{14}C]-acetate.[11] To correlate the acetate clearance kinetic with TCA cycle flux, the rate of oxidation of [^{14}C]-acetate and rate of venous efflux of [^{14}C]O_2 were compared with the rate of oxygen consumption calculated from the arteriovenous oxygen difference. Subsequent studies had to verify that the behavior of externally recorded [^{11}C]-acetate clearance paralleled the rate of efflux of total of [^{14}C]O_2 and oxygen consumption. Therefore, experiments were performed using simultaneous infusion of [^{11}C]-acetate and [^{14}C]-acetate, and external detection of [^{11}C]-acetate clearance was done by using gamma probes.[11,14] These measurements were performed under different workload and inotropic conditions. The results showed not only that the rate of total [^{14}C] efflux, [^{14}C]O_2 efflux, and oxygen consumption correlated well but also that [^{11}C]-acetate clearance faithfully reproduced [^{14}C]-acetate clearance.

Next, in vivo studies in anesthetized closed-chest dogs were

performed by using PET.[12,15] The animals were placed into a PET scanner, and external clearance of [^{11}C] radioactivity, blood [^{11}C] radioactivity, and [^{11}C]O_2 content were measured after intravenous injection of [^{11}C]-acetate. The results were compared with the maximum oxygen consumption (MVO_2) calculated from the arteriovenous difference obtained from coronary sinus blood sampling under various blood flows and metabolic conditions[3] and during several ischemic, hyperemic, and postischemic states. A similar linear relation was found between the monoexponential rate constant and MVO_2 as that previously demonstrated in vitro (Fig. 5-5). It was also shown that arterial lactate concentration and the amount of free fatty acid oxygen equivalents have only a small impact on the relation between the [^{11}C] rate constants and MVO_2.[3]

To mathematically confirm the empirically derived linear relation between [^{11}C]-acetate clearance rates and turnover rates of TCA, pool sizes, turnover rates and washout rates of labeled intermediates of [^{14}C]-acetate were determined in a Langendorff preparation of isolated working rat heart.[50] After bolus injection of [^{14}C]-acetate, the preparation was freeze-clamped and ^{14}C-radioactivity in amino acids and TCA-cycle intermediates was determined at various moments after bolus administration. The pool sizes, turnover rates, and washout rates of the labeled intermediates of [^{14}C]-acetate were determined under different normoxic, low-flow, and hypoxic conditions, and a six-compartment model was formulated that described the kinetics of [^{14}C]-labeled acetate in the myocardium. Although this model is too complex to be fitted with PET data, it could be fitted in the isolated heart model and correlated well with experimentally measured MVO_2. Simplification of the model also permitted the empirical determination of the relation between

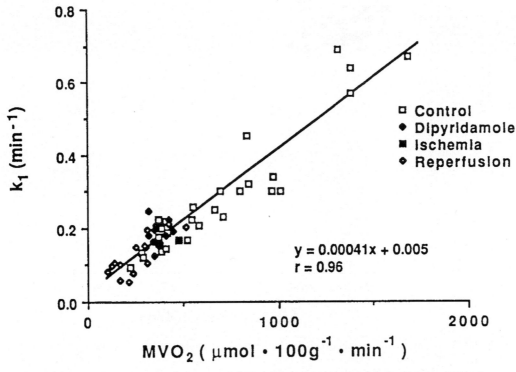

Fig. 5-5. Relation between oxygen consumption and the monoexponential clearance rate of carbon-11-acetate in dogs. (Reproduced with permission from Armbrecht JJ, Buxton DB, and Schelbert HR, et al: Validation of [1-11C]acetate as a tracer for noninvasive assessment of oxidative metabolism with positron emission tomography in normal, ischemic, postischemic, and hyperemic canine myocardium, *Circulation* 81:1594–1605, 1990.)

mono- or biexponential clearance of [^{11}C]-acetate and TCA flux.

Development of a tracer for myocardial extraction flow: [^{13}N]-ammonia

Conceptually, the simplest approach to quantifying myocardial blood flow is to label microspheres that are trapped in the myocardium. In this case, myocardial flow can be calculated using the formula

$$MBF \cdot E = C_m / \int C_a dt$$

where *MBF* is the myocardial blood flow, *E* is the extraction fraction, C_m is the myocardial tracer concentration, and $\int C_a$ is the integral of the arterial tracer concentration over time. Tracers for PET that were thought to mimic this extraction flow approach are [^{13}N]-ammonia and [^{82}Rb]-rubidium. The basic assumption needed for the use of an extraction flow tracer is that the extraction fraction remains constant over a large range of flows. Unfortunately, none of the current PET flow tracers has a constant extraction fraction, and corrections for decreasing extraction with increasing flow must be made. Alternatively, appropriate kinetic tracer models can be developed to faithfully describe the myocardial behavior of the tracer, such as in the case of [^{13}N]-ammonia.

After successful radiosynthesis of [^{13}N]-ammonia, high myocardial uptake of this tracer was observed in dogs and mice,[30,48] making it potentially useful for flow assessment. Once myocardial imaging using ^{13}N-ammonia and scintillation cameras became feasible in humans,[30,31] further studies[28,79] attempted to demonstrate that [^{13}N]-ammonia traced myocardial perfusion and showed the potential usefulness of [^{13}N]-ammonia to trace flow in a relative manner, as this was shown by comparing the uptake of [^{13}N]-ammonia measured by the PET scanner and by direct tissue sampling with microsphere retention in open-chest dogs.[58] A direct but nonlinear relation was found (Fig. 5-6).

To use [^{13}N]-ammonia as a quantitative blood flow tracer, the relation of extraction fraction to blood flow had to be delineated. Ideally, for a tracer to behave like radioactive microspheres, extraction should be maximal and constant under all physiologic flow rates. In isolated, retrogradely perfused rabbit hearts placed in coincidence counters, the extraction fraction of [^{13}N]-ammonia was determined under various flow rates and hypoxic and normoxic conditions.[5] It was found that the residual fraction did not directly correlate with coronary flow, as had been previously assumed. Furthermore, the residual fraction of ^{13}N-ammonia differed depending on tissue oxygenation. Because it was thought that retention of ^{13}N-ammonia depended on metabolic trapping by glutamine synthetase in the heart, the influence of methionine sulfoximine, a specific inhibitor of this enzyme, was investigated, resulting in a 60% decrease in myocardial retention and prolonged myocardial clearance of

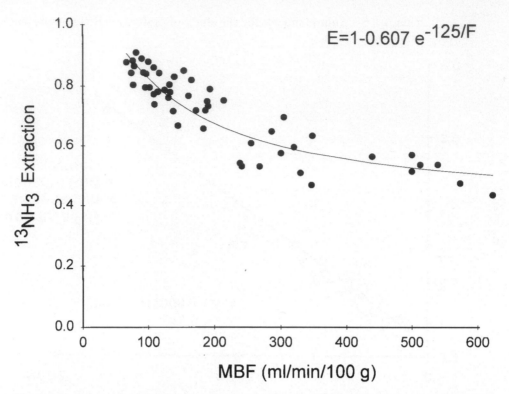

Fig. 5-6. Experimental relation between the first transit extraction fraction of nitrogen-13 ammonia and myocardial blood flow (MBF) in dogs. (Reproduced with permission from Schelbert HR, Phelps ME, Huang SC, et al: N-13 ammonia as an indicator of myocardial blood flow, *Circulation* 63:1259–1272, 1981.)

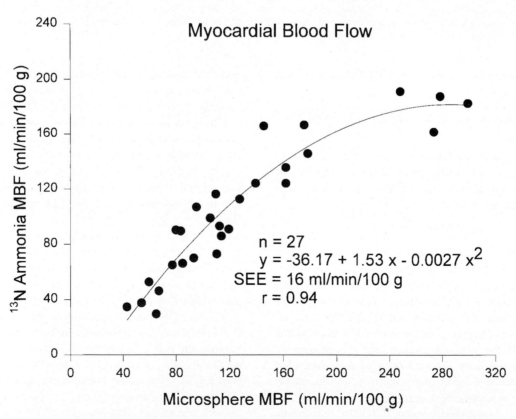

Fig. 5-7. Relation between regional myocardial blood flow (MBF) determined with the microsphere technique and with nitrogen-13 ammonia and positron emission tomography by using an extraction limited method in dogs. (Reproduced with permission from Shah A, Schelbert HR, Schwaiger M, et al: Measurement of regional myocardial blood flow with N-13 ammonia and positron-emission tomography in intact dogs, *J Am Coll Cardiol* 5:92–100, 1985.)

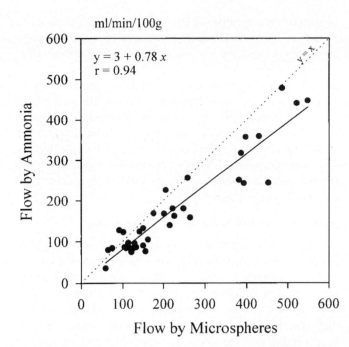

ml/min/100g

$y = 3 + 0.78\,x$
$r = 0.94$

Flow by Ammonia

Flow by Microspheres

Fig. 5-8. Relation between regional myocardial blood flow (MBF) determined with the microsphere technique and with nitrogen-13 ammonia and positron emission tomography by using a three-compartment model in dogs. (Reproduced with permission from Bol A, Malin JA, Vanoverschelde JL, et al: Direct comparison of [13N]ammonia and [15O]water estimates of perfusion with quantification of regional myocardial blood flow by microspheres, *Circulation* 87:512–525, 1993.)

13N-ammonia. These data indicated that 13NH3 was far from being an ideal extraction flow tracer, mainly because its extraction was dependent on metabolism. These observations were confirmed in vivo in dogs.[59]

The possibility of using a tracer with a flow-limited extraction in a way similar to microspheres was explored in closed-chest instrumented dogs.[66] Myocardial perfusion was simultaneously assessed by an injection of microspheres and by recording serial images by using dynamic imaging with PET after injection of 13NH3. Regional myocardial blood flow was calculated from the radioactivity in myocardial tissue at different times after tracer injection divided by the time integral of the input curve of the in vitro sampled arterial concentration of nitrogen-13. It was found that the overall relation between the blood flow measured by microspheres and that estimated by 13NH3 was nonlinear (Fig. 5-7) with a good correlation at low flow rates but increasing underestimation at high flow rates when the extraction fraction of 13N-ammonia decreased. To compensate for this underestimation, an empirical correction had to be proposed.[4]

To better understand these observations, Krivokapich et al[40] studied the retention of 13N-ammonia in isolated perfused rabbit septum after bolus injection under different flow rates. The resulting curves of activity retention of nitrogen-13 concentration were fitted to a weighted sum of exponential components to determine the number of compartments into which [13N] ac-

tivity was distributed. Three exponential components were identified. The biological half-time of the third compartment but not of the other two was dependent on temperature (and thus on metabolism). These data therefore suggested the existence of freely diffusible 13N-ammonia and of a metabolic compartment related to the definitive trapping of 13NH3 in the cell. This metabolic trapping could, in theory, be caused by any of the three metabolic pathways in mammalian cells that fix ammonia into organically bound nitrogen: that is, the carbamylphosphate-synthetase that ultimately results in production of urea, synthesis of basic amino acids (glutamic or aspartic acid), or synthesis of glutamine. To determine the mechanism responsible for trapping of 13N-ammonia in the myocardium of rabbit septum,[40] studies were repeated in the presence of specific inhibitors for glutamine synthetase (methionine sulfoximine), and γ-glutamyl cysteine synthetase (buthionine sulfoximine) after bolus injection of 13NH3 or [13N]-glutamine. Chemical analysis of tissue and effluent showed that the synthesis of glutamine catalyzed by glutamine synthetase was primarily responsible for retention of the 13N label.

Finally, because of the rapid metabolism of 13N-ammonia, it was important to know whether the arterial input function was contaminated by [13N]-labeled metabolites.[55] After injection of 13N-ammonia into dogs and humans, radio-HPLC of arterial blood confirmed the presence of contaminating metabolites in blood activity, mainly 13N-glutamine and urea, and emphasized the need to correct the arterial input function for their presence when quantifying myocardial blood flow. Taking into account these findings as well as the shortcomings of measuring myocardial blood flow by the net extraction method, two–[41] and three–kinetic compartment[36] models were developed in humans[36,41] and were validated in closed-chest dogs.[8,42,49] The agreement of blood flow estimations by all three approaches with microsphere flow was found to be excellent (Fig. 5-8).

ANIMAL MODELS USED TO STUDY THE PATHOPHYSIOLOGY OF MYOCARDIAL DISEASE

Positron emission tomography is becoming increasingly popular for studying of various myocardial disease states in intact animal models. This method has several advantages for the study of basic variables, such as perfusion and metabolism, compared with more invasive techniques (see box on p 64). Because it is noninvasive PET allows the design of long-term animal models without the risk of losing the animals to infection or traumatic injury. In contrast with studies with microspheres, PET yields immediate results of myocardial perfusion and does not necessitate sacrifice of the animal. In long-term studies, microspheres are lost from tissue with time,[20] which biases measurements from early injections. The number of microsphere injections into one animal is limited by available radioisotopes (usually less than six). Each injection of microspheres permanently alters the remaining tissue by obstructing part of the available capillaries. In contrast, measurements of perfusion or metabolism by PET can be repeated almost indefinitely and do not affect the tissue. Repeated readings in the same animal during different interventions or physiopathologic situations can also be made. Moreover, because different myocardial segments are studied simultaneously, regional differences can be assessed, and remote regions can serve as controls to different vascular territories. Use of the more indirect PET technique has potential limitations. Models of PET require steady states of flow and metabolism during scintigraphic examination. To fulfill the assumptions made for kinetic modeling, metabolic pools are not allowed to change in size during the study. In addition, PET often studies metabolic phenomena indirectly. For instance, glucose metabolism measured by PET necessitates incorporation of a correction factor that takes into account the distinctive affinity of the transport system for glucose and fluorodeoxyglucose (FDG) (lumped constant). Unfortunately, the lumped constant can change substantially with different metabolic conditions.[29] In addition to the potential errors arising from tracer kinetics, the limited spatial resolution of a PET scanner[35] may also introduce errors. Because of limited spatial resolution, PET measurements are confined to average transmural readings, precluding evaluation of differences between endocardial and epicardial regions. In certain cases, such as in perfusion measurements with [^{15}O] water, heterogeneity of tissue may introduce bias into the average readings given by the PET model.[33] Imperfections in PET readings arise also from the finite resolution that is dependent on wall motion. Ideally, gated dynamic studies should be performed to correct for effects of respiratory and cardiac motion, but these corrections are tedious to perform with current PET technology.

The following section reviews animal models that are potentially useful to study pathophysiologic mechanisms with PET. Given the importance of coronary artery disease in man, the animal models most studied with PET are those with ex-

perimental coronary disease. Because PET is used in humans to identify reversible ischemic dysfunction and because the mechanisms responsible for regional contractile dysfunction in humans are multiple and complex, particular interest was directed toward the development of representative animal models of ischemia, stunning, and hibernation. Studies using PET have permitted insight into the metabolic alterations present in stunned and chronically dysfunctional myocardium. Some PET studies have also been performed in other animal models focusing on alterations in chronic denervation, whereas experimental models for congestive heart failure have not yet been extensively studied with PET.

Acute myocardial ischemia and reperfusion

Models for ischemia and reperfusion are often to study PET tracers in animals because they mimic the physiopathologic situations encountered in humans with acute myocardial infarction. It became important to develop PET as a clinical tool to differentiate viable from nonviable myocardium after myocardial infarction and to characterize, on the basis of metabolism, irrecoverable necrotic tissue and reversibly jeopardized myocardial tissue. Experiments are usually performed in anesthetized open-chest dogs or pigs. Ischemia is usually induced by tightening snares or by inflating hydraulic occluders around the coronary arteries. Alternatively, it can be produced in closed-chest animals by inflating an angioplasty balloon catheter in a proximal coronary artery. Permanent occlusion of coronary arteries can be obtained by placing a copper coil inside the artery. Depending on the duration of ischemia, various results are achieved. Acute ischemia is a condition of low coronary blood flow associated with proportional reduction of contraction and a steady-state adjustment of energy supply and demand. Reperfusion after very short periods of ischemia (less than 2 minutes) usually results in rapid and complete restoration of contractile function. If ischemia is more prolonged (5 minutes to 15 to 20 minutes), postischemic dysfunction is more extensive and is termed stunning. Models of myocardial stunning will be discussed further below. A longer duration of ischemia results in irreversible cell damage, the ultrastructural characteristics of which include cellular swelling, contracture, and membrane rupture. Myocardial necrosis occurs first in the subendocardium; with longer ischemia, the necrotic zone expands towards the epicardium. Complete transmural necrosis occurs when ischemia continues for more than 3 hours. Thus, in models with ischemia between 20 minutes and 3 to 6 hours, normal, reversibly stunned cells and irreversibly necrotic injured cells may coexist in the same area, depending on the duration of ischemia.

During reperfusion of an established myocardial infarct, development of microvascular occlusion may result in regional hypoperfusion even when the infarct-related artery has become patent. This observation has been termed the *no-reflow phenomenon*.[38] Evidence indicates that this phenomenon may be caused by progressive microvascular occlusion by neutrophil leukocytes in postischemic myocardium.[25]

The no-reflow phenomenon and its time course were studied by Jeremy, Links, and Becker[37] in 12 anesthetized dogs in which the left anterior descending coronary artery (LAD) was occluded for 90 minutes, followed by full reperfusion. Serial PET studies of myocardial perfusion and microsphere blood flow were obtained after infusion of [82]Rb before and during occlusion and during a 4-hour reperfusion period. The no- reflow zone was determined after death by thioflavin staining. The study demonstrated that the no-reflow phenomenon could easily be observed in vivo. Immediately after reperfusion, the defect in [82]Rb perfusion observed during coronary occlusion resolved fully but reappeared progressively over the next 4 hours. A similar time-dependent decrease in microsphere flow in the LAD region was seen. Thus, this study demonstrated that the no-reflow phenomenon does not appear immediately on reperfusion but progressively develops during the first 4 hours thereafter.

Metabolic characterization of acutely ischemic tissue was performed with both ^{11}C]-palmitate and FDG. In a model of pacing-induced ischemia in dogs, Lerch et al[43] and Schelbert et al[60,61] demonstrated that the uptake and clearance of ^{11}C-palmitate were delayed and that FDG uptake was increased compared with that of controls. In closed-chest dogs with coronary occlusion induced by a thrombogenic copper coil, Bergmann et al[6] performed PET imaging immediately after occlusion and 90 minutes after thrombolysis induced with streptokinase. These authors observed that metabolic activity in the initially jeopardized regions increased after thrombolysis. Schwaiger et al[64] used PET in chronically instrumented dogs given 3-hour balloon occlusion of the LAD followed by complete reperfusion; the aim was to correlate metabolic findings soon after reperfusion with subsequent recovery of contractile function. In this model, regional function remained severely impaired early after reperfusion but improved over time. However, the amount of recovery of contractile function after reperfusion varied considerably among animals and was correlated with the amount of histologic necrosis. Animals with a large amount of necrotic tissue had poor functional recovery and had no uptake of ^{11}C]-palmitate or FDG early after reperfusion. On the other hand, animals with little necrosis had good functional recovery and had improved blood flow and ^{11}C]-palmitate uptake, reduced ^{11}C]-palmitate clearance, and a markedly increased FDG soon after reperfusion. The authors concluded that metabolic indices of ^{11}C]-palmitate kinetic and FDG uptake measured at the time of reperfusion could identify reversibly injured viable tissue before functional improvement.

In the dog model of 3 hours of balloon occlusion and 20 hours of reperfusion, Sochor et al[70] compared the amount of FDG uptake with microsphere blood flow and the extent of histologic necrosis. Reperfused myocardium had disproportionately higher rates of glucose utilization than did normal tissue. Uptake of FDG was highest in tissue with little or no necrosis compared with remote healthy tissue and drastically decreased as the fraction of necrotic cells exceeded 30%. Using D-6-[14C] glucose and L-U-[13C] lactate to determine the relative contributions of oxidative and nonoxidative glucose utilization and assessing myocardial glycogen content in tissue samples, Schwaiger et al[65] demonstrated that the increase in FDG uptake in reperfused myocardium corresponded to increased glycolytic flux and overall oxidative metabolism and to replenishment of glycogen stores. The metabolic abnormalities in reperfused myocardium were assessed quantitatively by Buxton et al[16,17] by using ^{11}C]-acetate, ^{13}N-ammonia, ^{11}C]-palmitate, and FDG. These experiments quantitatively clarified the time course of metabolic abnormalities and showed that after an initial reduction during ischemia, myocardial blood flow to reversibly injured myocardium returned to normal after 24 hours of reperfusion. Oxygen consumption was reduced during ischemia but not to the same extent as blood flow, remained depressed during reperfusion, and returned more slowly to normal tissue than blood flow. The time course of recovery of oxygen consumption paralleled that of regional wall motion. The glucose metabolic rate increased 24 hours after reperfusion in injured tissue compared with remote healthy tissue and was higher in reversibly damaged tissue than in permanently infarcted tissue. Palmitate time–activity curves were consistent with decreased fatty-acid oxidation and increased esterification in postischemic tissue.

These studies demonstrated the ability of PET to identify reversibly injured tissue early after acute myocardial ischemia and led to the clinical use of PET to identify viable myocardium after myocardial infarction in humans. These studies also aimed to delineate the underlying physiopathologic processes in reperfused myocardium. Unfortunately, these models studied a heterogeneous pattern of myocardial injury, and permanently injured tissue was produced. Another problem with these studies was the poor control of substrate availability and dietary state, which resulted in a variable pattern of glucose utilization in injured and remote normal tissue. Therefore, to study the underlying physiopathologic processes in dysfunctional but nonnecrotic tissue, more specific models must be designed. Such models are discussed in the following sections.

Myocardial stunning

Stunning is a form of reversible myocardial contractile dysfunction that occurs after restoration of myocardial blood flow following a relatively brief period of coronary occlusion.[72] Therefore, stunning represents a state of contraction–perfusion mismatch. Because myocardial stunning is believed to occur frequently in humans[9] after angioplasty and during attacks of unstable angina,[80] understanding its physiopathologic mechanisms is important. Stunning is thought to be a form of reperfusion injury whereby reintroduction of oxygen after a period of deprivation provokes transient calcium overload and damages the contractile machinery. Stunning is usually induced in open-chest or closed-chest animals after transient complete coronary occlusion and reperfusion. To obtain prolonged dysfunction, no-flow ischemia must last from 15 to 20 minutes. A longer duration of ischemia results in irreversible cell damage.

The severity of myocardial stunning depends markedly on the type of animal model used, the presence or absence of anesthetics, and body temperature.[75] Open-chest dogs anesthetized with barbiturates show greatly exaggerated severity and duration of myocardial stunning after 15 minutes of coronary occlusion that is approximately twice as severe as in the conscious dog. The time course of the recovery of contractile function is also quite different in the two models. In conscious dogs, recovery of function is gradual; it starts 1 hour after reperfusion and is almost complete after 4 hours of reperfusion. Open-chest dogs, however, have dysfunction that persists at almost the same level from 1 hour after reperfusion that lasts for several hours up to one day. Therefore, duration of ischemia must be long enough to perform PET studies in closed-chest animals to obtain a sustained period of dysfunction. Studies with PET of dysfunctional tissue performed in experimental models with prolonged coronary occlusion and reperfusion are not suitable for the study of myocardial stunning because the reperfused myocardium is composed of a mixture of permanently damaged and temporarily stunned myocardium. Furthermore, final recovery of function is incomplete.

Heyndrickx et al[72] postulated on the basis of their observations that a definite diagnosis of pure myocardial stunning implies gradual but complete recovery of function within days after full reperfusion and the absence of histologic evidence for myocardial necrosis. Studies using PET were performed in acutely stunned myocardium to understand metabolic utilization of substrate and the response to inotropic stimuli.

McFalls et al[46] studied acutely stunned myocardium in open-chest pigs by using [^{15}O]-water and FDG 2 and 24 hours after reperfusion following 20 minutes of occlusion of the LAD. Regional anterior wall motion was assessed by use of ultrasonic crystals, myocardial blood flow was quantified with the radioactive microspheres technique, and oxygen consumption was calculated from the arteriovenous difference in oxygen between arterial blood and the great cardiac vein. Uptake of FDG in acutely stunned myocardium was found to be decreased as compared with remote tissue 2 hours after reperfusion; that is, when MBF had already normalized. However, 24 hours after reperfusion, FDG uptake was found to be increased relative to perfusion. The ability of stunned myocardium to increase function under inotropic stimulation, such as paired pacing or β-agonist stimulation, has been used as a diagnostic procedure and serves as the basis for the dobutamine stress test, which is used to delineate viable myocardium.

Several studies aimed to determine the relation among flow, metabolism, and function in stunned myocardium and to assess regional myocardial efficiency. Bergmann et al[7] studied 12 closed-chest dogs kept under general anesthesia after 15 minutes of coronary occlusion by an angioplasty balloon catheter and subsequent reperfusion of the LAD. Measurements were performed 1 hour after reperfusion. Contractile function was assessed by two-dimensional echocardiography, perfusion was determined with the microsphere technique, and regional myocardial oxygen consumption was measured with [^{11}C]-acetate and PET. After baseline studies, hearts were subjected to in-

otropic stimulation by paired pacing from a bipolar pacing electrode placed at the apex of the right ventricle; stimulation was administered at a rate slightly faster than intrinsic heart rate. This procedure was chosen because it causes inotropy without altering systemic hemodynamics. Evaluation of two-dimensional echocardiograms showed severe hypokinesis or akinesis during the early reperfusion period. With paired pacing, wall motion substantially improved. At the time of dysfunction, myocardial blood flow had recovered to 83% ± 17% of the remote normal regions. With paired pacing, flow in both the reperfused and remote regions increased by 70%. Regional MVO$_2$ in reperfused regions averaged 71% ± 27% of that in remote myocardium at baseline. With paired pacing, oxidative metabolism almost doubled in reperfused myocardium. An index for regional myocardial efficiency was obtained from the calculated average wall thickening per unit of oxygen consumed. At rest, stunned myocardium operated inefficiently, using considerable amounts of oxygen for relatively little mechanical work. With pacing, efficiency improved to almost that observed in normal myocardium.

A similar study by Hashimoto et al[32] examined the effect of dobutamine on blood flow, oxygen consumption, and contractile function in stunned myocardium from 9 closed-chest dogs. Stunning was induced by 25 minutes of occlusion of the LAD by a balloon catheter followed by reperfusion. Microsphere flow and oxygen consumption were measured with [^{11}C]-acetate and contractile function was measured by two-dimensional echocardiography 2 hours after reperfusion; these measurements were repeated during dobutamine infusion adjusted to achieve a maximal steady-state rate–pressure product. Two hours after reperfusion, the myocardium remained hypokinetic or akinetic, whereas myocardial perfusion had already recovered, confirming the presence of myocardial stunning. However, this study found substantially lower myocardial perfusion in the postischemic myocardium than in remote control myocardium. During dobutamine infusion, contractile function of previously dysfunctional segments improved greatly. In contrast to the previous study, MVO$_2$ was decreased in stunned myocardium compared with normally contracting myocardium. Myocardial blood flow and MVO$_2$ increased greatly in remote and stunned myocardium under dobutamine infusion, with a greater increase in the stunned myocardium.

We recently investigated an alternative conscious model of provoking stunning in chronically instrumented dogs.[34] Instead of inducing ischemia by single or repeated episodes of total coronary occlusions of variable duration, we provoked a single 1-hour coronary artery stenosis by using a previously implanted hydraulic occluder. The dogs were studied 2 weeks after surgical instrumentation. Progressive inflation of the hydraulic cuff occluder was initiated, but complete coronary occlusion was avoided by monitoring a Doppler flow signal proximal to the occluder. The degree of stenosis was set so that it produced severe hypokinesia or akinesia in the posterior wall. The coronary stenosis was completely released after 1 hour. During cuff inflation, systolic wall thickening measured by using ultrasonic crystals in the ischemic zone was almost completely abolished and remained depressed, with progressive recovery during reperfusion. Systolic wall thickening was still depressed after 24 hours but recovered completely after 1 week. At the end of the experiments, the dogs were sacrificed, and the absence of necrosis in the dysfunctional region was confirmed. Another 18 dogs instrumented in a similar way were used to determine the time course of alterations in fatty-acid and oxygen metabolism in stunned myocardium. Dynamic PET using [^{11}C]-acetate and [^{11}C]-palmitate was performed at 6 hours (18 dogs), 12 hours (4 dogs), 24 hours (4 dogs), 1 week (8 dogs) and 2 weeks (4 dogs) after reperfusion. Although transmural microsphere flow did not differ between remote and stunned myocardial zones, significant prolongation of the ^{11}C-palmitate clearance half-time was found as early as 4 to 6 hours after reperfusion and persisted for up to 24 hours after reperfusion. The difference between postischemic and normal fatty-acid metabolism disappeared gradually with time and paralleled the recovery of function. Overall oxidative metabolism measured with [^{11}C]-acetate was found to be moderately reduced in stunned compared with remote myocardium.

In another 12 dogs, we studied oxidative metabolism and contractile function 4 to 8 hours after reperfusion and repeated this measurement during inotropic stimulation by norepinephrine infusion or chronotropic stimulation by rapid (195 ± 5 beats per minute [bpm]) right ventricular pacing. Norepinephrine increased contractile performance of normal and postischemic segments. On the contrary, right ventricular pacing (but not atrial pacing) decreased segmental wall thickening in stunned myocardium but did not change it in normal regions. Most important, despite these diverging mechanical responses, remote normal and postischemic segments showed a marked acceleration of [^{11}C]-acetate clearance, suggesting increased oxygen consumption. Calculated myocardial efficiency was lower in stunned myocardium than in normal myocardium but could be increased by administering norepinephrine.

Chronic regional ischemic contractile dysfunction in dogs

Chronic contractile dysfunction that is reversible upon reperfusion has been observed in persons with ischemic cardiomyopathy. This state has been termed *hibernating myocardium* by Diamond et al[21] and Rahimtoola.[52] According to Rahimtoola's hypothesis, hibernating myocardium results from a relatively uncommon response to reduced myocardial blood flow in which the heart downgrades its myocardial function so that blood flow and function are once again in equilibrium. As a result, neither myocardial necrosis nor ischemic symptoms are present. This type of low-flow state has been produced in animal models for short periods of time (up to several hours)[62] and was accompanied by sustained proportional reduction of contraction without myocardial necrosis. However, the animal models were very unstable: Superimposition of a chronotropic or inotropic stress increased lactate production, decreased high energy stores, and eventually caused myocardial necrosis.[63]

Until now, it has not been possible to develop a chronic animal model of hibernating myocardium; all models aimed at

producing chronic hypoperfusion have resulted in myocardial necrosis. Transient dysfunction in long-term animal models was observed in pigs after implantation of an ameroid occluder.[10,44] Implantation of a single ameroid occluder in dogs failed to produce contractile dysfunction because collateral circulation developed rapidly.[18,73,74] The underlying mechanism for the dysfunction seemed to involve repetitive episodes of myocardial stunning rather than a state of chronic hypoperfusion.[67]

Recently, we investigated a newly developed model aimed at inducing chronic contractile dysfunction in dogs.[27] Mongrel dogs were instrumented with ring occluders on the left anterior descending coronary artery (LAD) and two ameroid constrictors on the right coronary artery and left circumflex artery to produce a model of three-vessel disease and to reduce coronary flow reserve to a level at which collateral development would not prevent the appearance of dysfunction. To understand the physiopathology of the model, the animals were studied by PET and by M-mode echocardiography on 2 consecutive days before surgery and again at 6, 12, 18, and 24 weeks after implantation of the ameroid occluder. Resting transmural myocardial perfusion was assessed by using ^{13}NH$_3$, resting myocardial oxygen consumption was measured by using [^{11}C]-acetate, and resting glucose uptake was measured by using FDG under fasting conditions and under euglycemic hyperinsulinemic glucose clamp. Systolic wall thickening in the posterior wall (depending on collateral circulation) and interventricular septum (which was LAD dependent) was assessed by M-mode echocardiography at the time of PET. This model produced a substantially decreased thickening in the posterior wall (Fig. 5-9) of all instrumented dogs starting 6 weeks after ameroid occluder implantation, which decreased progressively with time and reached a minimum after 24 weeks at 36% + 12% of baseline values. Histologic observations at the end of the experi-

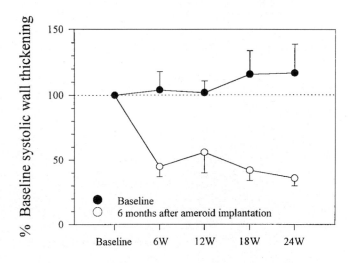

Fig. 5-9. Time course of development of myocardial dysfunction in a model of three-vessel disease in dogs after implantation of an ameroid occluder. (Courtesy of Gerber BL, Lock S, Melin JA, et al.)

ment confirmed the absence of myocardial infarction in all but one dog; this animal had a small subendocardial infarction that occupied only a small part of the dysfunctional region. Resting perfusion (Fig. 5-10), measured by ^{13}N-ammonia, and MVO$_2$, measured by [^{11}C]-acetate clearance, remained unchanged in the dysfunctional regions compared with the remote control region. The dogs showed a perfusion-contraction mismatch, demonstrated by the decreased function and maintained perfusion in the collateral-dependent region (Fig. 5-11). Glucose metabolism during fasting or under insulin stimulation remained similar in the dysfunctional compared with the normally contracting region. Flow reserve under adenosine infusion was assessed by using microsphere and ^{13}NH$_3$ flow at the end of the experiment (that is, 6 months after ameroid occluder implantation. Hyperemic blood flow was reduced in the collateral-dependent posterior wall compared with the interventricular septum both in the endocardium (206 ± 64 ml/min/100 g vs 529 ± 170 ml/min/100g, $p<0.05$) and the epicardium (359 ± 102 vs 663 ± 184 ml/min/100 g, $p<0.05$). The endocardial flow reserve was greatly lower than the epicardial flow reserve.

At the end of the experiment, the effect of dobutamine stimulation on contractile function, myocardial blood flow, and oxygen consumption was also assessed. A small amount of dobutamine infusion increased the rate pressure product approximately twofold, from 6200 ± 1680 to 12,992 ± 2617 ($p<0.001$). Thickening of the posterior wall substantially improved from 30% ± 8% to 69 ± 19%; values were similar to those in the interventricular septum. Myocardial perfusion increased from 57 ± 24 ml/min/100 g to 144 ± 30 ml/min/100 g in the posterior wall and from 56 ± 20 ml/min/100 g to 155 ± 42 ml/min/100 g in the interventricular septum; these values were not statistically significant. Oxygen consumption in the interventricular septum increased from 5.6 ± 1.6 ml/min/100g to 12.9 ± 3.8 ml/min/100 g) in the posterior wall and 5.6 ± 2.4 ml/min/100 g to 13.8 ± 3.7

ml/min/100 g; the p value was not significant compared with the posterior wall at rest and under the influence of dobutamine. Myocardial efficiency calculated from the ratio of calculated mechanical work to total oxygen consumption was decreased at rest in the dysfunctional segment and remained unchanged. Our investigation demonstrates that chronic localized hypokinesis of the posterior and lateral myocardial wall that is not related to infarction can develop in collateral-dependent myocardium in dogs. The data suggest the existence of a perfusion–contraction mismatch in this model. Resting perfusion and oxygen consumption remained normal, and flow reserve was reduced. The dysfunctional myocardium showed recruitable inotropic reserve when challenged with a low-dose dobutamine infusion. Thus, as previously observed in humans,[77] long-term collateral-dependent myocardium in dogs did not demonstrate chronic hypoperfusion at rest but did show reduced flow reserve. It can be assumed that the underlying physiopathologic mechanism for dysfunction in this model may be chronic repetitive stunning rather than chronic hypoperfusion.

Congestive heart failure

Spontaneously occurring cardiomyopathy[69] with silent left ventricular dysfunction as well as Duchenne's cardiomyopathy[47] have been observed in some dogs. However, these observations are too rare and too poorly documented to serve as models for congestive heart failure in man. Various experimental models of congestive heart failure have therefore been tried.[68] Models based on volume and pressure overload are technically complicated and yield unpredictable results. Today, the most widely used preparation is the model of rapid ventricular pacing in dogs[19,82] or pigs.[71] Very rapid ventricular pacing at rates of 240 to 280 bpm for 2 weeks produces hemodynamic and neurohumoral changes similar to those observed in humans with biventricular cardiac dysfunction. Left and right ventricu-

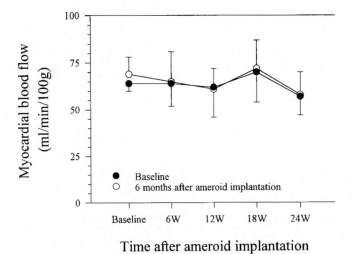

Fig. 5-10. Time course of myocardial perfusion measured by using positron emission tomography and nitrogen-13 ammonia in a model of three-vessel disease in dogs after implantation of an ameroid occluder. (Courtesy of Gerber BL, Lock S, Melin JA, et al.)

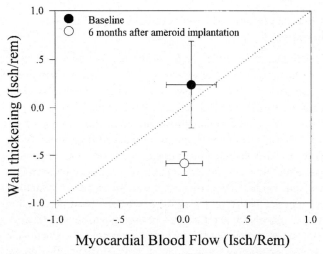

Fig. 5-11. Diagram illustrating the relation between reduction of perfusion and reduction of contraction in a model of three-vessel disease in dogs. The departure from the line clearly illustrates the existence of a perfusion–contraction mismatch. (Courtesy of Gerber BL, Lock S, Melin JA, et al.)

lar volumes are increased, cardiac output is increased, pulmonary wedge pressures are elevated, and left ventricular shortening is reduced. Pacing at high rates (260 bpm) cannot be maintained for more than 4 to 6 weeks because the animals rapidly die of pulmonary edema. At slightly lower pacing rates (220 to 240 bpm), moderate biventricular heart failure can be maintained for longer periods of time. Once pacing is discontinued, reduced cardiac output is observed for a short time, but pump function tends to recover. Although the mechanism underlying the dysfunction in this model is not entirely clear, it is assumed that it represents an abnormality of calcium metabolism or adenosine triphosphate (ATP) activity.

Another approach to producing congestive heart failure is by repeated microembolizations in dogs.[56] However, this procedure is technically demanding, relatively difficult to perform, and time consuming. Coronary microembolizations must be repeated five or six times during sequential cardiac catheterizations under general anesthesia over about 9 weeks to achieve a stable state of left ventricular dysfunction. After this time, hemodynamic and neurohumoral alterations slowly progress.

An approach to inducing left ventricular dysfunction is intravenous or intracoronary injection of Adriamycin.[45] This approach is preferable because it involves minimal systemic toxicity. Although such models of dilated cardiomyopathy would be good for repeated study by PET to assess the influence of medications[57] on oxygen consumption, blood flow, and receptor density, no such studies have been performed.

Denervated myocardium

Cardiac transplantation causes extrinsic cardiac denervation. Therefore, canine models of chronic denervated hearts can serve as models for alterations found in patients who have had heart transplantation.

Denervation of the canine heart can be obtained by different approaches, either surgically or chemically. The surgical approach has many variations.[22,53] Simple denervation of the sympathetic nerve system can be obtained by dissection and phenolization of the right and left stellate cervical ganglia. To denervate the parasympathetic nerve system, the vagal nerves are cut. For complete selective denervation of the myocardium without touching the nerve system of other organs, an intrapericardial technique can be used. Here, the connective tissue around the pulmonary artery is dissected and treated with phenol.[53] Denervation created by this procedure is complete; however, reinnervation of the atrium is noted 3 to 4 months after denervation. Nine to 14 months later, progressive ventricular sympathetic reinnervation occurs from the base to the apex. Regional sympathetic denervation of the heart can be obtained by touching the epicardial surface with phenol solution. The effect of chemical denervation is obtained by intravenous injection of 6-hydroxydopamine.[26] This compound selectively destroys sympathetic nerve endings and leaves vagal fibers unaffected. Because this compound produces a strong sympathomimetic effect, animals must be treated with propranolol and phentolamine.

Several metabolic modifications have been found after cardiac denervation. Stores of tissue catecholamines are depleted, and the heart develops supersensitivity to noradrenaline, probably because of lack of noradrenaline reuptake.[78] Myocardial oxygen consumption has been shown to be increased in vivo and Na$^+$,K$^+$ ATPase activity to be augmented in vitro.[13,24] However, under ischemic conditions the microregional heterogeneity of oxygenation in the ischemic heart is reduced, and ischemic injury is decreased.[1] In addition, glucose oxidation is inhibited.[3]

The function of a chronically denervated heart is normal except for blunted frequency response to changes in exercise level or other reflex demands on cardiac responsiveness.[22] Positron emission tomography studies using the false synthetic neurotransmitter [^{18}F]-fluorometariminol were performed in dogs that were chemically denervated with 6-hydroxydopamine or locally denervated with phenol. These studies showed reduced slow washout kinetics, indicating the inability of denervated neurons to retain this tracer. Adrenergic and muscarinic receptors were assessed by using ^{11}C-CPG1277 and ^{11}C-methylquinuclidinyl benzylate in surgically and chemically denervated dogs.[76] Measurements by PET were performed 3 to 7 weeks after denervation and were repeated 23 to 28 weeks thereafter. The study demonstrated prolonged upregulation of β-adrenergic receptors following heart denervation and absence of change in muscarinic receptor density after this procedure.

SUMMARY

This review aimed to inform the reader about the development and validation of PET tracers by using in vitro and in vivo models and to review models for different disease states that are used or are potentially useful for PET studies in large animals.

The basic procedures used to develop tracers for PET are discussed and are illustrated by four examples dealing with a metabolic tracer, a myocardial flow extraction tracer, a freely diffusible flow tracer, and a receptor tracer. The second part of the review discusses animal models that simulate various disease states in man, particularly acute ischemia and reperfusion, myocardial stunning, hibernating myocardium, congestive heart failure, and denervated myocardium. These examples show the usefulness of PET for the study of the pathophysiologic mechanisms of heart disease.

REFERENCES

1. Acad BA, Joselevitz-Goldman J, Scholz PM, et al: Improved distribution of regional oxygenation in denervated ischemic dog myocardium, *Circ Res* 62:1041–1048, 1988.
2. Allan RM et al: Myocardial metabolism of C11-acetate: Experimental and patient studies (abstract), *Circulation* 64 (suppl IV):75, 1981.
3. Armbrecht JJ, Buxton DB, and Schelbert HR: Validation of [$^{1-11}$C] acetate as a tracer for noninvasive assessment of oxidative metabolism with positron emission tomography in normal, ischemic, postischemic, and hyperemic canine myocardium, *Circulation* 81:1594–1605, 1990.
4. Bellina CR, Parodi O, Camici P, et al: Simultaneous in vitro and in vivo validation of nitrogen-13-ammonia for the assessment of regional myocardial blood flow, *J Nucl Med* 31:1335–1343, 1990.
5. Bergmann SR, Hack S, Tewson T, et al: The dependence of accumula-

tion of $^{13}NH_3$ by myocardium on metabolic factors and its implications for quantitative assessment of perfusion, *Circulation* 61:34–43, 1980.

6. Bergmann SR et al: Temporal dependence of beneficial effects of coronary thrombolysis characterized by positron tomography, *Medicine Sciences* 73:573–581, 1982.

7. Bergmann SR, Weinheimer CJ, Brown MA, et al: Enhancement of regional myocardial efficiency and persistence of perfusion, oxidative, and functional reserve with paired pacing of stunned myocardium, *Circulation* 89:2290–2296, 1994.

8. Bol A, Melin JA, Vanoverschelde JL, et al: Direct comparison of [^{13}N]ammonia and [^{15}O]water estimates of perfusion with quantification of regional myocardial blood flow by microspheres, *Circulation* 87:512–525, 1993.

9. Bolli R: Myocardial "stunning" in man, *Circulation* 86:1671–1691, 1992.

10. Bolukoglu H, Liedtke AJ, Nellis SH, et al: An animal model of chronic coronary stenosis resulting in hibernating myocardium, *Am J Physiol* 263(1 Pt 2):H20–H29, 1992.

11. Brown M, Marshall DR, Sobel BE, et al: Delineation of myocardial oxygen utilization with carbon-11-labeled acetate, *Circulation* 76:687–696, 1987.

12. Brown MA, Myears DW, and Bergmann SR: Noninvasive assessment of canine myocardial oxidative metabolism with carbon-11 acetate and positron emission tomography, *J Am Coll Cardiol* 12:1054–1063, 1988.

13. Butcher RG, Drake-Holland AJ, Wanless RB, et al: Effect of lack of noradrenaline on myocardial oxygen consumption in denervated dog hearts, *Cardiovasc Res* 21:515–520, 1987.

14. Buxton DR, Schwaiger M, Nguyen A, et al: Radiolabeled acetate as a tracer of myocardial tricarboxylic acid cycle flux, *Circ Res* 63:628–634, 1988.

15. Buxton DB, Nienaber CA, Luxen A, et al: Noninvasive quantitation of regional myocardial oxygen consumption in vivo with [1-11C]acetate and dynamic positron emission tomography, *Circulation* 79:134–142, 1989.

16. Buxton DB, Mody FV, Krivokapich J, et al: Quantitative assessment of prolonged metabolic abnormalities in reperfused canine myocardium, *Circulation* 85:1842–1856, 1992.

17. Buxton DB and Schelbert HR: Measurement of regional glucose metabolic rates in reperfused myocardium, *Am J Physiol* 261(6 Pt 2):H2058–H2068, 1991.

18. Canty JM Jr and Klocke FJ: Reductions in regional myocardial function at rest in conscious dogs with chronically reduced regional coronary artery pressure, *Circ Res* 61(5 Pt 2):II107–II116, 1987.

19. Coleman HN 3d, Taylor RR, Pool PE, et al: Congestive heart failure following chronic tachycardia, *Am Heart J* 81:790–798, 1971.

20. Consigny PM, Verrier ED, Payne BD, et al: Acute and chronic microsphere loss from canine left ventricular myocardium, *Am J Physiol* 242: H392–H404, 1982.

21. Diamond GA, Forrester JS, deLuz PL, et al: Post-extrasystolic potentiation of ischemic myocardium by atrial stimulation, *Am Heart J* 95:204–209, 1978.

22. Donald DE and Shepherd JT: Response to exercise in dogs with cardiac denervation, *Am J Physiol* 205:393–400, 1963.

23. Drake AJ, Papadoyannis DE, Butcher RG, et al: Inhibition of glycolysis in the denervated heart, *Circ Res* 47:338–345, 1980.

24. Drake AJ, Stubbs J, and Noble MIM: Dependence of myocardial blood flow and metabolism on cardiac innervation, *Cardiovasc Res* 12:69–80, 1978.

25. Engler RL, Schmid-Schonbein GW, and Pavelec RS: Leukocyte capillary plugging in myocardial ischemia and reperfusion in the dog, *Am J Pathol* 111:98–111, 1983.

26. Gauthier P, Nadeau R, and De Champlain J: Acute and chronic cardiovascular effects of 6-hydroxydopamine in dogs, *Circ Res* 31:207–217, 1972.

27. Gerber BL, Coycock S, Melin JA, et al: Physiopathological investiga-

tion of a canine model of dysfunctional myocardium, *Circulation* 92:I-314 (abstract), 1995.

28. Gould KL et al: Noninvasive assessment of coronary stenoses with myocardial perfusion imaging during pharmacologic coronary vasodilation. V. Detection of 47 percent diameter coronary stenosis with intravenous nitrogen-13 ammonia and emission-computed tomography in intact dogs, *Am J Cardiol* 43:200–208, 1979.

29. Hariharan R, Bray M, Ganim R, et al: Fundamental limitations of [^{18}F]2-deoxy-2-fluoro-D-glucose for assessing myocardial glucose uptake, *Circulation* 91:2435–2444, 1995.

30. Harper PV, Lathrop KA, Krizek H, et al: Clinical feasibility of myocardial imaging with 13 NH 3, *J Nucl Med* 13:278–280, 1972.

31. Harper PV, Schwartz J, Beck RW, et al: Clinical myocardial imaging with nitrogen-13 ammonia, *Radiology* 108:613–617, 1973.

32. Hashimoto T, Buxton DB, Krivokapich J, et al: Responses of blood flow, oxygen consumption, and contractile function to inotropic stimulation in stunned canine myocardium, *Am Heart J* 127(5):1250–1262, 1994.

33. Herrero P, Staudenherz A, Walsh JF, et al: Heterogeneity of myocardial perfusion provides the physiological basis of perfusable tissue index, *J Nucl Med* 36:320–327, 1995.

34. Heyndrickx GR, Wijns W, Vogelaers D, et al: Recovery of regional contractile function and oxidative metabolism in stunned myocardium induced by 1-hour circumflex coronary artery stenosis in chronically instrumented dogs, *Circ Res* 72:901–913, 1993.

35. Hoffmann EJ, Huang SC, and Phelps ME: Quantitation in positron emission tomography. 1. Effect of object size, *J Comput Assist Tomogr* 3:299–308, 1979.

36. Hutchins GD, Schwaiger M, Rosenspire KC, et al: Noninvasive quantification of regional blood flow in the human heart using N-13 ammonia and dynamic positron emission tomographic imaging, *J Am Coll Cardiol* 15:1032–1042, 1990.

37. Jeremy RW, Links JM, and Becker LC: Progressive failure of coronary flow during reperfusion of myocardial infarction: documentation of the no reflow phenomenon with positron emission tomography, *J Am Coll Cardiol* 16:695–704, 1990.

38. Kloner RA, Ganote CE, and Jennings RB: The "no-reflow" phenomenon after temporary coronary occlusion in the dog, *J Clin Invest* 54:1496–1508, 1974.

39. Krivokapich J, Huang SC, Phelps ME, et al: Dependence of $^{13}NH_3$ myocardial extraction and clearance on flow and metabolism, *Am J Physiol* 242:H536–H542, 1982.

40. Krivokapich J, Barrio JR, Phelps ME, et al: Kinetic characterization of $^{13}NH_3$ and ^{13}N-glutamine metabolism in rabbit heart, *Am J Physiol* 246(2 Pt 2):H267–H273, 1984.

41. Krivokapich J, Smith GT, Huang SC, et al: ^{13}N ammonia myocardial imaging at rest and with exercise in normal volunteers. Quantification of absolute myocardial perfusion with dynamic positron emission tomography, *Circulation* 80:1328–1337, 1989.

42. Kuhle WG, Porenta G, Huang SC, et al: Quantification of regional myocardial blood flow using ^{13}N-ammonia and reoriented dynamic positron emission tomographic imaging, *Circulation* 86:1004–1017, 1992.

43. Lerch RA, Ambos HD, Bergmann JR, et al: Localization of viable, ischemic myocardium by positron-emission tomography with ^{11}C-palmitate, *Circulation* 64:689–698, 1981.

44. Liedtke AJ, Renstrom B, Nellis SH, et al: Mechanical and metabolic functions in pig hearts after 4 days of chronic coronary stenosis, *J Am Coll Cardiol* 26:815–825, 1995.

45. Magovern JA, Christlieb IV, Badylale SF, et al: A model of left ventricular dysfunction caused by intracoronary adriamycin, *Ann Thorac Surg* 53:861–863, 1992.

46. McFalls EO, Ward H, Fashingbauer P, et al: Myocardial blood flow and FDG retention in acutely stunned porcine myocardium, *J Nucl Med* 36:637–643, 1995.

47. Moise NS, Valentine BA, Brown CA, et al: Duchenne's cardiomyopa-

thy in a canine model: electrocardiographic and echocardiographic studies, *J Am Coll Cardiol* 17:812–820, 1991.

48. Monahan WG, Tilbury RS, and Laughlin JS: Uptake of 13 N-labeled ammonia, *J Nucl Med* 13:274–277, 1972.

49. Muzik O, Beanlands RS, Hutchins GD, et al: Validation of nitrogen-13-ammonia tracer kinetic model for quantification of myocardial blood flow using PET, *J Nucl Med* 34:83–91, 1993.

50. Ng CK, Huang SC, Schelbert HR, et al: Validation of a model for [1-^{11}C]acetate as a tracer of cardiac oxidative metabolism, *Am J Physiol* 266(4 Pt 2):H1304–H1315, 1994.

51. Pike VW, Eakins MN, Allan RM, et al: Preparation of [1-11C]acetate—an agent for the study of myocardial metabolism by positron emission tomography, *Int J Appl Radiat Isot* 33:505–512, 1982.

52. Rahimtoola S: The hibernating myocardium, *Am Heart J* 117:211–221, 1989.

53. Randall WC, Kaye MP, Thomas JX, et al: Intrapericardial denervation of the heart, *J Surg Res* 29:101–109, 1980.

54. Randle PJ, England PJ, and Denton RM: Control of the tricarboxylate cycle and its interaction with glycolysis during acetate utilization in rat heart, *Biochem J* 117:677–695, 1970.

55. Rosenspire KC, Schwaiger M, Mangner TJ, et al: Metabolic fate of [^{13}N]-ammonia in human and canine blood, *J Nucl Med* 31:163–167, 1990.

56. Sabbah HN, Stein PD, Kono T, et al: A canine model of chronic heart failure produced by multiple sequential coronary microembolizations, *Am J Physiol* 260(4 Pt 2):H1379–1384, 1991.

57. Sabbah HN, Shimoyama H, Kono T, et al: Effects of long-term monotherapy with enalapril, metoprolol, and digoxin on the progression of left ventricular dysfunction and dilation in dogs with reduced ejection fraction, *Circulation* 89:2852–2859, 1994.

58. Schelbert HR, Phelps ME, Hoffman EJ, et al: Regional myocardial perfusion assessed with N-13 labelled ammonia and positron emission computerized axial tomography, *Am J Cardiol* 43:209–218, 1979.

59. Schelbert HR, Phelps ME, Huang SC, et al: N-13 ammonia as an indicator of myocardial blood flow, *Circulation* 63:1259–1272, 1981.

60. Schelbert HR, Henze E, Phelps ME, et al: Assessment of regional myocardial ischemia by positron-emission tomography, *Am Heart J* 103:588–597, 1982.

61. Schelbert HR, Henze E, Keen R, et al: C-11 palmitate for the noninvasive evaluation of region retention in myocardium, *Circulation* 63:1259–1272, 1981.

62. Schulz R, Guth BD, Pieper K, et al: Recruitment of an inotropic reserve in moderately ischemic myocardium at the expense of metabolic recovery. A model of short-term hibernation, *Circ Res* 70:1282–1295, 1992.

63. Schulz R, Rose J, Martin G, et al: Development of short-term myocardial hibernation. Its limitation by the severity of ischemia and inotropic stimulation, *Circulation* 88:684–695, 1993.

64. Schwaiger M, Schelbert HR, Ellison D, et al: Sustained regional abnormalities in cardiac metabolism after transient ischemia in the chronic dog model, *J Am Coll Cardiol* 6:336–347, 1985.

65. Schwaiger M, Neese RA, Araujo L, et al: Sustained nonoxidative glucose utilization and depletion of glycogen in reperfused canine myocardium, *J Am Coll Cardiol* 13:745–754, 1989.

66. Shah A, Schelbert HR, Schwaiger M, et al: Measurement of regional myocardial blood flow with N-13 ammonia and positron-emission tomography in intact dogs, *J Am Coll Cardiol* 5:92–100, 1985.

67. Shen YT and Vatner SF: Mechanism of impaired myocardial function during progressive coronary stenosis in conscious pigs. Hibernation versus Stunning? *Circ Res* 76:479–488, 1995.

68. Smith HJ and Nuttall A: Experimental models of heart failure, *Cardiovasc Res* 19:181–186, 1985.

69. Smucker M et al: Naturally occurring cardiomyopathy in the Doberman pinscher: a possible large animal model of human cardiomyopathy? *J Am Coll Cardiol* 16:200–206, 1990.

70. Sochor H, Schwaiger M, Schelbert HR, et al: Relationship between Tl-201, Tc-99m (Sn) pyrophosphate and F-18 2-deoxyglucose uptake in ischemically injured dog myocardium, *Am Heart J* 114:1066–1077, 1987.

71. Spinale F, Hendrick DA, Crawford FA, et al: Chronic supraventricular tachycardia causes ventricular dysfunction and subendocardial injury in swine, *Am J Physiol* 258(1 Pt 2):H218–H229, 1990.

72. Swain JA, Heyndrickx GR, Boettcher DH, et al: Prostaglandin control of renal circulation in the unanesthetized dog and baboon, *Am J Physiol* 229:826–830, 1975.

73. Tomoike H, Franklin D, Kemper WS, et al: Functional evaluation of coronary collateral development in conscious dogs, *Am J Physiol* 241:H519–H524, 1981.

74. Tomoike H, Li XY, Jamaluddin U, et al: Functional significance of collaterals during ameroid induced coronary stenosis in conscious dogs. Interrelationships among regional shortening, regional flow and grade of coronary stenosis, *Circulation* 67:1001–1008, 1983.

75. Triana JF, et al: Postischemic myocardial "stunning." Identification of major differences between the open-chest and the conscious dog and evaluation of the oxygen radical hypothesis in the conscious dog, *Circ Res* 69:731–747, 1991.

76. Valette H, DeLeuze P, Syrota A, et al: Canine myocardial beta-adrenergic, muscarinic receptor densities after denervation: a PET study, *J Nucl Med* 36:140–146, 1995.

77. Vanoverschelde JL, Wijns W, Depre C, et al: Mechanisms of chronic regional postischemic dysfunction in humans. New insights from the study of noninfarcted collateral-dependent myocardium, *Circulation* 87:1513–1523, 1993.

78. Vatner DE, Lavallee M, Amano J, et al: Mechanisms of supersensitivity to sympathomimetic amines in the chronically denervated heart of the conscious dog, *Circ Res* 57:55–64, 1985.

79. Walsh WF, Harper PV, Resnekov L, et al: Noninvasive evaluation of regional myocardial perfusion in 112 patients using a mobile scintillation camera and intravenous nitrogen-13 labeled ammonia, *Circulation* 54:266–275, 1976.

80. Wijns W, Vanoverschelde JL, Gerber DL, et al: Evidence that myocardial stunning occurs in humans following unstable angina, *J Am Coll Cardiol* 2:427A, 1995.

81. Williamson JR: Effects of insulin and starvation on the metabolism of acetate and pyruvate by the perfused rat heart, *Biochem J* 93:97–106, 1964.

82. Wilson JR, Douglas P, Hickey WF, et al: Experimental congestive heart failure produced by rapid ventricular pacing in the dog: cardiac effects, *Circulation* 75:857–867, 1987.

Chapter 6

Fatty acid analogs

Tsunehiko Nishimura

The main substrates of myocardial metabolism are glucose, fatty acids, and lactate. Long-chain fatty acids constitute the principal substrate for myocardial oxygen consumption and provide 60% to 80% of the energy utilized by the heart in the resting state.[61,63] Thus, assessment of fatty acid metabolism may help elucidate the causes of loss of myocardial function and cell death in coronary artery disease and cardiomyopathy. Furthermore, in clinical settings, delineation of metabolic changes may permit early recognition of cellular dysfunction in patients, improve disease management, and facilitate assessment of therapeutic effects.[53,69,70]

Accordingly, methods have been developed to assess the uptake and clearance of radiolabeled long-chain fatty acids to trace myocardial metabolism. The physiologic properties of ^{11}C-palmitate together with the intrinsic quantification characteristics of positron emission tomography (PET) have provided a promising approach that not only permits imaging of the myocardium but also may provide information on regional fatty acid metabolism noninvasively.[23,84] However, only institutions equipped with a PET scanner and in-house cyclotron can study myocardial fatty acid metabolism in humans; consequently, many attempts have been made to determine the metabolic integrity of myocardium with radioiodinated free fatty acids.

Myocardial imaging in humans with fatty acids was first demonstrated in 1965 by using ^{131}I iodine (I)-131–labeled oleic acid.[11] This approach did not gain widespread acceptance in part because of the relatively low extraction of the tracer compared with natural fatty acids.[71] The use of radioiodinated fatty acids for myocardial imaging has interested many investigators ever since these early studies were done. Radiolabeling with ^{123}I causes relatively modest structural alterations; moreover, because it has excellent imaging properties and there are many chemical methods available for attaching it to organic molecules, ^{123}I is the best radioisotope for fatty acid labeling in single-photon emission computed tomography (SPECT). Moreover, high-purity ^{123}I is routinely available, and decreasing cost is expected to increase availability and use.

Until the last decade, studies focused on ^{123}I-labeled iodoalkyl-substituted straight-chain fatty acids. These analogs are rapidly metabolized in the myocardium, resulting in the release of free radioiodine, and can be used for planar imaging. Terminal iodophenyl-substituted fatty acids illustrate a successful approach to stabilizing radioiodine to overcome the release of free iodine. Various modified straight-chain fatty acids have been developed and are now in clinical use for planar imaging and SPECT. Furthermore, the introduction of methyl branching is a major important approach to altering the tracer kinetics of radioiodinated free fatty acids by imaging myocardial retention. A key example of this class of compounds is 15-(p-iodophenyl)-3-R,S-methylpentadecanoic acid (BMIPP), an analog of 15-(p-iodophenyl) pentadecanoic acid (IPPA), in which methyl branching has been introduced into the β position of the carbon chain. Furthermore, the long period of tracer retention of these branched-chain fatty acids makes SPECT feasible.

Radioiodine-labeled fatty acids have therefore received the greatest attention among the candidates for application in SPECT as a means of investigating myocardial metabolism. In this chapter, the development of various radioiodinated fatty acids is reviewed and the effects of their molecular structure on myocardial uptake and release kinetics are related to clinical application.

MYOCARDIAL FATTY ACID METABOLISM

To accurately understand the tracer kinetics of various radioiodinated free fatty acids, it is necessary to briefly review a simplified scheme of myocardial lipid metabolism (Fig. 6-1).

Free fatty acids are transported in plasma that is loosely bound to serum albumin. Extraction of fatty acids by the myocardium is dependent on the ratio of free fatty acids to albumin, the length of the free fatty acid chain, and saturation of free fatty acids. The mechanism by which fatty acids cross the sarcolemma is not precisely known, but a concentration gradient between the interstitial and the cytoplasmic compartments is required.[63,70] This gradient is maintained by the steady supply of free fatty acids from the coronary circulation and removal of the cytoplasmic pool by metabolic reaction. Extracted fatty acids may diffuse back into the vascular space.[14,83]

The initial step in intracellular metabolism is thioesterification with coenzyme A (CoA). There are two major pathways for further metabolism of long-chain acyl CoA. The first pathway is transfer into the mitochondrial matrix mediated by the carnitine translocase system followed by β-oxidation and metabolism to carbon dioxide (CO_2) in the tricarboxylic acid (TCA) cycle. The second pathway involves incorporation into triglyceride or phospholipid. The relative size of the acyl CoA fraction channeled into oxidation compared with the fraction undergoing storage varies with the rate of oxidative phosphorylation, levels of myocardial acyl CoA, presence of alternative substrate, and availability of glycolytically produced α-glycerol phosphate for triglyceride synthesis. Accordingly, the oxidized fraction of extracted fatty acid depends on such factors as relative plasma concentration, work load, availability of oxygen, and hormonal influences.[62,63,69]

During fasting, free fatty acid accounts for 60% to 80% of total oxygen consumption. After feeding, insulin levels increase and plasma fatty acid levels decrease because of inhibition of lipolysis by insulin. The combination of a decrease in plasma free fatty acid levels and an increase in plasma glucose supply insulin levels leads to increased glucose utilization and decreased fatty acid utilization.[23]

During ischemia, the rate of myocardial β-oxidation decreases substantially according to the severity of flow reduction and duration of ischemia. This results from several factors. First, pyruvate is preferentially metabolized to lactate, increasing accumulation of pyruvate while simultaneously decreasing its availability from the TCA cycle. Together, these factors de-

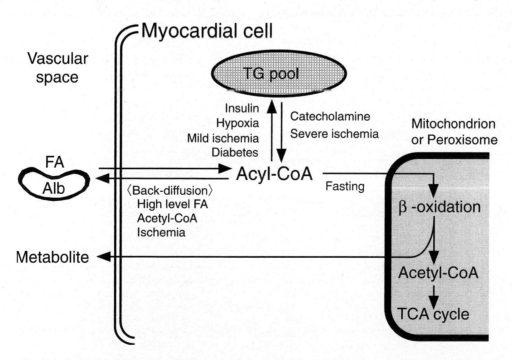

Fig. 6-1. Schema of free fatty acid metabolism. Free fatty acids *(FA)* are transported in plasma bound to serum albumin. The initial step in intracellular metabolism is thioesterification with coenzyme A *(CoA)*. There are two major pathways for further metabolism of long-chain acyl CoA: 1. Transfer into the mitochondrial matrix mediated by the carnitine translocase system followed by β-oxidation and metabolism to carbon dioxide in the tricarboxylic acid cycle. 2. Incorporation into triglyceride or phospholipid. The oxidized fraction of extracted fatty acid depends on such factors as plasma concentration, work load, availability of oxygen, and hormonal influences.

crease TCA cycle activity.[69,70] Furthermore, levels of free CoA are decreased, reducing thioesterification. High lactate levels also inhibit thiokinase.[83] These factors limit the ability of myocardium to extract and retain long-chain fatty acids, and decrease its ability to metabolize them once they are extracted. Early in ischemia, α-glycerol phosphate accumulates because of increased glycolytic flux, thereby enhancing the storage of free fatty acids in triglyceride form. Late in ischemia, α-glycerol phosphate levels decrease, inhibiting the trapping of free fatty acids in the myocardium.[69]

RADIOLABELED FATTY ACID ANALOGS

The chemical structures of the different types of radioiodinated fatty acids discussed in this chapter are illustrated in Table 6-1. There are iodoalkyl-substituted straight-chain fatty acid analogs, iodophenyl straight-chain fatty acid analogs, and iodophenyl methyl-branched fatty acid analogs.[44] The pharmacokinetics of representative radioiodinated fatty acid analogs are illustrated in Table 6-2. The effects of fatty acid structure on the kinetics of myocardial release of metabolites (time–activity curves) are illustrated in Fig. 6-2.

IODOALKYL-SUBSTITUTED STRAIGHT-CHAIN FATTY ACIDS

16-iodo-9-hexadecanoic acid

Iodoalkyl-substituted straight-chain fatty acids were developed to evaluate fatty acid metabolism by myocardial washout analysis with planar imaging. An early example of an iodoalkyl-substituted straight-chain analog is 16-[^{131}I]-iodo-9-hexadecanoic acid.[72] Although this fatty acid is rapidly degraded in the myocardium, it was used in early patient studies.[73]

Table 6-1. Chemical structure of representative iodine-123–labeled straight-chain and branched-chain fatty acid analogs

Iodoalkyl straight or methyl-branched chain fatty acids

IHA — 16-Iodo-9-hexadecanoic acid

IHDA — 17-Iodoheptadecanoic acid

IMHA — 16-Iodo-3-methylhexadecanoic acid

Iodophenyl straight-chain fatty acids

p-IPPA — 15-(p-Iodophenyl) pentadecanoic acid

o-IPPA — 15-(o-Iodophenyl) pentadecanoic acid

Iodophenyl methyl-branched chain fatty acids

BMIPP — 15-(p-Iodophenyl)-3-(R,S)-methylpentadecanoic acid

9MPA — 15-(p-Iodophenyl)-9-(R,S)-methylpentadecanoic acid

Table 6-2. Comparison of pharmacokinetic data for radioiodinated IHDA, IPPA, and BMIPP

Chemical name and structure	First-pass extraction fraction	Heart clearance, $T_{1/2}$ (min)	Myocardial catabolism	Oxidative fraction, %
IHDA $^{123}I\text{-}(CH_2)_{16}\text{-}COOH$	Dog[27]: ~0.50 Dog[86]: 0.54±0.12	Human[17]: 24±4.7 Dog[89]: 11.2 Dog[86]: 1st, 9.3±2.8; 2nd, 245±158	Inorganic I-123(iodide) is rapidly released by β-oxidation[33]	Dog[27]: ~75 Dog[86]: 45±22
IPPA $^{123}I\text{-}\langle\text{⬡}\rangle\text{-}(CH_2)_{14}\text{-}COOH$	Dog[3]: 0.72±0.06	Dog[3]: 13.2 Baboon[7]: 1st, 24.0±2.6; 2nd, 90.0±11.1 Human[97]: 1st; 35±27 2nd; 58±1	p-Iodobenzoic acid, ω-(p-iodophenyl)-propenoic acid and ω-(p-iodophenyl)-propionic acid are released by β-oxidation[10,85]	Human[29]: 14.2±5.8 (30 min) Human[6]: 17±2 (30 min) Baboon[7]: 47 (60 min)
BMIPP $^{123}I\text{-}\langle\text{⬡}\rangle\text{-}(CH_2)_{12}\text{-}\overset{\overset{\displaystyle CH_3}{\mid}}{CH}\text{-}CH_2\text{-}COOH$	Dog[21]: 0.740±0.107	Rat[61]: 152 Baboon[8]: 1st, 55.5±19.3; 2nd, 132.5±35.0	p-Iodophenyl-acetic acid and intermediary metabolites are released by initial α-oxidation and subsequent cycles of β-oxidation[98]	Human[58]: 13.0±1.0 (3 h) Human[4]: 18.2±7.5 (3 h) Baboon[8]: 10 (1 h)

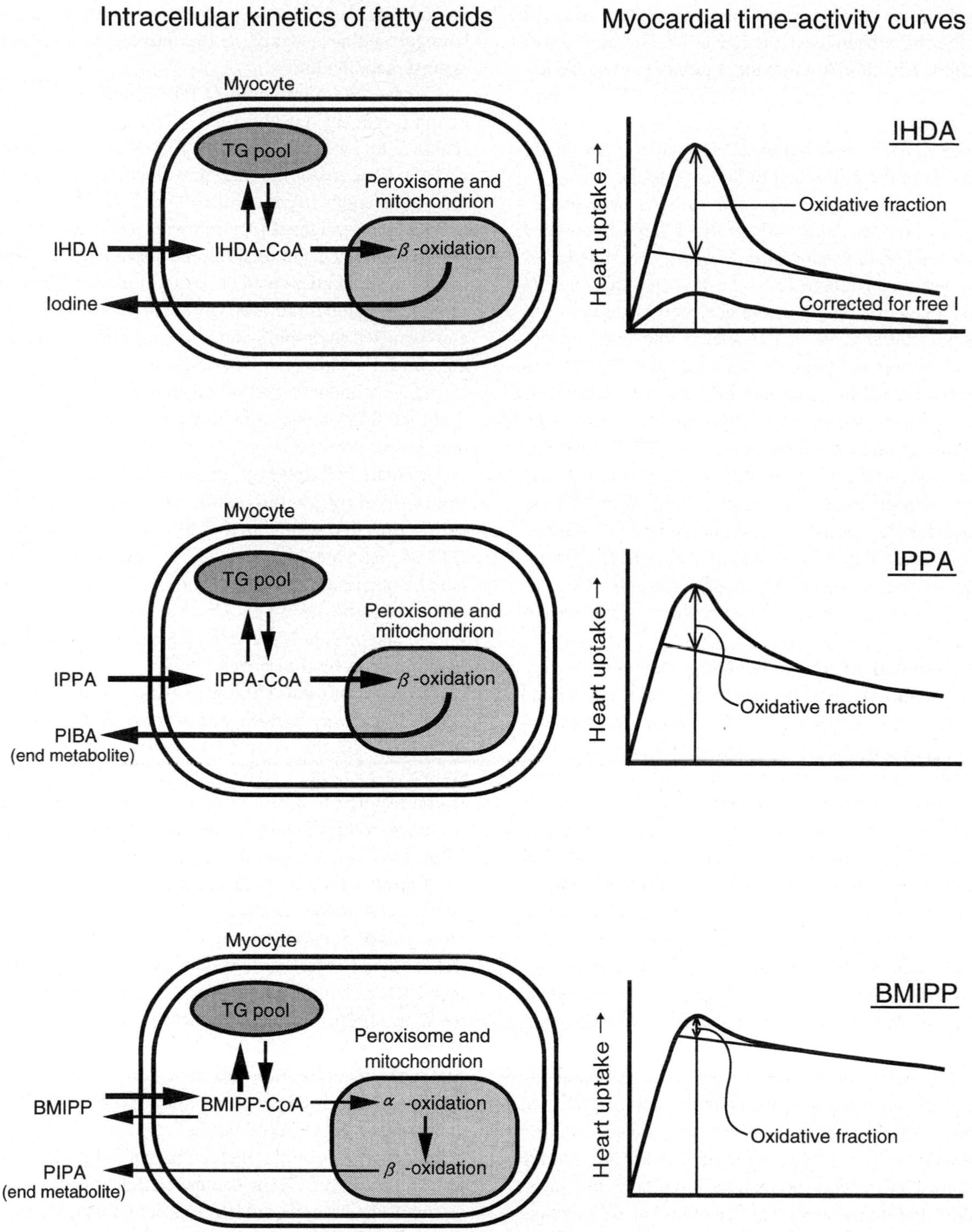

Intracellular kinetics of fatty acids

Myocardial time-activity curves

Fig. 6-2. Effects of structure modifications on intracellular fatty acid metabolism and the observed myocardial kinetics of fatty acid analogs.

17-iodoheptadecanoic acid (IHDA)

Cardiac metabolism of IHDA. The IHDA agent is an analog of stearic acid, because the terminal iodine substituent is about the same size as a methyl group.[17] Several animal studies indicated that a large fraction of the iodine is rapidly liberated in the myocardium after intravenous injection of IHDA. It was assumed that IHDA enhances the rate of transfer of fatty acids into β-oxidation in mitochondria compared with fatty acid uptake into complex lipids. The time–activity curve after correction for the relatively large amount of free myocardial iodine indicates uptake of labeled fatty acids into myocardial lipids and the rate of release from myocardial lipids.[86,89,94,96]

Although techniques to correct for free radioiodine released from catabolites have been used, the rate at which free ^{123}I was transported from mitochondria into the capillary system and appeared in circulating blood after β-oxidation of IHDA remained to be established.[22,27]

Dual-tracer analysis used IHDA labeled with ^{131}I in the ω-position and ^{14}C in the 1-position to investigate the rate of release of free iodine from myocardial cells into the capillary circulation.[12,33] The results demonstrated that a large fraction of injected IHDA is rapidly catabolized, with quick release of catabolically generated iodine from the myocardium into the venous blood together with CO_2 from the same substrate, without recognizable differences in the release rate over the observed period. Almost no iodine is liberated from IHDA without β-oxidation. Free iodine entering the coronary artery is initially distributed in the myocardium with a delayed release rate.

A proper correction technique was devised, and the resulting time–activity curve indicates uptake, peak accumulation, and substrate loss from the total of myocardial lipids with different turnover rates for the various lipid components.[17,34] Various methods of analyzing IHDA time–activity curves have been applied. Application of these methods to ischemic animal studies has revealed an altered oxidative–storage pattern on the basis of IHDA time–activity curve analysis.

IHDA in clinical practice. Several patient studies performed at rest with IHDA demonstrated decreased uptake and reduced clearance of radioactivity and decreased relative oxidative size or component ratios.[75,95] Thus, IHDA has been useful in diagnosing coronary artery disease on the basis of tracer kinetics.[17,18] Other investigators, however, found a weak relation between clearance rate and improvement in ventricular function in assessment of myocardial viability.[82,91] These conflicting results may be attributable to the inability of straight-chain fatty acids to differentiate between metabolism, which encompasses β-oxidation or incorporation into the lipid pool, and back-diffusion. Studies in patients with congestive cardiomyopathy done by using IHDA indicate that regional uptake is not homogenously reduced and that clearance from the myocardium is altered.[34,74]

Because IHDA has been a useful approach to metabolic imaging over the last 20 years, many investigators evaluated the metabolism of this tracer in animal and human studies. However, because of the inability to apply it to SPECT and the need for special correction procedures involving the intravenous administration of sodium [^{123}I] iodine to differentiate the myocardial mass from free blood activity, its use in clinical settings has decreased.

Iodophenyl straight-chain fatty acids

15-(p-iodophenyl) pentadecanoic acid (IPPA). To stabilize the ^{123}I attached to fatty acid and to overcome the rapid loss of free radioiodine, Machulla et al[54] developed IPPA as an alternative for myocardial metabolic studies. The development of a ω-phenyl–substituted straight-chain fatty acid involved attachment of radioiodine at the para-position of the terminal phenyl ring.[54,55] Because the carbon–iodine chemical bond is stronger, iodine attached in this manner is considered stable against deiodination.

Cardiac metabolism of IPPA. Rapid uptake of 4% to 5% of intravenously injected IPPA in rat myocardium was found within 2 to 3 minutes and was followed by rapid myocardial washout. The major cardiac lipid fractions are rapidly labeled after intravenous injection of IPPA.[80,81] Cardiac metabolism of IPPA was investigated together with a standard free fatty acid (^{14}C-palmitic acid) in dual-tracer experiments to compare both tracers in an identical metabolic environment.[79] The uptake and turnover of global radioactivity incorporated into myocardium and extracted hydrophilic and lipophilic metabolites correlated significantly. Thus, the kinetic behavior of IPPA in the myocardium is similar to that of the natural fatty acids.

Initial IPPA uptake is mainly governed by regional myocardial blood flow in normally perfused and acutely ischemic myocardium.[3,81] However, the rate of binding to CoA and the rate of tracer release through β-oxidation seemed to be slightly slower than that seen with ^{14}C-palmitate.[78] In the myocardium, IPPA is degraded to short-chain catabolites (mainly iodine-labeled benzoic acid) that are released rapidly from this tissue and excreted by the kidney. Catabolite recirculation is thus minimized and does not interfere with external local measurement of myocardial lipid turnover.[10,49,85]

IPPA in animal studies. Uptake of IPPA in reperfused myocardium was investigated in experiments in dogs.[87] Although all of the control dogs with permanent occlusion showed a concordant reduction of IPPA and flow tracer, reperfusion restored both IPPA and flow tracer compared with preocclusion values. Thus, sustained regional cardiac uptake of IPPA was found in potentially salvageable myocardium after short-term occlusion of a coronary artery. In addition, in a swine heart model perfused by using the Langendorff technique, myocardial free fatty acid utilization decreased during ischemia and increased considerably with reperfusion.[46] This increase was similar to the increase in glucose utilization. Furthermore, IPPA injected during reperfusion was retained in viable myocardium in relation to regional myocardial blood flow. Metabolic incorporation into myocardial lipids allowed clear discrimination among control tissue, reversibly ischemic tissue, and irreversible damaged tissue.[46]

Regional myocardial metabolism of IPPA has been assessed by means of SPECT in canine experiments.[77] Normal myocardium shows uniform left ventricular uptake and homogenous clearance. Myocardial infarcts are visualized as areas of deficient accumulation of radioactivity. Regional elimination, expressed in half-time of IPPA clearance as determined by SPECT, was substantially prolonged in reperfused myocardium. These findings suggest a potential role of IPPA in SPECT for noninvasive identification of reversible tissue injury in reperfused myocardium.

IPPA in clinical practice. Recent studies on the detection of coronary artery disease have used a maximal stress protocol to induce acute ischemia.[28] However, the results are somewhat disappointing, possibly because of increased serum lactate levels.[90] These factors initially suggested that a submaximal stress protocol could be used to enhance tracer uptake rather than to induce acute ischemia. Clinical use of this tracer has the added advantage that SPECT can be performed, although the timing of the tomographic period must be carefully controlled, especially during stress. Because of the convenience of using IPPA (there is no need to correct for catabolites) and the similarities in metabolism of ^{11}C-palmitate, IPPA has been more widely used clinically than IHDA, mainly to diagnose coronary artery disease.[30,58,97]

The sensitivity of this approach to the evaluation of tracer accumulation and turnover as a means of diagnosing coronary artery disease was found to be at least as good as exercise-redistribution thallium-201 (^{201}Tl) imaging.[6,35] Studies at rest have recently been suggested to be useful in conjunction with semiquantification for detection of myocardial viability or prediction of functional recovery after revascularization and in comparison with rest-redistribution ^{201}Tl imaging.[29,48] In these studies, myocardial uptake of IPPA was found to predict left ventricular function, and abnormalities in IPPA metabolism aided in predicting functional recovery. Recent studies have also demonstrated that IPPA more clearly visualizes areas of myocardial viability than does technetium-99m sestamibi.[46,50] The advantages of using IPPA over pure flow tracers include lower radiation dose and shorter examination time. Single-photon emission computed tomography with IPPA can also be used in patients who are unable to performance maximal exercise, for reliable diagnosis in high-risk patients, and for better specificity than can be obtained with [201]Tl. In addition, IPPA was used to evaluate alterations in fatty acid metabolism in cardiomyopathy patients.[93]

15-(o-iodophenyl) pentadecanoic acid (o-IPPA). *Cardiac metabolism of o-IPPA.* In o-IPPA, ^{123}I is introduced into the ortho-position rather than the para-position (as in IPPA). This analog shows rapid myocardial washout kinetics in rodents (half-time 8.6 minutes).[2] In pharmacokinetic studies using rodents, o-IPPA was found to enter the myocardium at a rate comparable to that of IPPA. In contrast to IPPA, however, o-IPPA was rapidly lost from the free fatty acid pool and almost none of it was converted to other lipid fractions. β-Oxidation was minimal. Thus, in rodents, o-IPPA quickly returned to circulating blood following myocardial accumulation. For this reason, o-IPPA was considered to have no clinical value.

The myocardial release kinetics of o-IPPA in human studies, however, are surprisingly different from the results observed in rodent studies.[1] This analog exhibits almost irreversible myocardial retention in humans (half-time >200 minutes). Studies in humans with dual-tracer techniques have involved the use of two isomers labeled on the phenyl ring with [131]I-(IPPA) and in position 1 with [14]C (o-IPPA).[7,36] The results of these studies confirmed that there is discrimination against o-IPPA entering the mitochondria after substrate accumulation in myocardial cells.

It is not known whether o-IPPA is retained in the human myocardial lipid pool. In concordance with the findings in the rat heart, it is speculated that the substrate is not readily converted into complex lipids but is held in the free fatty acid pool, a phenomenon that may be linked to storage proteins. If o-IPPA is released from the human myocardium, it is probably because of back-diffusion into the circulating blood rather than because of induction of transport into mitochondria or a nonspecific type of catabolism.

o-IPPA in clinical practice. Because o-IPPA accumulates and is retained in the human myocardium, it provides a timing advantage for SPECT. An initial study of patients with acute myocardial infarction compared ^{201}Tl with o-IPPA and ^{18}F-fluorodeoxyglucose (FDG) in evaluating myocardial viability. A substantial fraction of redistribution ^{201}Tl–defects exhibited uptake of o-IPPA and FDG, thus indicating the potential of o-IPPA to identify viable myocardium.[32] Another study addressed the relation between o-IPPA uptake and technetium-99m sestamibi uptake in SPECT after acute thrombolysis.[15] Areas of decreased o-IPPA activity were larger and more hypoactive than ^{99m}Tc sestamibi activity in successfully reperfused myocardium. The results of this study suggested that combined use of o-IPPA and ^{99m}Tc sestamibi may be useful as a means of showing the myocardial area at risk.

When applied sequentially in patients, the isomers have been used as metabolic probes to appraise the relative contribution of β-oxidation (with IPPA) and back-diffusion into the circulation (with o-IPPA) to the turnover of myocardial lipids.[7,36] Comparing the myocardial turnover rate of these two isomers promises to yield new information on intracardiac lipid metabolism that may be of diagnostic importance. Thus, for the first time, IPPA and o-IPPA were used in the dual-substrate approach in dilated cardiomyopathy.[13] Substantial alterations in myocardial lipid turnover were found in the cardiomyopathic patients. However, o-IPPA has not been widely used because of considerable difference between its pharmacokinetics in rodents and humans.

Radioiodinated methyl-branched fatty acid analogs

Substantial myocardial washout during the acquisition period must be minimized during the relatively long time periods required for camera rotation and data collection by SPECT. Because straight-chain fatty acids are rapidly metabolized by β-oxidation, various structural modifications have been introduced with fatty acid analogs to evaluate their inhibition of β-oxidation, thus delaying myocardial tracer clearance and relative regional distribution. The degree of branching and the length of the chain determine the myocardial uptake of these tracers.

Iodoalkyl-substituted analog. *16-[^{123}I]-iodo-3-methylhexadecanoic acid (IMHA).* The IMHA analog is an example of a methyl-branched analog in which ^{123}I has not been chemically stabilized on the fatty acid chain. Because it prevents β-oxidation, IMHA myocardial clearance is low enough to allow SPECT acquisition in human studies. Although SPECT with IMHA is associated with higher levels of background activity due to free iodine release, IMHA has been shown to yield satisfactory SPECT quality in clinical practice.

Recent reports have shown that resting SPECT with IMHA frequently reveals increased levels of uptake in areas with irreversible exercise defects on redistribution or rejection shown by ^{201}Tl on SPECT.[56,57] The mismatch pattern provided by a flow tracer (^{201}Tl) and a metabolic tracer (IMHA) may correspond to areas of ischemic but viable myocardium.[32]

15-(p-iodophenyl)-3-R,S-methylpentadecanoic acid (BMIPP).

Iodophenyl-substituted analogs. The analog in the 3-methyl-branched series, 15-(p-iodophenyl)-3-R,S-methylpentadecanoic acid (BMIPP), was developed and has been widely studied in animal models and in humans.[25,26,39,41] The BMIPP analog has the same 15-carbon-chain length as IPPA; the only structural change is the introduction of the methyl group in the 3 position (carbon-3). The corresponding 3,3-dimethyl analog, 15-(p-iodophenyl)-3,3-dimethylpentadecanoic acid (DMIPP), has also been evaluated.[41] Results of detailed triple-label studies comparing the relative uptake and clearance kinetics of IPPA, BMIPP, and DMIPP have clearly shown the expected effect of 3-methyl substitution in rat myocardium. Because BMIPP exhibits slow myocardial washout, the introduction of two methyl groups, such as DMIPP, was expected to inhibit β-oxidation more effectively and to prolong retention.[40,41,89] The 14-carbon-chain length analog of BMIPP, 14-(p-iodophenyl)-3-R,S-methyltertradec-anoic acid, has also been evaluated.[37]

Cardiac metabolism of BMIPP. Although the 3-methyl substituent was initially introduced to BMIPP to inhibit β-oxidation and block its metabolism, slow washout of BMIPP from the myocardium has been observed in animal and human studies. Water-soluble metabolites of BMIPP were also detected in the plasma and urine of animals and humans injected with BMIPP.[9,47] Two possible metabolic pathways have been proposed for myocardial oxidative degradation of BMIPP metabolism.[42–44] The first pathway is direct β-oxidation of BMIPP, which causes metabolic trapping of β-hydroxy-BMIPP in the myocardium. The second pathway consists of initial α-oxidation and the subsequent cycle of p-iodophenylacetic acid (PIPA) as the end-product, which was found to be the sole product in both plasma and urine (that is, as conjugate) after intravenous injection of BMIPP in rats, rabbits, and humans. However, these metabolites reflect only the overall catabolism of BMIPP throughout the entire body and do not necessarily indicate the metabolic fate of the tracer in the heart.[68] Recently, investigators detected an unidentified polar metabolite in the effluent of perfused rat hearts that had received BMIPP.[42,47] The metabolite was speculated to be β-hydroxy-BMIPP, but it was not identical to the authentic sample.

We evaluated cardiac metabolism of BMIPP by using an isolated rat heart and a perfusion system (Fig. 6-3). Rat hearts were perfused with 5 mmol/L of N-2-hydroxyethylpiperazine-N-2-ethanesulfonic acid buffer containing various energy sub-

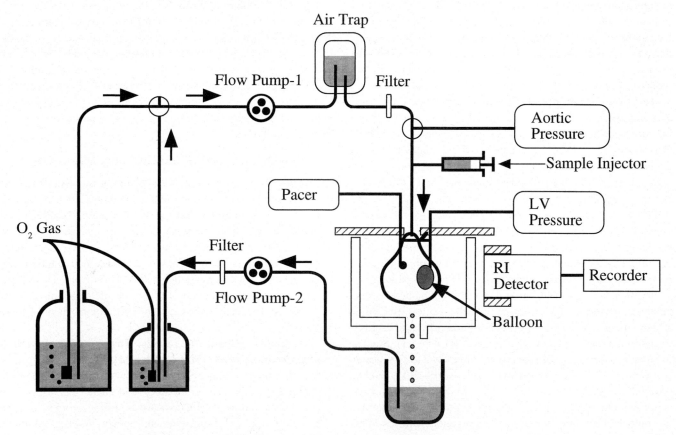

Fig. 6-3. Schematic diagram of perfusion system for an isolated rat heart. RI = radioactivity; LV = left ventricle. (Reprinted by permission of the Society of Nuclear Medicine, From Yamamichi Y, Kusuoka H, Morishita K, et al, *J Nucl Med* 36:1043-1050, 1995.)

strates and 1% bovine serum albumin. The buffer was recirculated for 4 hours after bolus injection of BMIPP. Heart time–activity curves were monitored externally. Radioactivity in the heart and levels of recirculated buffer were measured after perfusion, and the metabolites in the buffer were extracted. We performed high-performance liquid chromatography and thin-layer chromatography and detected a series of metabolites in the perfusate of isolated rat hearts recirculated after injection of BMIPP (Fig. 6-4). Three BMIPP metabolites, ^{123}I-α-methyl-(p-iodophenyl)-tetradecanoic acid (AMIPT), [123]I-(p-iodophenyl) decanoic acid (PIPC$_{12}$), and [123]I-(p-iodophenyl) acetic acid (PIPA), were identified.[98] These key compounds corroborate one of the metabolic pathways hypothesized for BMIPP. In the effluent, AMIPT was always the most abundant metabolite, strongly suggesting that BMIPP is first digested by α-oxidation similar to phytanic acid, an analog of natural fatty acids with β-methyl substituents.

Although BMIPP would be α-hydroxylated and then decarboxylated to AMIPT, α-hydroxylated intermediate (α-hydroxy-BMIPP) was not detected because of enzymatic channeling in the hydroxylation process. Therefore, AMIPT would subse-

quently be processed by classic β-oxidation because it would no longer be impeded by the branched-methyl group, now converted from the β-position to the α-position. As for PIPA, it could be the end product of AMIPT through successive β-oxidation cycles, which suggests the occurrence of complete chain shortening of BMIPP in the rat heart. The appearance of PIPC$_{12}$, which is generated from AMIPT by one cycle of the β-oxidation process, indicates that such intermediates permeate from myocardial cells, as AMIPT does. Thus, BMIPP is metabolized through initial α-oxidation and subsequent cycles of β-oxidation, yielding PIPA as its end product. On the other hand, β-hydroxy-BMIPP, a possible metabolic trapping product produced by direct β-oxidation of BMIPP, was not detected in the myocardial effluent of rats. More recently, this pathway was also confirmed in a canine open-chest model.[21]

We have also shown that BMIPP metabolism depends on energy substrates used in the heart.[98] Fig. 6-5 shows the influence of various energy substrates on BMIPP metabolism by using the amount of AMIPT and the sum of the amounts of the other metabolites as indices for the contributions of the α-oxidation and β-oxidation fraction, respectively. The total myo-

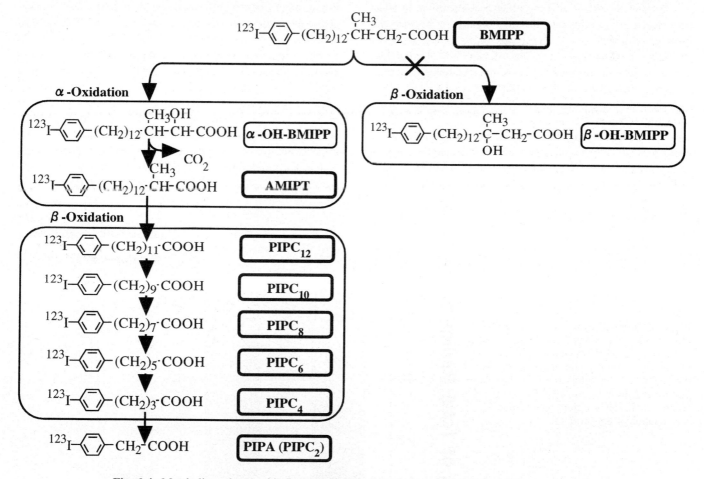

Fig. 6-4. Metabolic pathway of iodine-123 BMIPP (15-p-iodophenyl)-3-R,S-methylpentadecanoic acid) in the rat heart. Metabolites surrounded by a thick line were detected and were identified by high-performance liquid chromatography and thin-layer. Metabolites surrounded by a thin line have not yet been detected or identified but are expected to be formed during the catabolic process. (Reprinted by permission of the Society of Nuclear Medicine, From Yamamichi Y, Kusuoka H, Morishita K, et al, *J Nucl Med* 36:1043-1050, 1995.)

cardial uptake of BMIPP, defined by the sum of heart uptake, α-oxidation fraction, and β-oxidation fraction, was high in the oleate and glucose-insulin groups and low in the acetate group, with no difference between initial heart uptake in the two groups. Metabolism of BMIPP, however, was significantly different in these two groups, and oleate stimulated both α-oxidation and β-oxidation of BMIPP. In contrast, both the α-oxidation and β-oxidation were significantly smaller in the glucose-insulin group than in the oleate group. Moreover, the heart uptake of BMIPP in the glucose-insulin group was significantly greater than in the oleate group. These findings suggest that the glucose-insulin solution reduced fatty acid oxidation because of an increase in glucose consumption and that the decrease in both oxidation fractions resulted in increased heart retention. This is consistent with earlier observations with ^{11}C-palmitate and IHDA.[24,84] The acetate group showed moderate total myocardial uptake of BMIPP; despite low total uptake, the α-oxidation fraction was significantly larger compared with that of the oleate group. In contrast, the β-oxidation fraction was relatively inhibited. These findings suggest that acetate inhibits β-oxidation of fatty acids due to competition in acyl CoA formation but that α-oxidation is free of such competition. In addition, acetate may stimulate α-oxidation per se because the increase of α-oxidation fraction was much greater than expected when β-oxidation blockade is taken into consideration. These results indicate that analysis of the metabolite in plasma and urine as well as the myocardial time–activity curve may provide information on the metabolism of free fatty acids in the myocardium with different diseases.

We also evaluated the slow washout of BMIPP in normal rat hearts by analyzing the subcellular distribution and lipid classes on the basis of BMIPP metabolism (Fig. 6-6). The heart uptake of BMIPP was maximal at 5 minutes, and 41% of the radioac-

tivity disappeared within 120 minutes. Myocardial radioactivity was immediately distributed into the cytosolic, mitochondrial, microsomal, and nuclear fractions. The distribution (percentage) of each fraction was almost identical from 5 minutes through 120 minutes. The cytosolic fraction was always the major site of radioactivity deposition (60%), and the time–activity curve of the cytosolic fraction paralleled that of the whole heart throughout the 120-minute study period. Most of the radioactivity in the cytosolic fraction was incorporated into the triglyceride class, and the rest was present in the free fatty acid, phospholipid (phosphatidylcholine), and diglyceride classes. In the mitochondrial fraction, radioactivity was mostly incorporated into the phospholipid class (phosphatidylethanolamine), followed by free fatty acids. The final metabolite of BMIPP, PIPA, appeared first in the mitochondrial fraction as early as 1 minute and subsequently in the cytosolic fraction at 5 minutes. Another intermediary metabolite, $PIPC_{12}$, was found only in the mitochondrial fraction after 5 minutes. Our results suggest that slow washout kinetics of BMIPP from the myocardium mainly reflect the turnover rate of the triglyceride pool in the cytosol.[60] Metabolism of BMIPP was confirmed to be the same in vivo as in isolated perfuse rat hearts, and our data also suggested the participation of the mitochondria in BMIPP metabolism.[98]

The correlation between myocardial BMIPP uptake and levels of free adenosine triphosphate (ATP) is an important finding.[9,20] This relation has been investigated in normal and salt-sensitive Dahl-strain rats after administration of an inhibitor of mitochondrial carnitine acyltransferase (tetradecylglycidic acid). Initial myocardial uptake of BMIPP was uninfluenced by acute inhibition of β-oxidation by the inhibitor. Intracellular ATP levels correlating with BMIPP retention are interpreted as a reflection of cytosolic activation of BMIPP to BMIPP CoA

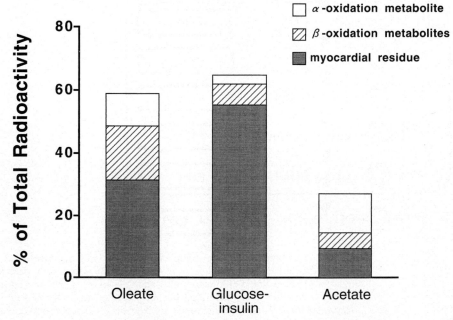

Fig. 6-5. Dependency of iodine-123 BMIPP (15-(*p*-iodophenyl)-3-R,S-methylpentadecanoic acid) metabolism on energy substrates utilized in isolated perfused rat hearts. The distribution of the radioactivity is classified into α- and β-oxidation metabolites, and retention in the myocardium after 4 hours of recirculation of the perfusate.

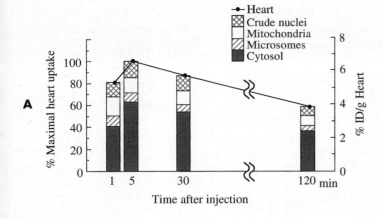

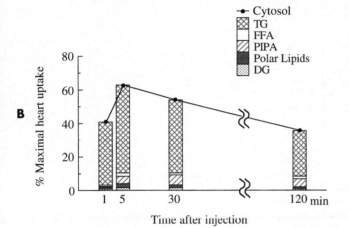

Fig. 6-6. A, Radioactivity changes in the subcellular distribution after injection of iodine-123 BMIPP (15-(*p*-iodophenyl)-3-R,S-methylpentadecanoic acid). **B,** Radioactivity changes in the lipid distribution of the cytosolic fraction. The myocardial radioactivity was immediately distributed into the cytosolic, mitochondrial, microsomal, and crude nuclear fraction. The distribution of each fraction was almost identical from 5 minutes through 120 minutes. The cytosolic fraction was the major site of radioactivity deposition. In the cytosolic fraction, most of the radioactivity was incorporated into the triglyceride *(TG)* classes. DG = diglycerides; FFA = free fatty acids; PIPA = *P*-iodophenylacetic acid.

with slow shunting into triglyceride storage products. A negative correlation was observed between ATP levels and severely compromised myocardial BMIPP in the hypertrophied hearts of Dahl rats. Differences in mitochondrial and cytosolic ATP pools may explain these results.[20]

BMIPP in animal studies. Recent work by Fujibayashi et al[21] revealed that the half-time of BMIPP myocardial washout was calculated as 138 minutes from the retention fraction at 30 minutes after injection. This value was similar to those previously reported after intravenous injection of BMIPP in animal models.[8,64] The fate of intracoronary BMIPP 30 minutes after injection is summarized in Fig. 6-7. This analog was largely extracted from the plasma into myocardium (74% of the injected dose) and substantially retained (65.3%). Washout of the retained radioactivity was rather low (8.7%), and most of the

washout consisted of α- and β-oxidation metabolites (2.3%, 2.9%, 1.4%), with little BMIPP itself (2.1%). Because of metabolic washout, BMIPP is not an ideal SPECT agent. Such degradation, however, is considered to be negligible in SPECT protocols. As Knapp Jr et al[44] pointed out, this metabolism might make BMIPP useful in delineating patients with heart disease. In fact, some clinical studies indicated that the difference between early and late BMIPP images provides useful diagnostic information in various diseases.[4,45,57]

A seemingly unique property of BMIPP is the mismatch often observed between metabolic tracer (BMIPP) and flow tracer ([201]T1), although it has not yet been firmly established.[43,76] Animal studies with BMIPP evaluated the regional myocardial distribution of this tracer in various cardiac disease models by using autoradiography and gamma-camera imaging. Significant differences have been found between flow tracer and methyl-branched fatty acid distribution in spontaneous hypertensive rats, hamster models of hypertrophic cardiomyopathy (Bio 14.6), and Adriamycin-induced cardiomyopathies.[51,67,99] We also demonstrated dissociations between uptake of BMIPP and [201]T1 in these animal models (Fig. 6-8).

The properties of BMIPP were also evaluated by using [201]T1 and BMIPP in an ischemic canine model.[59,64,65] In our studies, sequential gamma-camera images obtained after intravenous administration of [201]T1 and BMIPP were evaluated by using occlusion–reperfusion models. The hearts were also imaged after excision. Whereas all control dogs with longer occlusion showed persistent defects with BMIPP and [201]T1, 80% of the dogs with 3 hours of occlusion followed by 1 hour of reperfusion showed BMIPP–[201]T1 uptake mismatch.[65]

Regional mismatches of BMIPP uptake in comparison with flow tracer distribution may thus be expected to result from other factors unrelated to oxidative catabolism. Furthermore, the factors resulting in mismatch phenomena between BMIPP and flow tracer are probably unrelated to the formation of oxidative product. Rather, they are probably related to differences in cellular uptake compared with normal myocytes and cells that are viable but metabolically impaired.[43,76]

BMIPP in clinical practice. The first clinical study with BMIPP involved the use of planar imaging.[9] It was demonstrated that this agent has higher uptake and longer retention in normal myocardium. Because of these characteristics, current studies with BMIPP are mainly performed by using SPECT. Excellent delineation of the myocardium was revealed by SPECT. In addition, myocardial SPECT with BMIPP was applied to patients with ischemic heart disease and cardiomyopathy by combined use of BMIPP and [201]T1.[65,66]

We evaluated the relation between myocardial perfusion and free fatty acid metabolism by simultaneous BMIPP and [201]T1 myocardial SPECT in patients with acute myocardial infarction.[66] Dissociations between BMIPP and [201]T1 defects were frequently observed in patients with acute myocardial infarction on successful reperfusion. Uptake of BMIPP was impaired in salvaged myocardium immediately after successful reperfusion in which myocardial perfusion was established. These ar-

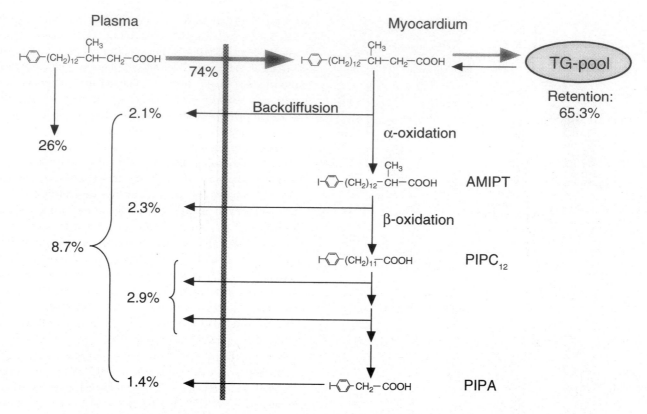

Fig. 6-7. The fate of intracoronary iodine-123-BMIPP (15-(*p*-iodophenyl)-3-R,S-methylpentadec-anoic acid) 30 minutes after injection. This agent was extensively extracted from the plasma into the myocardium (74% of the injected dose) and was substantially retained (65.3%). Washout of the retained radioactivity was low (8.7%), and most of the washout was as α- and β-oxidation metabolite (2.3%, 2.9%, 1.4%), with little BMIPP itself (2.1%). (From Fujibayashi Y, Nihara R, Hosokawa R, et al: Metabolism and kinetics of iodine-123-BMIPP in canine myocardium, *J Nucl Med* 37:757–761, 1996. Reprinted by permission of the Society of Nuclear Medicine.)

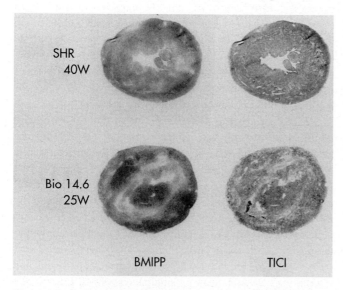

Fig. 6-8. Dual iodine-123-BMIPP (15-(*p*-iodophenyl)3-R,S-methylpentadecanoic acid) and thallium-201 (²⁰¹Tl) autoradio-grams in spontaneous hypertensive rat (*SHR*) and cardiomyopathic hamster (Bio 14.6). Dissociations between ¹²⁵I-BMIPP and ²⁰¹Tl uptake were clearly observed in both animal models. W = weeks of age.

eas showed gradual recovery during the chronic phase with functional recovery (Fig. 6-9). In contrast, in patients without reperfusion, BMIPP and ²⁰¹Tl defects were of similar size. These areas may present complete scar. Therefore, degree and improvement of perfusion and metabolism mismatch in acute myocardial infarction may reflect subsequent recovery from postischemic wall-motion abnormality. These procedures are valuable for patient management from the standpoint of myocardial viability assessment in emergency patients who had intracoronary thrombolysis.[16,31] More than 70% of patients with acute coronary syndromes, such as unstable angina, had BMIPP defects. Therefore, resting myocardial SPECT with BMIPP is very sensitive for detecting myocardial ischemia in clinical settings.[92] Myocardial SPECT with BMIPP is useful in identifying culprit regions in acute coronary syndromes and is thus valuable in patients undergoing emergency percutaneous transluminal coronary angioplasty.

The results of our study indicate that impairment of myocardial fatty acid metabolism in cardiomyopathy may precede the decrease in myocardial perfusion in hypertrophic myocardium, because decreased BMIPP uptake and normal ²⁰¹Tl

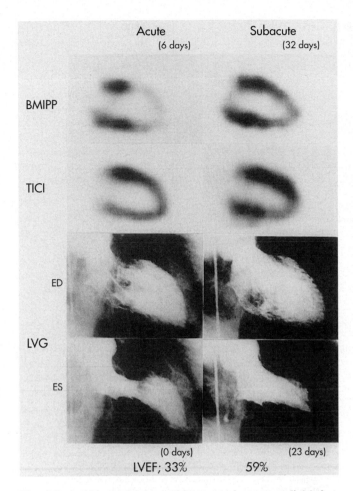

Fig. 6-9. A 46-year-old man with an anterior myocardial infarction. Single-photon emission computed tomography with BMIPP and thallium-201 (^{201}Tl) myocardial were performed simultaneously 6 days after percutaneous transluminal coronary angioplasty and 32 days later. Percutaneous transluminal coronary angioplasty resulted in prompt restoration of myocardial blood flow, as evidenced by improved regional ^{201}Tl uptake. However, BMIPP uptake and regional wall motion of the anteroseptal wall remained depressed. However, regional wall motion and BMIPP uptake showed gradual recovery during the chronic phase. Left ventricular ejection fraction (*LVEF*) showed substantial improvement, from 33% to 59%. ED = end-diastole; ES = end-systole; LVG = contrast left ventriculogram. (From Nishimura T, Uehara T, Shimonagata T, et al: *J Nucl Cardiol* 1:S65-S71, 1994.)

perfusion were frequently observed in hypertrophic cardiomyopathy (Fig. 6-10). The correlation between severity score and wall thickness of the septum was better with BMIPP SPECT than with ^{201}Tl SPECT, suggesting that BMIPP is more suitable for assessing myocardial integrity in hypertrophic cardiomyopathy.[66,67] Furthermore, the correlation between severity score and left ventricular function was better with BMIPP SPECT than with ^{201}Tl SPECT.[4,88]

The clinical results of myocardial SPECT with BMIPP in patients with myocardial infarction and hypertrophic car-

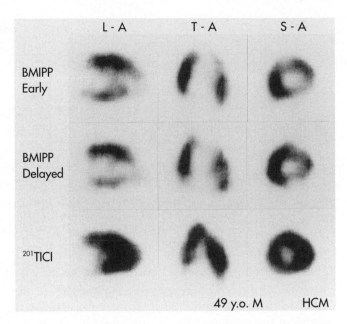

Fig. 6-10. A 49-year-old man with hypertrophic cardiomyopathy. Single-photon emission computed tomography with BMIPP and thallium-201 (^{201}Tl) myocardial were performed. Increased ^{201}Tl uptake was observed in the apical and posterolateral regions, whereas BMIPP myocardial uptake was reduced in the same segments in both early and delayed images. Dissociations of BMIPP and ^{201}Tl uptake were clearly demonstrated in the hypertrophic myocardium. (From Nishimura T, Uehara T, Shimonagata T, et al: *J Nucl Cardiol* 1:S65-S71, 1994.)

diomyopathy indicate that BMIPP is a suitable agent for the assessment of left ventricular functional integrity, because left ventricular wall motion is energy dependent and BMIPP may reflect an aspect of myocardial energy production. This agent may be useful as an alternative to PET studies for the early detection and management of various cardiac diseases.[38]

15-(*p*-iodophenyl)-9-R,S-methylpentadecanoic acid (9MPA). This analog is a modified long-chain (15 carbons) fatty acid that differs from BMIPP by having a methyl branch at the 9 carbon location. In rat myocardium, the mean percentage of uptake of an injected dose of IPPA, 9MPA, and BMIPP at 5 minutes was 2.65%, 2.60%, and 3.76%, respectively. Furthermore, the myocardial time–activity curve of 9MPA demonstrated washout between that of IPPA and that of BMIPP (Fig. 6-11). Combined 9MPA and ^{201}Tl studies were performed in coronary artery disease by using planar imaging. It was shown that 9MPA was suitable for myocardial imaging and correlated closely with ^{201}Tl for initial postexercise myocardial uptake and defect reversibility. Defect reversibility seems to result from deferential myocardial clearance in normal and ischemic regions.[5] On the basis of the results of these studies, 9MPA may serve as a probe for myocardial viability.

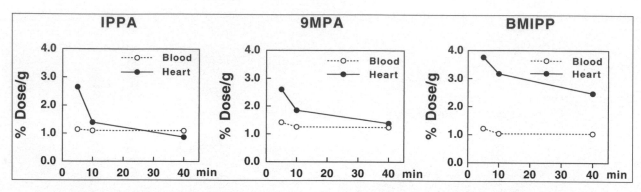

Fig. 6-11. Time–activity curves for IPPA (15-(*p*-iodophenyl) pentadecanoic acid), 9MPA (15-(*p*-iodophenyl)-9-R,S-methylpentadecanoic acid) and BMIPP in the myocardium and blood of four normal rats. The time–activity curve of 9MPA in the myocardium showed washout between that of IPPA and BMIPP.

Table 6-3. Summary of general structures and the characteristics of radioiodinated fatty acid analogs for clinical application

General structure	I—(CH$_2$)$_n$—COOH	I—⟨ ⟩—(CH$_2$)$_n$—COOH	I—⟨ ⟩—(CH$_2$)$_n$—CH—COOH (with CH$_3$)
Type	Iodoalkyl straight chain	Iodophenyl straight chain	Iodophenyl methyl-branched chain
Heart clearance	Rapid	Rapid	Slow (incorporation to triglyceride pool)
Metabolism	Rapid released of free iodine by β-oxidation	Rapidly metabolized by β-oxidation	Blockade of direct β-oxidation
Imaging	Planar	Planar/SPECT	SPECT

CONCLUSIONS

Fatty acid metabolism provides a major source of energy to the myocardium. It can be traced by SPECT with various radioiodinated fatty acid analogs, as can be done by PET with ^{11}C-palmitate. Table 6-3 summarizes some of the physiologic properties of radioiodinated fatty acids that are most extensively used clinically.

Since the introduction of interventional therapy, including percutaneous transluminal coronary angioplasty or coronary artery bypass surgery, it has been important to precisely evaluate myocardial viability in stunned or hibernating myocardium. Iodine-123 fatty acids are expected to provide an alternative to PET as a method of assessing myocardial viability. Studying more diverse populations with fatty acid analogs compared with PET metabolic imaging should increase insight into disease processes and enhance the ability to assess the effects of therapeutic interventions in various cardiac diseases.

REFERENCES

1. Antar MA, Spohn G, Herzog HH, et al: 15-(ortho-^{123}I-phenyl)-pentadecanoic acid, a new myocardial imaging agent for clinical use. *Nucl Med Commun* 7:683–696, 1986.
2. Beckurts TE, Shreeve WW, Schieren R, et al: Kinetics of different [123]I- and ^{14}C-labelled fatty acids in normal and diabetic rat myocardium in vivo. *Nucl Med Commun* 6:415–421, 1985.
3. Caldwell HJ, Martin GV, Link JM, et al: Iodophenylpentadecanoic acid-myocardial blood flow relationship during maximal exercise with coronary occlusion. *J Nucl Med* 30:99–105, 1990.
4. Chen SL, Vehara T, Morozumi T, et al: Myocardial metabolism of ^{123}I-BMIPP in patients with hypertrophic cardiomyopathy: assessment by radial long-axis SPECT. *Nucl Med Commun* 16:336–343, 1995.
5. Chouraqui P, Maddahi J, Henkin R, et al: Comparison of myocardial imaging with iodine-123-*p*-iodophenyl-9-methylpentadecanoic acid and thallium-201-chloride for assessment of patients with exercise-induced myocardial ischemia. *J Nucl Med* 32:447–452, 1991.
6. Corbett J: Clinical experience with iodine-123-iodophenylpentadecanoic acid. *J Nucl Med* 35 (4 Suppl):32S–37S, 1994.
7. Dormehl I, Feinendegen L, Hugo N, et al: Comparative myocardial imaging in the baboon with ^{123}I-labelled ortho and para isomers of 15-(iodophenyl)pentadecanoic acid (IPPA). *Nucl Med Commun* 14:998–1004, 1993.
8. Dormehl IC, Hugo N, Rossover D, et al: Planar myocardial imaging in the baboon model with iodine-123-15-(iodophenyl) pentadecanoic acid (IPPA) and iodine-123-15-(*p*-iodophenyl)-3-R,S-methylpentadecanoic acid (BMIPP), using time-activity curves for evaluation of metabolism. *Nucl Med Biol* 22:837–847, 1995.
9. Dudczak R, Schmoliner R, Angelberger P, et al: Structurally modified fatty acids: clinical potential as tracers of metabolism. *Eur J Nucl Med* 12 Suppl:S45–S48, 1986.
10. Eisenhut M, Lehmann WD, and Sutterle A. Metabolism of 15-(4'-^{123}I]iodophenyl)pentadecanoic acid (^{123}I]IPPA) in the rat heart; identification of new metabolites by high pressure liquid chromatography and fast atom bombardment-mass spectrometry. *Nucl Med Biol* 20:747–754, 1993.
11. Evans JR, Guntan RW, Baker RG, et al: Use of radioiodinated fatty acid for photoscans of the heart. *Circ Res* 15:1–10, 1965.
12. Feinendegen LE, Vyska K, Freundlieb C, et al: Non-invasive analysis of metabolic reactions in body tissues, the case of myocardial fatty acids. *Eur J Nucl Med* 6:191–200, 1981.
13. Feinendegen LE, Henrick MM, Kuikka JT, et al: Myocardial lipid

turnover in dilated cardiomyopathy: a dual in vivo tracer approach. *J Nucl Cardiol* 2:42–52, 1995.

14. Fox KAA, Abendschein DR, Ambos HD, et al: Efflux of metabolized and nonmetabolized fatty acid from canine myocardium. Implications for quantifying myocardial metabolism tomographically. *Circ Res* 57:232–243, 1985.

15. Franken PR, De Geeter F, Dendale P, et al: Regional distribution of ^{123}I-(ortho-iodophenyl)-pentadecanoic acid and ^{99m}Tc-MIBI in relation to wall motion after thrombolysis for acute myocardial infarction. *Nucl Med Commun* 14:310–317, 1993.

16. Franken PR, De Geeter F, Dendale P, et al: Abnormal free fatty acid uptake in subacute myocardial infarction after coronary thrombolysis: correlation with wall motion and inotropic reserve. *J Nucl Med* 35:1758–1765, 1994.

17. Freundlieb C, Hock A, Vyska K, et al: Myocardial imaging and metabolic studies with [17-^{123}I] iodoheptadecanoic acid. *J Nucl Med* 21:1043–1050, 1980.

18. Friedrich L, Pichler M, Gassner A, et al: Tracer elimination in ^{123}I-heptadecanoic acid: half-life, component ratio and circumferential profiles in patients with cardiac disease. *Eur Heart J* Suppl B:61–70, 1985.

19. Fujibayashi Y, Yonekura Y, Takemura Y, et al: Myocardial accumulation of iodinated beta-methyl-branched fatty acid analogue, iodine-125-15-(*p*-iodophenyl)-3-(R,S)methylpentadecanoic acid (BMIPP), in relation to ATP concentration. *J Nucl Med* 31:1818–1822, 1990.

20. Fujibayashi Y, Som P, Yonekura Y, et al: Myocardial accumulation of iodinated β-methyl-branched fatty acid analog, [^{125}I](*p*-iodophenyl-3-(R,S)-methylpentadecanoic acid (BMIPP), and correlation to ATP concentration—II. Studies in salt-induced hypertensive rats. *Nucl Biol Med* 20:163, 1993.

21. Fujibayashi Y, Nohara R, Hosokawa R, et al: Metabolism and kinetics of iodine-123-BMIPP in canine myocardium. *J Nucl Med* 37:757–761, 1996.

22. Garnier A, Dubois F, Keriel C, et al: Influence of fatty acid backdiffusion on compartmental analysis of external detection curves obtained with 123-iodohexadecanoic acid in isolated rat heart. *Nucl Med Biol* 20:297–306, 1993.

23. Geltman EM: Assessment of myocardial fatty acid metabolism with 1-^{11}C-palmitate. *J Nucl Cardiol* 1(2 Pt 2):S15–S22, 1994.

24. Ghezzi C, Keriel C, Pernin C, et al: Iodohexadecanoic acid as a tracer of myocardial metabolism. *Nuc Compact* 21:248–252, 1990.

25. Goodman MM, et al: New myocardial imaging agents: synthesis of 15-(*p*-iodophenyl)-3-R,S-methylpentadecanoic acid by decomposition of a piperidinyl triazene precursor. *J Org Chem* 49:2322–2325, 1984.

26. Goodman MM, Knapp FF Jr, Elmalch DR: Synthesis and evaluation of radioiodinated terminal *p*-iodophenyl-substituted α- and β-methyl-branched fatty acids. *J Med Chem* 27:390–397, 1984.

27. Groeneveld AB and Visser FC: Correlation of heterogenous blood flow and fatty acid uptake in normal dog heart. *Basic Res Cardiol* 88:222–232, 1993.

28. Hansen CL, Corbett JB, Pippin JJ, et al: Iodine-123 phenylpentadecanoic acid and single photon emission computed tomography in identifying left ventricular regional metabolic abnormalities in patients with coronary heart disease: comparison with thallium-201 myocardial tomography. *J Am Coll Cardiol* 12:78–87, 1988.

29. Hansen CL, Heo J, Oliner C, et al: Prediction of functional recovery with I-123 phenylpentadecanoic acid after coronary revascularization. *J Nucl Med* 35 (Suppl):49, 1994.

30. Hansen CL, Kulkarni PV, Ugolini V, et al: Detection of alterations in left ventricular fatty acid metabolism in patients with acute myocardial infarction by 15-(*p*-^{123}I-phenyl)-pentadecanoic acid and tomographic imaging. *Am Heart J* 129:476–481, 1995.

31. Hashimoto A, Nakata T, Tsuchihashi K, et al: Postischemic functional recovery and BMIPP uptake after primary percutaneous transluminal coronary angioplasty in acute myocardial infarction. *Am J Cardiol* 77:25–30, 1996.

32. Henrich MM, Vester E, von der Lohe E, et al: The comparison of 2-^{18}F-deoxyglucose and 15-(ortho-^{123}I-phenyl)-pentadecanoic acid uptake in persisting defects on thallium-201 tomography in myocardial infarction. *J Nucl Med* 32:1353–1357, 1991.

33. Henrich MM, Grossmann K, Motz W, et al: Beta-oxidation of 1-[^{14}C]- and 17-[^{131}I]-iodo-heptadecanoic acid following intracoronary injection in humans results in similar release of both tracers. *Eur J Nucl Med* 20:225–230, 1993.

34. Hock A, Freundlieb C, Vyska K, et al: Myocardial imaging and metabolic studies with (17-^{123}I) iodoheptadecanoic acid in patients with idiopathic congestive cardiomyopathy. *J Nucl Med* 24:22–28, 1983.

35. Iskandrian AS, Powers J, Cave V, et al: Assessment of myocardial viability by dynamic tomographic iodine 123 iodophenylpentadecanoic acid imaging: comparison with rest-redistribution thallium 201 imaging. *J Nucl Cardiol* 2(2 Pt 1):101–109, 1995.

36. Kaiser KP, Geuting B, Grossmann K, et al: Tracer kinetics of 5-(ortho-$^{123/131}$I-phenyl)-pentadecanoic acid (oPPA) and 15-(para $^{123/131}$I-phenyl)-pentadecanoic acid (pPPA) in animals and man. *J Nucl Med* 31:1608–1616, 1990.

37. Kariento AL, Livni E, Mattila S, et al: Comparative evaluation of [^{123}I] 14-*p*-iodophenyl-beta-methyltetradecanoic acid and thallium-201 in the detection of infarcted areas in the dog heart using SPECT. *Nucl Med Biol* 15:333–338, 1988.

38. Kawamoto M, Tamaki N, Yonekura Y, et al: Combined study with I-123 fatty acid and thallium-201 to assess ischemic myocardium: comparison with thallium redistribution and glucose metabolism. *Ann Nucl Med* 8:47–54, 1994.

39. Knapp FF Jr, Ambrose KR, Goodman MM: New radioiodinated methyl-branched fatty acids for cardiac studies. *Eur J Nucl Med* 12:S39–S44, 1986.

40. Knapp FF Jr, Goodman MM, Callahan AP, et al: Radioiodinated 15-(*p*-iodophenyl)-3,3-dimethylpentadecanoic acid: a useful new agent to evaluate myocardial fatty acid uptake. *J Nucl Med* 27:521–531, 1986.

41. Knapp FF Jr, Goodman MM, Ambrose KR, et al: *The development of radioiodinated 3-methyl-branched fatty acids for evaluation of myocardial disease by single photon tomography.* In: Van der Wall EE, ed. *Noninvasive imaging of cardiac metabolism.* Dordrecht: Martinus Nijhoff Publisher, pp 159–202, 1987.

42. Knapp FF Jr, Goodman MM, Reske SN, et al: Radioiodinated methyl-branched fatty acids—evaluation of catabolites formed in vivo. *Nuc Compact* 21:229–231, 1990.

43. Knapp FF Jr: Myocardial metabolism of radioiodinated BMIPP. *J Nucl Med* 36:1051–1054, 1995.

44. Knapp FF Jr and Kropp J: Iodine-123-labelled fatty acids for myocardial single-photon emission tomography: current status and future perspective. *Eur J Nucl Med* 22:361–381, 1995.

45. Kobayashi H, Asano R, Inoue S, et al: Simultaneous evaluation of myocardial perfusion and fatty acid metabolism using dynamic SPECT with single injection of ^{123}I-15-(*p*-iodophenyl)-3-methyl pentadecanoic acid (BMIPP). *Kaku Igaku* 32:19, 1995.

46. Kropp J, Jorgens C, Glanzer K, et al: Flow and viability of the myocardium detected by isonitriles (RP-30) and IPPA fatty acid in patients with coronary artery disease (CHD). *Eur J Nucl Med* 16:471, 1990.

47. Kropp J, Knapp FF Jr, Ambrose KR, et al: Release of an unexpected myocardial metabolite of radioiodinated 15-(*p*-iodophenyl)-3-R,S-methylpentadecanoic acid (BMIPP) from isolated rat hearts and canine hearts in vivo. *J Nucl Med* 31:896, 1990.

48. Kropp J, Likungu J, Kirchoff PG, et al: SPECT-imaging of myocardial oxidative metabolism with (I-123) IPPA in patients with coronary artery disease and aorto-coronary bypass graft surgery. *Eur J Nucl Med* 18:467–474, 1991.

49. Kropp J, Ambrose KR, Knapp FF Jr, et al: Incorporation of radioiodinated IPPA and BMIPP fatty acid analogues into complex lipids from isolated rat heart. *Nucl Med Biol* 19:283–288, 1992.

50. Kuikka JT, Mussalo H, Hietakorpi S, et al: Evaluation of myocardial viability with technetium-99m hexakis-2-methoxyisobutyl isonitrile

and iodine-123 phenylpentadecanoic acid and single photon emission tomography. *Eur J Nucl Med* 19:882–889, 1992.

51. Kurata C, Kobayashi A, and Yamazaki N: Dual tracer autoradiographic study with thallium-201 and radioiodinated fatty acid in cardiomyopathic hamsters. *J Nucl Med* 30:80–87, 1989.

52. Liedtke AJ, Nellis SH, and Whitesell LF: Effects of regional ischemia on metabolic function in adjacent aerobic myocardium. *J Mol Cell Cardiol* 14:195–205, 1982.

53. Machulla HJ, Stocklin G, Kupfernagel C, et al: Comparative evaluation of fatty acids labelled with C-11, Cl-34m, Br-77, and I-123 for metabolic studies of the myocardium: concise communication. *J Nucl Med* 19:298–302, 1978.

54. Machulla HJ, Marsmann M, and Dutsehka K: Biochemical concept and synthesis of a radioiodinated phenylfatty acid for in vivo metabolic studies of the myocardium. *Eur J Nucl Med* 5:171–173, 1980.

55. Marie PY, Olivier P, Angioi M, et al: Detection of myocardial viability in irreversible defects of exercise SPECT-[201]T1 with rest-injection by means of rest-SPECT with a methylated labeled free fatty acid. *J Nucl Cardiol* 2:S47, 1995.

56. Marie PY, Karcher G, Danchin N, et al: Thallium-201 rest-reinjection and iodine-123-MIHA imaging of myocardial infarction: analysis of defect reversibility. *J Nucl Med* 36:1561–1568, 1995.

57. Matsunari I, Saga T, Taki J, et al: Kinetics of iodine-123-BMIPP in patients with prior myocardial infarction: assessment with dynamic rest and stress images compared with stress thallium-201 SPECT. *J Nucl Med* 35:1279–1285, 1994.

58. Medolago G, Piti A, Tespili M, et al: Perfusion (^{99m}Tc-MIBI) and metabolic (^{123}I-IPPA) study in recent myocardial infarction by SPECT imaging. *Eur J Nucl Med* 16:471, 1990.

59. Miller DD, Gill JB, Livni E, et al: Fatty acid analogue accumulation: a marker of myocyte viability in ischemic-reperfused myocardium. *Circ Res* 63:681–692, 1988.

60. Morishita S, Kusuoka H, Yamamichi Y, et al: Kinetics of radioiodinated species in subcellular fractions from rat hearts following administration of iodine-123-labeled 15-(*p*-iodophenyl)-3(R,S)-methyl pentadecanoic acid (^{123}I-BMIPP). *Eur J Nucl Med* 23:383–389, 1996.

61. Neely JR, Rovetto MJ, and Oram JF: Myocardial utilization of carbohydrate and lipids. *Prog Cardiovasc Dis* 15:289–329, 1972.

62. Neely JR, Whitmer M, and Mochizuki S: Effects of mechanical activity and hormones on myocardial glucose and fatty acid utilization. *Circ Res* 38(5 Suppl 1): I22–I30, 1976.

63. Neely JR and Margan HE: Relationship between carbohydrate and lipid metabolism and the energy balance of heart muscle. *Annu Rev Physiol* 36:413–459, 1974.

64. Nishimura T, Sago M, Kihara K, et al: Fatty acid myocardial imaging using [123]I-*β*-methyl-iodophenyl pentadecanoic acid (BMIPP): comparison of myocardial perfusion and fatty acid utilization in canine myocardial infarction (occlusion and reperfusion model). *Eur J Nucl Med* 15:341–347, 1989.

65. Nishimura T, Vehard T, Shimonagata T, et al: Clinical experience of ^{123}I-BMIPP myocardial imaging for myocardial infarction and hypertrophic cardiomyopathy. *Ann Nucl Med* 7:SI35–SI39, 1993.

66. Nishimura T, Uehara T, Shimonagata T: Clinical results of β-methyl-*p*-(^{123}I) iodophenylpentadecanoic acid, single-photon emission computed tomography in cardiac disease. *J Nucl Cardiol* 1(2 Pt 2):S65–S71, 1994.

67. Ogata M, Kajiyama K, Yamaguchi Y, et al: BMIPP uptake in Adriamycin cardiomyopathic rat hearts. *J Mol Cell Cardiol* (Suppl 1–5), 28:1998.

68. Okano S, Yoshimura H, Okarro K, et al: Metabolite of 15-*p*-iodophenyl-3(R,S)-methylpentadecanoic acid (^{123}I) in blood and urine. *Kaku Igaku* 29:1489–1493, 1992.

69. Opie LH: Metabolism of the heart in health and disease. I. *Am Heart J* 76:685–698, 1968.

70. Opie LH: Effects of regional ischemia on metabolism of glucose and fatty acids. Relative rates of aerobic and anaerobic energy production

during myocardial infarction and comparison with effects of anoxia. *Circ Res* 38 (5 Suppl 1):I52–I74, 1976.

71. Poe ND, Robinson GD, MacDonald NS: Myocardial extraction of labeled long-chain fatty acid analogs. *Proc Soc Exp Biol Med* 148:215–218, 1975.

72. Poe ND, Robinson GD Jr, Graham LS, et al: Experimental basis of myocardial imaging with ^{123}I-labeled hexadecanoic acid. *J Nucl Med* 17:1077–1082, 1976.

73. Poe ND, Robinson GD Jr, Zielinski FW, et al: Myocardial imaging with ^{123}I-hexadecanoic acid. *Radiology* 124:419–424, 1977.

74. Rabinovitch MA, Kalff V, Allen R, et al: ω-^{123}I-hexadecanoic acid metabolic probe of cardiomyopathy. *Eur J Nucl Med* 10:222–227, 1985.

75. Railton R, Roger JC, Small DR, et al: Myocardial scintigraphy with I-123 heptadecanoic acid as a test for coronary heart disease. *Eur J Nucl Med* 13:63–66, 1987.

76. Reinhardt CP, Weinstein H, Marcel R, et al: Comparison of iodine-125-BMIPP and thallium-201 in myocardial hypoperfusion. *J Nucl Med* 36:1645–1653, 1995.

77. Rellas GS, Corbett JR, Kulkarni P, et al: Iodine-123 phenylpentadecanoic acid: detection of acute myocardial infarction and injuring in dogs using an iodinated fatty acid and single-photon emission tomography. *Am J Cardiol* 52:1326–1332, 1983.

78. Reske SN, Sauer W, Machulla HJ, et al: 15 (*p*-[123I]-Iodophenyl)pentadecanoic acid as tracer of lipid metabolism: comparison with 1[14C]-palmitic acid in murine tissues. *J Nucl Med* 25:1335–1342, 1984.

79. Reske SN: Viability as seen with radiolabelled fatty acids—a new approach to a challenging problem. *Eur J Nucl Med* 21:279–282, 1994.

80. Reske SN, Sauer W, Machulla HJ, et al: Metabolism of 15 (pI123 iodophenyl-) pentadecanoic acid in heart muscle and noncardiac tissues. *Eur J Nucl Med* 10:228–234, 1985.

81. Reske SN, Schon S, Schmitt W, et al: Effect of myocardial perfusion and metabolic interventions on cardiac kinetics of phenylpentadecanoic acid (IPPA). *Eur J Nucl Med* 12Suppl:S27–S31, 1986.

82. Roessler H, Hess T, Weiss M, et al: Tomographic assessment of myocardial metabolic heterogeneity. *J Nucl Med* 24:285–296, 1983.

83. Rose CP and Goresky CA: Constraints on the uptake of labeled palmitate by the heart. The barriers at the capillary and sarcolemmal surfaces and the control of intracellular sequestration. *Circ Res* 41:534–545, 1977.

84. Schelbert HR, Henze E, Schon HR, et al: C-11 palmitate for the noninvasive evaluation of regional myocardial fatty acid metabolism with positron computed tomography. III. In vivo demonstration of the effects of substrate availability on myocardial metabolism. *Am Heart J* 105:492–504, 1983.

85. Schmitz B, Reskes SN, Machulla HJ, et al: Cardiac metabolism of ω-(*p*-iodophenyl)-pentadecanoic acid: a gas-liquid chromatographic-mass spectrometric analysis. *J Lipid Res* 25:1102–1108, 1984.

86. Schon HR, Senekowitsch R, Berg D, et al: Measurement of myocardial fatty acid metabolism: kinetics of iodine-123 heptadecanoic acid in normal dog heart. *J Nucl Med* 27:1449–1455, 1986.

87. Schon S, Reske SN, Schmitt H, et al: Substantial I-131 phenylpentadecanoic acid uptake in salvaged myocardium [abstract]. *J Nucl Med* 25:80, 1984 (abstract).

88. Shimonagata T, Nishimura T, Uehara T, et al: Discrepancies between myocardial perfusion and free fatty acid metabolism in patients with hypertrophic cardiomyopathy. *Nucl Med Commun* 14:1005–1013, 1993.

89. Sloof GW, Visser FC, van Fenige MJ, et al: Comparison of uptake, oxidation and lipid distribution of 17-iodoheptadecanoic acid, 15-(*p*-iodophenyl)pentadecanoic acid and 15-(*p* iodophenyl)-3,3-dimethylpentadecanoic acid in normal canine myocardium. *J Nucl Med* 34:649–657, 1993.

90. Spitzer JJ: Effect of lactate infusion on canine myocardial free fatty acid metabolism in vivo. *Am J Physiol* 226:213–217, 1974.

91. Stoddart PGP, Papouchado M, Wilde P: Prognostic value of 123IODO-

heptadecanoic acid imaging in patients with acute myocardial infarction. *Eur J Nucl Med* 12:525–528, 1987.

92. Takeishi Y, Sukekawa H, Saito H, et al: Impaired myocardial fatty acid metabolism detected by ^{123}I-BMIPP in patients with unstable angina pectoris: comparison with perfusion imaging by ^{99m}Tc-sestamibi. *Ann Nucl Med* 9:125–130, 1995.

93. Ugolini V, Hansen CL, Kulkarni PV, et al: Abnormal fatty acid metabolism in dilated cardiomyopathy detected by iodine-123 phenylpentadecanoic acid and tomographic imaging. *Am J Cardiol* 62:923–928, 1988.

94. van Eenige MJ, Visser FC, Duwee CM, et al: Comparison of 17-iodine-131 heptadecanoic acid kinetics from externally measured time-activity curves and from serial myocardial biopsies in an open-chest canine model. *J Nucl Med* 29:1934–1942, 1988.

95. van Eenige MJ, et al: Clinical value of studies with radioiodinated heptadecanoic acid in patients with coronary artery disease. *Eur Heart J* 11:258–268, 1990.

96. Visser FC, van Eenige MJ, Westera G, et al: Metabolic fate of radioiodinated heptadecanoic acid in the normal canine heart. *Circulation* 72:565–571, 1985.

97. Wieler H, Kaiser KP, Kuikka JT, et al: Standardized noninvasive assessment of myocardial free fatty acid kinetics by means of 15-(*p*-iodo-phenyl) pentadecanoic acid (^{123}I-pPPA) scintigraphy: II. Clinical results. *Nucl Med Commun* 13:168–185, 1992.

98. Yamamichi Y, Kusuoka H, Morishita K, et al: Metabolism of iodine-123-BMIPP in perfused rat hearts. *J Nucl Med* 36:1043–1050, 1995.

99. Yamamoto K, Som P, Brill AB, et al: Dual tracer autoradiographic study of β-methyl-(1-^{14}C) heptadecanoic acid and 15-*p*-(^{131}I)-iodophenyl-β-methylpentadecanoic acid in normotensive and hypertensive rats. *J Nucl Med* 27:1178–1183, 1986.

Chapter 7

Nitroimidazoles for imaging hypoxic myocardium

H. William Strauss and Karen E. Linder

Adequate supplies of oxygen are a fundamental requirement for mammalian life. The ability of tissue to survive under circumstances of decreased oxygen delivery is determined by a complex balance between oxygen use for maintenance of cellular integrity and the oxygen use to allow the cell to perform its normal function. Myocardium responds to decreased oxygen delivery with prompt cessation of contractile function. Myocytes in this vegetative state require only about 15% of the oxygen necessary for the support of full contractile function. This hibernating state allows myocytes exposed to prolonged ischemia to survive and return to contractile function when oxygen is restored. Although it is not clear how long myocytes can remain in this state, recovery of function after months of decreased contractile performance has been reported. If oxygen delivery is reduced to the point that vegetative function cannot be maintained (<15% of normal levels), the cells die. From a clinical perspective, it is important to distinguish viable ischemic tissue from that which is irreversibly damaged. At present, perfusion imaging is the primary tool that has been employed, with glucose metabolic imaging serving as an alternative. Both techniques require great sophistication on the part of the person interpreting the procedure. If the tissue concentration of oxygen could be determined noninvasively, it could provide a direct method to identify the status of the myocardium.

Molecules containing a nitroimidazole moiety as part of their structure concentrate in tissues with decreased oxygen content. In the cell, these agents are reduced in a series of steps by such enzymes as xanthine oxidase; when intracellular oxygen levels are adequate (normoxic tissue), the molecule is reoxidized. The molecule is repetitively reduced and oxidized until it leaves the cell by diffusion, the same way in which it entered. In hypoxic tissue, reoxidation is not favored, allowing the reduced product to undergo additional reduction reactions to form products that diffuse from the cell slowly if at all. This preferential retention in hypoxic cells and diffusion out of normoxic cells forms the basis of the mechanism that allows imaging of hypoxia. In addition, localization of these tracers provides evidence of viability. Viability is required for the reductase enzymes to function, a key step in localization of the agent.

Nitroimidazole concentration in hypoxic tissue is specific not to a disease state but only to the oxygenation status of the tissue. As a result, these agents may be useful in characterizing the status of myocardial and cerebral ischemia or infarction, cancer, and peripheral vascular disease. Human clinical trials with iodinated and fluorinated nitroimidazole compounds have demonstrated localization in patients with peripheral vascular disease, small-cell lung cancer, soft-tissue sarcoma, and head and neck cancers. In this review, we discuss the behavior of this class of compounds under hypoxic and normoxic conditions in myocytes, isolated perfused hearts, and autoradiographic and gamma camera studies in animal models of cardiac pathology.

Major clinical decisions in patients with suspected or known coronary heart disease revolve around detection of ischemia and identification of viable ischemic myocardium. Because adequate tissue oxygen concentration is critical to maintaining contractile function, a direct measurement of tissue oxygen levels could offer important information about the status of the myocardium. Under normal circumstances, substrate delivery and utilization are closely coupled, making perfusion imaging clinically valuable as a means of estimating tissue oxygen status. Interpreting perfusion images, however, can be difficult. Attenuation artifacts and differentiation of subtle differences in perfusion to specific areas of myocardium can be challenging.

A deficiency of intracellular oxygen results in an immediate reduction in function, but cells will regain function with prompt restoration of oxygen in hypoxic myocardium. Prolonged hypoxia causes injury[12,14] followed ultimately by cell death. Normal myocardium has an extensive network of mechanisms to provide tight coupling between the requirements for oxygen and the amount of oxygen delivered.[5] Hyperlipidemia and coronary atheroma alter this coupling of the supply-demand relation. Atheromatous lesions limit maximal flow by the physical narrowing, and these vessels fail to dilate in response to increased demand[54] and may vasoconstrict instead. This combination limits the supply of blood that can be delivered to the tissue during peak demand and, in severe cases, in the basal state.

The intracellular partial pressure of oxygen (Po_2) ranges from 12 to 20 mm Hg in normal myocardium. This surprisingly low concentration is the end result of the process of oxygen delivery. No active transport system exists. Oxygen diffuses from erythrocytes, crosses the capillary endothelial barrier, traverses the extracellular fluid space, passes through the myocyte lipid bilayer to the intracellular environment, and finally crosses the mitochondrial membrane. At each step, the oxygen tension is reduced. In skeletal muscle, under conditions of severe exertion, intracellular oxygen levels can decrease to less than 5 mm Hg,* requiring the energy-yielding reactions in the cell to shift to anaerobic pathways for a limited time. However, in the myocardium, oxygen levels must be maintained for the cell to perform its contractile function; at levels below 10 mm Hg,[23] contractile functions decrease; below 5 mm Hg, they cease. For short periods (seconds), cellular work can exceed the oxygen supply, but the oxygen debt must be repaid.[6] Using microelectrodes, the extracellular fluid around specific cells has been sampled in animals breathing room air.[56] It was found that the left ventricular endocardium of normally contracting dog myocardium had a Po_2 of 14 to 17 Torr and the epicardium had a Po_2 of 27 to 31 Torr. An alternative approach to measuring local tissue Po_2 uses an instrument (the Oxyspot) sensitive to the phosphorescent lifetime of a palladium porphine compound, Pd-meso-tetra (4-carboxyphenyl) porphine. A solution of the palladium porphine and bovine serum albumin are injected intravenously, and capillary Po_2 values are determined by exciting the blood-borne compound with a laser. The decay of the resulting phosphorescent signal is inversely proportional to Po_2, as oxygen in the bloodstream quenches the phosphorescent signal. These techniques are useful for investigating open-chest animals but are not suitable for noninvasive studies.[45,59]

Perfusion tracers, such as sestamibi, injected at rest in conjunction with nitroglycerin[24,37] or thallium-201 rest-redistribution imaging[41] are useful techniques to identify hibernating myocardium. However, these techniques are not completely sensitive and often require great skill to detect slight differences in relative tracer concentration as an indication of hibernating tissue. Similarly, metabolic imaging with fluo-

*Many different units have been used for reporting oxygen concentration. The most common units are percentage, parts per million (ppm), and Torr ($\cong$mmHg = Po_2. Conversion rates are: room air = 20.5% O_2 = 205,000 ppm = 156 Torr).

rodeoxyglucose (FDG) is helpful for this purpose. Because normal myocardium also concentrates this substrate, the metabolic images must be compared with perfusion to detect viable ischemic tissue. In addition, to maximize the sensitivity of the procedure FDG images require careful control of the patient's glucose metabolic state before injection of the tracer and are probably best performed by using an insulin clamp. A single-tracer, single-imaging approach that provides a positive signal (increase in tracer localization) in the area of ischemic viable tissue would offer advantages in terms of sensitivity and certainty of interpretation.

Hypoxia-localizing radiopharmaceuticals, which require cellular metabolic activity for localization, would differentiate viable from irreversibly damaged tissue. Such agents would provide unique data about cellular metabolic integrity (measured by the ability of cells to reduce the agent) and the status of intracellular oxygen.

Historically, the concept of hypoxia-localizing agents begins in the 1950s, when a series of compounds containing nitroimidazoles were synthesized to treat anaerobic infections. In 1955 Nakamura discovered that a 5-nitroimidazole (azomycin) was active against infections associated with anaerobic conditions. This agent, once in the organism, was only effective if the intracellular oxygen concentration was extremely low. Over the next four decades, analogs were developed, with varying degrees of lipophilicity (solubility in fatty tissue, a variable that determines the relative concentration in tissue vs blood, route of excretion [bile vs urine], etc.) and degrees of reactivity (defining the degree of hypoxia required in the intracellular environment for the reduction reaction to take place). These antimicrobial agents are now an integral part of the treatment armamentarium for fungal infections. The idea that this mechanism might be adapted to allow visualization of hypoxic tissue in vivo was first suggested by Chapman, Franko, and Sharpman[10] in 1981, about 25 years after the initial discovery by Nakamura that reduction pathways of nitroimidazole compounds were influenced by intracellular Po_2.[57] It took several more years to develop the first generation of practical radiopharmaceuticals to test this hypothesis in animals and perform preliminary human studies. The utility of these agents as potential radiopharmaceuticals for imaging hypoxic tissue in a broad range of conditions was recently reviewed by Nunn, Linder, and Strauss.[40] Although several chemical classes of molecules have been synthesized, most of these new compounds contain a nitroimidazole moiety as part of their structure. When labeled with technetium-99m (^{99m}Tc), such compounds have been shown to localize preferentially in myocardium with an intracellular Po_2 less than 3 Torr (about 25% of the normal value). Such tissue has lost its contractile ability but maintained its ability to catabolize glucose.

When nitroimidazole-bearing compounds enter viable cells, they are reduced in a series of steps by nitroreductase enzymes, such as xanthine oxidase. In the presence of adequate intracellular oxygen levels (normoxic tissue), the first one-electron reduction step is reversible, and the molecule is reoxidized. These reactions are repeated until the intact molecule diffuses back out of the cell. However, in cells with reduced oxygen concentration, reoxidation to starting material is not favored, and the reduced product undergoes additional reduction reactions. The gain of these electrons alters the molecule in a manner that limits its diffusion from the cell. This preferential retention in hypoxic cells and diffusion out of normoxic cells is the mechanism that allows imaging of hypoxia.

Nitroimidazole compounds labeled with iodine or fluorine have been used in clinical trials for the assessment of hypoxia in peripheral vascular disease and in several cancers, including small-cell lung cancer, soft-tissue sarcoma, and head and neck cancers.[7,20,43,44] Results of limited human trials aimed at imaging of stroke with a Tc-labeled nitroimidazole were also recently reported.[4]

The usefulness of hypoxia-avid radiopharmaceuticals will be determined by various factors, including the contrast between the hypoxic tissue and background and the concentration of radiopharmaceuticals in tissue. If localization is fast, these agents may identify sites of transient ischemia.

MECHANISMS

The 2-nitroimidazole ring structure, shown schematically in Fig. 7-1, can accept up to six electrons in a series of steps under chemical or enzymatic-reducing conditions. The final product is the formation of an amine. The first step in this pathway, a one-electron reduction that leads to the formation of a nitro radical, is the only reversible step in the process. Many of the subsequent reduction products in this cascade are reactive or polar. These intermediates can bind to cellular components or can be trapped inside the cell because of decreases in permeability of the reduced products. It is likely that enzymatically catalyzed reduction of the 2-nitroimidazole moiety to these reactive intermediates is responsible for the preferential localization of nitroimidazole compounds in hypoxic cells.

However, if such a reduction is initiated in a normoxic cell, oxygen (a powerful oxidant) can reoxidize the initial one-electron radical product back to starting material. This redox cycle will be repeated until the starting compound diffuses back out of the cell. Because the rate of oxidation depends on the intracellular concentration of oxygen, the initial step in the pathway gives the reaction its oxygen sensitivity. The more hypoxic the cell is, the less likely it is that reoxidation to starting material will take place and the more likely it is that reactive reduced products will be formed. These compounds are summarized in Fig. 7-2. The cellular components with which these reduced products react have not been identified definitively. Experiments seeking the final species of nitroimidazole interaction have studied possible DNA adducts and proteins, but less than 2% of the compounds in any of these forms have been identified. For imaging purposes, the chemical form of the species is not as critical as the relative concentration of the material in the target tissue to that in the surrounding background. Formation of less permeable species, such as the amine, which is charged and therefore less likely to diffuse through the cell membrane, is as effective as covalent binding to macromolecules.

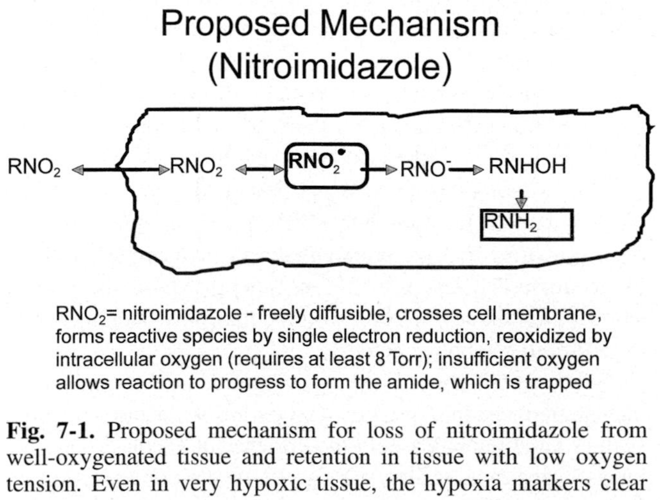

The specific enzyme or enzymes responsible for reduction of the molecule in mammalian cells has not been identified, but several enzymes capable of this reaction are known.[26] For example, xanthine oxidase, an enzyme found in many mammalian cells, is often used[15] as a test system in laboratory studies. It should be noted that in infarcted cells, reduction does not take place, because the enzymes that catalyze the reaction are no longer viable.

FACTORS AFFECTING LOCALIZATION

The absolute uptake of a nitroimidazole compound in hypoxic tissue will be determined by:

1. Severity and duration of ischemia. Because low oxygen tension is required to establish the intracellular circumstances required for trapping, severe ischemia or a prolonged insult favors localization of the compounds.
2. Delivery to the tissue. Rapid localization in areas of modest ischemia will permit these agents to be used in conjunction with stress tests, whereas a requirement for severe ischemia or slower localization will limit the application of these agents to persistent low-flow conditions, such as those that occur in patients with hibernating myocardium.
3. Permeability of the agent and its metabolites. Because these compounds must cross cell membranes to enter the cells where the enzymes required for trapping are located, molecules that are readily able to get into cells will, with a given concentration of agent in the blood stream, deliver more signal than those that are not readily permeable. The ability to cross lipid bilayers is determined by charge, molecular weight, and lipophilicity. Compounds that are neutral, of low molecular weight, and of intermediate lipophilicity seem best able to enter cells. When the compounds are metabolized it is important that the resulting metabolic product be unable to

Proposed Mechanism
(Nitroimidazole)

$RNO_2 \leftrightarrow RNO_2 \leftrightarrow \boxed{RNO_2^{\bullet}} \rightarrow RNO^- \rightarrow RNHOH$
$\rightarrow \boxed{RNH_2}$

RNO_2 = nitroimidazole - freely diffusible, crosses cell membrane, forms reactive species by single electron reduction, reoxidized by intracellular oxygen (requires at least 8 Torr); insufficient oxygen allows reaction to progress to form the amide, which is trapped

Fig. 7-1. Proposed mechanism for loss of nitroimidazole from well-oxygenated tissue and retention in tissue with low oxygen tension. Even in very hypoxic tissue, the hypoxia markers clear over time.

STRUCTURES OF SELECTED COMPOUNDS

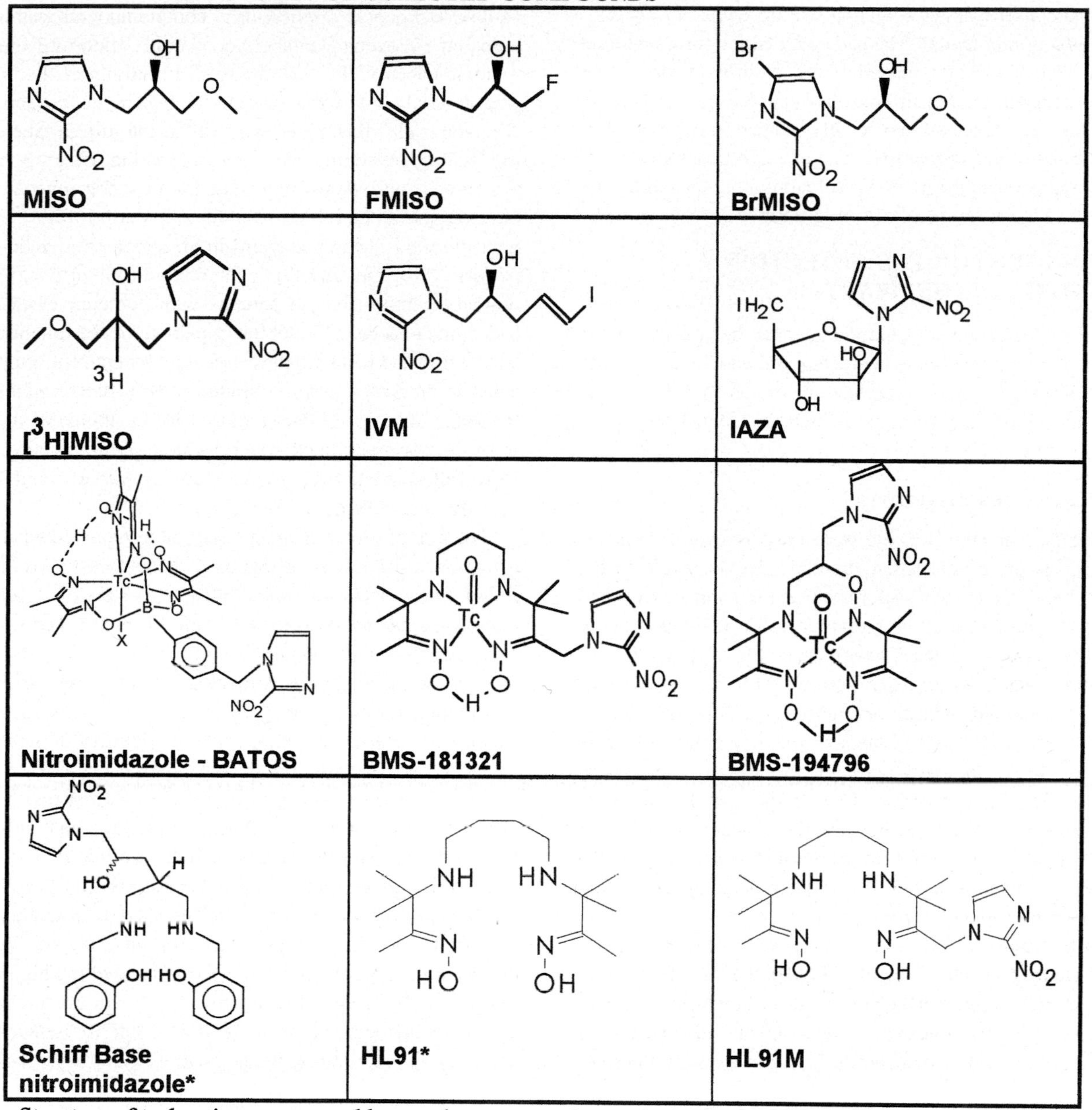

MISO   **FMISO**   **BrMISO**

[³H]MISO   **IVM**   **IAZA**

Nitroimidazole - BATOS   **BMS-181321**   **BMS-194796**

Schiff Base nitroimidazole*   **HL91***   **HL91M**

Structure of technetium compound has not been reported, so only the structure of the ligand used to make the compound is provided here.

Fig. 7-2. Structures of selected nitroimidazole compounds. BrMISO = brom-misonidazole; FMISO = fluoromisonidazole; IAZA = iodoazomycin arabinoside; IVM = iodovinylmisonidazole; MISO = misonidazole.

diffuse out of the cell quickly, because this will result in signal loss over time.

4. Blood clearance and biodistribution. Because these compounds must cross membranes to access the mechanisms required for trapping, charged compounds are unlikely to be useful. Agents that are rapidly cleared from the blood may have a shorter input function to the tissue than those that remain in the circulation for a longer time. Neutral, very polar compounds will usually be poorly extracted by most tissues; therefore, the potential input function for these agents from the blood may be greater than that for compounds that clear readily from the blood. However, because slow clearance from the blood is usually coupled with low permeability, the relative efficacy of two hypothetical agents (one with slow blood clearance but poor extraction vs one with rapid blood clearance but excellent myocardial extraction) must be empirically determined. Such characteristics as background levels in nontarget organs, such as

muscle and liver, will also determine the ability to obtain useful images of hypoxia in vivo.

5. Reduction potential. The ease with which the compound is reduced can be adjusted by the addition of substituents on the nitroimidazole ring. Compounds that are harder to reduce are not readily trapped in hypoxic tissue. However, compounds that are significantly easier to reduce than the prototypical compound misonidazole show significant localization in normoxic tissue as well.

AGENTS USED FOR THE DETECTION OF HYPOXIA IN THE HEART

Three major classes of compounds have been used for the assessment of hypoxia in the heart (Fig. 7-2 and Table 7-1): derivatives of the prototype compound misonidazole (MISO), Tc-labeled nitroimidazole derivatives, and Tc-labeled non-nitroimidazole compounds.

Misonidazole and derivatives

Derivatives of misonidazole were initially evaluated as radiosensitizers in cancer chemotherapy. To accomplish that function, these agents were administered in quantities of 0.5 to 1 mmol/kg. At that dose, the blood clearance is biphasic, with about 30% of the dose clearing with a half-life of about 30 minutes and the remainder clearing with a half life of 70 to 90 minutes.[11,22] Compounds with lipophilicity equal to or greater than that of misonidazole have a longer second component of clearance as the dose is increased, probably because of saturation of the metabolizing enzymes for these compounds. Lower doses have faster blood clearance. Because the lowest doses used for radiosensitization are orders of magnitude greater than those proposed for imaging studies, tracer quantities may have much faster blood clearance.

Both brominated (^{77}Br and ^{82}Br-misonidazole)[22,25] and iodinated (iodovinyl misonidazole [IVM]) derivatives of misonidazole have been synthesized; to date, however, no information on the usefulness of these agents in myocardial ischemia is available. However, the positron-emitting fluorine-labeled compound ^{18}F-fluoromisonidazole has been studied for cardiac and cancer applications. This compound was initially prepared by exchange labeling of cold ^{18}fluoromisonidazole with radioactive ^{18}F; thus, the specific activity of this material was relatively low. When prepared in higher specific activity by Grierson et al,[20] this material as well as the tritium-labeled analog ^{3}H-fluoromisonidazole was successful in detecting hypoxic tumors [43,44] and identifying ischemia in a dog myocardial infarct model. Although several clinical studies with ^{18}F-misonidazole and ^{123}I-iodinated nitroimidazole derivative have been performed for the detection of hypoxia in tumors[21,28,29,55] preliminary human trials in patients with coronary disease have had limited success.[8] Potential explanations for imaging problems with ^{18}F-MISO are the relatively low concentration of the agent in the lesion and the limited photon flux available after the delay of several hours required for clearance of the agent from the normoxic background tissue and the blood (contrast between lesion and background is usually <2:1 at about 90 minutes after injection).

The rate of blood clearance will be a major factor defining the potential usefulness of hypoxia agents for in vivo imaging. Rapid blood clearance limits delivery to sites of low flow. If blood clearance is slow, as it is with ^{18}F-misonidazole, higher concentrations can potentially be delivered to low-flow areas (by diffusion through the extracellular fluid space) but the time between injection and imaging is prolonged. This slow blood clearance is one of the reasons that the delivery of antimyosin, an agent used to detect acute myocardial necrosis, achieves highest tissue concentrations in zones of lowest flow.[27] However, slow blood clearance will also create low contrast between the blood pool and the organs of interest soon after injection. Even with high-resolution positron emission tomography, this combination of circumstances makes successful evaluation of hypoxic lesions a challenge. The 110-minute physical half-life of ^{18}F limits the time after injection during which high-quality images can be recorded to about 3 to 4 hours. As a result, images must be recorded when significant activity remains in the normoxic tissue, limiting image contrast in the myocardium.

Table 7-1. Retention of compounds in hypoxic and normoxic myocytes

Compound	Log k′ value	Normoxic cells at 60 minutes, %	Hypoxic cells at 60 minutes, %	Ratio of hypoxic to normoxic myocytes
^{3}H-fluoromisonidazole	−0.7	3	8	2.6
Tc-PnAO-6-amide-(2-nitroimidazole)	−0.45	10	18	1.8
^{131}I-iodovinyl misonidazole	−0.19	12	26	2.2
Tc-PnAO-1-(-4-nitroimidazole)	0.16	23	40	1.7
Tc-PnAO-1-(-2-nitroimidazole) (BMS-181321)	0.31	22	50	2.3
BMS-194796*		9	52	5.8
Control—Tc-PnAO-6-Me (non-nitroimidazole)	0.31	17.4	22.7	1.3

*First column only—Reprinted by permission of the Society of Nuclear Medicine. Data from Wedeking P, Yost F, Wen M, et al: Comparison of the biological activity of the isomers of the Tc-99m-nitroimidazole complex BMS-194796. *J Nucl Med* 36(5):17P, 1995.

All other data from Rumsey WL, Patel B, Kuczynski B, et al: Potential of nitroimidazoles as markers of hypoxia in heart. In Vaupel P, et al, eds: *Oxygen transport to tissues*, New York, 1994, Plenum Press.

Technetium derivatives

Coupling oxygen-sensitive moieties to Tc should permit administration of higher doses and provide higher-quality images. Initial attempts at the design of Tc-based hypoxia imaging agents aimed at molecules with a blood clearance half-time of 15 minutes or less to permit imaging within about 1 hour while increasing the delivery to sites of markedly decreased flow. The earliest attempts at the design of Tc-based nitroimidazoles were based on the lipophilic and highly extractable class of BATO (boronic acid adduct of Tc dioximes) class of compounds.[33] However, although these molecules were recognized and reduced by nitroimidazole reductase enzymes in vitro, preliminary evaluations in isolated perfused hearts and in vivo were disappointing because the compounds did not cross cell membranes to access the enzymatic trapping mechanisms inside the cell. Schiff-base derivative of Tc were explored,[38] but these compounds also failed to show promise in studies with isolated myocytes because of high lipophilicity coupled with low diffusibility through cell membranes.[42]

Greater success was obtained with Tc compounds that cross cell membranes readily, and, in 1992, ^{99m}Tc-labeled nitroimidazole, [99m]TcO (PnAO-1-(2-nitroimidazole) (BMS-181321), was described that had in vivo kinetics that were potentially suitable for detection of hypoxic myocardium. The agent BMS-181321 is a 2-nitroimidazole derivative of the well known class of technetium(V) oxo-propylene-amine-oxime (PnAO) complexes.[32] It passes readily through bovine brain endothelial cells with a permeability that is about 60% of that of water. Laboratory studies have demonstrated preferential binding of BMS-181321 to hypoxic myocytes and isolated perfused hearts in vitro and to ischemic myocardial tissue in laboratory animals. Preferential uptake in hypoxic tumors, both in vitro and in vivo,[3] and in animal models of stroke[16] have been reported. This agent has also been used to evaluate hypoxia in stroke in patients with cerebrovascular disease.[4]

It seems that BMS-181321 localizes in hypoxic tissue by forming a polar species,[9] with only a small fraction of the dose bound to protein in the cell. These findings are in keeping with postulates in the literature about the trapping mechanism of nitroimidazoles. Most metabolites were low-molecular-weight polar products that did not pass readily from the cytosol into the extracellular medium.

Several derivatives of BMS-181321 were studied, and structure–activity relationships were developed.[34] From this work, a second-generation Tc-labeled nitroimidazole, BMS-194796, based on an oxa-amine-oxime ligand core, was designed.[58] In comparison with BMS-181321, this compound has improved stability, clears more completely from the blood, is less active in the liver, and has more rapid clearance through the GI tract. The compound has been evaluated in vitro in isolated myocytes and tumor cells, and in dog and swine models of myocardial ischemia. These studies demonstrate faster trapping kinetics and higher hypoxic-to-normoxic ratios for BMS-194796 than BMS-181321. It is hoped that these improved properties will lead to a more efficacious agent for clinical use.

Non–nitroimidazole-containing chelates

A recent patent application reports that some Tc metal chelates without an appended nitro-containing group show some specificity for hypoxic tissue.[1] In an isolated buffer-perfused rat heart model, compounds such as HL91, a Tc complex of the butane-amineoxime ligand BnAO, showed high hypoxic-to-normoxic ratios. The mechanism of localization of these non-nitro complexes is unclear but seems to be an intrinsic property of the Tc complex itself. In vitro uptake of this compound in tumor cells at markedly reduced oxygen concentrations (ranging from 0% to 20%) showed that the highest retention occurs at the lowest oxygen concentrations. However, after 4.5 hours of incubation, the uptake of HL91 in completely anoxic cells was only about 5.5% of that of ^{3}H-misonidazole in the same system.[2] This may be due to the hydrophilicity of the compound, which prevents ready diffusion of the compound across cell membranes, or the fact that retention requires some form of energy, which is not maintained as the hypoxic cells die. The distribution of ^{99m}Tc-HL91 in human tumors was recently compared to that of [18]FDG.[4]

Following is a summary of the current state of information available with nitroimidazole and non–nitroimidazole-based hypoxia localizing agents in the heart.

- Myocytes: Studies in isolated cardiac myocytes allow determination of uptake of putative hypoxia imaging agents under carefully controlled oxygen levels in the absence of confounding factors that may affect distribution, such as blood flow. However, care must be taken when comparing values obtained from different groups, because minor differences in isolation and the washing procedures used after incubation can affect the final values. For example, Biskupiak et al[7] compared the retention of F-misonidazole and IVM in separated adult rat myocytes. After 1 hour, IVM had an anoxic-to-normoxic ratio of 9.6. By 3 hours, this value had increased to 22.0 and was similar to that of F-misonidazole (20.3). In contrast, Rumsey et al (Table 7-1) obtained an anoxic-to-normoxic ratio of 2.2 for IVM after 1 hour, but they used a different workup procedure.

  Retention in both normoxic and anoxic cells seems to depend in part on the lipophilicity of the complexes. Rumsey et al[47] noted that the absolute uptake in both normoxic and hypoxic cells increased with log k′ (a measure of lipophilicity). ^{3}H-Fluoromisonidazole, the least lipophilic compound tested (log k′ = −0.7), had the lowest level of uptake (3% in normoxic cells and 8% in hypoxic cells), whereas BMS-181321, the most lipophilic compound tested, had retention of 22% in normoxic cells and 50% in hypoxic cells after 1 hour of incubation. Uptake in normoxic cells reached a plateau within 1 minute, suggesting that this activity was nonspecifically bound rather than metabolically trapped. In contrast, activity levels in hypoxic myocytes increased over a 60-minute period. Most of the compounds tested had hypoxic-to-normoxic ratios of about 2:1 in this system. In this respect, BMS-194796 was anomalous, with a hypoxic-to-normoxic ratio of 5:1.

- Isolated perfused hearts: Shelton et al[51] determined the retention of ^{18}F-misonidazole in hypoxic, ischemic, and normal hearts and in hearts subjected to ischemia and reperfusion before injection. They found about 200% greater retention in the hypoxic and ischemic hearts compared with the controls and the ischemic–reperfused hearts. Even under these optimized circumstances, nonischemic tissue retained about 20% of the initially administered tracer. Although ischemic hearts had longer retention time and the ischemic-to-normal tissue ratio was borderline for imaging, these investigators demonstrated the feasibility of imaging with this agent in a series of five dogs with experimental ischemia.

Retention of BMS-181321 in buffer-perfused rat hearts was 2.5 to about 10 times higher under hypoxic than normoxic conditions.[27,32] The second phase of clearance of activity (retained after 2 minutes) had a half-time of 170 ± 30 minutes in normoxic hearts, whereas the hearts perfused with hypoxic buffer had a clearance half-time of 604 ± 112 minutes. In normoxic hearts, only 33% of the peak activity remained after 40 minutes of clearance. In contrast, 65% of peak activity was retained in the hypoxic hearts.

When oxygen levels in perfusate were reduced from 544 to 29 Torr in graded intervals, each decrease in perfusate Po_2 caused an increase in the level of BMS-181321 retention, and a very strong correlation between the level of retention of BMS-181321 and the cytosolic [lactate]/[pyruvate] ratio was seen.[49] Similarly, the studies of Shi et al[52] in the dog demonstrated the correlation of lactate production retention. The inverse relation between Po_2 and retention of BMS-181321 in the experiments of Rumsey et al was best described by a linear equation (retained radioactivity = $58.1 - 0.55 \times$ perfusate oxygen (Torr); $R^2 = 0.948$). If a constant was added to the equation to allow for the non-zero retention observed during perfusion with fully oxygenated buffer, the fit found by Ng et al[39] was more appropriately described as sigmoidal, indicating that a threshold level of hypoxia is needed for significant uptake of the tracer. Tissue retention varied from $0.61\% \pm 0.14\%$ in normoxia to $5.94\% \pm 1.16\%$ under the most severe hypoxic conditions. These results were mirrored by those of Kusuoka et al,[31] who also studied the retention of BMS-181321 in isolated perfused rat hearts under normoxic, hypoxic, or no-flow ischemia followed by reperfusion. Under normoxic conditions, BMS-181321 was injected and allowed to wash out of the heart. After 10 minutes, absolute retention in the heart was <1% ID/g wet wt. In contrast, when hypoxic buffer was used at similar flow rates, retention in the heart at 10 minutes was four times higher.

The normalized retention and hypoxic-to normoxic ratio

for the non-nitroimidazole Tc complex HL91 was compared to that of ^{3}H-misonidazole, iodine-labeled iodoazomycin arabinoside (IAZA), and BMS-181321 in the isolated perfused heart. In these studies, ^{3}H-MISO was used as an internal standard. Data are shown in Table 7-2. Hypoxic-to-normoxic ratios for HL91 (54:1) were significantly higher than any other value that has been reported for a hypoxia localizing agent. However, absolute uptake of the compound was similar to that of misonidazole and IAZA. The agent BMS-181321 showed about 3.6-fold greater absolute retention than HL91 in this model. The high hypoxic-to-normoxic ratio observed by Archer et al[2] for HL91 has not reproduced by others, although substantial retention in these models was noted. Fukuchi et al[18] compared the distribution of coinjected HL91 and ^{14}C-deoxyglucose in isolated perfused rat hearts by autoradiography by studying three conditions. In the first, the left circumflex artery (LCA) was occluded for 15 min, the vessel was reperfused for 30 minutes and tracer was injected, followed by sacrifice after 30 minutes. Under these conditions, no preferential localization of HL91 was noted. However, if the LCA was occluded for 60 minutes instead of 15 minutes, localization in the reperfused territory was noted, with an LCA-to-septum ratio of about 3:1. If the LCA was completely occluded and tracer was injected after 1 hour of a 1.5-hour occlusion, no ^{14}C-deoxyglucose or HL91 activity was noted in the occluded territory, but hyperactivity was seen in the border zone, with LCA-to-septum activity ratios of about 5:1 (HL91) or 3:1 (^{14}C-deoxyglucose). The border zone for HL91 was significantly smaller than that of the ^{14}C compound, similar to data seen previously with BMS-181321.[17]

• Experimental studies in vivo: Garrecht and Chapman[19] observed about twice as much misonidazole retention in the myocardium of mice treated with isoproterenol to induce myocardial ischemia compared with controls. Retention of IVM in the myocardium of dogs after partial left anterior descending coronary artery (LAD) stenosis with or without demand ischemia was examined by Martin et al.[35] Increased retention of radioactivity was seen in areas with reduced blood supply. Retention increased linearly as the blood flow in the tissue decreased below 30% of the baseline value, in association with decreased contractile function shown by sonomicrometry. These areas of increased retention should have consisted of viable tissue because contractile function returned with relief of ischemia. Additional studies demonstrated retention of IVM in animals with severe stenosis and ischemia due to increased demand. The maximal ratio of is-

Table 7-2 Retention of nitroimidazole and non-nitroimidazole compounds in isolated perfused heart

Compound	Hypoxic-to-normoxic ratio	Normalized retention relative to ^{3}H-misonidazole
Misonidazole*	10:1	1
HL91*	54:1	2.3:1
Iodoazomycin arabinoside*	~10	2.8:1
BMS-181321†	10	8.4:1

*Data from Archer, Edwards B, Kelly JD, et al: Technetium labeled agents or imaging tissue hypoxia in vivo. In Nicolini M, Bandoli G, and Mazzi V, et al, eds: *Technetium and rhenium in chemistry and nuclear medicine,* Padova, Italy, 1995, SG Editorali.
†Data from WO95/04552 patent application.

chemic tissue to blood in the myocardium was 3.2 at 4 hours after injection. Unfortunately, these investigators did not include attempts to obtain images of the myo-cardium.

DiRocco et al[17] coinjected BMS-181321 with ^{14}C-deoxyglucose or ^{14}C-MISO in rabbits 20 minutes after ligation of the LAD.[17] Double-label autoradiography revealed a similarity in the distribution of the Tc and ^{14}C agents in the border zone of the ischemic LAD territory, with an isch-emic-to-nonischemic ratio of 3:1 at 30 minutes.

Open-chest dogs were injected with BMS-181321 after the LAD was partially occluded and isoproterenol was infused or pacing was used to induce ischemia, with epicardial P_{O_2} reduced from the normal value of 20 to 25 Torr to 2 to 5 Torr. Uptake was seen in both planar and SPECT images with isoproterenol but was only seen on the ex vivo SPECT images with pacing.[52] Autoradiography revealed marked retention of activity in the LAD territory, with an optical density ratio of 4:1 between the ischemic and nonischemic territories. Pronounced uptake was seen in the endocardium and the mesocardium, with little activity on the epicardium. Rumsey et al found that in vivo planar[45] and SPECT[46] images can be obtained in an open-chest dog model. Images can be obtained at 2 hours after injection of BMS-181321 (planar imaging), and the lesion could be detected in vivo with SPECT as early as 14 minutes after injection. Clearance from the blood was rapid; because the liver was the main source of excretion, uptake was greater in the liver than in the myocardium. The rapid visualization of the lesions contrasts with the 2 to 4 hours that is necessary to wait after injection of ^{18}F-misonidazole.[55]

The myocardial kinetics of BMS-181321 in open-chest swine[53] was studied in a model in which flow through the LAD was reduced by 50% to 80%. Initial planar imaging revealed a homogenous distribution, but washout from normoxic tissue was more rapid ($T_{1/2} = 1.0 + 0.1$ h) than that from the ischemic LAD territory ($T_{1/2} = 2.0 + 0.1$ h), allowing visualization of the hypoxic LAD territory at the end of the reperfusion. Tissue activity of BMS-181321 was found to be inversely related to blood flow, as determined by using microspheres. In this model, BMS-194796 was also studied[53] by doing dual-isotope studies in which BMS-194796 was labeled with ^{99m}Tc and BMS-181321 was labeled with [96]Tc. Injections were performed after 30 minutes of ischemia. Ten minutes later, the LAD bed was reperfused for 70 minutes, and regional uptake in the ischemic region could be seen with planar imaging. A significant inverse correlation was seen between flow and uptake of both agents, but clearance from venous blood was enhanced for BMS-194796. The washout half-time for the slow phase of clearance of activity in the LAD was also faster for BMS-194796 (1.4 ± 0.1 h) than for BMS-181321.

The relative kinetics of trapping of BMS-181321 and BMS-194796 were also compared in an open-chest dog model by using the LAD partial occlusion model.[48] The tracer was injected, and the LAD was fully occluded 28 seconds later for a period of 1, 2, 3, or 10 minutes and then released, restoring P_{O_2} to its original value. Neither compound localized in the ischemic lesion after 1 minute of occlusion. After 2 or 3 minutes of no flow followed by reperfusion, the lesion could be visualized with BMS-194796 but not by

BMS-181321, with which good visualization of the lesion required 10 minutes of occlusion. Autoradiographic analysis of tissue slices, obtained after 70 minutes of reperfusion, showed that the ischemic-to-non-ischemic ratio for BMS-194796 was 2.1 ± 0.5 for 2 minutes of no flow and increased to 3.2 ± 0.8 after 3 minutes of occlusion. At 3 hours after injection, liver retention of BMS-194796 (16.7% ± 1.8%) was markedly reduced compared with retention of BMS-181321 (32.6% ± 6.8%) The improved clearance of BMS-194796 from liver and normal tissue and the improved trapping kinetics relative to BMS-181321 should enhance the ability to visualize hypoxia.

The distribution of BMS-194796 was compared with that of Tl in a dual-isotope study in open-chest dogs.[30] The P_{O_2} value in the LAD bed was reduced to 2 to 6 Torr for about 10 to 20 minutes before coinjection of ^{201}Tl and BMS-194796. Ischemic lesions were well visualized by using SPECT from 40 to 120 minutes after injection. Analysis of the hearts ex vivo after about 2 hours after injection showed a lesion-to-normal tissue ratio of 2.7 ± 0.76 for BMS-194796. Ratios of normal tissue-to-lesion for the corresponding Tl ex vivo images were 1.23 ± 0.13. The extent of the jeopardized region was easily delineated with BMS-194796.

Archer et al[2] studied HL91, HL91M, and BMS-181321 in a dog stenosis model. Partial stenosis (75% to 90% occlusion) of the left circumflex artery was used. Planar images were obtained for 4 hours. All three agents localized, but clearer images of the heart were obtained with HL91 and HL91M than with BMS-181321 because of better background clearance. Ex vivo images showed clear localization in the stenotic region, but no in vivo images were presented. Limited biodistribution data were obtained on blood and liver activity in these dogs at 4 hours. Activity in the liver for HL91 was significantly lower (5%) than for BMS-181321 (34%) because clearance of HL91 occurs primarily through the renal system. It is not yet clear whether the decrease in liver background activity is offset by a parallel decrease in the uptake in hypoxic regions of the heart, a result that would be predicted from in vitro studies described earlier. To date, no in vivo images have been presented, although ex vivo autoradiographic slices through the LAD bed reveal good lesion-to-nonlesion contrast.

THE IDEAL AGENT

An optimal agent should localize in the tissue of interest quickly, with a target-to-background ratio of more than 3:1, and provide sufficient photon flux to record high-quality images in a short time at an acceptable radiation burden to the patient. Ischemic tissue usually has decreased perfusion, which limits first-pass delivery of the tracer to the cells of interest. To optimize delivery, blood clearance should be relatively long compared with a perfusion agent.[50] Contrast is determined by the relative retention in ischemic tissue and clearance from normoxic tissue. Optimal imaging time will be determined by the balance between the target-to-background ratio and clearance from the site of ischemia. The biological characteristics of the radiopharmaceutical should have clearance from normal tissue that parallels that of the blood. If the desired delivery to ischemic tissue and clearance can be accomplished, high-quality images could be recorded about 45 to 60 minutes after injection.

POTENTIAL APPLICATIONS

To the extent that the criteria for an ideal agent are met, the agent should be useful in the following situations:

- To evaluate patients admitted as "rule-out myocardial infarction"
- To identify the territory at risk in patients with unstable angina
- After thrombolytic therapy in patients with pain or ST changes that are slow to resolve
- To delineate hibernating myocardium in patients with markedly reduced contractile function
- During episodes of transient ischemia (if trapping is sufficient and blood clearance is fast enough)

Unfortunately, the known kinetics of delivery and nitroimidazole reduction make it unlikely that BMS-181321 would be useful for the detection of transient ischemia. Two recent studies point out the difficulties of using this agent for identification of brief episodes of ischemia. Ng et al[39] used the isolated perfused heart to demonstrate that severe ischemia is required for trapping, and Shi et al[52] found that although localization of BMS-181321 in acute ischemia induced by stenosis of the LAD and pacing was seen in ex vivo images of the heart, the lesion was difficult to see on in vivo planar images (because of high concentration of tracer in the liver). Because it has been determined that the trapping kinetics of this agent[48] are faster than those of BMS-181321, BMS-194796 may prove more suitable for such studies.

When low flow is persistent, which is the problem in identifying viable ischemic tissue in patients with infarction, these agents may play a major role. Optimal preservation of cardiac function requires restoration of perfusion to all viable tissue. After treating chest pain and arrhythmias and achieving hemodynamic stabilization, major management decisions concern the effectiveness of thrombolysis and whether additional mechanical intervention, such as angioplasty or coronary artery bypass graft surgery, is necessary. If reperfusion was successful or if the tissue is dead, further efforts to revascularize the tissue are unnecessary. However, if the tissue remains ischemic, additional intervention is warranted.

CONCLUSION

At present, no human trials of ^{99m}Tc nitroimidazoles have been conducted in patients with coronary disease. Therefore, it is difficult to predict exactly how these agents may be used in clinical decision making. From a realistic perspective, it is likely that the current generation of agents could be useful in patients with stable, severe, persistent ischemia. Even the most pessimistic considerations suggest that we have a new class of agents in our armamentarium. If the current agents are not up to the task, it is likely that some innovative chemistry will be called on to correct the deficiencies and provide the type of agents we will need to determine intracellular Po_2 in vivo.

REFERENCES

1. Archer C, Burke JF, Canning LR, et al: International patent application WO 95/04552, February 1995.
2. Archer CM, Edwards B, Kelly JD, et al: *Technetium labeled agents for imaging tissue hypoxia in vivo.* In Nicolini M, Bandoli G, and Mazzi U, eds: *Technetium & rhenium in chemistry & nuclear medicine,* Padova, 1995, SG Editoriali.
3. Ballinger JR, Kee JWM, and Rauth AM: In vitro and in vivo evaluation of a technetium 99m-labeled 2-nitroimidazole (BMS-181321) as a marker of tumor hypoxia. *J Nucl Med* 37:1023–1031, 1996.
4. Barron B, Grotta J, Lamki L, et al: Preliminary experience with technetium-99m BMS-181321, a nitroimidazole, in the detection of cerebral ischemia associated with acute stroke. *J Nucl Med* 37:272, 1996 (abstract).
5. Berne RM and Levy MN: *The peripheral circulation and its control.* In Berne RM amd Levy MN, eds: *Physiology,* ed 3, St. Louis, 1993, Mosby.
6. Berne RM and Levy MN: *Skeletal physiology.* In Berne RM and Levy MN, eds: *Physiology,* ed 3, St. Louis, 1993, Mosby.
7. Biskupiak JE, Grierson JR, Rasey JS, et al: Synthesis of an (Iodovinyl) misonidazole derivative for hypoxia imaging. *J Med Chem* 34:2165–2168, 1991.
8. Caldwell JH, Revenaugh JR, Martin GV, et al: Comparison of fluorine-18-fluorodeoxyglucose and tritiated fluoromisonidazole uptake during low-flow ischemia. *J Nucl Med* 36:1633–1638, 1995.
9. Chan YW, Romero V, Linder KE, et al: In-vitro studies on the hypoxia retention of a novel technetium-99m labeled nitroimidazole in rat heart. *J Nucl Med* 35:152, 1994 (abstract).
10. Chapman JD, Franko AJ, and Sharplin J: A marker for hypoxic cells in tumors with potential clinical applicability. *Brit J Cancer* 43:546–550, 1981.
11. Chin JB and Rauth AM: The metabolism and pharmacokinetics of the hypoxic cell radiosensitizer and cytotoxic agent, misonidazole in C3H mice. *Radiat Res* 86:341–357, 1981.
12. Connet RG, Honig CG, Gayeski E, et al: Defining hypoxia: a systems view of VO_2, glycolysis, energetics and intracellular Po_2. *J Appl Physiol* 68:833–842, 1990.
13. Cook GJR, Barrington S, Houston S, et al: HL91, a new Tc-99m labeled agent with potential for identifying tumore hypoxia: correlation with FDG PET. *J Nucl Med* 37:87P, 1996 (abstract).
14. Contran RS, Kumar V, and Robbins SL: *Cellular injury and death.* In Cotran RS, Kumar V, Robbins SL, eds: *Robbins pathologic basis of disease,* ed 4, Philadelphia, 1989, WB Saunders and Co.
15. deJong JW, van der Meer P, Nieukoop AS, et al: Xanthine oxidoreductase activity in perfused hearts of various species, including humans. *Circ Res* 67:770–777, 1990.
16. DiRocco RD, Kuczynski BL, Pirro JP, et al: Imaging ischemic tissue at risk of infarction in stroke. *J Cerebral Blood Flow and Metab* 13:755–762, 1993.
17. DiRocco RJ, Bauer A, Kuczynski BL, et al: Imaging regional hypoxia with a new technetium-labeled imaging agent in rabbit myocardium after occlusion of the left anterior descending coronary artery. *J Nucl Med* 33:865P, 1992 (abstract).
18. Fukuchi K, Kusuoka K, Yutani K, et al: Assessment of reperfused myocardium using new hypoxia avid imaging agent Tc-99m HL91. *J Nucl Med* 37:94P, 1996 (abstract).
19. Garrecht BM and Chapman JD: The labeling of EMT-6 tumors in BALB/C mice with ^{14}C-misonidazole. *Brit J Radiol* 56:745–753, 1983.
20. Grierson JR, Link JM, Mathis CA, et al: A radiosynthesis of fluorine-18 fluoromisonidazole. *J Nucl Med* 30:343–350, 1989.
21. Groshar D, McEwan AJB, Parliament MB, et al: Imaging tumor hypoxia and tumor perfusion. *J Nucl Med* 34:885–888, 1993.

22. Grunbaum Z, Freauff SJ, Krohn KA, et al: Synthesis and characterization of congeners of misonidazole for imaging hypoxia. *J Nucl Med* 28:68–75, 1987.

23. Guyton AC: *Transport of oxygen and carbon dioxide in the blood and body fluids.* In *Textbook of physiology,* Philadelphia, 1981, WB Saunders and Co.

24. Hendel RC:Single-photon perfusion imaging for the assessment of myocardial viability. *J Nucl Med* 35(4 Suppl):23S–31S, 1994.

25. Jette DC, Wiebe LI, and Chapman JD: Synthesis and in vivo studies of the radiosensitizer 4-[BR]bromomisonidazole. *Int J Nucl Med Biol* 10:205–212, 1983.

26. Kedderris GL and Miwa GT: The metabolic activation of nitroheterocyclic therapeutic agents. *Drug Metab Rev*19:33–62, 1998.

27. Khaw BA, Strauss HW, Moore R, et al: Myocardial damage delineated by Indium-111 antimyosin FAB and technetium-99m pyrophosphate. *J Nucl Med* 28:76–82, 1987.

28. Koh WJ, Bergman KS, Rasey JS, et al: Evaluation of oxygenation status during fractionated radiotherapy in human nonsmall cell lung cancers using [F-18]fluoromisonidazole positron emission tomography. *Int J Radiat Oncol Biol Phys* 33:391–398, 1995.

29. Koh WJ, Rasey JS, Evans ML, et al: Imaging of hypoxia in human tumors with [F-18]fluoromisonidazole. *Int J Radiat Oncol Biol Phys* 22:199–212, 1991.

30. Kuczynski B, Linder K, Patel B, et al: Dual isotope imaging of Tc-99m (BMS-194796) and Tl-201 in dog coronary artery stenosis model. *J Nucl Cardiol* 2(2 Part 2)S28, 1995 (abstract).

31. Kusuoka B, Hashimoto K, Fukuchi K, et al: Kinetics of a putative hypoxic tissue marker, techetium-99m-nitroimidazole (BMS-181321), in normoxic, hypoxic, ischemic and stunned myocardium. *J Nucl Med* 35:1371–1376, 1994.

32. Linder KE, Chan YW, Cyr JE, et al: ^{99}TcO(PnAO-1-2-nitroimidazole) [BMS-181321], a new technetium-containing nitroimidazole complex for imaging hypoxia: synthesis, characterization and xanthine oxidase-catalyzed reduction. *J Med Chem* 37:9, 1994.

33. Linder K, Chan YW, Cyr JE, et al: Synthesis, characterization and in vitro evaluation of nitroimidazole BATO complexes: new technetium compounds designed for imaging hypoxic tissue. *Bioconjug Chem* 4:326–333, 1993.

34. Linder KE, Cyr JE, Chan YW, et al: Effect of substituents on physiochemical and biological behavior of Tc-PnAO nitroimidazoles. *J Nucl Med* 35:18P, 1994 (abstract).

35. Martin GV, Biskupiak JE, Caldwell JH, et al: Characterization of iodovinylmisonidazole as a marker for myocardial hypoxia. *J Nucl Med* 34:918–923, 1993.

36. Martin GV, Caldwell JH, Graham MN, et al: Non-invasive detection of hypoxic myocardium using fluorine-18-misonidazole and positron emission tomography. *J Nucl Med* 33:2202–2208, 1992.

37. Maurea S, Cuocolo A, Soricelli A, et al: Enhanced detection of viable myocardium by technetium-99m-MIBI imaging after nitrate administration in chronic coronary artery disease. *J Nucl Med* 36:1945–1952, 1995.

38. Neumeier R, Kramp W, and Maecke HR:*European Patent Application* EP417,870:1991.

39. Ng C, Sinusas AJ, Zaret BL, Soufer R: Kinetic analysis of technetium-99m labeled nitroimidazole (BMS-181321) as a tracer of myocardial hypoxia. *Circulation* 92:1261–1268, 1995.

40. Nunn A, Linder K, Strauss HW: Nitroimidazoles and imaging hypoxia: a review. *Eur J Nucl Med* 22:265–280, 1995.

41. Pontillo D, Carboni GP, Capezzuto A, et al: Identification of viable myocardium by nitrate echocardiography after myocardial infarction: comparison with planar thallium reinjection scintigraphy. *Angiology* 47:437–464, 1996.

42. Ramalingam K, Raju N, Nanjappan P, et al: The synthesis and in vitro evaluation of a ^{99m}technetium-nitroimidazole complex based on a bis(amine-phenol) ligand: comparison to BMS-181321. *J Med Chem* 37:4155–4163, 1994.

43. Rasey JS, Grunbaum Z, Magee S, et al: Characterization of radiolabeled fluoromisonidazole as a probe for hypoxic cells. *Radiat Res* 111:292–304, 1987.

44. Rasey JS,Koh WJ, Grierson JR: Radiolabeled fluoromisonidazole as an imaging agent for tumor hypoxia. *Int Radiat Oncol Biol Phys* 17:985–991, 1989.

45. Rumsey WL, Kuczynski B, and Patel B: Detecting hypoxia in heart using phosphorescence quenching and ^{99m}technetium-nitroimidazoles. In Hogan et al, eds: *Oxygen transport to tissue XVI,* New York, 1994, Plenum Press.

46. Rumsey WL, Kuczynski B, Patel B, et al: SPECT imaging of ischemic myocardium using a technetium-99m-nitroimidazole ligand. *J Nucl Med* 36:1445–1450, 1995.

47. Rumsey WL, Patel B, Kuczynski BL, et al: *Potential of nitroimidazoles as markers of hypoxia in heart.* In Vaupel P, et al, eds: *Oxygen transport to tissue,* New York, 1994, Plenum Press.

48. Rumsey WL, Patel B, Kuczynski BL, et al: Comparison of two novel technetium agents for imaging ischemic myocardium. Anaheim, 1995 (abstract).

49. Rumsey WL, Patel B, and Linder KE: Effect of graded hypoxia on the retention of a novel technetium-99m-nitroheterocycle in perfused rat heart. *J Nucl Med* 36:632–636, 1995.

50. Sapirstein LA: Regional blood flow by the fractional distribution of indicators. *Am J Physiol* 193:161–168, 1958.

51. Shelton ME, Dence CS, Hwang DR, et al: Myocardial kinetics of fluorine-18 misonidazole: a marker of hypoxic myocardium. *J Nucl Med* 30:351–358, 1989.

52. Shi C, Sinusas AJ, Dione DP, et al: Technetium-99m-nitroimidazole (BMS 181321): a positive imaging agent for detecting myocardial ischemia. *J Nucl Med* 36:1078–1086, 1995.

53. Stone CK, Mulnix T, Nickles RJ, et al: Myocardial kinetics of a putative hypoxic tissue marker, ^{99m}Tc-labeled nitroimidazole (BMS-181321), after regional ischemia and reperfusion. *Circulation* 92:1246 1253, 1995.

54. Treasure C, Klein JL, Weintraub WS, et al: Beneficial effects of cholesterol-lowering therapy on the coronary endothelium in patients with coronary artery disease. *N Engl J Med* 332:481–487, 1995.

55. Valk PE, Mathis CA, Prados MD, et al: Hypoxia in human gliomas: a demonstration by PET with fluorine-18-fluoromisonidazole. *J Nucl Med* 33:2133–2137, 1992.

56. Vanderkooi JM, Erecinska M, and Silver IA: Oxygen in mammalian tissue: methods of measurement and affinities of various reactions. *Am J Physiol* 260(6 Part 1):C1131–1150, 1990.

57. Webster LT: *Drugs used in chemotherapy of protozoal infections.* In Gilman AG, Rall TW, Nies AS, et al, eds: *The pharmacological basis of therapeutics,* New York, 1990, Pergamon Press.

58. Wedeking P, Yost F, Wen M, et al: Comparison of the biological activity of the isomers of the Tc-99m-nitroimidazole complex BMS-194796. *J Nucl Med* 36:17P, 1995 (abstract).

59. Wilson DF, Rumsey Wl, Green TJ, et al: The oxygen dependence of mitochondrial oxidative phosphorylation measured by a new optical method for measuring oxygen concentration. *J Biol Chem* 263:2712–2718, 1988.

INSTRUMENTATION

Future developments in single-photon emission computed tomography quantification and display

Tracy L. Faber, Ernest V. Garcia, and **C. David Cooke**

Myocardial perfusion imaging is the most frequently used study in nuclear cardiology. In the past two decades, major advancements in automated quantification and display, along with better hardware and camera technology and new radiotracers, have improved greatly the quality of the images obtained and the ability to glean clinically useful information from them. Changes will continue to be made, and the future is likely to bring more automation, leading eventually to completely automatic reconstruction, reslicing, quantification, and high-level analysis of results. New databases consistent with the types of studies being performed, including dual-isotope and attenuation-corrected images, will be developed and made commercially available. Three-dimensional displays of quantitated perfusion will be more common and will be used in conjunction with the original slices for patient evaluation. Automated interpretation of quantitative information in the form of expert systems or neural nets will become available to help train new nuclear medicine physicians, to aid in the analysis of complex cases, or to act as a second opinion. Finally, explicit integration of perfusion data with other methods will become a standard way to combine and compare the information in each system; the automation of this process will complement the implicit integration of information that the cardiologist performs mentally. In short, the future will bring more automation to more types of studies, thereby objectifying and standardizing analysis, display, integration, and interpretation of myocardial perfusion.

OBLIQUE REORIENTATION AND RESLICING

Most cardiac images are viewed in a standard format: short-axis, horizontal long-axis, or vertical long-axis slices. Short-axis slices are also necessary for some automatic perfusion quantification algorithms. These standard sections have been generated interactively from the original transaxial images, a method that requires the user to mark the location of the left ventricular axis. In the past few years, some automatic techniques for performing this task have been described and are or will be commercially available.[21-38]

In two of these automatic approaches,[21,30] the left ventricular region is identified in the transaxial images by using a threshold-based approach that includes knowledge about the expected position, size, and shape of the left ventricle. Once the left ventricular region is isolated, the approach described by Germano et al[21] uses the original data to refine the estimate of the myocardial surface. Normalization to an ellipsoid fit to the left ventricular region is used to resample the myocardium; a Gaussian function is fit to the profiles obtained at each sample. The best-fit Gaussian is used to estimate the myocardial center for each profile, and after further refinement on the basis of image intensities and myocardial smoothness, the resulting midmyocardial points are fitted to an ellipsoid whose long axis is used as the final left ventricular long axis. This method was tested on 400 patient images, and the result was similar to interactively denoted long axes. Failure of the method was defined as not localizing the left ventricle, presence of substantial hepatic or intestinal activity in the "left ventricular" region of the image, or a greater than 45° difference between automatically and interactively determined axes. With these criteria, the method was successful in 394 of the 400 cases. Fig. 8-1 shows typical results.

Mullick and Ezquerra[30] used a more complex heuristic technique to determine the optimal left ventricular threshold and isolate it from other structures. After this was accomplished, they used the segmented data directly to determine the long axis. The binary image was tessellated into triangular plates, and the normal of each plate on the endocardial surface was used to point to the long axis of the left ventricle. The intersection (or near-intersection) of these normals were collected and fitted to a three-dimensional straight line, which was then returned as the left ventricular long axis. This method was tested

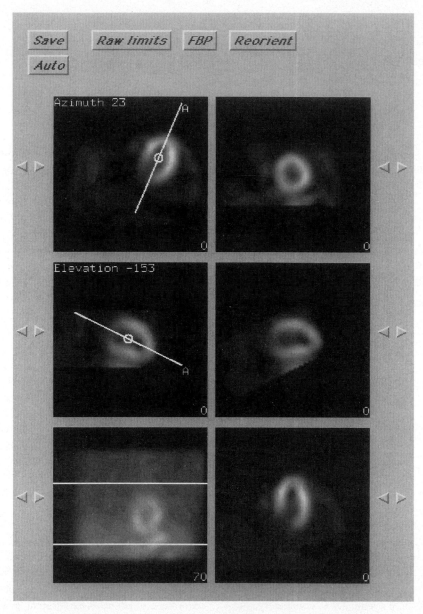

Fig. 8-1. Example of the display screen and results of an automatic reorientation method. *Upper left*, the long axis detected on an original transaxial slice; *middle left*, the long axis detected on a sagittal image. The reoriented short axis, vertical long axis, and horizontal long axis sections are shown on the right from top to bottom, respectively. Automatically determined bounds for reconstruction are shown on a planar projection in the bottom left. (Reprinted by permission of the Society of Nuclear Medicine. From Germano G, Kavanagh PB, Chen J, et al: Operator-less processing of myocardial perfusion SPECT studies. *J Nucl Med* 36:2127–2132, 1995. Used with permission.)

on 124 patient data sets, and the automated long-axis orientation was compared with interactively determined angles. Failure was defined as a failure to isolate the left ventricle. This method succeeded in 116 of 124 cases.

Slomka et al[38] took a different approach to automated reorientation. Their method registers the original image data to a template image in which the orientation of the left ventricle is known and standardized. The template is created by averaging a large number of registered, normal patient data sets; separate templates are created for men and women. Registration is done by first translating and scaling the image on the basis of principal axes. The match is then refined by minimizing the sum of the absolute differences between the template and the image being registered. This method was not compared with interactively reoriented images; however, it was evaluated visually for 38 normal and 10 abnormal patients and was found to be successful for all.

AUTOMATED PERFUSION QUANTIFICATION

Data-based methods for identifying myocardial perfusion abnormalities from thallium-201(^{201}Tl) single-photon emission computed tomography (SPECT) studies were developed and commercialized by investigators at Cedars-Sinai Medical Center[20] and Emory University[3] and results were reported as early as 1985. These methods used a statistically defined database of normal patients to be used as a comparison group against patients with possible coronary artery disease. Although these methods have been extensively validated[3-41] and proven to be clinically valuable[42] in standardizing and objectifying myocardial perfusion scans, they have several deficiencies.

Five major limitations have been identified with these early approaches. First, extensive operator interaction occurs, which results in a reduced objectivity and reproducibility of the program. By automating the process, this limitation has been overcome. Second, these methods fail to sample the count distribution perpendicular to the myocardial wall, particularly at the apex. This usually results in artifactually increasing the counts from the apical region. Third, we lack databases for perfusion tracers other than ^{201}Tl. Comparison of data acquired with different tracers or different protocols with the ^{201}Tl database often leads to incorrect identification of abnormalities. Fourth, these data-based approaches cannot compensate for attenuation in a patient who has much more attenuating tissue (such as breast and diaphragm) than do normal patients selected for the normal database. This almost always leads to the artifactual definition of these photopenic regions as hypoperfused myocardium. Finally, the polar map display cannot represent accurately the true extent and location of an abnormality because of the warping created by transforming a three-dimensional distribution into a two-dimensional polar map. This results in underestimation of the extent of hypoperfused apical regions and overestimation of the extent of hypoperfused basal regions.

More recently, investigators at Emory University and Cedars-Sinai Medical Center developed[16] and extensively validated[40] a new, data-based quantitative package known as CEqual (Cedars–Emory quantitative analysis), which is designed to overcome the aforementioned limitations.

Methods

The CEqual quantitative method uses several image identification techniques (such as image clustering, filtered thresholding, and specified threshold constraints) for isolation of the left ventricular myocardium from the remainder of the image.[5] Once the left ventricular myocardium is identified, the apical and basal image slices, the (x, y) coordinates of the central axis of the ventricular chamber, and a limiting radius for the maximum count circumferential profile search are determined automatically. In most cases, operator interaction is required only for verification of automatically determined features. If at any time the program fails to locate any of the features, it will branch to an interactive mode and require the operator to select the variables manually.

The CEqual technique was developed to generate count profiles from a hybrid, two-part, three-dimensional sampling scheme of stacked short-axis slices. In this approach the apical region of the myocardium is sampled by using spherical coordinates and the rest of the myocardium is sampled by using cylindrical coordinates. This approach promotes a radial sampling that is mostly perpendicular to the myocardial wall for all points and thus results in more accurate representation of the perfusion distribution with minimal sampling artifacts. After operator verification of the automatically derived features, the three-dimensional maximum-count myocardial distribution is extracted from all stacked short-axis tomograms.[16] Maximum-count circumferential profiles, each comprising 40 points, are automatically generated from the short-axis slices by using this two-part sampling scheme. These profiles are generated for stress and rest myocardial perfusion distributions. A normalized percent change between stress and rest is also calculated as a reversibility circumferential profile.[27] The most normal region of the stress distribution is used for normalizing the rest distribution to the stress distribution.

New databases

By using the CEqual approach, normal limits were defined from a group of patients with less than 5% probability of coronary artery disease. Gender-matched normal databases have been defined[39] and validated for the following SPECT protocols:

1. Low-dose rest, high-dose stress, one-day technetium-99m (^{99m}Tc) sestamibi (Cardiolite) protocol[40]
2. High-dose stress and rest two-day ^{99m}Tc sestamibi protocol
3. Stress-redistribution ^{201}Tl protocol
4. Rest ^{201}Tl–stress ^{99m}Tc sestamibi dual-isotope protocol[13]
5. Low-dose stress, high-dose rest ^{99m}Tc tetrofosmin (Myoview) one-day protocol.

All protocols used treadmill exercise to stress the patients.

For each of these protocols, the normal database criteria for abnormality and prospective validation were defined in a standardized approach.[39] From the low-likelihood patients, the normal mean and standard deviation for each myocardial sample were determined. The objective criteria for abnormality were defined from expert visual interpretation of normal and hypoperfused regions. These criteria are based on how many standard deviations below the mean normal distribution constitute an abnormality for each myocardial wall. This must be established because these counts are not distributed in a Gaussian distribution or Bell-shaped curve. Once the normal database and criteria for abnormality are determined, they are tested by using a prospective population in which each patient has undergone coronary catheterization. By using angiography as a gold standard, the accuracy of the method and protocols are established.

The choice of radiopharmaceutical or protocol is more of a clinical question or a question of laboratory logistics and is beyond the scope of this chapter. However, many questions related to these normal databases are often asked that merit further discussion.

One concern is whether the normal databases developed by using patients stressed with exercise can be used for patients undergoing pharmacologic stress. It is evident by looking at these studies that patients who undergo imaging after pharmacologic stress have more background activity and more myocardial activity than patients who undergo treadmill exercise. Nevertheless, the relative distribution in normal patients and patients with coronary artery disease is sufficiently similar that when the same normal database is used for both forms of stress, similar diagnostic accuracy results.[4] Although it would be ideal to have separate databases for protocols using pharmacologic stress, the development cost would be prohibitive.

A second concern is whether the normal database developed for ^{201}Tl stress and redistribution studies may be used for stress and reinjection protocols. The stress protocol is the same for both studies; thus, no new errors should be introduced. However, reinjection images do look different from the redistribution images. Nevertheless, in the CEqual program, the resting distribution is not quantified; rather, the reversibility or change between rest and stress is analyzed. Because reinjection is supposed to result in a more marked difference between the two physiologic states, it is actually easier for the program to detect this difference in the form of defect reversibility. Thus, the stress and redistribution ^{201}Tl normal database may be used to quantify stress/reinjection studies.

The last concern is whether the normal database for ^{99m}Tc sestamibi protocols may be used for ^{99m}Tc tetrofosmin studies and vice-versa. Although there are subtle differences in how these two radiopharmaceuticals are distributed in the body, the main variables driving the final count distributions in the images are the type of collimators and filters used for a given count distribution. It seems that these normal databases are interchangeable, but additional studies are required to confirm these observations.

Compensation for physical effects and implication on quantification

Algorithms that compensate for photon attenuation, scatter effects, and collimation effects in SPECT imaging have been developed over the last 20 years and are well understood.[15–26] Although these compensations are not exact analytic corrections, as in positron emission tomography (PET), preliminary results indicate that their use should improve myocardial perfusion images.[12]

These improvements are expected to result in increased accuracy for detecting coronary artery disease, particularly in improving specificity through correction of diaphragm and breast attenuation artifacts. Application of these compensations will result in a concomitant shift in the normal myocardial tracer distribution previously found by experts, which could have a temporary confounding effect. Moreover, because experts who have learned to read around these artifacts from noncompensated studies have a high accuracy rate for diagnosing coronary artery disease, these compensations are expected to most help researchers with more limited expertise.

Commercial implementations of compensations vary among manufacturers. The main differences are related to the geometry of the way in which the transmission and emission images are generated (parallel vs converging); the degree, if any, to which the algorithms compensate for attenuation, scatter effects, and collimation effects; and the exact mathematical formulation of the algorithms used to reconstruct and correct the images. A concern is that variations in the implementation of these compensations may create variation in the expected normal tracer distribution among systems by different manufacturers or among patients with different anatomy. These variations can complicate image interpretation and comparison with a normal database. Large, prospective clinical trials are needed to document the advantages and limitations of the different approaches. It is expected that as more data become available, manufacturers will find a common approach for image compensation, thus facilitating visual interpretation and image quantification.

DISPLAY

Once perfusion has been quantified, the quantitative data must be displayed. In planar perfusion imaging, myocardial samples are often displayed as a graph of relative counts compared with angle (around the left ventricle). Perfusion data from SPECT require more complex methods of display to present the larger amount of information clearly and logically. Polar maps were developed to display the quantified perfusion data of the entire left ventricle in a single picture. More recently, three-dimensional displays have been adopted by many researchers, hospitals, and manufacturers as a more natural way to present information.

Polar maps

Polar maps, or bulls-eye displays, are the standard for viewing circumferential profiles. They allow a quick and comprehensive overview of the circumferential samples from all slices by combining the samples into a color-coded image. The points of each circumferential profile are assigned a color based on normalized count values, and the colored profiles are shaped into concentric rings. The most apical slice processed with circumferential profiles forms the center of the polar map, and each successive profile from each successive short-axis slice is displayed as a new ring surrounding the previous one until the most basal slice of the left ventricle makes up the outermost ring of the polar map. Fig. 8-2 shows polar maps created by applying the CEqual quantification method to a ^{99m}Tc sestamibi study.

In addition, the use of color can help identify abnormal areas at a glance. Abnormal regions from the stress study can be assigned a black color, thus creating a blackout map. Blacked-out areas that normalize at rest can be color-coded white, thus creating a whiteout reversibility map.[27] This effect can be seen in Fig. 8-2, A. Additional maps, such as a standard deviation map that shows the number of standard deviations below normal of each point in each circumferential profile, can aid in evaluation of the study by indicating the severity of abnormality.

Although polar maps offer a comprehensive view of the quantitation results, they distort the size and shape of the myocardium and any defects. Many improvements have been made in the basic polar map display to help overcome some of these problems.[16] For instance, in distance-weighted maps, each ring

is the same thickness. These maps have been shown to be useful for accurate localization of abnormalities. In volume-weighted maps, the area of each ring is proportional to the volume of the corresponding slice. This type of map has been shown to be best for estimating defect size. However, more realistic displays have been introduced that do not have the distortions of polar maps.

Three-dimensional displays

Three-dimensional graphic techniques can be used to overlay results of perfusion quantification onto a representation of a patient's left ventricle. This representation is generated by using endocardial or epicardial surface points extracted from the perfusion data.

For example, the method used at Emory University for detecting the surface of the myocardium starts with the coordinates of the maximal myocardial count samples created during perfusion quantification.[8] The coordinates of each sampled point are filtered to remove noise. By assuming that the myocardium is 1 cm thick at end diastole, an estimate of the endocardial surface can be generated by subtracting a distance of 5 mm from the myocardial center point. Adding 5 mm estimates the epicardial surface. Other investigators have also used the surface model for displaying myocardial perfusion. Faber et al[7,10] used a surface detection process very different from the previous example.

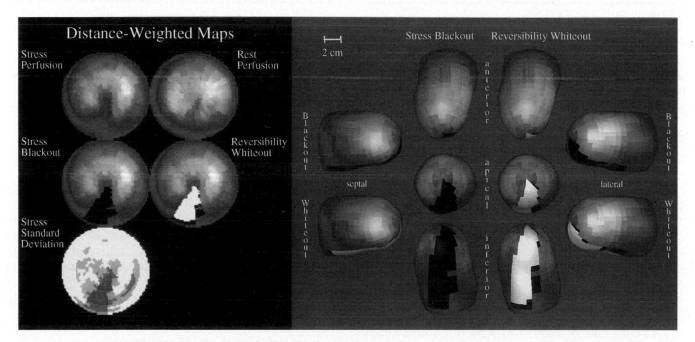

Fig. 8-2. A, Polar maps displaying the results of perfusion quantification. The top row shows the quantitated stress and rest perfusion. The middle row shows the stress blackout map *(left)* and the whiteout reversibility map *(right)*. The bottom left map displays the number of standard deviations below normal of each myocardial sample of the stress perfusion. This patient had a completely reversible inferior perfusion defect. **B,** Three-dimensional displays of the stress blackout and reversibility whiteout information from the same patient. Clockwise from the top are shown an anterior, lateral, inferior, and septal views. An apical view is shown in the middle of the display.

Once extracted, boundary points can be connected into triangles or quadrilaterals, which are in turn connected into a polygonal surface representing the endocardial or epicardial surface. Once a surface is generated, perfusion is shown by assigning to each triangle or quadrilateral a color corresponding to the counts extracted from the myocardium at that sample during a quantification process. Colors can be interpolated between triangles to produce a continuum of colors across the myocardium, or the triangles can be left as patches of distinct color. Fig. 8-2, B shows the same information seen in the polar maps in Fig. 8-2, A with the three-dimensional representation described by Faber et al.[8]

Surface models can usually be displayed by using standard computer graphics packages that allow rotations and translations of the model, positioning of one or more light sources, and adjustment of the model's opacity (the amount of light shining through the model) or reflectance (the amount of light reflecting off of the model). The speed of a three-dimensional surface model display depends greatly on the type and number of individual elements from which the model is composed. In general, however, surface model displays are fast and often can be rotated and translated interactively. The accuracy of such displays depends primarily on the surface detection and the mapping of function onto the surface. They have the advantage of showing the actual size and shape of the left ventricle and the extent and location of any defect in a realistic manner. Preliminary studies have demonstrated that such three-dimensional displays are equivalent to or better than polar maps or the original slice-by-slice displays for estimating the size and location of defects.[2,35]

The biggest disadvantage of three-dimensional displays is that they require more computer screen space (and therefore more film or paper for hard copies) than polar maps. The entire left ventricle can be visualized in a single circular polar map, but only one side of the left ventricle can be seen when it is displayed by using three-dimensional graphics.

A second approach to creating three-dimensional displays from cardiac SPECT generates the myocardial boundaries directly from image voxels (volume elements). These methods originated from those used to generate three-dimensional displays of bony surfaces from computed tomography[23] and require segmentation and boundary tracking. Segmentation is the process of separating the myocardium from the background and can be accomplished by using various methods, such as tracing the myocardium by hand in every slice or by using a thresholding technique in which pixels with values greater than the threshold are assumed to be part of the myocardium and all other pixels are assumed to be background. The goal of segmentation is to produce a binary dataset in which myocardial voxels have a value of 1 and background voxels have a value of 0. A boundary-tracking algorithm is then used to identify the surface of the myocardium as the boundary between 1s and 0s. As a result, a set of triangles usually composes the surface of the left ventricle, which can be rendered in three dimensions as described above. For example, Slomka et al[38] registered and compared test images with normal templates to determine

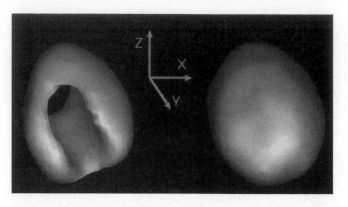

Fig. 8-3. A three-dimensional display of quantitated stress *(left)* and rest *(right)* perfusion. This is approximately a left anterior oblique view of the left ventricle. The display was created by first averaging the registered, standardized images of 10 men with disease of the left anterior descending coronary artery and comparing the result to the normal template image. Only pixels with an intensity above that of the normal template are displayed; in this case, the hole in the anterior wall in the stress image on the left is attributable to the anterior perfusion defects in these subjects. The average rest study *(right)* demonstrates no defects. (Reprinted by permission of the Society of Nuclear Medicine. From Slomka PJ, Hurwitz GA, Stephenson J, Cradduck T: Automated alignment and sizing of myocardial stress and rest scans to three-dimensional normal templates. *J Nucl Med* 36:1115–1122, 1995.)

which left ventricular pixels are normal and which are abnormal. Normal pixels can be assigned a value of 1, and abnormal pixels can be assigned a value of 0, so that the three-dimensional display depicts a hole in the left ventricle where a perfusion abnormality is located (Fig. 8-3). This approach for segmenting the left ventricle before boundary tracking is the only quantitative one described thus far; surface shaded displays are usually generated by having the user set a qualitative threshold.[24] Without quantitative analysis, however, improper segmentation can easily result and produce an erroneous picture of myocardial perfusion.

ARTIFICIAL INTELLIGENCE TECHNIQUES APPLIED TO SINGLE-PHOTON EMISSION COMPUTED TOMOGRAPHY

Interpretation of medical images by decision-support systems has made great progress in recent years, mostly because of the implementation of artificial intelligence techniques. Several major application areas are associated with artificial intelligence:[1,31] natural language processing, problem solving, planning, computer vision, expert systems, and neural computing (neural networks). Expert systems and neural networks are currently being applied to nuclear medicine.

Expert system analysis of perfusion tomograms

Expert systems attempt to capture the knowledge or expertise of the human domain expert. Thus expert systems are becoming commercially popular because they are designed to circumvent the problem of having few experts in areas where many are needed.

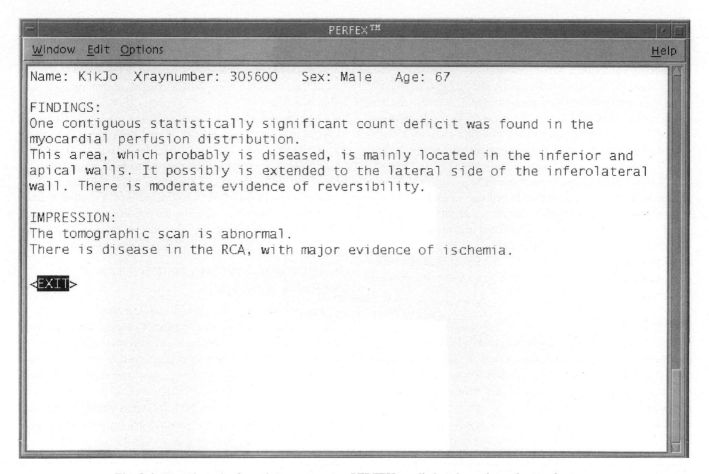

Fig. 8-4. Textual results from the expert system PERFEX, applied to the patient whose polar maps are shown in Fig. 8-2, A.

An example of the power of expert systems is found in PER-FEX (Perfusion expert), a preliminary system that was developed to assist in diagnosing coronary artery disease by using ^{201}Tl three-dimensional myocardial distributions.[6,18] This type of approach has the potential for standardizing the image interpretation process. After reviewing 291 studies in patients with angiographically documented coronary artery disease, heuristic rules were derived that best correlated the presence and location of perfusion defects on ^{201}Tl SPECT studies with the presence and location of coronary lesions. These rules operate on data that are entered in the expert system from the CEqual SPECT quantification process, which identifies defects as portions of the myocardium in which normalized perfusion falls below a predetermined number of standard deviations when compared with a gender-matched normal file. Reversibility is defined as defects at stress that improve at rest. An automatic feature extraction program then describes the location, size, shape, and severity of each defect or reversibility. The location is expressed in the form of 32 possible descriptors and is defined by coordinates of depth (basal, medial, distal–apical, and proximal–apical) and angular location (eight subsets of the septal, inferior, lateral, and anterior myocardial walls). Severity is expressed in terms of certainty factors that range from −1 to +1

(−1 means there is definitely no disease, +1 means there is definitely disease, and the range from −0.2 to +0.2 means an equivocal or indeterminable state). This information is used to "fire" or execute the 253 heuristic rules to produce new facts or draw new inferences. A certainty factor is assigned for each input variable and for each rule; these factors are used to determine the certainty of the identification and location of a coronary lesion. The polar maps for an example patient with documented right coronary artery (RCA) disease is shown in Fig. 8-2, A, and the results of the expert system interpretation, which correctly identified disease, are shown in Fig. 8-4.

The PERFEX system has undergone extensive validation. Sixty prospective patients examined with ^{99m}Tc sestamibi (30 underwent angiographic correlation; 40 had coronary disease and 20 were normal) were first used to validate the clinical efficacy of the CEqual/PERFEX program for detecting and localizing coronary artery disease.[17] The results showed excellent agreement between PERFEX and the human expert for detecting the presence (95%) and localizing coronary artery disease to the left anterior descending (LAD) artery (92%), left circumflex coronary (LCX) artery (100%), and the RCA (96%) vascular territories. The results were good but less impressive for detecting the absence of coronary artery disease (50%)

overall or in the LAD (46%), LCX (71%), and RCA (76%) regions. These disagreements were concluded to be due mostly to the inherent limitation of not taking into account all of the clinical variables as experts do.

A second study[19] was conducted to validate PERFEX by doing a large prospective study consisting of 150 stress and delayed ^{201}Tl studies and 138 rest and stress ^{99m}Tc sestamibi myocardial perfusion studies in patients who also underwent coronary angiography. The visual interpretations of slices and maps by a human expert, vessel stenosis on coronary angiography, and PERFEX interpretations were accessed automatically from databases and used to automatically generate intercomparisons. In this study, PERFEX had a higher sensitivity and, correspondingly, a lower specificity than visual interpretation by human experts for identifying the presence and location of coronary artery disease. In addition, the agreement between PERFEX and the human expert was better than those compared with coronary angiography.

Neural networks

Neural networks were developed as an attempt to simulate the highly connected biological system found in the brain through the use of computer hardware or software. In the brain, a neuron receives input from many different sources. It integrates all of these inputs and "fires" (sends a pulse down the nerve to other connected neurons) if the result is greater than a set threshold. In the same way, a neural network has nodes (the equivalent of a neuron) that are interconnected and receive input from other nodes. Each node sums or integrates its inputs and uses a linear or nonlinear transfer function to determine whether the node should fire.

A neural network can be arranged in many different ways. For example, it can have one or more layers of nodes, it can be fully connected (in which every node is connected to every other node), or it can be partially connected. In addition, it can have feedforward processing (in which processing only travels one direction) or it can have feedback processing (in which processing travels both ways).

Another important aspect of neural networks is their ability to "learn" from input patterns. A neural network (or "net") can be trained in a supervised or unsupervised mode. In the supervised mode, the net is trained by presenting it with input and the desired output. The error between the output of the net and the desired output is then propagated backward through the net, adjusting the weights of the inputs of all the nodes so that the desired output is achieved. This is repeated for many input sets of training data and for multiple cycles per training set. Once the net has converged (that is, once the weights change very little for additional training sets or cycles), it can be tested with prospective data. This kind of training system is very useful for finding patterns out of a known collection of patterns.

Unsupervised training is similar to supervised training, but instead of providing the net with the desired output, it is free to find its own output. This type of training system can be useful for finding patterns in data for which no set of existing patterns

is known. The main advantage of a neural net is the ability to solve a problem that can be represented by some sort of training data without the need for an expert. However, if the training data is not complete or if a problem is presented to the network that it has not been trained to solve, it may not give reliable answers.

With careful training, neural networks can provide a unique approach to solving problems. Neural networks have already been used by three groups in nuclear cardiology to identify which coronary arteries are expected to have stenotic lesions for a specific hypoperfused distribution.[14,22,34] These methods vary on the number of input and output nodes used. The more training data available, the better the possibility for more nodes. The output of these systems can be as simple as a single node signifying that a lesion is present in the myocardium.

INTEGRATION OF MULTIMODALITY CARDIAC IMAGERY

Often, more than one type of imaging procedure is used to evaluate patients for cardiac disease. Coronary angiography is the gold standard for diagnosis of coronary artery stenosis, magnetic resonance imaging is performed to determine gross anatomy, and SPECT is used to evaluate myocardial perfusion. There are major advantages to automatically reorienting and rescaling multimodality images so that they are in the same position and orientation and so that they display their information in a unified manner. This process is termed *multimodality registration, fusion,* or *unification.* Although physicians frequently perform this image integration mentally, automating the processes may improve their ability to assimilate the large amount of data and draw meaningful conclusions from it. After automatic unification, comparisons between information contained in the studies are straightforward because cardiac structures can be viewed in the same orientation or sliced in the same manner. Cause-and-effect relations may be more obvious, and anatomy and physiology may be more easily compared. In the following sections, four approaches to automatic integration of images from cardiac nuclear medicine with other modality data are described.

Registration of myocardial perfusion and magnetic resonance images

Registration of SPECT perfusion images with magnetic resonance (MR) images from the same patient was first demonstrated by Faber et al.[9] This method requires that endocardial surfaces be detected in both sets of images.[7] The end-diastolic and end-systolic frames are then determined by using the chamber volumes computed from those surfaces. A cost function consisting of the distance of the MR end-diastolic surface from the SPECT end-diastolic surface plus the distance of the MR end-systolic surface from the SPECT end-systolic surface is minimized over translation and rotation in three dimensions. This approach is similar to that described by Pelizzari et al[33] for registration of brain images. The resulting transformation is then applied to the SPECT image itself, along with an interpolation between frames, so that the images match in both time

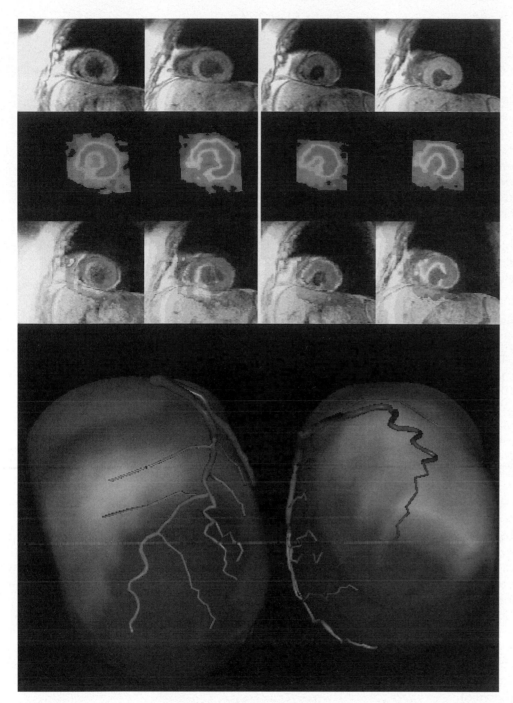

Fig. 8-5. Multimodality registration. **A,** Cardiac metabolism information in positron emission tomograms (PET) created by using fluoro-deoxyglucose, registered with anatomic magnetic resonance (MR) images of the same patient. From top to bottom, MR images, registered PET, and unified MR images and PET. The first two columns show two short-axis slices at end diastole; the final two columns show the same short-axis slices at end systole. **B,** Demonstration of unifying three-dimensional coronary artery trees with single-photon emission computed tomography perfusion images. The left side is approximately a septal view; the right view is approximately lateral. Perfusion is color-coded onto the left ventricular epicardial surface; the blacked-out region indicates an anterior or apical perfusion defect. The lighter portion of the left anterior descending coronary artery indicates the segment of the artery distal to the stenosis. Note the overlap between the stenosed artery and the perfusion defect. (Courtesy of Dr. Shantanu Sinha, University of California, Los Angeles.)

and space. Therefore, myocardial thickening observed in MR images can be directly compared with perfusion information from the SPECT images in the same areas of the heart. In clinical tests using these methods, left ventricular and right ventricular walls in SPECT were aligned well with those in MR images, and areas of decreased perfusion in SPECT images were aligned with areas of decreased myocardial thickening in MR images.

More recently, a report describing alignment of cardiac MR and PET images was published.[37] In this study, the left ventricular boundaries were detected interactively by using morphologic and linear filtering tools. The surface-fitting technique of

Pelizzari et al[33] was used to determine the best linear transformation that would align the left ventricular boundaries. By combining this transformation with the known pixel sizes and temporal resolution, either of the four-dimensional image sets could be transformed into the spatial and temporal coordinates of the other. This method was validated by calculating the difference between user-identified landmarks in the two images after transformation by using six MR–PET image pairs and an average of 14 landmarks per pair. The accuracy was determined to be 1.3 ± 1.1 mm for the end-diastolic images, and 1.95 ± 1.6 for end-systolic images. Fig. 8-5, A shows the latest results of applying this technique.

Registration of echocardiographic and metabolism images

Cardiac ultrasound images have also been aligned to PET images of glucose metabolism. In the study by Savi et al,[36] anatomic landmarks were interactively chosen in short-axis echocardiograms and short-axis PET images. In particular, the two papillary muscles and the inferior junction of the right ventricle were identified in short-axis images acquired by using both methods. Registration was performed in the plane defined by the three landmarks; a least-squares minimization was performed to determine the best rotation, scaling, and translation to transform one set of x,y coordinates into the other. This technique was demonstrated on two case studies. Although this work is still in a preliminary stage, it is important, given the high availability and use of echocardiography. If it is found to be useful, it could easily be extended to process high-resolution SPECT images and perhaps be automated to improve its usability and reproducibility.

Registration of SPECT and coronary angiographic data

Ideally, accurate assessment of the extent and severity of coronary artery disease requires the integration of physiologic information derived from SPECT perfusion images and anatomic information derived from coronary angiography. This integration has been performed by registering a three-dimensional left ventricular model representing myocardial perfusion with the patient's own three-dimensional coronary artery tree and presenting both in a single unified display. The patient-specific coronary artery tree is obtained from a three-dimensional geometric reconstruction performed on simultaneously acquired digital biplane angiographic projections or from two single-plane projections acquired at different angles.[32] The three-dimensional reconstructed artery tree is approximated by successive conical segments and is scaled and rotated to fit onto the myocardial surface. The left or right coronary arteries are registered with the myocardial perfusion surface model by automatically minimizing a cost function that describes the relation of the coronary artery tree to the interventricular and atrioventricular groove and the surface of the myocardium. Fig. 8-5, B illustrates this unified display. Recent reports have described preliminary validations of this technique in animal studies[11]; human studies are being performed.

Krause et al[28] have reported similar work. Three-dimensional models of the left ventricular epicardium were generated by SPECT and were aligned with three-dimensional models of the left coronary artery tree created from angiograms. In this work, however, the alignment was performed by using acquisition features for SPECT and angiography to determine the patient coordinates of the two models. Once these coordinates were known, the models could be easily aligned, and a simple translation between the two models was applied if necessary to refine the match. A display was generated by reprojecting both three-dimensional models into the desired view angle.

CONCLUSIONS

Perfusion quantification methods will continue to evolve and adapt to the demands of nuclear cardiology, specific physicians, nuclear medicine technology, and the health care system. The high level of automation already achieved in myocardial perfusion imaging is unmatched by any other cardiac imaging method and continues to be a major strength. In addition, strong statistical evaluations of the accuracy and validity of the various techniques have been made possible by great objectivity and standardization in the automated processes. These strengths should be built upon and enhanced to demonstrate the value of nuclear cardiology in patient management, and, most important, to maintain the highest quality in clinical care.

REFERENCES

1. Anderson JA and Rosenfeld E, eds: *Neurocomputing: foundations of research*, Cambridge, Mass., 1988, MIT Press.
2. Cooke CD, Vansant JP, Krawczynska E, et al: Clinical validation of 3-d color-modulated displays of myocardial perfusion, *J Nucl Cardiol* 4:108–116, 1997.
3. DePasquale EE, Nody AC, DePuey EG, et al: Quantitative rotational thallium-201 tomography for identifying and localizing coronary artery disease, *Circulation* 77:316–327, 1988.
4. DePuey EG, Krawcynska EG, D'Amato PH, et al: Thallium-201 single photon emission computed tomography with intravenous dipyridamole to diagnose coronary artery disease, *Coron Artery Dis* 1:75–82, 1990.
5. Ezekiel A, Van Train KF, Berman DB, et al: *Automatic determination of quantitation parameters from Tc-sestamibi myocardial tomograms.* In *Computers in cardiology*, Los Alamitos, Calif., 1991, IEEE Computer Society.
6. Ezquerra NF and Garcia EV: Artificial intelligence in nuclear medicine imaging. *Am J Cardiac Imaging* 3:130–141, 1989.
7. Faber TL, Akers MS, Peshock RM, et al: Three-dimensional motion and perfusion quantification in gated single-photon emission computed tomograms, *J Nucl Med* 32:2311–2317, 1991.
8. Faber TL, Cooke CD, Peifer JW, et al: Three-dimensional displays of left ventricular epicardial surface from standard cardiac SPECT perfusion quantification techniques, *J Nucl Med* 36:697–703, 1995.
9. Faber TL, McColl RW, Opperman R, et al: Spatial and temporal registration of cardiac SPECT and MR images: Methods and evaluation, *Radiology* 179:857–861, 1991.
10. Faber TL, Stokely EM, Peshock RM, et al: A model-based four dimensional left ventricular surface detector, *IEEE Trans Med Imaging* 10:321–329, 1991.
11. Faber TL, Klein JL, Folks RD, et al: *Automated unification of three-dimensional models of the left ventricular epicardium and coronary artery tree*, In *Computers in Cardiology*, Los Alamitos, Calif., 1996, IEEE Computer Society.
12. Ficaro EP, Fessler JA, Shreve PD, et al: Simultaneous transmission/emission myocardial perfusion tomography. Diagnostic accuracy of attenuation-corrected ^{99m}Tc-sestamibi single-photon emission computed tomography, *Circulation* 93:463–473, 1996.
13. Folks R, Garcia E, Van Train K, et al: Quantitative two-day Tc-99m sestamibi myocardial SPECT: multicenter trial validation of normal limits, *J Med Tech* 24:158, 1996.
14. Fujita H, Katafuchi T, Uehara T, et al: Application of artificial neural network to computer-aided diagnosis of coronary artery disease in myocardial SPECT bull's-eye images, *J Nucl Med* 33:272–276, 1992.
15. Garcia EV: Quantitative myocardial perfusion single-photon emission computed tomographic imaging: quo vadis? (Where do we go from

here?), *J Nucl Cardiol* 1:83–93, 1994.

16. Garcia EV, Cooke CD, Van Train KF, et al: Technical aspects of myo-cardial perfusion SPECT imaging with technetium-99m sestamibi, *Am J Cardiol* 66:23E–31E, 1990.

17. Garcia EV, Cooke CD, Krawczynska E, et al: Expert system interpre-tation of technetium-99m sestamibi myocardial perfusion tomograms: enhacements and validation, *Circulation* 92:I-10, 1995.

18. Garcia EV, Herbst MD, Cooke CD, et al: *Knowledge-based visualiza-tion of myocardial perfusion tomographic images. In Proceedings of the first conference on visualization in biomedical computing.* Atlanta, 1990, IEEE Press..

19. Garcia EV, Krawczynska EG, Folks RD, et al: Expert system interpre-tation of myocardial perfusion tomograms: validation using 288 prospective patients, *J Nuc Med* 37:48P, 1996.

20. Garcia EV, Van Train K, Maddahi J, et al: Quantification of rotational thallium-201 myocardial tomography, *J Nucl Med* 26:17–26, 1985.

21. Germano G, Kavanagh PB, Su HT, et al: Automatic reorientation of three-dimensional, transaxial myocardial perfusion SPECT images, *J Nucl Med* 36:1107–1114, 1995.

22. Hamilton D, Riley PJ, Miola UJ, et al: A feed forward neural network for classification of bull's-eye myocardial perfusion images, *Eur J Nucl Med* 22:108–115, 1995.

23. Herman GT: Computerized reconstruction and 3-d imaging in medi-cine, *Ann Rev Comput Sci* 1:153–179, 1986.

24. Nowak D: Method for producing 3-d images from nuclear data. US patent number 4,879,652.

25. King MA, Tsui BMW, Pan T-S: Attenuation compensation for cardiac SPECT imaging: Part 1. Impact of attenuation and methods of esti-mating attenuating maps, *J Nucl Cardiol* 2:513–524, 1995.

26. King MA, Tsui BMW, Pan T-S, et al: Attenuation compensation for cardiac single-photon emission computed tomographic imaging: Part 2. Attenuation compensation algorithms, *J Nucl Cardiol* 3:55–64, 1996.

27. Klein JL, Garcia EV, DePuey EG, et al: Reversibility bull's-eye: a new polar bull's-eye map to quantify reversibility of stress-induced SPECT thallium-201 myocardial perfusion defects, *J Nucl Med* 31:1240–1246, 1990.

28. Krause T, Fischer R, Solzback U, et al: 3-D fusion of myocardial per-fusion scintigraphy and coronary angiography. *J Nucl Med* 37:218P, 1996 (abstract).

29. Maddahi J, Van Train K, Prigent F, et al: Quantitative single photon

emission computerized thallium-201 tomography for the evaluation of coronary artery disease: optimization and prospective validation of a new technique, *J Am Coll Cardiol* 14:1689–1699, 1989.

30. Mullick R and Ezquerra NF: Automatic determination of left ventricu-lar orientation from SPECT data, *IEEE Trans Med Imag* 14:88–99, 1995.

31. Nilsson N: *Principles of artificial intelligence,* 1980, Palo Alto, Calif., Tioga Publishing.

32. Peifer JW, Ezquerra NF, Cooke CD, et al: Visualization of multi-modality cardiac imagery, *IEEE Trans Biomed Eng* 37:744–756, 1990.

33. Pelizzari C, Chen G, Spelbring D, et al: Accurate three-dimensional registration of CT, PET, and/or MR images of the brain, *J Comput As-sist Tomogr* 13:20–26, 1989.

34. Porenta G, Dorffner G, Kundrat S, et al: Automated interpretation of planar thallium-201-dipyridamole stress-redistribution scintigrams us-ing artificial neural networks, *J Nucl Med* 35:2041–2047, 1994.

35. Quaife RA, Faber TL, and Corbett JR: Visual assessment of quantita-tive three-dimensional displays of stress thallium-201 tomograms: comparison with visual multislice analysis, *J Nucl Med* 32:1006P, 1991 (abstract).

36. Savi A, Gilardi MC, Rizzo G, et al: Spatial registration of echocardio-graphic and positron emission tomographic heart studies, *Eur J Nucl Med* 22:243–247, 1995.

37. Sinha S, Sinha U, Czernin J, et al: Noninvasive assessment of myocar-dial perfusion and metabolism: feasibility of registering gated MR and PET images, *Am J Roentgenol* 164:301–307, 1995.

38. Slomka PJ, Hurwitz GA, Stephenson J, et al: Automated alignment and sizing of myocardial stress and rest scans to three-dimensional normal templates using an image registration algorithm, *J Nucl Med* 36:1115–1122, 1995.

39. Van Train KF, Areeda J, Garcia EV, et al: Quantitative same-day rest-stress technetium-99m-sestamibi SPECT: definition and validation of stress normal limits and criteria for abnormality, *J Nucl Med* 34:1494–1502, 1993.

40. Van Train KF, Garcia EV, Maddahi J, et al: Multicenter trial validation for quantitative analysis of same-day rest-stress technetium-99m-ses-tamibi myocardial tomograms, *J Nucl Med* 35:609–618, 1994.

41. Van Train KF, Maddahi J, Berman DS, et al: Quantitative analysis of tomographic stress thallium-201 myocardial scintigrams: a multicenter trial, *J Nucl Med* 31:1168–1179, 1990.

42. Wackers FJT: Science, art, and artifacts: how important is quantifica-tion for the practicing physician interpreting myocardial perfusion studies? *J Nucl Cardiol* 1(5 Pt 2):S109–S117, 1994.

Chapter 9

Recent advances in cardiac positron emission tomography

Stephen L. Bacharach

In recent years, several new developments in positron emission tomography (PET) have had or are expected to have a clinical impact on cardiac PET. For example, gated PET is now possible, which allows simultaneous measurement of metabolism and global and regional ventricular function. So-called three-dimensional PET may result in a large increase in detection sensitivity, permitting lower doses to be used or imaging of tracers with low uptake. Advances in cardiac image registration may increase patient throughput, simplify data analysis, and reduce transmission scan time. Finally, new instrumentation developments may permit true coincidence PET to be performed with slightly modified dual-headed gamma cameras; this may greatly expand the use of cardiac PET.

Proper use of these advances often requires at least a basic understanding of the underlying principles involved. In addition, many of these developments put further demands on the instrumentation, demands that often require the clinician to use the PET scanner at the limit of its capabilities. Under these circumstances, it is essential to understand not just how these new applications of PET work, but also the way in which the physical characteristics of the PET scanner may limit the clinical use of these applications. Such an understanding is essential if one wishes to properly acquire and interpret the image data made possible by these advances in PET.

This chapter reviews several of the recent technical advances made in cardiac imaging with PET. A basic description of the underlying principles of these advances is presented, along with an outline of the clinical uses of the techniques and the limitations and difficulties that may be encountered when using these new methods.

LEFT VENTRICULAR FUNCTION FROM GATED PET IMAGING

It is now possible to make simultaneous measurements of left ventricular myocardial metabolism and left ventricular regional and global function by use of gated PET. Measurement of global function is often based directly on detection of the motion of endocardial borders. Measurement of regional function, however, often requires more accurate determination of endocardial and epicardial borders than is necessary for measurement of global function. It is not yet clear that such accuracy is achievable with gated PET (or, in fact, with gated nuclear imaging of any kind). To this end, another method has recently been investigated that relies on the so-called partial volume effect, a phenomenon that is usually considered deleterious to the imaging process but that, in the case of gated imaging, can be turned to clinical advantage.

Partial volume effects

When imaging an object of uniform activity concentration whose dimensions are comparable to or less than the resolution of the imaging device, the measured activity concentration may be erroneously underestimated. This is called the *partial volume effect* and is well known and documented.[28] This effect is important in cardiac imaging[6] because the walls of the myocardium are usually only about 10 mm thick in normal persons and are often much thinner in persons with certain cardiac diseases (such as coronary artery disease). Typical reconstructed in-plane resolutions for cardiac imaging with PET scanners are about 6 mm with modern scanners and about 10 mm for older machines. In these circumstances, the partial volume effect can cause substantial misestimates of myocardial activity. For example, consider a uniform circular shell (representing the myocardium) that contains a uniform concentration of activity (such as 100 nCi/cc). Figure 9-1, A shows a simulated short-axis myocardium (10-mm wall thickness), imaged with a scanner with a resolution of 7 mm at the full width of the photopeak measured at half the maximal count (FWHM). Superimposed on this image is a region of interest of exactly the anatomic dimensions of the myocardium (in this case, 10 mm thick). Figure 9-1, B shows how the measured activity concentration, determined by the average counts within this region of interest, depends on the reconstructed resolution of the scanner and on the wall thickness. This dependence differs depending on the size of the region of interest used. The ordinate in Fig. 9-1, B shows the measured activity concentration, with 100 nCi/cc as the "true" value. The abscissa shows the resolution of the scan-

ner measured in FWHM divided by the myocardial wall thickness. This means that if the wall under consideration were 10 mm thick, an abscissa value of 1.0 would represent a scanner with 10 mm FWHM resolution and an abscissa of 0.5 would represent a FWHM resolution of 5 mm. Similarly, if the myocardial wall were 6 mm and the scanner had a resolution of 7.2 mm, this would correspond to an x-axis value of 1.2 mm (resolution ÷ wall thickness [7.2 mm ÷ 6 mm] = 1.2 mm). The x-axis is plotted with these seemingly strange units so that this one curve can be used to estimate the partial-volume recovery coefficient (that is, fraction of true activity that is measured by the scanner) for all scanner resolutions and all wall thicknesses.

In Fig. 9-1, triangles represent a region of interest that is exactly equal to the anatomical size of the myocardium (if one

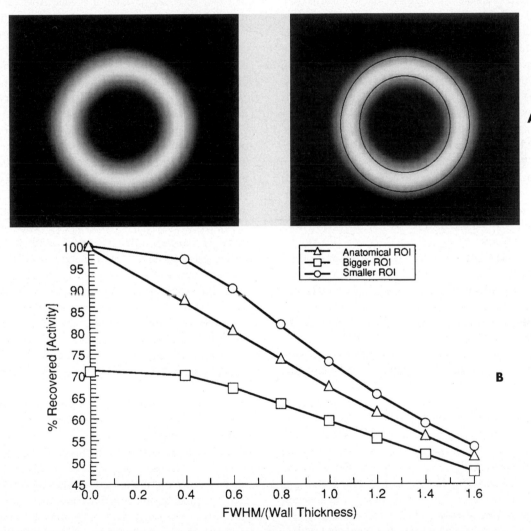

Fig. 9-1. A, A stimulated myocardial short-axis slice *(left)*, with region of interest *(right)* drawn at exactly the anatomic borders of the myocardium. Because of imperfect resolution, some counts blur outside the borders of the region of interest. **B,** Loss of counts in the myocardial region of interest as a function of wall thickness and resolution. The three curves show the loss for an anatomically perfect region of interest and for regions of interest that are 20% larger and 20% smaller. True myocardial activity is 100 nCi/cc, uniformly distributed around the myocardium. No account has been taken of thickening or motion of the heart. This figure can be used for any scanner by converting the x axis in the following way: take the resolution of the scanner in question in millimeters and divide by the values shown on the x axis. The new x-axis scale is the wall thickness in millimeters.

had used a region of interest size based on a magnetic resonance imaging scan). Even a 4-mm FWHM scanner imaging a 10-mm-thick wall (x-axis value of 4/10 = 0.4) would measure only about 88 nCi/cc rather than the correct value of 100 nCi/cc, for a recovery coefficient of 88%. Increases in full width of the photo peak would further reduce the measured activity. The circles represent a region of interest that is 10% smaller in its inner and outer radius than the true anatomical wall (for example, an 8-mm-thick region of interest on a 10-mm-thick wall or a 4.8-mm thick region of interest on a 6-mm-thick wall). Initially, there is very little reduction in measured activity concentration with increasing scanner FWHM. At around 4 or 5 mm (with a 10-mm-thick wall), the recovered activity concentration decreases rapidly with increasing FWHM. Finally, the squares represent a region of interest that is 10% bigger in inner and outer diameter than the anatomical size of the myocardium. Even a scanner with a FWHM far smaller than the wall thickness would give a measured activity concentration reduced by almost 30%. However, this value falls off much more slowly with worsening resolution (or decreasing wall thickness).

If one knew the actual myocardial thickness, one could attempt to correct for these partial volume effects.[6] Several authors have used such corrections in their analysis of PET data. Conversely, it would be possible to use the change in recovered counts with changing wall thickness to estimate the magnitude of thickening directly from gated PET images. This has been attempted with single-photon emission computed tomography (SPECT) images[17,26,35] and is also possible with gated PET, as will be described below.

Unfortunately the model on which Fig. 9-1 is based is overly simplistic. First, it ignores myocardial thickening during systole. This thickening blurs the image because of motion and alters the thickness and, therefore, the operating point. Second, true myocardial motion (apart from thickening) often occurs during contraction and relaxation, causing further image blurring. These effects have been the subject of speculation and observation on the part of many investigators.[6,10,26] Finally, Fig. 9-1 treats the problem in only 2 dimensions. In a true PET scan, data in the axial direction must also be considered. Data from adjacent slices will contribute some events to the slice in question, and the slice under study may lose some of its activity to adjacent slices. This is especially critical for the transaxial slices usually obtained in PET. In the transaxial orientation, the myocardium of one slice may be blurred with the overlying or underlying left ventricular cavity or lung tissue. The situation cannot be corrected by simply reslicing the transaxially acquired data along the short axis because the data are blurred at the time of acquisition, independent of any after-the-fact reslicing.

All these additional sources of image blurring have been quantitatively assessed in a study in which images obtained through gated magnetic resonance imaging (MRI) were used.[6] In this study, a multislice set of gated MRI images was collected, and the myocardium in each was set to a uniform value of 100. These images were subsequently blurred in all three spatial directions according to the resolution of the actual PET scanner for which partial volume corrections were desired, then blurred in the temporal dimension according to the true wall thickening and motion exhibited by the particular patient under consideration, as determined from the gated MRI scans. The resultant blurred image represents what a PET scan of a particular patient would look like had the activity uptake in the myocardium been uniform. Unlike data from simulation studies, these data are based on the actual observed thickening and wall motion from human studies. The first column of Fig. 9-2 shows such a PET image (three transaxial slices) from a volunteer with no known cardiac disease. The actual underlying activity distribution is perfectly uniform (and set artificially to a value of 100 in these images), but it is clear from the images in column 1 that the *measured* distribution is far from uniform.

These nonuniformities are caused by the partial volume effects related to scanner resolution, wall motion, and wall thickening. Analysis of images from a series of normal patients indicated that substantial artifactual reduction in measured counts can occur, especially at the apex. In addition, it was found that inhomogeneities, such as erroneous free wall-to-septum ratios, can be induced by variations in thickening, thickness, and motion of the wall, even for a scanner with a reconstructed resolution of approximately 7 mm. Clearly, such effects might have important clinical ramifications. Unless care was taken to compensate for these effects, one might falsely conclude that changes in metabolism or flow had occurred when, in reality, such changes were caused by changes in wall motion and thickening. The second and third columns of Fig. 9-2 show the same images gated at end diastole and end systole. By gating the images, the effects of wall motion and thickening are eliminated, leaving only the partial volume effects associated with the finite wall thickness at end diastole or end systole relative to the scanner resolution (7 mm in planar resolution and 12.5 mm in axial resolution). Again, inhomogeneities are present, especially at end diastole (where the wall is thinnest).

All of the partial volume effects discussed have primarily involved the loss of events from a bright homogeneous region into surrounding regions. In cardiac imaging, the converse is more likely to be a problem. Frequently, the clinical finding of interest is a defect: that is, a reduction in tracer uptake in a region of the myocardial wall. In this case, the partial volume effect reduces the magnitude of the defect (that is it, increases the apparent counts in the defect) by blurring counts from neighboring regions of higher activity into the defect. This may be part of the reason that supposedly nonviable tissue is still observed to have nonzero uptake of fluorine-18 fluorodeoxyglucose (FDG) and nonzero perfusion.

Myocardial thickening

The partial volume effects described above are, in general, deleterious to image interpretation and analysis. However, in recent years, it has been proposed that this effect may be put to beneficial use in estimating myocardial thickening. The idea

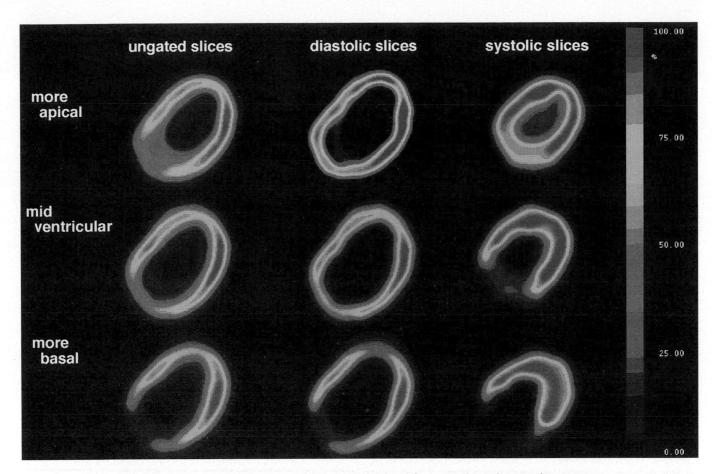

Fig. 9-2. Positron emission tomographic images simulated from actual gated magnetic resonance images of a human subject by setting the myocardium uniformly to a value of 100 and blurring according to 7 mm in plane resolution and 12.5 mm in axial resolution. Each row shows images from a different level in the heart. The columns (left to right) show ungated images, gated end diastole images, and gated end systole images, respectively. The underlying activity distribution is perfectly homogeneous. The inhomogeneities are produced by imperfect resolution and motion blurring.

would be to gate the myocardial images and look for changes in image intensity over the cardiac cycle.[7,11,17,35] Of course, the actual activity concentration in the myocardium remains constant over the cardiac cycle. Changes in image intensity are caused by the partial volume effect, the magnitude of which varies over the cardiac cycle as the myocardium thickens and thins with time.

Consider one small region of the myocardium. At end diastole, when this section of the myocardium is thinnest, the recovery coefficient is smallest, resulting in the smallest value of measured counts (and an image which is least bright).[9] At end systole, the myocardium is thickest and the counts and image brightness are correspondingly greater. Fig. 9-3 plots the peak brightness (in relative units) for any section of the myocardium as a function of myocardial thickness for two different in-plane resolutions (7 mm FWHM on the left and 14 mm FWHM on the right). The solid lines are the theoretical predictions, and the circles are the measured data (based on blurred MRI images as described previously). Using Fig. 9-3 B (14-mm resolution) as an example, a 4-mm-thick section of myocardium that thickens during systole to 6 mm will

result in a change in peak brightness, a change that is much smaller than that which would be obtained if a 7-mm resolution scanner had been used. In other words, the slope at low thickness is much greater with high resolution (as might be obtained with a current-generation PET scanner) than with lower resolution (as might be obtained with a current-generation SPECT scanner). This has clinical importance: Thin regions of myocardium that are thickening only slightly will be much easier to observe with PET than with SPECT. On the other hand, with a 7-mm resolution PET scanner, the curve in Fig. 9-3, A flattens out when the wall thickness is normal (10 mm) or thicker. That is, when the wall thickness is great compared with the resolution, peak brightness changes little with increasing thickness; the counts recovery approaches 100% and cannot get any larger. Clinically, this means that at PET resolutions, regions of myocardium that are of normal or greater thickness at end diastole will not brighten appreciably at end systole, even if they thicken normally. At the lower resolution associated with SPECT (14 mm), the curve flattens out less but, of course, is less steep to begin with. This suggests that gated PET studies at high resolution (7 mm) are best for

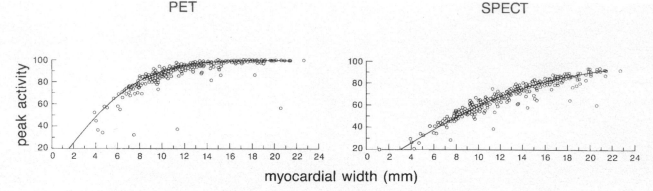

Fig. 9-3. Percentage of recovered activity versus myocardial thickness for a 7-mm resolution positron emission tomography (PET) scanner *(left)* and a 14-mm scanner typical of single-photon emission computed tomography or older PET *(right)*. The image data were derived from actual gated magnetic resonance images of human subjects. Solid lines represent theoretical predictions of recovered counts; open circles represent data derived from the study subjects.

determining whether thin regions of myocardium are thickening, whereas for persons in whom the myocardium is thick, it may be desirable to smooth the gated set first.

Instead of using maximum brightening of the images, it would in theory be possible to measure thickening directly by measuring the edges of the myocardium directly from the images. One interesting modification of such geometric-based methods assumes that the underlying myocardial activity concentration is a square-wave function convolved with the imaging system resolution.[37] Such edge detection schemes may be possible when measuring global left-ventricular function (as will be discussed below). However, when endocardial and epicardial edge detection has been used to measure thickening, only limited success has been achieved, even with such high-resolution methods as gated MRI cardiac images. Edge detection is even less likely to succeed with gated PET data. The reason for the difficulty is that the myocardial thickening is relatively small. For example, consider the potentially clinically important situation described above in which viability is assessed in a thin (4 mm thick) region. This region was observed to thicken vigorously from 4 mm to 6 mm—a thickening of 50%. However, even a 1-mm uncertainty in myocardial edge definition would cause a huge error in the measurement of thickening: That is, because the thickening is only 2 mm to begin with, a 1-mm error in measurement would mean a 50% relative error, possibly too large to be of clinical use. This problem is most severe in regions for which accurate thickening measurements are most needed—for distinguishing viable from nonviable tissue in often thin, potentially severely ischemic regions of the myocardium.

As shown above, measuring thickening by observing brightening is problematic at large thicknesses, whereas measuring thickness geometrically (that is, by edge detection) is difficult at low thicknesses. An alternative approach has recently been proposed[11] that combines these two techniques. This hybrid method is based on the profile of myocardial counts from en-

docardium to epicardium. Instead of using the maximum of this profile (maximum brightening) or an edge-based width of the profile, the hybrid method uses the change in integrated counts from end diastole to end systole within a width under the profile. In this way, changes in counts are combined with width measurements, yielding an index of thickening that seems to be relatively linear over a wide range of thicknesses and seems less susceptible to error than pure edge-based methods. Even with this hybrid method, however, it is uncertain whether sufficiently accurate regional measures of fractional thickening can be made. Nonetheless, it is hoped that such measurements will permit accurate categorization of myocardial segments into a few broad categories of thickening, which may be sufficient to justify clinical use of the technique.

Global function from gated PET

Recent studies have shown that it may be possible to determine global left ventricular function (ejection fraction) from gated SPECT perfusion studies.[20,27,31] These methods have been based primarily on edge detection of the endocardial borders. In regions that are poorly perfused, smoothing or interpolation across the low count regions has been proposed. Although edge detection methods may be inadequate for measurements of regional thickening, preliminary studies indicate that such methods may prove adequate for measurement of global function, where small regional variations in edge determinations are unimportant, as long as the overall changes in volume are reflected accurately. For such indices as ejection fraction, only relative changes in volume need be accurate; a less stringent requirement than that needed for accurate measurement of absolute volumes. It may prove possible to use edge-based techniques to make clinically useful measures of absolute volumes, but considerable effort will be needed to provide adequate validation. Most of the early studies of global function have been made from gated SPECT, not gated myocardial PET.

Two opposing factors should be considered in terms of the feasibility of such measurements by PET. The higher resolution of PET should make it easier to make accurate edge determinations. However, despite the higher efficiency of PET compared to SPECT, the total counts per transaxial slice of a typical 25-mCi gated MIBI study are larger than those of many typical 5-mCi gated PET studies (normalized to the same slice thickness). Therefore, the statistical fluctuations of a 5 mCi PET study (in standard two-dimensional acquisition) may be similar to those of a 25-mCi MIBI study, although the PET data will have considerably better resolution. Nonetheless, it is likely that the same techniques that are applicable for global function measurements with SPECT will also be applicable (with slight modification) for PET.[42]

THREE-DIMENSIONAL (SEPTA-OUT) PET

In SPECT, a collimator is used to define the projection line along which the photon traveled. This collimator accepts only photons perpendicular to the camera crystal face; therefore, most of the photons emitted by the body are left out. In PET, coincidence detection defines the projection line, and a collimator is not needed. Thus, in theory, PET should have a much larger sensitivity than SPECT. However, until recently, most PET scanners used a coarse collimator in the form of lead septa between one or two rings of detectors and the next ring or set of rings. The septa excluded all photons except those in the plane of the imaging ring or adjacent rings. Again, sensitivity is reduced, although not nearly as much as with a gamma camera collimator.

The reason for the septa is twofold. First, and most important, they reduce the fraction of scattered photons. Second, until recently, no practical method was available to make use of the photons that produced coincidences between remote crystal rings. Scanners for PET in which the septa are removable and practical three-dimensional data reconstruction methods are now available.[15,19,23,29] When the septa are in the withdrawn position, the scanner is said to be operating in three-dimensional mode, meaning that photons from all angles are being used in the reconstruction. In this sense, it is not really three-dimensional because the finite axial field of view allows the use of only a relatively small range of angles. Nonetheless, even if only ±11 planes are used, sensitivity can increase up to a factor of seven. Scatter fraction also increases and is typically about 60% for a cardiac study acquired in three-dimensional mode compared with about 12% for the same scan in two-dimensional mode (that is, with the septa in place). These realistic scatter fractions are much larger than those frequently quoted for the National Electrical Manufacturers Association (NEMA) standard 20-cm phantom due to the large size of the chest.

Unfortunately, the greatest benefits of three-dimensional imaging are achievable only at very low injected activities. This is because when the septa are removed, the singles rates seen by each of the detectors increases dramatically. This causes a corresponding dramatic increase in the fraction of counts that are random and an increase in system deadtime. Evaluation of the performance of individual scanners when operating in three-dimensional mode has only recently been undertaken,[32,42] and seems to vary greatly among manufacturers. Although large increases in sensitivity can be achieved by having the septa out, many of the extra counts are random and scattered events and others are lost to deadtime.

Correction for random events and scatter adds noise to the images. Therefore, even if a three-dimensional study of a patient produces more true coincident counts than does a two-dimensional study for the same acquisition time, the three-dimensional study may or may not have better image quality (that is, less noise and better contrast). Noise in a three-dimensional image, despite increased total counts, may actually be worse than the noise in an equivalent two-dimensional image, depending on the activity in the field of view. Therefore, total true coincident counts is not a useful variable for assessment of the benefits of three-dimensional imaging compared with two-dimensional imaging. Instead, a variable called the *noise equivalent count (NEC)*[34] is usually used. This variable reflects the statistical quality of the image after correction for random events and scatter. For very low activities in the field of view, doubling the activity may double both the true coincidences and the NEC, indicating that the relative statistical fluctuations in the image would go down by the expected factor of square root of 2. At higher activities in the field of view, however, an increase in activity might increase the true coincidence counts but might cause the noise equivalent count to drop. This implies that although the extra activity produces extra total true coincidences, it also produces additional extra randoms, so that after correction for randoms and scatter, the resultant image actually has more noise than the lower activity image. Thus, two images with the same NEC have similar noise properties, even though one image might have been reconstructed from more total coincident counts than the other.

Figure 9-4 compares three-dimensional with two-dimensional imaging in terms of variance in the myocardium[30] for a General Electric Advance scanner (the data in this figure are highly scanner dependent).[36] An elliptical chest phantom with lungs and a cardiac insert was filled so that it mimicked typical distributions of activity that might be obtained after FDG injection. Rather than compute the NEC from theoretical grounds, the actual variance of counts within the myocardium was measured by acquiring a gated study of the phantom at 40 time points. Because the phantom's heart did not beat, this produced 40 replicate images from which the variance of any structure, including the myocardium, could be accurately measured.

Figure 9-4, A plots the decrease in variance over the myocardium as a function of activity in the field of view. In a scanner with a 15-cm axial field of view, a 5-mCi injection of FDG typically produces about 0.75 to 1 mCi in the field of view. Figure 9-4 can therefore be used to compare the efficacy of three-dimensional imaging versus that of two-dimensional imaging for a 5-mCi injection and the savings in imaging time (or improvement in image quality) that may be obtained by increasing the injected dose from 5 mCi to 10 mCi can be computed. From Fig. 9-4, A, a 5-mCi injection (assumed to yield 1 mCi in the field of view) yields a relative variance in the myocardium of 0.8 in three-dimensional imaging and about 2.0 in two-dimensional imaging. Because the y axis of Fig. 9-4 is variance, it is also proportional to the relative imaging time. Therefore, at a 5-mCi injected dose (1 mCi in the field of view), a scanner operating in three-dimensional mode will produce the same quality image as in two-dimensional mode in a factor of 0.4 (0.8/2) of the time. In other words, a scan that takes 10 minutes in two-dimensional mode would take only 4 minutes in three-dimensional mode. At very low activities the gain in imaging time approaches a factor of 4; that is, at very low activities, a three-dimensional scan will produce the same image quality in one quarter the time as a two-dimensional scan for the same dose.

The ratio of two-dimensional to three-dimensional imaging time to produce the same quality scan (called the *three-dimensional sensitivity advantage*) is plotted in Fig. 9-4, B. As activity in the field of view increases, the advantage of three-dimensional over two-dimensional imaging diminishes, until at about 3.4 mCi in the field, the two methods produce the same variance. Further increases in activity cause three-dimensional imaging to be worse than two-dimensional imaging—the extra noise produced by the random events correction more than offsets the extra activity. Furthermore, when imaging in three dimensions, the curve shown in Fig. 9-4, A becomes flat after about 1.2 mCi in the field of view (about 6 mCi injected), then increases. Therefore, further increases in injected activity above 6 mCi will increase the dose to the patient, but will not improve the image quality in three-dimensional imaging—in fact, image quality will actually degrade. This contrasts with two-dimensional imaging, in which further increases in activity substantially improve image quality for the same imaging time up to a fairly high activity level. Ultimately, the minimum variance is smaller in two-dimensional imaging (that is, the image quality is ultimately better) than in three-dimensional imaging by a factor of about 1.7. However, this gain is achieved only with a factor of five or greater increase in the dose to the patient.

Curves such as those in Fig. 9-4, A are very dependent on the characteristics of the scanner being used. Preliminary evidence indicates that different scanners may produce similar curves, but they are shifted to the left: that is, the gain of three-dimensional versus two-dimensional imaging is lost at much earlier activities. Obviously, having data such as those in Fig. 9-4 is crucial to determine whether to image in three dimensions or two dimensions and to determine reasonable injected doses to use when imaging in three dimensions.

Figure 9-4 was produced by using a cardiac chest phantom. In actual patients, activity outside the field of view (such as the bladder) may produce extra random events when three-dimensional, septa out mode is used. This plus the additional scatter would have the effect of shifting the curves in Fig. 9-4 to the left. Preliminary investigations of the effects of out-of-field activity have been made.[5,18] Slight shielding redesign may reduce

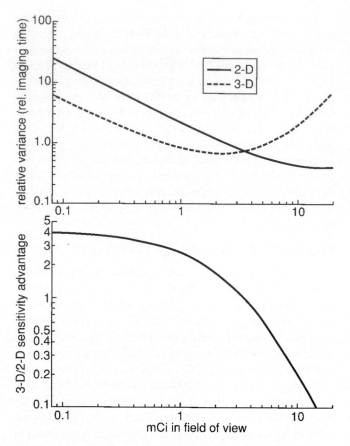

Fig. 9-4. Comparison of noise characteristics of a three-dimensional and a two-dimensional positron emission tomography cardiac imaging system (General Electric Advantage). Data were derived from a cardiac chest phantom with lung and cardiac inserts. *(top)*, Relative variance for three-dimensional and two-dimensional cardiac imaging versus activity in the field of view (for fluorodeoxyglucose and ammonia, a 5-mCi injected dose results in roughly 0.75 to 1 mCi in the field of view). The ordinate of **A** may also be considered the relative two-dimensional and three-dimensional imaging times necessary to achieve the same quality image for the same dose. *(bottom)*, the ratio of two-dimensional to three-dimensional imaging time necessary to achieve the same image quality compared with activity in the field of view. The ordinate is the effective sensitivity advantage of three-dimensional over two-dimensional imaging. A value of 2 would imply that it would take twice as long in two-dimensional mode as in three-dimensional mode to achieve the same image quality.

these effects, permitting more effective use of three-dimensional imaging.

In addition to difficulties with large activities in the field of view, three-dimensional has other disadvantages. First, because so many different lines of coincidence are possible in three-dimensional imaging, the data sets produced are huge compared with those produced by two-dimensional imaging. For example, a typical 35-slice sinogram from a two-dimensional scan might occupy 3 or 4 megabytes of disk storage, whereas a three-dimensional sinogram set might occupy 25 megabytes. This has important ramifications for disk storage and for reconstruction times. If a dynamic study (for example, ammonia or water) were acquired in three dimensions, it might typically produce almost 0.5 gigabyte of disk storage per study. Reconstruction times, which can be less than 30 seconds per 35 slices in two dimensions, are often as long as 5 or 6 minutes per set of 35 slices in three dimensions. This difference can be substantial when reconstructing dynamic sets of data: For example, a 16–time point set of three-dimensional data would take 80 to 100 minutes to reconstruct compared with only about 8 minutes for two-dimensional data. Recent studies have investigated methods to reduce the storage and reconstruction times.

In addition, resolution is reduced in three-dimensional images, primarily in the axial direction. The amount is very dependent on scanner design and reconstruction method but might be 4 mm FWHM in axial resolution in two dimensions compared with 6 mm FWHM in three dimensions. Although this is fractionally a large difference, it is probably not important for cardiac imaging and may result in more uniform in-plane or axial resolution.

The most important disadvantage of three-dimensional imaging is scatter. Scatter fractions of about 30% are typical in three-dimensional imaging when NEMA phantoms are used. In actual cardiac studies, however, scatter of 60% is not uncommon. Much progress has been made in accurate correction for scatter in the brain. For the chest, the situation is more difficult, and much work remains to be done to ensure that accurate scatter correction can be performed. The situation is worse if the arms are in the field of view, because many scatter correction schemes depend on the presence of a region devoid of scattering material (which is usually not true if arms are in the field) or on a more geometrically simple scattering medium than is present when the arms are in the field. In any case, having the arms in the field can produce subtle but large artifacts when performing attenuation correction and should probably be avoided.

Despite the difficulties, three-dimensional imaging may prove important in many cardiac applications, most notably for cardiac receptor imaging (in which sensitivity is critical and activities are, in general, low), and in gated FDG imaging.

CARDIAC PET IMAGE REGISTRATION

There are many clinically important reasons to want to align PET scans with other PET images or with images from other imaging methods. For example, when looking for match or mismatch between PET flow and metabolism, one would ideally have perfectly aligned images to ensure that the flow and metabolism values came from the same region. One may wish to increase patient throughput by realigning a patient data set to a previously acquired attenuation scan. Or, one may want to align a PET scan with a scan from another imaging method—SPECT, MRI or echocardiography—for image fusion or for correction of partial volume effects through knowledge of wall thickness from the other method (as with MRI or echocardiography).

Although considerable effort has been expended on aligning brain PET images between and across imaging methods, methods for alignment of cardiac images are less well developed.

Some applications for image alignment are described below, along with some of the more promising new methods.

An earlier approach to cardiac PET image alignment was alignment of two PET transmission scans.[4,8] This alignment may be useful in its own right, or, if the transmission scan is assumed to be aligned with the associated emission scan, as a method of aligning emission scans. Transmission-to-transmission alignment can be used in and of itself to reduce the time spent for acquisition of transmission scan in patients who must undergo more than one PET scan. This alignment method can also be used for post-injection attenuation correction, permitting correction with an uncontaminated transmission scan, as follows. First, a high-quality transmission scan is performed as usual. This scan can be done immediately before injection of the emission pharmaceutical earlier in the day, or on a previous day. When the next emission scan is to be performed, a very short (2- to 3-minute) transmission scan is acquired. This second scan may or may not be contaminated with emission counts (that is, they may precede or follow emission scanning) and is inadequate in performance of attenuation correction. However, it has been shown that it can be accurately aligned to the original high-quality transmission scan, even in the presence of emission contamination.[12] Therefore, any subsequent emission scan can be corrected by using the original high-quality transmission scan by first obtaining a very short, possibly contaminated transmission scan (which is assumed to be already aligned with the emission data) for alignment purposes. Attenuation scan alignment has been described and validated in three dimensions by using correlation methods[4,21] or in two dimensions by using cross correlation.[8] Alignment must be very accurate to permit good attenuation correction,[33] but the required degree of accuracy has been shown to be attainable.

Alignment of PET emission data with subsequent PET emission scans is clearly important. As has been noted elsewhere,[2] accurate emission scan alignment would permit a region of interest drawn on one scan (such as a metabolic scan) to be applied to a second scan (such as a perfusion scan). The single region of interest would correspond to the same myocardial tissue within the accuracy of the alignment method. Analysis of interventional studies (such vasodilation and angioplasty) would be greatly facilitated by such alignment. Similarly, patients who are being followed over time would benefit greatly from such alignment.

As mentioned above, if the transmission data are assumed to be perfectly aligned with the emission data (a necessary assumption for accurate attenuation correction), attenuation scan alignment can be used to align emission data. Some work has been done to investigate the more difficult problem of aligning emission data with emission data. This alignment task is more difficult because emission data, even from the same pharmaceutical, may vary from one scan to the next.

Clearly, metabolic images and flow images with a mismatch pattern would also be difficult to align. Nonetheless, several different methods (some of which have been successful in aligning brain PET images) have been tried on cardiac PET images with varying degrees of success. Water and acetate realignments were investigated by using edge information and image similarity methods.[1] A thorax phantom was used to test the alignment accuracy with a sum of absolute differences method,[22] and manual realignment by using laser markers[43] has been shown to achieve 3-mm or less misalignment in more than 80% of cases. Echocardiographic images have been aligned with images obtained through FDG PET by using homologous anatomic landmarks visible on both image sets (papillary muscles and the inferior junction of the right ventricle),[40] and it has been proposed that similar techniques may be applicable to other acquisition methods (such as MRI).

Despite many advances in alignment techniques, much work remains to be done in the field of emission-to-emission alignment and alignment to other modalities, before these techniques can be widely used clinically. Alignment of PET transmission scans with SPECT transmission scans or with CT may be an exception because by appropriately scaling the data, these images portray the identical underlying data, and because alignment of transmission-to-transmission data sets is well validated.

ATTENUATION EFFECTS

All radionuclide imaging techniques are deleteriously affected by attenuation. The only radionuclide imaging method in which the effects of attenuation can, in theory, be exactly compensated for before reconstruction is PET. Attenuation correction in SPECT is also possible,[3] but because it is a nonlinear process it requires an iterative reconstruction techniques. Even attenuation correction in PET requires considerable care to achieve good accuracy in the correction process, especially when imaging the thorax. This is because the large size and inhomogeneous nature of the chest results in attenuation factors that are very large and that vary rapidly over the chest cavity. At first, one might think that the higher energy of the annihilation photons (0.511 MeV) would make the attenuation effects in PET much smaller than those in SPECT. In fact, attenuation effects are often larger in PET than in SPECT because PET requires the simultaneous detection of both annihilation photons. Therefore, the net attenuation in PET is that of the entire thickness of the body, whereas in SPECT, the attenuation is determined only by the distance from the radioactive source in the myocardium to the detector. For most projection angles, the increased thickness encountered by the dual photons in a PET scan more than compensates for the slightly lower attenuation coefficient. The 0.511 annihilation photons have an attenuation coefficient of 0.096 cm^{-1}, whereas m for technetium-99m is about 0.15 cm^{-1} (excluding scatter effects) and 0.18 cm^{-1} for thallium. Because the length of the path traversed by the coincident 511-KeV photons is often greater than twice that in SPECT, the product of an attenuation coefficient and distance is often greater in PET than in SPECT.

The rotating rod method of attenuation correction[2,3,13,39] is now the standard method for attenuation correction in most commercial PET scanners (except for those using large crystal area detectors, such as gamma camera–based PET or devices similar to the "PENN-PET" scanner.[25,30] By electronically eliminating all coincidences that are not collinear with the rotating rod source, most scatter and random events are eliminated. Because the rod is very close to the crystals, count rate performance of the PET scanner is critical.

Attenuation correction in PET by using measured transmission data always adds some noise to the corrected emission image. However, in many modern PET scanners, it is possible to keep this added noise below clinically significant levels by using only an 8-minute attenuation acquisition. This assumes a camera with good count rate characteristics and two 5-mCi rod sources. For scanners that have poorer count-rate performance, or that use fewer rods, or that have a wider acceptance angles, substantially longer acquisition times may be necessary (many older scanners require transmission times of 30 minutes or longer to keep noise at clinically acceptable levels in the corrected emission image). A method to determine the appropriate attenuation scanning time for any particular PET scanner has been described in detail elsewhere.[2]

More research is needed in attenuation correction of three-dimensional (septa-out) data sets. Currently, most scanners use conventional two-dimensional (septa-in) attenuation acquisition to correct a three-dimensional emission study. Two-dimensional data can be used to perform three-dimensional attenuation correction by reprojecting the attenuation data along the nontransaxial projection lines and using those data to correct the corresponding three-dimensional projecting lines. Some commercial PET scanners simply ignore the obliquity of the nontransaxial projection lines and correct oblique emission projection lines with the most central transaxial attenuation lines under the assumption that the oblique lines are at such small angles that their obliquity does not matter. The most straightforward way to correct a three-dimensional emission scan for attenuation would seem to be to acquire a transmission scan in three dimensions. However, no scanner is able to perform such an acquisition as of now. Presumably, this is in part related to the fact that with the septa out, the rod source might produce a singles count rate beyond the capabilities of the scanner.

Postinjection attenuation correction

It is often desirable or necessary to perform a transmission scan after the patient has been injected with the radiopharmaceutical. For example, if one is performing a simple, static FDG uptake study, it is awkward and inefficient (and increases the likelihood of patient motion) to require the patient to lie motionless on the scan table for the 30 minutes between injection and the start of imaging. One approach to this problem has already been discussed: use of a second short transmission scan immediately before the emission scan followed by transmission scan alignment. Several other approaches have also recently been investigated, most of which involve performance of an attenuation scan after the patient has been injected with isotope. In this case, the transmission scan will be slightly contaminated with emission counts (the amount of contamination will depend in part on the degree of electronic collimation used with the rod source). In general, accurate transmission scan imaging cannot be performed when there is even a small amount of activity in the patient, because even a few emission photons will distort the apparent attenuation measured by the transmission scan.

Several studies have shown that, for brain PET, correction of this contamination can be accurately performed[14] by using an emission scan acquired immediately before or after the attenuation scan. The use of this technique for cardiac PET is not as thoroughly documented. Other approaches involve attempting to use the emission contaminated transmission scan for segmentation purposes. By segmenting the attenuation scan into regions of supposedly uniform attenuation (such as soft tissue or lungs), one could presumably assign the correct value of attenuation to pixels within these regions, obviating the need to accurately measure attenuation values by instead assigning pixels to predetermined values. The underlying assumption is that one set of predetermined values of μ are applicable to lungs or soft tissue, for example, for all patients.

Subtraction of emission from contaminated transmission scans presents special difficulties when doing three-dimensional (septa-out) emission scanning. Because the transmission scan is performed in two-dimensional (septa-in) mode on many scanners, a two-dimensional emission scan must also be used to do the subtraction. However, a two-dimensional scan is not available if the emission data are acquired in three dimensions. Correction of the two-dimensional transmission scan therefore requires separate acquisition of two-dimensional scan emission, which adds considerable time to the procedure and thereby offsets some of the advantages of the three-dimensional emission scan. More research is needed to permit the acquisition of accurate attenuation scans in three dimensions or to develop methods to use three-dimensional emission scans for subtraction of emission counts from two-dimensional transmission data.

Reducing the time needed for transmission scanning

Transmission scans can substantially increase the total time during which the patient must remain motionless on the scanning table. Too short a transmission scan can compromise the quality of the emission scan by increasing noise in the corrected image. Using a higher activity rod source can, in theory, reduce transmission scan time, but this approach is of limited value. Because the rod is so close to the detectors, random events and deadtime set an upper limit[2] on the amount of activity that one should put in the rod. Beyond this limit, increases in rod activity will increase rather than decrease the noise in the corrected emission data.

Several other methods exist for reducing the time needed to perform a transmission scan. When sequential scanning is being performed, one can use very short attenuation scans to align with a long, high statistics scan, as described above. More commonly, however, smoothing of the transmission scan is used. Because the raw transmission data are relatively noisy, even a small amount of smoothing is usually beneficial, and the technique has been almost universally adopted.

The question arises as to how much smoothing can be tolerated before the beneficial noise-reducing effects of smoothing are offset by potential deleterious effects. Studies indicate that if the emission data do not have the same resolution as the transmission data—a resolution mismatch caused, for example, by excessive smoothing of the transmission data—bias in the resultant corrected emission scan can result.[24,34] The magnitude of this bias for cardiac scans has been measured, and data are now available that permit an appropriate trade-off to be made between reduction in transmission imaging time and bias due to resolution mismatch.

A second approach to reducing the time needed to acquire an attenuation scan (that is, reduction of the transmission scan time without an increase in the noise in the emission corrected image) is to segment the transmission scan into lung tissue, soft tissue, and air (the region outside the body) and to assign uniform attenuation values to each of these three segments. The segmenting can be done manually or automatically. The resulting attenuation image is then reprojected and used to perform the attenuation correction. Because each of the three segments is assigned a uniform value-of-attenuation coefficient, no additional noise is added to the emission scan when attenuation correction is performed. In addition, the transmission scan could presumably be contaminated with emission counts, because each segment will be assigned the "correct" attenuation value. The effects of the scanning bed must also be accounted for by manually or automatically positioning a standardized "bed" value of attenuation or by using the measured data. The transmission scan need only have good enough statistics that the segmentation itself is accurate. The more robust the segmentation method, the shorter the attenuation scan can be.

Data are limited on the effects of inaccurate segmentation. One potential objection to the method is that it assumes that all lung and other tissue from all patients has the same attenuation values, which may not be true. In addition, it is unclear what the effect of liver tissue might be as it begins to appear in the lung field. Several approaches have been taken to deciding what value to assign to each of the segments—theoretically derived values or empirical values derived from many patients or values derived from average values in the transmission scan of each patient. Nonetheless, because the reduction in emission scan noise is so great, the method bears further consideration. Smoothing may still be required with segmentation methods; even if the edge borders were perfect, they mismatch the emission scan resolution and, in theory, should be blurred to the emission scan resolution.

One final scheme has been proposed that attempts to combine the best features of measured and segmented transmission scans.[38] This method keeps the underlying philosophy of segmentation while eliminating the need to define borders or decide on appropriate attenuation values to assign. A histogram of attenuation values is made from the transmission scan. In general, this histogram has three broad peaks which presumably correspond to lung, soft tissue, and air. The width of these peaks is caused by true variations in attenuation values over the tissue; noise; and, secondarily, scanner resolution effects. Because the noise characteristics can be estimated and the scanner resolution is known, the peaks in the histogram can, in principle, be "sharpened"—that is, reduced to the width that would be obtained only from true variations in attenuation values—by one of several mathematical techniques. Initial results seem promising, but further work will be needed before it is known how well the method will work in clinical practice.

Patient motion

Patient motion may occur between the time of the attenuation scan and the time of the emission scan. This is especially likely in scans that require a prolonged uptake. For example, the patient must usually wait 30 minutes between injection and the start of imaging in an [18]FDG scan. If the patient shifts position during this time, the attenuation correction factors would not be applied to the proper regions of the emission image because the transmission scan would no longer be aligned with the emission scan. The question arises as to what effect such misalignment would have on the resulting emission image.

McCord et al[33] found that the effects of such misalignment on cardiac PET emission imaging could be severe. Not only did errors occur in the absolute values of activity concentration measured but regional effects occurred. Misalignment was shown to produce apparent activity increases in some portions of the myocardium and decreases in other regions. For a 1-cm lateral shift, the septal wall remained almost unaffected, whereas the free wall increased or decreased (depending on the direction of the shift) by about 15%. Similar inhomogeneities were found for z-axis shifts and for the less probable anterior–posterior patients shifts. Such regional effects could certainly affect clinical interpretations made from the images.

It is easy to understand why small patient motions can cause regional changes in apparent myocardial uptake. Consider two positron decays, one emanating from the lateral free wall of the heart and the other emanating from the septum. Imagine that both pairs of photons are detected by crystals anterior and posterior to the patient. These photons travel through a certain path-length of tissue, primarily myocardial tissue and blood as well as chest wall. The attenuation correction factor for this anterior–posterior projection is calculated during the transmission scan. If, after the transmission scan, the patient moved 1 cm to the left, the lateral myocardial wall tissue would move into a position occupied by lung in the attenuation scan. Anterior–posterior projections from photons emitted by the lateral wall would, after this shift in position, falsely be assumed to pass mostly through lung tissue and would be undercorrected. The septal wall, however, would remain within the cardiac structures after the 1-cm shift, and its attenuation correction factors would not change appreciably. One cm of motion to the patient's left therefore results in an undercorrection of the free wall, which in turn causes an erroneous decrease in the free-wall activity whereas that of the septal wall remains more

or less constant. Regional inhomogeneity is thereby introduced. The situation for motions to the patient's right is similar but reversed: The lateral wall will show erroneously increased activity and the septal wall will remain almost unchanged.

One centimeter of motion may seem unreasonably large. With the usual head-holder schemes used during a brain scan, the head would rarely, if ever, move that much. When imaging the chest, however, the patient is usually immobilized far less rigorously than is the head during a brain scan. In addition, the cardiac patient is usually in an uncomfortable position, often with arms extended above the level of the shoulders. In addition, the outer wall of the thorax is (especially in mildly obese persons) a rather plastic structure. For these reasons, shifts of 1 cm or more during a 1-hour scan are plausible. It is surprising that the same amount effort put into developing head immobilization systems has not been expended to develop a chest immobilization system. It is hoped that a comfortable, reliable chest immobilizer will be developed and widely used. Alteration in PET camera gantry designs may reduce the angle at which patients must extend their arms. Until such changes occur, patient motion may cause considerable variation in the levels of observed activity uptake around the myocardium. Recent studies have indicated that respiratory motion can also play a role in cardiac motion (and, presumably, in variability in measured uptake); such effects clearly need further study.[9]

NEW PET CAMERA DESIGNS

Many developments have been made in the design of crystal and photomultiplier tubes and in the use of potentially new important scintillation materials (such as lutetium ortho-silicate, a fast crystal with a stopping power greater than bismuth germanate, but with a light output almost as great as that of sodium–iodide). In addition, many exciting advances have been made in small-animal PET cameras, devices with very small fields of view but exquisitely high resolution that may considerably advance pharmaceutical development and research in basic physiology.[16]

A detailed description of such developments is outside the scope of this text. One development (or, rather, a revisitation of a very old idea) is worth briefly discussing, as it could have a broad clinical impact in the near future. This development involves the use of two almost conventional gamma cameras, placed 180 degrees apart and operating in coincidence, to perform positron emission tomography. Such a device, operating without a collimator or with coarse scatter-reducing collimation similar to the septa in a conventional ring PET scanner, could, in principle, permit positron tomography to be performed by using the hardware in a SPECT camera system.

The addition of coincidence circuitry is simple and relatively inexpensive. However, several other problems remain to be solved, most notably the problem of being able to handle the very high singles count rates produced in each gamma camera when the collimator is removed. When the collimator is removed from a gamma camera, its sensitivity increases dramatically (for example, a typical technetium collimator might reduce the counting rate for a technetium source by a factor of 1000).

High count rates are also a problem in ring-type PET scanners. These scanners are made up of hundreds or thousands of small separate crystals. Each crystal is connected to its own photomultiplier or, more commonly, small groups of crystals share a photomultiplier tube so that the total singles count rate is divided among the separate crystals and electronic elements. In a gamma camera–based PET scanner two huge crystals are used, one for each of the two opposing gamma cameras. Although many photomultiplier tubes may view this crystal, a large fraction of these tubes view the light produced by every event that strikes the crystal. Therefore, the number of photons seen by the photomultiplier tubes and the associated electronics could be much greater for gamma camera–based PET than for ring-based PET. In addition, just as with three-dimensional ring–based PET, gamma camera–based PET without a collimator requires special three-dimensional reconstruction software and, more important, may have very high scatter fractions. As of now its clinical use is still under investigation, but it has shown promise for imaging low-level activity distributions. Advancements in gamma-camera count rate performance may soon broaden its clinical utility.

REFERENCES

1. Anderson JL: A rapid and accurate method to realign PET scans utilizing image edge information, *J Nucl Med* 36:657–669, 1995.
2. Bacharach SL: *Attenuation correction: practical considerations.* In Schwaiger M, ed: *Cardiac positron emission tomography,* Kluwer Academic Publishers, Boston, 1996.
3. Bacharach SL and Buvat I: Attenuation correction in cardiac positron emission tomography and single-photon tomography, *J Nucl Cardiol* 2:246–255, 1995.
4. Bacharach SL, Douglas MA, Carson RE, et al: Three dimensional registration of cardiac positron emission tomography attenuation scans. *J Nucl Med* 34:311–321, 1993.
5. Bailey DL, Miller MP, Spinks TJ, Bloomfield PM, Livieratos L, Young HE, and Jones T: Experience with fully 3D PET and implications for future high resolution 3D tomographs, *Phys Med Biol,* 1998 (in press).
6. Bartlett ML, Bacharach SL, Voipio-Pulkki LM, et al: Artifactual inhomogeneities in myocardial PET and SPECT scans in normal subjects, *J Nucl Med* 36:188–195, 1995.
7. Bartlett ML, Buvat I, Vaquero JJ, et al: Measurement of myocardial wall thickening from PET/SPECT images: comparison of two methods, *J Comput Assist Tomogr* 20:473–481, 1996.
8. Bettinardi V, Gilardi MC, Lucignani G, et al: A procedure for patient repositioning and compensation for misalignment between transmission and emission data in PET heart studies, *J Nucl Med* 34:137–142, 1993.
9. Budinger T, Klein CJ, Reed JH, et al: Compensation for respiratory motion in cardiac PET—a feasibility study, *J Nucl Med* 37:130P, 1996.
10. Budinger TF: Medical criteria for the design of a dynamic positron tomograph for heart studies, *IEEE Transactions in Nuclear Science* 29:488, 1982.
11. Buvat I, Bartlett ML, Kitsiou AN, et al: A "hybrid" method for measuring myocardial wall thickening from gated PET/SPECT images, *J Nucl Med* 38:324–329, 1997.
12. Buvat I, Freedman NMT, Dilsizian V, et al: Realignment of emission contaminated attenuation maps with uncontaminated attenuation maps for attenuation correction in PET, *J Comput Assist Tomogr* 20:848–854, 1996.

13. Carroll LR, Kertz P. and Orcut G: *The orbiting rod source: improving performance in PET transmission correction scans.* In *Emission computed tomography—current trends,* 1983.
14. Carson RE, Daube-Witherspoon ME, and Green MV: A method for postinjection PET transmission measurements with a rotating source, *J Nucl Med* 29:1558–1567, 1988.
15. Cherry SR, Dahlbom M, and Hoffman EJ: 3D PET using a conventional multislice tomograph without septa, *J Comput Assist Tomogr* 15:655–668, 1991.
16. Cherry SR, Shao Y, Silverman RW, et al: Micropet - a high resolution PET scanner for imaging small animals, *IEEE Transaction on Nuclear Science* 44:1161–1166, 1997.
17. Cooke CD, Garcia EV, Cullom SJ, et al: Determining the accuracy of calculating systolic wall thickening using a fast Fourier transform approximation: a simulation study based on canine and patient data, *J Nucl Med* 35:1185–1192, 1994.
18. Daube-Witherspoon ME, Green SL, Bacharach SL, and Carson RE: Influence of activity outside the field-of-view on 3-D PET imaging, *J Nucl Med* 36:184P, 1995.
19. Defrise M, Geissbuhler A, and Townsend DW: A performance study of 3D reconstruction algorithms for positron emission tomography, *Phys Med Biol* 39:305–320, 1994.
20. DePuey EG, Nichols K, and Dobrinsky C: Left ventricular ejection fraction assessed from gated technetium-99m-sestamibi SPECT, *J Nucl Med* 34:1871–1876, 1993.
21. Douglas MA, Bacharach SL, and Kalkowski PJ: Alignment of cardiac PET attenuation images, *IEEE Computers in Cardiology* 249–252, 1991.
22. Eberl S, Kanno I, Fulton RR, et al: Automated interstudy image registration technique for SPECT and PET, *J Nucl Med* 37:137–145, 1996.
23. Erlandsson K and Strand SE: A new approach to 3-dimensional image-reconstruction in PET, *IEEE Transactions on Nuclear Science* 39:1438–1443, 1992.
24. Freedman NMT, Bacharach SL, Carson RE, et al: Effect of smoothing during transmission processing on quantitative cardiac PET. *J Nucl Med* 37:690–694, 1996.
25. Freifelder R, Karp JS, Geagan M, et al: Design and performance of the head PENN-PET scanner, *IEEE Transactions on Nuclear Science* 41:1436–1440, 1994.
26. Galt J, Garcia E, and Robbins W: Effects of myocardial wall thickness on SPECT quantification, *IEEE Trans Med Imag* 9:144–150, 1990.
27. Germano G, Kiat H, Kavanagh PB, et al: Automatic quantification of ejection fraction from gated myocardial perfusion SPECT, *J Nucl Med* 36:2138–2147, 1995.
28. Hoffman EJ, Huang S-C, and Phelps ME: Quantitation in positron emission computed tomography: 1. Effect of object size, *J Comput Assist Tomogr* 3:299–308, 1979.
29. Johnson CA, Yan YC, Carson RE, et al: A system for the 3D reconstruction of retracted-septa PET data using the EM algorithm, *IEEE Transactions on Nuclear Science* 42:1223–1227, 1995.
30. Karp JS and Muehllehner G: Standards for performance measurements of PET scanners: evaluation with the UGM PENN-PET 240H scanner, *Med Prog Technol* 17:173–187, 1991.
31. Kouris K, Abdel-Dayem HM, Taha B, et al: Left ventricular ejection fraction and volumes calculated from dual gated SPECT myocardial imaging with 99Tcm-MIBI, *Nucl Med Commun* 13:648–655, 1992.
32. Lewellen TK, Kohlmyer SG, Miyaoka RS, et al: Investigation of the performance of the General Electric ADVANCE positron emission tomograph in 3D mode, *IEEE Transactions in Nuclear Science* 43:2199–2206, 1996.
33. McCord ME, Bacharach SL, Bonow RO, et al: Misalignment between PET transmission and emission scans: its effect on myocardial imaging, *J Nucl Med* 33:1209–1214; discussion 1214–1215, 1992.
34. Meikle SR, Dahlbom M, and Cherry S: Attenuation correction using count-limited transmission data in positron emission tomography, *J Nucl Med* 34:143–150, 1993.

35. Mok DY, Bartlett ML, Bacharach SL, et al: Can partial volume effects be used to measure myocardial thickness and thickening? *IEEE Computers in Cardiology* NA: 195–198, 1992.

36. Pajevic S, Daube-Witherspoon ME, Bacharach SL, Carson RE: Noise characteristic of 3-D and 2-D PET images. *IEEE Trans Med Imaging* 17:9–23, 1988.

37. Porenta G, Kuhle W, Sinha S, et al: Parameter estimation of cardiac geometry by ECG-gated PET imaging: validation using magnetic resonance imaging and echocardiography, *J Nucl Med* 36:1123–1129, 1995.

38. Price JC, Bacharach SL, et al: Noise reduction in PET attenuation correction by maximum likelihood histogram sharpening of attenuation images. *J Nucl Med* 37(5):786–794, 1996.

39. Ranger NT, Thompson CJ, and Evans AC: The application of a masked orbiting transmission source for attenuation correction in PET, *J Nucl Med* 30:1056–1068, 1989.

40. Savi A, Gilardi MC, Rizzo G, et al: Spatial registration of echocardiographic and positron emission tomographic heart studies, *Eur J Nucl Med* 22:243–247, 1995.

41. Strother SC, Casey ME, and Hoffman EJ: Measuring PET scanner sensitivity: relating count rates to image signal-to-noise ratios using noise equivalent counts, *IEEE Transactions in Nuclear Science* 37:783–788, 1990.

42. Wienhard K, Eriksson L, Grootonk S, et al: Performance evaluation of the positron scanner ECAT EXACT, *J Comput Assist Tomogr* 16:804–813, 1992.

43. Yamashita K, Tamaki N, Yonekura Y, et al: Quantitative analysis of regional wall motion by gated myocardial positron emission tomography: validation and comparison with left ventriculography, *J Nucl Med* 30:1775–1786, 1989.

44. Yu JN, Fahey FH, Harkness BA, et al: Evaluation of emission-transmission registration in thoracic PET, *J Nucl Med* 35:1777–1780, 1994.

Chapter 10

Correction of attenuation and scatter for single-photon emission computed tomography

Michael A. King, Benjamin M.W. Tsui, and **Tinsu Pan**

Numerous factors can cause artifacts in cardiac single-photon emission computed tomography (SPECT).[15] Among these factors are the attenuation and scattering of the photons in the patient's tissues. The emergence of commercially available hardware and software additions to SPECT systems to correct for attenuation and scatter has created a need for the understanding of the degradations caused by these phenomena and the alternatives available to correct them. This chapter provides a survey of the physics underlying attenuation and scatter and a summary of methods for correction of scatter, estimation of patient-specific attenuation maps, and performing attenuation correction. Other recent reviews on these subjects have been published by Bacharach and Buvat[3] and King et al.[41-43]

EFFECT OF ATTENUATION AND SCATTER ON CARDIAC SPECT IMAGING

Interactions and exponential attenuation

For a photon, whether a gamma ray from technetium-99m (^{99m}Tc) or X-ray after decay of thallium-201 (^{201}Tl), to become part of a cardiac image, it must first escape the body (Fig. 10-1, A). The chances of this occurring are reduced in proportion to the likelihood that the photon will interact in the patient's body before it can escape. At the photon energies used in nuclear cardiology, the major interactions in tissues are Compton scattering and photoelectric absorption.[1,71] In Compton scattering, a photon interacts with an electron that is loosely bound compared with the photon's energy. As a result, the electron is ejected from the atom and a new photon with a lower energy and different direction is created (Fig. 10-1, B, C). The probability of interaction per unit path length (characterized by the linear attenuation coefficient for Compton scattering) depends on the tissue density (number of electrons per gram) and decreases slowly with increasing photon energy. In photoelectric absorption, the photon imparts all of its energy to an electron that is subsequently ejected from the atom. The ejected photoelectron carries a kinetic energy that is equal to the energy of the incident photon minus the binding energy with which it was held to the atom. No scattered photon is emitted in the photoelectric interaction (Fig. 10-1, D). However, characteristic radiation will probably be emitted when the electrons of the atom rearrange to fill the vacancy left by the photoelectron. The linear attenuation coefficient for photoelectric absorption increases as the cube of the atomic number of the atom, depends on tissue density, and decreases as the inverse cube of the photon energy.

Mathematically, the fraction of photons that will be transmitted through an attenuator (the transmitted fraction [TF]) is given by:

$$TF = e^{-\mu x} \tag{1}$$

where μ is the linear attenuation coefficient (sum of all of the coefficients for individual interactions), and x is the thickness

The contents of this chapter are solely the responsibility of the authors and do not necessarily represent the official views of the National Heart, Lung, and Blood Institute.

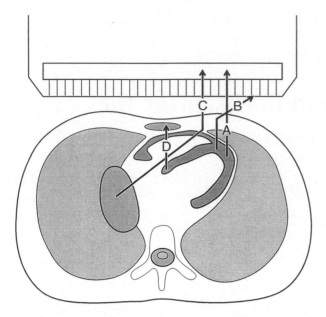

Fig. 10-1. Photon interactions of interest in patient for cardiac imaging: **A,** Transmitted photon originating in myocardium; **B,** Compton-scattered photon originating in myocardium, which the collimator stops from striking the crystal; **C,** Compton-scattered photon originating in the liver, which the collimator allows to pass, resulting in detection of an event that apparently originated in the myocardium; **D,** Photon that is photoelectrically absorbed in bone, which originated in myocardium.

of the attenuator the photons pass through. If the attenuator is made up of many materials of various compositions, the product μx in Equation 1 is replaced by a sum of the attenuation coefficients for each material multiplied by the thickness of that material which the transmitted photons pass through (path length of the travel of the photons in the material). Because the attenuation coefficient varies according to type of tissue, the transmitted fraction will vary with the materials traversed even if the total patient thickness between the site of emission and the camera is the same. Thus, one must have patient-specific information on the spatial distribution of attenuation coefficients (an attenuation map) to calculate the attenuation that will decrease the probability of photon detection.

Attenuation artifacts

The change in transmitted fraction with direction of the photons and among different locations in the patient results in variation in sensitivity with site of emission. This can be visualized in planar images as, for example, breast shadows (Fig. 10-2, *top*) or decreased posterior apical counts in the presence of an elevated diaphragm. In SPECT slices, these artifactual shadows are difficult to recognize (Fig. 10-2, *middle*); however, a pattern of altered relative counts appears that is consistent with the influence of attenuation in the mean bull's-eye polar maps of patients with a low likelihood of coronary artery disease (Fig. 10-2, *bottom*). Eisner et al[16] reported decreased relative counts in the anterior wall of ^{201}Tl polar maps for women because of breast attenuation and a relative decrease in the inferior wall of men, which may be caused by diaphragmatic attenuation. The

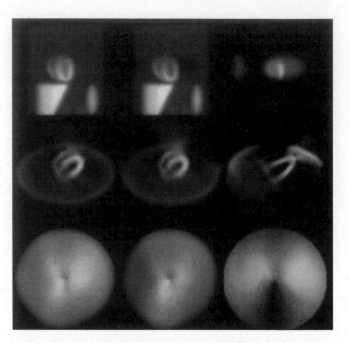

Fig. 10-2. Monte Carlo simulated images of the MCAT phantom modeling technetium-99m sestamibi distribution, showing some of the artifacts encountered with breast attenuation. The top row shows left anterior oblique planar images. The middle row shows selected 180° filtered back-projection transverse slices. The bottom row shows bull's-eye polar maps obtained from the filtered back-projection reconstructed slices. The images on the left are for an attenuation distribution that does not include breasts. The images in the middle are for the same source and attenuator distribution to which breast attenuation has been added. The images on the right are the images in the left column minus the images in the middle column; thus, they show where count losses have occurred as a result of breast attenuation.

location, extent, and severity of these reduced count regions varies from patient to patient as a function of the patient's anatomy.[76] Thus, the variation in the pattern of apparent localization in disease-free patients is increased, resulting in more false-positive results (lower specificity) at any given level of true-positive results (sensitivity).

Variation in transmitted fraction also results in inconsistent projection data, which can cause distortions in the reconstructed slices. Geometrical distortion manifests itself as alterations of the size and shape of cardiac structures and lesions (note the change in shape of the heart with the addition of breast attenuation in Fig. 10-2, *middle*), and artifacts in the regions surrounding "hot" structures (note the apparent location of counts past the anterior surface of the patient with breast attenuation in Fig. 10-2, *middle*). Because of the greater inconsistencies in the emission profiles in the absence of averaging by combining conjugate views, geometrical distortion will be greater for 180° than 360° reconstruction.[44] The positive and negative tails from hot sources, which result from the incomplete cancellation of inconsistent data in the emission profiles, can also lead to serious distortions in cardiac wall counts when substantial extracardiac localization occurs, such as with hepatic uptake. Germano et al[26] showed in phantom studies that

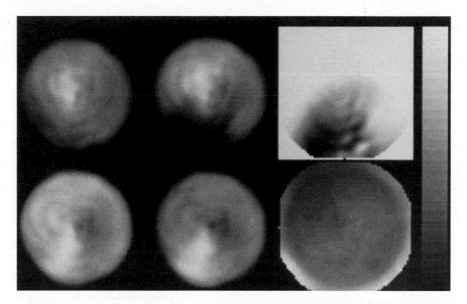

Fig. 10-3. Bull's-eye polar maps of the technetium-99m sestamibi counts at the center of the left ventricle wall for 180°, 30-iteration maximum-likelihood expectation maximization (MLEM) reconstructions of simulated projections of the mathematical cardiac–torso phantom modeling technetium-99m sestamibi localization. *Top left,* map for reconstruction with only the heart present. Included is influence of attenuation and distance-dependent spatial resolution but not scatter. *Top center,* map for hepatic uptake at twice the heart concentration additionally present. *Top right,* map for the percentage change in heart counts with the presence of the liver. Note the decrease in counts especially in the posterior wall. *Lower left,* map from attenuation-corrected slices when both cardiac and hepatic uptake are present, but not scatter. *Lower center,* map with scatter included in the simulation but not corrected for prior-to-attenuation correction in MLEM reconstruction. *Lower right,* map for the percentage change in heart counts as a result of including scatter in the simulation. Maps where the heart is present were lower thresholded at 50% of their maximum value to present changes with greater contrast. The shade of gray around the outside of the polar map represents zero counts, and shades of gray darker than this shade in the top right map represent a negative contribution of the liver to the polar map.

an apparent reduction in counts occurs with the presence of a hot liver in the slices with the heart. Nuyts et al observed that use of 360° as opposed to 180° with filtered back-projection reconstruction reduced the magnitude of the artifact. The artifact was further reduced by use of attenuation compensation with maximum-likelihood expectation maximization (MLEM) reconstruction. The artifact and its reduction by use of MLEM reconstruction are shown in the polar maps of Fig. 10-3 for 180° MLEM reconstruction of Monte Carlo simulations[54] of the three-dimensional mathematical cardiac–torso (MCAT) phantom developed at the University of North Carolina at Chapel Hill.[76]

Figure 10-3, *top right*, shows a polar map of the percentage change in cardiac wall counts with the addition of hepatic activity in the slices. The percentage change is defined as:

$$\% \text{ change} = [(HL - H)/H] \cdot 100\% \qquad (2)$$

where *HL* is the map count when both heart and liver activity are present and *H* is the map count when heart activity alone is present.

Broad-beam attenuation and scatter

Equation 1 is accurate only for a beam of photons with the same energy and under the good-geometry condition[1,71] that as

soon as a photon undergoes any interaction, it is no longer counted as a member of the beam. Attenuation coefficients that are measured under these conditions are good-geometry attenuation coefficients. Compton scattered photons, even though they are reduced in energy, are not necessarily excluded from the image because of the finite width of the energy windows, which are caused because of the finite energy resolution of the cameras (Fig. 10-4). In fact, the ratio of scattered photons included in the energy window to primary photons in the energy window (scatter fraction) is typically 0.34 for ^{99m}Tc[14] and 0.95 for ^{201}Tl[31] for cardiac SPECT. Thus, to match the broad-beam attenuation that actually occurs in emission imaging, Equation 1 must be modified by inclusion of the buildup factor, *B,* which is dependent on both μ and *x.* The result is:[1,71]

$$TF = B(\mu, x) \, e^{-\mu x} \qquad (3)$$

Numerically, the buildup factor is the ratio between the sum of primary and scatter counts over the primary counts only or the relative increase in counts due to the inclusion of scattered photons. It therefore depends on such variables as location in the attenuator, geometry and composition of the attenuator, energy of the photon, energy resolution of the camera, and energy window used in imaging.

When scatter is not removed from the emission profiles be-

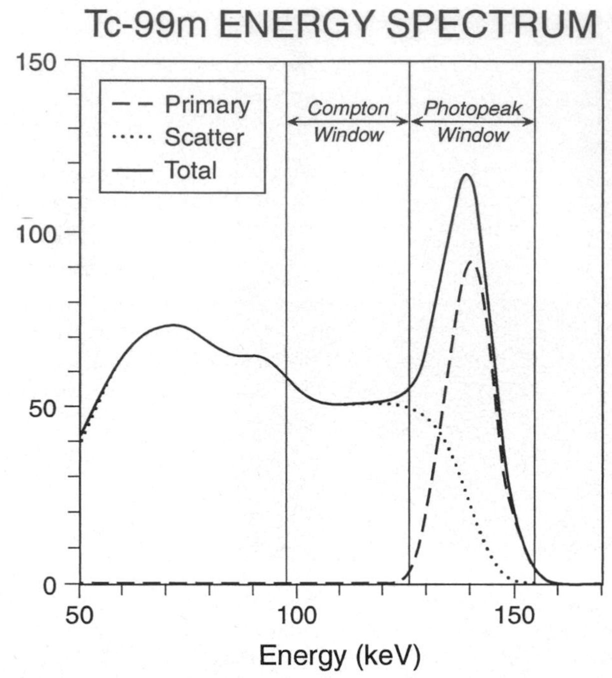

Tc-99m ENERGY SPECTRUM

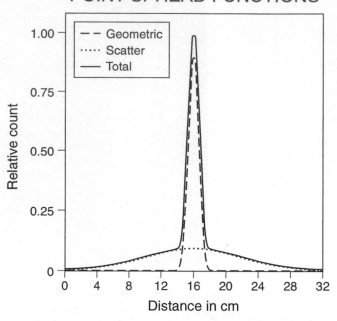

Fig. 10-4. Energy distribution of primary and scattered photons for a technetium-99m point source in an attenuating medium. Shown also are the locations of the photopeak and Compton scatter windows.

POINT SPREAD FUNCTIONS

Fig. 10-5. Geometric, scatter, and total point spread function for a technetium-99m point source in an attenuating medium.

fore reconstruction or when its presence is incorporated into the reconstruction process itself, overcorrection will occur. This is illustrated by the polar maps in Fig. 10-3, *bottom*. The polar map at the lower left is for ideal scatter correction (scattered photons were not included in the Monte Carlo simulated emission profiles that were reconstructed) coupled with attenuation correction. The polar map in the center shows the changes that occur when scatter is included in the simulated slices without correction and when attenuation correction with good-geometry attenuation coefficients is performed. The polar map at the right is the percentage change in the polar map at the left by the addition of scatter. The total change in counts in the polar map with the addition of scatter is 31.3%. Of note, all pixels of the polar map are increased to some extent, and in the percentage change map, the event gradually increases as one proceeds from the apex to base. The increase is larger in the posterior wall than the anterior wall because the posterior wall is generally deeper. This is a reversal of the pattern seen in the absence of attenuation correction and is a manifestation of the overcorrection that occurs when attenuation correction alone is applied. The increase in counts in the posterior wall is larger also because it is closer to hepatic activity.[42]

SCATTER CORRECTION METHODS

As will be seen in the next section, the methods for estimating attenuation maps that are becoming available commercially provide estimates of good-geometry attenuation maps. In the past, Equation 3 has been approximated by using an effective (reduced) attenuation coefficient that undercorrects the

primary content of the emission projections, so that a flat reconstruction of a tub uniformly filled with activity results.[32] Thus, one way to diminish overcorrection would be to use attenuation maps that comprise effective attenuation coefficients. This would only be an approximate solution because the scatter detected as arising from a site depends not only on the attenuator but also on the distribution of the source. In addition, it would not correct for the degradation of contrast caused by inclusion of scattered photons in the imaging window. The best way to reduce the effect of scatter would be to improve the energy resolution of the imaging systems by using an alternative to sodium–iodine (NaI)(Tl) scintillation detection.[71] For such a system, the Gaussian function representing the distribution of primary photons with energy in Fig. 10-4 would shrink to a single vertical line; as a result, very few scattered photons would be included in the energy window.

Alternatively, for the NaI(Tl)-based imaging systems usually used in SPECT, many scatter correction methods have been proposed. These can generally be divided into spatial distribution–based or energy distribution–based methods.

Spatial distribution–based methods

When a point source is imaged, the resulting distribution of counts around the projected location of the point is called the *point-spread function* (Fig. 10-5). The point-spread function shows how the point is spread out during imaging. When the point source is in an attenuating medium, the point-spread function has at least two components. The first is the geometrical point-spread function, which characterizes the spatial resolution of the system for the distance of the point source from the camera. The second is scatter point-spread function caused by the imaging of such photons as those in Fig. 10-1. Both the shape and number of counts in the scatter point-spread function relative to the attenuated geometrical point spread function (the scatter fraction) are needed to fully characterize the point-spread function. Spatial distribution methods seek to estimate the scatter contamination of the images on the basis of the acquired photopeak window data, which serves as an estimate of the source distribution, and a model of the blurring of the source into the scatter distribution (the scatter point-spread function). The model may additionally require knowledge of the attenuation map (map of likelihood of photons scattering) of the patient.

An early example of a spatial distribution method for scatter compensation in SPECT is the investigation of Axelsson et al.[2] They modeled the scatter function as decreasing exponentially from its center maximum value. The center value and slope of the exponential were obtained from measurements made with a line source. This function was convolved (blurred) with the acquired projection data, and the result was used as an estimate of the scatter distribution in the projection. The estimated distribution was subtracted from the original data to yield scatter-corrected projection data. One problem with this method was that it assumed that the scatter model did not change with location. To overcome this problem, Monte Carlo methods were used to generate a set of scatter responses that were interpolated in estimating the scatter distribution.[55] Both of these approaches used scatter line-spread functions instead of point-spread functions. That is, the source modeled was of a finite length line and was not a point. Convolution was performed one-dimensionally in the plane of the slice to be reconstructed. Scatter originating outside the plane was assumed to be included by the use of the finite length line.

Msaki et al[61] modeled the two-dimensional (across-plane and within-plane) scatter point-spread function and performed two-dimensional convolution to account for across-plane scatter. Meikle et al[59] further refined this technique by adapting the scatter point-spread function for the individual patient by using the measured photon transmission. Convolution subtraction methods offer a fast and reasonably accurate way of correcting for scatter. Their main disadvantages are that subtraction of the scatter estimate elevates noise in the primary estimate, the accuracy with which the scatter point-spread function is modeled varies, and estimation of scatter from sources not within the field of view of the camera poses a problem (for example, ^{99m}Tc sestamibi imaging with substantial hepatic uptake with the liver only partially in the field of view).

Modeling of the nonstationary scatter spread function can be built into the reconstructions process.[6,20,21] The resulting iterative reconstructions have a lower magnitude of image noise than those that are obtained when convolution subtraction is used. However, the processing time is greatly increased.

Energy distribution–based methods

The detected energy spectrum (Fig. 10-4) is made up of 1) the photopeak distribution of each energy photon emitted, which is Gaussian in shape (the width of the Gaussian is dependent on the energy resolution of the detector system); 2) the distribution of photons detected after scattering; and 3) the Compton plateau for each energy photon emitted (not a significant factor for photon energies less than 250 keV).[71] Energy distribution–based methods seek to estimate the number of scatter counts in a pixel from the variation in counts for that pixel within two or more energy windows (the detected-photon energy distribution). Because this is done for each pixel in the image, the result is an image of the scatter distribution that can be subtracted from the acquired image containing primary counts and scatter.

The Compton window subtraction method of Jaszczak et al[37] is the classic example of this strategy. In this method, a second energy window placed below the photopeak window (Fig. 10-4) is used to record an image consisting of scattered photons. This image is multiplied by a scaling factor, *k*, and is subtracted from the acquired image to yield a scatter-corrected image. This method assumes that the spatial distribution of the scatter within the Compton scatter window is the same as that within the photopeak window and that once it is determined from a calibration study, a single scaling factor holds true for all applications on a given system. That the distribution of scatter between the two windows differs can be seen by noting that the average angle of scattering (and, hence, the degree of blurring) changes with energy.

The difference in the distribution of scatter with energy can be minimized by making the scatter window smaller and placing it just below the photopeak window. With this arrangement, one obtains the two energy-window variant of the triple energy-window scatter-correction method of Ogawa et al[64] as applied to [99m]Tc. When downscatter (scattered photons from a higher energy emission) is present, a third small window is added above the photopeak; scatter is estimated as the area under the trapezoid between the two narrow windows on either side of the photopeak.[63] In this way, triple energy-window scatter correction can be used with radionuclides, such as ^{201}Tl, that emit photons of multiple energies, or for scatter correction when imaging multiple radionuclides. Ljungberg et al[52] compared Compton window subtraction, triple energy-window scatter correction, and other methods in a recent review.

Energy distribution–based methods that use a limited number of energy windows to estimate the primary counts do not completely compensate for scatter. Performance can be improved through the use of more windows. Examples of multi-window approaches include the investigations of Koral et al,[45] Gagnon et al,[24] and Haynor et al.[33] Buvat et al[7] compared nine scatter correction methods based on spectral analysis in a recent investigation. The problems with methods that require more than a few energy windows are that the required number of windows is not available on many SPECT systems and dividing the spectrum up into a large number of windows decreases the detected counts in each window, thus increasing the noise in the windows.

ESTIMATION OF PATIENT-SPECIFIC ATTENUATION MAPS

Combined transmission and emission imaging on the same SPECT system is the currently favored method of estimating patient-specific attenuation maps that are registered with the emission data. Transmission imaging consists of positioning a source of radiation on one side of the patient and a detector on the other side to measure the transmitted intensity. By taking the ratio of the transmitted intensity to the intensity without the patient present, the transmitted fraction of Equation 1 is determined. Because we wish to estimate μ, Equation 1 can be rearranged to solve for it, as follows:

$$\mu = [\ln(1/TF)]/x \qquad (4)$$

An estimate of the attenuation map is obtained by reconstruction of attenuation profiles in which each pixel has first been transformed as in Equation 4. Reconstruction can be done through filtered back-projection or an iterative algorithm.

Basic transmission configurations

The basic transmission source and camera collimator configurations are summarized in Fig. 10-6 for a 40-cm field of view, single-headed SPECT system imaging a patient 50 cm in diameter. The first configuration, illustrated in Fig. 10-6, A, is that of a sheet transmission source opposite a parallel hole collimator on the camera head. Many investigators used this

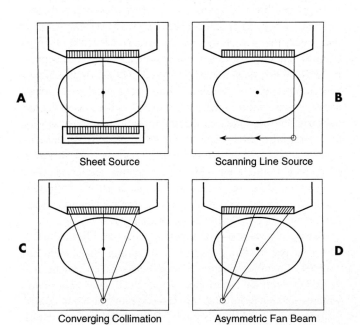

A Sheet Source

B Scanning Line Source

C Converging Collimation

D Asymmetric Fan Beam

Fig. 10-6. Four configurations of transmission sources and collimators for use in transmission imaging. In each case, a 40-cm camera field of view is shown imaging a patient with a 50-cm major axis. Truncation will vary with camera field of view, patient size, and focal distance for converging collimation.

method to estimate attenuation maps.[4,9,25,29,73] The advantages of this method are as follows.

1. The entire field of view of the camera is used for transmission imaging; thus, the attenuation maps are truncated only to the same extent as the emission slices that they will be used to correct.
2. If no source collimation is used, the transmission source is not required to be at a fixed distance from a parallel hole collimator as it would be with a convergent collimator; thus, the source does not have to be moved radially to compensate for radial motion of the camera head in a body-contouring acquisition.
3. Because the whole field of view is covered by the planar source, no lateral motion of this source is required.

The disadvantages of this configuration include:

1. The sheet source requires the addition of a holder that will keep the source opposite the camera collimator. Such an arrangement is cumbersome when used clinically.
2. The attenuation coefficients measured are broad-beam coefficients, because the geometry of imaging leads to substantial inclusion of scattered transmission photons in the transmission energy window.
3. The sheet source can be collimated to reduce the patient exposure to transmission photons that would not be transmitted through the camera collimator, can reduce the imaging of scattered transmission photons so that values of the attenuation coefficients closer to good geometry are determined, and can improve spatial resolution. However, this adds to the weight of the transmission source unit, which must be rigidly supported opposite the camera head.
4. For multiple-headed SPECT systems, the sheet source could partially or wholly block the other heads.
5. If a transmission source with a short half-life is used (^{99m}Tc or ^{201}Tl), the source must be prepared each day, which requires time and exposure to radiation on the part of the technologist.

A variation on this method that overcomes some of its disadvantages is to use several stationary, long-lived line sources.[48]

As shown in Fig. 10-6, B, the sheet transmission source can also be replaced by a scanning line source.[72] The camera head opposite the line source is electronically windowed to store only the events detected in a narrow region opposite the line source in the transmission image. This results in substantial reduction in the amount of scattered transmission radiation to the extent that good-geometry attenuation coefficients are obtained. It also decreases (but does not eliminate) cross-contamination from emission photons because only the portion of the camera face on which it is highly likely that a transmission photon will be detected is used to form the transmission image.

The emission images can also be electronically windowed to store counts in the emission image only when the transmission source is not opposite the location of the detected event. This simplifies the correction for downscatter from a higher energy transmission source to a lower energy emission source window if different radionuclides are used or provides self correction if the same radionuclide is used for emission and transmission imaging. This configuration also has the further advantages:

1. The entire camera field of view is used for transmission imaging.
2. The line source is not required to be at a fixed distance, because parallel collimators are used.
3. Only a line source needs to be filled, stored, shielded, or mounted on the system, thus making handling more manageable and reducing personnel exposure.
4. Scatter can be easily reduced by collimating the line source.
5. The scanning line source and assembly is lightweight compared with a sheet source with assembly and collimator, making the line source easier to support.

The scanning line source has the disadvantage of requiring modification of the system to mechanically move the source and to perform electronic windowing to accept into the transmission image only the region of the camera face opposite the line. On modern SPECT systems, these difficulties have been overcome, and commercial SPECT systems with transmission imaging based on scanning line sources are now available. In addition, the transmission images are of lower spatial resolution than those acquired by using convergent collimation, but the lower spatial resolution is compatible with the emission images and is adequate for attenuation correction purposes.

The need for lateral motion of the transmission source can be avoided without using a cumbersome sheet source if convergent collimation is used. Figure 10-6, C depicts the use of a fan-beam collimator with a line transmission source at its focal distance.[13,38,40,77] This configuration has the following advantages.

1. It obtains almost good geometry attenuation coefficients, because the collimator acts as an antiscatter grid.[53]
2. Because this method gives computed tomography–like imaging geometry, attenuation maps with spatial resolution superior to that of emission images acquired through the same collimator can be reconstructed.
3. Convergent collimators provide a better spatial resolution–sensitivity combination for small structures, such as the heart, than can be achieved with parallel collimation for emission imaging.
4. As noted above, only line or point sources need to be handled, shielded, or mounted on the system.

The potential disadvantages of this configuration are:

1. An increased truncation of the field of view compared with that of parallel collimation on the same camera head.
2. Lack of electronic windowing to assist in correction of cross-contamination between emission and transmission imaging.
3. Need to keep the source at the focal distance of the collimator. To overcome this difficulty, the transmission source can be mounted on the system with motorized computer control to move the source radially in relation to motion of the opposed camera head, thereby maintaining the source in focus.

With sequential transmission and emission imaging, correction of the emission images for the presence of the transmission source is not necessary, and images acquired in the transmission window during emission imaging can be used to estimate the contamination of the transmission images with transmission source present by the emission photons. Methods have been developed to estimate the contamination of emission and transmission images by the other source of radiation when simultaneous emission and transmission imaging is used.[13,23,38,77] Thus, the influence of cross-contamination can be greatly reduced.

The major remaining problem with using convergent collimation for estimation of attenuation maps is truncation. Truncation of attenuation profiles creates estimated attenuation maps that show the "cupping artifact"—a pileup of information that occurs in the truncated region near its edge when the reconstruction is limited to only the region within the field of view (FOV) at very angle. If the reconstruction is not limited to the fully sampled region, the area outside of the fully sampled region is distorted and the area inside of it is slightly reduced in value. Great improvement can be obtained by constraining the reconstruction to the actual area of the attenuator.[13,38,77] Because the goal of transmission imaging is to estimate attenuation maps for correction of attenuation in the emission images, the important question is not whether the maps are distorted by truncation but whether the correction of attenuation is degraded by truncation.

It has been reported that even though the attenuation map is significantly distorted outside the fully sampled region, the attenuation sums (exponentials of the sums of the attenuation coefficients multiplied by path lengths) for locations in the fully sampled regions are estimated fairly accurately by iterative reconstruction.[58,77] This is because iterative reconstruction algorithms force the total attenuation across the maps to be consistent with the measured attenuation profiles and because all locations are viewed at least part of the time. Thus, for such structures as the heart, which are within the fully sampled region, reasonably accurate attenuation correction can be obtained. Recently, it has been shown in receiver-operating characteristics (ROC) studies that truncation affects the detection of cardiac lesions and that addition of knowledge of the patient's body outline obtained independently to the reconstruction of the attenuation maps essentially removes the loss in lesion detection accuracy.[30]

Use of body outline and other information obtained by using parallel hole collimators in addition to convergent collimators to image the patient can be used to improve the accuracy of estimating the attenuation maps in the region truncated by convergent collimators.[10,19,57,65] Truncation can be reduced by using collimators with longer focal length so that the field of view of the collimator covers more of the patient.[38] This requires that the other two heads be backed away from the patient so that they do not block the field of view of the first collimator. Truncation can also be reduced by performing two transmission acquisitions with the patient moved laterally between the two collimators or by extrapolating the transmission profiles.[39] A third way to reduce truncation is the use of asymmetric fan-beam collimators[11] shown in Fig. 10-6, D. By rotating the collimator 360° around the patient, conjugate views will fill in the region truncated by each other to such an extent that a fully sampled region equivalent to that of imaging with a parallel hole collimator can be obtained.

Transmission sources

Many potential transmission sources are available for use with ^{99m}Tc or ^{201}Tl as the emission source.[4,18,22,23,38,72,77,79] Table 10-1, adapted from data in Ficaro et al,[79] summarizes the physical properties of several of these sources. If simultaneous transmission and emission imaging are to be used, the ideal transmission source would have the following properties.

1. It would emit monoenergetic photons of an energy lower than that of the photons of the emission source to avoid contamination of the emission images by the transmission source.
2. It would emit photons with energy sufficiently close to that of the emission source that the magnitude of the correction required to convert the attenuation map measured at the transmission photon energy to that of the emission photon energy would be reduced.
3. It would have a long half-life so that the transmission source will require replacement infrequently.
4. It would not be expensive to manufacture.

On the basis of these requirements, gadolinium-153 (^{153}Gd),

with its two photons at 97.4 and 103.2 keV, is a good choice for use as a transmission source for ^{99m}Tc emission imaging. For ^{201}Tl, americium-241 (^{241}Am), with its 59.4-keV photons, is an excellent choice; however, care must be taken not to over estimate the attenuation coefficient of bones, because at 59.4 keV, the photoelectric effect has a much larger linear attenuation coefficient than it does at the energies of the x-rays emitted subsequent to the decay of ^{201}Tl. When using a sequential imaging protocol or with correction of the emission image for the transmission source, ^{153}Gd, cobalt-57, and ^{99m}Tc are suitable transmission sources for ^{201}Tl. The problems of cross-contamination between emission and transmission can be reduced by using a scanning line source and electronic windowing and sequential as opposed to simultaneous transmission and emission imaging. The major problem with sequential imaging is the added imaging time and, therefore, the increased likelihood of patient or physiologic motion that causes the attenuation map to not be truly registered with the emission data. Fast transmission imaging reduces this added time and, hence, the potential for this problem.

Noise in the estimated attenuation map

The concept of fast imaging leads to the question of how noise in the attenuation map may affect the noise level in the emission slices reconstructed from the maps. In a comprehensive study, Tung and Gullberg[78] showed that the statistical noise in the slices was dominated by the noise in the emission profiles for transmission count levels that were typical of that used with simultaneous emission and transmission imaging on a three-headed SPECT system with fan-beam collimators. This is because the noise in the attenuation maps is averaged out in the process of calculating attenuation correction factors (sums of coefficient multiplied by distance) from them. As the number of counts in the transmission profiles decrease, a point is reached at which not only does the noise in the attenuation map increase but the measured attenuation coefficients start to show a bias. This bias is due to the decrease in counts that causes the expected counts in locations of the transmission profiles to approach or fall below 1 during the imaging period.[75] This results in projections with zero counts at locations, even after smoothing. However, say that no counts make it through the attenuator is a powerful statement in the case of exponential attenuation, in which a

Table 10-1. Physical characteristics of the common emission and transmission radionuclides

Radionuclide	Technetium-99m	Thallium-201	Gadolinium-153	Cobalt-57	Americium-241
Gamma Rays	140.5	167.4	97.4	122	59.4
Energy, keV	89	10	28	86	36
Abundance, %			103.2	136.5	
			20	10	
X-Rays		68.9–82.6	40.9–48.3		
Energy, keV	–			–	–
Abundance, %	–	94	119		
Half-Life	6 hours	73 hours	242 days	272 days	432 years

very small but finite possibility of transmission always exists. The result is an overestimate of the amount of attenuation in the slices on reconstruction.

Transmission imaging time could be substantially reduced without a decrease in counts in the transmission projections by increasing the activity of the transmission source. However, the limited performance in high counting rate of older SPECT systems results in substantial count loss and degradation in image quality if the count rate becomes too large. With proper shielding to limit exposure to personnel and patients, increasing the activity of the transmission would not increase the radiation dose to the patients as long as imaging time was similarly reduced. With the advent of camera technology with high-counting-rate capability, transmission imaging time can be performed with higher transmission source strengths.

ATTENUATION CORRECTION METHODS

Both the ability to estimate attenuation maps and the ability to perform correction of attenuation once the attenuation maps are estimated have improved greatly. This is in part because of the great changes in computing power available with computers in the clinic, making computations that could only be performed as research exercises 10 years ago practical. It is also because of improvements in the algorithms used for correction and the efficiency of their implementation. An example is the development of ordered subset or block-iterative algorithms for use with the statistically based reconstruction methods discussed below.[8,36] Several algorithms have been developed for compensation of attenuation. Other reviews contain more details and other algorithms.[3,43] We focus on the group of methods most likely to replace filtered back-projection.

Statistically based reconstruction methods

Statistically based reconstruction algorithms start with a model for noise in the emission data and derive an estimate of the source distribution on the basis of some statistical criterion. In MLEM,[47,68] the noise fluctuations in the projection data are modeled as following a Poisson distribution; the criterion is to determine the source distribution that most likely gave rise to the emission projection data (mode of the probability distribution). The expectation-maximization algorithm is used to find the source distribution with which the highest likelihood resulted in the projection data. The success of this method of reconstruction is reflected by the fact that it is the standard against which other reconstruction methods are compared.

The MLEM algorithm works as follows. First an initial estimate of the slices is made. This is usually a uniform count in each slice volume element (voxel) equal to the average count to be back-projected per voxel. Next, each voxel estimate is updated according to the following equation:

$$\mathrm{Voxel}_i^{\text{new}} = \frac{\mathrm{Voxel}_i^{\text{old}}}{\sum\limits_{j}^{\text{All Pixels}} B(\mathrm{Voxel}_t, \mathrm{Pixel}_j)} \sum\limits_{j}^{\text{All Pixels}} B(\mathrm{Voxel}_t, \mathrm{Pixel}_j) \frac{\mathrm{Projection\ Data}_j}{\sum\limits_{k}^{\text{All Voxels}} P(\mathrm{Pixel}_j, \mathrm{Voxel}_k)\mathrm{Voxel}_k^{\text{old}}} \tag{5}$$

where *voxel* refers to radioactivity in three-dimensional locations in the slices being estimated, *Pixel* refers to counts detected at two-dimensional locations in the emission profiles, $B(\mathrm{Voxel}_i, \mathrm{Pixel}_j)$ is the back-projection operation from emission profile pixels to slice voxels, $P(\mathrm{Pixel}_j, \mathrm{Voxel}_k)$ is the projection operation from slice voxels to counts in the emission profile pixels, and *Projection Data*$_j$ are the counts in the actual emission profiles in pixel *j*. On the right is the ratio of the actual counts in pixel *j* (*Projection Data*$_j$) over the counts estimated to be in pixel *j* by imaging all of the old estimates of the voxel estimates. If the ratio is greater than 1, the current estimate of the counts from the slices is too low and should be increased (that is, the estimates in the voxels should be larger). If the ratio is less than 1, the voxel estimates should be decreased. If the ratio is 1, the voxel estimates are just right, and no change should be made.

These ratios are summed by the back-projection operator to arrive at a final multiplier to update the old voxel value to become the new estimate. The back-projection operator weights the pixels *j* by the likelihood they were actually contributed to by voxels *i*. This step is repeated until a set number of iterations has been performed.

The advantages of MLEM reconstruction are:[5,60,80]

1. It has a good theoretical basis.
2. It is known that the method converges.
3. It readily lends itself to incorporation of the physics of imaging[27,35,50,66,74,81] (that is, one can include knowledge of nonuniform attenuation, nonstationary spatial resolution, scatter, septal penetration, and motion into *P* and *B* of Equation 5).
4. The standard deviation in voxel counts resembles the image itself; therefore, the lower count areas have low noise magnitude compared with higher count areas. This is unlike filtered back-projection, in which the noise from high count areas spreads into low count areas.[5]
5. Because of its slow convergence, it is less sensitive to the exact stopping point than other iterative algorithms.

The disadvantages of MLEM are:

1. The processing time for 128 × 128 images, gated studies, or dynamic studies can still be excessive, especially if three-dimensional distance-dependent spatial resolution is included in the projection and back-projection operations.
2. There is some debate about the best method of controlling noise.[17,28,34,46,49,56,60,69,70]
3. Although compensation for attenuation seems to be achieved in a limited number of iterations, resolution continues to change for many more iterations and varies across the image, being worst in the center.[51,60]
4. Recovery of image features is faster for lower than for higher spatial frequencies.
5. The final estimate can be dependent on the initial estimate if high frequency components are included in it.

6. The local rate of convergence or improvement in resolution depends on what is in the image with it; for example, a hot liver slows the recovery of counts within the cardiac walls.[42,62]

The debate about how best to control noise in MLEM reconstruction is reminiscent of a similar debate about which filter to use with filtered back-projection. Candidates for noise control include stopping at a subjectively chosen number of iterations, use of a statistical rule to determine when to stop iteration, or use of regularization (filters or noise penalty functions inside the MLEM algorithm) to iterate until convergence.

In the past, the major disadvantage of MLEM has been processing time. Algorithms and techniques have been developed to speed the inclusion of nonuniform attenuation in the reconstruction process and decrease the number of iterations required in reconstruction.[8,12,36,67] One of the most successful techniques to accomplish the latter is the method of ordered subsets.[36] By updating the estimate of the slices in Equation 5 for only a well-chosen subset of the acquired data at one time instead of all the angles, an order of magnitude decrease in the computational time needed to obtain comparable MLEM reconstructions is obtained compared with updating by the projection data from all angles each time. Byrne[8] showed that ordered-subset MLEM reconstruction converges only in the case of subset balance (that is, when the normalization sum below the voxel value being updated is the same for all subsets). He also showed that ordered-subset MLEM was a special case of a formulation that he called *rescaled block-iterative MLEM,* which converges in the absence of subset balance.

Figure 10-7 shows a comparison of the transverse slices and polar maps for reconstructions of simulations of the MCAT phantom.[76] In the first row on the right, the selected image slice and polar map are for the case of inclusion of solely distance-dependent spatial resolution in the simulated projections. It therefore represents the case of ideal attenuation correction of note. The counts in the left ventricular wall are not uniform, nor are the counts in the polar map. The nonuniformities reflect the impact of the partial volume effect on maximal wall counts when the wall is not of constant thickness. The variation in wall thickness arises at the joining of the ventricles and is caused by the inclusion of apical thinning. Thus, even with ideal attenuation correction, one should not expect to obtain uniform counts in the polar maps. The second row shows the result of inclusion of attenuation when simulating the projections. The counts fall off substantially as one moves basally (deeper in the patient). The second row shows how well the significant nonuniformity in counts created by the addition of attenuation to the simulation is corrected by 30 and 100 iterations of MLEM, which accounts for the presence of the attenuation. At 100 iterations, the noise increased slightly. However, somewhat better resolution is apparent in the transverse slice, and the polar map is slightly less uniform than at 30 iterations. The latter effect is probably because of the better resolution.

CONCLUSIONS

Extensive clinical trials, such as those reported by Ficaro et al,[19] are needed to determine whether the anticipated increased specificity with attenuation and scatter compensation will be achieved. These compensation methods are technically demanding, and many of the issues brought up in this review are

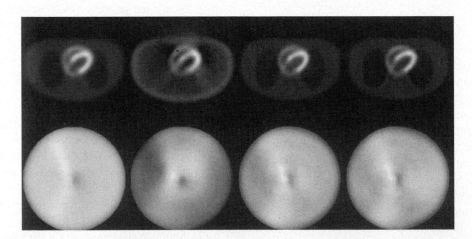

Fig. 10-7. Comparison of transverse slices *(top row)* and maximum count polar maps *(bottom row)* of mathematical cardiac–torso (MCAT) phantom simulations. *Left,* slice and polar map for filtered back-projection reconstruction without attenuation correction of MCAT phantom simulations that included only the influence of distance-dependent resolution. It represents ideal attenuation correction. *Left middle,* slice and polar map for filtered back-projection reconstruction without attenuation correction when simulation included the influence of distance-dependent resolution and attenuation. It represents how reconstruction is typically performed presently. *Right middle,* slice and polar map for 30 iterations of MLEM reconstruction that included modeling of attenuation in projection and back-projection. *Right,* slice and polar map for 100 iterations of MLEM reconstruction.

still under investigation. In addition, it is unlikely that attenuation and scatter compensation will result in uniform left ventricular wall counts in normal patients because variations will still be caused by the nonstationary spatial resolution of the imaging system, cardiac and respiratory motion that causes more blurring of the wall counts in some regions than others, and variation in wall thickness coupled with the partial volume effect.

ACKNOWLEDGMENTS

This work was supported in part by U.S. Public Health grant HL50349 of the National Heart, Lung, and Blood Institute.

This work is based on a series of two review papers previously published in the *Journal of Nuclear Cardiology*. The authors thank the editor of that journal for permission to republish, in part, those reviews, including several of the figures.

REFERENCES

1. Attiax H: *Introduction to Radiological Physics and Radiation Dosimetry,* New York, 1986:38–60, 124-159, John Wiley and Sons.
2. Axelsson B, Msaki P, and Israelsson A: Subtraction of Compton-scattered photons in single-photon emission computerized tomography, *J Nucl Med* 25:490-494, 1984.
3. Bacharach SL and Buvat I: Attenuation correction in cardiac positron emission tomography and single-photon emission computed tomography, *J Nucl Cardiol* 2:246-255, 1995.
4. Bailey DL, Hutton BF, and Walker PJ: Improved SPECT using simultaneous emission and transmission tomography, *J Nucl Med* 28:844-851, 1987.
5. Barrett HH, Wilson DW, and Tsui BMW: Noise properties of EM algorithm: I. Theory, *Phys Med Biol* 39:833-846, 1994.
6. Beekman F, et al: Object shape dependent PSF model for SPECT imaging, *IEEE Transactions on Nuclear Science* 40:31-39, 1993.
7. Buvat I, Rodriguez-Villafuerte M, Todd-Pokropck A, et al: Comparative assessment of nine scatter correction methods based on spectral analysis using Monte Carlo simulations, *J Nucl Med* 36:1476-1488, 1995.
8. Byrne CL: Block-iterative methods for image reconstruction from projections, *IEEE Trans Imag Proc* 5:792-794, 1996.
9. Cao Z and Tsui BMW: Performance characteristics of transmission imaging using a uniform sheet source with a parallel-hole collimator, *Med Phys* 19:1205-1212, 1992.
10. Case JA, Pan T-S, King MA, Lao D-S, Penney BC, Rabin MSZ: Reduction of truncation artifacts in fanbeam transmission imaging using a spatially varying gamma prior, *IEEE Transactions on Nuclear Science* 42:2260-2265, 1995.
11. Chang W, Loncaric S, Huang G, et al: Asymmetrical fan transmission CT on SPECT systems. *Phys Med Biol* 40:913-928, 1995.
12. Clinthorne NH, Pan T-S, Chiao PC, et al: Preconditioning methods for improved convergence rates in iterative reconstructions. *IEEE Trans Med Imaging* 12:78-83, 1993.
13. Datz FL, Gullberg GT, Zeng GL, et al: Application of convergent-beam collimation and simultaneous transmission emission tomography to cardiac single-photon emission computed tomography, *Semin Nucl Med* 24:17-37, 1994.
14. deVries DJ and King MA: Window selection for dual photopeak window scatter correction in Tc-99m imaging, *IEEE Transactions on Nuclear Science* 41:2771-2778, 1994.
15. DePuey EG and Garcia EV: Optimal specificity of thallium-201 SPECT through recognition of imaging artifacts, *J Nucl Med* 30:441-449, 1989.
16. Eisner RL, Tamas ML, Cloninger K, et al: Normal SPECT thallium-201 bull's-eye display: gender differences, *J Nucl Med* 29:1901-1909, 1988.

17. Fessler JA and Hero AO: Penalized maximum-likelihood image reconstruction using space-alternating generalized EM algorithms. *IEEE Trans Med Imaging* 4:1417-1429, 1995.
18. Ficaro EP, Fessler JA, Rogers WL, et al: Comparison of americium-241 and technetium-99m as transmission sources for attenuation correction of thallium-201 SPECT imaging of the heart. *J Nucl Med* 35:652-663, 1994.
19. Ficaro EP, Fessler JA, Shreve PD, et al: Simultaneous transmission/emission myocardial perfusion tomography. Diagnostic accuracy of attenuation-corrected 99mTc-sestamibi single-photon emission computed tomography, *Circulation* 93:463-473, 1996.
20. Floyd CE, Jaszczak RJ, and Coleman RE: Inverse Monte Carlo: a unified reconstruction algorithm. *IEEE Transactions on Nuclear Science* 32:779-785, 1985.
21. Frey E and Tsui BMW: A practical method for incorporating scatter in a projector-backprojector for accurate scatter compensation in SPECT. *IEEE Transactions on Nuclear Science* 40:1107-1116, 1993.
22. Frey EC and Tsui BMW: A comparison of Gd-153 and Co-57 as transmission sources for simultaneous TCT and Tl-201 SPECT. *IEEE Transactions on Nuclear Science* 42:1201-1206, 1995.
23. Frey EC, Tsui BMW, and Perry JR: Simultaneous acquisition of emission and transmission data for improved thallium-201 cardiac SPECT imaging using a technetium-99m transmission source. *J Nucl Med* 33:2238-2245, 1992.
24. Gagnon D, Todd-Pokropek A, Arsenault A, Dapras G: Introduction to holospectral imaging in nuclear medicine for scatter subtraction. *IEEE Trans Med Imaging* 8:245-250, 1989.
25. Galt JR, Cullom J, and Garcia EV: SPECT quantitation: a simplified method of attenuation and scatter correction for cardiac imaging, *J Nucl Med* 33:2232-2237, 1992.
26. Germano G, Chua T, Kiat H, et al: A quantitative phantom analysis of artifacts due to hepatic activity in technetium-99m myocardial perfusion SPECT studies, *J Nucl Med* 35:356-359, 1994.
27. Gilland DR, Jaszczak RJ, Wang H, et al: A 3D model of non-uniform attenuation and detector response for efficient iterative reconstruction in SPECT, *Phys Med Biol* 39:547-561, 1994.
28. Green PJ: Bayesian reconstructions from emission tomography data using a modified EM algorithm, *IEEE Trans Med Imaging* 9:84-93, 1990.
29. Greer KL, Harris CC, Jaszczak RJ, et al: Transmission computed tomography data acquisition with a SPECT system. *J Nucl Med Technol* 15:53-56, 1987.
30. Gregoriou GK, Tsui BMW, and Gullberg GT: Effect of truncated projections on defect detection in attenuation compensated fanbeam cardiac SPECT, *J Nucl Med* 39:166-175, 1998.
31. Hademenous GJ, King MA, and Ljungberg M: A scatter correction method for T1-201 images: a Monte Carlo investigation, *IEEE Transactions on Nuclear Science* 30:1179-1186, 1993.
32. Harris CC, Greer KL, Jaszczak RJ, et al: Tc-99m attenuation coefficients in water-filled phantoms determined with gamma cameras. *Med Phys* 11:681-685, 1984.
33. Haynor DR, Kaplan MS, Miyaoka RS, et al: Multiwindow scatter correction techniques in single-photon imaging. *Med Phys* 22:2015-2024, 1995.
34. Hebert TJ and Leahy R: A generalized EM algorithm for 3-D Bayesian reconstruction from Poisson data using Gibbs priors. *IEEE Trans Med Imaging* 8:194-202, 1989.
35. Hebert TJ and Leahy R: Fast methods for including attenuation in EM algorithm. *IEEE Transactions on Nuclear Science* 37:754-758, 1990.
36. Hudson HM and Larkin RS: Accelerated image reconstruction using ordered subsets of projection data. *IEEE Trans Med Imaging* 13:601-609, 1994.
37. Jaszczak RJ, Greer KL, Floyd CE Jr, et al: Improved SPECT quantification using compensation for scattered photons. *J Nucl Med* 25:893-900, 1984.
38. Jaszczak RJ, Gilland DR, Hanson MW, et al: Fast transmission CT for

determining attenuation maps using a collimated line source, rotatable air-copper-lead attenuators and fan-beam collimation. *J Nucl Med* 34:1577-1586, 1993.

39. Kadrmas DJ, Jaszczak RJ, McCormick JW, et al: Truncation artifact reduction in transmission CT for improved SPECT attenuation compensation. *Phys Med Biol* 40:1085-1104, 1995.

40. Kemp BJ, Prato FS, Nicholson RL, et al: Transmission computed tomography imaging of the head with a SPECT system and a collimated line source. *J Nucl Med* 36:328-335, 1995.

41. King MA, Tsui BM, Pan T-S, et al: Attenuation compensation for cardiac single-photon emission computed tomographic imaging: Part 2. Attenuation compensation algorithms, *J Nucl Cardiol* 3:55-64, 1996.

42. King MA, Xia W, deVries DJ, et al: A Monte Carlo investigation of artifacts caused by liver uptake in single-photon emission computed tomography perfusion imaging with technetium 99m-labeled agents, *J Nucl Cardiol* 3:18-29, 1996.

43. King MA, Tsui BMW, and Pan T-S: Attenuation compensation for cardiac single-photon emission tomographic imaging: Part 1. Impact of attenuation and methods of estimating attenuation maps, *J Nucl Cardiol* 2:513-524, 1995.

44. Knesaurek K, King MA, Glick SJ, et al: Investigation of causes of geometrical distortion in 180 degrees and 360 degrees angular sampling SPECT, *J Nucl Med* 30:1666-1675, 1989.

45. Koral KF, Wang XQ, Rogers WL, et al: SPECT Compton-scattering correction by analysis of energy spectra, *J Nucl Med* 29:195-202, 1988.

46. Lalush DS and Tsui BMW: Simulation evaluation of Gibbs prior distributions for use in maximum a posteriori SPECT reconstructions, *IEEE Trans Med Imaging* 11:267-275, 1992.

47. Lange K and Carson R: EM reconstruction algorithms for emission and transmission tomography, *J Comput Assist Tomogr* 8:306-316, 1984.

48. Larsson SA, Kimiaei S, and Ribbe T: Simultaneous SPECT and CT with shutter controlled radionuclide line sources and parallel collimator geometry, *IEEE Transactions on Nuclear Science* 40:1117-1122, 1993.

49. Levitan E and Herman GT: A maximum a posteriori probability expectation maximization algorithm for image reconstruction in emission tomography, *IEEE Trans Med Imaging* 6:185-192, 1987.

50. Liang Z, Turkington TG, Gilland JR, et al: Simultaneous compensation for attenuation, scatter and detector response for SPECT reconstruction in three dimensions, *Phys Med Biol* 37:587-603, 1992.

51. Liow JS and Strother SC: The convergence of object dependent resolution in maximum likelihood based tomographic image reconstruction, *Phys Med Biol* 38:55-70, 1993.

52. Ljungberg M, King MA, Hademenos GJ, et al: Comparison of four scatter correction methods using Monte Carlo simulated source distributions, *J Nucl Med* 35:143-151, 1994.

53. Ljungberg M, Strand SE, Rajeevan N, and King MA: Monte Carlo simulation of transmission studies using a planar source with a parallel collimator and a line source with a fan-beam collimator, *IEEE Transactions on Nuclear Science* 41:1577-1584, 1994.

54. Ljungberg M and Strand S-E: A Monte Carlo program for the simulation of scintillation camera characteristics, *Comput Methods Programs Biomed* 29:257-272, 1989.

55. Ljungberg M and Strand S-E: Attenuation and scatter correction in SPECT for sources in nonhomogeneous object: a Monte Carlo study, *J Nucl Med* 32:1278-1284, 1991.

56. Llacer J and Veklerov E: Feasible images and practical stopping rules for iterative algorithms for emission and transmission tomography, *IEEE Trans Med Imaging* 6:106-114, 1987.

57. Loncaric S, Chang W, and Huang G: Using simultaneous transmission and scatter SPECT imaging from external sources for the determination of the thoracic u-map, *IEEE Transactions on Nuclear Science* 41:1601-1606, 1994.

58. Manglos SH, Gagne GM, and Bassano DA: Quantitative analysis of image truncation in focal-beam CT, *Phys Med Biol* 38:1443-1457, 1993.

59. Meikle SR, Hutton BF, and Bailey DL: A transmission-dependent method for scatter correction in SPECT, *J Nucl Med* 35:360-367, 1994.

60. Miller TR and Wallis JW: Clinically important characteristics of maximum-likelihood reconstruction, *J Nucl Med* 33:1678-1684, 1992.

61. Msaki P, Axelsson B, Dahl CM, et al: Generalized scatter correction method in SPECT using point scatter distribution functions, *J Nucl Med* 28:1861-1869, 1987.

62. Nuyts J, Dupont P, Van den Maegdenbergh V, et al: A study of the liver-heart artifact in emission tomography, *J Nucl Med* 36:133-139, 1995.

63. Ogawa K, Harata Y, Ichihara T, et al: A practical method for position dependent Compton-scatter correction in single photon emission CT, *IEEE Trans Med Imaging* 10:408-412, 1991.

64. Ogawa K, Ichihara T, and Kubo A: Accurate scatter correction in single photon emission CT, *Ann Nucl Med* 7:145-150, 1994.

65. Pan T-S, et al: Reduction of truncation artifacts in fan beam transmission by using parallel beam emission data, *IEEE Transaction on Nuclear Science* 42:1310-1320, 1995.

66. Pan T-S, Luo D-S, and King MA: *Design of an efficient 3D projector and backprojector for SPECT: In Proceedings of 1995 International Meeting on Fully Three-Dimensional Image Reconstruction in Radiology and Nuclear Medicine,* 1995.

67. Rajeevan N, Rajgopal K, and Krishna G: Vector-extrapolated fast maximum likelihood estimation algorithms for emission tomography. *IEEE Trans Med Imaging* 11:9-20, 1992.

68. Shepp LA and Vardi Y: Maximum likelihood reconstruction for emission tomography, *IEEE Trans Med Imaging* 1:113-121, 1982.

69. Snyder DL, et al: Noise and edge artifacts in maximum-likelihood reconstructions for emission tomography, *IEEE Trans Med Imaging* 6:228-238, 1987.

70. Snyder DL and Miller MI: The use of sieves to stabilize images produced with the EM algorithm for emission tomography, *IEEE Transaction on Nuclear Science* 32:3864-3872, 1985.

71. Sorenson JA and Phelps ME: *Physics in Nuclear Medicine,* ed 2, Orlando, 1987, Grune and Stratton, Inc, 178-196.

72. Tan P, Bailey DL, Meikle SR, et al: A scanning line source for simultaneous emission and transmission measurements in SPECT, *J Nucl Med* 34:1752-1760, 1993.

73. Tsui BMW, Gullberg GT, Edgerton ER, et al: Correction of nonuniform attenuation in cardiac SPECT imaging, *J Nucl Med* 30:497-507, 1989.

74. Tsui BMW, Frey EC, Zhao X, et al: The importance and implementation of accurate 3D compensation methods for quantitative SPECT, *Phys Med Biol* 39:509-530, 1994.

75. Tsui BMW, Zhao XD, Lalush DS, et al: Pitfalls of attenuation compensation and their remedies in cardiac SPECT, *J Nucl Med* 35:115P, 1994.

76. Tsui BMW, Zhao XD, Gregoriou GK, et al: Quantitative cardiac SPECT reconstruction with reduced image degradation due to patient anatomy, *IEEE Transactions on Nuclear Science* 41:2838-2848, 1994.

77. Tung C-H, Gullberg GT, Zeng GL, et al: Nonuniform attenuation correction using simultaneous transmission and emission converging tomography, *IEEE Transactions on Nuclear Science* 39:1134-1143, 1992.

78. Tung C-H and Gullberg GT: A simulation of emission and transmission noise propagation in cardiac SPECT imaging with nonuniform attenuation correction, *Med Phys* 21:1565-1576, 1994.

79. Welch A, Gullberg GT, Christian DE, et al: A comparison of Gd/Tc versus Tc/T1 simultaneous transmission and emission imaging using both single and triple detector fan-beam SPECT systems, *IEEE Transactions on Nuclear Science* 41:2779-2786, 1994.

80. Wilson DW, Barrett HH, and Tsui BMW: Noise properties of EM algorithm: II. Monte Carlo simulations, *Phys Med Biol* 39:845-871, 1994.

81. Zeng GL, Gullberg GT, Tsui BMW, et al: Three-dimensional iterative reconstruction algorithms with attenuation and geometric point response correction, *IEEE Transactions on Nuclear Science* 38:693-702, 1991.

Chapter 11

Dynamic cardiac single-photon emission computed tomography

Grant T. Gullberg, Ronald H. Huesman, Steven G. Ross, Edward V. R. Di Bella,
Gengsheng L. Zeng, Bryan W. Reutter, Paul E. Christian, and **Stefano A. Foresti**

The measurement of perfusion and metabolism is important in the diagnosis and management of coronary artery disease. The use of multidetector single-photon emission computed tomography (SPECT) systems is showing[32,119,193,194] that dynamic cardiac SPECT imaging of thallium-201 (^{201}Tl) or technetium-99m (^{99m}Tc)–labeled teboroxime can measure perfusion in myocardial tissue. Because SPECT is more widely available than positron emission tomography (PET), researchers are investigating whether dynamic cardiac SPECT can be used to extract physiologic values of perfusion and metabolism in a manner similar to that of dynamic PET. An open question is whether similar results are possible in the measurement of glucose metabolism with 2-[^{18}F]fluorodeoxyglucose (^{18}FDG) and the measurement of fatty acid metabolism with such agents as ^{123}I-labeled iodophenylpentadecanoic acid (^{123}IPPA). A body of knowledge is growing to help answer these questions.

Research in dynamic cardiac SPECT draws heavily upon developments in PET, especially in the work that has been accomplished in modeling the kinetics of perfusion of rubidium-82 (^{82}Rb),* nitrogen-13 ammonia (^{13}NH$_3$),† and oxygen-15 water (H$_2$^{15}O).‡ Results have shown that a physiologically appropriate one-compartment model can quantify regional myocardial blood flow by using ^{82}Rb; this model is less complicated than the two-compartment model required to measure myocardial blood flow by using ^{13}NH$_3$. The myocardial uptake and retention of ^{82}Rb, a cationic tracer, is dependent upon active transport and is therefore affected by the metabolic status of the myocardium. In contrast, H$_2$^{15}O, which is also used to measure myocardial blood flow, is a freely diffusible tracer. Its myocardial kinetics seem to be related solely to flow and are not altered by changes in metabolism.[36] The disadvantage of using H$_2$^{15}O is that it requires that a cyclotron be nearby during the administration of the radiopharmaceutical. Moreover, because of its fast kinetics, large doses requiring extremely fast

---

*References 18, 21, 24, 26, 42, 49, 71, 73, 74, 91, 93, 100, 105, 147, 152, 157, 158, 215, 222, 229.
†References 13, 26, 37, 47, 49, 82, 93, 108, 110, 129-132, 160, 161, 165, 180, 184, 188, 215.
‡ References 4, 14, 15, 90, 97, 109, 116-118, 213.

counting rates must be administered. It is anticipated that future developments in dynamic SPECT metabolic imaging will draw upon previous work in PET.*

Many of the data analysis challenges faced in dynamic cardiac PET are also found in dynamic cardiac SPECT. However, in SPECT, more complicated imaging physics related to attenuation, poor statistics, and poor spatial and timing resolution exacerbate the problems. Many of the solutions implemented in PET are nonetheless still applicable to SPECT. First, tissue contamination of the blood input function obtained from a time–activity curve generated from a region of interest in the left ventricular cavity occurs.[192] This problem has led several researchers[4,15,97,116,117,118] to investigate the use of $C^{15}O$ (a substance that remains intravascular because of hemoglobin binding) for correction of spillover from tissue to blood. This work with $C^{15}O$ suggests the use of an intravascular tracer, such as radiolabeled albumin or erythrocytes, in dynamic SPECT to correct for tissue-to-blood contamination. It may also be possible to include the spillover as an unknown fraction in the model.[64] Second, the partial volume effect has an impact on the bias of estimated parameters.[219] We have found the work of Hutchins et al[108] to be useful for developing a strategy of sampling the myocardium to minimize the partial volume effect in SPECT. An intravascular tracer can also eliminate partial volume effects in SPECT,[112] much as $C^{15}O$ has been used to correct for partial volume effects in PET.[178,197] Third, problems with retention of the tracer in the blood occur.[183,192] Work in PET, in which measurements of metabolites of $^{13}NH_3$ in the blood[132,160,180] have been used to obtain a more accurate blood input function in the compartment modeling of myocardial perfusion, suggests techniques that could be used to measure retention of ^{99m}Tc teboroxime in the blood. Finally, input function shape, timing resolution of the SPECT system, and intervals between samples affect the bias and precision of the kinetic parameters.[182] In PET, this problem has been investigated in some detail.[152,171] A great difference in SPECT is the changing of the pharmaceutical distribution during the acquisition of the rotating detectors.[145,182,204] This has led us and others to develop methods that estimate kinetic model parameters directly from projection measurements.[33,34,106,144,227]

The results obtained[32,119,193,194] by using multidetector SPECT systems indicate that dynamic cardiac SPECT[19] can be used to estimate physiologic kinetic parameters of the myocardial tissue. On the basis of work performed on a ring-detector SPECT system,[201] it was hypothesized that dynamic SPECT and kinetic modeling of the rapid washin and washout kinetics of ^{99m}Tc teboroxime could be used to estimate myocardial blood flow. Original work with multidetector (three-detector) systems concentrated on relatively long acquisition times to obtain estimates of the washout of ^{99m}Tc teboroxime from the myocardium. Nakajima et al.[162,163] were the first to use a commercial three-detector SPECT system to obtain 360° tomographic acquisitions every 1 minute for 15 minutes by using continuous rotation. Dynamic reconstructed data were obtained of the ^{99m}Tc teboroxime washout phase from the heart, which was fit to a biexponential function to measure reperfusion after an ischemic insult. Chua et al[38,39] used a similar protocol to obtain a relative measure of the washout kinetics of ^{99m}Tc teboroxime. The original work of Budinger et al[20] showed that a three-detector system could acquire dynamic cardiac SPECT data of 360° of angular sampling every 5 seconds, which could be used to measure the kinetics of ^{99m}Tc pertechnetate. Our research[193,194] built on this discovery to demonstrate that 5-second and 10-second tomographic acquisitions could be acquired for estimating the washin and washout of ^{99m}Tc teboroxime in dogs by using kinetic compartment modeling techniques. Chiao et al[32] later showed that this was possible in humans.

Another interesting application of dynamic cardiac SPECT is the measurement of perfusion of ^{201}Tl and its distribution volume in the heart. Iida et al[119] published results from canine studies in which good correlation of flow values with microspheres was demonstrated. It is hypothesized that the distribution volume of ^{201}Tl in cardiac tissue, which is obtained from estimating the ratio of the kinetic parameters of the compartment model, is a good indicator of tissue viability. In this chapter, we present preliminary results obtained in our laboratory.

Compartment models that describe the kinetics of four myocardial agents will also be discussed in this chapter: a one-compartment model for ^{201}Tl and a one-compartment model for ^{99m}Tc teboroxime cardiac perfusion, a two-compartment model of the uptake and metabolism of the glucose analogue ^{18}FDG, and a three-compartment model of the uptake and metabolism of the fatty acid $^{123}IPPA$. More experience has accumulated for dynamic SPECT with ^{201}Tl and ^{99m}Tc teboroxime than with the other two agents. The ^{99m}Tc teboroxime radiopharmaceutical was developed to replace ^{201}Tl for imaging myocardial ischemia,* but its usefulness has not been realized because imaging and data analysis techniques were not able to handle its fast clearance from the myocardium (half-life in the myocardium, 10 to 15 minutes[138,139]; 90% first-pass extraction). It is anticipated that use of dynamic SPECT could make ^{99m}Tc-teboroxime more useful as a flow agent and will better use ^{201}Tl as a marker of viability. In fact, dynamic SPECT may provide advantages to using ^{201}Tl over ^{99m}Tc-teboroxime; ^{201}Tl may enable better measurement of both perfusion and viability because teboroxime does not seem to be hindered by the shutdown of active transport mechanisms.

The use of such agents as ^{18}FDG and fatty acids with dynamic cardiac SPECT may also be useful for assessing myocardial viability. The quantification of uptake and metabolism of ^{18}FDG has been accomplished by using PET[95,120] and is expected to work with dynamic SPECT. This expectation is based on work that has demonstrated that SPECT can identify viable

---

*References 25, 31, 36, 84, 95, 96, 120, 124, 169, 172, 185, 196.

*References 16, 44, 45, 55, 57, 70, 75, 85-87, 122, 138-141, 148, 151, 167, 170, 183, 186, 187, 200, 201, 216, 217, 225.

myocardial tissue in regions of perfusion defects by using 511-keV collimators with simultaneous imaging of [18]FDG and ^{99m}Tc-labeled sestamibi.[48] On the other hand, it may be more difficult to extract the kinetics of fatty acid metabolism with SPECT than with PET[95] because of the more complex biochemical pathways. In this chapter, we present preliminary results of the use of dynamic SPECT to extract the kinetics of the fatty acid [123]IPPA, which has been used with planar and static SPECT for diagnosis of coronary artery disease[2,3,35,40,81,143,146,159,173–175,190] but has not previously been used with dynamic SPECT.

Successful extraction of time–activity curves for regions of interest in the blood and heart tissue is a critical component in the analysis of dynamic cardiac SPECT data. If the blood input function is not physically sampled, its time–activity curve must be derived from the acquired data, usually in an intraventricular region. Partial volume effects, cardiac motion, lung motion, and patient motion tend to mix the blood and tissue in the input blood region of interest. Recently, Wu et al.[220] extracted input functions from dynamic PET studies by using a factor analysis approach. The results obtained in this manner correlated highly with region-of-interest measurements. It is anticipated that the blood input function can be improved by combining regions of interest and a factor analysis approach.[89] It may also be possible to obtain input functions that have been derived from a model[62] or from a sampling of a patient population.[59] A semiautomatic technique was shown to be able to generate time–activity curves from optimally selected regions of interest.[52] Simulation studies have shown that with noise comparable to typical dynamic SPECT studies, this approach gives parameter estimates similar to those obtained from manually chosen regions of interest.

Kinetic modeling of dynamic SPECT data involves a complex multivariable nonlinear estimation problem.[28] Efforts are being made to develop mathematical tools that can be used to obtain accurate and precise estimates of kinetic parameters of compartment models. Most of this work involves developing techniques that fit time–activity curves sampled from dynamic tomographic reconstructions. Iterative reconstruction algorithms are usually performed to reconstruct each dynamic three-dimensional distribution. These algorithms correct for attenuation, scatter, and the spatially varying geometric point response. The iterative approach makes it difficult to obtain estimates of the reconstructed errors. Kinetic parameters and errors are more accurate when the full covariance matrix of the sampled data (including reconstructed sampled blood and tissue data) is used as a weighting matrix than when errors are ignored and a weighting matrix of equal errors in the fitting procedure is used.[105] Knowledge of the full covariance matrix is essential to obtain confidence estimates of the appropriateness of the model. A better but more computationally intensive approach is to use direct matrix inversion for reconstruction. This provides a direct estimate of all variances and covariances of the reconstructed estimates. With today's computers, it is possible to obtain 64 × 64 reconstructions and error estimates from direct matrix inversion by using singular value decomposition (SVD) of 4096 × 4096 matrices.[78]

A better approach to analyzing dynamic cardiac SPECT data may be to estimate the regions of interest or kinetic parameters directly from the projection data.[33,34,106,144,227] This would reduce bias by more accurately modeling the change in the concentration of the radiopharmaceutical from sampled projection to sampled projection, thus improving the temporal resolution. One approach is to directly calculate activities for regions of interest; the results are then used to generate time–activity curves from which kinetic parameters are estimated.[27,66] Another approach is to estimate kinetic parameters directly from the projection data, where it is assumed that the regions of interest are specified and that expressions between the compartment model parameters and the dynamically acquired projections can be formulated in a chi-square formulation.[106,227] Chiao et al[33,34] refined this approach by estimating kinetic parameters and registration parameters of region-of-interest boundaries from projections and auxiliary boundary information. They showed that biases of estimates are reduced by including region-of-interest specification inaccuracy. We demonstrated improvement in bias by estimating kinetic parameters directly from projections for a 3 × 3 computer-simulated image array.[227] In this chapter, results of similar improvement for a 64 × 64 computer simulation are presented and in a recent publication, results are presented for cone beam tomography.[106]

The physics of the imaging detection process in dynamic SPECT is complicated by the degradation of images because of scatter, attenuation, spatially varying geometric point response, poor statistics, and poor spatial resolution.* It is likely that SPECT will never be able to match the physical imaging characteristics of PET. At present, dynamic SPECT imaging has poorer statistics, poorer spatial and temporal resolution, and more difficulty in correcting for attenuation. However, computer simulations[90] have demonstrated that the compartment modeling approach is less sensitive to most physical sources of error than to timing discrepancies, especially discrepancies between the arterial input function and the tissue time–activity curve. This is encouraging because improvements have been and will continue to be made in temporal resolution in SPECT. Using computer simulations, investigations into the optimal timing resolution (acquisition interval) and input function shape in dynamic SPECT[182] show that current SPECT systems are adequate to follow the kinetics of cardiac tracers. Nevertheless, the physical effects of image detection are important. Partial volume effects are as important in SPECT as in dynamic PET,[94,108] and the problem is worse with SPECT because of poorer resolution. Because of its poorer resolution, dynamic SPECT seems to be less sensitive to cardiac motion[181]; respiratory motion may be more of a problem, as is the case in PET.[205]

In this chapter, we summarize recent developments in dynamic cardiac SPECT and provide insight into the unique features of dynamic SPECT that differentiate it from PET, such as

---

*References 12, 67, 77, 94, 121, 126, 127, 181, 202, 207-211, 218, 228.

the process of extracting similar information from data that have more statistical noise and poorer spatial and timing resolution. First, compartment modeling techniques are discussed. Examples of one-, two-, and three-compartment models for dynamic cardiac SPECT applications are given. Second, data segmentation techniques for extracting time–activity curves are described. Then, new methods for estimating the kinetic parameters from dynamic reconstructions and directly from projections are presented. Third, the effects of the physical aspects of the image detection on the bias and variance of the estimated parameters are discussed. Finally, results of canine studies are presented.

PRINCIPLES OF TRACER KINETIC MODELING

Tracer kinetic modeling is used in several areas of biological research to follow dynamic processes of blood flow, tissue perfusion, transport, metabolism, and receptor binding.* The principles are based on the early work of Fick[65] and Stewart,[198,199] and, later, of Hamilton et al.[80] Meier and Zierler developed equations for many of these original principles in the 1950s[153] and in the 1960s.[230] They formulated general equations for estimating flow using tracers for the inflow injection/outflow technique and the inflow injection/residue detection technique.[10] The latter term applies when external detection is used to measure the time sequence of tracer content in an organ, as is done with dynamic PET and dynamic SPECT. The modeling of tracer kinetics relies on the principle of indicator dilution, whereby models are developed that compartmentalize the dilution of the tracer. This compartmentalization allows the use of dynamic SPECT to measure flow and metabolism for the myocardium from the time sequence of tomographic acquisition of tracer activity.

Tracer kinetic techniques use a measurable tracer that is introduced in the biological system under study to follow the physiologic or biochemical process of a particular biochemical substance.[95] Upon introduction, the tracer distributes throughout the sample. Measurements of the tracer are taken as a function of time. The chosen tracer must follow the dynamic process of interest; thus, the tracer must be structurally related to the natural biochemical substance involved in the dynamic process under study or have similar transport properties. The tracer must be measurable and distinguishable from the natural substance that it mimics. The tracer is given in a trace amount, so that the tracer does not perturb the process being measured. To better measure the dynamic process, some compartmentalization is imposed on the basis of a priori knowledge of structural or configurational information about the process or the organ system.

A compartment model is a mathematical description of the pathways and dynamic behavior of the tracer in the biological tissue of interest. A compartment is the volume or space in which the tracer is uniformly distributed.[95] It may have an ob-

*References 9, 10, 25, 65, 79, 80, 95, 125, 133, 135, 153, 179, 198, 199, 212, 230.

vious physical interpretation, such as the blood, an entire organ, or a space separated by a membrane. The compartment could also, for example, represent one of the chemical species of the tracer in a catabolic or anabolic process of metabolism.

A compartmental model is represented by several compartments linked by arrows indicating transport between the compartments. The arrows indicate the pathways that the tracer can follow. In our application, the amount of tracer leaving a compartment is assumed to be proportional to the total amount in the compartment. The constant of proportionality (the rate constant) has the unit of inverse time and denotes the fraction of total tracer that will leave the compartment per unit time. The kinetics between compartments are described by a system of differential equations.

For example, consider a blood compartment with concentration $B(t)$ and an extravascular compartment with concentration $C_2(t)$. The rate equation for the extravascular space is

$$\frac{d}{dt}C_2(t) = -\frac{P_{12}S}{V_2}C_2(t) + \frac{P_{21}S}{V_2}B(t) \tag{1}$$

where V_2 is the volume of the extravascular compartment, P_{12} and P_{21} (in cm/min) are the permeability coefficients for flux out of and into the capillary, respectively, and S (in cm^2) is the surface area of the capillary in the sampled volume element (voxel). Setting $k_{21} = (P_{21}S)/V_2$ and $k_{12} = (P_{12}S)/V_2$, the rate constants in and out of the extravascular compartment are expressed in units of per minute per extravascular volume (V_2). Substituting k_{21} and k_{12} into Equation 1, the differential equation describing the exchange between the intravascular and extravascular compartments can be rewritten as

$$\frac{d}{dt}C_2(t) = -k_{12}C_2(t) + k_{21}B(t) \tag{2}$$

where the rate of change in and out of the extravascular compartment is proportional to the concentration in the blood and the concentration in the extravascular compartment, respectively.

For the models presented in this chapter, it is assumed that $B(t)$ is known, either by sampling the image-derived reconstruction or by measuring plasma samples. In this case, we have a one-compartment model instead of a two-compartment model because the kinetics of the blood compartment is known from an independent measurement. Thus, Equation 2 completely describes the kinetics of the model.

The amount of tracer in a volume of tissue may deviate greatly in value from the chemical concentration in individual spaces if the tracer does not distribute uniformly over all the spaces in the tissue. Thus, the distribution volume V_d is defined as the fractional space of volume V_2 that a tracer would occupy in the tissue extravascular space with the same concentration as in the blood B[95]:

$$V_d = \frac{\text{(amount of tracer/ml of tissue)}}{\text{(amount of tracer/ml of blood)}} \tag{3}$$

If we assume equilibrium, we can set Equation 2 to zero, which implies that $k_{21}B(\infty) = k_{12}C_2(\infty)$ or the distribution volume $V_d = C_2(\infty)/B(\infty) = k_{21}/k_{12}$. The definition of the partition coefficient is precisely the ratio of the tracer concentration in tissue to that in blood at equilibrium. Thus, the distribution volume and partition coefficient have identical value but different conceptual meanings. The term *partition coefficient* implies that the tracer can distribute over the entire tissue space, but because the capillary wall forms a partition, the tracer concentration on the two sides need not be equal. In contrast, the distribution volume implies that some limited volume exists in which the tracer can distribute. In reality, a tracer does not distribute uniformly over the entire tissue space, nor does it have the same concentration in tissue as in blood. Therefore, strictly speaking, one should think of distribution volume or partition coefficient only in terms of the definition given in Equation 3.

In dynamic cardiac SPECT, compartment modeling techniques are used to measure myocardial perfusion and metabolism. Measures of the tracer concentration curves as a function of time are obtained by using fixed ring or rotating gamma-camera SPECT systems (Fig. 11-1). These data represent the distribution of the tracer through various compartments as a function of time. Estimates of the compartment model rate constants are determined by fitting these data with an estimation procedure. If a rotating gamma camera SPECT system is used to measure the injected tracer, the detectors (Fig. 11-1) must rotate fast enough so that the reconstruction adequately measures the changes of the concentration as a function of time. In dynamic mode, tomographic projection sets of 120 projection angles can be acquired in as little as 5 seconds.[193] A series of tomographic projections are reconstructed to give a three-dimensional distribution of the radiolabeled tracer at every time interval. From the serial three-dimensional reconstructions, time–activity curves of the blood input in the left ventricular

cavity and myocardial tissue are generated (Fig. 11-1). These curves are fit to a compartment model representing the tracer kinetics by using a fitting routine, such as RFIT (region-of-interest fitting).[104] In discussing the models presented in this section, it is assumed that a blood input function can be determined. This function can be obtained from the reconstructed images by drawing a region of interest in the atrium or the left ventricular cavity or may be determined by withdrawing blood and counting the blood samples in a well counter. Other possibilities for defining the input function are discussed in a later section.

In this section, we look at three different compartment models used to measure cardiac function: a one-compartment perfusion model that can be used to follow the dynamics of ^{201}Tl or ^{99m}Tc teboroxime, a two-compartment model that describes the uptake and phosphorylation of ^{18}FDG, and a three-compartment model that follows the uptake and metabolism of ^{123}IPPA.

One-compartment model for measuring cardiac perfusion of thallium-201 and technetium-99m–labeled teboroxime

A one-compartment model that can be used to model ^{201}Tl and ^{99m}Tc-labeled teboroxime kinetics in the heart has been developed. Although it has been proposed[119] that a two-compartment model may be a more appropriate model for ^{201}Tl kinetics, we present results obtained by using a one-compartment model.

Thallium-201 is often considered to be an analog of potassium. Thus, it is actively transported across the cell membrane. Uptake of ^{201}Tl implies an intact cell membrane and some

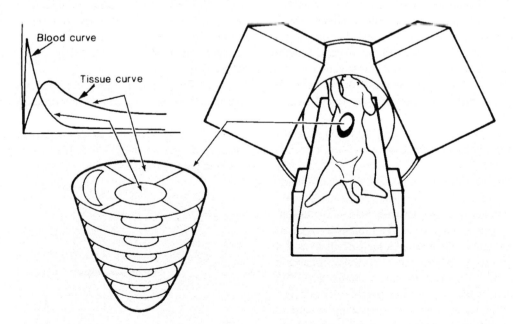

Fig. 11-1. Dynamic cardiac single-photon emission computed tomography is performed by using rapidly rotating gamma cameras to obtain projection measurements, which are used to reconstruct time–activity curves for a blood region of interest and tissue regions of interest. Compartment model parameters are estimated by fitting the time–activity curves to a mathematical model.

metabolic activity. Thallium-201 is widely used for determining regional myocardial blood flow and viability. Its initial uptake correlates highly with myocardial blood flow, and it redistributes relatively slowly over time in normal myocardium. Defects in ischemic regions generally resolve, indicating viable tissue. Necrotic tissue is usually not perfused, and even if flow to the region is high, the ^{201}Tl leaks out of the cells. However, Tl differs from potassium in many ways.[69] Up to only half of Tl uptake by myocardial cells can be inhibited by metabolic poisons. In addition, ouabain and hypoxia have only minor effects on uptake and retention of ^{201}Tl by the myocardium. Moreover, the distribution of ^{201}Tl is a dynamic process, although it is on a very different time scale than that of ^{99m}Tc teboroxime.

Technetium-99m teboroxime (Cardio-Tec, Bracco) is a boronic acid adduct of technetium dioxime complex that is stable, neutral, and lipid soluble. Technetium-99m teboroxime is more diffusible and has a faster clearance time from the myocardium (half-life of 10 to 15 minutes)[138,139] than ^{201}Tl or ^{99m}Tc sestamibi and has the least degree of sensitivity to cellular dysfunction compared with these substances. It is 80% to 90% extracted in the first pass.[138] Use of ^{99m}Tc teboroxime may result in images that more consistently display effects of blood flow as opposed to possible enhancements or depression of uptake related to cellular dysfunction, reperfusion, or shutdown of adenosine triphosphate–facilitated transport mechanisms.[44] Compared with PET analogues, one would conclude that ^{99m}Tc teboroxime is more similar to $H_2^{15}O$ than it is to ^{82}Rb.

Technetium-99m teboroxime is an excellent agent for measuring flow but may not be as useful in the study of tissue viability. Work by Heller et al[85] indicates that the uptake of ^{99m}Tc teboroxime in rabbits correlates with the flow that is measured by using microspheres and is not related to viability. Maublant et al[151] showed that for cells in culture, ^{99m}Tc teboroxime had the lowest sensitivity to metabolic impairment compared with ^{201}Tl and ^{99m}Tc sestamibi. In contrast, Serafini et al[187] in humans showed that further investigation of the ability of ^{99m}Tc teboroxime to distinguish between ischemic and infarcted myocardium is warranted. They found significant differences between ^{201}Tl and ^{99m}Tc teboroxime in classifying infarct and infarct or ischemia; ^{99m}Tc teboroxime detected a larger percentage of infarct or infarct and ischemia defects than did ^{201}Tl.

Initially, ^{99m}Tc-teboroxime was evaluated for cardiac imaging with static techniques, in which it was assumed that the radiolabeled tracer did not wash out or redistribute during the duration of the scan. This assumption is valid for such tracers as ^{201}Tl and ^{99m}Tc sestamibi, which have biological half-lives of 4 and 6 hours, respectively. Teboroxime is attractive because it can be labeled with ^{99m}Tc, which is more desirable than ^{201}Tl because of its better photon energy for gamma-camera detection. Technetium-99m teboroxime is also appealing because of its high extraction and rapid washout; in combination with the better radiation dosimetry of ^{99m}Tc, these factors permit the injection of 10 times as much radioactivity compared with ^{201}Tl. Promising results were reported for planar imaging of swine,[75] dogs,[200] and humans.[45] However, because ^{99m}Tc teboroxime is

rapidly cleared from the myocardium and typical SPECT scans take 20 to 40 minutes, interest in use of ^{99m}Tc teboroxime for static SPECT imaging has waned. However, dynamic SPECT has recently shown potential for imaging ^{99m}Tc teboroxime in canine studies reported by Smith et al[193,194] and human studies reported by Chiao et al[32] and Chua et al.[38,39]

The kinetics of ^{201}Tl or ^{99m}Tc teboroxime in the myocardium are modeled by a simple one-compartment model (Fig. 11-2). It is assumed that the blood concentration measured in the left ventricular cavity represents the blood concentration of the particular radiopharmaceutical available to the myocardium. One point of caution must be noted. Even though ^{99m}Tc teboroxime is highly extracted on the first pass, the work of Rumsey et al[183] indicated that extraction from subsequent passes may be affected by binding of ^{99m}Tc teboroxime to blood cells and plasma proteins. Smith et al[192] reported on the effect of this on the bias of the model estimates. Here, it is assumed that the percentage of binding is small.

Each data point from the blood and tissue time–activity curves represents an accumulation of counts from the radioactive emissions of the radioisotope (^{201}Tl or ^{99m}Tc) over the acquisition time Δt. The accumulation of counts in the tissue is modeled as

$$A_T(t_k) = (1 - f_v) \int_{t_k - \Delta t}^{t_k} C_2(t)dt + f_v \int_{t_k - \Delta t}^{t_k} B(t)dt \qquad (4)$$

where A_T is the model of the measured myocardial tissue activity concentration acquired between the time $t_k - \Delta t$, and t_k in the region of interest, f_v is the vascular fraction of blood in the tissue, Δt is the acquisition time of the tomographic data set, $B(t)$ is the measured activity concentration from the blood compartment at time t, $C_2(t)$ is the activity concentration from the extravascular compartment at time t, and $(1 - f_v)$ is the fractional blood volume of the extravascular space. The blood activity concentration $B(t)$ is measured by using a region of interest drawn inside the left intraventricular cavity.

The activity concentration $C_2(t)$ from the extravascular compartment is given by the first-order ordinary differential equation in Equation 2, which describes the kinetic exchange between the blood and the extravascular space for the compartment model shown in Fig. 11-2. If everything is zero at $t = 0$, the solution to Equation 2 is

$$C_2(t) = k_{21} \int_0^t e^{-k_{12}(t-\tau)} B(\tau)d\tau \qquad (5)$$

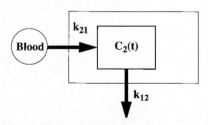

Fig. 11-2. One-compartment model for technetium-99m teboroxime. The rate constants k_{21} and k_{12} are given in (ml/min)/ml of extravascular space.

The parameters k_{21} and k_{12} are the washin and washout rate constants, respectively, of ^{99m}Tc teboroxime. The units of k_{21} and k_{12} are (ml/min)/(ml of extravascular space), but k_{21} and k_{12} are commonly given in min^{-1}.

The one-compartment model shown in Fig. 11-2 has the following four assumptions:

1. The time–activity curve of the blood compartment can be measured independently of the extravascular compartment of the myocardial tissue.

2. All myocardial tissue regions exchange with the same blood time–activity curve.

3. The distribution of the tracer is homogeneous throughout the region of interest.

4. The tissue region of interest contains only regions from the blood and extravascular compartments.

Figure 11-3 depicts results of an analysis of the sensitivity of the tissue curve to changes in k_{21}, k_{12}, and f_v. A finite difference technique was used to solve the differential equation for the model. Five simulations were run for each parameter. In each simulation, the value of one variable was changed by 20% while the other two remained fixed. The values were chosen from estimates obtained from actual canine data. Parameter f_v is the least sensitive, whereas k_{21} (the washin) substantially affects the peak of the tissue activity curve and k_{12} affects its washout phase.

In dynamic cardiac SPECT, the kinetic variables are esti-

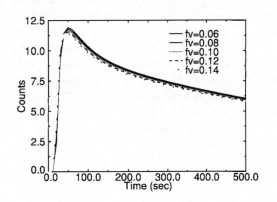

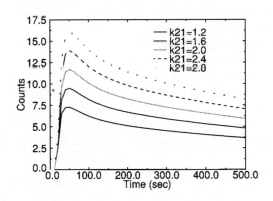

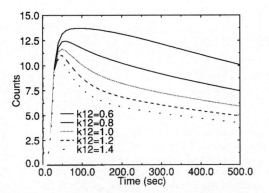

Fig. 11-3. Illustration of output as a function of parameter change (one plot for each parameter). (Published with permission of Dr. Anne Smith.)

mated for multiple three-dimensional regions in the left ventricular myocardium. The vector $\theta_1 = (f_v, k_{21}, k_{12})$ is used to denote the kinetic parameters, where f_v, k_{21}, and k_{12} are vectors with components f_v^s, k_{21}^s, and k_{12}^s for each tissue region s. Methods for estimating these compartment model parameters and results from dynamic SPECT canine studies are presented later.

Two-compartment model for measuring cardiac glucose metabolism of 2-[^{18}F]fluorodeoxyglucose

The tracer 2-[^{18}F]fluorodeoxyglucose[113] is used in PET studies to isolate the transport and phosphorylation steps from the complicated pathway of glucose metabolism.[95] This allows the formulation of simple tracer kinetic models for estimation of exogenous glucose use.[196] Deoxyglucose[196] is an analog of glucose in which the hydroxyl group on the second carbon has been replaced by hydrogen. In the formation of ^{18}FDG, this hydrogen is substituted with the positron emitter ^{18}F. The agent is transported into tissue and phosphorylated to ^{18}FDG-6-phosphate (^{18}FDG-6-P), which is catalyzed by hexokinase, in the same manner as deoxyglucose or glucose. However, because of the substitution in the second carbon position, ^{18}FDG-6-P does not continue to the next reaction step in the glycolytic pathway. Furthermore, ^{18}FDG-6-P is not a substrate for glycogen synthesis or the pentose shunt. It can leave the cell only through slow hydrolysis back to free ^{18}FDG, which can then be transported to plasma or be rephosphorylated.

Fluorodeoxyglucose is similar to glucose in its transport from plasma to tissue and its phosphorylation. After injection, ^{18}FDG is cleared by the kidneys and extracted by various tissues to produce a relatively rapid decline of ^{18}FDG in the blood. However, free ^{18}FDG in tissue decreases rather slowly (a 4-minute to 5-minute half-time in the tissue precursor pool of the human brain).[169] The transport of glucose or ^{18}FDG across the cell membrane is assumed to be fast compared with the transport across the capillary wall and the phosphorylation reaction.

A two-compartment model (Fig. 11-4) proposed by Sokoloff et al.[196] is used to represent the kinetics of ^{18}FDG in the myocardium. The model has a washin of ^{18}FDG from the blood to the extravascular space and washout similar to the one-compartment model discussed in the previous section as well as an additional compartment representing phosphorylation of ^{18}FDG to ^{18}FDG-6-P in the myocardial cell. The hydrolyzation of ^{18}FDG-6-P back to ^{18}FDG is slow, and for some modeling applications, one might eliminate this pathway.

The accumulation of counts from emissions of ^{18}FDG located in myocardial tissue is modeled as

$$A_T(t_k) = (1 - f_v) \int_{t_k - \Delta t}^{t_k} \left(C_2(t) + \frac{1}{\beta} C_3(t) \right) dt + f_v \int_{t_k - \Delta t}^{t_k} B(t) dt \quad (6)$$

where A_T is the model of the measured myocardial tissue activity concentration acquired between the time $t_k - \Delta t$ and t_k in the region of interest, f_v is the vascular fraction of blood in the tissue, Δt is the acquisition time of the tomographic data set, $B(t)$ is the measured activity concentration from the blood compartment at time t, $C_2(t)$ is the activity concentration of ^{18}FDG in the extravascular compartment at time t, $C_3(t)$ is the activity concentration of phosphorylated ^{18}FDG (^{18}FDG-6-P) in the extravascular compartment at time t, $(1 - f_v)$ is the fractional volume of extravascular space, and β is the ratio V_2/V_3 of the extravascular volume V_2 and the distribution volume V_3 of ^{18}FDG-6-P. The blood activity concentration $B(t)$ is measured by using a region of interest drawn inside the left intraventricular cavity or from plasma samples.

The activity concentrations $C_2(t)$ and $C_3(t)$ in the two extravascular compartments are given by the following two first-order ordinary differential equations:

$$V_2 dC_2(t)/dt = P_{21}SB(t) - (P_{12}S + P_{32}S')C_2(t) + P_{23}S'C_3(t) \quad (7)$$

and

$$V_3 dC_3(t)/dt = P_{32}S'C_2(t) - P_{23}S'C_3(t) \quad (8)$$

where P_{21} and P_{12} are the permeability coefficients for flux out of and into the capillary with a total surface area S within the voxel and P_{32} and P_{23} are the permeability coefficients for flux between ^{18}FDG and ^{18}FDG-6-P with a total pseudo–surface area S' within the voxel. Setting $k_{21} = (P_{21}S)/V_2$, $k_{12} = (P_{12}S)/V_2$, $k_{32} = (P_{32}S')/V_2$, and $k_{23} = (P_{23}S')/V_2$, we have

$$dC_2(t)/dt = k_{21}B(t) - (k_{12} + k_{32})C_2(t) + k_{23}C_3(t) \quad (9)$$

and

$$dC_3(t)/dt = \beta k_{32}C_2(t) - \beta k_{23}C_3(t) \quad (10)$$

which describe the kinetic exchange between the compartments for the model shown in Fig. 11-4. Four rate constants are given: k_{21} (washin of glucose from the blood), k_{12} (washout of nonphosphorylated glucose), k_{32} (rate of phosphorylation by the enzyme hexokinase), and k_{23} (rate of dephosphorylation). The three-dimensional distribution of model variables is denoted by the vector $\theta_2 = (f_v, k_{21}, k_{12}, k_{32}, k_{23})$, where f_v, k_{21}, k_{12}, k_{32}, and k_{23} are vectors with components f_v^s, k_{21}^s, k_{12}^s, k_{32}^s, and k_{23}^s corresponding to each tissue region s.

The utilization rate of glucose ($MRGlc$) in the myocardium can be calculated from the rate constants as $MRGlc =$

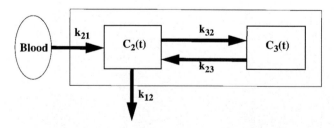

Fig. 11-4. Two-compartment model for [^{18}F]fluorodeoxyglucose. A compartmental representation of the Sokoloff model with four rate constants: k_{21} = uptake rate of fluorodeoxyglucose from the blood pool; k_{12} = washout rate of nonphosphorylated fluorodeoxyglucose; k_{32} = rate of phosphorylation; and k_{23} = rate of dephosphorylation.

$(C_p/LC)((k_{21}k_{32})/(k_{12} + k_{32}))$, where C_p is the glucose concentration in plasma and LC is a lumped constant that calibrates the difference in transport and phosphorylation rates between ^{18}FDG and glucose.[95]

The two-compartment model to study the kinetics of ^{18}FDG has been used in dynamic PET studies for years. Results with dynamic SPECT have only recently been obtained. Computer simulations[53] have been performed to study the feasibility of fitting ^{18}FDG data acquired with dynamic SPECT to the same two-compartment model. These studies used an anatomically realistic software phantom and incorporated noise and geometric response. It seems that obtaining the input function from the images may not be practical because of too few counts detected in the short acquisition time necessary to sample the rapidly changing input function. However, the simulations indicate the possibility of accurate fits from longer (60-second) tomographic acquisitions and arterial sampling. To reduce bias due to the long acquisitions, it may be necessary to estimate the variables directly from the projection measurements, as we will discuss in a later section.

Three-compartment model for measuring cardiac fatty acid metabolism of iodine-123–labeled iodophenylpentadecanoic acid

Iodine-123–labeled iodophenylpentadecanoic acid (^{123}IPPA) is a radiolabeled synthetic fatty acid with kinetics similar to that of palmitate.[35,174,175] Iodine-123 is a 159-keV gamma emitter with a half-life of 13 hours. The agent ^{123}IPPA is metabolized by the heart in a manner similar to other fatty acids. A previous investigation[35] demonstrated that ^{123}IPPA metabolism follows a biexponential washout pattern, with the first, rapid phase reflecting β-oxidation and a second, slower phase reflecting the turnover in triglyceride pools.

Under normal resting aerobic conditions, ^{123}IPPA is β-oxidized to iodobenzoic acid and washes out of the myocardium without iodine dissociation.[3,146] Fatty acid uptake and β-oxidation are reduced during ischemia,[2] and transient ^{123}IPPA accumulation can occur.[173] The ischemic regions take up less tracer because the muscle switches to glucose for its energy supply. However, the defects in such regions will resolve, because washout from ischemic regions is slower than from normal tissue. Similarly, ^{123}IPPA uptake and clearance are reduced in myocardial infarction.[173] A recent study by Shi et al[190] showed a correlation with ^{18}FDG, suggesting that ^{123}IPPA may serve as a marker for viability. Studies with planar imaging of ^{123}IPPA[159] and two static SPECT ^{123}IPPA acquisitions[40] report that imaging with ^{123}IPPA is similar to imaging with ^{201}Tl. Sequentially acquired studies have also been compared to angiographic data,[81] with promising results.

The three-compartment model shown in Fig. 11-5 is used to represent the kinetics of ^{123}IPPA in the myocardium. The model assumes that the metabolite of β-oxidation (iodobenzoic acid) that is released into the blood is taken up almost immediately by the kidney and is thus not available for reintroduction into the myocardium.

The accumulation of counts from emissions of ^{123}IPPA in the myocardium is modeled as

$$A_T(t_k) = (1 - f_v) \int_{t_k - \Delta t}^{t_k} \left(C_2(t) + \frac{1}{\beta_1} C_3(t) + \frac{1}{\beta_2} C_4(t) \right) dt + f_v \int_{t_k - \Delta t}^{t_k} B(t) dt \quad (11)$$

where A_T is the model of the measured myocardial tissue activity concentration acquired between the time $t_k - \Delta t$ and t_k in the regions of interest, f_v is the vascular fraction of blood in the tissue, Δt is the acquisition time of the tomographic data set, $B(t)$ is the measured activity concentration from the blood compartment at time t, $C_2(t)$ is the activity concentration in the extravascular compartment of ^{123}IPPA at time t, $C_3(t)$ is the activity concentration in the extravascular compartment of ^{123}I-labeled triglycerides and lipids at time t, $C_4(t)$ is the activity concentration in the extravascular compartment of ^{123}I-benzoic acid at time t, $(1 - f_v)$ is the fractional volume of extravascular space in the tissue, β_1 is the ratio V_2/V_3 of the extravascular volume V_2 and distribution volume V_3 of triglycerides and lipids, and β_2 is the ratio V_2/V_4 of the extravascular volume V_2 and distribution volume V_4 of ^{123}I-benzoic acid. The blood activity concentration $B(t)$ is measured by using a region of interest drawn inside the left intraventricular cavity or by using blood samples.

The activity concentrations $C_2(t)$, $C_3(t)$, and $C_4(t)$ in the extravascular compartments are given by three first-order ordinary differential equations:

$$V_2 dC_2(t)/dt = P_{21}SB(t) - (P_{12}S + P_{32}S' - P_{42}S^*)C_2(t) + P_{23}S'C_3(t) \quad (12)$$

$$V_3 dC_3(t)/dt = P_{32}S'C_2(t) - P_{23}S'C_3(t) \quad (13)$$

$$V_4 dC_4(t)/dt = P_{42}S^*C_2(t) - P_{14}SC_4(t) \quad (14)$$

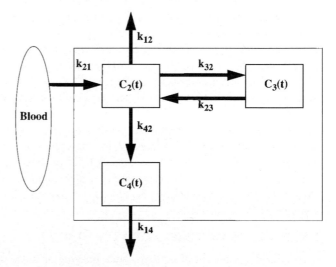

Fig. 11-5. Three-compartment model for a [^{123}I]-labeled fatty acid. A compartmental representation with six rate constants: k_{21} = rate of uptake of iodine-123 iodophenylpentadecanoic acid (^{123}IPPA) from the blood pool; k_{12} = washout rate of nonmetabolized ^{123}IPPA; k_{42} = rate of beta-oxidation of ^{123}IPPA to iodobenzoic acid; k_{14} = rate of washout of iodobenzoic acid; k_{32} = rate of accumulation of labeled triglycerides and lipids; and k_{23} = rate of breakdown of triglycerides to labeled fatty acid.

where P_{21} and P_{12} are the permeability coefficients for flux out of and into the capillary with a total surface area S within the voxel, P_{32} and P_{23} are the permeability coefficients for flux between [123]IPPA and triglycerides with a total pseudo–surface area S' within the voxel, and P_{42} and P_{24} are the permeability coefficients for flux between [123]IPPA and its β-oxidized product iodobenzoic acid with a total pseudo–surface area S^* within the voxel. Setting $k_{21} = (P_{21}S)/V_2$, $k_{12} = (P_{12}S)/V_2$, $k_{32} = (P_{32}S')/V_2$, $k_{23} = (P_{23}S')/V_2$, $k_{42} = (P_{42}S^*)/V_2$, $k_{24} = (P_{24}S^*)/V_2$, we have

$$dC_2(t)/dt = k_{21}B(t) - (k_{12} + k_{32} + k_{42})C_2(t) + k_{23}C_3(t) \quad (15)$$

$$dC_3(t)/dt = \beta_1 k_{32}C_2(t) - \beta_1 k_{23}C_3(t) \quad (16)$$

$$dC_4(t)/dt = \beta_2 k_{42}C_2(t) - \beta_2 k_{14}C_4(t) \quad (17)$$

which describe the kinetics of the exchange between the compartments shown in Fig. 11-5. There are six rate constants: k_{21} (washin of [123]IPPA from the blood), k_{12} (washout of nonmetabolized [123]IPPA), k_{42} (rate of β-oxidation of [123]IPPA to iodobenzoic acid), k_{14} (washout of iodobenzoic acid), k_{32} (rate of accumulation of labeled triglycerides and lipids), and k_{23} (rate of breakdown of labeled triglycerides to labeled fatty acid). The three-dimensional distribution of model parameters is denoted by the vector $\theta_3 = (f_v, k_{21}, k_{12}, k_{32}, k_{23}, k_{42}, k_{14})$, where f_v, k_{21}, k_{12}, k_{32}, k_{23}, k_{42}, and k_{14} are vectors with components f_v^s, k_{21}^s, k_{12}^s, k_{32}^s, k_{23}^s, k_{42}^s, and k_{14}^s for each tissue region s.

Results from dynamic SPECT have only recently been obtained. Using compartment modeling, attempts are being made to simultaneously obtain a measure of regional myocardial blood flow in terms of the rate constant k_{21}^s and metabolism. It is uncertain whether all parameters of the model are identifiable by using data acquired with the poor statistics and low resolution of SPECT systems. Myocardial ischemia inhibits β-oxidation. This causes a relative increase in the proportion of fatty acids in the more slowly metabolized triglyceride pool and results in a decrease in fatty acid metabolism.[159] Numerous investigations have established that ischemia reduces washout of fatty acids in animal models.[159] Therefore, it may be critical to be able to separate the compartments to differentiate viable tissue from mere uptake and exchange with triglyceride pools. The ability to use [123]IPPA with dynamic SPECT to show differences in metabolism may help clarify which regions are ischemic and ultimately identify patients who are most likely to benefit from revascularization.

EXTRACTION OF TIME–ACTIVITY CURVES

A critical component of most dynamic imaging methods is the extraction of myocardial tissue time–activity curves for estimating kinetic parameters. If the input function is not physically sampled, its time–activity curve must also be found from the acquired data. These time–activity curve extractions can be considered a segmentation problem: The goal is to find and localize the appropriate time–activity curves. This segmentation problem is difficult to address in dynamic emission tomography

imaging, especially in dynamic cardiac SPECT. Partial volume effects, system resolution, cardiac motion, and thorax motion tend to mix the background, blood, normal tissue, and abnormal tissue components. The very low number of detected counts also impedes delineation of regions. Some of the difficulties in accurately generating time–activity curves can be appreciated by looking at images in Fig. 11-6. These images are representative of canine cardiac ^{99m}Tc teboroxime data sets. Several approaches for extracting time–activity curves by using segmentation techniques will be discussed in this section.

Manual region-of-interest selection

The most straightforward segmentation approach is to choose regions of interest manually and use the average counts sampled over voxels in the region at each time point to compose the time–activity curve for that region. Specification of the tissue and blood regions of interest boundaries is simplest from short-axis slices. Registration with microspheres and clinical use of the data are also easier from short-axis slices. Septal, anterior, lateral, and inferior regions can be readily identified. Evidence suggests, as well, that the oblique nature of transaxial slices results in greater variation in myocardial wall thicknesses[132] than do short-axis slices. Reorientation offers potentially more accurate partial volume correction, as was demonstrated for dynamic PET imaging of ammonia.[132] Almost all dynamic cardiac SPECT research reported to date includes reorientation of the transaxial reconstructions as an explicit step before selection of the region of interest. Tissue regions are typically selected to cover the inferior, septal, anterior, and lateral areas in each short-axis slice of interest.[32,38,193,219] Regions in separate slices may then be combined to form larger regions. The blood region of interest is formed from delineation of the blood pool in several basal short-axis slices.

Considerable research has been done with planar imaging of ^{99m}Tc teboroxime,[16,45,75,141,170,200,216] in which the images have

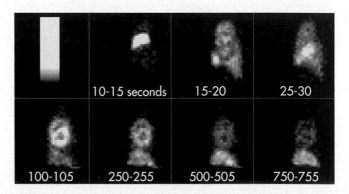

Fig. 11-6. Sequential images of one short-axis slice from a canine dynamic ^{99m}Tc teboroxime acquisition. (5-second acquisition times are labeled in seconds). The injected bolus is seen first in the right ventricle, then in the left ventricle, before distributing to the myocardium. The same grayscale *(upper left)* is used for all of the images. (From Di Bella EVR, Gullberg GT, Barclay AB, Eisner RL: Automated region selection for analysis of dynamic cardiac SPECT data, *IEEE Trans on Nucl Sci* 44:1355-1361.)

also been segmented by choosing regions of interest manually. However, researchers using planar imaging typically do not fit to compartment models. Washout ratios or ischemic zone–to–normal zone ratios are calculated instead, and results similar to those found with planar ^{201}Tl imaging are frequently reported.

Regardless of the method used to select the region of interest, interoperator and intraoperator variability can confound the results. In addition, selection of the region of interest is difficult and tedious. As discussed for dynamic PET[108] and for dynamic SPECT,[219] small position differences (0.7 cm for SPECT) can lead to substantially different fits. In particular, even small background components within the regions can bias the kinetic estimates considerably. To reduce bias, regions should be chosen close to the endocardial surface. The trade-off for reduced bias is the increase in variance of the washin and washout rate constants as the fraction of blood in the region of interest increases. In several of the canine experiments conducted in our laboratory, we found that the regions of interest must be drawn a second time to achieve reasonable kinetic parameters.

Region size

The size of the region of interest is also an issue. How many voxels should the operator include in a region? A larger region is easier to register with microspheres and offers a better signal-to-noise ratio but may obscure small defects. The size of regions used in single slices of previously reported dynamic PET studies ranges from 0.3 cm^{2,220} to 1.8 cm^{2,41} for the blood pool and from 0.5 cm^{2,41} to 1.1 cm^{2,108} for tissue regions of interest. In planar dynamic scintigraphy, most reports do not quantitate the regions of interest sizes. A few works[193,219] in dynamic cardiac SPECT with ^{99m}Tc teboroxime report that 2×2 intraslice regions of interest were selected, giving a volume of 1.43 cm^3. Some investigators found[193] that the smallest regions that correlated well to blood flow measured with microspheres were those that encompassed all of the septal, anterior, inferior, or lateral midventricular slices (8.6 cm^3). The most apical and basal slices were not used because of partial volume effects secondary to cardiac motion.

Automatic region selection

In line with seeking optimal time–activity curves to proffer to fitting programs, we have developed a semiautomatic approach to generate regions of interest.[52] Given a point near the center of the short-axis slices, the data are converted to polar coordinates. The location of the maximum along each ray can be found but is subject to constraints, such as being approximately circular and having a time–activity curve more like that of myocardial tissue than that of liver. These constraints are often necessary because of the proximity and high count emission of the liver, the high level of noise in the data, and the possibility of defects in the myocardium. Pixels radially adjacent to the location of the maximum along each ray are considered part of the region of interest (approximate size, 3.6 cm^3). Kinetic pa-

rameter estimates from the semiautomatically generated regions are similar to estimates from manually selected regions in dynamic cardiac SPECT studies of dogs with ^{99m}Tc teboroxime.

Other segmentation methods

Alternatives to manual tracing of the region of interest include thresholding, a widely applicable image segmentation method. Other methods used in nuclear medicine may also be directly applicable, even if they are not specifically intended for use in dynamic cardiac SPECT. For example, edge detection in planar scintigraphy has been studied to automate ejection fraction calculations. Germano et al[68] used a robust edge discriminator to calculate ejection fractions in gated SPECT images. Second derivative (Laplacian) techniques and relaxation labeling[60,61] have been used to segment scintigraphic images. Population modeling has also shown promising results in dynamic PET imaging.[149] A relatively large number of potentially correct time–activity curves are generated, and the curve that has the highest correlation with the measured data is selected. Hebert et al[88] also investigated region growing for automatic delineation of the blood pool in radiolabeled erythrocyte studies.

Another segmentation approach was developed by Chiao et al[34] for use in dynamic cardiac PET or SPECT. The endocardial and epicardial radii were considered as additional parameters to be estimated. All parameters were jointly estimated by maximizing a likelihood function with a nonlinear technique similar to Newton's method. Time–activity curves were extracted simultaneously with estimation of the kinetic parameters. Here, the line is blurred between estimation of the parameters directly from the projections and explicit region-based estimation. Relevant schemes for estimating parameters directly from projections without explicit reconstruction are covered in a later section. Chiao et al[34] proposed that if the model-based estimation method failed for studies with poor statistics, some regularization could be used, such as combining a priori boundary information from computed tomography or magnetic resonance imaging.

Factor analysis of dynamic structures

A potentially powerful segmentation approach is to find a few basic curves that include within their span the pure tissue and blood time–activity curves. The blood and tissue curves are then found by iteratively choosing linear combinations of the basis curves that satisfy a priori constraints, such as nonnegativity. This approach assumes that the time sequence of images is a linear combination of several homogeneous components, such as blood, tissue, and background and that there is no motion.

The method begins by using principal components analysis. The principal components are the eigenvectors of the covariance matrix of the time–activity curves. Most of the energy in the signal is usually in a few components; the rest of the eigenvectors are discarded. Principal component analysis promises to best represent the data in a mean square error sense for a given number of components. The components are not physiologically meaningful; to satisfy the eigenvector orthogonality condition, some components must contain negative values. Factor analysis of dynamic structures (FADS) iteratively rotates the retained principal components until all of the time–activity values and their coefficients are positive.[6] Although the result is not unique, this approach correlates highly with region-of-interest measurements in reports on planar imaging from numerous authors. However, some authors have reported failure of FADS to produce meaningful results in certain cases.[166]

Recently, the input functions from dynamic PET studies were extracted by using FADS.[220,221] Instead of using the iterative method recommended by Di Paola et al,[54] a constrained optimization routine was used to solve for the factors while the factors and factor coefficients were constrained to be positive. Additional constraints or modifications of the objective function by, for example, maximizing entropy[164] may improve the implementation of the oblique rotation step of FADS. However, solving the equations given by Wu et al[220] still does not result in a unique solution, but the results correlate with measurements from manually chosen regions of interest for simulations and [18]FDG PET patient studies. Moreover, studies using small hearts can produce poor results. Incorporation of additional information about the input function enables FADS to extract useful blood curves, even in small hearts.[221]

The advantages of FADS include automatic generation of time–activity curves and generation of "true" underlying curves (spillover, the fact that many pixels are a combination of blood, tissue, and other components, is eliminated). It is not known whether the higher noise levels and poor resolution of dynamic cardiac SPECT data will cause FADS to be ineffective. Preliminary research in our laboratory has shown that the blood time–activity curve could be extracted from dynamic ^{99m}Tc teboroxime data acquired from dogs when a modified version of FADS is used.[51] The method works well if the first step of determining the principal components is eliminated, where instead the FADS are estimated directly from the dynamic data. This is especially effective if a maximum entropy prior is used to select a unique solution. We have also demonstrated that FADS can be used to extract time–activity curves separately for normal and abnormal tissue regions.

O'Sullivan[168] reported a method similar to FADS in that underlying time–activity curves are extracted automatically. The mixture analysis model involves finding the same data representation as FADS but does not explicitly compute principal components. Promising results from the complex mixture analysis procedure were shown for [18]FDG PET brain imaging.

Accurate regional time–activity curves that are simple and sufficiently robust are important for compartmental modeling in dynamic cardiac SPECT. The regions selected must be chosen so that they do not bias the fits. Background should not be included in the region of interest, and an appropriate mix of blood and tissue should be in the region. If these methods are to be used in clinical settings, it is critical to automate the process and to understand the possible shortcomings of different data segmentation methods. An alternative is to incorporate the region selection into the fitting algorithm by estimating time–activity curves directly from projections[191] or to estimate parameters directly from projections. In such cases, the kinetics must still be mapped back to reconstructed slices to localize the defect.

ESTIMATION OF KINETIC PARAMETERS

The goal of parameter estimation in dynamic cardiac SPECT is to mathematically extract physiologic information about cardiac function from dynamically measured data. Parameter estimation is a branch of mathematics and statistics[7,11,17,50,56,58,224] that involves the development of methods that make efficient use of data in the process of estimating parameters of mathematical models. The process of parameter estimation involves the interplay between experimental design, model specification, and techniques of data collection.[28] The collected data are used in the estimation process to produce parameter estimates of the model. On the basis of a statistical model of the data, the estimation procedure produces parameter estimates and statistical measures of their accuracy. Careful statistical analysis and hypothesis testing of the results provide a feedback mechanism whereby the model, the data collection protocol, and the parameter estimation process can be evaluated and modified.

As we already saw, the model is a mathematical formulation that uses a set of parameters reflecting local rates of physiologic transport and biochemical reactions. Because of physical complications in the image detection process, the models used in dynamic cardiac SPECT must be relatively simple. The aim is to estimate values for the model parameters from dynamically acquired SPECT data.

Data are collected by using either rotating gamma cameras or fixed-ring systems. After the projection data are reconstructed by using an iterative reconstruction algorithm, a set of regions of interest are usually defined on the summed image and time–activity curves are generated for each region. Model parameters are estimated individually from a tissue curve of a particular region of interest. There is concern that during the acquisition of one tomographic data set, the distribution of the tracer in the myocardium will change. Thus, in dynamic SPECT, methods must be developed that can estimate the model parameters directly from the projections.

Both the image reconstruction and the process of determining the kinetic parameters of compartment models are parameter estimation problems. Ideally, to obtain efficient estimates of kinetic parameters, a measure of the statistics of the reconstructed estimates is required to calculate the statistics of the time–activity curves. Determining the characteristics of these statistics is more difficult in dynamic SPECT than in PET: In SPECT, a large system of linear equations must be solved, whereas in PET a direct filtered back-projection reconstruction algorithm is used. With matrix inversion reconstruction techniques, one can obtain estimates of the reconstructed errors; however, this is usually solved by using iterative reconstruction algorithms. The reconstruction problem is a linear estimation problem, whereas the process of estimating kinetic parameters of the compartment model is a nonlinear estimation problem.[7,50] An iterative algorithm, such as that found in the computer software package RFIT,[104] is used to fit the model parameters so that the sampled time–activity curves in the tissue regions of interest fit the predicted time–response curves of the model. The program estimates the model parameters and the statistical errors.

Careful analysis of the parameter estimates provides useful information on the appropriateness of the entire estimation process.[28] Goodness-of-fit tests can be used to determine whether the model has captured all of the deterministic characteristics of the data.[17,56,58,224] One quick and easy test is to determine whether the chi-square of the fit is equal to the number of degrees of freedom. More sophisticated hypothesis testing may be needed to answer some crucial questions: Are there enough compartments and parameters? Is the model overspecified for the level of noise and sampling resolution of data so that the data cannot differentiate the compartments? Is the assumed statistical nature of the data appropriate? (Analysis of residuals can validate the assumptions regarding the nature of the measurement noise.[58]) Does the data acquisition adequately capture the dynamics of the physiologic process?

We present a fairly detailed development of the mathematics used in dynamic cardiac SPECT to obtain estimates of the reconstruction and the compartment model parameters. The mathematics are particular to the dynamic SPECT problem. In PET, filtered back-projection reconstruction is used; this is not accurate in SPECT because the method cannot adequately compensate for attenuation. Therefore, iterative and direct matrix inverse reconstruction techniques, which model the attenuation in projection and back-projection equations, are used. Great attention is given to direct matrix inverse reconstruction in the hope that these techniques can provide error estimates that can be used in the estimation of model parameters. Because of the low counts in dynamic SPECT, this may be important to produce more efficient estimates with minimum bias.

Two approaches for estimating kinetic parameters in dynamic cardiac SPECT are discussed. The first approach is to estimate the kinetic parameters from the three-dimensional reconstructed dynamic data. The second approach is to estimate the kinetic parameters directly from the projection data.

Estimation of kinetic parameters from dynamic reconstructed images

Estimation of kinetic parameters from dynamic reconstructed images is a two-step process that differs from the one-step approach of estimating them directly from projections (see later discussion). The projections are first reconstructed for each complete projection data set, giving a set of K three-dimensional reconstructions sequenced in time. The blood and various tissue regions of interest are determined from a summed image of the dynamic set, and time–activity curves are generated. The kinetic parameters are estimated for each region

of interest. In the two-step approach, the reconstruction algorithm is a complicating aspect of the kinetic parameter estimation process.

Reconstruction algorithms. Iterative and matrix inversion reconstruction algorithms are used to reconstruct the dynamically acquired projections. Matrix inversion techniques have the advantage that weighting can be included in estimating the reconstructed images. In addition, they can obtain estimates of the reconstructed errors. Knowledge of the statistical errors of the reconstruction allows one to obtain weighted least-square estimates of the kinetic parameters and an estimate of the chi-square value from which one can evaluate the appropriateness of the kinetic model.

Iterative reconstruction. Iterative reconstruction uses an iterative algorithm, such as conjugate gradient,[102] maximum-likelihood expectation maximization (ML-EM),[134,189] or ordered-subset expectation maximization (OSEM),[98] to obtain reconstruction from each tomographic data set. The disadvantage of using iterative reconstruction algorithms for kinetic modeling is that estimates of reconstructed errors are difficult to obtain; however, estimates can be approximated.[8] On the other hand, because of the size of the reconstruction problem, it is not always possible to use matrix inversion approaches; inevitably, some type of iterative reconstruction technique must be used.

Matrix inversion reconstruction using singular value decomposition. A matrix inversion reconstruction algorithm uses singular value decomposition (SVD) to invert the matrix.[5,72] The physical effects of attenuation, geometric response, and scatter are incorporated into the matrix projection operator F, which is used to describe the imaging process. We assume that the imaging model is $P = FX$, where X is the source distribution vector, P is the projection vector, and F is the $N \times L$ projection operator (N is the number of projection samples for all projection angles and L is the total number of pixels reconstructed).

Least-squares reconstruction. The least-squares solution for X is the solution of the matrix equation $F^T P = MX$, where $M = F^T F$ and F^T is the transposed matrix of F. The estimate of the source distribution X is then $X = M^+(F^T P)$, where M^+ is the generalized inverse of M. To evaluate M^+, the SVD of M is first determined: $M = U\Lambda U^T$, where U is an orthogonal matrix and $\Lambda = \mathrm{diag}\{\lambda_1, \lambda_2, \ldots, \lambda_L\}$ is a diagonal matrix of singular values, with $\lambda_1 \geq \lambda_2 \geq \ldots \geq \lambda_L$. A diagonal matrix is defined as $\Lambda^+ = diag\{1/\lambda_1, 1/\lambda_2, \ldots, 1/\lambda_r, 0, \ldots, 0\}$, where r is determined by regularization. The generalized inverse of M is then $M^+ = U\Lambda^+ U^T$. The reconstructed source distribution is given by $X = U\Lambda^+ U^T (F^T P)$, that is, $X = \sum_{m=1}^r [u_m^T(F^T P)/\lambda_m] u_m$, where u_m is the mth column vector of U and u_m^T is the mth column vector of U^T.

The estimated reconstructed source value for the ith pixel is

$$\hat{x}_i = \sum_{n=1}^N \sum_{l=1}^L \sum_{m=1}^r \frac{u_{im} u_{lm} f_{nl} p_n}{\lambda_m} \qquad (18)$$

where $\hat{x}_i$ is the ith element of the vector X; u_{im} is the (i,m)th and u_{lm} is the (l,m)th element of the matrix U; f_{nl} is the (n,l)th element of the matrix F; and p_n is the nth projection sample, which is the nth element of the vector P. It is assumed that the sampled projection bin values are independent random variables; thus, the covariance between the ith image pixel and the jth image pixel is given by

$$cov(\hat{x}_i, \hat{x}_j) = \sum_{n=1}^{N} \sum_{l=1}^{L} \sum_{m=1}^{r} \sum_{l'=1}^{L} \sum_{m'=1}^{r} \frac{u_{im}u_{lm}f_{nl}}{\lambda_m} \frac{u_{jm'}u_{l'm'}f_{nl'}}{\lambda_{m'}} \sigma_n^2 \quad (19)$$

where σ_n^2 is the variance of the sampled projection p_n. The covariance is location and projection-data dependent.

In the modeling of dynamic cardiac SPECT data, two types of regions of interest are delineated: a heart tissue region and a blood-pool region specified in the left ventricular cavity. We define

$$\alpha_s = \sum_{i \in \text{heart region s}} \hat{x}_i \quad (20)$$

and

$$\beta = \sum_{j \in \text{blood}} \hat{x}_j \quad (21)$$

to be the total counts in each region. The covariance between the two random variables, α_s and β, is

$$cov(\alpha_s, \beta) = \sum_{i \in \text{heart region s}} \sum_{j \in \text{blood}}$$
$$\left(\sum_{n=1}^{N} \sum_{l=1}^{L} \sum_{m=1}^{r} \sum_{l'=1}^{L} \sum_{m'=1}^{r} \frac{u_{im}u_{lm}f_{nl}}{\lambda_m} \frac{u_{jm'}u_{l'm'}f_{nl'}}{\lambda_{m'}} p_n \right) \quad (22)$$

This assumes that the variance σ_n^2 is equal to the counts in the projection: $\sigma_n^2 = p_n$. Similarly, the variances of α_s and β are given by

$$\sigma^2(\alpha_s) = \sum_{i \in \text{heart region s}} \sum_{i' \in \text{heart region s}}$$
$$\left(\sum_{n=1}^{N} \sum_{l=1}^{L} \sum_{m=1}^{r} \sum_{l'=1}^{L} \sum_{m'=1}^{r} \frac{u_{im}u_{lm}f_{nl}}{\lambda_m} \frac{u_{i'm'}u_{l'm'}f_{nl'}}{\lambda_{m'}} p_n \right) \quad (23)$$

$$\sigma^2(\beta) = \sum_{j \in \text{blood}} \sum_{j' \in \text{blood}}$$
$$\left(\sum_{n=1}^{N} \sum_{l=1}^{L} \sum_{m=1}^{r} \sum_{l'=1}^{L} \sum_{m'=1}^{r} \frac{u_{jm}u_{lm}f_{nl}}{\lambda_m} \frac{u_{j'm'}u_{l'm'}f_{nl'}}{\lambda_{m'}} p_n \right) \quad (24)$$

The least-squares reconstruction of a dynamic sequence requires one SVD calculation for each transaxial slice reconstructed. For a 64×64 transaxial slice, this requires an SVD calculation of a 4096×4096 matrix. On a SPARCcenter 2000 (4 SuperSPARC 167-Mhz processors, 1 Gbyte RAM), the computation time is approximately 20 hours. It will be shown in the next section that a weighted least-squares approach requires an SVD calculation for each transaxial slice in the dynamic sequence because the projection errors must be included in each matrix that is to be inverted.

Weighted least-squares reconstruction. The weighted least-squares solution for X is the solution of the matrix equation: $F^T\Phi^{-1}P = M_W X$, where $M_W = F^T\Phi^{-1}F$, F^T is the transposed matrix of F, and $\Phi = \text{diag}\{\sigma_1^2, \sigma_2^2, \ldots, \sigma_L^2\}$ is a diagonal matrix of projection measurement errors. The weighted least-squares estimate of the source distribution X is then $X^W = M_W^+ (F^T\Phi^{-1}P)$, where M_W^+ is the generalized inverse of M_W. To

evaluate M_W^+, the SVD of M_W is determined by $M_W = U_W\Lambda_W U_W^T$, where U_W is an orthogonal matrix and $\Lambda_W = \text{diag}\{\lambda_1^W, \lambda_2^W, \ldots, \lambda_L^W\}$ is a diagonal matrix of singular values, with $\lambda_1^W \geq \lambda_2^W \geq \ldots \geq \lambda_L^W$. A diagonal matrix is defined as $\Lambda_W^+ = \text{diag}\{1/\lambda_1^W, 1/\lambda_2^W, \ldots, 1/\lambda_r^W, 0, \ldots, 0\}$, where r is determined by regularization. The generalized inverse of M_W is then $M_W^+ = U_W\Lambda_W^+ U_W^T$. The reconstructed source distribution is given by $X^W = U_W\Lambda_W^+ U_W^T (F^T\Phi^{-1}P)$: that is, $X^W = \sum_{m=1}^{r} [{}^W u_m^T (F^T\Phi^{-1}P)/\lambda_m^W]u_m^W$, where u_m^W is the mth column vector of U_W and ${}^W u_m^T$ is the mth column vector of U_W^T.

The estimated reconstructed source distribution for the ith pixel is

$$\hat{x}_i^W = \sum_{n=1}^{N} \sum_{l=1}^{L} \sum_{m=1}^{r} \frac{u_{im}^W u_{lm}^W f_{nl} p_n}{\lambda_m^W \sigma_n^2} \quad (25)$$

or

$$\hat{x}_i^W = \sum_{n=1}^{N} \sum_{l=1}^{L} \sum_{m=1}^{r} \frac{u_{im}^W u_{lm}^W f_{nl}}{\lambda_m^W} \quad (26)$$

A more compact form of Equation 26 is $\hat{x}_i^W = \sum_{n=1}^{N} \sum_{l=1}^{L} (M_W^+)_{il}f_{nl}$. The singular values λ_m^W of the matrix M_W are dependent on the measurement errors σ_n^2.

It is assumed that the sampled projection bin values are independent random variables; thus, the covariance between the ith image pixel and the jth image pixel is given by

$$cov(\hat{x}_i^W, \hat{x}_j^W) = \sum_{n=1}^{N} \sum_{l=1}^{L} \sum_{m=1}^{r} \sum_{l'=1}^{L} \sum_{m'=1}^{r} \frac{u_{im}^W u_{lm}^W f_{nl}}{\lambda_m^W} \frac{u_{jm'}^W u_{l'm'}^W f_{nl'}}{\lambda_{m'}^W} \frac{1}{\sigma_n^2} \quad (27)$$

$$= (M_W^+)_{ij} = \sum_{m=1}^{r} \frac{u_{im}^W u_{jm}^W}{\lambda_m^W} \quad (28)$$

The covariance between the random variables ${}_w\alpha_s$ and ${}_w\beta$ is

$$cov({}_w\alpha_s, {}_w\beta) = \sum_{i \in \text{heart region s}} \sum_{j \in \text{blood}} \sum_{m=1}^{r} \frac{u_{im}^W u_{jm}^W}{\lambda_m^W} \quad (29)$$

Similarly, the variances of ${}_w\alpha_s$ and ${}_w\beta$ are given by

$$\sigma^2({}_w\alpha_s) = \sum_{i \in \text{heart region s}} \sum_{i' \in \text{heart region s}} \sum_{m=1}^{r} \frac{u_{im}^W u_{i'm}^W}{\lambda_m^W} \quad (30)$$

$$\sigma^2({}_w\beta) = \sum_{j \in \text{blood}} \sum_{j' \in \text{blood}} \sum_{m=1}^{r} \frac{u_{jm}^W u_{j'm}^W}{\lambda_m^W} \quad (31)$$

A dynamic weighted least-squares reconstruction of the entire heart may require a 4096×4096 SVD calculation for as many as 180 (time frames) multiplied by 20 (slices) matrices. This requires fast computing and optimized code if the calculations are to be done in a reasonable time. It may be possible to provide a fairly accurate estimate of the errors by scaling the errors from frame to frame by a single constant. If this can be done, only one SVD needs to be calculated to obtain a weighted least-squares estimate of one transaxial slice for all time frames.

The errors in the projection measurements σ_n^2 do not appear explicitly in the expressions of Equations 28 through 31. Instead, the errors are incorporated in the matrix M_W for which the SVD is performed. Thus, the singular values are a function of the measurement errors. We use the notation λ^W to indicate this dependency.

Parameter estimation with noisy input function. The second step in the estimation procedure is to estimate compartment model parameters from time–activity curves generated from the dynamic reconstructions. The projections are reconstructed for each complete dynamic projection data set, creating a set of K three-dimensional reconstructions sequenced in time. Blood and tissue time–activity curves are generated from the sequence of dynamic reconstructions described in an earlier section. As we will see, the compartment model depends upon a blood input function. Because this function is known only from its measurements of the dynamic reconstructions, it is noisy (that is, it has statistical fluctuations). The kinetic parameters are estimated for each region of interest by fitting the measured tissue data to a model of the dynamic emission tomographic reconstructions with a noisy input function.

The vascular compartment concentration $B(t)$ in the heart is the input function to the compartment models and the extravascular tracer concentration, denoted by $C(t)$, is

$$C(t) = \sum_{q=2}^{Q} C_q(t) \qquad (32)$$

where the compartment functions $C_q(t)$ are the solutions to the system of differential equations described earlier for the one-compartment ($Q = 2$), two-compartment ($Q = 3$), and three-compartment ($Q = 4$) models. Equation 32 describes the concentration of tracer in the extravascular compartment as a function of time, which is simply the blood input concentration function $B(t)$ convolved with an exponential function:

$$C(t) = \int_0^t h_{n_c}(\theta_{n_c}, \tau)B(t - \tau)dt \qquad (33)$$

where $h_{n_c}(\theta_{n_c}, \tau)$ is the exponential system transfer function for $n_c = 1, 2, 3$ compartments and θ_{n_c} is the vector of model parameters. In the data analysis, $B(t)$ is usually measured directly from image-derived data (that is, the reconstructions), but it may be obtained from samples of drawn blood or from intraarterial catheters shunted for external counting.

By using regions in the left ventricular cavity and over the myocardial tissue, dynamic reconstructions can provide time–activity curves for the blood tracer concentration $B(t)$ and tissue activity concentration $A_T(t)$ accumulated over time intervals $[t_{k-1}, t_k]$, where $k = 1, \ldots, K$. The activity in the heart tissue region is a vascular fraction f_v added to an extravascular fraction $(1 - f_v)$:

$$a_k = (1 - f_v) \int_{t_k - \Delta t}^{t_k} C(t)dt + f_v b_k \qquad (34)$$

where a_k is the sampled tissue activity accumulated over $[t_{k-1}, t_k]$:

$$a_k = \int_{t_k - \Delta t}^{t_k} A_T(t)dt \qquad (35)$$

and b_k is the sampled blood activity accumulated over $[t_{k-1}, t_k]$:

$$b_k = \int_{t_k - \Delta t}^{t_k} B(t)dt \qquad (36)$$

The activity concentration $A_T(t)$ can be written in a more compact form as

$$A_T(t) = \int_0^t h_{n_c}(\theta_{n_c}, \tau)B(t - \tau)d\tau \qquad (37)$$

where, for example, in the case of the one-compartment model,

$$h_1(\theta_1, t) = f_v\delta(t) + (1 - f_v)k_{21}\exp(-k_{12}t) \qquad (38)$$

where $\delta(t)$ is the impulse function. Substituting Equation 37 into Equation 35, a_k can be rewritten as

$$a_k = \int_{t_k-1}^{t_k} A_T(t)dt = \int_{t_k - \Delta t}^{t_k} \left(\int_0^t h_{n_c}(\theta_{n_c}, \tau)B(t - \tau)d\tau \right)dt \qquad (39)$$

Because the integral of a convolution of two functions is the convolution of either of the functions with the integral of the other, Equation 39 can be rewritten as

$$a_k = \int_0^{t_k} h_{n_c}(\theta_{n_c}, t_k - \tau)\left(\int_0^\tau B(t)dt \right)d\tau - \int_0^{t_{k-1}} h_{n_c}(\theta_{n_c}, t_{k-1} - \tau)\left(\int_0^\tau B(t)dt \right)d\tau \qquad (40)$$

By using Equation 36, the integrals of $B(t)$ in Equation 40 can be written as

$$\int_0^\tau B(t)dt = \sum_{j=1}^{k-1} b_j + \int_{t_{k-1}}^\tau B(t)dt \qquad t_{k-1} \leq \tau \leq t_k \quad k > 1 \qquad (41)$$

To estimate the model-predicted values for a_k from the blood input function integrals b_k, we use the following linear interpolation:

$$\int_0^\tau B(t)dt \approx \begin{cases} \left(\dfrac{\tau}{t_1}\right)b_1 & 0 \leq \tau \leq t_1 \\ \displaystyle\sum_{j=1}^{k-1} b_j + \left(\dfrac{\tau - t_{k-1}}{t_k - t_{k-1}}\right)b_k & t_{k-1} \leq \tau \leq t_k \quad k > 1 \end{cases} \qquad (42)$$

Substituting Equation 42 into Equation 40, we see that a_k can be expressed as a linear combination of b_j:

$$a_k = \sum_{j=1}^{k} H_{kj}b_j \qquad (43)$$

where

$$H_{kj} = \begin{cases} \displaystyle\int_{t_{j-1}}^{t_j} \left(\dfrac{\tau - t_{j-1}}{t_j - t_{j-1}}\right)[h_{n_c}(\theta_{n_c}, t_k - \tau) - h_{n_c}(\theta_{n_c}, t_{k-1} - \tau)]d\tau + \int_{t_{k-1} - t_j}^{t_k - t_j} h_{n_c}(\theta_{n_c}, \tau)d\tau & j < k \\[2ex] \displaystyle\int_{t_{k-1}}^{t_k} \left(\dfrac{\tau - t_{k-1}}{t_k - t_{k-1}}\right)h_{n_c}(\theta_{n_c}, t_k - \tau)d\tau & j = k \\[2ex] 0 & j > k \end{cases} \qquad (44)$$

In vector notation, Equation 43 is expressed as

$$A(\theta_{n_c}) = H(\theta_{n_c})B \qquad (45)$$

where the tissue activities a_k are elements of the vector $A(\theta_{n_c})$, the blood activities b_k are elements of the vector B, and $H(\theta_{n_c})$ is a matrix that depends on the model parameters θ_{n_c}. Therefore, by using linear interpolation to approximate $B(t)$, Equation 39 can be reduced to the linear form in Equation 45.[105]

Let α_{sk} ($k = 1, \ldots, K$) be the experimental measurements of a_k (the model-predicted values of the tissue data) for region of interest s and β_k, the experimental measurement of b_k (the model-predicted values of the blood data) at the time index k. The residuals, which are the difference between the tissue region-of-interest data and the model-predicted values, are given by $(\alpha_{sk} - a_k)$. The estimates of β_k and α_{sk} are obtained by an iterative reconstruction algorithm or by matrix inversion to obtain weighted $_w\beta_k$, $_w\alpha_{sk}$ or unweighted β_k, α_{sk} estimates. In addition, in actual practice, it is assumed that the model-predicted values A are related to the measured input function β: $A = H\beta$.

Because the model-predicted values $A = H\beta$ are related to the measured input function β, a correlation between the input function and the model-predicted values is imposed. If measurements β_k of the blood input function b_k are achieved by using the reconstructed region of interest of the dynamic SPECT data, α_{sk} and β_k are correlated by the reconstruction process. In addition, because the model-predicted values a_k are computed through the convolution operation by using the same blood data (Equation 37), the values for a_k have correlations between them. These correlations lead to covariances in the residuals. We denote the $K \times K$ matrix Ψ to be the covariance matrix of the residuals ($\alpha_{sk} - a_k$).

It is assumed that the residuals are normally distributed (where $\alpha_s - A$ is a vector with the elements $\alpha_{sk} - a_k$). The elements α_{sk} are the weighted $_w\alpha_{sk}$ or unweighted α_{sk} estimates for the region of interest s at time k. Therefore, to determine parameter estimates $\hat{\theta}_{n_c}$ and uncertainties, we minimize the chi-square function χ^2, defined as:

$$\chi^2(\theta_{n_c}) = (\alpha_s - A)^T \Psi^{-1} (\alpha_s - A) \tag{46}$$

where[105]

$$\Psi = \text{cov}(\alpha_s - A) = \text{cov}(\alpha_s, \alpha_s) + H\,\text{cov}(\beta, \beta)H^T - H\,\text{cov}(\alpha_s, \beta) - \text{cov}(\alpha_s, \beta)^T H^T \tag{47}$$

Notice that Ψ depends on the actual model parameter values and that the derivatives of Ψ^{-1} must be included in the fitting procedure. To minimize χ^2, a modified Newton–Raphson algorithm is used in RFIT,[104] in which the first-order and second-order derivatives of χ^2 with respect to the parameters are computed by using a central difference operator. For example, values of a_k and Ψ^{-1} are computed for small increments of one or two parameters and are used to estimate χ^2 derivatives.

The parameters θ_1, θ_2, and θ_3 for the one-, two-, and three-compartment models described earlier are estimated for the myocardium by using the appropriate tracer. Of interest, one could include in the estimation procedure the estimation of the blood input function b_k. It is shown in[101] that this least-squares problem is equivalent to that given above. Therefore, one will obtain the same result for the compartment parameters whether the estimation problem includes or does not include the estimation of the input function. This, of course, assumes that tissue contamination has not occurred in the blood samples.

Modeled input function. The potential for finding techniques other than use of the reconstructed image to determine the input function is of interest. One possibility is sampling of blood, a technique that is very accurate but invasive. Another proposed technique is use of a population-based input function,[59] in which the input function is specified from samples of the patient population. One could use the mean time series of these samples normalized by taking one blood sample as Iida et al[115] did in ^{123}I-labeled IMP dynamic SPECT studies. Representation of the population from its spectral decomposition might also be considered. Yet another approach is development of a model of the input based on a physioanatomic compartmentalized model that represents the tracer behavior in the circulatory system, similar to that in the investigation into the use of [18]FDG.[62]

An important factor in obtaining a good input function is the need to obtain a pure input. Some investigators suggested that it is important to only sample plasma that is independent of erythrocytes. Other researchers found it difficult to obtain a pure blood sample from a reconstructed region in the left ventricular cavity because of contamination from the myocardial tissue. Others have included this tissue-to-blood contamination in the model for the input function.[64] Another approach that we mentioned in the introduction uses an intravascular tracer to better identify the vasculature component.

Efficient estimation of kinetic parameters. Considering the low counts obtained in dynamic cardiac SPECT, it is important to know whether more efficient estimates of kinetic parameters can be made. It is known in estimation theory that weighted least-squares estimation using weights equal to the measurement errors uses the available data most efficiently. This means that for our problem the dynamic sequence of reconstructions should first be estimated using weighted least-squares, then the kinetic parameters should be estimated from the weighted least-squares estimates of the reconstructed dynamic sequence.[78] This is done by using weighted least-squares with weights equal to the errors estimated in the first step to obtain the dynamic sequence of weighted reconstructions. A computer simulation of dynamic cardiac SPECT data intended to represent ^{99m}Tc teboroxime kinetics in the myocardium is presented to demonstrate that more efficient estimates of kinetic parameters can be obtained by using weighted least-squares in both steps. The mathematics presented in the previous sections were used to determine weighted least-squares estimates for the sequence of dynamic reconstructions and the estimation of the kinetic parameters.

Computer simulation. Dynamic cardiac SPECT data were simulated assuming a fixed-ring system. Complete tomographic data sets were generated at 5-second intervals. In each 5-second segment, 120 attenuated projections of the mathematical cardiac–torso (MCAT) phantom[206] were produced over 360 degrees. The attenuation and emission distributions of the phantom are shown in Fig. 11-15. The uptake in the blood and in the tissue corresponded to ^{99m}Tc teboroxime kinetics, with $k_{21} = 0.8$ min[-1], $k_{12} = 0.4$ min[-1], and $f_v = 0.15$ for the one-compartment model in Fig. 11-2. The blood input function was the same as that given in Equation 81. Fan-beam (65-cm focal length) projections of 128 projection bins were generated from a 128×128 image matrix of the MCAT phantom by using PLFA in the RECLBL Library.[102] The 128 projection bins were rebinned into 64 projection bins for reconstruction. Poisson noise was added to the projection data to simulate counts equal to approximately 10 times that of a normal ^{99m}Tc teboroxime dynamic SPECT scan. Fifty complete tomographic projections were simulated.

Each of the dynamic tomographic projection sets were reconstructed into 64×64 transaxial images. Only a central circular region of 3228 pixels was reconstructed. In one case, least-squares estimates of the reconstructions were obtained for the entire sequence of dynamic reconstructions by using Equation 18 and calculating only one 3228×3228 SVD of $M = F^T F$ for the entire sequence. In the second case, weighted least-squares estimates of the reconstructions were obtained by using Equation 26 and calculating a separate SVD of $M_W = F^T \Phi^{-1} F$ for each 64×64 transaxial slice reconstructed in the time sequence. The errors in the projections were assumed to be equal to the true value generated by the projection operation (PLFA). In the third case, weighted least-squares estimates of the reconstructions similar to that in the second case were obtained, but the errors were assumed to be equal to the sampled noisy projections (as one would assume in an actual experiment). Attenuation factors were included in the projection equations.

Time–activity curves for a manually selected blood region inside the left ventricle and a cardiac tissue region (10 pixels in each region) were generated from the attenuation-corrected transaxial reconstructions by using Equations 20 and 21. These time–activity curves were fitted to the one-compartment model shown in Fig. 11-2. For the unweighted least-squares reconstructions, the covariance $cov(\alpha_{(s=1)}, \beta)$ (s was just one region) between the heart and the blood regions was calculated by using Equation 22, and the variances $\sigma^2(\alpha_{(s=1)})$ and $\sigma^2(\beta)$ were calculated by using Equations 23 and 24. RFIT[104] determined the weighted least-squares estimates of the kinetic parameters f_v, k_{21}, and k_{12} by minimizing the chi-square function $\chi^2(f_v, k_{21}, k_{12}) = (A_T - \alpha_{(s=1)})^T \Psi^{-1} (A_T - \alpha_{(s=1)})$, where the diagonal elements of Ψ were the reconstructed values. The activity $A_T(t)$

in the heart tissue region was modeled as a vascular fraction f_v added to an extravascular fraction $(1 - f_v)$: $A_T(t) = f_v B(t) + (1 - f_v) C_2(t)$, where the extravascular concentration $C_2(t)$ was given by Equation 5 and $B(t)$ was assumed to be equal to the sampled blood time–activity curve. For the weighted least-squares reconstructions, the covariance $cov(_w\alpha_{(s=1)}, _w\beta)$ between heart and blood regions was calculated by using Equation 29, and variances $\sigma^2(_w\alpha_{(s=1)})$ and $\sigma^2(_w\beta)$ were calculated by using Equations 30 and 31. By using the weighted least-squares reconstructions, RFIT determined the weighted least-squares estimates of the kinetic parameters f_v, k_{21}, and k_{12} by minimizing the same chi-square function above, except that Ψ was calculated by using Equation 47. In one case, the measurement errors σ_n^2 were equal to the true projection value, and in the other case, the measurement errors were approximated from the noisy projection value.

It would be ideal to evaluate efficiency only for unbiased estimators. However, in SPECT, most estimators are biased because of model mismatches between projection measurements and the model used to reconstruct the data. When dealing with biased estimators, it is preferable to base efficiency comparisons on $E[(\hat{\theta} - \theta)^2]$, where θ is the true value instead of $var(\hat{\theta}) = E[(\hat{\theta} - \bar{\theta})^2]$, where $\bar{\theta}$ is the estimated mean. An unbiased estimator of a parameter is said to be most efficient if its variance is at least as small as that of any other unbiased estimator of the parameter. In our analysis, we considered an estimator to be more efficient than another estimator if its $(var(\hat{\theta}) + bias(\hat{\theta})^2)^{1/2}$ was smaller.

Results. The result of the first nineteen 5-second frames of the reconstructed transaxial slice is shown in Fig. 11-7. A weighted least-squares reconstruction (in which the measured

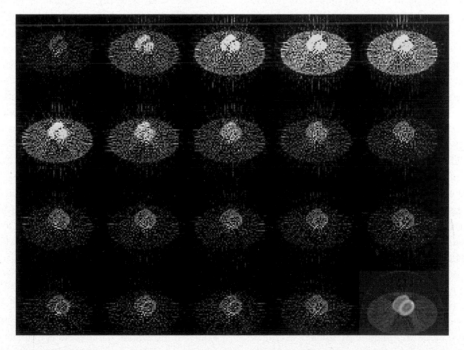

Fig. 11-7. The first 19 5-second reconstructed frames of the transaxial slice used in the simulation study. The last frame is the composite of all 50 5-second frames used in the study.

Table 11-1. Results of weighted least-squares estimates of washin (k_{21}), washout (k_{12}), and tissue vascular fraction (f_v) from weighted and unweighted least-squares reconstructions*

Variables	Actual values	Unweighted least-squares estimate	Weighted least-squares estimate (estimated measurement errors)	Weighted least-squares estimate (actual measurement errors)
k_{21}	0.800	0.7498 ± 0.0599 (0.0782)	0.7684 ± 0.0635 (0.0709)	0.7648 ± 0.0618 (0.0711)
k_{12}	0.400	0.3833 ± 0.0551 (0.0576)	0.4164 ± 0.0586 (0.0609)	0.3924 ± 0.0559 (0.0564)
f_v	0.150	0.1309 ± 0.0496 (0.0532)	0.1548 ± 0.0497 (0.0499)	0.1607 ± 0.0493 (0.0504)
χ^2	DF = 48	42.448	42.503	49.294

*For the weighted case, estimates calculated by using the actual known projection errors are compared with those calculated by estimating the errors from a noisy simulated realization. The number of unknowns equals 3228. The number of singular terms equals 3228 for both the weighted and unweighted reconstructions. The number of degrees of freedom (DF) equals 48. The efficiency measure, $(var(\hat{\theta}) + bias(\hat{\theta})^2)^{1/2}$, is given in parentheses.

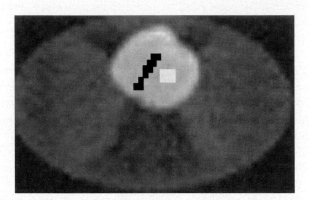

Fig. 11-8. One tissue region and one blood region of 10 voxels each were identified to generate time–activity curves for the compartment model fitting.

projection values were used as the measurement errors in the weighting matrix Ψ^{-1}) was obtained by using Equation 26, which required that 50 SVDs be calculated for the entire reconstructed time sequence. Each reconstruction in the sequence was obtained by using the 3228 singular values with corresponding eigenvectors. No regularization was used. The composite transaxial slice for all 50 frames is shown in the last frame of Fig. 11-7.

The reconstructed composite transaxial slice was used to identify one tissue region of interest and one blood region of interest, shown in Fig. 11-8. The tissue region contained 10 voxels in the septal wall, and the blood region contained 10 voxels in the intraventricular cavity. For the blood and tissue regions, time–activity curves sampled at 5-second intervals (Fig. 11-9) were generated from the reconstructed time sequence corresponding to the transaxial slice. Variance time curves for the selected tissue region and the selected blood region and the covariance time curve for the covariance between blood and tissue regions were also generated (Fig. 11-10).

By using both the tissue and blood time–activity curves in Fig. 11-9 and the variance and covariance time–activity curves in Fig. 11-10, RFIT produced weighted least-squares estimates of the kinetic parameters for the left ventricular tissue region. The results are shown in Table 11-1 in the column labeled

Weighted least-squares estimate (estimated measurement errors). These results were compared with results obtained from the weighted least-squares reconstruction in which true projection values were used as the measurement errors in the weighting matrix Ψ^{-1} and with results obtained from the unweighted least-squares reconstruction using Equation 18.

The weighted least-squares reconstructions provided more efficient estimates for all parameters as measured by $(var(\hat{\theta}) + bias(\hat{\theta})^2)^{1/2}$ than did the unweighted reconstruction, except for k_{12}. Using the true projection error estimates gave a χ^2 value that was closest to the number of degrees of freedom. This is what one would expect in that a knowledge of the true measurement errors would give the lowest model mismatch in the estimation procedure.

For the weighted case, fifty 3228 × 3228 SVDs had to be calculated; for the unweighted case, only one SVD had to be calculated. The 50 SVDs were obtained in 27.5 hours (33 minutes per SVD) by using a 75-mHz Silicon Graphics, Inc. (SGI) PowerChallenge. All reconstructions used 3228 singular terms.

This simulation demonstrated that more efficient estimates of dynamic cardiac SPECT kinetic parameters can be determined by using weighted least-squares fitting that incorporates the variance and covariance of dynamic weighted least-squares reconstructions. The simulation assumed better statistics than one would obtain clinically. This was because of concern that poor statistics would amplify any numerical errors in the SVD, producing erroneous results. Further investigation is needed to determine whether the SVD approach can be used with data with substantially higher levels of noise.

Computer speed has developed to a degree that makes it possible to estimate reconstruction errors in SPECT reconstructions by inverting matrices as large as 4096 × 4096. However, the computational speed is still not fast enough to be clinically feasible.

Compensation of inconsistent projection data due to time-varying activity during camera rotation

An important issue to address when obtaining unbiased estimates of the kinetic parameters is to insure that projection samples are consistent in each complete rotation of the gantry. For a single detector and for multiple detector SPECT systems, the

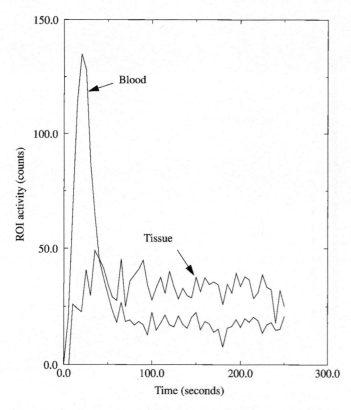

Fig. 11-9. Time–activity curves for the blood and tissue regions of interest shown in Fig. 11-8.

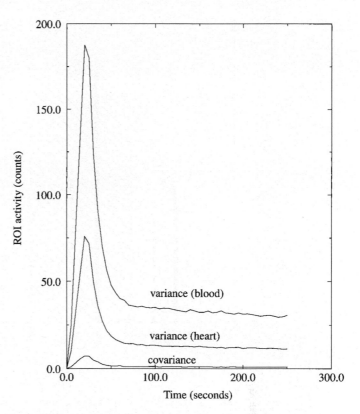

Fig. 11-10. Variance time sequences for the blood and tissue regions of interest shown in Fig. 11-8 and time sequence for covariance between blood and tissue regions of interest.

distribution of tracer activity in the tissues changes while the detector rotates during acquisition of a complete tomographic projection data set. This inconsistency in the projections produces artifacts in the dynamic reconstructions that lead to biases in kinetic parameters. Various methods have been proposed to compensate for the resulting inconsistent projection data sets.

To obtain a consistent set of projections for a particular time interval, all projections acquired during a tomographic acquisition interval must be interpolated. This is done so that all projections correspond to the same time interval within the tomographic acquisition interval of a complete rotation of the camera. Therefore, a projection at a particular angle for the desired time period is calculated by interpolating between samples of the particular projection angle taken at adjacent tomographic acquisitions (before and after). The interpolation of all projections to a particular time interval becomes a problem of defining the best interpolation scheme for sparse time samples. Various schemes have been examined.[137,214]

The simplest interpolation scheme is linear interpolation (Fig. 11-11). The projection data, integrated over a particular time frame $[\tau_a, \tau_b]$ are estimated. The curves in Fig. 11-11 show the evolution of the time–activity curve for projection bin i at two detector positions, j and j'. The time interval between τ_a and τ_b is chosen as the time interval for which it is desired to know the total integrated counts accumulated for projection bin i and all bins at the jth view and for all bins at all views of the complete tomographic acquisition. One criterion for establishing the chosen interval may be use of the total tomographic acquisition interval, which can be anywhere from 5 seconds to more than 1 minute. Other criteria that may allow for changes in width and sampling at irregular intervals over the time of the study may be used to establish the chosen interval. The total counts in the interval are calculated by assuming linear variation in the time activity between the samples. A projection sample in bin i at the jth view, which lies within the interval, is selected. The projection sample (activity in counts/sec) for the jth view at time $t_{(k-1)j}$ during the previous rotation and the sample at time t_{kj} is linearly interpolated to obtain the area for the first segment. The same process is used to obtain the area for the next segment by linearly interpolating between the sample at time t_{kj} and the sample at time $t_{(k+1)j}$ during the next rotation. The area segments are added together and divided by the time difference between τ_a and τ_b to obtain the average count rate for the projection bin i at projection view j during this same time interval. The process is repeated for the integral between τ_a and τ_b for another projection at the detector position j', and so on for every projection in one complete tomographic acquisition. This procedure is continued for every tomographic data set throughout the entire study.

Linear interpolation is relatively inaccurate for certain shapes of the time–activity distribution function. An alternative approach, based on the integration of overlapped parabolas, has

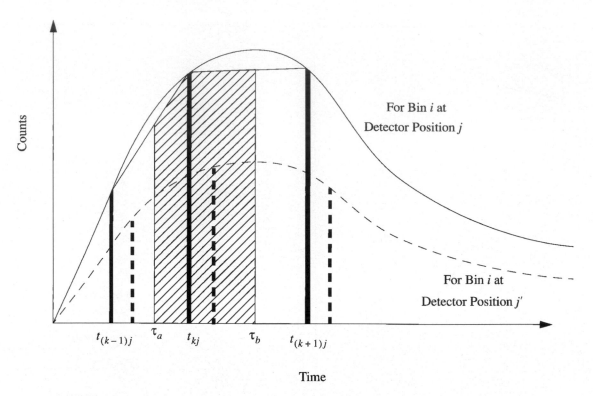

Fig. 11-11. Linear interpolation of time–activity curves to obtain consistent tomographic projection data sets. The areas under the time–activity curve between τ_a and τ_b for bin i at view j, view j', and other views in the tomographic acquisition are calculated by linear interpolation. A projection sample in bin i at the jth view that lies within the interval is selected. The projection activity (counts/s) for the jth view at time $t_{(k-1)j}$ during the previous rotation and the sample at time t_{kj} are linearly interpolated to obtain the area for the first segment. The same process is performed to obtain the area for the next segment by linearly interpolating between the sample at time t_{kj} and the sample at time $t_{(k+1)j}$ during the next rotation. The area segments are added together and divided by the time difference between τ_a and τ_b to obtain the average count rate for the projection bin i at projection view j during this time interval. The same calculation is done to find the integral between τ_a and τ_b for another projection at the detector position j', and for every other projection in one complete tomographic acquisition. (Adapted from Lau CH et al: Technique for image reconstruction and kinetic modelling from rotating camera systems, submitted to *IEEE Trans Med Imaging,* 1997.)

also been investigated.[137,214] These methods are computationally less intensive than those that we will discuss later, in which the kinetic parameters are estimated directly from each projection sample without interpolation.

Estimation of kinetic parameters directly from projections

Because acquisition of SPECT data involves movement of the detectors (Fig. 11-1) and because the distribution of radiopharmaceutical changes during the acquisition, the image reconstruction step can produce erroneous results that lead to biases in the estimated kinetic parameters. To overcome this problem, we are investigating the estimation of the kinetic parameters directly from the projection data by using a model-based, a spectral-based, or a weighted integration approach. To model the data acquisition accurately, the spatial and temporal distribution of the radiopharmaceutical within the SPECT field of view must be parameterized. It is hypothesized that by esti-

mating directly from projections instead of from reconstructed time–activity curves, the model parameters that describe the time-varying distribution of radiopharmaceutical can be estimated without bias.

Research along this line first pursued the estimation of only the region-of-interest time–activity curve from projections without reconstructing the region of interest. This was fairly easy to do with PET data in which a convolution backprojection algorithm was used: Huesman[100] described a method to estimate the average activity in a two-dimensional region of interest. Defrise et al[46] extended these ideas to three-dimensional regions of interest. To compensate for physical factors, such as attenuation and detector resolution, maximum-likelihood techniques had to be used. Carson[27] described a method to estimate uniform activities in a set of regions of interest assuming a Poisson distribution; Formiconi[66] did the same assuming a Gaussian distribution.

Later, attempts were made to eliminate the step of estimating time–activity curves by directly estimating the model parameters from the measured projections. This pursuit has become an active area of research. At the University of Michigan, Chiao et al[33,34] performed estimates of region-of-interest kinetic parameters for a one-compartment model and estimates of boundary parameters for the regions from simulated transaxial PET measurements. They demonstrated that the biases in the kinetic parameter estimators were reduced by allowing for estimators of the boundary of the region of interest to be included in the estimation process. At the University of British Columbia, Limber et al.[144] fit the parameters of a single exponential decay (to model fatty acid metabolism in the heart) directly from simulated projections acquired with a single rotating detector SPECT system.

Recent efforts have been made to develop a more general parameterization of the kinetics independent of any particular compartment model: for example, by allowing for a spectrum of exponential terms in time. The spectral-based approach builds on the early work of Cunningham and Jones,[43] who suggested that instead of estimating the kinetic parameters of models, one could estimate the coefficients of a predefined spectrum of exponentially decaying factors. Efforts are being made to calculate these coefficients directly from projections. This has been done for two[83] and for several spectral terms.[150]

For some parameter estimation problems, the parameters can be calculated by weighted integration of the time–activity curves.[29,114] This method eliminates the need to collect and store dynamic data. The kinetic parameters are calculated from the weighted integrals of the projection data, which are adequate for measuring the time-varying activity changes during the projection sampling provided that the integrals are calculated with sufficient numeric accuracy.

We look first at a model-based approach for estimating kinetic parameters directly from projections. We then show how the model-based approach can be used as a spectral formulation whereby coefficients of spectral components can be estimated for each pixel directly from the projection data. Finally, we illustrate how the processing for a one-compartment model can be simplified to calculating only a few weighted integrals of the total time–activity without having to store the entire time sequence of data.

A model-based approach. The work presented here builds on our earlier research[227] in which the parameters of a one-compartment model were fitted directly from projection measurements of a 3×3 image. It was shown that biases in estimates from the time–activity curves generated from the reconstructions were eliminated by estimating the parameters directly from the projections. The estimation from projections was performed in two steps. The multiplicative factors were estimated by using a linear estimation technique. The exponential factors were estimated by reducing the nonlinear estimation problem to a linear estimation problem by using linear time-invariant system theory: The estimation was performed on the sum of the counts in a projection. Here, the problem is formulated as a minimization of a weighted sum of squared differ-

ences between the projection data (not the sum of the projection data) and the model predicted values. A one-compartment model is assumed for the simulated myocardium tissue, and the blood input function is assumed to be known. For four regions of interest, a 64×64 simulation is used to compare the direct estimation from parallel projections with estimates from time–activity curves generated from the reconstructions and with estimates from reconstructed time–activity curves.[66] The same evaluation has also been performed for cone-beam projections.[106]

The parameters are determined from a model of the projection data that assumes a one-compartment kinetic model (Fig. 11-2) for each tissue type. The expression for uptake in tissue type s is

$$A_T^s(t) = f_v B(t) + \hat{k}_{21}^s \hat{C}^s(t) \tag{48}$$

where $\hat{k}_{21}^s = (1 - f_v^s) k_{21}^s$, k_{21}^s is the washin parameter, f_v^s is the fraction of vascular blood in the tissue, $B(t)$ is the known blood input function, and $\hat{C}^s(t)$ is given by

$$\hat{C}^s(t) = \int_0^t B(\tau) e^{-k_{12}^s(t-\tau)} d\tau \tag{49}$$

where k_{12}^s is the washout parameter.

The estimation process begins with an image segmented into blood pool, S tissue types of interest, and background, as schematically shown in Fig. 11-12 with attenuator shown in Fig. 11-13. To obtain tissue boundaries, the patient is assumed to be motionless during data acquisition, and a reconstructed image (for example, obtained through the projections at the time of strongest signal or through the summed projections) is segmented to provide anatomic structure. The image intensity at each segmented region is not used. A model of the attenuation distribution is created from the segmented image, and the attenuated unit activity projections of the blood pool, tissue,

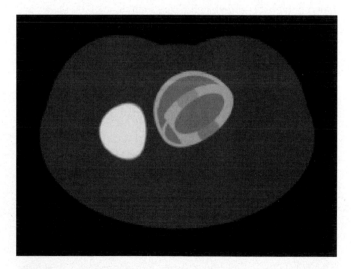

Fig. 11-12. The emission mathematical cardiac–torso phantom used in the simulation study that estimated the kinetic parameters directly from the projections. Dynamic data were generated for background, liver, myocardial blood pool, normal myocardium, and septal and lateral wall defects seen with lower intensity.

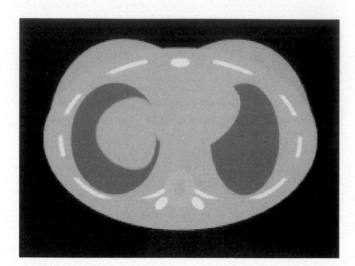

Fig. 11-13. The mathematical cardiac–torso phantom attenuator used in the simulation study that estimated the kinetic parameters directly from the projections.

and background regions are calculated for each projection ray of each projection angle. In other words, the number of events that would be detected from each region, given a unit concentration of activity within the region, is calculated for each projection ray of each projection angle. With no attenuation, the unit activity projections correspond to the lengths of the blood pool, tissue, and background regions along each projection ray of each projection angle. The number of projection rays per projection angle is denoted by I, the number of projection angles per rotation is denoted by J, and the number of rotations is indicated by K. Thus, a total of IJK projection rays are distributed in time and space. For a typical projection ray at angle j and position i, the attenuated unit activity projections of the blood pool, background, and tissue s are denoted by u_{ji}, v_{ji}, and w_{ji}^s, respectively. The background is assumed to be proportional to the blood activity, where the proportionality constant is g.

The projection equations are expressed as:

$$p_{kji} = u_{ji} \int_{t_{kj}-\Delta t}^{t_{kj}} B(t)dt + v_{ji}g \int_{t_{kj}-\Delta t}^{t_{kj}} B(t)dt + \sum_{s=1}^{S} w_{ji}^s \int_{t_{kj}-\Delta t}^{t_{kj}} A_T^s(t)dt \quad (50)$$

where the time t_{kj} is proportional to $j + (k-1)J$ (if the time per view is Δt, the proportionality constant is Δt). Substituting the expression in Equation 48 for $A_T^s(t)$ gives

$$p_{kji} = u_{ji} \int_{t_{kj}-\Delta t}^{t_{kj}} B(t)dt + v_{ji}g \int_{t_{kj}-\Delta t}^{t_{kj}} B(t)dt + \sum_{s=1}^{S} w_{ji}^s \int_{t_{kj}-\Delta t}^{t_{kj}} [\hat{k}_{21}^s \hat{C}^s(t) + f_v^s B(t)]dt \quad (51)$$

and

$$p_{kji} = u_{ji}b_{kj} + v_{ji}gb_{kj} + \sum_{s=1}^{S} w_{ji}^s [\hat{k}_{21}^s \hat{c}_{kj}^s + f_v^s b_{kj}] \quad (52)$$

The constants u_{ji}, v_{ji}, and w_{ji}^s are pure geometrical weighting factors for blood, background, and tissue s, respectively. These equations are linear in the unknowns g, $\hat{k}_{21}^s$, and f_v^s. The nonlinear parameters k_{12}^s are contained in $\hat{c}_{kj}^s$. If the washout parameters k_{12}^s associated with a one-compartment model for the

S tissue types are known, we can estimate straightforwardly the multiplicative parameters associated with the model by using linear estimation methods.

We reformulate Equation 52 as a matrix equation. The washout parameters are elements of the vector

$$\boldsymbol{\lambda} = [k_{12}^1 \ldots k_{12}^S]^T \quad (53)$$

and the multiplicative parameters are elements of the vector

$$\boldsymbol{\mu} = [g, \hat{k}_{21}^1, \ldots, \hat{k}_{21}^S, f_v^1, \ldots, f_v^S]^T \quad (54)$$

From the segmented image, the attenuated activity projections of the blood pool, tissue, and background regions along each projection ray for each projection angle are calculated. At a particular time t_m (corresponding to a particular projection angle acquired during a particular rotation—the index m is a contraction of the indices kj used above), we denote the attenuated activity projections of the blood pool, background, and tissue type s along each of the I projection rays by the vectors

$$\boldsymbol{u}(t_m) = [u_1(t_m) \ldots u_I(t_m)]^T \quad (55)$$

$$\boldsymbol{v}(t_m) = [v_1(t_m) \ldots v_I(t_m)]^T \quad (56)$$

$$\boldsymbol{w}^s(t_m) = [w_1^s(t_m) \ldots w_I^s(t_m)]^T \quad (57)$$

respectively. Note that $\boldsymbol{u}(t)$, $\boldsymbol{v}(t)$, and $\boldsymbol{w}^s(t)$ are periodic with period $t_{J+1} - t_1$.

We denote the projections acquired at time t_m by the vector

$$\boldsymbol{p}(t_m) = [p_1(t_m) \ldots p_I(t_m)]^T \quad (58)$$

Thus, we can write the set of $I \cdot J \cdot K = I \cdot M$ equations

$$R\boldsymbol{\mu} = \hat{\boldsymbol{p}} \quad (59)$$

where

$$R = \begin{bmatrix} \boldsymbol{v}(t_1)\boldsymbol{b}_1 & \boldsymbol{w}^1(t_1)\hat{c}_1^1 & \ldots & \boldsymbol{w}^S(t_1)\hat{c}_1^S & \boldsymbol{w}^1(t_1)\boldsymbol{b}_1 & \ldots \boldsymbol{w}^S(t_1)\boldsymbol{b}_1 \\ \cdot & \cdot & \cdot & \cdot & \cdot & \cdot \\ \cdot & \cdot & \cdot & \cdot & \cdot & \cdot \\ \boldsymbol{v}(t_M)\boldsymbol{b}_M & \boldsymbol{w}^1(t_M)\hat{c}_M^1 & \ldots & \boldsymbol{w}^S(t_M)\hat{c}_M^S & \boldsymbol{w}^1(t_M)\boldsymbol{b}_M & \ldots \boldsymbol{w}^S(t_M)\boldsymbol{b}_M \end{bmatrix} \quad (60)$$

and

$$\hat{\boldsymbol{p}} = \begin{bmatrix} \boldsymbol{p}(t_1) - \boldsymbol{u}(t_1)\boldsymbol{b}_1 \\ \cdot \\ \cdot \\ \boldsymbol{p}(t_M) - \boldsymbol{u}(t_M)\boldsymbol{b}_M \end{bmatrix} \quad (61)$$

To determine estimates of the model parameter vectors $\boldsymbol{\lambda}$ and $\boldsymbol{\mu}$, the weighted sum of squares is minimized:

$$\chi^2(\boldsymbol{\lambda}, \boldsymbol{\mu}) = (\hat{\boldsymbol{p}} - R\boldsymbol{\mu})^T W(\hat{\boldsymbol{p}} - R\boldsymbol{\mu}) \quad (62)$$

where the matrix W contains the weighting factors. Typically, W is the inverse of the covariance matrix for the residual vector $\hat{\boldsymbol{p}} - R\boldsymbol{\mu}$ or an identity matrix (for an unweighted least-squares fit). The value of $\chi^2(\boldsymbol{\lambda}, \boldsymbol{\mu})$ is minimized for

$$\boldsymbol{\mu} = (R^T W R)^{-1} R^T W \hat{\boldsymbol{p}} \quad (63)$$

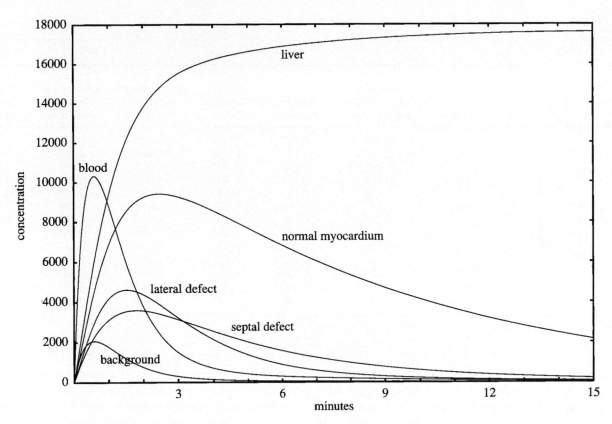

Fig. 11-14. The time–activity curves for blood, background, liver, and three myocardial tissue regions of interest: normal myocardium, lateral defect, and septal defect.

yielding, for symmetric W,

$$\chi^2(\lambda) = \chi^2(\lambda, (R^T W R)^{-1} R^T W \hat{p}) \qquad (64)$$

$$= \hat{p}^T W \hat{p} - \hat{p}^T W R (R^T W R)^{-1} R^T W \hat{p} \qquad (65)$$

Thus, the criterion $\chi^2(\lambda)$ can be used to optimize a fit based explicitly on the model washout parameters. If desired, the criterion $\chi^2(\lambda, \mu)$ can be used to optimize a fit based on all of the model parameters.

Computer simulation. We performed a simulation to evaluate the ability to estimate kinetic parameters directly from projection data.

The 256×256 computer generated image shown in Fig. 11-12 was used in the simulation. The simulation contained myocardial tissue, liver, blood, and background regions. The emission distribution was assumed to be attenuated by using the attenuation distribution in Fig. 11-13, calculated for 140 keV. The blood input function and simulated tissue-activity curves for blood, liver, background, normal myocardium, lateral defect, and septal defect are shown in Fig. 11-14. The blood input function was assumed to be known, and one-compartment models were used in the liver and the three regions of interest of the simulated transverse slice of the myocardium. Boundaries of the myocardial regions were assumed to be known, and background activity was proportional to the input

function. The parmeter g was the ratio of background to blood. Thirteen parameters were estimated: the amplitudes, decay rates, and vascular fractions for the liver and the three myocardial regions and the amplitude of the background. By using these 13 parameters and the known input function, a dynamic sinogram was formed that represented the attenuated projections of the six constituent components (blood, normal myocardium, septal defect, lateral defect, liver, and background) that compose the image volume. The 15-minute data acquisition protocol consisted of 15 revolutions of a single-detector SPECT system, acquiring 120 angles of parallel projections per revolution and 64 projection samples per angle. Estimates of the kinetic parameters directly from the projection data for the simulation were obtained by minimizing a weighted sum of squared differences between the projection data and the model predicted values (Equation 62). The estimation from projections was compared with estimation from dynamic reconstructions. Fifteen 41×41 attenuation-corrected reconstructions were formed by using 30 iterations of the conjugate gradient algorithm.[102] The pixel width was equal to 1.5 that of the bin width. Line-length weighting was used in the formulation of the projections. The estimation from projections was also compared with the direct estimation of region time–activity curves by using the method proposed by Formiconi.[66] Neither scatter nor geometric point response was included in the simulation.

Table 11-2. Results of estimating parameters directly from projections*

Tissue types in the image slice	Parameter	Simulated	Estimate					
			Noiseless Conventional (10.5 mm pixels)	Noiseless Formiconi	Noiseless Direct	Direct Uncertainties for 500,000 events	Noiseless Conventional (consistent projections)	Noiseless Formiconi (consistent projections)
Normal	$\hat{k}_{21}$	0.700	0.665	0.767	0.700	0.009	0.669	0.700
	k_{12}	0.150	0.149	0.162	0.150	0.002	0.152	0.150
	f_v	0.150	0.160	−0.032	0.150	0.022	0.187	0.150
Septal defect	$\hat{k}_{21}$	0.300	0.112	0.314	0.300	0.060	0.291	0.300
	k_{12}	0.300	0.116	0.286	0.300	0.048	0.279	0.300
	f_v	0.100	0.394	0.110	0.100	0.097	0.134	0.100
Lateral defect	$\hat{k}_{21}$	0.500	0.218	0.096	0.500	0.126	0.480	0.500
	k_{12}	0.600	0.247	0.214	0.600	0.105	0.467	0.600
	f_v	0.100	0.278	0.199	0.100	0.115	0.137	0.100
Liver	$\hat{k}_{21}$	0.900	0.924	0.888	0.900	0.005	0.923	0.900
	k_{12}	0.0020	0.0020	0.0006	0.0020	0.0006	0.0020	0.0020
	f_v	0.200	0.236	0.325	0.200	0.012	0.198	0.200
Background	g	0.200	0.200	0.201	0.200	0.001	0.199	0.200

*Rate constants are given in min^{-1}.

Results. The results of the simulation are given in Table 11-2. Parameter estimates (4th column) obtained using the conventional method (estimating parameters from time–activity curves generated from reconstructed projections) applied to noiseless simulated data had significant biases (ranging from 1% to 60% in the uptake and washout parameters for the three myocardial regions). Significant bias occurred in the lateral and septal defects. The large biases are not unexpected considering the long tomographic acquisition time of 1 minute. The estimates obtained by using Formiconi's method (5th column) had less bias in the septal defect and more bias in the normal myocardium and in the lateral defect compared with the conventional method. For all cases, the estimates of the kinetic parameters directly from the noiseless projection data (6th column) equaled the simulated value for the significant number of digits shown. The estimates were unbiased as expected, because the model used for fitting was faithful to the simulation. The 7th column gives the parameter uncertainties for the direct estimates assuming 500,000 total events for one transaxial slice summed over the entire dynamic scan, as would be expected for a dynamic cardiac SPECT scan using ^{99m}Tc teboroxime. Parameter uncertainties ranged from 1% to 18% for myocardial washout parameters and 1% to 25% for myocardial washin parameters. The uncertainties in the parameter estimates are especially large for the septal and lateral defects. The biases in the parameter estimates improved substantially for the conventional approach (8th column) and were eliminated for Formiconi's approach (9th column) when the projections were consistent over the 1-minute time frame of dynamic data acquisition, as would be the case with a PET scanner or a fixed-ring SPECT scanner. The results show how poorly the kinetics are represented in dynamic reconstructions if these reconstructions

are formed from inconsistent projections due to time–activity changing over the acquisition frame.

In summary, the combination of gantry motion and the time-varying nature of the radionuclide distribution being imaged results in inconsistent projection data sets. Estimating kinetic parameters from reconstructed time–activity curves results in biases. Estimating the kinetic parameters directly from projections removes all biases.

A spectral-based approach. Another approach to parameterizing the kinetics of radiopharmaceutical distribution in tissue is to represent the time–activity as a series of exponentials as opposed to assuming an a priori compartment model.[43] The decay constants for the exponentials are assumed to span some physiologically reasonable range and to be predefined with fine enough sampling to adequately represent the kinetics of the tracer.

We expand the development in the previous section so that each voxel is a tissue region. Projections will be formed by summing over all voxels in the image.

The tissue time–activity curve $A_T^s(t)$ for the voxel s is modeled as a fraction f_v^s of the arterial blood time–activity function $B(t)$ plus a linear combination of single exponential basis functions in time, convolved with the same arterial blood function $B(t)$. The expression for uptake in voxel s is

$$A_T^s(t) = f_v^s B(t) + \sum_{q=1}^{Q} \gamma_q^s \hat{C}^q(t) \qquad (66)$$

where $\hat{\gamma}_q^s = (1 - f_v^s)\gamma_q^s$ and $\hat{C}^q(t)$ is given by

$$\hat{C}^q(t) = \int_0^t B(\tau)e^{-\lambda_q(t-\tau)}d\tau \qquad (67)$$

The coefficients $\hat{\gamma}_q^s$ of the basis functions are all greater than or equal to 0; $\hat{\gamma}_q^s \geq 0$, the decay constants, are bounded below by the decay constant λ of the radioisotope, $\lambda \leq \lambda_q \leq 1$ (upper limit somewhat arbitrary); and Q is the maximum number of basis functions allowed in the model. The problem is determining the values of $\hat{\gamma}_q^s$ that best fit the measured data given predefined values for λ_q.

The camera is assumed to rotate as the activity is changing. At each projection j during the kth rotation, counts are accumulated between the time interval $[t_{kj} - \Delta t, t_{kj}]$ in the time evolution of the distribution. The projection equations for activity accumulated over $[t_{kj} - \Delta t, t_{kj}]$ are expressed as:

$$p_{kji} = \sum_{s=1}^{S} w_{ji}^s \int_{t_{kj}-\Delta t}^{t_{kj}} A_T^s(t)dt \tag{68}$$

Substituting the expression for $A_T^s(t)$ in Equation 66 into Equation 68, we obtain the following projection value for the ith projection bin at time t_{kj}:

$$p_{kji} = \sum_{s=1}^{S} w_{ji}^s \int_{t_{kj}-\Delta t}^{t_{kj}} \left(f_v^s B(t) + \sum_{q=1}^{Q} \hat{\gamma}_q^s \hat{C}^q(t) \right)dt \tag{69}$$

where p_{kji} is the number of counts recorded for the interval $[t_{kj} - \Delta t, t_{kj}]$ in projection bin i at time t_{kj}, w_{ji}^s is the probability of a photon emitted from pixel s being recorded in bin i and projection angle j, $\hat{\gamma}_q^s$ is the spectral coefficient for the qth spectral component for the pixel s, and λ_q is the decay constant for the qth spectral component.

Rewriting Equation 69 by performing the integral over the interval $[t_{kj} - \Delta t, t_{kj}]$, we have

$$p_{kji} = \sum_{s=1}^{S} w_{ji}^s \left[\gamma_0^s \hat{c}_{kj}^0 + \sum_{q=1}^{Q} \hat{\gamma}_q^s \hat{c}_{kj}^q \right] \tag{70}$$

where

$$\hat{c}_{kj}^q = \int_{t_{kj}-\Delta t}^{t_{kj}} \hat{C}^q(t)dt \tag{71}$$

$$\hat{c}_{kj}^0 = \int_{t_{kj}-\Delta t}^{t_{kj}} B(t)dt \tag{72}$$

$$\hat{\gamma}_0^s = f_v^s \tag{73}$$

and

$$\hat{\gamma}_q^s = \hat{\gamma}_q^s(1 - f_v^s) \tag{74}$$

The expression in Equation 70 can be written as the following summation from $q = 0$:

$$p_{kji} = \sum_{s=1}^{S} w_{ji}^s \sum_{q=0}^{Q} \hat{\gamma}_q^s \hat{c}_{kj}^q \tag{75}$$

In matrix notation, this is

$$P = \Omega\Gamma \tag{76}$$

where elements of Ω are $\omega_{kji,\,sq} = w_{ji}^s \hat{c}_{kj}^q$ and q is indexed from 0 to Q. The problem, one of linear estimation, is to solve for Γ.

Solution Γ must be positive. It can be determined by a non-negative least-squares technique[154,155] or by using the ML-EM algorithm,[134,189] such as the one suggested by Matthews et

al.[150] The formulation in Equation 76 determines the spectral components for every pixel in the image directly from the projections. This is a large problem in terms of computation. It can be broken up by determining spectral components for each projection sample,[154,155] then reconstructing the spectral components for each pixel from the spectral components of the ray sums. Instead of using an exponential decomposition, one can use another parametric decomposition[150] or best-fit model.[99,111]

Because this process is a large reconstruction problem, it is useful to consider the application of the OSEM algorithm.[98,99] A procedure for the maximum-likelihood expectation maximization (ML-EM) algorithm that has been laid out by Mathews et al.[150] could easily be adapted for the OSEM algorithm. Much of the algorithm development for the spectral approach is based on the early work of Carson and Lange.[30] The drawback of a spectral-based approach is that it is computationally intensive.

A weighted-integration approach. Most methods used for calculating kinetic parameters from PET data are based on fitting a compartment model to the change in the tracer concentration in tissue regions over time. Most of those methods demand dynamic data acquisition after tracer administration and a nonlinear least-squares fitting to estimate the kinetic parameters. Several image reconstructions are required from several data sets, all of which must be archived. A weighted-integration technique was proposed by Carson et al.[29] and implemented by Alpert et al.[1] to minimize the data processing time in generating functional maps of cerebral blood flow and distribution volume for $H_2^{15}O$ administration studies. In this technique, the dynamic frame images are integrated after multiplication by two time-dependent weight functions, and two functional parameters are calculated by means of a table look-up procedure for each image pixel.

The following equations illustrate the theory for calculating the rate constants for the one-compartment model (Fig. 11-2) from the time-weighted integrated data. The differential equation for the tissue compartment in the one-compartment model is described as

$$\frac{d}{dt}C_2(t) = -k_{12}C_2(t) + k_{21}B(t) \tag{77}$$

Solving Equation 77 gives

$$C_2(t) = k_{21}\int_0^t e^{-k_{12}(t-\tau)}B(\tau)d\tau \tag{78}$$

Multiplying both sides of Equation 78 by two time-dependent weight functions $W_1(t)$ and $W_2(t)$ gives

$$\frac{\int_0^T W_1(t)C_2(t)dt}{\int_0^T W_2(t)C_2(t)dt} = \frac{\int_0^T W_1(t)\left(\int_0^t e^{-k_{12}(t-\tau)}B(\tau)d\tau\right)dt}{\int_0^T W_2(t)\left(\int_0^t e^{-k_{12}(t-\tau)}B(\tau)d\tau\right)dt} \tag{79}$$

where the weight functions $W_1(t) = 1$ and $W_2(t) = t$ were used by Alpert et al.[1] to specify the kinetics of $H_2^{15}O$. First k_{12} is estimated by generating a table of the ratio of integrals on the right side of Equation 79 as a function of k_{12} for the measured input function, $B(t)$. Using the table generated, k_{12} is estimated at each pixel element by matching the ratio of the two weighted-integrated images on the left side of Equation 79 against the ratio of integrals on the right side of Equation 79 entered in the table. Once k_{12} is determined, then the functional image of k_{21} can be calculated by using

$$k_{21} = \frac{\int_0^T W_1(t)C_2(t)dt}{\int_0^T W_1(t)\left(\int_0^t e^{-k_{12}(t-\tau)}B(\tau)d\tau\right)dt} \qquad (80)$$

A data acquisition system has been developed in which multiple time-weighted integrated sinograms can be acquired to generate multiple time-weighted integrated reconstructed images without acquiring the total set of dynamic frames.[114] The system can calculate up to six independent weighted-integrated sinograms. Values from the weighted-integrated sinograms are inserted into operation equations, such as Equation 80, to generate functional parameter images for $H_2^{15}O$ and ^{18}FDG. The two-compartment model of ^{18}FDG uses three independent time-weighted integrated images that are inserted into the operation equations. Carson et al.[29] studied the optimization of the choice of the weight function.

The use of weighted integration to solve kinetic equations is suitable for certain models, such as one-, two-, and three-compartment models.[114] The solution requires integration of the acquired counts over time. The time points for the acquired samples need not be at the same time for each projection, which accommodates the rotation of the camera. Application of weighted integration has been explored in dynamic SPECT.[203] The advantage of the weighted-integration approach is that it provides a straightforward solution calculated directly from projections that, assuming adequate numerical integration, are independent of the sampling limitations.

EFFECTS OF THE PHYSICAL ASPECTS OF IMAGE DETECTION

Many techniques for estimating compartment model parameters with dynamic cardiac SPECT data were reviewed earlier. The accuracy of estimating these parameters is impaired by degrading physical aspects associated with dynamic cardiac SPECT. These aspects include inadequate spatial resolution, cardiac motion, inadequate temporal sampling, poor photon statistics, detector motion, and photon attenuation. We describe computer simulations conducted to investigate the effect of these factors on kinetic parameter estimates. Additional factors, such as scatter and lung motion, affect the bias of parameter estimates; these are being investigated in ongoing research.

Partial volume

Major causes of contamination in tissue and blood regions are blurring from the collimator geometric point response, cardiac wall thickening, and wall motion during myocardial contraction. Because kinetic parameters are obtained by using compartment models that include a convolution of the tissue response with a noisy blood input function, it is important that accurate blood and tissue time–activity curves are sampled. These activity curves are usually obtained from blood and tissue regions drawn on reconstructed images. Partial volume effects cause the myocardial tissue regions to be contaminated with blood and background activity. Spatial resolution (typically 15 mm) is a critical aspect of the partial volume effect. In addition, varying wall thickness and wall motion of the myocardium during the cardiac cycle contribute to the overall partial volume effect.

The partial volume effect[94] results in a reduction of the measured signal if the object being imaged only partially occupies the sensitive volume of the measuring instrument because the object is spatially blurred or because the object moves in and out of the sensitive volume. The combined factors of spatial resolution, wall thickening, and wall motion make it difficult to quantify myocardial uptake, especially because the low count rate in dynamic SPECT studies makes gated acquisition impractical. We look at the effects of collimator response on the bias of the estimated kinetic parameters and examine the effects of wall motion.

We investigated the effect of finite geometric response on the dynamic parameter estimates by using computer-simulated projection data generated from an anatomically realistic phantom, MCAT,[206] shown in Fig. 11-15. The phantom was generated by using a code that subdivides each image voxel into eight subvoxels. The phantom was defined to give three images: the myocardial tissue, blood pool, and uniform background. The location of each subvoxel within the torso was calculated, and the appropriate activity concentration was added to the voxel.

Unattenuated fan-beam projection data were simulated with and without depth-dependent geometric response by using a ray-driven projector. To simulate a perfect detector geometry, the projection data were taken as the line integral of the activity along a ray from the focal line to the center of the projection bin. For the simulation of depth-dependent geometric response, projection data were formed by integrating the activity along a weighted cone of lines for each projection bin.[228] This cone was consistent with a collimator with circular holes of 2.7 cm in length and 0.07 cm in radius. Time-varying tracer activity was simulated by varying the myocardial, blood pool, and background activity concentration in the phantom with samples taken every 0.03125 second from blood and tissue time–activity curves consistent with canine studies.[194] The blood activity concentration resulting from a bolus infusion of ^{99m}Tc teboroxime was modeled as

$$B(t) = \begin{cases} 450\,t/20 & t \leq 20 \\ 400\,e^{-0.1(t-20)} + 50\,e^{-0.100(t-20)} & t > 20 \end{cases} \qquad (81)$$

The time activity in the myocardial tissue was calculated using

$$A(t) = (1 - f_v)k_{21}\int_0^t e^{-k_{12}\tau}B(t - \tau)d\tau + f_v B(t) \qquad (82)$$

with kinetic parameters $f_v = 0.15$, $k_{21} = 0.8$ min^{-1}, and $k_{12} = 0.4$

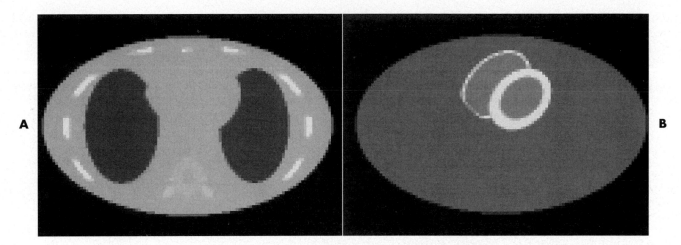

Fig. 11-15. A single slice of the mathematical cardiac–phantom used in the simulation studies of the physical effects of the image detection process. **A,** Attenuator; **B,** emission distribution.

min⁻¹. The background activity was taken to be 0.2 times the blood activity at all points.

A three-detector continuous rotation SPECT scanner, which acquires 60 projection views per acquisition, was simulated. Sixty projection angles were acquired in 10 seconds, and 50 complete projection data sets were acquired dynamically over 500 seconds. Continuous rotation was simulated by moving the three detectors in steps of 0.375 degrees. The tracer activity in the organs was also changed with each step of the detectors or once every 0.03125 second. The projections used for reconstruction were formed by integrating the subprojections formed every 0.375 degree over 6 degrees.

The projection data were reconstructed by using 25 iterations of the ML-EM algorithm. The images were rotated in three dimensions to produce short-axis slices through the heart. The kinetic parameters were calculated from regions of interest drawn over the myocardium and left ventricle blood pool. The myocardium region was defined as a $2 \times 2 \times 2$ array of voxels, which was moved across the images as shown in Fig. 11-16. The percentage of blood pool, background, and myocar-

dial tissue in each of the five regions is shown in Table 11-3 along with the fraction of blood, f_v, in each region.

The blood and tissue time–activity curves were fitted to the one-compartment model to obtain the exchange parameters k_{21} and k_{12} and the blood volume fraction f_v by using RFIT.[104] The

Table 11-3. Percentage of blood pool, background, and myocardial tissue in each of the five tissue regions shown in Fig. 11-16 along with the fraction of blood, f_v, in each region. (Published with permission of *Medical Physics*.)

Region number	Blood pool	Background	Myocardium	Fraction of blood f_v
	%			
1	95	0	5	0.961
2	58	0	42	0.644
3	13	9	78	0.263
4	0	52	48	0.176
5	0	93	7	0.197

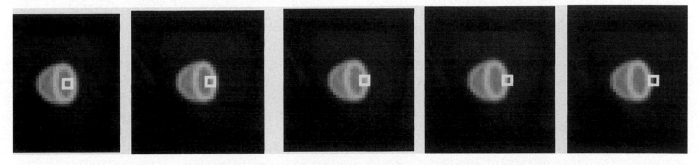

Fig. 11-16. Location of the five myocardial regions of interest used for analysis of the simulated dynamic images. Left to Right, Region 1 through Region 5. (Reprinted with permission from Welch AE, Smith AM, Gullberg GT: An investigation of the effect of finite system resolution and photon noise on the bias and precision of dynamic cardiac SPECT parameters, *Med Phys* 22:1829-1836, 1995.)

Table 11-4. Kinetic parameters k_{21}, k_{12}, and f_v for the five tissue regions, extracted from the noise-free data, for perfect and typical single-photon emission computed tomography (SPECT) resolution

Region number	Perfect SPECT resolution				Typical SPECT resolution			
	k_{21}*	k_{12}†	f_v‡	Average bias	k_{21}*	k_{12}†	f_v‡	Average bias
1	0.745	0.428	0.952	0.028	0.784	0.453	0.931	0.033
2	0.798	0.413	0.711	0.027	0.763	0.445	0.698	0.045
3	0.721	0.391	0.387	0.071	0.644	0.427	0.429	0.116
4	0.459	0.386	0.214	0.131	0.423	0.417	0.259	0.159
5	0.156	0.404	0.193	0.217	0.186	0.419	0.213	0.216

*True value, 0.8 min^{-1}.
†True value, 0.4 min^{-1}.
‡True value given in Table 11-3.
(Reprinted with permission from Welch AE, Smith AM, Gullberg GT: An investigation of the effect of finite system resolution and photon noise on the bias and precision of dynamic cardiac SPECT parameters, *Med Phys* 22:1829-1836; 1995.)

results, given in Table 11-4, demonstrate that the kinetic parameter estimates are sensitive to background contamination. As background contamination increases, estimates of k_{21} decrease. Estimates of k_{12} are not affected as severely. The main effect of geometric response is the reduction of the value of k_{21} for regions containing mostly myocardium (that is, regions 2 to 4). The inclusion of geometric response in the simulation has little effect on the parameters f_v and k_{12}.

The parameter k_{21} is reduced because the size of the myocardium is of the order of the geometric resolution of the SPECT system, whereas the blood pool is substantially larger. Therefore, inclusion of geometric response in the simulation reduces the concentration in the center of the myocardium with respect to the concentration in the center of the blood pool. Because the parameter k_{21} is effectively a scaling factor in the model equations, this reduction in concentration leads to a reduction in k_{21}. The most accurate estimates were obtained in region 2 because of the limited background activity. This region was contaminated with blood, but because blood was accounted for in the model, the contamination did not result in a large level of bias. However, it was subsequently shown that as the tissue region was contaminated with blood, variance in the estimates in the presence of photon noise increased substantially.[192] Thus, the trade-off between bias and variance must be considered when drawing regions of interest.

In PET studies, efforts have been made to solve the partial volume effect problem (including the effects of wall thickening and wall motion) by using an intravascular tracer.[197] Efforts have also been made to address the problem of identifying the myocardial wall when there is only partial tracer uptake because of infarction.[118]

It has been proposed that an intravascular tracer be used in SPECT studies to eliminate partial volume effects so that exact myocardial uptake can be measured.[112] This method relies on the presence of identical partial volume effects for transmission and emission data. Extravascular density can be estimated by using a combination of transmission data and emission data from an intravascular study.[178] The tissue density distribution is

obtained from the transmission study, which provides an image of tissue density. The blood volume distribution is obtained by performing an emission scan with the injection of a tracer that remains totally intravascular. The extravascular tissue density distribution is then obtained by subtracting the normalized blood volume scan from the normalized transmission scan. From this information, the uptake of a perfusion agent into the extravascular tissue can be estimated.[112]

An absolute distribution of the fractional blood content (in ml [blood] cm^{-3}) can be obtained if the concentration of the intravascular tracer in the blood (BP) is known. This assumes that there is a linear relationship between tomographic picture element counts and isotope concentration, such as in the equation:

$$\text{element counts (cts/s/pixel)} = k_E \times \text{isotope concentration } (\mu\text{Ci cm}^{-3}) \tag{83}$$

where k_E is the calibration factor. Venous blood samples taken from a peripheral site during the emission scan are used to measure the whole blood concentration C_{BP} (in μCi cm^{-3}). The product of the blood concentration and k_E results in an image pixel count (cts/s/pixel), provided that there is no partial volume effect. The blood density scan D_V (in ml [blood] cm^{-3}) is then obtained by dividing each element count density of the emission scan (S_{BP}) by the calculated whole-blood pixel count:

$$D_v = S_{BP}/(k_E C_{BP}) \tag{84}$$

This fraction can be converted to ml/cm^3 or to blood density equivalents (that is, 1 blood density equivalent = 1.06 g cm^{-3}).

The density distribution (vascular and extravascular) is obtained from the transmission scan, which is taken through the same plane as the emission scan. Each pixel in the transmission scan is divided by a calibration factor (k_T) that relates transmission pixel counts (counts pixel^{-1}) to blood density equivalents. This calibration factor is derived from the transmission scan itself and is the mean pixel count within the boundary of the heart chamber. This region should have values of unity in the blood density scan. Denoting the original transmission scan as

S_T and the normalized tissue density scan (vascular plus extravascular) as $D_{(V + EV)}$, we obtain:

$$D_{(V + EV)} = S_T / k_T \tag{85}$$

The extravascular density distribution (D_{EV}) is obtained by subtracting the blood density scan from the normalized tissue density scan:

$$D_{EV} = D_{(V + EV)} - D_V \tag{86}$$

$$D_{EV} = \frac{S_T}{k_T} - \frac{S_{BP}}{k_{BP} C_{BP}} \tag{87}$$

The result is a density distribution expressed as blood density equivalents. It can be converted to g cm^{-3} by multiplying each pixel in the scan by the numeric value for the density of blood.

If a scan is performed with a perfusion agent, the regional uptake per gram of tissue of the perfusion agent can be obtained[112]:

$$\text{regional uptake } (\mu\text{Ci/g of tissue}) = [S_P/k_P] / \left(\frac{S_T}{k_T} - \frac{S_{BP}}{k_{BP} C_{BP}} \right) \tag{88}$$

where the calibration factor k_P converts the element count density S_P to microcuries per gram of tissue.

Cardiac motion

The previous section showed that background contamination of the region of interest introduces bias into estimates of kinetic parameters. An important factor that contributes to background contamination is cardiac motion. A beating version of the three-dimensional MCAT phantom described in the previous section was used to investigate the effects of cardiac motion on bias in kinetic estimates. The entire cardiac cycle was simulated with 16 intermediate cardiac frames. Three different simulations were used to investigate the effects of cardiac motion. The first used only the diastolic frame of the cardiac cycle, the second used only the systolic frame, and the third simulated the entire cardiac cycle by using 16 cardiac frames to represent a heart rate of 60 beats per minute.

Simulated dynamic projection sets were formed to coincide with 10-second acquisitions over 500 seconds as described in the previous section. Projection data were formed by using a three-dimensional collimator response consistent with a collimator with hexagonal holes 2.7 cm in length and 0.14 cm in flat-to-flat diameter.[228] In addition, a second set of projection data was formed that included collimator response and photon noise. Photon noise was added to the projection data to simulate the counts observed when a 30-mCi injection of ^{99m}Tc teboroxime is administered to a 35-kg dog. This resulted in approximately 1,200,000 total counts summed over all projections in the maximum 10-second 360° projection set and represented approximately 10 slices with no liver activity. Fifty realizations of the noisy projection data were generated. The resulting 60 angular projection sets were reconstructed with 25 iterations of the ML-EM algorithm. The images were reoriented to obtain short-axis slices of the heart. Septal, anterior, lateral, and inferior tissue regions ranging from 2.17 cm^3 in the apex to 5.06 cm^3 in the base were drawn on apical, midventric-

ular, and basal regions of the heart (Fig. 11-17) and a blood region of 4.33 cm^3 was drawn in the left ventricle. Blood and tissue time–activity curves were generated and submitted to RFIT, which estimated the kinetic parameters.

Figure 11-18 shows a plot of estimates of k_{21} and k_{12} generated with noise-free projection data for the different regions. The estimates were obtained at end systole, end diastole, and during continuous heartbeating. Cardiac motion introduces significant bias in the apical regions of the heart. This bias is greatest at the end systolic frame because of background contamination in the regions of interest. Estimates in the basal regions show less bias from motion. Figure 11-19 shows the mean and standard deviations of estimates of k_{21} and k_{12} with photon noise included in the projection data. As one would expect, this figure looks very similar to Fig. 11-18 but has error bars. When estimating k_{21} in the basal and midventricular regions of the heart, bias and variance from noise and collimator response tend to overwhelm effects from cardiac motion. In the apical regions, cardiac motion introduces additional bias in k_{21} estimates, even in the presence of noise. The large difference in bias levels within each slice is due to background contamination in the regions. The septal regions have the least bias because background contamination is much lower in this region than in the anterior, lateral, and inferior regions. In PET, techniques for eliminating the effects of cardiac motion rely on gating the acquisition relative to the cardiac cycle.[22,128] However, this is difficult to accomplish in dynamic cardiac SPECT because of the low count densities.

Detector motion

In most dynamic SPECT acquisitions, the projection data are obtained by rotating one or more detectors around the patient. The projection data are inconsistent because each angular sample is produced from photons that are detected from activity in the body, which is changing rapidly as the data are acquired. This differs from dynamic PET studies, in which static-ring detectors are usually used.

The next series of simulations addresses the effects of detector motion and varying acquisition intervals by using computer simulations. Results were obtained by modeling the three-detector rotating SPECT system with an acquisition of 60 projection sets as it rotates over 360 degrees. Varying acquisition intervals were simulated by varying the number of subprojections in each six-degree angular sample. That is, each subprojection was obtained every 0.03125 second, but the number of subprojections per six-degree angular sample was varied. Thus, a 5-second image acquisition used 8 subprojections, a 10-second acquisition used 16 subprojections, a 20-second acquisition used 32 subprojections, and a 40-second acquisition used 64 subprojections per six-degree angular sample. A fixed-ring detector SPECT system was also modeled, which acquired 60 projection sets with no rotation. In these simulations, no attenuation was simulated.

Figure 11-20, A shows estimates of washin compared with iteration number of the ML-EM algorithm for the fixed detec-

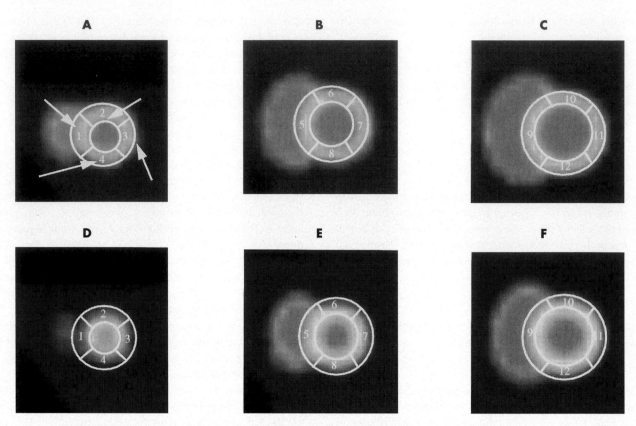

Fig. 11-17. Short-axis slices of the beating mathematical cardiac–torso phantom (original phantom, not reconstructions) at end diastole (**A,** apex; **B,** mid-ventricle; **C,** base) and at end systole (**D,** apex; **E,** mid-ventricle; **F,** base). The regions are numbered for later reference. The actual regions chosen are similar to those shown above. (From Ross SG, Gullberg GT, Huesman RH: The effect of heart motion on kinetic parameter estimates for dynamic cardiac SPECT, *IEEE Trans on Nucl Sci* 44:1409-1416, 1997.)

tor with a bolus infusion and 5-second, 10-second, 20-second, and 40-second acquisition intervals. The estimates obtained using the static detector system reached convergence at approximately 50 iterations. Results obtained with filtered back-projection are shown at iteration number zero and compare well with those obtained with the ML-EM results as it asymptotically approaches convergence.

Figure 11-20, *B* shows estimates of washin for the moving detector system. Unlike for the static detector, estimates of washin do not converge as the iteration number increases. The rate of divergence is smallest for a 5-second acquisition. Estimates obtained with filtered back-projection show relatively small levels of bias for all acquisition intervals. Filtered back-projection is not used in practice because of the need for attenuation correction.

Input function shape and acquisition interval

The need to match the shape of the input function to the frequency response of the organ system with good statistics during critical phases (fast varying) of time–activity curves of the dynamic system makes it difficult to select an optimal input function. It also makes it difficult to find an acquisition interval long enough to maximize statistics but short enough to capture the timing resolution necessary to reproduce accurately the time variation in the time–activity curves and to obtain samples taken at intervals that minimize the data storage but retain the full information content of the time-varying dynamic system. Various investigations in PET and SPECT have been performed to clarify this important problem.[136,142,152,171,182] These studies addressed the question of number of samples and optimal choice of sample period (which may be irregular).[142,171,182] Lau et al[136] suggested a sampling scheme for [201]Tl. Our group[182] addressed the question of optimal choice of sample period in connection with the duration of the input function. We present computer simulations that show how sampling and input function shape affect bias and variance.

In the computer simulation, a three-detector camera is rotated at high rates of speed, with the maximum rotation rate giving 360 degrees of coverage in 5 seconds. Although this has the advantage of tracking the temporal variations in the tracer, it results in poor photon statistics. For example, in a dog weighing approximately 30 kg, a 15-mCi bolus injection of ^{99m}Tc-labeled teboroxime yields approximately 320,000 counts summed over all projections in the maximum 5-second projection set (64 × 64 × 120 angles).

It has been demonstrated[219] that bias and variance are in-

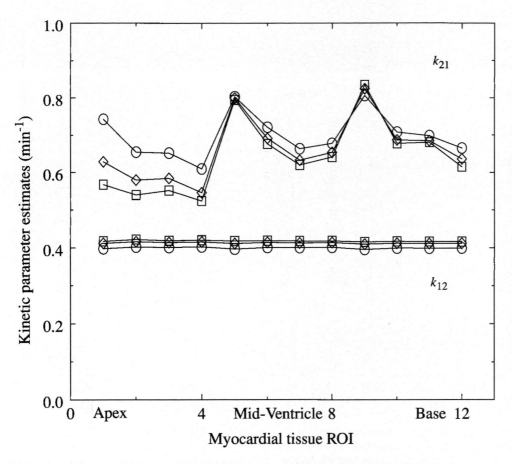

Fig. 11-18. Plots of estimates of k_{21} and k_{12} obtained from images reconstructed from noise-free projection data formed with geometric collimator response. $\bigcirc$ = end diastole, $\square$ = end systole, and $\diamondsuit$ = beating. Actual values are $k_{21} = 0.8$ min^{-1} and $k_{12} = 0.4$ min^{-1}. Numbering of the region of interest corresponds to that in Fig. 11-17. (From Ross SG, Gullberg GT, Huesman RH: The effect of heart motion on kinetic parameter estimates for dynamic cardiac SPECT, *IEEE Trans on Nucl Sci* 44:1409-1416, 1997.)

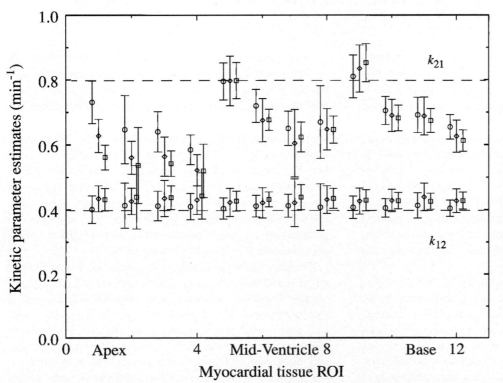

Fig. 11-19. Plots of estimates of k_{21} and k_{12} obtained from images reconstructed from projection data generated with geometric collimator response and photon noise. $\bigcirc$ = end diastole, $\square$ = end systole, and $\diamondsuit$ = beating. Actual values are $k_{21} = 0.8$ min^{-1} and $k_{12} = 0.4$ min^{-1}. Numbering of the regions of interest corresponds to that in Fig. 11-17.

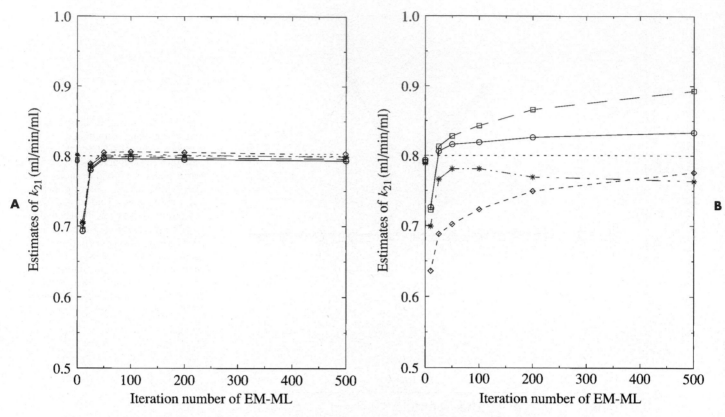

Fig. 11-20. Estimates of k_{21} for varying iteration number of the maximum-likelihood expectation maximizations algorithm. Iteration zero corresponds to estimates obtained using filtered back-projection. **A,** Fixed detector and bolus infusion; **B,** moving detector and bolus infusion. ○ = 5-second acquisition, □ = 10-second acquisition, ◇ = 20-second acquisition, * = 40-second acquisition, and ---------- = actual value of k_{21}. (From Ross SG, Welch A, Gullberg GT, Huesman RH: An investigation into the effect of input function shape and image acquisition interval on estimates of washin for dynamic cardiac SPECT, *Phys Med Biol* 42:2193-2213, 1997. Reproduced with permission from IOP Publishing Limited.)

creased substantially when photon counts are reduced to levels typically observed in dynamic cardiac SPECT. It was also shown that a slight improvement in count levels (from 320,000 counts to 640,000 counts in the maximum 5-second projection set) greatly decreases bias and variance in the kinetic parameter estimates. This effect has also been observed in ongoing canine studies, such as those discussed later, which show that bias and variance in the parameter estimates are substantially reduced by increasing the injection of ^{99m}Tc teboroxime from 15 mCi to 30 mCi. Of course, the maximum allowable levels of the injected radioactive-labeled tracer; the maximum count rate capability of the camera; and count-limiting factors, such as body attenuation, impose practical limits on the maximum counting rate.

Counts in the maximum tomographic acquisition depend on the gantry rotation acquisition interval and duration of the injection. By increasing the gantry rotation acquisition interval, more counts are obtained in the projection sets and errors in kinetic parameter estimates are reduced. However, the gantry acquisition interval cannot be increased indefinitely because temporal resolution is adversely affected by inadequate sampling of

the time-varying dynamics of the tracer. To compensate for this, the injection of the tracer can be slowed, thus reducing the high frequency components. However, this results in a reduced peak projection set, which results in larger errors in the param-eter estimates. It is therefore important to optimize both the input function shape and the image acquisition rate to obtain maximum projection counts and provide sufficient temporal resolution. The effects of input function shape and acquisition interval have been studied in dynamic PET.[152,171] However, because of the poor photon statistics associated with dynamic cardiac SPECT and its sequential projection acquisition, protocols that produce optimal kinetic parameter estimates in PET may produce suboptimal estimates in dynamic SPECT.

The effect of input function shape and acquisition interval on parameter estimates was studied with the MCAT phantom already described. Geometric point response and attenuation were not included in the projection data. The acquisition intervals were varied as already described. Blood time–activities were generated to correspond to a bolus infusion and 30-second, 60-second, and 90-second infusions. The myocardial tissue activity was simulated with two different kinetic models

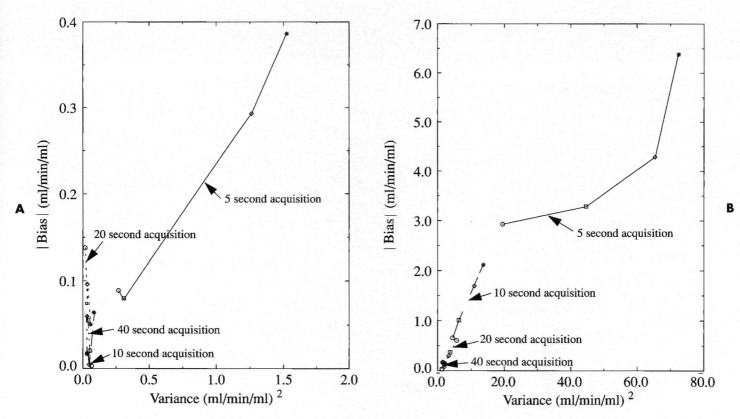

Fig. 11-21. Variance compared with absolute bias with noise simulating a 15-mCi injection of technetium-99m teboroxime into a 35-kg dog. **A,** Resting kinetic parameters; **B,** vasodilated kinetic parameters. $\bigcirc$ = Bolus infusion, $\square$ = 30-second infusion, $\diamond$ = 60-second infusion, and $*$ = 90-second infusion. (From Ross SG, Welch A, Gullberg GT, Huesman RH: An investigation into the effect of input function shape and image acquisition interval on estimates of washin for dynamic cardiac SPECT, *Phys Med Biol* 42:2193-2213, 1997. Reproduced with permission from IOP Publishing Limited.)

that were based on canine studies reported by Smith et al[193,194] as well as in our ongoing studies. The first model was typical of those found at baseline in a dog and had parameters f_v = 0.15, k_{21} = 0.8 min^{-1}, and k_{12} = 0.4 min^{-1}. Kinetic parameters typical of those observed in a dog vasodilated with adenosine were used in the second model; parameters were f_v = 0.15, k_{21} = 4.0 min^{-1}, and k_{12} = 2.0 min^{-1}. Dynamic reconstruction were obtained using 25 iterations of the ML-EM algorithm. A single reconstructed transaxial slice was used to draw blood and tissue regions of interest of 7.2 cm^3 and 4.2 cm^3, respectively. From these regions time–activity curves were generated and kinetic parameters were estimated using these curves.

The results of this study are shown in Fig. 11-21 and Fig. 11-22. The plots show the variance in estimates of washin compared with absolute bias in estimates of washin for each acquisition interval. The variances are based on a simulation of 100 realizations.

The plot in Fig. 11-21, A corresponds to resting kinetic parameters with noise simulating injection of 15 mCi of ^{99m}Tc teboroxime into a 35-kg dog. The largest variance occurs for a 5-second acquisition interval. Variance for the 5-second acqui-

sition interval is reduced by using a sharper input function. Variance levels decrease when 10-second, 20-second, and 40-second acquisition intervals are used. The smallest amount of bias is observed with a 10-second acquisition and a bolus infusion. The greatest amount of bias (ignoring 5-second acquisitions) is observed with a 20-second acquisition and a bolus infusion. This is probably attributable to integration effects that can cause the time–activity curves to be misrepresented. This occurs most often when the time from the injection to the peak of the time–activity curve corresponds to one acquisition interval. This effect is also observed when a 40-second acquisition interval is used with a 30-second and a 60-second infusion.

The results in Fig. 11-21, B correspond to vasodilated kinetic parameters with noise simulating 15 mCi injection of ^{99m}Tc teboroxime into a 35-kg dog. Variance levels are much larger than those observed for resting kinetics. Variance consistently decreases as the acquisition interval is lengthened. Along with variance levels, bias is also decreased as the acquisition interval is lengthened. This suggests that when kinetics are increased, count levels become more critical than with resting kinetics. The reduction in aliasing and, subsequently, in bias, that

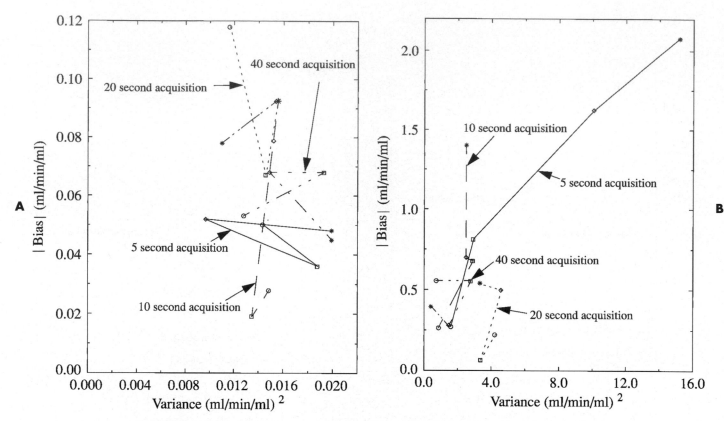

Fig. 11-22. Variance compared with absolute bias with noise simulating a 30-mCi injection of technetium-99m teboroxime into a 35-kg dog. **A,** Resting kinetic parameters; **B,** vasodilated kinetic parameters. O = Bolus infusion, □ = 30-second infusion, ◇ = 60-second infusion, and * = 90-second infusion. (From Ross SG, Welch A, Gullberg GT, Huesman RH: An investigation into the effect of input function shape and image acquisition interval on estimates of washin for dynamic cardiac SPECT, *Phys Med Biol* 42:2193-2213, 1997. Reproduced with permission from IOP Publishing Limited.)

is produced with 5-second acquisition, is not noticeable because of the high levels of variance. Bias and variance are less sensitive to input function shape than to acquisition interval. For 5- and 10-second acquisitions, the smallest amount of bias and variance was observed with shorter infusion rates. This trend was reversed with 20-second acquisition. A 40-second acquisition had the smallest amount of bias when 30-second and 60-second infusions were used. In general, as the acquisition interval was increased and count levels were subsequently increased, the input function shape had a less noticeable effect.

The results in Fig. 11-22, A correspond to resting kinetic parameters with noise simulating injection of 30 mCi of ^{99m}Tc teboroxime into a 35-kg dog. The higher photon count rates result in much smaller levels of variance than those observed for resting parameters in Fig. 11-21, A. Bias is also much lower with better photon statistics, with variance levels approximately one order of magnitude smaller than the bias levels. The results show that the effect of acquisition interval is much less distinct when count levels are increased. The minimum levels of variance for the estimates are observed with a 5-second acquisition and a 60-second infusion, although the differences in variance are not large for any of these esti-

mates. The plot shows no distinct trends, with the smallest amount of bias arising with a 10-second acquisition and a bolus infusion.

The results in Fig. 11-22, B correspond to vasodilated kinetic parameters with noise simulating injection of 30 mCi of ^{99m}Tc teboroxime into a 35-kg dog. Variance levels are now more sensitive to acquisition interval than they were with the resting parameters. Five-second acquisitions give high levels of variance when 60- and 90-second infusion rates are used. However, the variance levels are substantially lower than those observed when the injection was only 15 mCi. Levels of variance for 10-second acquisition are less sensitive to input function shape than those for 5-second acquisition, although variance is slightly reduced when a bolus infusion is used. Bias is greatly reduced by using a sharper input function for 5- and 10-second acquisitions. The results suggest that the acquisition interval is more critical than the infusion length, particularly when photon statistics are low.

Table 11-5 summarizes the optimal estimates obtained with each simulated protocol. The results imply that the input function shape and acquisition interval must be selected carefully depending on the count levels and kinetics associated with the

Table 11-5. Summary of results from simulations of various input functions and acquisition intervals with photon noise (100 realizations).* (From Ross SG, Welch A, Gullberg GT, Huesman RH: An investigation into the effect of input function shape and image acquisition interval on estimates of washin for dynamic cardiac SPECT, *Phys Med Biol* 42:2193-2213, 1997. Reproduced with permission from IOP Publishing Limited.)

	Simulation			
Protocol	15 mCi, resting	15 mCi, vasodilated	30 mCi, resting	30 mCi, vasodilated
Minimum bias	Bolus infusion 10-second acquisition	30-second infusion 40-second acquisition	30-second infusion 10-second acquisition	30-second infusion 20-second acquisition
Minimum variance	Bolus infusion 20-second acquisition	30-second infusion 40-second acquisition	60-second infusion 5-second acquisition	90-second infusion 40-second acquisition
Minimum $\sqrt{bias^2 + variance}$	Bolus infusion 40-second acquisition	30-second infusion 40-second acquisition	30-second infusion 10-second acquisition	90-second infusion 40-second acquisition

*Changes in estimates of wash in for different input function shape and image acquisition interval are not always significant. Figures 11-21 and 11-22 should be addressed to best interpret the data.

protocol. However, careful analysis of the results shown in Figs. 11-21 and 11-22 shows that in some cases, kinetic parameter estimates differ little for different input function shapes and image acquisition intervals. Longer acquisition intervals result in the most accurate estimates of kinetic parameters when vasodilated kinetics are assumed. When resting kinetics are assumed with a 15-mCi injection of ^{99m}Tc-labeled teboroxime into a 35-kg dog, a bolus infusion always provided optimal estimates of kinetic parameters. The smallest amount of bias was observed with a 10-second acquisition, the smallest amount of variance was seen with a 20-second acquisition, and the estimates with the least total $\sqrt{bias^2 + variance}$ were obtained with a 40-second acquisition. When the count rates were doubled, longer infusions and shorter acquisitions provided more accurate estimates of kinetic parameters when resting kinetics were simulated. When kinetics were increased to simulate vasodilated parameters, longer acquisition resulted in better estimates. This indicates that better signal-to-noise ratios are required when fast kinetics are to be estimated.

Attenuation

Photon attenuation is particularly important in dynamic SPECT. Unlike in PET, attenuation correction in SPECT is not achieved by a simple multiplicative correction of the data.[23] A method for correcting artifacts from attenuation described by Gullberg et al[77] is used here to examine the benefits of attenuation correction for dynamic cardiac SPECT.

The MCAT phantom described earlier is used to investigate the effects of attenuation. The attenuation and emission distributions are shown in Fig. 11-15, A and B. Geometric point response and photon noise were not included in these simulations. Ten-second intervals were used to acquire the dynamic projection data. A bolus infusion was used to model the blood time–activity; tissue activity corresponded to rate constants with $f_v = 0.15$, $k_{21} = 0.8$ min^{-1}, and $k_{12} = 0.4$ min^{-1}. A blood region was drawn in the left ventricle, and two tissue regions were drawn in the septal and lateral regions of the myocardial

Table 11-6. Comparison of kinetic parameter estimates obtained with and without attenuation correction

Type of correction	Kinetic parameter estimate with $k_{21} = 0.8$ ml/min/ml		Kinetic parameter estimate with $k_{12} = 0.4$ ml/min/ml	
	Septal region	Lateral region	Septal region	Lateral region
No correction	0.8920	1.008	0.377	0.410
Attenuation correction	0.838	0.868	0.381	0.413

tissue. Kinetic parameter estimates were obtained from time–activity curves by using RFIT. The results show that attenuation significantly biases k_{21} estimates (Table 11-6). In addition, attenuation correction has been shown to have significant effects on the accuracy of results in canine studies.

Other physical factors in image detection

The effect of other physical factors of dynamic cardiac SPECT on the accuracy and precision of estimated kinetic parameters has not yet been determined. Among these factors are scatter and lung motion. It may be possible to use methods that are currently being investigated in PET,[103,176,177] in which gating is used to correlate the data acquisition with the respiratory cycle. It may be easier to use this technique in dynamic cardiac SPECT than to use cardiac gating because the respiratory cycle is longer than the cardiac cycle and thus allows for better counting statistics. Dispersion of the tracer from the sample of the input function to the point of measurement has also not been studied.[156] If the left ventricular cavity is used to determine the input function, dispersion may not be a problem. However, if arterial or venous blood samples are taken, dispersion and knowledge of the arrival time can be a substantial problem.

The ultimate goals are to achieve a point-by-point measure of the absolute myocardial activity and to know its variation as a function of time. To do this, all of the physical aspects of dynamic cardiac SPECT must be fully investigated.

ESTIMATION OF MODEL PARAMETERS IN DOGS

Throughout this chapter, we have used computer simulations to illustrate many concepts that relate to dynamic cardiac SPECT. Computer simulations are particularly effective in helping to understand the effects of partial volume, cardiac motion, detector motion, input function shape, acquisition interval, and attenuation. However, because the image detection process and the physiologic processes associated with myocardial function are complex, animal studies are necessary to obtain realistic information on the usefulness of dynamic cardiac SPECT. Canine studies[193,194] have demonstrated that ^{99m}Tc teboroxime has the potential to quantitatively measure myocardial perfusion. Further work is needed to determine the effectiveness of dynamic cardiac SPECT in a clinical setting, and, in particular, to determine whether dynamic cardiac SPECT is a more quantitative technique than the nuclear cardiology procedures currently used. We present results of canine studies that evaluated the usefulness of dynamic cardiac SPECT in the kinetic analysis of ^{201}Tl, ^{99m}Tc teboroxime, ^{18}FDG, and ^{123}IPPA.

Motivation

The first objective of the canine studies was to determine whether measurement of the kinetics of ^{99m}Tc teboroxime with dynamic cardiac SPECT is a more sensitive indicator of ischemia than static SPECT imaging with ^{201}Tl. The second objective was to determine whether measurement of the kinetics of ^{18}FDG and ^{123}IPPA can be used to simultaneously determine perfusion and viability. Other issues addressed in the studies included the effect of photon statistics on variability of estimates of washin, the effect of cardiac motion on parameter estimates, the effect of partial volume on parameter estimates, the variability of flow in the myocardium, and the variability of microsphere trapping in the myocardium.

Animal preparation

In each study, a dog weighing approximately 30 kg was initially sedated with 5 mg/kg of telazol and attached to a ventilator dispensing oxygen and halothane (1% to 10%). The chest was opened at the fourth left intercostal space, and the heart was suspended in a pericardial cradle. An ultrasonic flow probe was placed on the left anterior descending artery. A second flow probe was placed over the aorta to measure cardiac output. On each dog, an occlusion study or a nonocclusion study was performed. During occlusion studies, a vascular occluder (In Vivo Metrics, Healdsburg, California) was placed distal to the flow probe. A catheter was placed in the left atrium for injection of microspheres, and the chest was closed with nonmetallic sutures. The abdominal cavity was opened, and the liver was physically pushed away from the heart and supported with gauze. This was done to avoid contamination of the myocardial tissue region with liver activity. A shunt was made from one of the femoral arteries to the femoral vein. A gamma-radiation detector was placed over the shunt to measure radiation in the arterial blood during the study. An intravenous drip was placed in an antecubital vein in the foreleg, and a catheter was placed in the left femoral artery to measure blood pressure. The lungs were tucked below the heart, the pericardial cradle was left intact, and the chest wall was closed. Blood pressure, electrocardiogram, and blood gases were monitored to ensure normal physiologic conditions. After preparation, the dog was transferred to the three-detector SPECT system for imaging.

Data acquisition

Protocol 1. Static ^{201}Tl imaging was compared with dynamic SPECT using ^{99m}Tc teboroxime. A three-detector SPECT scanner (PRISM 3000XP, Picker International, Cleveland, Ohio) was used to perform the scans. The dogs were placed on their right sides and positioned so that the heart was in the center of the field of view. High-resolution fan-beam collimators with a focal length of 65 cm were used. First, the transmission scan was performed for each dog using a gadolinium line source for 15 minutes; during this time, 120 angles were acquired over 360 degrees by using step-and-shoot mode. The dog was not moved during or after this scan. Immediately after the transmission scan, a 10-mmol/L adenosine and saline mixture was infused into an artery. The flow in the left anterior descending coronary artery (LAD) was raised to approximately three times the baseline flow. Once the flow seemed to have reached a constant value, the adenosine infusion was reduced and maintained at a constant level.

Next, the stress ^{201}Tl scan was begun. This scan was performed by using a continuous circular orbit that acquired 120 angles over 360 degrees with a 20% energy window centered at 80 keV. Approximately 2 mCi of ^{201}Tl was injected through an antecubital vein in the foreleg of the dog. In occlusion studies, a second ^{201}Tl scan was performed at rest. Adenosine administration was terminated and blood flow was returned as near as possible to the baseline. A second ^{201}Tl scan was then performed with approximately 4 mCi of ^{201}Tl.

Next, two ^{99m}Tc teboroxime dynamic SPECT scans were done. If occlusion was being performed (flow was at baseline for the last ^{201}Tl scan), a rest ^{99m}Tc teboroxime scan was followed by a stress ^{99m}Tc teboroxime scan. If no occlusion was being performed (flow was vasodilated for the second ^{201}Tl scan), a stress ^{99m}Tc teboroxime scan was followed by a rest ^{99m}Tc teboroxime scan. In the first scan, approximately 15 mCi of ^{99m}Tc teboroxime was injected as a bolus. Five-second dynamic projection sets were acquired for 15 minutes. In the second scan, approximately 30 mCi of ^{99m}Tc teboroxime was injected as a bolus, and five-second dynamic projection sets were acquired for 15 minutes. During each scan, a radiation monitor was placed over the arterioventricular shunt to monitor the activity in the blood. The data from the monitor could then be used as a separate measure of blood activity to compare with the image-derived activity.

At the start of each scan, microspheres were injected according to the methods of Heymann et al.[92] to serve as a gold standard for blood flow. At the end of the study, the dog was sacrificed and the heart was excised. The heart was cut into uniform sections for counting of the microspheres.

Protocol 2. The kinetics of ^{201}Tl, ^{18}FDG, and ^{123}IPPA were compared in a single dog. The standard imaging procedures described above were used, with the following modifications. A transmission scan was performed first, followed by a ^{201}Tl dynamic SPECT study; a ^{123}IPPA dynamic SPECT study; and, finally, a ^{18}FDG dynamic SPECT study. Between the ^{123}IPPA and ^{18}FDG study, collimators were changed from low-energy, high-resolution fan-beam collimators to ultra–high-energy parallel-hole collimators to image the 511-keV photons of ^{18}FDG. Projections of 120 angles sampled over 360 degrees were acquired after an injected dose as follows: ^{201}Tl, 30 $\times$ 10 seconds followed by 25 $\times$ 60 seconds = 30 minutes total (dose, 3 mCi); ^{123}IPPA, 60 $\times$ 10 seconds followed by 50 $\times$ 60 seconds = 60 minutes (dose, 11 mCi); and ^{18}FDG, 60 $\times$ 10 seconds followed by 50 $\times$ 60 seconds = 60 minutes (dose of 17 mCi).

Data analysis

Protocol 1. The 180 dynamic projection sets were reconstructed by using 25 iterations of ML-EM with attenuation correction. The voxel dimensions were 0.712 cm in the x, y, and z directions. All but the first 30 reconstructed images were summed to create an image with sufficient quality to draw regions of interest. Regions were drawn on short-axis slices in the left ventricle blood pool and in the myocardial tissue as shown in Fig. 11-23. The blood regions were generally drawn from three slices located in the left ventricle with a volume of approximately 4.33 cm^3. The myocardial tissue regions were drawn in six or seven short-axis slices. Each region was 7 mm thick and varied in size from 4 cm^3 to 7 cm^3. Kinetic parameters were then estimated by using RFIT.

Protocol 2. The dynamic projection sets were reconstructed by using 25 iterations of the ML-EM algorithm to ob-

tain attenuation-corrected dynamic reconstructions. No attenuation correction was performed for the ^{18}FDG reconstructions. Time–activity curves of the blood and myocardial tissue were generated. For the blood, a 4-cm^3 region in the left ventricular cavity was selected, except in the ^{18}FDG study, in which plasma samples were used instead. The entire left ventricle was selected for the generation of the tissue time–activity curves. The ^{201}Tl time–activity curves were fitted to a one-compartment model (Fig. 11-2), the ^{18}FDG time–activity curves were fitted to a two-compartment model (Fig. 11-4) with $\beta = 1$, and the ^{123}IPPA time–activity curves were fitted to a three-compartment model (Fig. 11-5) with $\beta_1 = \beta_2 = 1$. The results were compared with ^{99m}Tc teboroxime time–activity curves generated from another study performed on a separate day. The ^{99m}Tc teboroxime time–activity curves were also fitted to a one-compartment model (Fig. 11-2).

Initial results

Technetium-99m teboroxime dynamic SPECT compared with static thallium-201 imaging. Estimates of the washin of ^{99m}Tc teboroxime are compared with relative intensity measurements of ^{201}Tl for each region of interest. Table 11-7 shows the correlation coefficient of estimates of washin compared with ^{201}Tl intensity for six dogs. It can be seen that washin correlates well with ^{201}Tl intensity. In addition, washin provides a measure of perfusion times extraction. This is shown in Fig. 11-24, in which estimates of washin are compared with microsphere flow measurements in regions of interest (corresponding to Fig. 11-23) for a dog with occlusion. Figure 11-24, A shows a regression plot of microsphere flow compared with estimates of washin of ^{99m}Tc teboroxime from a stress scan, and Fig. 11-24, B shows results as a plot of heart region compared with microsphere flow and estimates of washin. Figure 11-24, C shows a regress plot of microsphere flow compared with measures of ^{201}Tl intensity from the baseline scan, and Fig. 11-24, D shows the same results as a plot of heart region compared with microsphere flow and measurements of ^{201}Tl intensity.

The results indicate a strong correlation between ^{99m}Tc teboroxime washin and ^{201}Tl intensity. In addition, ^{201}Tl and ^{99m}Tc teboroxime correlated with the microsphere data. The re-

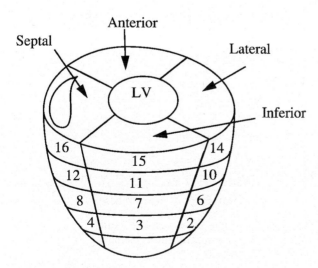

Fig. 11-23. Diagram indicating the position of the myocardial tissue regions of interest.

Table 11-7. Correlation of technetium-99m teboroxime washin to thallium-201 static intensities in canine studies

Canine study	Correlation (washin to ^{201}Tl)
No occlusion	
1	0.713
2	0.735
3	0.837
Occlusion	
4	0.754
5	0.842
6	0.943

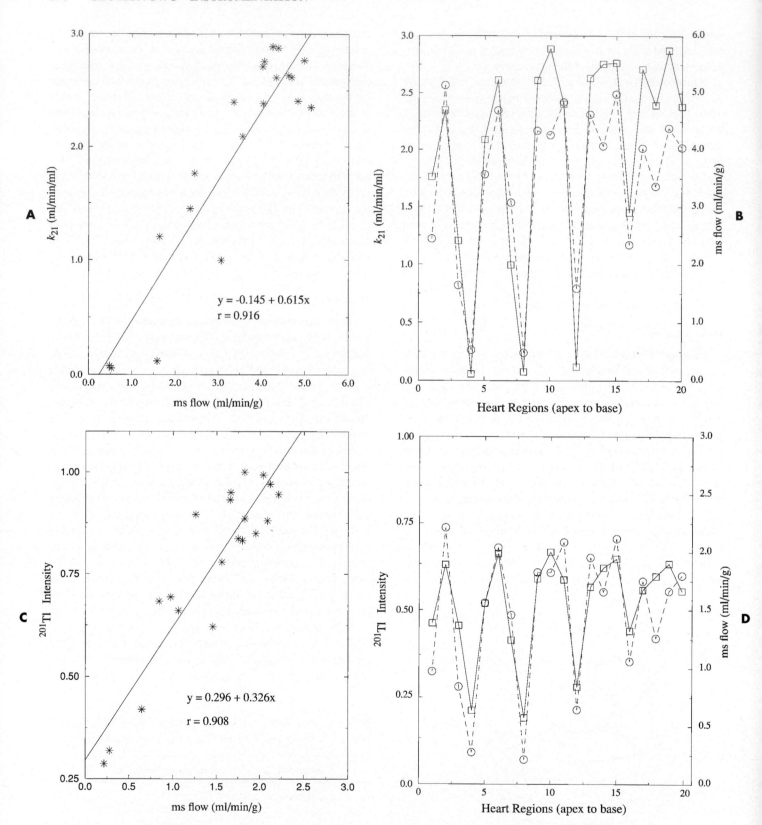

Fig. 11-24. Results from an occluded canine study. **A,** Microsphere *(ms)* flow vs estimates of washin (k_{21}); **B,** heart region vs microsphere flow and estimates of washin; **C,** microsphere flow vs thallium-201 intensity; **D,** heart region vs microsphere flow and thallium-201 intensity.

sults suggest that estimates of the washin of ^{99m}Tc teboroxime can provide relative flow measurements with a sensitivity similar to that of ^{201}Tl.

Dynamic SPECT comparison of the kinetics of thallium-201, technetium-99m teboroxime, fluorine-18 fluorodeoxyglucose, and iodine-123 iodophenylpentadecanoic acid. Comparison of the kinetic parameters for ^{201}Tl, ^{99m}Tc teboroxime, ^{123}IPPA, and ^{18}FDG are presented in Table 11-8. The estimates of the kinetic parameters were obtained from the time–activity curves shown in Fig. 11-25. Flow-times-extraction value (washin, k_{21}) is greatest for ^{99m}Tc teboroxime; that of ^{99m}Tc teboroxime is greater than that of ^{123}IPPA; it is about equal for ^{123}IPPA and ^{201}Tl; and that of ^{201}Tl is greater than that of ^{18}FDG. For ^{99m}Tc teboroxime, the large flow-times-extraction value is indicative of an excellent flow tracer. The slower flow-times-extraction for ^{201}Tl and the washout rate constant may be indicative of active transport. Thus, ^{201}Tl dynamic SPECT may be useful for viability. The ^{123}IPPA blood curve does not clear as one would expect, indicating that some metabolites in the blood were not modeled or that the myocardium preferentially metabolizes glucose instead of fatty acids. For ^{18}FDG, it is important to correct for geometric point response to avoid bias and to minimize tissue contamination in the blood caused by partial volume effects. As expected, the tissue curves for ^{18}FDG show a continual increase because phosphorylated ^{18}FDG is trapped in the cell mitochondria. It was pointed out by Stefan Eberl [private communication] that our distribution volume (k_{21}/k_{12}) for ^{201}Tl was an order of magnitude lower than from their experience. It could be that we did not collect the ^{201}Tl dynamic data long enough to adequately sample the washout of ^{201}Tl from the myocardium. It has been suggested that samples should be taken for several hours at hourly intervals after the initial rapid sampling of the uptake and initial washout phase.

Data visualization

Clinical use of kinetic parameters may require the development of new and unique methods for summarizing the information. For example, the k_{21} parameters from one of the dynamic SPECT ^{99m}Tc teboroxime canine studies performed in our laboratory are shown in Table 11-9 for 24 manually selected regions. The parameters correspond to regions drawn over the septal, lateral, inferior, and anterior short-axis regions described earlier. In the table, slice 1 refers to the most apical short-axis slice used and slice 6 refers to the most basal short-axis slice used. The same data are plotted in Fig. 11-26, in which the washin variability is more clearly seen.

The data can also be viewed by using polar bull's-eye plots. This type of data representation has greatly enhanced the reading and use of myocardial perfusion data in static SPECT and PET. Similar representation of kinetic parameters may offer improvements in dynamic SPECT and PET. Tables of kinetic parameters, such as Table 11-9, are dense, making the detection of trends difficult. The data are easier to digest by matching them to the regions of the myocardium that they represent, as in bull's-eyes. To create a bull's-eye plot, the image of the heart is warped into a standard format when fits are done for regions. The relative value of the k_{21} parameter appears as an intensity in each region. Parametric bull's-eye plots for adenosine stress and rest canine ^{99m}Tc teboroxime studies are shown in Fig. 11-27. The images are individually scaled to bring out variability and patterns. The plot (Fig. 11-26) is perhaps more useful for visualizing the level of differences as opposed to the pattern of differences. Error bull's-eyes, for example, would be so dim that no detail could be seen compared with k_{21} polar plots. A study with an occlusion of the LAD is shown in Fig. 11-28. The occlusion is easily identified from the bull's-eye. The wash-out (k_{12}) and fraction of blood in the tissue (f_v) show more variability, and the occlusion is more difficult to detect when examining the polar plots for f_v and k_{12}. This follows from the work of Smith et al,[193] who found that the washin correlates more highly with flow than does washout (k_{12}) or f_v. Ischemic zones typically do not wash out as quickly. Washout is flow dependent, so if flow is equalized after stress, delayed ^{99m}Tc teboroxime images may display fixed (ischemic) defects.

Another important step is the creation of normal files to assess when areas of low kinetic parameter values correspond to low flow rather than to variability caused by noise and the imaging and fitting process. Normal files may be created in tabular or plot type form, but are often easier to interpret in the

Table 11-8. Comparison of kinetic rate parameters for thallium-201, technetium-99m teboroxime, fluorine-18 fluorodeoxyglucose, and iodine-123 iodophenylpentadecanoic acid

Radionuclide	k_{21}	k_{12}	k_{32}	k_{23}	k_{42}	k_{54}	f_v
Thallium-201*	0.44	0.27	–†	–†	–†	–†	0.23
Technetium-99m teboroxime*	0.94	0.38	–†	–†	–†	–†	0.41
Fluorine-18 fluorodeoxyglucose‡	0.21	1.42	0.13	0.001	–†	–†	0.13
Iodine-123 iodophenylpentadecanoic acid§	0.47	0.22	–3.2	0.013	3.3	0.013	0.40
Iodine-123 iodophenylpentadecanoic acid‡	0.49	0.25	–0.01	0.03	–†	–†	0.39

*Fitted to a one-compartment model.
†The rate constant was not included in the model.
‡Fitted to a two-compartment model.
§Fitted to a three-compartment model.

Table 11-9. Kinetic parameter k_{21} (washin) from a dynamic SPECT canine study using ^{99m}Tc teboroxime*

Physiological condition	Slice																							
	1				**2**				**3**				**4**				**5**				**6**			
									REGION															
	S	A	L	I	S	A	L	I	S	A	L	I	S	A	L	I	S	A	L	I	S	A	L	I
Stress	2.3	2.6	2.8	2.8	2.7	2.2	3.3	2.9	2.7	2.6	3.3	3.0	2.5	2.4	3.2	3.0	2.2	2.3	3.1	2.9	1.6	2.3	2.3	2.1
(Error)	.10	.15	.12	.14	.15	.11	.17	.14	.15	.15	.17	.16	.15	.14	.17	.17	.15	.16	.20	.24	.15	.17	.13	.14
Rest	.83	.91	1.0	.98	.97	.84	1.1	1.0	.98	.97	1.2	1.1	1.0	.92	1.2	1.1	.95	.99	1.2	1.1	.88	.97	.94	1.0
(Error)	.04	.04	.04	.04	.06	.04	.04	.04	.06	.05	.06	.05	.07	.05	.05	.05	.08	.06	.06	.06	.09	.06	.04	.05

* Error values reflect the standard deviations estimated for each k_{21} fit.
S, septal region; A, anterior region; L, lateral region; I, inferior region.

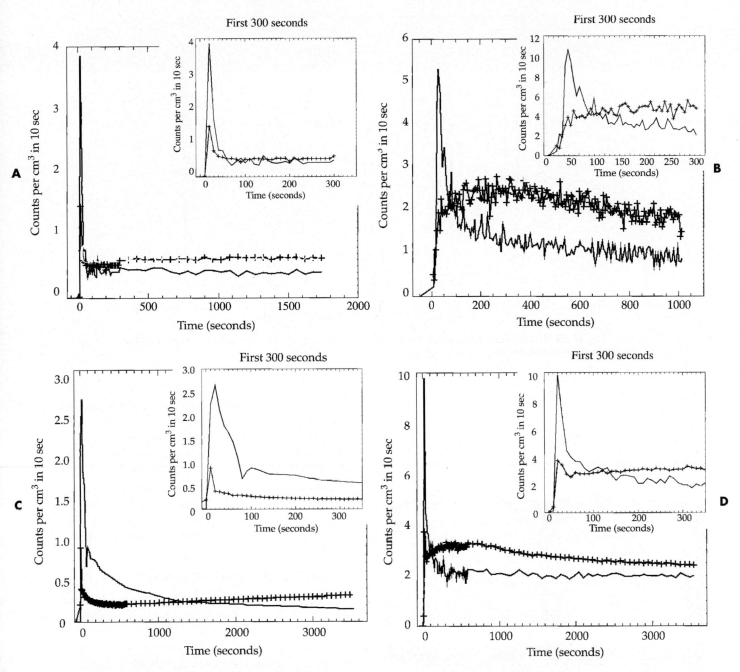

Fig. 11-25. Time–activity curves generated from canine dynamic single-photon emission computed tomography studies. **A,** thallium-201; **B,** technetium-99m teboroxime; **C,** 2-[^{18}F] fluorodeoxyglucose; **D,** iodine-123 iodophenylpentadecanoic acid.

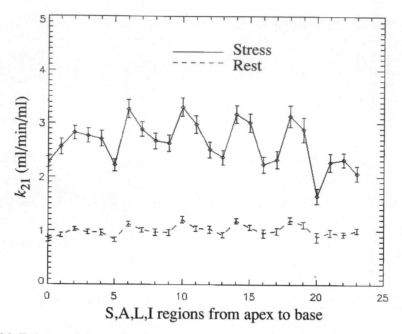

Fig. 11-26. Estimates of the washin rate parameter k_{21} from one canine study using technetium-99m teboroxime with adenosine stress and rest.

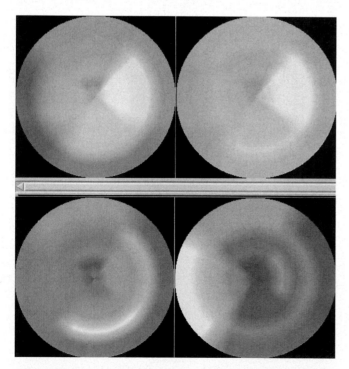

Fig. 11-27. Bull's-eye plots for the washin parameter k_{21} *(top)* and error estimates for the k_{21} parameters *(bottom)* from a technetium-99m-teboroxime canine study.

bull's-eye format. Making a diagnosis without normal files is almost impossible—if the normal files are not given explicitly, they are stored in the clinician's mind as the result of clinical experience. Registration with microspheres is somewhat simplified when represented in bull's-eye form. One can rapidly assess whether a rotation would better align the data sets.

Further work in processing and displaying dynamic cardiac SPECT data is needed to make timely and accurate clinical decisions. The bull's-eye promises to aid in the use of kinetic parameter estimates.

SUMMARY AND FUTURE DIRECTIONS

This chapter highlights some of the important compartment modeling and data processing aspects of dynamic cardiac SPECT. It shows how dynamic cardiac SPECT builds on much of the work in dynamic PET. However, key differences between these methods are noted, particularly in the areas of instrumentation and the physics of the image detection process. Specifically, SPECT has poorer spatial resolution and poorer statistics than PET, factors that have motivated research on automated extraction of time–activity curves that are reproducible, efficient, and accurate. The poor statistics associated with dynamic cardiac SPECT have also spurred the development of methods that can be used to estimate compartment model parameters that more efficiently use data. In most applications of dynamic cardiac SPECT, problems with detector movement occur during the transit of the radiopharmaceutical through the myocardium. This movement produces inconsistent equations for tomographic reconstruction and has directed research toward estimating kinetic parameters directly from projection data. In general, the model of the image detection

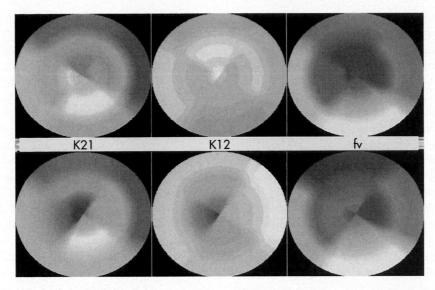

Fig. 11-28. Parametric bull's-eye plots. *Top row,* Baseline study of a dog. *Bottom row,* With occlusion of the left anterior descending coronary artery. *Left to right,* Washin (k_{21}), washout (k_{12}), and fraction of blood in tissue (f_v).

process is more complicated with SPECT; specifically, the attenuation problem in SPECT is much more complicated to compensate for than that in PET. Because of the resulting algorithm complications, it is difficult to obtain reconstructions in a timely manner and to obtain error estimates that are useful for evaluation of the appropriateness of the compartment models for representing the kinetics of the tracer. These difficulties associated with modeling of the SPECT imaging physics have led us to investigate the use of SVDs to solve large systems of linear equations. However, even with these difficulties, the results of compartment modeling applied in three applications are exciting. Results of canine experiments were presented that demonstrate that dynamic cardiac SPECT can obtain estimates of flow kinetics by using ^{99m}Tc teboroxime and ^{201}Tl, metabolism of glucose by using ^{18}FDG, and the potential for estimating metabolism of fatty acids by using ^{123}IPPA in myocardial tissue.

Data segmentation techniques are vital for the processing of dynamic SPECT data. Because of the large amount of data, automatic or semiautomatic approaches are essential for minimizing operator involvement and for efficient production of accurate and reproducible results within a study as well as between studies performed at other times. It is difficult for a user to reliably differentiate and select blood and tissue regions when there is significant statistical noise and poor region delineation due to poor resolution. It is anticipated that automated methods of selecting regions of interest will produce more accurate and reliable kinetic parameter estimates than those that are obtained with user interaction. Automatic methods can be optimized to minimize the tissue contamination in the blood pool and the background contamination in the tissue regions of the myocardium, thereby reducing the bias in parameter estimates. The use of factor analysis methods may be useful in separating regions on the basis of the characteristics of their known time–activity curves. For instance, the myocardium time–activity curve may be separated from background time–activity curves or liver time–activity curves. A model-based or population-based description of the input function may also be useful to obtain a more accurate and reproducible definition of the input function for the study by aiding in the segmentation of the blood region. It also may be helpful in specifying the input function, thereby obviating the need to obtain the information from image-derived reconstructions. As discussed earlier, segmentation plays a role in the estimation of parameters from projections as well.

The efficient use of noisy data obtained from a dynamic cardiac SPECT study is crucial in obtaining meaningful estimates of kinetic parameters for small tissue regions in the myocardium. The mathematics developed in this chapter is presented with this goal in mind. First, the estimation of reconstructed regions of activity was discussed. The use of matrix inversion reconstruction to solve a large linear estimation problem illustrated a means for estimating reconstruction errors and covariances between regions of interest. Estimates of correlations between regions must be calculated to obtain weighted least-squares estimates of the compartment kinetic parameters because the tissue model and the blood input obtained from the dynamic reconstructions are correlated by the assumed model. Second, by using the reconstructed error estimates, it was shown how compartment model parameters were estimated from time–activity curves generated from reconstructed regions of interest. In addition, a computer simulation showed that the use of weighted least-squares in both the reconstruction and the estimates the parameters gave lower variance plus square of the bias, demonstrating the possibility that data may be used more efficiently. A true knowledge of the errors in the estimates is also necessary when evaluating the appropriateness of the model for the kinetics of the pharmaceutical that one is attempting to model. Biases are an indicator of model mismatch that stems from the reconstruction process and estimates of compartment model parameters that model the tracer kinetics. Unfortunately, calculating SVDs to invert the 3228×3228 matrices requires 33 minutes on an SGI Power-Challenge (75 Mhz processors with 64-bit registers and 2 Gbyte of memory) for one transaxial slice. For 20 slices of 180 dynamic reconstructions, this would take approximately 1980 hours (83.5 days) of computational time, which would not be feasible on a routine basis with present computer technology.

The use of estimation of kinetic parameters from projections may enable dynamic SPECT to be performed at most SPECT facilities. The results presented in this chapter indicate that unbiased estimates are obtained from tomographic acquisitions of 1 minute, which is much longer than the 5-second acquisitions used in our dynamic SPECT studies with a three-detector SPECT system. Thus, single-detector SPECT systems (with arterial blood sampling) may be used instead of multiple-detector systems. This would significantly reduce the cost of this procedure. However, a single-detector system cannot provide the higher quality statistics that can be obtained with a multiple-detector SPECT system. An important aspect of estimating kinetic parameters from projections is the development of techniques to segment such regions as ventricular blood, myocardial tissue, background, and liver, to form the projection equations for the various desired regions of interest. Currently, these estimations cannot be obtained with dynamic cardiac SPECT. This will probably have to be done by first obtaining an estimate of the regions from the three-dimensional reconstruction of the inconsistent projections. It may also be necessary to develop models for large regions, such as the background, that can have many spectral components that represent the kinetics for several tissue types. Also, of interest is the possibility of estimating multiple spectral components for each pixel directly from the projection data.

The estimation of kinetic parameters directly from the projections may be computationally intensive. It may be necessary to develop more efficient methods for calculating kinetic parameters from rotating-detector SPECT systems. Better interpolation schemes will help improve the inconsistent projection data caused by the rotating SPECT camera. The possibility of using weighted integration to estimate kinetic parameters for certain compartment models is especially appealing. This approach would be extremely efficient and would greatly reduce data storage requirements. Experiments with PET have shown that much of the data processing can be accomplished in hardware.

Accurate modeling of the physics of the image detection process is critical to making dynamic cardiac SPECT a clinical reality. The model mismatch is complicated by two levels of parameter estimation: estimation of the reconstructed dynamic images and estimation of the compartment model parameters. Results from computer simulations illustrate the effects of partial volume, cardiac motion, detector motion, input function shape and acquisition interval, and attenuation on the bias and variance of model parameter estimates. Scatter and lung motion were not addressed in this chapter but are also important. Specifically, partial volume has a substantial effect on the estimated kinetic parameters, necessitating careful selection of regions of interest. The improvement in bias with correction for the geometric response and scatter is being investigated.

There is concern about data storage and data processing if dynamic cardiac SPECT is to become a routine clinical procedure. A typical study will acquire as much as 2×180 (stress/rest) Mbytes of data (120 64×64 projections for each of the 180 dynamic tomographic data sets). Because iterative or matrix inversion reconstructions are used to correct for attenuation, geometric response, and scatter, the computation time is lengthy. The present reconstruction time to perform 25 iterations with attenuation correction for one dynamic study of 180 43×43 three-dimensional reconstructions (each with 34 transaxial slices) from 120 projection angles is 20 hours on a SUN ULTRA Enterprise 3000 (4 167-MHz Ultra SPARC processors). Future computers with 500-MHz and, eventually, 1000-MHz processors will reduce this processing time considerably. The processing time to perform matrix inversion would require much longer time.

The results presented in this chapter show that ^{99m}Tc teboroxime is an excellent marker of flow. The results of canine studies show that the estimated washin and washout rate constants in a one-compartment model correlate with flow and that the washin parameter k_{21} is a more sensitive measure of flow than is k_{12}. It is anticipated that the estimation of kinetic parameters will yield more dynamic range than the mapping of flow based on the intensity uptake of the radiopharmaceutical from a static study, the method used when using ^{201}Tl to detect ischemia or infarct. It is known that ^{99m}Tc teboroxime follows flow linearly over a longer range of flows than does ^{201}Tl or ^{99m}Tc sestamibi. This means that the use of dynamic SPECT with ^{99m}Tc teboroxime may be better for predicting flow reserve between a rest and a stress study. However, this hypothesis has not yet been proven. More investigation is needed to verify that ^{99m}Tc teboroxime is metabolized and retained in the blood as are labeled metabolites of ^{13}N-ammonia[132,160,180] when using ^{13}NH$_3$ in PET blood flow studies. More study is needed to evaluate whether dynamic SPECT imaging with ^{99m}Tc teboroxime is a more sensitive marker of ischemia or viability than is ^{201}Tl or ^{99m}Tc sestamibi.

The study performed with ^{201}Tl was encouraging in that the results from estimates of the kinetic model parameters seemed to represent what is known of the kinetics of ^{201}Tl in myocardial tissue. The washin rate constant was half of that of teboroxime. However, this smaller flow-times-extraction may indicate that the distribution of ^{201}Tl is facilitated by active transport and, thus, that ^{201}Tl is useful for evaluation of perfusion and viability. Research is ongoing in this area with the aim of measuring both myocardial perfusion and volume of distribution, which is believed to be directly linked to viability. Our results and those of Iida et al[119] demonstrate that ^{201}Tl correlates well with flow. Iida et al[119] suggested that a two-compartment model is more appropriate for measuring the kinetics of ^{201}Tl than the one-compartment model that was used to fit our data presented in this chapter. They also stressed the importance of sampling blood that is devoid of erythrocytes to obtain an input function from counting only plasma samples.

The SPECT NaI(Tl) detector is not the optimal detector for imaging ^{18}FDG. However, ^{18}FDG has high affinity for viable myocardial tissue because of ^{18}FDG's utility as a marker of metabolism. Preliminary canine results presented in this chapter show that dynamic SPECT can obtain data of sufficient quality (statistical, temporal, and spatial resolution) to track the kinetics of ^{18}FDG, yielding reasonable estimates of the rate of myocardial uptake and the rate of metabolism. This could have significant use for evaluating myocardial viability but needs further evaluation. It can be difficult to resolve tissue from the ventricular blood pool in the dynamic reconstructions because of the poor spatial resolution (2 to 2.5 cm in the myocardium). This is because of the thick septa that are used to stop the high-energy 511-keV photons in combination with the large holes that are needed to obtain photon efficiency. The myocardium and blood pool are much better resolved if a proper point response correction is used in the reconstruction.

Application of dynamic SPECT may be necessary in some cases in which ^{123}IPPA is used to determine viable myocardium. It may be important to differentiate metabolism from uptake in triglyceride pools. Because both β-oxidation and triglyceride exchange may be measured with dynamic SPECT, dynamic cardiac SPECT may be necessary when using ^{123}IPPA to identify viable myocardium. An additional consideration in using dynamic SPECT with metabolic agents is the potential for obtaining flow and metabolism while using only one tracer. With static imaging techniques, simultaneous imaging of two tracers—a flow agent and a metabolic agent—is required to obtain flow and metabolism data.

As we mentioned earlier the ultimate goal is to achieve a point-by-point measure of the absolute activity and its variation in time. However, several influencing factors have yet to be fully addressed. Important developments have included simultaneous measurement of transmission and emission data so that attenuation correction can be achieved in a clinical setting as well as development of corrections for scatter and depth-dependent resolution with inclusion in iterative reconstruction algorithms. Much work still needs to be done in investigating problems associated with attenuation, scatter, and partial volume effects (caused by collimator response, motion of the myocardium, and lungs). Developing better models for the physics of the image detection process will help improve the bias of the estimated kinetic parameters by improving the model mismatch. These models must be implemented efficiently so that variance in the estimated parameters is minimized. The acceleration of these algorithms so that they are clinically feasible will also be important.[111] The OSEM algorithm will be useful in speeding up the calculations of the estimated parameters. There is also interest in developing list-mode expectation maximization algorithms for more accurate and efficient use of the data.[195]

In summary, SPECT has become an important diagnostic tool in cardiovascular nuclear medicine, and the role of radionuclide procedures using SPECT for diagnosis and therapeutic planning continues to grow. Dynamic SPECT potentially improves diagnostic accuracy over conventional SPECT at little, if any, increased cost. Because cardiovascular disease continues to be prevalent in the U.S. population, tests that allow noninvasive assessment of cardiac function, such as those involving dynamic cardiac SPECT, will continue to play an important role in clinical nuclear medicine. The results presented in this chapter increased our enthusiasm for dynamic cardiac SPECT imaging for three reasons. First, current three-detector systems can acquire data quickly enough to extract kinetic information with a spatial resolution useful for clinical diagnosis. Second, the physiologic properties of ^{201}Tl, ^{99m}Tc teboroxime, ^{18}FDG, and ^{123}IPPA make them excellent markers of flow and metabolism, which is valuable in the diagnosis of ischemia and viability. Finally, mathematical tools have demonstrated the ability to make efficient use of dynamic data to obtain accurate and precise estimates of kinetic parameters. These mathematical tools are essential for making dynamic cardiac SPECT a viable clinical tool and are useful in the application of dynamic SPECT to other organ systems, such as the kidney[76] and the brain.[115,223] The development of new mathematical tools, such as linear system theory for converting a large nonlinear estimation problem to a linear estimation problem,[63] is appealing. Some of these developments may also have significant implications for application to other imaging methods, such as the analysis of MRI kinetic data of the perfusion of endogenous excited protons.[79]

The results presented here are preliminary, and the clinical efficacy of dynamic SPECT imaging still awaits a thorough investigation of the utility of the technique. However, with proper attention to experimental design and processing of dynamic data, information about kinetic parameters can be obtained from noisy data sets; this will make dynamic SPECT a useful tool in clinical nuclear cardiology.

ACKNOWLEDGMENT

The research presented in this chapter was partially supported by National Institutes of Health grant no. RO1-HL-39792. The authors thank Brian Hutton for providing many helpful comments that have been incorporated into the text and Sean Webb for carefully proofreading the manuscript.

REFERENCES

1. Alpert NM, Eriksson L, Chang JY, et al: Strategy for the measurement of regional cerebral blood flow using short-lived tracers and emission tomography, *J Cereb Blood Flow Metab* 4:28–34, 1984.
2. Antar M: *Radiolabeled fatty acids for myocardial studies.* In: Spencer RP, ed: *New procedures in nuclear medicine,* Boca Raton, Fla, 1989, CRC Press, pp 95–126.
3. Antar M: Radiopharmaceuticals for studying cardiac metabolism, *Int J Rad Appl Instrum [B]* 17:103–128, 1990.
4. Araujo LI, Lammertsma AA, Rhodes CG, et al: Noninvasive quantification of regional myocardial blood flow in coronary artery disease

with oxygen-15-labeled carbon dioxide inhalation and positron emission tomography, *Circulation* 83:875–885, 1991.

5. Atkinson KE: *An introduction to numerical analysis,* 2, New York, 1989, John Wiley and Sons.

6. Barber DC: The use of principal components in the quantitative analysis of gamma camera dynamic studies, *Phys Med Biol* 25: 283–292, 1980.

7. Bard Y: *Nonlinear parameter estimation,* New York, 1974, Academic Press.

8. Barrett HH, Wilson DW, Tsui BMW: Noise properties of the EM algorithm: I. Theory, *Phys Med Biol* 39:833–846, 1994.

9. Bassingthwaighte JB: A concurrent flow model for extraction during transcapillary passage, *Circ Res* 35:483–503, 1974.

10. Bassingthwaighte JB, Raymond GM, Chan JI: *Principles of tracer kinetics.* In Zaret BL, Beller GA, eds: *Nuclear cardiology: state of the art and future directions,* St. Louis, 1993, Mosby, pp 3–23.

11. Beck JV, Arnold KJ: *Parameter estimation in engineering and science,* New York, 1977, John Wiley and Sons.

12. Beekman FJ, Kamphuis C, Viergever MA: Improved SPECT quantitation using fully three-dimensional iterative spatially variant scatter response compensation, *IEEE Trans Med Imaging* 15:491–499, 1996.

13. Bellina CR, Parodi O, Camici P, et al: Simultaneous in vitro and in vivo validation of nitrogen-13-ammonia for the assessment of regional myocardial blood flow, *J Nucl Med* 31:1335–1343, 1990.

14. Bergmann SR, Fox KAA, Rand AL, et al: Quantification of regional myocardial blood flow in vivo with $H_2^{15}O$, *Circulation* 70:724–733, 1984.

15. Bergmann SR, Herrero P, Markham J, et al: Noninvasive quantitation of myocardial blood flow in human subjects with oxygen-15-labeled water and positron emission tomography, *J Am Coll Cardiol* 14:639–652, 1989.

16. Bontemps L, Geronicola-Trapali X, Sayegh Y, et al: Technetium-99m teboroxime scintigraphy. Clinical experience in patients referred for myocardial perfusion evaluation, *Eur J Nucl Med* 18: 732–739, 1991.

17. Brownlee KA: *Statistical theory and methodology in science and engineering* ed 2, Malabar, Fla, 1984, Robert E. Krieger Publishing Company, Inc.

18. Budinger TF: *Physiology and physics of nuclear cardiology.* In Willerson JT, ed: *Nuclear cardiology,* Philadelphia, 1979, F.A. Davis & Co., pp. 9–77.

19. Budinger TF: *Dynamic SPECT opens new horizons for technetium radiopharmaceutical applications and new challenges for ligand designs.* In Nicolini M, Bandoli G, Mazzi U, eds: *Technetium and rhenium in chemistry and nuclear medicine,* 4th International Symposium on Technetium Chemistry and Nuclear Medicine, Bressanone, Italy, 1995, pp 475–489.

20. Budinger TF, Araujo L, Ranger N, et al: Dynamic SPECT feasibility studies, *J Nucl Med* 32:955, 1991 (abstract).

21. Budinger TF, Derenzo SE, Huesman RH, et al: Medical criteria for the design of a dynamic positron tomograph for heart studies, *IEEE Trans Nucl Sci* NS-29:488–492, 1982.

22. Budinger TF, Derenzo SE, Huesman RH, et al: Quantitative myocardial flow-extraction data using gated ECT, *J Nucl Med* 21:P16, 1980 (abstract).

23. Budinger TF, Gullberg GT, Huesman RH: *Emission computed tomography.* In Herman GT, ed: *Image reconstruction from projections: implementation and applications,* New York, 1979, Springer-Verlag, pp 147–246.

24. Budinger TF, Huesman RH: Ten precepts for quantitative data acquisition and analysis, *Circulation* 72(5 Pt 2):IV53–IV62, 1985.

25. Budinger TF, Huesman RH, Knittel B, et al: *Physiological modeling of dynamic measurements of metabolism using positron emission tomography.* In Greitz T, Ingvar DH, Widen L, eds: *The metabolism of the human brain studied with positron emission tomography,* New York, 1985, Raven Press, pp 165–183.

26. Budinger TF, Yano Y, Hoop B: A comparison of $^{82}Rb^+$ and $^{13}NH_3$ for myocardial positron scintigraphy, *J Nucl Med* 16:429–431, 1975.

27. Carson RE: A maximum likelihood method for region-of-interest evaluation in emission tomography, *J Comput Assist Tomogr* 10:654–663, 1986.

28. Carson RE: *Parameter estimation in positron emission tomography.* In Phelps ME, Mazziotta J, Schelbert H, eds: *Positron emission tomography and autoradiography: principles and applications for the brain and heart,* New York, 1986, Raven Press, pp 347–390.

29. Carson RE, Huang SC, Green MV: Weighted integration method for local cerebral blood flow measurements with positron emission tomography, *J Cereb Blood Flow and Metab* 6:245–258, 1986.

30. Carson RE, Lange K: The EM parametric image reconstruction algorithm, *J Amer Statist Assoc* 80:20–22, 1985.

31. Chan SY, Brunken RC, Phelps ME, et al: Use of the metabolic tracer carbon-11-acetate for evaluation of regional myocardial perfusion, *J Nucl Med* 32:665–672, 1991.

32. Chiao P-C, Ficaro EP, Dayanikli F, et al: Compartmental analysis of technetium-99m-teboroxime kinetics employing fast dynamic SPECT at rest and stress, *J Nucl Med* 35:1265–1273, 1994.

33. Chiao P-C, Rogers WL, Clinthorne NH, et al: Model-based estimation for dynamic cardiac studies using ECT, *IEEE Trans Med Imaging* 13:217–226, 1994.

34. Chiao P-C, Rogers WL, Fessler JA, et al: Model-based estimation with boundary side information or boundary regularization, *IEEE Trans Med Imaging* 13:227–234, 1994.

35. Chien KR, Han A, White J, et al: In vivo esterification of a synthetic ^{125}I-labeled fatty acid into cardiac glycerolipids, *Am J Physiol* 245:H693–H697, 1983.

36. Choi Y, Hawkins RA, Huang S-C, et al: Parametric images of myocardial metabolic rate of glucose generated from dynamic cardiac PET and 2-[^{18}F]Fluoro-2-deoxy-d-glucose studies, *J Nucl Med* 32: 733–738, 1991.

37. Choi Y, Huang S-C, Hawkins RA, et al: A simplified method for quantification of myocardial blood flow using nitrogen-13-ammonia and dynamic PET, *J Nucl Med* 34:488–497, 1993.

38. Chua T, Kiat H, Germano G, et al: Technetium-99m teboroxime regional myocardial washout in subjects with and without coronary artery disease, *Am J Cardiol* 72:728–734, 1993.

39. Chua T, Kiat H, Germano G, et al: Rapid back to back adenosine stress/rest technetium-99m teboroxime myocardial perfusion SPECT using a triple-detector camera, *J Nucl Med* 34:1485–1493, 1993.

40. Corbett J: Clinical experience with iodine-123-iodophenylpentadecanoic acid, *J Nucl Med* 35(4 Suppl):32S–37S, 1994.

41. Coxson PG, Brennan KN, Huesman RH, et al: Variability and reproducibility of rubidium-82 kinetic parameters in the myocardium of the anesthetized canine, *J Nucl Med* 36:287–296, 1995.

42. Coxson PG, Salmeron EM, Huesman RH, et al: Simulation of compartmental models for kinetic data from a positron emission tomograph, *Comput Methods and Programs in Biomed* 37:205–214, 1992.

43. Cunningham VJ, Jones T: Spectral analysis of dynamic PET studies, *J Cereb Blood Flow Metab* 13:15–23, 1993.

44. Cuocolo A, Pace L, Ricciardelli B, et al: Identification of viable myocardium in patients with chronic coronary artery disease: comparison of thallium-201 scintigraphy with reinjection and technetium-99m-methoxyisobutyl isonitrile, *J Nucl Med* 33:505–511, 1992.

45. Dahlberg ST, Weinstein H, Hendel RC, et al: Planar myocardial perfusion imaging with technetium-99m-teboroxime: comparison by vascular territory with thallium-201 and coronary angiography, *J Nucl Med* 33:1783–1788, 1992.

46. Defrise M, Townsend D, Geissbuhler A: Implementation of three-dimensional image reconstruction for multi-ring positron tomographs, *Phys Med Biol* 35:1361–1372, 1990.

47. Delbeke D, Lorenz CH, Votaw JR, et al: Estimation of left ventricular mass and infarct size from nitrogen-13-ammonia PET images

based on pathological examination of explanted human hearts, *J Nucl Med* 34:826–833, 1993.

48. Delbeke D, Videlefsky S, Patton JA, et al: Rest myocardial perfusion/metabolism imaging using simultaneous dual-isotope acquisition SPECT with technetium-99m-MIBI/fluorine-18-FDG, *J Nucl Med* 36:2110–2119, 1995.

49. Demer LL, Gould KL, Goldstein RA, et al: Noninvasive assessment of coronary collaterals in man by PET perfusion imaging, *J Nucl Med* 31:259–270, 1990.

50. Deutsch R: *Estimation theory,* Englewood Cliffs, NJ, 1965, Prentice-Hall, Inc.

51. Di Bella EVR, Gullberg GT: Extraction of the input function in cardiac dynamic SPECT using factor analysis, *J Nucl Med* 38:8P–9P, 1997 (abstract).

52. Di Bella EVR, Gullberg GT, et al: Automated region selection for analysis of dynamic cardiac SPECT data, *IEEE Trans Nucl Sci,* 44:1355–1361, 1997.

53. Di Bella EVR, Gullberg GT, Ross SG, Christian PE: Compartmental modeling of ^{18}FDG in the heart using dynamic SPECT. In 1997 IEEE Nuclear Science Symposium Conference Record, Nov. 9–15, 1997, Albuquerque, New Mexico, CD-ROM.

54. Di Paola R, Bazin JP, Aubry F, et al: Handling of dynamic sequences in nuclear medicine, *IEEE Trans Nucl Sci* 29: 1310–1321, 1982.

55. Di Rocco RJ, Rumsey WL, Kuczynski BL, et al: Measurement of myocardial blood flow using a co-injection technique for technetium-99m-teboroxime, technetium-96-sestamibi and thallium-201, *J Nucl Med* 33:1152–1159, 1992.

56. Dixon WJ, Massey FJ: *Introduction to statistical analysis,* New York, 1969, McGraw-Hill.

57. Drane WE, Keim S, Strickland P, et al: Preliminary report of SPECT imaging with Tc-99m teboroxime in ischemic heart disease, *Clin Nucl Med* 17:215–225, 1992.

58. Draper NR, Smith H: *Applied regression analysis,* New York, 1966, John Wiley and Sons.

59. Eberl S, Anayat AR, Fulton RR, et al: Evaluation of two population-based input functions for quantitative FDG PET studies, *Eur J Nucl Med* 24:299–304, 1997.

60. Faber TL, Akers M, Peshock RM, et al: Three-dimensional motion and perfusion quantification in gated single-photon emission computed tomograms, *J Nucl Med* 32:2311–2317, 1991.

61. Faber TL, Stokely EM, Peshock RM, et al: A model-based four-dimensional left ventricular surface detector, *IEEE Trans Med Imaging* 10:321–329, 1991.

62. Feng D, Huang SC, Wang X: Models for computer simulation studies of input functions for tracer kinetic modeling with positron emission tomography, *Int J Biomed Comput* 32:95–110, 1993.

63. Feng D, Huang SC, Wang Z, et al: An unbiased parametric imaging algorithm for nonuniformly sampled biomedical system parameter estimation, *IEEE Trans Med Imaging* 15:512–518, 1996.

64. Feng D, Li X, Huang SC: A new double modeling approach for dynamic cardiac PET studies using noise and spillover contaminated LV measurements, *IEEE Trans Biomed Engin* 43:319–327, 1996.

65. Fick A: *Sitzungsb. der Phys.-Med. Ges. zu Wurzburg,* 1870.

66. Formiconi AR: Least squares algorithm for region-of-interest evaluation in emission tomography. *IEEE Trans Med Imaging* 12:90–100, 1993.

67. Frey EC, Ju ZW, Tsui BMW: A fast projector-backprojector pair modeling the asymmetric, spatially varying scatter response function for scatter compensation in SPECT imaging, *IEEE Trans Nucl Sci* NS-40:1192–1197, 1993.

68. Germano G, Kiat H, Kavanaugh PB, et al: Automatic quantification of ejection fraction from gated myocardial perfusion SPECT, *J Nucl Med* 36:2138–2147, 1995.

69. Gewirtz H: *Present status and future directions for nuclear cardiology: observations derived from intact animal models.* In Zaret BL,

Beller GA, eds: *Nuclear cardiology: state of the art and future directions,* St. Louis, 1993, Mosby-Year Book, pp 53–61.

70. Glover DK, Ruiz M, Bergmann EE, et al: Myocardial technetium-99m-teboroxime uptake during adenosine-induced hyperemia in dogs with either a critical or mild coronary stenosis: comparison to thallium-210 and regional blood flow, *J Nucl Med* 36:476–483, 1995.

71. Goldstein RA, Mullani NA, Marani SK, et al: Myocardial perfusion with rubidium-82. II. Effects of metabolic and pharmacologic interventions, *J Nucl Med* 24:907–915, 1983.

72. Golub GH, Van Loan CF: *Matrix computation,* ed. 2, Baltimore, 1989, The Johns Hopkins University Press.

73. Gould KL: PET perfusion imaging and nuclear cardiology, *J Nucl Med* 32:579–606, 1991.

74. Gould KL, Goldstein RA, Mullani NA, et al: Noninvasive assessment of coronary stenoses by myocardial perfusion imaging during pharmacologic coronary vasodilation. VIII. Clinical feasibility of positron cardiac imaging without a cyclotron using generator-produced rubidium-82, *J Am Coll Cardiol* 7:775–789, 1986.

75. Gray WA, Gewirtz H: Comparison of ^{99m}Tc-teboroxime with thallium for myocardial imaging in the presence of a coronary artery stenosis, *Circulation* 84:1796–1807, 1991.

76. Gullberg GT: *Kidney compartment model.* Lawrence Berkeley Laboratory Report No. 2896, Berkeley, CA, 1976.

77. Gullberg GT, Huesman RH, Malko JA, et al: An attenuated projector-backprojector for iterative SPECT reconstruction. *Phys Med Biol* 30:799–816, 1985.

78. Gullberg GT, Huesman RH, Zeng GL, et al: *Efficient estimation of dynamic cardiac SPECT kinetic parameters using weighted least squares estimates of dynamic reconstructions.* In *1995 IEEE nuclear science symposium and medical imaging conference record,* San Francisco, 1995, IEEE, pp 1684–1688.

79. Gullberg GT, Ma X, Parker DL, et al: An MRI perfusion model incorporating nonequilibrium exchange between vascular and extravascular compartments, *Magn Reson Imaging* 9:39–52, 1991.

80. Hamilton WF, Moore JW, Kinsman JM, et al: Simultaneous determination of the pulmonary and systemic circulation times in man and of a figure related to the cardiac output, *Am J Physiol* 84:338–344, 1928.

81. Hansen CL: Preliminary report of an ongoing phase I/II dose range, safety and efficacy study of iodine-123-phenylpentadecanoic acid for the identification of viable myocardium, *J Nucl Med* 35(4 Suppl): 38S–42S, 1994.

82. Hara T, Michihata T, Yokoi F, et al: Quantitative measurement of regional myocardial blood flow in patients with coronary artery disease by intravenous injection of ^{13}N-ammonia in positron emission tomography, *Eur J Nucl Med* 16:231–235, 1990.

83. Hebber E, Oldenburg D, Farnocombe M, et al: Direct estimation of dynamic parameters in SPECT tomography, *IEEE Trans Nucl Sci* 44:2425–2430, 1997.

84. Heiss W-D, Pawlik G, Herholz K, et al: Regional kinetic constants and cerebral metabolic rate for glucose in normal human volunteers determined by dynamic positron emission tomography of [^{18}F]-2-fluoro-2-deoxy-D-glucose, *J Cereb Blood Flow Metab* 4:212–223, 1984.

85. Heller LI, Villegas BJ, Reinhardt CP, et al: Teboxime is a marker of blood flow following reperfusion of a myocardial infarction, *J Nucl Med* 34:14P–15P, 1993 (abstract).

86. Hendel RC, McSherry B, Karimeddini M, et al: Diagnostic value of a new myocardial perfusion agent, teboroxime (SQ30217), utilizing a rapid planar imaging protocol: preliminary results, *J Am Coll Cardiol* 16:855–861, 1990.

87. Henzlova MJ, Machac J: Clinical utility of technetium-99m-teboroxime myocardial washout imaging, *J Nucl Med* 35:575–579, 1994.

88. Hebert TJ, Moore WH, Dhekne RD, et al: Design of an automated algorithm for labeling the cardiac blood pool in gated SPECT images of radiolabeled red blood cells, *IEEE Trans Nucl Sci* 43:2299–2305, 1996.

89. Hermansen F, Bloomfield PM, Ashburner J, et al: Linear dimension reduction of sequences of medical images: II. Direct sum decomposition, *Phys Med Biol* 40:1921–1941, 1995.

90. Herrero P, Markham J, Bergmann SR: Quantitation of myocardial blood flow with H$_2$^{15}O and positron emission tomography: assessment and error analysis of a mathematical approach, *J Comput Assist Tomogr* 13:862–873, 1989.

91. Herrero P, Markham J, Shelton ME, et al: Implementation and evaluation of a two-compartment model for quantification of myocardial perfusion with rubidium-82 and positron emission tomography, *Circ Res* 70:496–507, 1992.

92. Heymann MA, Payne BD, Hoffman JIE, et al: Blood flow measurements with radionuclide-labeled particles, *Prog Cardiovas Dis* 20:55–79, 1977.

93. Hicks K, Ganti G, Mullani N, et al: Automated quantitation of three-dimensional cardiac positron emission tomography for routine clinical use, *J Nucl Med* 30:1787–1797, 1989.

94. Hoffman EJ, Huang S-C, Phelps ME: Quantitation in positron emission computed tomography: 1. Effect of object size, *J Comput Assist Tomogr* 3:299–308, 1979.

95. Huang S-C, Phelps ME: *Principles of tracer kinetic modeling in positron emission tomography and autoradiography*. In Phelps ME, Mazziotta J, Schelbert H, eds: Positron *emission tomography and autoradiography: principles and applications for the brain and heart*, New York, 1986, Raven Press, pp. 287–346.

96. Huang SC, Phelps ME, Hoffman EJ, et al: Noninvasive determination of local cerebral metabolic rate of glucose in man, *Am J Physiol* 238:E69–E82, 1980.

97. Huang SC, Schwaiger M, Carson RE, et al: Quantitative measurement of myocardial blood flow with oxygen-15 water and positron computed tomography: an assessment of potential and problems, *J Nucl Med* 26:616–625, 1985.

98. Hudson HM, Larkin RS: Accelerated image reconstruction using ordered subsets of projection data, *IEEE Trans Med Imaging* 13:601–609, 1994.

99. Hudson HM, Walsh C: *Density deconvolution using spectral mixture models. In Computational statistics and data analysis,* Proceedings of the Second World Congress of the IASC, Pasadena, Calif., 1997 Feb 19–22, pp. 593–599.

100. Huesman RH: A new fast algorithm for the evaluation of regions of interest and statistical uncertainty in computed tomography, *Phys Med Biol* 29:543–552, 1984.

101. Huesman RH: Equivalent methods to analyze dynamic experiments in which the input function is noisy, *Phys Med Biol* 42:147–153, 1997.

102. Huesman RH, Gullberg GT, Greenberg WL, et al: *Users manual—Donner algorithms for reconstruction tomography,* Lawrence Berkeley Laboratory Publication, PUB-214, Berkeley, CA, 1977.

103. Huesman RH, Klein GJ, Reutter BW: Respiratory compensation in cardiac PET using doubly-gated acquisitions, *J Nucl Med* 38:114P, 1997 (abstract).

104. Huesman RH, Knittel BL, Mazoyer BM, et al: *Notes on RFIT: a program for fitting compartment models to region-of-interest dynamic emission tomography data,* Lawrence Berkeley Laboratory Report No. LBL-37621, version 4.3, Berkeley, CA, 1995.

105. Huesman RH, Mazoyer BM: Kinetic data analysis with a noisy input function, *Phys Med Biol* 32:1569–1579, 1987.

106. Huesman RH, Reutter BW, Zeng GL, Gullberg GT: Kinetic parameter estimation from SPECT cone-beam projection measurements, *Phys Med Biol* 44:973–982, 1998.

107. Huesman RH, Reutter BW, Zeng GL, Gullberg GT: Kinetic parameters estimation from SPECT cone-beam projection measurements, *Phys Med Biol* 44:973–982, 1998.

108. Hutchins GD, Caraher JM, Raylman RR: A region of interest strategy for minimizing resolution distortions in quantitative myocardial PET studies, *J Nucl Med* 33:1243–1250, 1992.

109. Hutchins GD, Hichwa RD, Koeppe RA: A continuous flow input function detector for H$_2$^{15}O blood flow studies in positron emission tomography, *IEEE Trans Nucl Sci* NS-33:546–549, 1986.

110. Hutchins GD, Schwaiger M, Rosenspire KC, et al: Noninvasive quantification of regional blood flow in the human heart using N-13 ammonia and dynamic positron emission tomographic imaging, *J Am Coll Cardiol* 15:1032–1042, 1990.

111. Hutton BF, Hudson HM, Beekman FJ: A clinical perspective of accelerated statistical reconstruction, *Eur J Nucl Med* 24:797–808, 1997.

112. Hutton BF, Osiecki A: Correction of errors due to partial volume effects including contractile movement in resting myocardial SPECT, *J Nucl Med* 37:215P, 1996 (abstract).

113. Ido T, Wan CN, Casella V, et al: Labeled 2-deoxy-D-glucose analogs: ^{18}F-labeled 2-deoxy-2-fluoro-D-glucose, 2-deoxy-2-fluoro-D-mannose, and ^{14}C-2-deoxy-2-fluoro-D-glucose, *J Label Compds Radiopharm* 14:175–183, 1978.

114. Iida H, Bloomfield PM, Miura S, et al: Effect of real-time weighted integration system for rapid calculation of functional images in clinical positron emission tomography, *IEEE Trans Med Imaging,* 14:116–121, 1995.

115. Iida H, Itoh H, Bloomfield PM, et al: A method to quantitate cerebral blood flow using a rotating gamma camera and iodine-123 iodoamphetamine with one blood sampling, *Eur J Nucl Med* 21:1072–1084, 1994.

116. Iida H, Kanno I, Takahashi A, et al: Measurement of absolute myocardial blood flow with H$_2$^{15}O and dynamic positron-emission tomography. Strategy for quantification in relation to the partial-volume effect, *Circulation* 78:104–115, 1988.

117. Iida H, Rhodes CG, de Silva R, et al: Use of the left ventricular time-activity curve as a noninvasive input function in dynamic oxygen-15-water positron emission tomography, *J Nucl Med* 33:1669–1677, 1992.

118. Iida H, Rhodes CG, De Silva R, et al: Myocardial tissue fraction—correction for partial volume effects and measure of tissue viability, *J Nucl Med* 32:2169–2175, 1991.

119. Iida H, Eberl S: Quantitative assessment of regional myocardial blood flow with thallium-201 and SPECT, *J Nucl Card* 5:313–331, 1998.

120. Jagust WJ, Budinger TF, Huesman RH, et al: Methodologic factors affecting PET measurements of cerebral glucose metabolism, *J Nucl Med* 27:1358–1361, 1986.

121. Jaszczak RJ, Floyd CE, Coleman RE: Scatter compensation techniques for SPECT, *IEEE Trans Nucl Sci* NS-32:786–793, 1985.

122. Johnson G 3d, Glover DK, Hebert CB, et al: Early myocardial clearance kinetics of technetium-99m-teboroxime differentiate normal and flow-restricted canine myocardium at rest, *J Nucl Med* 34:630–636, 1993.

123. Juni JE: SPECT of rapidly cleared tracers: imaging a cheshire cat, *J Nucl Med* 33:1206–1208, 1992 (editorial).

124. Kalff V, Schwaiger M, Nguyen N, et al: The relationship between myocardial blood flow and glucose uptake in ischemic canine myocardium determined with fluorine-18-deoxyglucose, *J Nucl Med* 33:1346–1353, 1992.

125. Kety SS, Schmidt CF: The nitrous oxide method for the quantitative determination of cerebral blood flow in man: Theory, procedure, and normal values, *J Clin Invest* 27:476–483, 1948.

126. King MA, Tsui BMW, Pan T-S: Attenuation compensation for cardiac single-photon emission computed tomographic imaging: Part 1. Impact of attenuation and methods of estimating attenuation maps, *J Nucl Cardiol* 2:513–524, 1995.

127. King MA, Tsui BMW, Pan T-S, et al: Attenuation compensation for cardiac single-photon emission computed tomographic imaging: Part 2. Attenuation compensation algorithms, *J Nucl Cardiol* 3:55–64, 1996.

128. Klein GJ, Reutter BW, Huesman RH: Non-rigid summing of gated PET via optical flow, *IEEE Trans Nucl Sci,* 44:1509–1512, 1997.

129. Krivokapich J, Huang S-C, Phelps ME, MacDonald NS, Shine KI: Dependence of $^{13}NH_3$ myocardial extraction and clearance on flow and metabolism, *Am J Physiol* 242:H536–H542, 1982.

130. Krivokapich J, Smith GT, Huang S-C, et al: ^{13}N ammonia myocardial imaging at rest and with exercise in normal volunteers. Quantification of absolute myocardial perfusion with dynamic positron emission tomography, *Circulation* 80:1328–1337, 1989.

131. Krivokapich J, Stevenson LW, Kobashigawa J, et al: Quantification of absolute myocardial perfusion at rest and during exercise with positron emission tomography after human cardiac transplantation, *J Am Coll Cardiol* 18:512–517, 1991.

132. Kuhle WG, Porenta G, Huang S-C, et al: Quantification of regional myocardial blood flow using ^{13}N-ammonia and reoriented dynamic positron emission tomographic imaging, *Circulation* 86:1004–1017, 1992.

133. Lambrecht RM, Rescigno A: *Tracer kinetics and physiologic modeling,* New York, 1983, Springer-Verlag.

134. Lange K, Carson R: EM reconstruction algorithms for emission and transmission tomography, *J Comput Assist Tomogr* 8:306–316, 1984.

135. Lassen NA, Perl W: *Tracer kinetic methods in medical physiology,* New York, 1979, Raven Press.

136. Lau CH, Eberl S, Feng D, et al: Optimized acquisition time and image sampling for dynamic SPECT of thallium-201, *IEEE Trans Med Imaging* 17:334-343, 1998.

137. Lau CH, Feng D, Hutton BF, et al: Technique for image reconstruction and kinetic modelling from rotating camera systems, submitted to *IEEE Trans Med Imaging,* 1997.

138. Leppo JA, DePuey EG, Johnson LL: A review of cardiac imaging with sestamibi and teboroxime, *J Nucl Med* 32:2012–2022, 1991.

139. Leppo JA, Meerdink DJ: Comparison of the myocardial uptake of a technetium-labeled isonitrile analogue and thallium, *Circ Res* 65:632–639, 1989.

140. Leppo JA, Meerdink DJ: Comparative myocardial extraction of two technetium-labeled BATO derivatives (SQ30217, SQ32014) and thallium, *J Nucl Med* 31:67–74, 1990.

141. Li Q-S, Solot G, Frank TL, et al: Tomographic myocardial perfusion imaging with technetium-99m-teboroxime at rest and after dipyridamole, *J Nucl Med* 32:1968–1976, 1991.

142. Li X, Feng D, Chen K: Optimal image sampling schedule: a new effective way to reduce dynamic image storage space and functional image processing time, *IEEE Trans Med Imaging* 15:710–719, 1996.

143. Liedtke A: Alterations of carbohydrate and lipid metabolism in the acutely ischemic heart, *Prog Cardiovasc Dis* 23:321–336, 1981.

144. Limber MA, Limber MN, Celler A, et al: Direct reconstruction of functional parameters for dynamic SPECT, *IEEE Trans Nucl Sci* 42:1249–1256, 1995.

145. Links JM, Frank TL, Becker LC: Effect of differential tracer washout during SPECT acquisition, *J Nucl Med* 32:2253–2257, 1991.

146. Machulla H, Knust E, Vyska K: Radioiodinated fatty acids for cardiological diagnosis, *Int J Rad Appl Instrum [A]* 37:777–788, 1986.

147. MacIntyre WJ, Go RT, King JL, et al: Clinical outcome of cardiac patients with negative thallium-201 SPECT and positive rubidium-82 PET myocardial perfusion imaging, *J Nucl Med* 34:400–404, 1993.

148. Marshall RC, Leidholdt EM Jr, Zhang D-Y, et al: The effect of flow on technetium-99m-teboroxime (SQ30217) and thallium-201 extraction and retention in rabbit heart, *J Nucl Med* 32:1979–1988, 1991.

149. Matthews J, Ashburner J, Bailey D, et al: The direct calculation of parameter images from raw PET data using maximum likelihood iterative reconstruction. *In 1995 IEEE Nuclear science symposium and medical imaging conference record,* San Francisco, 1995, pp. 3311–1315.

150. Matthews J, Bailey D, Price P, et al: The direct calculation of parametric images from dynamic PET data using maximum-likelihood iterative reconstruction, *Phys Med Biol* 42:1155–1173, 1997.

151. Maublant JC, Moins N, Gachon P, et al: Uptake of technetium-99m-teboroxime in cultured myocardial cells: comparison with thallium-201 and technetium-99m-sestamibi, *J Nucl Med* 34:255–259, 1993.

152. Mazoyer BM, Huesman RH, Budinger TF, et al: Dynamic PET data analysis, *J Comput Assist Tomogr* 10:645–653, 1986.

153. Meier P, Zierler KL: On the theory of the indicator-dilution method for measurement of blood flow and volume, *J Appl Physiol* 6:731–744, 1954.

154. Meikle SR, Matthews JC, Cunningham VJ, et al: *Spectral analysis of PET projection data.* In *1996 IEEE Nuclear science symposium and medical imaging conference record,* Anaheim, Calf., 1996, pp. 1888–1892.

155. Meikle SR, Matthews JC, Cunningham VJ, et al: Parametric image reconstruction using spectral analysis of PET projection data, *Phys Med Biol* 43:651–666, 1998.

156. Meyer E: Simultaneous correction for tracer arrival delay and dispersion in CBF measurements by the $H_2^{15}O$ autoradiographic method and dynamic PET. *J Nucl Med* 30:1069–1078, 1989.

157. Mullani NA, Goldstein RA, Gould KL, et al: Myocardial perfusion with rubidium-82. I. Measurement of extraction fraction and flow with external detectors, *J Nucl Med* 24:898–906, 1983.

158. Mullani NA, Gould KL: First-pass measurements of regional blood flow with external detectors, *J Nucl Med* 24:577–581, 1983.

159. Murray GL, Schad NC, Magill HL, et al: Myocardial viability assessment with dynamic low-dose iodine-123-iodophenylpentadecanoic acid metabolic imaging: comparison with myocardial biopsy and reinjection SPECT thallium after myocardial infarction, *J Nucl Med* 35 (4 Suppl):43S–48S, 1994.

160. Muzik O, Beanlands RSB, Hutchins GD, et al: Validation of nitrogen-13-ammonia tracer kinetic model for quantification of myocardial blood flow using PET, *J Nucl Med* 34:83–91, 1993.

161. Muzik O, Beanlands R, Wolfe E, et al: Automated region definition for cardiac nitrogen-13-ammonia PET imaging, *J Nucl Med* 34:336–344, 1993.

162. Nakajima K, Shuke N, Taki J, et al: A simulation of dynamic SPECT using radiopharmaceuticals with rapid clearance, *J Nucl Med* 33:1200–1206, 1992.

163. Nakajima K, Taki J, Bunko H, et al: Dynamic acquisition with a three-headed SPECT system: application to technetium 99m-SQ30217 myocardial imaging, *J Nucl Med* 32:1273–1277, 1991.

164. Nakamura M, Suzuki Y, Kobayashi S: A method for recovering physiological components from dynamic radionuclide images using the maximum entropy principle: a numerical investigation, *IEEE Trans Biomed Eng* 36:906–917, 1989.

165. Nienaber CA, Ratib O, Gambhir SS, et al: A quantitative index of regional blood flow in canine myocardium derived noninvasively with N-13 ammonia and dynamic positron emission tomography, *J Am Coll Cardiol* 17:260–269, 1991.

166. Nijran KS, Barber DC: Factor analysis of dynamic function studies using a priori physiological information, *Phys Med Biol* 31:1107–1117, 1986.

167. O'Connor MK, Cho DS: Rapid radiotracer washout from the heart: effect on image quality in SPECT performed with a single-headed gamma camera system, *J Nucl Med* 33:1146–1151, 1992.

168. O'Sullivan F: Imaging radiotracer model parameters in PET: A mixture analysis approach, *IEEE Trans Med Imaging* 12:399–412, 1993.

169. Phelps ME, Huang SC, Hoffman EJ, et al: Tomographic measurement of local cerebral glucose metabolic rate in humans with (F-18)2-fluoro-2-deoxy-D-glucose: validation of method, *Ann Neurol* 6:371–388, 1979.

170. Pieri P, Yasuda T, Fischman AJ, et al: Myocardial accumulation and clearance of technetium 99m teboroxime at 100%, 75%, 50%, and zero coronary blood flow in dogs, *Eur J Nucl Med* 18:725–731, 1991.

171. Raylman RR, Caraher JM, Hutchins GD: Sampling requirements for dynamic cardiac PET studies using image-derived input functions, *J Nucl Med* 34:440–447, 1993.

172. Reivich M, Alavi A, Wolf A, et al: Use of 2-deoxy-D-[1-^{11}C]glucose for the determination of local cerebral glucose metabolism in humans: variation within and between subjects, *J Cereb Blood Flow Metab* 2:307–319, 1982.

173. Reske S, Knapp FF Jr, Winkler C: Experimental basis of metabolic imaging of the myocardium with radioiodinated aromatic free fatty acids, *Am J Physiol Imaging* 1:214–229, 1986.

174. Reske SN: ^{123}I-phenylpentadecanoic acid as a tracer of cardiac free fatty acid metabolism. Experimental and clinical results, *Eur Heart J* 6 Suppl B:39–47, 1985.

175. Reske SN, Sauer W, Machulla HJ, et al: 15(p-[I-123]Iodophenyl)pentadecanoic acid as a tracer of lipid metabolism: comparison with [1-^{14}C] palmitic acid in murine tissues, *J Nucl Med* 25:1335–1342, 1984.

176. Reutter BW, Klein GJ, Huesman RH: Automated 3-D segmentation of respiratory-gated PET transmission images, *IEEE Trans Nucl Sci* 44:2473–2476, 1997.

177. Reutter BW, Klein GJ, Huesman RH: Respiration-compensated cardiac PET attenuation correction via automated 4-D segmentation of gated transmission images, *J Nucl Med* 38:203P, 1997 (abstract).

178. Rhodes CG, Wollmer P, Fazio F, et al: Quantitative measurement of regional extravascular lung density using positron emission and transmission tomography, *J Comput Assist Tomog* 5:783–791, 1981.

179. Rose CP, Goresky CA, Bach GG: The capillary and sarcolemmal barriers in the heart. An explanation of labeled water permeability, *Circ Res* 41:515–533, 1977.

180. Rosenspire KC, Schwaiger M, Mangner TJ, et al: Metabolic fate of [^{13}N]ammonia in human and canine blood, *J Nucl Med* 31:163–167, 1990.

181. Ross SG, Gullberg GT, Huesman RH: The effect of heart motion on kinetic parameter estimates for dynamic cardiac SPECT, *IEEE Trans Nucl Sci* 44:1409–1416, 1997.

182. Ross SG, Welch A, Gullberg GT, Huesman RH: An investigation into the effect of input function shape and image acquisition interval on estimates of washin for dynamic cardiac SPECT, *Phys Med Biol* 42:2193–2213, 1997.

183. Rumsey WL, Rosenspire KC, Nunn AD: Myocardial extraction of teboroxime: effects of teboroxime interaction with blood, *J Nucl Med* 33:94–101, 1992.

184. Schelbert HR, Phelps ME, Huang S-C, et al: N-13 ammonia as an indicator of myocardial blood flow, *Circulation* 63:1259–1272, 1981.

185. Schwaiger M, Hicks R: The clinical role of metabolic imaging of the heart by positron emission tomography, *J Nucl Med* 32:565–578, 1991.

186. Seldin DW, Johnson LL, Blood DK, et al: Myocardial perfusion imaging with technetium-99m SQ30217: comparison with thallium-201 and coronary anatomy, *J Nucl Med* 30:312–319, 1989.

187. Serafini AN, Topchik S, Jimenez H, et al: Clinical comparison of technetium-99m-teboroxime and thallium-201 utilizing a continuous SPECT imaging protocol, *J Nucl Med* 33:1304–1311, 1992.

188. Shah A, Schelbert HR, Schwaiger M, et al: Measurement of regional myocardial blood flow with N-13 ammonia and positron-emission tomography in intact dogs, *J Am Coll Cardiol* 5:92–100, 1985.

189. Shepp LA, Vardi Y: Maximum likelihood reconstruction for emission tomography, *IEEE Trans Med Imaging* 1:113–122, 1982.

190. Shi CQ, Daher E, Young LH, et al: [^{123}I] Iodophenyl-pentadecanoic acid (p-[^{123}I]PPA) a noninvasive marker of ischemic viable myocardium: correlation of myocardial p-[^{123}I]PPA retention with [^{18}F] fluorodeoxyglucose accumulation during experimental low flow ischemia, *Circulation*, (submitted).

191. Sitek A, Di Bella EVR, Gullberg GT: Direct extraction of tomographic time activity curves from dynamic SPECT projections using factor analysis, *J Nucl Med* 39:144P, 1998.

192. Smith AM, Gullberg GT: Dynamic cardiac SPECT computer simulations for teboroxime kinetics, *IEEE Trans Nucl Sci* 41:1626–1633, 1994.

193. Smith AM, Gullberg GT, Christian PE: Experimental verification of technetium 99m-labeled teboroxime kinetic parameters in the myocardium with dynamic single-photon emission computed tomography: reproducibility, correlation to flow, and susceptibility to extravascular contamination, *J Nucl Cardiol* 3:130–142, 1996.

194. Smith AM, Gullberg GT, Christian PE, et al: Kinetic modeling of teboroxime using dynamic SPECT imaging of a canine model, *J Nucl Med* 35:484–495, 1994.

195. Snyder DL: Parameter estimation for dynamic studies in emission-tomography systems having list-mode data, *IEEE Trans Nucl Sci* NS-31:925–931, 1984.

196. Sokoloff L, Reivich M, Kennedy C, et al: The [^{14}C]deoxyglucose method for the measurement of local cerebral glucose utilization: theory, procedure and normal values in the conscious and anesthetized albino rat, *J Neurochem* 28:897–916, 1977.

197. Spinks TJ, Araujo LI, Rhodes CG, et al: Physical aspects of cardiac scanning with a block detector positron tomograph, *J Comput Assist Tomog* 15:893–904, 1991.

198. Stewart GN: Researches on the circulation time and on the influences which affect it: IV. The output of the heart, *J Physiol* 22:159–183, 1897.

199. Stewart GN: Researches on the circulation time and on the influences which affect it: V. The circulation time of the spleen, kidney, intestine, heart (coronary circulation) and retina, with some further observations on the time of the lesser circulation, *Am J Physiol* 58:278–295, 1921.

200. Stewart RE, Heyl B, O'Rourke RA, et al: Demonstration of differential post-stenotic myocardial technetium-99m-teboroxime clearance kinetics after experimental ischemia and hyperemic stress, *J Nucl Med* 32:2000–2008, 1991.

201. Stewart RE, Schwaiger M, Hutchins GD, et al: Myocardial clearance kinetics of technetium-99m-SQ30217: a marker of regional myocardial blood flow, *J Nucl Med* 31:1183–1190, 1990.

202. Tan P, Bailey DL, Meikle SR, et al: A scanning line source for simultaneous emission and transmission measurement in SPECT, *J Nucl Med* 34:1752–1760, 1993.

203. Tan K, Hutton BF, Feng D: A new approach for parameter estimation in SPECT dynamics using a rotating camera, *Eur J Nucl Med* 21:S29, 1994 (abstract).

204. Tan K, Hutton BF, Feng DD: *Assessment of errors due to changing activity during kinetic SPECT acquisition.* In *Proceedings of the 17th annual international conference of IEEE engineering in medicine and biology society,* Montreal, Canada, Sept. 20–23, 1995, Piscataway, NJ, IEEE Service Center, pp 527–528.

205. Ter-Pogossian MM, Bergmann SR, Sobel BE: Influence of cardiac and respiratory motion on tomographic reconstructions of the heart: implications for quantitative nuclear cardiology, *J Comput Assist Tomogr* 6:1148–1155, 1982.

206. Terry JA, Tsui BMW, Perry JR, et al: *The design of a mathematical phantom of the upper human torso for use in 3-D SPECT imaging research.* In *Biomedical engineering: opening new doors (proceedings of the 1990 fall meeting of the biomedical engineering society),* Blacksburg, VA, Oct. 21–24, 1990, New York University Press, pp. 185–190.

207. Tsui BMW, Gullberg GT: The geometric transfer function for cone and fan beam collimators, *Phys Med Biol* 35:81–93, 1990.

208. Tsui BMW, Gullberg GT, Edgerton ER, et al: Correction of nonuniform attenuation in cardiac SPECT imaging, *J Nucl Med* 30:497–507, 1989.

209. Tsui BMW, Hu HB, Gilland DR, et al: Implementation of simultaneous attenuation and detector response correction in SPECT, *IEEE Trans Nucl Sci* 35:778–783, 1988.

210. Tsui BMW, Zhao XD, Gregoriou GK, et al: Quantitative cardiac SPECT reconstruction with reduced image degradation due to patient anatomy, *IEEE Trans Nucl Sci* 41:2838–2844, 1994.

211. Tung C-H, Gullberg GT, Zeng GL, et al: Nonuniform attenuation correction using simultaneous transmission and emission converging tomography, *IEEE Trans Nucl Sci* 39:1134–1143, 1992.

212. Von Hevesy G: *Selected papers of George Hevesy,* London, 1967, Pergamon Press.

213. Walsh MN, Geltman EM, Steele RL, et al: Augmented myocardial perfusion reserve after coronary angioplasty quantified by positron emission tomography with $H_2^{15}O$, *J Am Coll Cardiol* 15:119–127, 1990.

214. Wang Z, Feng D: Continuous-time system modelling using the weighted-parabola-overlapping numerical integration method, *Int J Systems Sci* 23:1361–1369, 1992.

215. Weinberg IN, Huang S-C, Hoffman EJ, et al: Validation of PET-acquired input functions for cardiac studies, *J Nucl Med* 29:241–247, 1988.

216. Weinstein H, Dahlberg ST, McSherry BA, et al: Rapid redistribution of teboroxime, *Am J Cardiol* 71:848–852, 1993.

217. Weinstein H, Reinhardt CP, Leppo JA: Teboroxime, sestamibi, and thallium-201 as markers of myocardial hypoperfusion: comparison by quantitative dual-isotope autoradiography in rabbits, *J Nucl Med* 34:1510–1517, 1993.

218. Welch AE, Gullberg GT, Christian PE, et al: A transmission-map-based scatter correction technique for SPECT in inhomogeneous media, *Med Phys* 22:1627–1635, 1995.

219. Welch AE, Smith AM, Gullberg GT: An investigation of the effect of finite system resolution and photon noise on the bias and precision of dynamic cardiac SPECT parameters, *Med Phys* 22:1829–1836, 1995.

220. Wu H-M, Hoh CK, Choi Y, et al: Factor analysis for extraction of blood time-activity curves in dynamic FDG-PET studies, *J Nucl Med* 36:1714–1722, 1995.

221. Wu H-M, Huang S-C, Allada V, et al: Derivation of input function from FDG-PET studies in small hearts, *J Nucl Med* 37:1717–1722, 1996.

222. Yano Y, Chu P, Budinger TF, et al: Rubidium-82 generators for imaging studies, *J Nucl Med* 18:46–50, 1977.

223. Yokoi T, Iida H, Itoh H, et al: A new graphic plot analysis for cerebral blood flow and partition coefficient with iodine-123-iodoamphetamine and dynamic SPECT validation studies using oxygen-15-water and PET, *J Nucl Med* 34:498–505, 1993.

224. Zar JH: *Biostatistical analysis,* ed 2, Englewood Cliffs, N.J., 1984, Prentice-Hall, Inc.

225. Zaret BL, Beller GA, eds: *Nuclear cardiology: state of the art and future directions,* St. Louis, Missouri, 1993, Mosby-Year Book.

226. Zeng GL, Gullberg GT, Bai C, et al: Iterative reconstruction of fluorine-18 SPECT using geometric point response correction, *J Nucl Med* 39:124–130, 1998.

227. Zeng GL, Gullberg GT, Huesman RH: Using linear time-invariant system theory to estimate kinetic parameters directly from projection measurements, *IEEE Trans Nucl Sci* 42:2339–2346, 1995.

228. Zeng GL, Gullberg GT, Tsui BMW, et al: Three-dimensional iterative reconstruction algorithms with attenuation and geometric point response correction, *IEEE Trans Nucl Sci* 38:693–702, 1991.

229. Ziegler WH, Goresky CA: Kinetics of rubidium uptake in the working dog heart, *Circ Res* 29:208–220, 1971.

230. Zierler KL: Equations for measuring blood flow by external monitoring of radioisotopes, *Circ Res* 16:309–321, 1965.

VENTRICULAR
FUNCTION

Chapter 12

Monitoring of left ventricular function with miniaturized non-imaging detectors

Barry L. Zaret and **Diwakar Jain**

Nuclear cardiology has in part been defined by a sophisticated technology that involves increasingly complex and larger instrumentation. As the field enters a new era in which critical documentation of the added value of all procedures is needed and cost-effectiveness is emphasized, it is worth considering the potential advantages of miniaturized detector systems and their suitability for providing relevant clinical data. In addition, the ability to monitor relevant clinical physiologic variables over longer periods of time than can be done routinely in the exercise laboratory can provide important relevant clinical data, as has been demonstrated with ambulatory electrocardiographic and blood pressure monitoring.[9,25]

In nuclear cardiology, similar efforts have resulted in the development of miniaturized nonimaging detectors suitable for evaluation of left ventricular function in patients. This technology offers the possibility of obtaining new insights into cardiac performance on a sequential basis in patients during activities of daily life or during hospitalization in an acute care environment. Such data can provide new directions for clinical understanding of silent myocardial ischemia, acute myocardial infarction, unstable angina pectoris, congestive heart failure, and the impact of mental stress on cardiac function.

It is clear from studies in experimental animal models and in humans that left ventricular functional assessment provides a highly sensitive means of defining myocardial ischemia that may have substantial added value over conventional clinical assessment or electrocardiography. Consequently, evaluation of ventricular function seems to be an appropriate way to approach specific problems relating to the occurrence of myocardial ischemia with or without symptoms. In addition, an understanding of how left ventricular function relates to the pathophysiology of other conditions can allow further understanding of these conditions and their appropriate therapy. This chapter will review the instrumentation used for these evaluations as well as their current clinical investigative applications. Although this technology has not yet had the broad use of other nuclear methods, it has the potential for much wider clinical application now and in the future.

INSTRUMENTATION

Ambulatory and continuous monitoring of ventricular function is done using the basic principles of equilibrium blood pool imaging. By virtue of its positioning and collimation, a nonimaging, high-sensitivity radiation detector used for this purpose continuously acquires counts from the left ventricular blood pool. Changes in counts represent cyclic changes in left ventricular blood volume. From these counts, a time–activity curve is generated; this provides indices of systolic and diastolic function and relative cardiac output. Global left ventricular ejection fraction is the most commonly used index. A major limitation of the technique is its inability to define regional function. Two prominent devices have been developed and used: the c-VEST and the Cardioscint.

c-VEST

The c-VEST, a ventricular scintigraphic monitoring instrument, was initially described in 1983.[40] This miniature device is portable and suitable for use in ambulatory patients (Fig. 12-1). It has undergone many improvements and iterations since its introduction, and a further iteration is currently under active consideration and should be available shortly.[2] In its present form, the device comprises a nonimaging detector; a semi-rigid, plastic, vest-like garment with a bracket to hold the

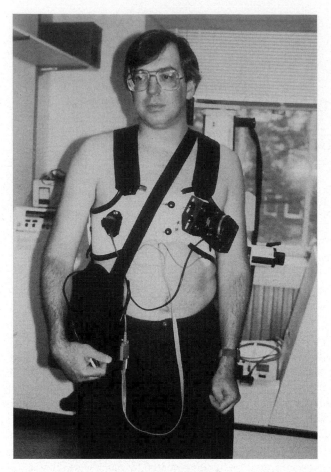

Fig. 12-1. Patient wearing the c-VEST ventricular scintigraphic imaging device. The detector is mounted in a plastic vest-like garment. The electronics are in a shoulder-strap bag, which the patient carries easily.

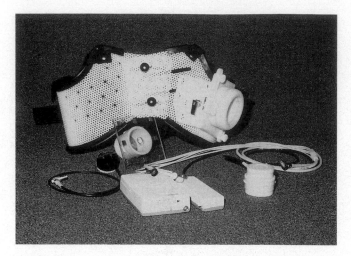

Fig. 12-2. Initial version of c-VEST *(background)* juxtaposed with the newer miniaturized prototype *(foreground)*. The latest version represents a substantial size reduction.

detector on the chest; two echocardiography (ECG) channels; and a modified Holter monitor that records scintigraphic and ECG data on ordinary magnetic tape for several hours. The nuclear data are in the form of sequential gamma counts obtained at 32 x/s. Analysis is done offline.[41]

The nonimaging detector is a sodium iodide crystal, 5.5 cm in diameter, that is equipped with a parallel-hole collimator. In its current version, the detector weighs about 1.5 lbs. This will be substantially miniaturized in the next iteration. A smaller cadmium telluride detector may be used to monitor background activity over the lung field. The plastic garment currently used to mount the device on the chest weighs 1.5 lbs. The associated electronics and recorder are placed in a lightweight shoulder strap bag that weighs approximately 4.5 lbs and is carried by the patient. A much smaller next-generation system has been modeled in prototype form (Fig. 12-2). This will enhance ease of operation and patient use.[2]

The c-VEST is best used in conjunction with gamma-camera imaging. After labeling of the blood pool with technetium-99m, conventional left anterior oblique gamma-camera imaging is done to visualize the left ventricle and to assess ejection fraction. This information is used to position the detector over the left ventricle. A positioning target with several lead markers that fits into the detector bracket is used to define the optimal position and angulation of the instrument (Fig. 12-3). After appropriate positioning, the device is activated to continuously monitor left ventricular activity and perform ECG.[19] Patients can be monitored for 2 to 6 hours with this device. For longer monitoring, augmented blood-pool labeling with additional injection of radionuclide is required.

The gated radionuclide data are summed for 15 to 60 seconds and are displayed in graphic form. Left ventricular ejection fraction measured by using this technique correlates well with conventional gamma-camera measures (Fig. 12-4). Studies have been obtained at rest and during treadmill exercise, mental stress, and other physiologic maneuvers. In general, a decrease of 0.05 ejection fraction units or more that lasts for at least 1 minute is considered abnormal. These values take into account the inherent variability of the measurement with respect to magnitude and duration of the abnormality.

Cardioscint

The Cardioscint is a smaller, light detector only 48 mm in diameter and 39 mm in height.[5,12] Its total weight is 0.14 kg. Instead of having a photomultiplier tube, this instrument contains a cesium iodide scintillation crystal (14 × 14 × 48 mL) equipped with a converging collimator 1 cm long. The crystal is optically coupled to a photodiode. The nuclear data and ECG are interfaced to a microcomputer for online analysis. The data can be displayed in real time or in beat-to-beat mode. Data can also be averaged over 10 to 300 seconds. This detector may be positioned with the assistance of a gamma camera or blindly using position algorithms similar to those developed previously for the nuclear stethoscope.[3] Background may be determined automatically or manually. Reasonably good correlations have been noted between ejection fraction measured with this device

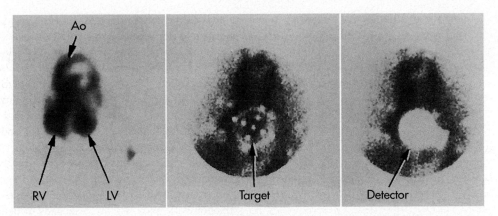

Fig. 12-3. Static imaging in left anterior oblique position demonstrating positioning of c-VEST. *Left,* blood pool image shows aorta (*Ao*), right ventricle (*RV*), and left ventricle (*LV*). The blood pool appears dark, and the interventricular septum appears as a light structure between the right and left ventricles. *Middle,* the positioning target is seen over the left ventricular blood pool. The target consists of two lines of 1-cm lead markers that are 1 cm apart and are arranged to form a cross. The target is centered over the left ventricle by angulating and moving the mounting bracket. The target fits into the same bracket as the detector and can be removed and replaced with the actual detector without changing the position or orientation of the mounting bracket. *Right,* the target has been replaced by the detector and is seen over the left ventricular blood pool, obscuring underlying blood pool radioactivity. (From Kayden DS, et al: *J Am Coll Cardiol* 15:1500, 1990. With permission of the American College of Cardiology.)

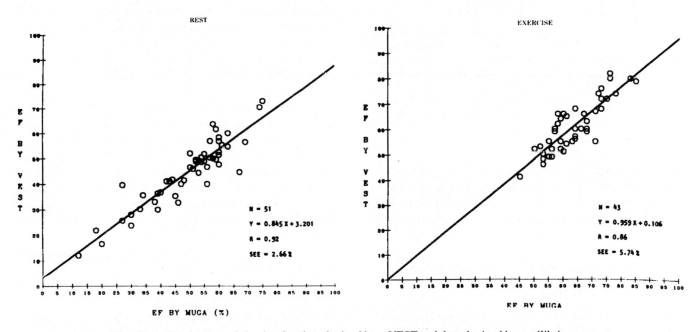

Fig. 12-4. Comparison of ejection fraction obtained by c-VEST and that obtained by equilibrium radionuclide studies. Data are shown at rest in left panel and during exercise in right panel. (From Tamaki N, et al: *J Am Coll Cardiol* 12:669, 1988. With permission of the American College of Cardiology.)

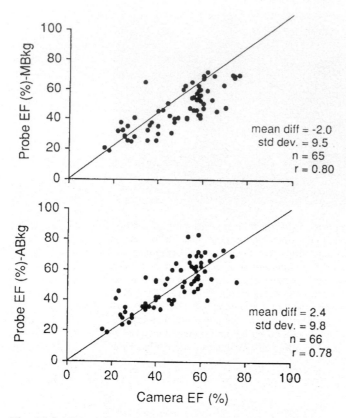

Fig. 12-5. Comparison of ejection fraction measured by gamma camera with that obtained with Cardioscint (probe). Data are shown for manually derived background *(top)* and automatically determined background *(bottom)*. (From Broadhurst P, et al: Clinical validation of a miniature nuclear probe system for continuous on-line monitoring of cardiac function and ST segment, *J Nucl Med* 32:37, 1991. With permission of the American College of Cardiology.)

and that obtained with gamma cameras[5,12] (Fig. 12-5). Variability over time has also been assessed. This device can only be used in recumbent patients; consequently, it is not applicable to the ambulatory patient and is most suitable for studies performed in intensive care units. An ongoing limitation of this device is the lack of a reliable external system to hold it in place in a constant position over an extended period of time.

VALIDATION STUDIES

Data obtained with these non-imaging probes correlate reasonably well with scintillation camera data. This has been demonstrated under conditions of exercise stress, in the resting state, and with pharmacologic agents.[27,38] It has also been shown that these devices are sensitive for detecting acute changes in ventricular function, such as those that can occur with transient myocardial ischemia. To demonstrate this in humans, studies using the coronary angioplasty model to produce myocardial ischemia were undertaken in the cardiac catheterization laboratory.[22] In this study, only left anterior descending angioplasties were evaluated. The c-VEST detector was positioned on the patient's chest, and ventricular function was monitored during acute coronary occlusion with the balloon angioplasty catheter as well as during the recovery period. In a total of 18 inflations in 12 patients, substantial abnormality in global left ventricular function was detected promptly (Fig. 12-6). Baseline ejection fraction decreased by approximately 25 units on average, and a decrease of at least 10 units was noted in 17 of 18 inflations. The change in ejection fraction was associated with a minimal but significant increase in end-diastolic volume of 4% ± 3%, and a substantial increase in end-systolic volume of 69% ± 43%. Of note, chest pain occurred in only 10 of 18 inflations, and ST-segment depression in the electrocardiogram was seen in only 7 of 18 inflations. The decrease in ejection fraction was noted within 15 seconds of balloon inflation and generally antedated the occurrence of chest pain. The maximum decrease in ejection fraction occurred approximately 40 seconds after inflation, and complete recovery was noted approximately 40 seconds after balloon deflation.

Other researchers have studied the effects of routine activities on ventricular function as measured with c-VEST. In 18 patients, Tamaki et al[37] noted that standing increased the ejection fraction by 3 units, routine walking increased it by 10 units, and climbing stairs increased it by 18 units. Exposure to a cold environment resulted in a prompt decrease in ejection fraction of 5 units. Bairey et al[1] evaluated a group of normal persons during routine activities.[1] They noted ejection fraction variability at rest to be low. Exercise uniformly increased ejection fraction; the increase was dependent on the intensity of the effort. Of note, 4 of 18 persons in their study had a decrease in ejection fraction associated with mental stress. Mortelmans et al[29] evaluated various activities of normal persons[29] and noted a prompt increase in ejection fraction in association with effort. Assuming the Trendelenburg position resulted in increasing ventricular end-diastolic volume, whereas administration of nitrates and inflation of thigh cuffs resulted in decreases in ventricular volumes. Imbriaco et al[11] evaluated the reproducibility of c-VEST measurements in response to different stimuli.[11] They found good reproducibility for measuring left ventricular functional responses to such stimuli as isometric hand grip, administration of nitroglycerin, and changes of position. Other investigators found that the c-VEST can be used to define optimal atrioventricular delay for dual-chambered pacemakers.[30]

Myocardial infarction

Several studies demonstrated that ambulatory assessment of ventricular function can provide relevant clinical information in patients with acute myocardial infarction. Breisblatt et al[4] evaluated a cohort of 35 patients with acute myocardial infarction during routine activities, exercise, and mental stress.[4] These patients did not receive thrombolytic therapy and were evaluated before hospital discharge. Twenty-three of the 35 patients manifested transient left ventricular dysfunction during exercise, mental stress, and routine activities. Of note, 75% of these episodes occurred in the absence of symptoms, and only 39% were associated with ECG changes.

Patients undergoing thrombolytic therapy also have been

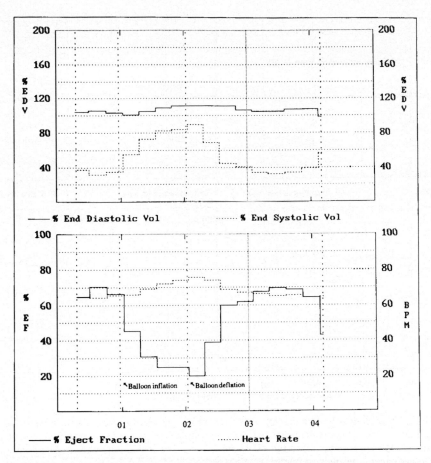

Fig. 12-6. Display of serial measurements obtained during coronary angioplasty. *Lower panel,* Ejection fraction and heart rate data; *upper panel,* relative end-diastolic and end-systolic volumes. During balloon inflation the ejection fraction abruptly decreases within the first 15 seconds of inflation. Onset of ejection fraction recovery occurs within 15 seconds after balloon deflation. While the ejection fraction is reduced, end-diastolic volume increases slightly and end-systolic volume increases substantially. (From Kayden DS, et al: Validation of continuous radionuclide left ventricular function monitoring, *Am J Cardiol* 67:339, 1991. With permission from Excerpta Medica, Inc.)

evaluated by this technique. Kayden et al[21] studied 33 patients who were monitored for approximately 3 hours before hospital discharge.[21] All patients received thrombolytic therapy with or without subsequent angioplasty. Twelve of the 33 patients experienced periods of transient left ventricular dysfunction. Only one of these episodes was associated with chest pain or ECG changes. Of note, patients with an abnormal response had a highly significant occurrence of subsequent cardiac events. No such relation to outcome was noted with exercise equilibrium radionuclide studies or perfusion imaging, which were performed according to protocol in the same patient cohort. The exact mechanism responsible for these abnormalities and how it relates to outcomes is not clear. Such spontaneous episodes of transient left ventricular dysfunction, detected over a relatively short period of time, may reflect instability of plaque, transient platelet plug formation, or abnormal coronary vasomotion.

In another study, ambulatory monitoring was carried out in a cohort of patients with unstable angina or non–Q wave myocardial infarction approximately 3 days after hospital admis-

sion.[18] These patients represent a clinical continuum. Patients were evaluated in the stepdown unit or the coronary care unit. Sixty-eight percent of patients experienced episodes of transient left ventricular dysfunction, which occurred in the absence of ECG changes in all but two instances. Only one patient experienced chest pain, and more than half of the episodes occurred at rest. Episodes were associated with such activities as eating (4%) or urination/defecation (22%) and lasted approximately 9 minutes. The decrease in ejection fraction averaged 8 units (Fig. 12-7).

Stable coronary artery disease

Several investigators have noted transient abnormalities in global left ventricular function in stable coronary patients. Tamaki et al,[38] using the c-VEST, evaluated 39 ambulatory patients during hospitalization. Sixteen of these patients manifested abnormal responses. Two thirds of the episodes occurred without symptoms or ECG changes. In 10 of the 12 symptomatic episodes, ventricular dysfunction occurred 30 to 90 sec-

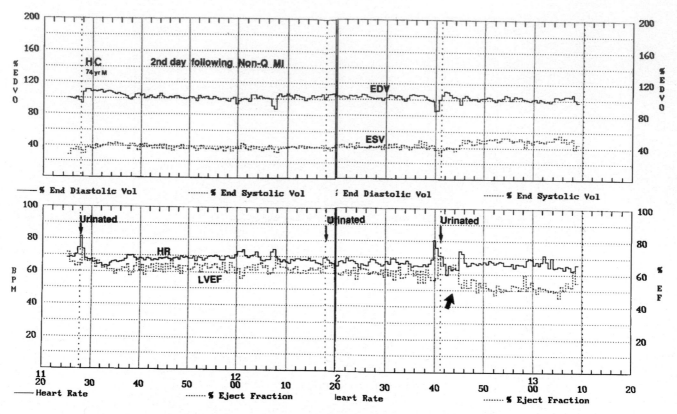

Fig. 12-7. Trended data from a patient with a recent non–Q wave myocardial infarction who was monitored for almost 2 hours. Relative end-diastolic volumes *(EDV)* and end-systolic volumes *(ESV)* are shown in the upper panel; heart rate *(HR)* and left ventricular ejection fraction *(LVEF)* are shown in the lower panel. The ejection fraction *(arrow)* decreased substantially almost 15 minutes after urination. Here, end-diastolic volume remains relatively constant, whereas end-systolic volume increases.

onds before onset of symptoms. Other investigators have found similar results when monitoring patients under various circumstances, including shoveling snow or physical exercise in challenging environments.

Vassiliadis et al[39] also noted transient left ventricular dysfunction during routine daily activities, such as walking, urinating, or eating, in patients with stable coronary disease. They found no relation between these events and the patient's symptomatic state, but noted that transient left ventricular dysfunction was more common in persons who had manifested exercise-induced abnormalities on other studies.

Mohiuddin et al[28] assessed the temporal relation among symptoms, ECG events, and ventricular dysfunction using the c-VEST.[28] They evaluated 27 patients with stable coronary disease who experienced 17 episodes of exercise-induced decrease in left ventricular ejection fraction. Of these episodes, 8 (47%) were electrocardiographically silent and 12 (71%) were asymptomatic. When the temporal sequence was evaluated, ejection fraction abnormalities were noted first, followed by ST-segment depression on ECG and symptoms. After discontinuation of exercise stress, ejection fraction returned to normal sooner than symptoms or ECG changes.

In patients with chronic stable coronary disease, this technique might prove suitable for evaluating therapeutic efficacy.

Preliminary studies have demonstrated its suitability for assessing effects of nitroglycerin or calcium-channel blockers.[22] As might be expected, effective revascularization surgery should alter stress-induced responses.[34]

Mental stress

A major potential use of ambulatory function involves studying patients during laboratory-induced and spontaneous mental stress. The efficacy of this approach for evaluating mental stress–related events has been demonstrated. In an initial study, 15 of 30 patients with evidence of myocardial ischemia on other studies showed mental stress–induced abnormalities in the laboratory in response to arithmetic problem solving or a structured interview[6] (Fig. 12-8). Patients with an abnormal response had a psychological profile consistent with type A behavior patterns of augmented anger, hostility, and inability to control anger. The episodes of mental stress induced a decrease in ejection fraction in the absence of symptoms or ECG changes. No differences were noted in any clinical characteristics between the groups with and without mental stress–induced ventricular dysfunction, including blood pressure response to mental stress, type and extent of medical therapy, extent of coronary disease, and degree of ischemia noted on perfusion imaging. The only char-

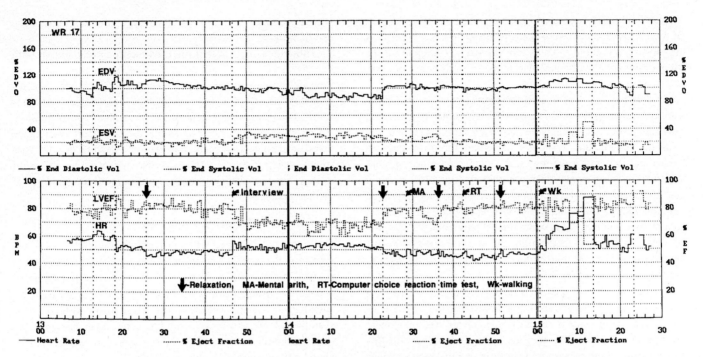

Fig. 12-8. Trended study over 2.5 hours in a patient undergoing a mental stress protocol. Ejection fraction *(LVEF)* and heart rate *(HR)* are shown in the lower panel, and relative end-systolic *(ESV)* and end-diastolic *(EDV)* volumes are shown in the upper panel. Arrows indicate time of specific interventions. After a period of stabilization, the patient underwent psychiatric interview to determine the psychological profile. The interview was associated with an increase in heart rate and end-systolic volume and a decrease in ejection fraction. Doing mental arithmetic *(MA)* produced similar changes. In contrast, computer choice reaction time *(RT)* produced no change. Likewise, walking *(Wk)* resulted in a marked increase in heart rate but no change in ejection fraction.

acteristics that distinguished patients from with patients without mental stress–induced left ventricular function were the type A behavior score and the component scores related to anger and hostility.

This study highlights the importance of behavioral and physiologic factors in mental stress–induced left ventricular dysfunction. As has been noted in other study subsets, both ECG changes and clinical manifestations are not common. The 30 patients were followed over 2 years, during which an increased number of cardiac events in patients with mental stress–induced left ventricular dysfunction was noted[15] (Fig. 12-9). These events involved myocardial infarction or unstable angina requiring hospitalization. No deaths occurred in either group. Differences persisted over the second year of follow-up.[15] The finding of prognostic significance of mental stress–induced left ventricular dysfunction is consistent with those of a recent study that used scintillation camera data in a much larger patient cohort.[20] In other studies, mental stress–induced left ventricular dysfunction has been associated with a greater prevalence of silent myocardial ischemia on ambulatory electrocardiographic monitoring.[10]

The issue of longer-term reproducibility of mental stress–induced left ventricular dysfunction has been investigated. In one investigation, patients were studied on two occasions 4 to 8 weeks apart with no change in medication. Overall, left ven-

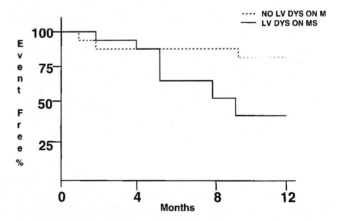

Fig. 12-9. Cardiac event–free survival in patients with no left ventricular dysfunction *(LV DYS)* on mental stress testing *(MS)* compared with patients with coronary disease and left ventricular dysfunction on mental stress. Many patients with mental stress–induced left ventricular dysfunction developed cardiac events during the 1 year follow-up. (From Jain D et al: Prognostic significance of mental stress induced left ventricular dysfunction in patients with coronary disease, *Am J Cardiol* 76:31, 1995. With permission from Excerpta Medica, Inc.)

tricular functional response to mental stress was reproducible. Of the various mental stress tasks, response to anger recall was the most reproducible.[13] Thus, this approach is suitable for the study of therapeutic efficacy over longer periods and is not limited to acute intervention studies.

Studies have also evaluated the affect of antianginal medication on mental stress–induced left ventricular dysfunction. This has important therapeutic implications because it is not clear that therapeutic responses designed for effort-induced angina and ischemia have the same therapeutic effect on mental stress–induced events. In a preliminary study, it was noted that treatment with a calcium-channel antagonist improved ischemic indices on treadmill exercise testing but did not affect mental stress–induced left ventricular dysfunction.[14] Thus, the effects of antianginal medications on exercise-induced versus mental stress–induced myocardial ischemia may be discordant. This topic merits further investigation.

Further studies are clearly necessary to define the mechanism for mental stress induced–left ventricular dysfunction. To this end, a preliminary pilot study was carried out to evaluate the effect of sympathetic nervous system interaction on this phenomenon. Endoscopic transthoracic sympathectomy was performed in patients with severe coronary artery disease and intractable angina.[24] Patients who underwent ambulatory left ventricular function monitoring with mental stress testing before and after endoscopic transthoracic sympathectomy had a substantial reduction in mental stress–induced left ventricular dysfunction before the intervention. This suggests that sympathetic nerve traffic may play a major role in the mental stress phenomenon. In addition, regional central nervous system activation and various centrally mediated effects may mechanistically affect this phenomenon.[33] The role of coronary flow–related ischemia compared with increased afterload-related ventricular dysfunction must also be defined. Data from our laboratory and others suggest that major changes in peripheral vascular resistance and afterload occur during mental stress, raising the possibility of the primacy of peripheral responses in this phenomenon.[8,17]

After cardiac transplantation

After successful cardiac transplantation, most patients have subnormal exercise capability despite normal left ventricular dysfunction. The cause of this limitation is not known. This issue was addressed in 11 patients undergoing cardiac transplantation an average of 2 years earlier.[16] Patients were monitored during level walking at a brisk pace for 7 to 10 minutes. This activity resulted in symptoms of shortness of breath and fatigue. Left ventricular function monitoring showed a marked increase in left ventricular ejection fraction (averaging 16 units) that was accompanied by a prompt marked increase in relative end-diastolic volume of approximately 8% and a marked reduction of end-systolic volume of 12%. Cardiac output increased 1.8-fold. Changes in ventricular volumes and output were maximal in the first 3 to 4 minutes, then remained at a plateau. In contrast, the heart rate increase was more gradual,

with a maximum increase of 20 beats per minute seen near the end of walking.

These data suggest that the increase in cardiac output with exercise occurs as a result of an increase in left ventricular volume and stroke volume without an appropriate chronotropic response. This effect would not be unexpected given the autonomic interruptions associated with cardiac transplantation. These findings may be responsible for the effort intolerance noted in cardiac transplantation patients despite normal ventricular function at rest. The study also indicates how this technology may be used in complex physiologic assessments of cardiac patients.

In patients with Parkinson disease

Nappi et al[31] studied left ventricular function of blood pressure in patients with Parkinson disease and with and without postural hypotension.[31] In patients with postural hypotension, change in posture from the supine to the upright position resulted in a substantial decrease in end-diastolic volume, end-systolic volume, stroke volume, left ventricular ejection fraction, and cardiac output. This change in posture was also associated with a great reduction in peripheral vascular resistance. In patients without postural hypotension, ejection fraction increased when the upright position was assumed, but ventricular volumes and output did not change. Therefore, abnormalities in peripheral vascular reactivity during postural changes may result in abnormal cardiac function in patients with Parkinson disease.

Miscellaneous studies

Conditions other than routine coronary disease have also been evaluated with the c-VEST. Patients have been evaluated during hemodialysis,[32] during which asymptomatic episodes of decrease in ejection fraction were commonly observed. These episodes were associated with an increase in end-systolic volume and no change in blood pressure or diastolic volume. Changes in ECG were rarely evident. These data indicate the potential value of ambulatory monitoring in the assessment of patients for prolonged periods of time while they are undergoing potentially deleterious interventions.

Another laboratory situation in which altered ventricular function has been noted involves sleep apnea.[7] In the laboratory, Garpestad et al[7] noted significant alterations in ventricular function associated with apneic periods. Abrupt decreases in left ventricular stroke volume and cardiac output at apnea termination occurred simultaneously with the nadir of oxygen saturation. On the basis of these observations, sleep apnea left ventricular dysfunction may be associated with further compromise tissue oxygen delivery in these patients. Other investigators have studied patients with syndrome X and hypertrophic cardiomyopathy.[35,36]

FUTURE DIRECTIONS

Ambulatory left ventricular function monitoring seems to have potential for the study of a broad spectrum of patients with and without coronary artery disease. Just as one would not treat hypertension without monitoring of the blood pressure, monitoring of ventricular function under various circumstances may be equally relevant for determining the optimal therapy. Ambulatory ventricular function may be particularly suitable for the study of patients with mental stress. Evaluating persons only in the exercise laboratory may not be adequate to define the true nature of the ischemic burden. Furthermore, definition of the exact potential triggering events for acute coronary syndromes may require mental stress testing on a broader basis.[23,26] New generations of equipment, which should be available shortly, should make this technology far more user friendly and accessible. At this point in time, the technology, if it is to have a role, must pass from the curiosities of the research laboratory to the practicalities of clinical care.

REFERENCES

1. Bairey CN, de Yang L, Berman DS, et al: Comparison of physiologic ejection fraction responses to activities of daily living: implications for clinical testing, *J Am Coll Cardiol* 16:847–854, 1990.
2. Bede J. Personal communication.
3. Berger HJ, Davies RA, Batsford WP, et al: Beat-to-beat left ventricular performance assessed from equilibrium cardiac blood pool using a computerized nuclear probe, *Circulation* 63:133–142, 1981.
4. Breisblatt WM, Weiland FL, McLain JR, et al: Usefulness of ambulatory radionuclide monitoring of left ventricular function early after acute myocardial infarction for predicting residual myocardial ischemia, *Am J Cardiol* 62:1005–1010, 1988.
5. Broadhurst P, Cashman P, Crawley J, et al: Clinical validation of a miniature nuclear probe system for continuous on-line monitoring of cardiac function and ST-segment, *J Nucl Med* 32:37–43, 1991.
6. Burg MM, Jain D, Soufer R, et al: Role of behavioral and psychological factors in mental stress-induced silent left ventricular dysfunction in coronary artery disease, *J Am Coll Cardiol* 22:440–448, 1993.
7. Garpestad E, Katayama H, Parker JA, et al: Stroke volume and cardiac output decrease at termination of obstructive apneas, *J Appl Physiol* 73:1743–1748, 1992.
8. Goldberg AD, Becker LC, Bonsall R, et al: Ischemic, hemodynamic, and neurohormonal responses to mental and exercise stress. Experience from the Psychophysiological Investigations of Myocardial Ischemia Study (PIMI), *Circulation* 94:2402–2409, 1996.
9. Gottlieb SO, Gottlieb SH, Achuff SC, et al: Silent ischemia on Holter monitoring predicts mortality in high-risk postinfarction patients, *JAMA* 259:1030–1035, 1988.
10. Gullette ECD, Blumenthal JA, Babyak M, et al: Effects of mental stress on myocardial ischemia during daily life, *JAMA* 277:1521–1526, 1997.
11. Imbriaco M, Cuocolo A, Pace L, et al: Repeatability of haemodynamic responses to cardiac stimulations by ambulatory monitoring of left ventricular function, *J Nucl Biol Med* 37:238–244, 1993.
12. Jain D, Allam AH, Wackers FJ, et al: Validation of a new non-imaging miniature probe for serial on-line left ventricular ejection fraction, *J Nucl Med* 32(Suppl):1038, 1991 (abstract).
13. Jain D, Burg M, Soufer R, et al: Day to day reproducibility of mental stress induced LV dysfunction, *J Am Coll Cardiol* 27(Suppl):240A, 1996 (abstract).
14. Jain D, Burg M, Soufer R, et al: Discordant effects of amlodipine on exercise-induced vs mental stress induced myocardial ischemia in patients with angina, *J Nucl Med* 37:59P, 1996 (abstract).
15. Jain D, Burg M, Soufer R, et al: Prognostic significance of mental stress-induced silent left ventricular dysfunction in patients with stable angina pectoris, *Am J Cardiol* 76:31–35, 1995.
16. Jain D, Lee FA, Revkin J, et al: Reduced exercise capacity in patients

17. following cardiac transplantation: Excellent ventricular function—a primary Starling effect but inadequate heart rate response during exercise, *J Nucl Med* 33:939, 1992 (abstract).
17. Jain D, Shaker SM, Burg M, et al: Effects of mental stress on left ventricular and peripheral vascular performance in patients with coronary artery disease. *J Am Coll Cardiol* 31:1314, 1998.
18. Jain D, Vita NA, Wackers FJ, Zaret BL: Transient silent left ventricular dysfunction in non-Q wave myocardial infarction and unstable angina, *J Nucl Med* 32(Suppl):938, 1991 (abstract).
19. Jain D, Zaret BL: *Ambulatory left ventricular function.* In Gerson M, ed: Cardiac nuclear medicine, ed 3, New York, 1996, McGraw-Hill.
20. Jiang W, Babyak M, Krantz DS, et al: Mental stress–induced myocardial ischemia and cardiac events, *JAMA* 275:1651–1656, 1996.
21. Kayden DS, Wackers FJ, Zaret BL: Silent left ventricular dysfunction during routine activity after thrombolytic therapy for acute myocardial infarction, *J Am Coll Cardiol* 15:1500–1507, 1990.
22. Kayden DS, Remetz MS, Cabin HS, et al: Validation of continuous radionuclide left ventricular function monitoring in detecting silent myocardial ischemia during balloon angioplasty of the left anterior descending artery, *Am J Cardiol* 67:1339–1343, 1991.
23. Leor J, Poole WK, Kloner RA: Sudden cardiac death triggered by an earthquake, *N Engl J Med.* 334:413–419, 1996.
24. Lomsky M, Jain D, Claes G, et al: Endoscopic transthoracic sympathecotomy protects against mental stress induced LV dysfunction in patients with severe angina. Pilot study results, *Circulation* 92:I–677, 1995 (abstract).
25. Millar-Craig MW, Bishop CN, Raftery EB: Circadian variation of blood pressure, *Lancet* 1:795–797, 1978.
26. Mittleman MA, Maclure M, Tofler GH, et al: Triggering of acute myocardial infarction by heavy physical exertion. Protection against triggering by regular exertion. Determinants of Myocardial Infarction Onset Investigators, *N Engl J Med* 329:1677–1683, 1993.
27. Mohiuddin IH, Kambara H, Ohkusa T, et al: Clinical evaluation of cardiac function by ambulatory ventricular scintigraphic monitoring (VEST): validation and study of the effects of nitroglycerin and nifedipine in patients with and without coronary artery disease, *Am Heart J* 123:386–394, 1992.
28. Mohiuddin IH, Tamaki N, Kambara H, et al: Detection of exercise induced silent ischemia and the sequence of ischemic events in coronary artery disease by radionuclide ambulatory ventricular function monitoring, *Jpn Circ J* 58:689–697, 1994.
29. Mortelmans L, Cabrera EZ, Dorny N, et al: Left ventricular function changes during pharmacological and physiological interventions and routine activities monitored in healthy volunteers by a portable radionuclide probe (VEST), *Int J Card Imaging* 7:79–87, 1991.
30. Mortelmans L, Vanhecke W, Mertens D, et al: Assessment of the optimal atrioventricular delay in dual chamber-paced patients by a portable scintillation probe (VEST), *J Nucl Cardiol* 3:321–326, 1996.
31. Nappi A, Cuocolo A, Iazzetta N, et al: Ambulatory monitoring of left ventricular function in patients with Parkinson's disease and postural hypotension, *Eur J Nucl Med* 21:1312–1317, 1994.
32. Singh N, Langer A, Freeman MR, et al: Myocardial alterations during hemodialysis: insights from new noninvasive technology, *Am J Nephrol* 14:173–181, 1994.
33. Soufer R, Bremmer D, Arrighi JA, et al: Cerebral cortical hyperactivation in response to mental stress in patients with heart disease, *Proc Natl Acad Sci U S A* 95:6454–6459, 1998.
34. Taki J, Muramori A, Nakajima K, Bunko H, et al: [Cardiac response to exercise before and after coronary artery bypass grafting: evaluation by continuous ventricular function monitor], *Kaku Igaku* 28:1313–1320, 1991.
35. Taki J, Nakajima K, Muramori A, et al: Left ventricular dysfunction during exercise in patients with angina pectoris and angiographically normal coronary arteries (syndrome X), *Eur J Nucl Med* 21:98–102, 1994.

36. Taki J, Nakajima K, Shimizu M, et al: Left ventricular functional reserve in nonobstructive hypertrophic cardiomyopathy: evaluation by continuous left ventricular function monitoring, *J Nucl Med* 35:1937–1943, 1994.

37. Tamaki N, Gill JB, Moore RH, et al: Cardiac response to daily activities and exercise in normal subjects assessed by an ambulatory ventricular function monitor, *Am J Cardiol* 59:1164–1169, 1987.

38. Tamaki N, Yasuda T, Moore RH, et al: Continuous monitoring of left ventricular function by an ambulatory radionuclide detector in patients with coronary artery disease, *J Am Coll Cardiol* 12:669–679, 1988.

39. Vassiliadis IV, Machac J, Sharma S, et al: Detection of silent left ventricular dysfunction during daily activities in coronary artery disease patients by the nuclear VEST, *J Nucl Biol Med* 37:198–206, 1993.

40. Wilson RA, Sullivan PJ, Moore RH, et al: An ambulatory ventricular function monitor: validation and preliminary clinical results, *Am J Cardiol* 52:601–606, 1983.

41. Zaret BL, Jain D: *Continuous monitoring of left ventricular function with miniaturized nonimaging detectors.* In Zaret BL, Beller GA, eds: *Nuclear cardiology: state of the art and future directions,* St. Louis, 1993, Mosby–Year Book.

Chapter 13

Measurement of ventricular function and volume

Jeffrey S. Borer

It is more than 35 years since the first report by Folse and Braunwald[40] of a nonimaging method for evaluating cardiac function and volumes with radioisotopes after administration of tracer directly into the left ventricle and 30 years since this invasive and relatively imprecise method was followed by development of a noninvasive approach to the same end by Hoffmann and Kleine[55] at the University of Fribourg. Hoffmann and Kleine's nonimaging radionuclide probe for defining variations in intraventricular blood volumes was a watershed discovery, but because it was published only in a German-language journal, it was little appreciated at a time when international communication was less well developed than it is today. In addition, application and validation efforts were minimal, in part because the device could not provide images that assured correct data collection.

Soon, efforts by other investigators provided the requisite images, first with radioisotope administered directly into the left ventricle during catheterization[71] and later noninvasively when Strauss et al[91] reported their first radioisotope angiocardiogram obtained with intravenous administration of a technetium-99m (^{99m}Tc)–labeled tracer. This early procedure did not involve dynamic data acquisition. Therefore, definition of cardiac function from temporal volume variations required a method for collection of data only from a relatively short period including end diastole and during another short period including end systole. Such a "gating" device was needed to enable superimposition of photon information collected from many cardiac cycles to provide total counts sufficient for statistically reliable volume determinations. To assure constancy of isotope concentration in the blood pool during the extended period of imaging, equilibration of isotope was allowed before data collection. Electrocardiographic signals provided the systolic time interval information needed to operate the gate (although other physiologic signals can and have been used) The result was relatively coarse temporal resolution and, consequently, imprecise end-diastolic and end-systolic volumes and ejection fractions. These early studies emulated contrast angiography by applying geometric formulae to images acquired in the right anterior oblique position to calculate volumes. However, with isotope equilibrated in the blood pool, right ventricular and left ventricular blood pools were superimposed, and the resulting edge overlap limited accuracy. Subsequent investigations by Parker et al[78] in 1972 demonstrated the feasibility of count-based determination of ejection fraction from gated studies on the basis of inherent proportionality between background-corrected photons and cardiac-chamber blood volumes. For this approach, data were collected in the left anterior oblique position, enabling visual separation of the cardiac chambers.

The next step, which began by two different routes in 1971 and culminated in clinical application in 1976, involved dynamic acquisition of sequential images throughout the cardiac cycle. This technique afforded time–volume curves for individual or superimposed sequential cardiac cycles. Application of this method, particularly when associated with simultaneously obtained hemodynamic information, permitted precise definition of a wide variety of functional descriptors and of relatively instantaneous volumes. One of the routes used a high-sensitivity multicrystal radiation detector. This device enabled collection of sufficient photons to provide statistically reliable time–volume curves for each of the few cardiac cycles that occur during a single passage of an intravenous isotope bolus through the heart. However, the sensitivity of the detector allowed only relatively coarse temporal resolution. This "first-pass" method, preliminarily reported by Jones, Howe, and Goodrich[62] in 1976, provided high-quality images in the right anterior oblique position. The precision of count-based methods was not sacrificed because residence of isotope in the superimposed ventricles was temporally separated.

The second route, conceived by physicist Michael Green, did not require temporal separation of right-ventricular and left-ventricular isotope residence. Instead, it made use of newly emerging computer methods to superimpose time–volume information from many sequential cardiac cycles by digitizing and storing information on spatial location and time of collection of emitted photons.[46-48] When this approach was rendered serviceable for real-time display by Bacharach et al,[4,5] it could be applied not only to resting studies, as earlier methods had been, but also to assessments performed during exercise, as first reported by Borer et al[20,21] in 1976. (The events leading to the development of exercise radionuclide cineangiography illustrate the serendipitous nature of some medical discoveries and are presented elsewhere.[29]) The usefulness of the latter development was confirmed by other investigators,[13,60,62,83] and a new era of physiologic measurement of cardiac volumes and function during stress had begun. Application of radionuclide-based measurements of ventricular volumes and function during exercise has been critically important in defining the pathophysiology of many heart diseases and has provided diagnostic and prognostic information that forms the basis for current management strategies in patients with coronary, valvular, and myopathic heart diseases.

By 1980, computer methods permitted three-dimensional display of data obtained simultaneously or sequentially from multiple angles. This method, which used both dual-photon (positron emission tomography [PET]) and single-photon (single-photon emission tomography [SPECT]) approaches, provided perfusion scintigraphic data of relatively high precision and diagnostic and pathophysiologic utility. With appropriate isotopes, these approaches quickly were applied to blood-pool imaging to assess volumes and function.[8,87] However, the cost and cumbersome nature of PET precluded its practical application for determination of volume and function. In addition, the time required to obtain blood-pool images by using SPECT has limited the practical use of this approach (see below). Moreover, during the early years of SPECT perfusion scintigraphy, the isotope used to define perfusion was thallium-201 (^{201}Tl), the physical characteristics of which are suboptimal for precise blood-pool scintigraphy or assessment of regional function from wall motion. During the past decade, several ^{99m}Tc-labeled tracers have been developed and used in perfusion scintigraphy; in theory, these agents enable function and perfusion studies to be obtained after a single administration of isotope.

To capture the prognostic and additional diagnostic value of left ventricular function determination during perfusion scintigraphic studies, two approaches have been adopted. First-pass blood-pool scintigraphy is performed immediately after intravenous administration of the perfusion agent and before extraction of the agent by the myocardium and subsequent collection of the perfusion image.[31,59,93] This approach enables application of count-based methods of global and regional ventricular volumes and function. The second approach abandons count-based methods; instead, it uses geometry-based formulae for assessment of ventricular volumes and function from images obtained after extraction of isotope by the myocardium (that is, subsequent to clearing of the blood pool).[39,92] Images of the perfused myocardium also have been used for additional functional assessments based on regional wall thickening[102]; this is not possible with blood-pool imaging but is commonly obtained by echocardiography.

TECHNICAL CONSIDERATIONS

Since the introduction of radionuclide cineangiography in 1976, this method generally has been accepted as the preferred noninvasive approach for assessing cardiac volumes and function, whether by blood-pool imaging using either first-pass or equilibrium methods or by imaging perfused myocardium after the blood pool has cleared. Technical considerations include selection, preparation, and administration of the radiopharmaceutical; photon collection systems and associated computer-data management algorithms; acquisition protocols; and data analysis and interpretation.

The radiopharmaceutical and its administration

First pass. For this application, the radiopharmaceutical must reside in the blood pool only for the relatively short time necessary for the bolus to pass through the heart once. During this period, isotope that is sufficiently mixed and adequately concentrated for reliable imaging resides in each ventricle for approximately five to six cardiac cycles. In theory, any pharmaceutical can be used for first-pass imaging unless, when passing through the lungs, the molecule is retained in the pulmonary vasculature (such as ^{99m}Tc-labeled macroaggregated albumin), is excreted (such as krypton-81m and xenon-127), or is otherwise extracted. A radiopharmaceutical that is retained would be adequate only for right ventricular assessment and would provide no left ventricular data.[63,84] However, if rest and exercise studies are to be performed the radiopharmaceutical administered during the initial study must be largely or completely cleared from the blood pool before the second study is performed. Therefore, radiopharmaceuticals that are rapidly cleared by the reticuloendothelial system, such as ^{99m}Tc sulfur colloid, have been widely employed.[10,90] However, the close proximity of the liver (a clearing site) and the heart can result in suboptimal resolution of the basal heart border in the second study. Technetium-99m diethylenetriamine pentaacetic acid is rapidly cleared by the kidneys,[51] thus avoiding this problem. Currently, the first-pass method is most commonly used in association with SPECT perfusion scintigraphy with such ^{99m}Tc-labeled agents as 2-methoxyisobutyl isonitrile (MIBI),[31] other isonitriles,[59] or tetrofosmin.[93] For this purpose, rest and exercise studies can be separated by sufficient time to permit clearance and decay of the relatively short-lived isotope (6-hour half-life). Because 2-day protocols are cumbersome, are inconvenient, and permit physiologic variation, which may confound study interpretation, rest and exercise studies often are performed in one session. The exercise assessment is undertaken immediately after the rest perfusion study, approximately 1 hour after rest ventriculography. To minimize the impact of residual background activity from the rest images on the exercise study, isotope doses can be adjusted; for this purpose, activity administered before the second study commonly is threefold that of the initial study.[31] When first-pass blood-pool and perfusion imaging are integrated, study interpretation can be confounded by spontaneous physiologic variation in ejection fraction during the 1 hour that separates the rest and exercise studies. To avoid this, the perfused myocardium itself can be used for closely sequenced functional assessments in a manner analogous to that used during equilibrium blood-pool imaging.[39,92]

Isotopes other than ^{99m}Tc have been used in first-pass imaging, particularly those with short half-lives, which permits high doses and excellent counting statistics without exceeding safe radiation exposures. Such agents include gold-195m,[97] tantalum-178,[56] and iridium-191m.[95]

First-pass blood-pool imaging requires maintenance of the bolus configuration of the injectate to avoid superimposition of labeled cardiac chambers during the transit of isotope through the heart. Thus, relatively large-bore cannulae inserted into large veins (external jugular or antecubital) are necessary and activity must be highly concentrated (bolus <1 ml).

Equilibrium. In contrast to first-pass methods, equilibrium methods require that the isotope remain in the intravascular blood pool for as long as possible to minimize both the rate of activity loss (with attendant loss of statistical precision) and development of extravascular background activity. For equilibrium studies, ^{99m}Tc is bound to an agent with long intravascular residence, such as human serum albumin (which is suboptimal because its metabolism begins relatively quickly) or erythrocytes (as is now the common practice). Erythrocyte binding is mediated by the reducing agent stannous pyrophosphate, which binds to erythrocyte surface receptors and to ^{99m}Tc. Erythrocyte binding can be achieved in vivo by intravenous administration of stannous pyrophosphate, in vitro by removing blood from the patient and causing the reaction among erythrocytes, stannous pyrophosphate, and Tc pertechnetate to occur in a test tube, or by a modified in vitro approach (ex vitro) involving intravenous administration of the binder, withdrawal of blood, and mixing of the stannous pyrophosphate–treated cells with Tc pertechnetate in a test tube.[35,52,79,94] Labeling efficiency approaches 90% with these methods, and the biological half-life of the labeled erythrocyte exceeds the physical half-life of the isotope.

Because equilibration of the tracer in the blood pool is required, there is no need for attention to bolus characteristics during intravenous administration. However, polyethylene intravenous lines seem to adsorb the injected radiopharmaceutical; direct administration from a syringe through a needle is therefore preferred.

When myocardium that is isotopically labeled with perfusion agents is used for geometric calculation of volumes and function,[39,92] bolus administration is not a concern. In addition, residence time within the myocardium is of only secondary concern, because outlining of the ventricular borders does not require proportionality between activity and blood volume. Duration of residence in the myocardium must be considered in defining imaging protocols if wall thickness is to be calculated,[102] because precision in such determinations depends in part on counting statistics.

Photon collection systems

First pass. Data can be collected only from the initial passage of isotope through the heart. Therefore, radiation detection must be highly efficient to assure statistically reliable volume determinations. For this purpose, the standard single crystal Anger camera is suboptimal. A multicrystal camera, in which each small crystal is separated from other crystals by photon-blocking septae and is connected to photomultiplier tubes by light pipes (recently superceded by more advanced techniques), provides adequate efficiency for quantitative accuracy. The spatial coarseness of images produced by the original multicrystal cameras has been minimized and the counting efficiency has been increased to linear responsiveness at >400,000 counts/sec. In some cases, counts that greatly exceed this lower limit have been achieved by increasing the number of crystals, reducing the size of individual crystals, eliminating light pipes, and improving circuitry. In addition, modification of computer methods to allow for identification of a second, distant point source of radiation has enabled image position correction from frame to frame to accurately register sequential images during exercise-induced movement. This development has increased the practicality of performing blood-pool imaging during the first passage of isotope administered for perfusion scintigraphy while the patient continues to exercise on an upright treadmill or bicycle.

Although multicrystal cameras provide the high counting efficiency necessary for first-pass imaging, digital single-crystal cameras have increased the efficiency of these better-resolved implements.[42] Consequently, they too can be effectively applied for first-pass imaging.

Because statistically reliable data are available from each cardiac cycle in first-pass collections, images are displayed sequentially and do not require superimposition within the computer. Therefore, computer requirements for data acquisition are relatively modest, and the appropriate algorithm can be inferred from the more complex collection algorithm used for equilibrium studies (see below). Usually, first-pass studies are collected in frame mode, in which photon-location data are compartmentalized and stored sequentially in segments of predetermined duration. The apparent data density of first-pass studies can be enhanced by using a gating device and superimposing sequential cycles in the computer to provide a composite of five or six cardiac cycles. Given the high data acquisition rates now possible with multicrystal cameras, the gated first-pass approach usually is unnecessary and has the potential disadvantage of loss of temporal resolution associated with superimposition of cycles of slightly varying duration. The latter problem can be obviated if data are collected in list mode (described below) for poststudy reformatting.

Equilibrium. The mainstay of equilibrium methods is the standard Anger camera equipped with a single Tl-activated sodium iodide crystal. This device has the advantage of relatively high spatial resolution compared with multicrystal detectors. However, it is considerably less efficient because dead time after photon capture affects the entire crystal rather than only one of many small crystals in the multicrystal camera. In addition, a collimator must be placed between the patient and the crystal to maximize the accuracy with which the position of incident photons can be tracked back to their source in a two-dimensional plane. The multicrystal camera obviates the need for a collimator because, in general, photons incident on each crystal originate from a relatively small subtended solid angle.

Patient fatigue or other symptoms and the need to maintain relative constancy of physiologic variables limit the time available for imaging during maximal exercise to no more than 2 to 3 minutes. During this time, sufficient radioactive emissions must be collected to ensure precise volume calculations (in practice, at least 2,000,000 counts from the heart and immediately surrounding thorax and diaphragm or at least 100,000 to 150,000 counts per composite movie frame). Therefore, low-energy, high-sensitivity collimators or the somewhat less sensitive low-energy, all-purpose collimators are used. If resting studies alone are performed, time is not a practical limitation, and it is reasonable to seek maximal resolution with low-energy, high-resolution collimation. In the course of developing exercise radionuclide cineangiography, my coworkers and I found that for a 2-minute collection during exercise, use of a high-sensitivity collimator caused a 15% loss in resolution compared with a high-resolution collimator when analyzed by line-spread function. However, this loss was more than compensated, visually and in quantitative precision of left ventricular ejection fraction determination, by the 250% increase in count-detection efficiency that resulted.

The limitations imposed by the standard single-crystal Anger camera include dead time, maximal crystal thickness (proportional to sensitivity) necessary to achieve acceptable resolution (inversely proportional to thickness), and need for collimation. Because of these limitations, near-linear proportionality between photon density incident on the collimator and photon density transmitted to the computer can be maintained only in the range of 30,000 counts/sec on older models and 80,000 counts/sec (advertised by some newer nondigital cameras). This rate may be exceeded if digital cameras are used.

Therefore, to collect sufficient counts for precise volumetric data from equilibrium studies, generally it is necessary to superimpose data collected from sequential cardiac cycles. This can be done with the frame mode approach, which requires the operator to select the expected maximal heart rate before data collection and requires division of the corresponding cardiac cycle lengths into equal segments, or frames. The number of frames depends on the amount of computer memory allocated for the task. Thus, in this mode, frame duration is a function of heart rate. However, particularly at heart rates achieved during exercise, accurate assessment of systolic function generally requires frame durations of no more than 40 msec, and diastolic function assessment often requires greater temporal resolution.[6] Therefore, frame duration in frame mode may be inadequate for optimal quantitation of ventricular function in some cases.

To avoid this problem, data can be collected in list mode, in which each data point receives a spatial address in computer memory, a temporal address, and an address indicating the cardiac cycle length at the time of collection. Determination of frame duration can be defined after the study is completed on the basis of heart rates known to have been achieved and on the requirements of the specific variables to be measured.

For each of these appoaches, a gating device triggered by a physiologic signal (usually the R-wave of electrocardiograph) is used to identify the onset of each new cardiac cycle so that sequential frames can be superimposed in perfect temporal registration. Because many cycles need to be collected and because errors in gating due to noisy signals or premature beats can be expected from time to time, a method for beat rejection is necessary. In frame mode, this is done on the fly with predetermined temporal or signal characteristic features that can be used to identify cycles that probably are inappropriate for collection. In list mode, a cycle-length histogram is constructed after completion of data collection. From the histogram, premature cycles can be identified and eliminated and the heart rate range or series of ranges to be analyzed in study can be defined.[46]

Acquisition protocols

First pass. During first-pass studies, isotopic labeling of cardiac-chamber blood occurs sequentially. Thus, labeling of the right ventricle is temporally separated from that of the left ventricle, and for a short period during the sequence of bolus progression, each chamber can be isolated at any angle of observation. However, the desired position must be determined before isotope administration, when the spatial orientation of the heart is not completely known.[82,83] Transmission scintigraphy of the heart often is used immediately before camera positioning to aid this process.

When exercise data are required, bicycle exercise can be performed both supine and upright; in the latter case, the patient is positioned with arms firmly holding the camera. When a noncardiac point source is used to aid in registration of successive images, treadmill exercise also can be used.[82]

Equilibrium. In contrast to first-pass studies, at equilibrium, all cardiac chambers simultaneously are filled with isotope-labeled blood. Therefore, quantitation of ventricular volumes and function can be performed only in the left anterior oblique position, in which the right ventricle and left ventricle do not overlap. Optimal ventricular separation can be achieved by imaging with a persistence oscilloscope during camera positioning. Because the temporal window for imaging after isotope administration is measured in hours and studies require only minutes, malpositioned studies can be repeated if necessary. Generally, adequate positioning is achieved in the 45° left anterior oblique position with a 15° caudal tilt to account for the orientation of the long axis of the ventricle within the chest. For qualitative wall motion assessment, other positions, including the anterior view (for anterolateral and apical motion and, sometimes, for the inferior wall), the steep left anterior oblique view, left lateral view, or the left posterior oblique views (all for the inferior wall) can be used. In general, it is impractical to perform more than one exercise test during a single study session; therefore, most exercise studies are obtained only in the left anterior oblique position to permit quantitation. However, reports have been published describing exercise studies performed in multiple positions[74] or repeated in a single position before and after pharmacologic intervention.[22]

When it was first developed, exercise radionuclide cineangiography was performed supine with bicycle exercise to minimize patient motion under the camera.[21] The feasibility of upright bicycle exercise since has been well demonstrated.[70] Be-cause patient motion occurs during exercise, the problem of adequate registration of hundreds of heartbeats during treadmill exercise has limited the application of the equilibrium method for this type of data acquisition.

Many exercise protocols have been used in association with radionuclide angiography. Unless a specific question can be best answered with submaximal exercise, most protocols continue until they are limited by symptoms (such as angina, dyspnea, or fatigue) or some prespecified event (such as arrhythmia). Responses of left ventricular ejection fraction have been defined in normal persons for submaximal exercise heart rates, providing a basis for comparison in clinical studies in which maximal exercise occurs at heart rates below those that might be expected in a normal person of similar age.[26] Stress also has been applied by cold temperature stimulation[99] and with pharmacologic agents,[29,37,41] but standards for the use of these stressors have not been well established.

Data analysis and interpretation

First pass. A region of interest is placed over the heart, and a low-frequency time–activity curve (temporal resolution of 0.5 seconds) is generated by summing collected counts sequentially (Fig. 13-1). Because right ventricular and left ventricular blood-pool labeling are temporally separated, this curve has two distinct areas of maximal oscillation. The first defines pas-

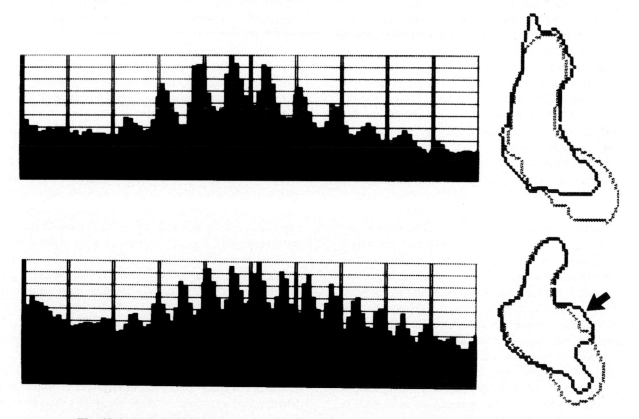

Fig. 13-1. Typical first-pass time–activity curve with associated end-diastolic and end-systolic images. (Reprinted from Port SC: Recent advances in first-pass radionuclide angiography, *Cardiol Clin* 12:359-372, 1994, W.B. Saunders, with permission.)

sage of the bolus through the right ventricle and the second shows its passage through the left ventricle. High-frequency time–activity curves then are constructed for the ventricular collections, and regions of interest are defined for each ventricle to maximize precision of subsequent volumetric calculations.

Although background radioactivity is considerably lower during first-pass studies than during equilibrium collections, approximately 20% to 30% of the total activity is background during the left ventricular phase. Background can be identified with a region of interest defined immediately outside the apical perimeter of the left ventricle, quantified for each frame, and subtracted from total counts before calculation of absolute or relative volumes. Alternatively, the cycle immediately preceding the identifiable entry of isotope into the left ventricle can be selected from the time–activity curve and subtracted from subsequent frames used to define left ventricular volume variations. Finally, a standard background subtraction constant can be determined by a variety of algorithms.[82]

For the right ventricle, background determination is more complex. In many views, the right ventricular region contains no background immediately before isotope entry into the ventricle. Effective spatial separation of the right ventricle and the pulmonary artery is possible, but complete separation of the right ventricle and the right atrium is difficult. Therefore, a background region of interest comprising a rim of pixels that define the overlap of the right atrium and the right ventricle can be applied to the frame immediately before isotope entry into the right ventricle, and the result can be subtracted from all frames comprising the right ventricular time–activity curve.[11]

Both first-pass and equilibrium radionuclide angiograms provide ejection fraction of either ventricle by application of the equation EF = [ED counts-ES counts]/[ED counts-BKG counts], where *ED* is end diastole, *ES* is end systole, and *BKG* is background. For this calculation, relative volumes are defined by the count densities within the ventricular regions of interest. Absolute left ventricular volumes can be defined from first-pass studies by outlining the left ventricle and performing geometric calculations.[83] Irregular chamber shape precludes accurate application of this approach to the right ventricle.

Other measures of left ventricular function, such as peak systolic ejection rate, peak diastolic filling rate, and time to peak filling rate, can be determined from the time–activity curves of individual cycles,[82] but the limitation in available counts minimizes the precision of these determinations. Superimposition of sequential cycles by gating can enhance such calculations,[82] but beat-to-beat variability in cycle length leads to imprecision in determination of the diastolic values. In theory, this problem could be minimized by list-mode data collection and backward framing, in which sequential beats from end diastole are aligned, as is done in the method developed for equilibrium studies.[6,47] However, this approach has generated little interest because of the limited number of cycles (and, hence, data) available for analysis.

Calculation of absolute volumes enables determination of

contractility measures (such as single-point pressure–volume ratios) in some patient subsets, but their usefulness is potentially limited by the imprecision of the volume determination.

Regional ventricular function or wall motion can be assessed visually with geometric calculations or with count-based regional ejection fractions. However, the inherent limitations in count rate and spatial resolution render regional assessment relatively imprecise. Shunt lesions also can be evaluated from first-pass studies by placing the region of interest over a lung region and analyzing the resulting pulmonary transit curve in a manner like that used for dye-dilution curves in the catheterization laboratory.[3] In recent years, this application has been largely obviated by improvements in echocardiographic methodology.

Equilibrium. The major strength of the equilibrium study compared with the first-pass study is count density and resulting volumetric precision (Fig. 13-2). Therefore, it is not surprising that ejection fraction usually is determined by count-based methods. For the left ventricle, the region of interest can be defined in end diastole and fixed in this configuration throughout systole (thereby relatively underestimating ejection fraction if background structures enter the region of interest during systole), or the region of interest can vary throughout the cardiac cycle on the basis of manual, semiautomated, or automated edge-detection algorithms applied to each frame.[21,32,50] In either case, the relation between radionuclide angiographic left ventricular ejection fraction and the corresponding contrast angiographic value is excellent both at rest and during exercise.[44]

Right ventricular ejection fraction is more difficult to determine with equilibrium studies because overlap of right heart structures invariably occurs during systole in any view. However, at end diastole, right atrial counts are minimal. Therefore, in the left anterior oblique view, in which only overlap of the right atrium and the right ventricle is of concern and the relatively posterior position of the right atrium minimizes contribution from that chamber, the effect of the right atrium can be disregarded. At end systole, separation of the right atrium and right ventricle generally is sufficient to permit spatial distinction of the two chambers. Therefore, definition of separate right ventricular end-diastole and end-systole regions of interest enables reasonably accurate measurement of right ventricular ejection fraction,[68] compared with first-pass[68] or contrast[44] standards. Full time–activity curves cannot be defined from equilibrium studies, potentially limiting the complement of physiologic information that can be obtained. Moreover, in practice, accurate definition of right ventricular ejection fraction by using equilibrium methods requires frequent repetition to assure consistency in identification of valve planes.

Background accounts for 35% to 60% of total counts in equilibrium studies. Therefore, inconsistencies in background determination can result in relatively large variations in ejection fraction. The preferred background region of interest is a crescent of pixels close to the periphery of the left ventricular apex and free wall. Other background regions of interest have

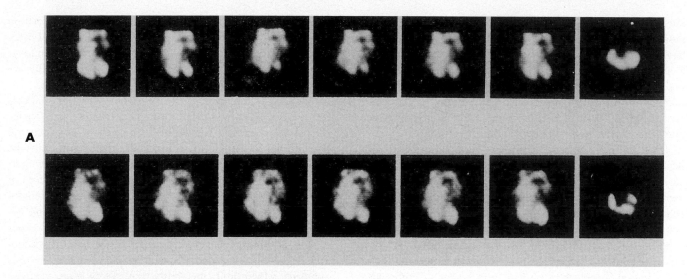

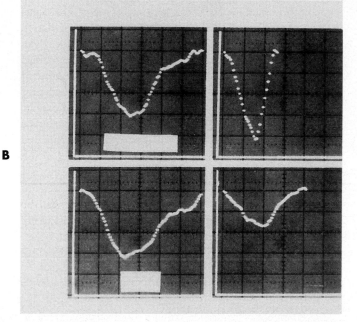

Fig. 13-2. A, Representative images from a multi-image, gated equilibrium radionuclide cineangiogram obtained at rest and during exercise in a patient with coronary artery disease (the first such series ever published). **B,** Time–activity curves from the studies shown in A along with a normal comparator. (Reprinted from Borer JS, Bacharach SL, Greene MV, et al: Real-time radionuclide cineangiography in the noninvasive evaluation of global and regional left ventricular function at rest and during exercise in patients with coronary artery disease, *N Engl J Med* 296:839-844, 1977, with permission.)

included those defined automatically or semiautomatically. The left ventricular background region also usually is used to determine right ventricular ejection fraction, although a background region of interest for the right ventricle can be determined.

With count densities achieved at equilibrium, regional time–activity curves can provide precise regional left ventricular ejection fraction and evidence of temporal asynchrony when the left ventricle is divided into wedges or grids.[34,53,57,69] Because this determination can be performed only in the left anterior oblique position, regions of interest often include the overlapping distributions of two or more coronary arteries. Therefore, these determinations may not precisely define the effect of lesions in any single artery. Although this is a limitation in assessing the functional severity of specific coronary obstructions in patients with multivessel disease, it is not an important limitation in evaluating the effects of pharmacologic or other therapies.

Absolute volumes can be determined geometrically in the lateral view.[2] However, volume determinations usually are performed by a count-based approach in the left anterior oblique view. For the latter, ventricular counts usually are corrected for attenuation[89] and are normalized for duration of collection and for counts in a blood sample drawn from the patient. Counts in the blood sample are also normalized for duration of collection.[65] If the time between blood collection and imaging is long, correction for decay also is necessary. Volume determination also can be performed without attenuation correction, and if the associated mathematical formulation accounts for the ratio of total counts to peak pixel counts in the left ventricle (which is a function of left ventricular volume), the need for blood sampling is avoided, simplifying the procedure considerably.[72]

Because of the relatively high count density and temporal resolution of equilibrium images, ejection rates and diastolic performance indices (peak filling rate and time to peak filling rate) obtained from time–activity curves are more reliable than those obtained with first-pass methods. Diastolic assessments have proven useful in diagnosis of coronary artery disease and evaluation of drug effects,[15,17,80] particularly when precision is optimized by backward framing (done to maximize temporal registration) of the list-mode data acquisitions[6,15] that make possible the 10-msec or finer temporal resolution needed to define diastolic function accurately at rapid heart rates.[6]

Like first-pass studies, equilibrium studies can be used in defining left ventricular contractility indices (for example, pressure–volume relations, such as the peak systolic pressure/left ventricular end-systolic volumes index). In combination with echocardiographic data, rest and exercise contractility can be defined by normalizing left ventricular ejection fraction for left ventricular end-systolic stress, a method which has proven particularly useful in prognostication among patients with aortic regurgitation.[27] Indices of pulmonary vascular pressures also have been obtained during equilibrium radionuclide cineangiography; these are based on activity in regions of interest placed over lung regions at rest and during exercise or in apical and basal lung segments.[77] With the increasing use of Doppler echocardiography, these methods are seldom used clinically. However, right ventricular ejection fraction is inversely related to pulmonary artery pressures[54] and may serve as a useful index of these values in clinical settings where right ventricular ejection fraction determination otherwise is applicable, as in mitral regurgitation.

Because of the high count density of the composite images, single functional images can be created. These images display regional count variation data in a format that can simplify identification of regional abnormalities. The first functional image was the subtraction image or stroke volume map, in which the end-systolic frame is subtracted from the end-diastolic frame with the amplitude of resulting pixels set proportional to the change from end-diastole to end-systolic. Thus, an akinetic region would appear as a black hole and a normally ejecting region as white area, with gradations in between. Normalization of the stroke volume map for the end-diastolic image results in an ejection fraction image. Further refinement of this procedure can be introduced by transforming the raw two-dimensional spatial images into spatial frequency components relating the rapidity of change in counts in each pixel. These frequency components are defined in terms of their amplitude and phase. A technique known as Fourier transformation is used to define spatial information in the frequency domain. The time–activity curve of each pixel can be approximated as a sinusoidal wave, the lowest frequency of which (the fundamental frequency) is defined by the heart rate.[7,33,66] Harmonics of this fundamental frequency can be defined mathematically. From this family of harmonics, each pixel within the region of interest can be related in terms of amplitude (a function of stroke volume) and alignment or phase angle; the latter defines the delay in emptying from one pixel to the next. With this analytic tool, it is possible to characterize contraction patterns and, thus, to identify conduction or contraction abnormalities. The latter information can serve as a useful adjunct to other methods of regional function assessment and can be used to maximize precision in identifying the demarcation between structures that normally are out of phase, such as the left atrium and the left ventricle.

For equilibrium studies, the size of the data set of total collected counts is limited only by computer memory size. Therefore, if collection time is unlimited, the precision of volumetric and functional data from radionuclide angiograms must be greater when the equilibrium approach rather than the first-pass approach is used. If similar imaging systems are used, it can be demonstrated mathematically that even for the temporally limited aquisition during exercise, precision of volume determination is greater with the equilibrium approach.[45] Other relative advantages and disadvantages of the two approaches include the inherently poorer spatial resolution of the first-pass approach, which limits the ability to precisely assess regional function. However, the limitation in available views and superimposition of isotope-filled structures limits regional function assessment with the equilibrium method. The ability to analyze individual cardiac cycles may be advantageous in some settings and is afforded by the first-pass approach, but the composite of hundreds of cycles obtained with the equilibrium approach provides a more representative and precise assessment of cardiac volumes and function. When using blood-pool scintigraphy for count-based assessments in combined perfusion and function studies, the first-pass method is the only practical choice; use of the equilibrium analog of geometry-based volume assessment is practical but sacrifices one of the inherent benefits of radionuclide angiography (the independence of results from the effect of geometric irregularities) while adding the ability to analyze wall thickness variation. Ultimately, the selection of approach must depend on the information required and the clinical setting in which the test is used.

CLINICAL APPLICATIONS

Measurement of ventricular volumes and function is useful in almost every clinical setting. Consequently, radionuclide-based determinations have been used in almost every area of cardiac disease. However, nuclear methods lack the spatial resolution of echocardiography, X-ray contrast angiography, or magnetic resonance imaging. Therefore, in settings that require precise anatomic detail (such as coronary arteriography, diagnosis of congenital heart diseases, or etiologic assessment of valvular diseases), radionuclide angiography has limited clinical value. Conversely, for functional determinations, radionuclide-based methods are less affected by the motion of exercise or by anatomic irregularities than other imaging techniques and have proven extraordinarily powerful in guiding therapeutic management decisions, particularly in coronary artery disease, regurgitant valvular diseases, and certain heart failure settings, and in assessing the effects of therapy for heart diseases or noncardiac diseases treated with potentially cardiotoxic agents.

Coronary artery disease

Diagnosis. This area has been extensively studied and recently reviewed.[29] Reported accuracy for diagnosis of chronic stable disease varies widely with study population selection and diagnostic criteria. Sensitivity and specificity have reached 100% in some studies, but a reasonable synthesis of published studies suggests an average sensitivity of about 90% and specificity of about 85%. Lack of absolute accuracy is not surprising: neither global nor regional ventricular dysfunction is biologically specific for coronary artery disease, and anatomic coronary obstruction need not result in regional dysfunction because regional dysfunction is affected by such factors as magnitude of obstruction, adequacy of collateral flow, and intrinsic myocardial metabolic characteristics. Moreover, functional variables can be affected by associated factors, including cardioactive drugs and noncoronary heart diseases. Currently, there is a growing trend toward identifying relative ischemia severity in different coronary artery territories (a process requiring three-dimensional or tomographic data display) to plan coronary angioplasty procedures. Because of this need as well as the relative lack of specificity of radionuclide angiography, dependence on radionuclide ventriculography for diagnosis has progressively decreased in favor of SPECT perfusion scintigraphy. Nonetheless, radionuclide cineangiography remains a viable diagnostic method for coronary artery disease when used alone and adds substantially to the diagnostic information available from myocardial perfusion scintigraphy when the methods are used together.[12,59] Used alone or in combination with other nonimaging noninvasive techniques,[100] radionuclide cineangiography is highly efficient in identifying the presence of multivessel coronary artery disease.

Descriptors of ventricular function and volume cannot discriminate independently between recent and remote impairment. Therefore, this approach has little value for diagnosis of acute myocardial infarction, for which more specific methods are available. However, the regional impairment associated with myocardial infarction can be well delineated,[96] and functional assessment can be useful in identifying right ventricular involvement when acute myocardial infarction is diagnosed by other means.[88] Despite recent improvements in echocardiographic imaging, radionuclide angiography may be unexcelled in diagnosis by functional assessment.

Prognosis and management decision making. The ease and accuracy of quantitation of the functional concomitant of ischemia with radionuclide ventriculography have led to evolution of the method primarily as a prognostic tool[29] and, therefore, as a basis for definition of management strategy. The prognostic value of ventriculography is based on the empirical observation that the functional effects of coronary lesions as they exist at the time of the test provide a statistically valid index of the likelihood of subsequent ischemic events. Currently, there is no better method for prognostication, including anatomic definition of the coronary lesion by coronary angiography.[29] In a recent study by Wallis et al,[101] in which 192 patients first studied after coronary bypass grafting were followed for an average of 9 years, the change in left ventricular ejection fraction from rest to exercise provided the best prediction of infarction or death during follow-up and was superior to indices of coronary anatomy, graft number, or other variables[101] (Fig. 13-3). Most important, the quantitative characteristics of ventriculography lend themselves to determination of relative risk when different management strategies are compared. Early work by Jones et al[61] suggested a variation in outcome ascribable to bypass grafting among surgical and nonsurgical patients with similar left ventricular functional characteristics. In more recent work preliminarily presented by Supino et al,[29] patients with three-vessel disease were categorized on the basis of left ventricular ejection function from rest to exercise before bypass grafting or prolonged medical therapy. The benefits of surgery compared with medical therapy were directly and quantitatively related to the extent of exercise-induced ischemia at index study, providing a matrix for decision making based on precise risk-to-benefit assessment.[29]

Despite its utility in prognostication, the relation between cardiac dysfunction, either at rest or unmasked by exercise, and

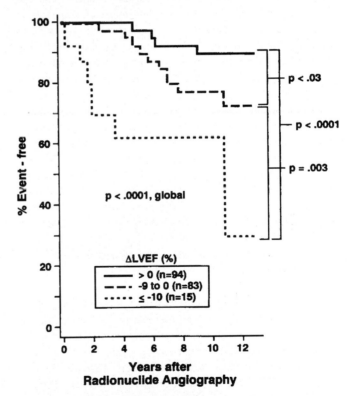

Fig. 13-3. Relation between survival after coronary bypass grafting (ordinate) and time (abscissa) as a function of the change (Δ) in left ventricular ejection fraction from rest to exercise as determined by radionuclide cineangiography. (Reprinted from Wallis JB, Supino PG, Borer JS, et al: Prognostic value of left ventricular ejection fraction response to exercise during long-term follow-up after coronary bypass graft surgery, *Circulation* 88(5Pt2):II99-II109, 1993, with permission from the American Heart Association, Dallas, Texas.)

ischemic events is largely by chance. Patients do not die or sustain infarction because of ischemia measured during exercise testing nor because of the lesion that causes such dysfunction. Instead, major ischemic events result from sudden structural change in the lesion underlying ischemic dysfunction and, often, because of sudden change in a hemodynamically modest lesion that may fail to cause ischemia with exercise. Thus, although exercise testing provides information on relative risk that justifies management decisions,[29] the accuracy of absolute risk determination is modest, primarily because the biological relation between test and event is tenuous at best. Improvement in prognostication and management decision making awaits application of radiolabeled metabolites or ligands that can define lesion biology to distinguish lesions imminently likely to rupture from those with equivalent hemodynamic and functional effects.[19]

Radionuclide-based ventricular function studies provide effective prognostication in the setting of myocardial infarction, both in the acute and recovery phases. Many studies have documented the ability of left ventricular ejection fraction at rest measured early during infarction to predict in-hospital outcome.[29,49] Perhaps more important, survival after hospital discharge also can be predicted from left ventricular function at rest, both without thrombolysis[29,75] and with thrombolysis. In the postthrombolytic era, left ventricular ejection fraction at rest remains the most powerful predictor of outcome but is importantly modified by age and the behavior of ST segment and chest pain during thrombolysis, factors that were not relevant before the availability of thrombolysis.[85] Moreover, radionuclide-based quantitation of regional left ventricular ejection fraction at rest after thrombolysis is a highly accurate index of sustained reperfusion of the infarct-related artery.[98]

Prediction of posthospital survival after infarction can be further enhanced by exercise assessment.[28,29,36] The utility of this approach is supported by recent studies of patients who have undergone thrombolysis,[38] although the relation between specific predictive indices and the outcomes they predict may differ among patients who have undergone thrombolysis and among those who have not.

Assessment of pharmacologic and mechanical interventions. In patients with coronary artery disease, study of the effects of drugs, surgery, and angioplasty on left ventricular volumes and function has been undertaken with radionuclide angiography at rest and during exercise. Mitigation of ischemic left ventricular dysfunction by nitroglycerin first was demonstrated in 1978.[22] The effects of other drugs have not been as clear: some anti-ischemic agents, such as β-blockers and calcium-channel blockers, have direct negative inotropic and peripheral vascular effects in addition to direct antiischemic actions, and the result of such complex actions is not easily predicted. However, assessment of effects on diastolic phase indices can be useful, for example, in distinguishing among the effects of different calcium-channel blocking drugs.[29] Unlike most drugs, mechanical revascularization affects only myocardial blood flow, resulting in enhancement of left ventricular

function at rest (if hibernating myocardium is present) or during exercise. Therefore, radionuclide cineangiography, alone or in combination with perfusion scintigraphy,[36] has been widely used to evaluate such therapy[29] and to prognosticate in postoperative patients.[58,101]

Valvular diseases

Nonischemic valvular heart diseases are among the most important causes of heart failure and sudden death. Radionuclide ventriculography does not permit the measurements necessary for diagnosis of stenotic conditions and lacks the precision of echocardiography in quantifying the severity of valvular regurgitation. Moreover, although it is useful in elucidating the pathophysiology of aortic[25,30] and mitral[30,73] stenosis and in evaluating the effects of surgery, radionuclide angiography has no clear role in management decision making for patients with these conditions. In contrast, the ability of radionuclide-based measures of ventricular performance, size, and function to predict outcome in patients with regurgitant valvular diseases is proven.[85]

Aortic regurgitation

Left ventricular ejection fraction at rest long has been a primary determinant of operability in aortic regurgitation[14,18] on the basis of demonstration of relatively poor long-term postoperative survival among patients with subnormal left ventricular ejection fraction before surgery. Several studies defining natural history in the unoperated patient with aortic regurgitation,[16,24,27,30] have shown that radionuclide cineangiography can be useful in selecting patients for valve replacement even if the patients are asymptomatic and have normal left ventricular ejection fraction at rest.[24,27] Studies by Borer et al[24,27] have shown that combination of echocardiographic wall thickness data and radionuclide-based volumes and left ventricular ejection fraction at rest and during exercise provides maximal prognostic power in aortic regurgitation, and can identify asymptomatic patients with measurable risk for sudden death.[24,27] Definition of the natural history of left ventricular function after surgery also has been undertaken with radionuclide cineangiography.[23] Elucidation of the 3-year course of full functional recovery after surgery has necessitated revision of previously held ideas about the cellular pathophysiology of this disease.

Mitral regurgitation

Radionuclide angiography is uniquely suited to use in mitral regurgitation.[30] This disease affects both ventricles directly, and although left ventricular performance carries important prognostic information, considerable data indicate the utility of assessing right ventricular performance at rest and during exercise in defining management strategies.[54,86] These data reveal that imminent mortality risk is relatively high, even in the absence of symptoms, when right ventricular ejection fraction is subnormal at rest[54] and that heart failure is best predicted by the absence of augmentation of right ventricular ejection fraction during exercise[86] (Fig.13-4). Among the methods available for

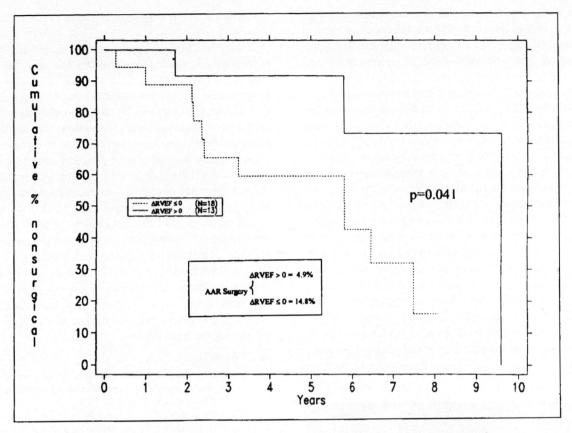

Fig. 13-4. Relation between development of congestive heart failure (percentage of nonsurgical patients, ordinate) and time as a function of right ventricular ejection fraction in patients with mitral regurgitation. (Reprinted from Rosen SE, Borer JS, Hochreiter C, et al: Natural history of the asymptomatic/minimally symptomatic patient with normal right and left ventricular performance and severe mitral regurgitation due to mitral valve prolapse, *Am J Cardiol* 74:374-380, 1994. The Cahners Publishing Co., with permission.)

the repeated applications necessary for surveillance in this chronic disease, only radionuclide angiography enables accurate determination of left ventricular and right ventricular performance at rest and during exercise. Both left ventricular ejection fraction[81] and right ventricular ejection fraction[30] are useful in predicting the long-term outcome of mitral valve surgery; similar parallel data have been reported for mitral regurgitation and aortic regurgitation combined.[76]

Myocardial diseases

Ventricular size and function as assessed by radionuclide angiography have been useful in making management decisions in several myocardial diseases. Selection of patients for cardiac transplantation has been made in part on the basis of serial radionuclide cineangiographic determinations of left ventricular ejection fraction among patients with congestive heart failure.[18] In this setting, left ventricular structural irregularities are common and militate against reliance on geometry-based measurements available with echocardiography.

Similarly, the cardiotoxic effects of therapies for non-cardiac conditions have been elucidated with radionuclide angiography.[1,43,64] The usefulness of this application has been particularly apparent in guiding antineoplastic therapy with Adriamycin.[1,43] Individualization of Adriamycin therapy with predose left ventricular ejection fraction determinations has allowed safe administration of doses well beyond those conventionally recommended on the basis of patient size characteristics alone. Individualization of antineoplastic therapy may be the primary current clinical application of radionuclide-based determination of left ventricular ejection fraction at rest. Although left ventricular ejection fraction defined during exercise can unmask abnormalities in patients with normal left ventricular ejection fraction at rest who are undergoing antineoplastic therapy, no clear evidence shows that exercise-induced abnormalities add substantially to management decision making information available from left ventricular ejection fraction at rest.[43]

FUTURE DIRECTIONS

Radionuclide-based assessment of ventricular volumes and function has been a standard evaluative procedure in cardiology for 20 years. The usefulness of this method is well established for diagnosis in coronary artery disease and, more important, for prognostication and management decision making in various cardiac conditions. However, all evaluation strategies must be tailored to answer questions that aid selection among currently available therapies. Complete revascularization for prolongation of life and relief of ischemic symptoms in patients with coronary artery disease has been supplemented with partial revascularization by catheter-based percutaneous angioplasty techniques and by minimally invasive percutaneous bypass grafting procedures for symptom relief alone. Sequential partial revascularization has been offered (without supporting data) as an alternative to complete revascularization surgery to minimize morbidity associated with surgical therapy. Such therapy is, by definition, regional; prediction of its likely outcome and determination of its anti-ischemic effectiveness require evaluation by techniques that can define regional characteristics. For example, SPECT perfusion scintigraphy is well suited to this purpose. To optimally supplement and amplify the diagnostic information available from perfusion scintigraphy, radionuclide angiography must make full use of the three-dimensional information available from scintigraphy (Fig. 13-5). When applied for this purpose,[67] SPECT radionuclide angiographic assessment of left ventricle aneurysm function has enabled prognostication among patients undergoing ventricular aneurysmectomy. This determination is not possible with the

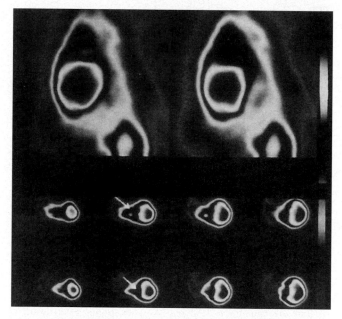

Fig. 13-5. Comparison of 70° left anterior oblique planar end-diastolic *(ED)* and end-systolic *(ES)* views from a standard radionuclide cineangiogram compared with selected ED and ES views of sections of the same study collected by single-photon emission computed tomography and reconstructed by computer in tomographic display. This study was obtained in a patient with a left ventricular aneurysm and illustrates the added information available from tomographic reconstruction. (Reprinted from Lu P, Liu X, Shi R, et al: Comparison of tomographic and planar radionuclide ventriculography in assessment of regional left ventricular function in patients with left ventricular aneurysm before and after surgery, *J Nucl Cardiol* 1:537-545, 1994. American Society of Nuclear Cardiology, with permission.)

two-dimensional display of conventional radionuclide cineangiography.

Currently, clinical application of tomographic blood-pool scintigraphy is limited primarily by the need for relatively lengthy data acquisition, which precludes evaluation of the effects of stress. Efforts now are under way to shorten acquisition time and improve accuracy[9] to enable application in the context of short-term pharmacologic interventions. The ability to assess regional function precisely also promises to enhance the value of radionuclide angiography for directing newer pharmacologic therapies on the basis of increasingly sophisticated knowledge of the importance of regional variations in myocardial cell biology in various disease states.

Enhanced speed of data acquisition, possibly coupled with use of relatively short-lived isotopes, may permit increasingly accurate assessment of regional wall thicknesses by tomographic SPECT, holding promise for precision in contractility assessments from radionuclide angiography in conjunction with perfusion scintigraphy. If the latter can be achieved, important improvements can be expected in management strategies for various heart diseases.

REFERENCES

1. Alexander J, Dainiak N, Berger HJ, et al: Serial assessment of doxorubicin cardiotoxicity with quantitative radionuclide angiocardiography, *N Engl J Med* 300:278–283, 1979.
2. Ashburn WL, Kostuk WJ, Karliner JS, et al: Left ventricular volume and ejection fraction determination by radionuclide angiography, *Semin Nucl Med* 3:165–176, 1973.
3. Askenazi J, Ahnberg DS, Korngold E, et al: Quantitative radionuclide angiography: detection and quantitation of left to right shunts, *Am J Cardiol* 37:382–387,1976.
4. Bacharach SL, Green MV, Borer JS, et al: Real-time scintigraphic cineangiography. *Computers in Cardiology (IEEE)* 45–48, 1976.
5. Bacharach SL, Green MV, Borer JS, et al: A real-time system for multi-image gated cardiac studies, *J Nucl Med* 18:79–84, 1997.
6. Bacharach SL, Green MV, Borer JS, et al: Left ventricular peak ejection rate, filling rate and ejection fraction: frame rate requirements at rest and exercise, *J Nucl Med* 20:189–193, 1979.
7. Bacharach SL, Green MV, Vitale D, et al: Optimum Fourier filtering of cardiac data: a minimum-error method, *J Nucl Med* 24:1176–1184, 1983.
8. Barat J-L, Brendel J, Colle J-P, et al: Quantitative analysis of left-ventricular function using gated single photon emission tomography, *J Nucl Med* 25:1167–1174, 1984.
9. Bartlett MC, Srinivasan G, Barker WC, et al: Left ventricular ejection fraction: comparison of results from planar and SPECT gated blood-pool studies, *J Nucl Med* 37:1795–1799, 1996.
10. Berger HJ, Gottschalk K, Zaret BL. *First pass radionuclide angiocardiography for evaluation of right and left ventricular performance: computer applications and technical considerations.* In Sorensen JA, ed: *Nuclear cardiology: selected computer aspects,* New York, Society of Nuclear Medicine, 1978.
11. Berger HJ, Matthay RA, Loke J, et al: Assessment of cardiac performance with quantitative radionuclide angiocardiography: right ventricular ejection fraction with reference to findings in chronic obstructive pulmonary disease, *Am J Cardiol* 41:897–905, 1978.
12. Berman DS, Kiat H, Germano G, et al: *99m-Tc-sestamibi SPECT.* In DePuey EG, Berman DS, Garcia EV, eds: *Cardiac SPECT imaging,* Raven Press (New York) 1995, pp. 121–146.
13. Bodenheimer MM, Banka VS, Fooshee CM, et al: Comparative sensitivity of the exercise electrocardiogram, thallium imaging and stress

radionuclide angiography to detect the presence and severity of coronary heart disease, *Circulation* 60:1270–1278, 1979.

14. Bonow RO: Asymptomatic aortic regurgitation: indications for operation, *J Card Surg* 9(2 Suppl):170–173, 1994.

15. Bonow RO, Bacharach SL, Green MV, et al: Impaired left ventricular diastolic filling in patients with coronary artery disease: assessment with radionuclide angiography, *Circulation* 64:315–323, 1981.

16. Bonow RO, Lakatos E, Maron BJ, et al: Serial long-term assessment of the natural history of asymptomatic patients with chronic aortic regurgitation and normal left ventricular systolic function, *Circulation* 84:1625–1635, 1991.

17. Bonow RO, Leon MB, Rosing DR, et al: Effects of verapamil and propranolol on left ventricular systolic function and diastolic filling in patients with coronary artery disease: radionuclide angiographic studies at rest and during exercise, *Circulation* 65:1337–1350, 1982.

18. Borer JS: *Prognostication strategies in heart failure and valvular heart diseases: current concepts and their support.* In Yacoub M, ed: *Annual of cardiac surgery,* London, 1989, Current Science.

19. Borer JS: Atherosclerosis imaging: pathophysiological assessment for a new era. *J Nucl Med* 34:1321–1325, 1993.

20. Borer JS, Bacharach SL, Green MV, et al: Rapid evaluation of left ventricular function during exercise in patients with coronary artery disease, *Circulation* 54(Suppl II):II–6, 1976 (abstract).

21. Borer JS, Bacharach SL, Green MV, et al: Real-time radionuclide cineangiography in the noninvasive evaluation of global and regional left ventricular function at rest and during exercise in patients with coronary-artery disease, *N Engl J Med* 296:839–844, 1977.

22. Borer JS, Bacharach SL, Green MV, et al: Effect of nitroglycerin on exercise-induced abnormalities of left ventricular regional function and ejection fraction in coronary artery disease. Assessment by radionuclide cineangiography in symptomatic and asymptomatic patients, *Circulation* 57:314–320, 1978.

23. Borer JS, Herrold EM, Hochreiter C, et al: Natural history of left ventricular performance at rest and during exercise after aortic valve replacement for aortic regurgitation, *Circulation* 84(5Suppl):III133–III139, 1991.

24. Borer JS, Hochreiter C, Herrold EM, et al: Prediction of indications for valve replacement among asymptomatic or minimally symptomatic patients with chronic aortic regurgitation and normal left ventricular performance, *Circulation* 97:525–534, 1998.

25. Borer JS, Jason M, Devereux RB, et al: Function of the hypertrophied left ventricle at rest and during exercise. Hypertension and aortic stenosis. *Am J Med* 75(3A):34–39, 1983.

26. Borer JS, Kent KM, Bacharach SL, et al: Sensitivity, specificity and predictive accuracy of radionuclide cineangiography during exercise in patients with coronary artery disease. Comparison with exercise electrocardiography. *Circulation* 60:572–580, 1979.

27. Borer JS, Kligfield P: Aortic regurgitation: making management decisions, *American College of Cardiology Journal Reviews* 4:30–32, 1995.

28. Borer JS, Miller D, Schreiber T, et al: Radionuclide cineangiography in acute myocardial infarction: role in prognostication, *Semin Nucl Med* 17:89–94, 1987.

29. Borer JS, Supino P, Wencker D, et al: Assessment of coronary artery disease by radionuclide cineangiography. History, current applications, and future directions, *Cardiol Clin* 12:333–357, 1994.

30. Borer JS, Wencker D, Hochreiter C: Management decisions in valvular heart disease: the role of radionuclide-based assessment of ventricular function and performance, *J Nucl Cardiol* 3:72–81, 1996.

31. Borges-Neto S, Coleman RE, Jones RH: Perfusion and function at rest and treadmill exercise using technetium-99m-sestamibi: comparison of one- and two-day protocols in normal volunteers, *J Nucl Med* 31:1128–1132, 1990.

32. Bourguignon MH, Douglass KH, Links JM, et al: Fully automated data acquisition, processing, and display in equilibrium radioventriculography, *Eur J Nucl Med* 6:343–347, 1981.

33. Brateman L, Buckley K, Keim SG, et al: Left ventricular regional wall motion assessment by radionuclide ventriculography: a comparison of cine display with Fourier imaging, *J Nucl Med* 32:777–782, 1991.

34. Caldwell JH, Williams DL, Kennedy JW, et al: Quantitative, semi-automated radionuclide technique for determination of regional left ventricular function during rest and exercise, *J Nucl Med* 19:710, 1978 (abstract).

35. Callahan RJ, Froelich JW, McKusick KA, et al: A modified method for the in vivo labeling of red blood cells with Tc-99m: concise communication, *J Nucl Med* 23:315–318, 1982.

36. Candell-Riera J, Permanyer-Miralda G, Castell J, et al: Uncomplicated first myocardial infarction: strategy for comprehensive prognostic studies, *J Am Coll Cardiol* 18:1207–1219, 1991.

37. Cates CU, Kronenberg MW, Collins HW, et al: Dipyridamole radionuclide ventriculography: a test with high specificity for severe coronary artery disease, *J Am Coll Cardiol* 13:841–851, 1989.

38. Cerqueira MD, Maynard C, Ritchie JL, et al: Long-term survival in 618 patients from the Western Washington Streptokinase in Myocardial Infarction Trials. *J Am Coll Cardiol* 20:1452–1459, 1992.

39. DePuey EG, Nichols K, Dobrinsky C: Left ventricular ejection fraction assessed from gated technetium-99m-sestamibi SPECT, *J Nucl Med* 34:1871–1876, 1993.

40. Folse R, Braunwald E: Determination of fraction of left ventricular volume ejected per beat and of ventricular end-diastolic and residual volumes, *Circulation* 25:674–684, 1962.

41. Freeman ML, Palac R, Mason J, et al: A comparison of dobutamine infusion and supine bicycle exercise for radionuclide cardiac stress testing, *Clin Nucl Med* 9:251–255, 1984.

42. Gelfand MJ, Thomas SR: *Acquisition and processing—two-dimensional studies.* In Gelfand MJ, ed: *Effective use of computers in nuclear medicine: practical clinical applications in the imaging laboratory,* New York, 1988, McGraw-Hill.

43. Gerling B, Gottdiener J, Borer JS: *Cardiovascular complications of the treatment of Hodgkin's disease.* In Lacher MJ, Redman JR, eds: *Hodgkin's disease: the consequences of survival,* Philadelphia, 1989, Lea & Febiger.

44. Goldberg HL, Herrold EM, Hochreiter C, et al: Videodensitometric determination of right ventricular and left ventricular ejection fraction, *Am J Non-Invasive Cardiol* 1:18–23, 1987.

45. Green MV, Bacharach SL, Borer JS, et al: A theoretical comparison of first-pass and gated equilibrium methods in the measurement of systolic left ventricular function, *J Nucl Med* 32:1801–1807, 1991.

46. Green MV, Bacharach SL, Douglas MA, et al: The measurement of left ventricular function and the detection of wall motion abnormalities with high temporal resolution ECG-gated scintigraphic angiocardiography, *IEEE Transactions on Nuclear Science* 23:1257–1263, 1976.

47. Green MV, Bailey JJ, Ostrow HG, et al: Computerized EKG-gated radionuclide angiocardiography: a non-invasive method for determining left ventricular volumes and focal myocardial dyskinesia, *Computers in Cardiology (IEEE)* 137–141, 1975.

48. Green MV, Ostrow HG, Doulas MA, et al: *Scintigraphic cineangiography of the heart. Proceedings of MEDINFO 74,* Amsterdam, 1974, North Holland Publishing Co.

49. Griffin BP, Shah PK, Diamond GA, et al: Incremental prognostic accuracy of clinical, radionuclide and hemodynamic data in acute myocardial infarction, *Am J Cardiol* 68:707–712, 1991.

50. Hains ADB, Al-Khawaja I, Hinge DA, et al: Radionuclide left ventricular ejection fraction: a comparison of three methods, *Br Heart J* 57:242–246, 1987.

51. Hauser W, Alkins HL, Nelson KG, et al: Techetium 99m DTPA: a new radiopharmaceutical for brain and kidney scanning, *Radiology* 94:679–684, 1970.

52. Hegge FN, Hamilton GW, Larson SM, et al: Cardiac chamber imaging: a comparison of red blood cells labelled with Tc-99m in vitro and in vivo, *J Nucl Med* 19:129–134, 1978.

53. Hinge DA, Lahiri A, Rodrigues RA, et al: A quantitative method for estimating regional left ventricular systolic and diastolic function, *Nucl Med Comm* 8:254, 1987 (abstract).

54. Hochreiter C, Niles N, Devereux RB, et al: Mitral regurgitation: relationship of noninvasive descriptors of right and left ventricular performance to clinical and hemodynamic findings and to prognosis in medically and surgically treated patients, *Circulation* 73:900–912, 1986.

55. Hoffmann G, Kleine N: The method of radiographic functional analysis, *Nucl Med (Stuttg)* 7:350–370, 1968.

56. Holman BL, Neirinckx RD, Treves S, et al: Cardiac imaging with tantalum-178, *Radiology* 131:525–526, 1979.

57. Holman BL, Wynne J, Idoine J, et al: Disruption in the temporal sequence of regional ventricular contraction. I. Characteristics and incidence in coronary artery disease, *Circulation* 61:1075–1083, 1980.

58. Iskandrian AS, Hakki AH, Goel IP, et al: The use of rest and exercise radionuclide ventriculography in risk stratification in patients with suspected coronary artery disease, *Am Heart J* 110:864–872, 1985.

59. Iskandrian AS, Heo J, Kong B, et al: Use of technetium-99m isonitrile (RP-30A) in assessing left ventricular perfusion and function at rest and during exercise in coronary artery disease, and comparison with coronary arteriography and exercise thallium-201 SPECT imaging, *Am J Cardiol* 64:270–275, 1989.

60. Jengo JA, Oren V, Conant R, et al: Effects of maximal stress on left ventricular function in patients with coronary artery disease using first pass radionuclide angiography: a rapid, noninvasive technique for determining ejection fraction and segmental wall motion, *Circulation* 59:60–65, 1979.

61. Jones RH, Floyd RD, Austin EH, et al: The role of radionuclide angiography in the preoperative prediction of pain relief and prolonged survival following coronary artery bypass grafting, *Ann Surg* 197:743–754, 1983.

62. Jones RH, Howe WR, Goodrich JK: Assessment of left ventricular function by a single radionuclide transit through the heart, *J Nucl Med* 17:556, 1976 (abstract).

63. Knapp WH, Helus F, Lambrecht RM, et al: Kr-81m for determination of right ventricular ejection fraction (RVEF), *Eur J Nucl Med* 5:487–492, 1980.

64. Leon MB, Borer JS, Bacharach SL, et al: Detection of early cardiac dysfunction in patients with severe beta-thalassemia and chronic iron overload, *N Engl J Med* 301:1143–1148, 1979.

65. Links JM, Becker LC, Shindledecker JG, et al: Measurement of absolute left ventricular volume from gated blood pool studies, *Circulation* 65:82–91, 1982.

66. Links JM, Douglass KH, Wagner HN Jr: Patterns of ventricular emptying by Fourier analysis of gated blood pool studies, *J Nucl Med* 21:978–982, 1980.

67. Lu P, Liu X, Shi R, et al: Comparison of tomographic and planar radionuclide ventriculography in the assessment of regional left ventricular function in patients with left ventricular aneurysm before and after surgery, *J Nucl Cardiol* 1:537–545, 1994.

68. Maddahi J, Berman D, Matsuoka DT, et al: A new technique for assessing right ventricular ejection fraction using rapid multiple gated equilibrium cardiac blood pool scintigraphy. Description, validation and findings in chronic coronary artery disease, *Circulation* 60:581–589, 1979.

69. Maddox DE, Wynne J, Uren R, et al: Regional ejection fraction: a quantitative radionuclide index of regional left ventricular performance, *Circulation* 59:1001–1009, 1979.

70. Manyari DE, Kostuk WJ: Left and right ventricular function at rest and during bicycle exercise in the supine and sitting positions in normal subjects and patients with coronary artery disease. Assessment by radionuclide ventriculography *Am J Cardiol* 51:36–42, 1983.

71. Mason DT, Ashburn WL, Harbert JC, et al: Rapid sequential visualization of the heart and great vessels in man using the wide-field Anger scintillation camera. Radioisotope-angiography following the injection of technetium-99m. *Circulation* 39:19–28, 1969.

72. Massardo T, Gal RA, Grenier RP, et al: Left ventricular volume calculation using a count-based ratio method applied to multigated radionuclide angiography, *J Nucl Med* 31:450–456, 1990.

73. Morise AP, Goodwin C: Exercise radionuclide angiography in patients with mitral stenosis: value of right ventricular response, *Am Heart J* 112:509–517, 1986.

74. Morris DD, Rozanski A, Berman DS, et al: Non-invasive prediction of the angiographic extent of coronary artery disease following myocardial infarction: comparison of clinical, exercise electrocardiographic, and ventriculographic parameters, *Circulation* 70:192–201, 1984.

75. Risk stratification and survival after myocardial infarction. *N Engl J Med* 309:331–336, 1983.

76. Niles N, Borer JS, Kamen M, et al: Preoperative left and right ventricular performance in combined aortic and mitral regurgitation and comparison with isolated aortic or mitral regurgitation, *Am J Cardiol* 65:1372–1378, 1990.

77. Okada RD, Osbakken MD, Boucher CA, et al: Pulmonary blood volume ratio response to exercise; a noninvasive determination of exercise-induced changes in pulmonary capillary wedge pressure, *Circulation* 65:126–133, 1982.

78. Parker JA, Secker-Walker R, Hill R, et al: A new technique for the calculation of left ventricular ejection fraction, *J Nucl Med* 13:649–651, 1972.

79. Pavel DG, Zimer AM, Patterson VN: In vivo labeling of red blood cells with 99mTc: a new approach to blood pool visualization, *J Nucl Med* 18:305–308, 1977.

80. Perrone-Filardi P, Bacharach SL, Dilsizian V, et al: Impaired left ventricular filling and regional diastolic asynchrony at rest in coronary artery disease and relation to exercise-induced myocardial ischemia, *Am J Cardiol* 67:356–360, 1991.

81. Phillips HR, Levine FH, Carter JE, et al: Mitral valve replacement for isolated mitral regurgitation: analysis of clinical course and late postoperative left ventricular ejection fraction, *Am J Cardiol* 48:647–654, 1981.

82. Port SC: Recent advances in first-pass radionuclide angiography, *Cardiol Clin* 12:359–372, 1994.

83. Rerych SK, Scholz PM, Newman GE, et al: Cardiac function at rest and during exercise in normals and in patients with coronary heart disease: evaluation by radionuclide angiocardiography, *Ann Surg* 187:449–464, 1979.

84. Rodrigues EA, Lahiri A, Hinge DA, et al: A new method for imaging the right ventricle using peripheral vein infusion of xenon 127, *Eur J Nucl Med* 12:617–619, 1987.

85. Rogers WJ, Papapietro SE, Wackers FJT, et al: Variables predictive of good functional outcome following thrombolytic therapy in the Thrombolysis in Myocardial Infarction phase II (TIMI II) pilot study, *Am J Cardiol* 63:503–512, 1989.

86. Rosen SE, Borer JS, Hochreiter C, et al: Natural history of the asymptomatic/minimally symptomatic patient with severe mitral regurgitation secondary to mitral valve prolapse and normal and left ventricular performance, *Am J Cardiol* 74:374–380, 1994.

87. Schelbert HR, Henze E, Phelps ME: Emission tomography of the heart, *Semin Nucl Med* 10:355–373, 1980.

88. Starling MR, Dell'Italia LJ, Chaudhuri TK, et al: First transit and equilibrium radionuclide angiography in patients with inferior transmural myocardial infarction: criteria for the diagnosis of associated hemodynamically significant right ventricular infarction, *J Am Coll Cardiol* 4:923–930, 1984.

89. Starling MR, Dell'Italia LJ, Walsh RA, et al: Accurate estimates of absolute left ventricular volumes from equilibrium radionuclide angiographic count data using a simple geometric attenuation correction, *J Am Coll Cardiol* 3:789–798, 1984.

90. Strauss HW, Pitt B: Evaluation of cardiac function and structure with radioactive tracer technique, *Circulation* 57:645–654, 1978.

91. Strauss HW, Zaret BL, Hurley PJ, et al: A scintiphotographic method

for measuring left ventricular ejection fraction in man without cardiac catheterization, *Am J Cardiol* 28:575–580, 1971.

92. Szulc M, Herrold EM, Zanzonico P, et al: Left ventricular ejection fractions from technetium MIBI perfusion scintigrams: computer-based method and validation, *Computers in Cardiology* IEEE publication 0276–6547/95:521–524, 1995.

93. Takahashi N, Tamaki N, Tadamura E, et al: Combined assessment of regional perfusion and wall motion in patients with coronary artery disease with technetium 99m tetrofosmin, *J Nucl Cardiol* 1:29–38, 1994.

94. Thrall JH, Freitas JE, Swanson D, et al: Clinical comparison of cardiac blood pool visualization with technetium-99m red blood cells labeled in vivo and with technetium-99m human serum albumin, *J Nucl Med* 19:796–803, 1978.

95. Treves S, Cheng C, Samuel A, et al: Iridium-191 angiocardiography for the detection and quantitation of left-to-right shunting, *J Nucl Med* 21:1151–1157, 1980.

96. Underwood SR, Walton S, Laming PJ, et al: Differential sensitivity of radionuclide ventriculography for the detection of anterior and inferior infarction, *Br Heart J* 60:411–416, 1988.

97. Wackers FJ, Giles RW, Hoffer PB, et al: Gold-195m, a new generator-produced short-lived radionuclide for sequential assessment of ventricular performance by first pass radionuclide angiocardiography, *Am J Cardiol* 50:89–94, 1982.

98. Wackers FJ, Terrin ML, Kayden DS, et al: Quantitative radionuclide assessment of regional ventricular function after thrombolytic therapy for acute myocardial infarction: results of phase I Thrombolysis in Myocardial Infarction (TIMI) trial, *J Am Coll Cardiol* 13:998–1005, 1989.

99. Wainwright RJ, Brennand-Roper DA, Cucni TA, et al: Cold pressor test in detection of coronary heart-disease and cardiomyopathy using technetium-99m gated blood-pool imaging, *Lancet* 2:320–323, 1979.

100. Wallis JB, Borer JS: Identification of "surgical" coronary anatomy by exercise radionuclide cineangiography, *Am J Cardiol* 68:1150–1157, 1991.

101. Wallis JB, Supino PG, Borer JS: Prognostic value of left ventricular ejection fraction response to exercise during long-term follow-up after coronary bypass graft surgery, *Circulation* 88(5 Pt 2):II99–II109, 1993.

102. Wisenberg G, Schelbert HR, Hoffman EJ, et al: In vivo quantitation of regional myocardial blood flow by positron-emission computed tomography, *Circulation* 63:1248–1258, 1981.

Chapter 14

Regional and global ventricular function analysis with SPECT perfusion imaging

Kenneth Nichols and **E. Gordon DePuey**

The high count density of technetium-99m (^{99m}Tc) sestamibi myocardial perfusion images affords the ability to obtain gated images that are synchronized to the patient's electrocardiogram and maintain adequate count density of individual cardiac frames.[52] This feature, in conjunction with the excellent spatial and contrast resolution provided by ^{99m}Tc sestamibi, allows simultaneous assessment of myocardial perfusion and ventricular function. Both wall motion and wall thickening can be evaluated, the former by excursion of the endocardial limits of the ventricle[7,12] and the latter by the increase in myocardial intensity during systole.[8]

GATED SPECT ACQUISITION

Myocardial perfusion images obtained after exercise or resting tracer injection can be gated. However, because gated images are acquired with the patient at rest, only resting ventricular function can be evaluated. The only method currently available to evaluate exercise ventricular function with ^{99m}Tc sestamibi is exercise first-pass radionuclide ventriculography.

As in the case with gated blood-pool imaging, there is a trade-off between the temporal resolution of gated ^{99m}Tc sestamibi images and the count density of each individual frame. To maintain adequate count density for single-photon emission computed tomography (SPECT) images obtained using a single-headed camera, no more than 8 frames per cycle are usually acquired. With multiheaded SPECT systems, which can obtain higher count density images with no increase in acquisition time, more frames per cardiac cycle can be acquired.

Image acquisition time is not usually increased by gating. In patients with arrhythmias, the R-R interval acceptance window can be increased to 100% (mean R-R interval ± 50%). By this method, most cardiac cycles are accepted. To reject arrhythmic beats and thereby increase (in theory) the accuracy of quantitative functional values derived from end-diastolic and end-systolic images, a narrower R-R interval acceptance window (20%) can be selected by using special software. With this option, the acquisition time of each individual projection image is increased appropriately so that an equal number of cardiac cycles is accepted for each projection image. For SPECT studies, processing time is increased by a factor equivalent to the number of gated frames acquired. Therefore, for slower computers, image processing time is a limiting factor for gated SPECT studies. With state-of-the-art nuclear medicine computers (1994 or later), the additional processing time is insignificant; only a few minutes are added to standard SPECT myocardial perfusion image processing. Because a scan can be processed while another is being acquired, no substantial additional camera, computer, or technologist time is required to perform gated SPECT.

We use the following protocol (Box 14-1) for acquisition and processing of gated ^{99m}Tc sestamibi studies (General Electric XCT camera and 3000 computer). Although this technique has not been clinically validated for ^{99m}Tc tetrofosmin and ^{99m}Tc furofosmin, it should also be applicable to these newer

---

Protocol for acquisition and processing of gated technetium-99m sestamibi studies

Dose

22–30 mCi stress, single or separate day protocol
22 mCi rest, separate day protocol
9 mCi rest, single day rest/stress protocol

Injection to imaging interval

Exercise: 30 minutes
Dipyridamole: 60 minutes

Acquisition

High-resolution parallel-hole collimator
Step-and-shoot, circular, patient-centered orbit
Imaging arc: 180° (45° right anterior oblique to 45° left posterior oblique)
No zoom
Eight frames per cardiac cycle
Rhythm acceptance: 100%*
At the end of the acquisition, eight data sets of tomograms will have been created, each representing an interval that is one eighth of the cardiac cycle. These data are reconstructed in two ways:

1. They are summed and processed as a single ungated SPECT study
2. They are processed individually as separate gated cardiac frames and displayed in cinematic or multiframe format

SUMMED FRAMES

Pre-filtering: Butterworth, 0.52 cutoff frequency, power of 5.0 for stress
Butterworth, 0.40 cutoff frequency, power of 10.0 for rest
X-plane filter: ramp
Slice reconstruction: 1 pixel thick
Slice display: 6.4 mm single or 12.8 staggered [1 + 2, 2 + 3, . . . , (n − 1) + n]

GATED FRAMES

Pre-filtering: Butterworth, 0.40 cutoff frequency, power of 10.0 regardless of dose
X-plane filter: ramp
Slice reconstruction: 1 pixel thick (6.4 minutes)
Slice display: 12.8 mm staggered [1 + 2, 2 + 3, . . . , (n − 1) + n], cinematic

---

Accepts beats 150% <100% <50% of the average R-R interval

radiopharmaceuticals. Gated SPECT may be done using the stress or the rest dose, but with either method, only resting ventricular function will be assessed.[62] In general, it is preferable to use the higher dose study for gating, because myocardial count density and gated image quality will be better. Precise protocols depend on the recommendations of the individual manufacturers of cameras and computers.

In patients with marked arrhythmias, images may be suboptimal. Rotating planar images sum to flash because a different number of cycles is accepted for each frame; thus, the count density of frames will vary.

As stated above, it is generally preferable to use the higher dose study, usually the stress scan, for gated acquisition. However, it was recently found that in a few patients with stress-induced ischemia, results of the poststress gated study may not truly represent resting ventricular function but may instead reflect in part stress-induced functional abnormalities, even though the stress scan acquisition is delayed for 30 minutes or more after the termination of exercise or pharmacologic stress. Johnson et al[43] reported that 60% of patients with stress-induced ischemia had left ventricular functional abnormalities in stress studies that were not present in separate scans performed after tracer injection with the patient at rest. In a similar study, DePuey et al[11] noted that only 12% of patients with stress-induced ischemia demonstrated such a difference. In that report, patients with normal perfusion or only fixed defects were also studied, all of whom had identical global and regional function in stress and rest gated SPECT studies.

QUANTITATIVE ANALYSIS OF GATED SPECT DATA

Data preprocessing

For all of the methods that compute ejection fraction from ^{99m}Tc 2-methoxyisobutyl isonitrile (MIBI)–gated tomograms, data preprocessing is required to reduce the data for input to algorithms that model the ventricle. Gated tomograms may be collected in several formats, but a widely used procedure is to acquire 8 separate tomograms, one for each gating interval. The original 8 separate gated tomograms are summed in time at each projection angle to provide time-averaged myocardial perfusion images. These summed tomograms are identical to ungated tomograms, provided that no counts are lost because of arrhythmic gating errors. The summed tomogram is prefiltered, usually with Butterworth filters, and an x-plane transaxial filter may also be used. In general, transaxial images are constructed, followed by selection of left ventricular anterior, inferior, septal, and lateral limits and identification of approximate left ventricular symmetry axes. These choices are needed to generate vertical long-axis slices, and it is necessary to identify the midventricular slice along with the approximate left ventricular symmetry axis, anterior and inferior limits, and apex-to-base length. These definitions are sufficient to produce the horizontal long-axis and short-axis sections. Some methods require that these axes and limit choices be performed manually,[83] although success has been reported in automating some or all of these decisions.[29,57,76]

Once the above steps have been applied to summed data, each of the 8 sets of projection data is treated as if it were a separate data acquisition. Because each set of projection data contains only one eighth of total counts, the filters applied to each data set are smoother than those used for ungated tomograms. In addition, time-smoothing is usually used among the different data subsets. After the 8 separate transaxial tomograms are reconstructed, the same left ventricular axes and limits are applied to each gated transaxial data set. At a minimum, the midventricular vertical long-axis and horizontal long-axis cinematic tomograms[13,45,59,70,86] and usually at least three short-axis cines are produced. Some gated SPECT ejection fraction algorithms require the complete set of all gated short-axis tomograms.[21,31,40,88]

Dodge–Sandler analogs

To compute left ventricular volumes or ejection fractions from any type of medical image, a conceptual model of the ventricle must be formed. Much of the literature on gated SPECT has proceeded from assumptions made for previous imaging methods. The simplest of these, requiring the minimum amount of gated tomographic input data, is use of the midventricular ^{99m}Tc MIBI vertical long-axis cinematic tomogram as an analog to a radiographic contrast ventriculogram acquired in the right anterior oblique-30-degree projection[45,70,88] (Fig. 14-1). The Dodge–Sandler formula, widely used in radiographic contrast angiography, assumes that the endocardial borders are seen at the most abrupt contrast change of cinefluoroangiograms during dye injection.[16] This formula has been applied to gated equilibrium blood-pool data[2] and radionuclide first-pass images.[53] When the formula is applied to gated SPECT data, the endocardial border seen from the midventricular end-diastolic vertical long-axis image is assumed to represent the endocardium. The Dodge–Sandler area–length method computes end-diastolic (ED) volume (V) from end-diastolic outlines drawn manually[45,74,76] or automatically.[75,88]

$$V = \frac{EDArea^2}{EDLength} \tag{1}$$

Left ventricular ejection fraction is computed from the differences between end-diastolic volume and end-systolic (ES) volumes:

$$LVEF = \frac{EDV - ESV}{EDV} \tag{2}$$

This simple method allows direct comparison with contrast angiography. It has the disadvantage of embodying the most restrictive assumptions about cardiac shape.

Simpson rule analogs

A more realistic cardiac model has been used in echocardiographic[81] and magnetic resonance imaging (MRI)[17] by using paired biplane midventricular tomographic sections. The method assumes that each short-axis slice is an ellipsoidal solid and divides the volume into slices of equal thickness T corresponding to the digitization dimension (5 to 7 cm/pixel) (Fig. 14-2). All short-axis slices are sampled simultaneously by

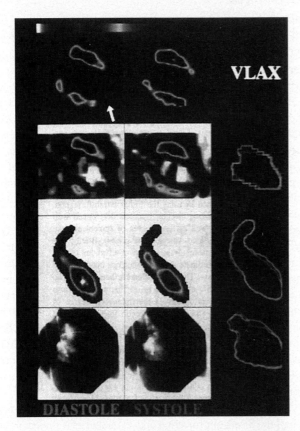

Fig. 14-1. Dodge–Sandler analog method for one patient. **A,** Technetium-99m sestamibi midventricular gated tomographic sections; **B,** the inverse of the images in A; **C,** first-pass radionuclide images; **D,** radiographic contrast angiograms. The left column shows the heart at end diastole, the middle column shows end systole, and the right column shows the outlines used for volume calculations. (From Williams KA, Taillon LA: Left ventricular function in patients with coronary artery disease assessed by gated tomographic myocardial perfusion images: Comparison with assessment by contrast ventriculography and first-pass radionuclide angiography, *J Am Coll Cardiol* 27:173-181, 1996. By permission of Elsevier Science, Inc.)

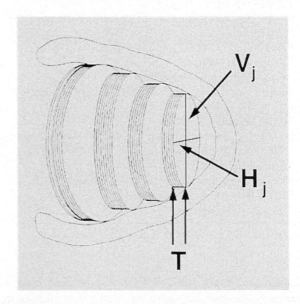

Fig. 14-2. A schematic of the Simpson rule method shows the thickness (T), vertical height (V), and horizontal width (H) taken from endocardial borders of paired tomograms for each of the elliptical slices summed to compute ventricular volume. (From DePuey EG, Nichols KN, Dobrinsky C: Left ventricular ejection fraction from gated Tc-99m sestamibi SPECT, *J Nucl Med* 34:1871-1876, 1993. By permission of the Journal of Nuclear Medicine.)

viewing orthogonal vertical long-axis and horizontal long-axis images. Labeling each of the short-axis slices by index j, starting from the first slice at the apex for $j = 1$ and proceeding to the last slice at the base for $j = N$, the vertical extent of each ellipsoid is V_j, and is the number of pixels measured from the anterior endocardial border to the inferior endocardial border on the vertical long-axis image (Fig. 14-2). The horizontal extent of the same ellipsoidal slice is the number of pixels H_j between the septal and lateral endocardial borders of the horizontal long-axis image. Volumes are computed by adding together the volumes of all the ellipsoidal cylinders with the Simpson rule formula, in which the volumes of the elliptical cylindrical slices are summed from the left ventricular apex to base for N slices:

$$V = \sum_{j=1}^{N} (\pi/4) H_j \times V_j \times T \tag{3}$$

It is assumed that drawing outlines according to a suggested percentage of contrast threshold will trace the endocardial border. Thus, the perfusion edge is identified as coinciding with the true endocardial edge. This technique, as adopted for processing ^{99m}Tc MIBI tomograms, uses midventricular vertical long-axis and horizontal short-axis cinematic tomograms. Originally, a group of cardiologists manually drew the endocardial borders that they perceived on the gated tomograms.[13] It was found that they followed a 34% contrast threshold on average. Phantom studies were then performed to find the amount of linear offset from a 34% edge to the true, known phantom endocardial wall.[12] This offset is applied to all clinical drawings. After the approach was developed from the drawings of experts, it was automated by emulating all choices made by expert observers in identifying the left ventricular cavity center, end-diastolic and end-systolic frames, and endocardial borders[59] (Fig. 14-3). The technique is conceptually simple and is relatively undemanding of computer resources. Although a disadvantage of the method is the conjecture that each short-axis slice is an ellipse, MRI studies have verified that this is a robust assumption.[17]

Relaxation labeling

More computer-intensive models require as input all levels of short-axis gated tomograms from apex to base.[21,25] The relaxation labeling approach assumes that a cone-shaped object is imbedded in a time-varying set of three-dimensional count distributions. The challenge is to locate this target structure. This model is used in the framework of hybrid coordinate systems, which are cylindrical near the base and spherical near the apex in many cardiographic imaging models.[50,83] Each volume element (voxel) of the set of all η_i three-dimensional voxels is assigned an initial probability $p_i(\lambda_j)$ that it belongs to the myocardium, where λ_j is labeled 1 for "myocardium" and 0 for "not myocardium." Initial probabilities are taken to be the normalized image count densities, and count changes are taken to be initial probabilities for voxels located on an epicardial or endocardial edge. Cross-correlation coefficients $c_{ik}(\lambda_j, \lambda_l)$ are included so that voxels labeled as myocardial points probably have neighboring myocardial voxels. An iterative relaxation labeling algorithm[72] is performed until convergence is achieved on the most probable myocardial edges:

$$p_i^{m+1}(\lambda_j) = \frac{p_i^m(\lambda_j)[1 + q_i^m(\lambda_j)]}{\sum_j p_i^m(\lambda_j)[1 + q_i^m(\lambda_j)]} \tag{4}$$

where m is the iteration number and weighting coefficients $q_i^m(\lambda_j)$ are:

$$q_i^m(\lambda j) = \sum_{k,l} c_{i,k}(\lambda_j, \lambda_i) p_i^m(\lambda_j) \tag{5}$$

This method was used manually at first, requiring the observer to define approximate left ventricular symmetry axes and to mark myocardial points of several normal ^{99m}Tc MIBI gated SPECT studies to derive cross-correlation coefficients[25] (Fig. 14-4).

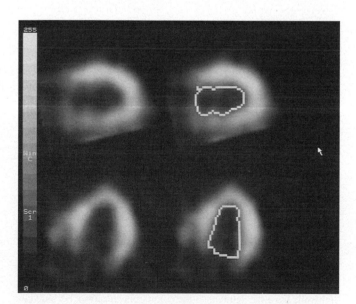

Fig. 14-3. Automated endocardial borders in the Simpson rule method are shown for the end-diastole midventricular vertical long-axis image *(top)* and horizontal long-axis image *(bottom)*.

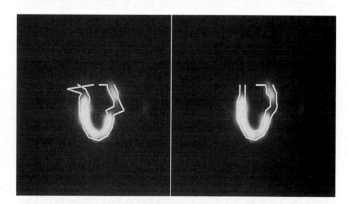

Fig. 14-4. Initial *(left)* and final *(right)* myocardial borders resulting from iteration of the relaxation labeling technique are depicted for the midventricular horizontal long-axis image. (From Faber TL et al: A model-based four-dimensional left ventricular surface detector, *IEEE Trans Med Imaging* 10:321-329, 1991. By permission of the IEEE.)

Gaussian midmyocardial detection

The relaxation labeling technique has been criticized on the basis that Equation 5 may not converge; if this occurs, the ventricle cannot be modeled from the input scintigraphic data. To circumvent this possibility, a different computationally intensive method has been used that requires all short-axis gated tomograms to be resident in computer memory at the same time.[31] It begins with a cluster analysis technique that labels each voxel of the summed tomogram above a 50% count threshold of maximum counts as 1 and sets all other voxels to 0. An algorithm then determines which labeled voxels are most likely to form connected clusters, raises the count threshold as necessary, and discards voxel clusters that are probably too small to represent myocardium. The most probable single cluster among occurrences of multiple surviving clusters is selected on the basis of reasonable physiologic criteria (Fig. 14-5). Circles are fit to short-axis clusters to form a nest of circular cylinders; maximum counts are found near these cylinders, which are taken to be locations of the midmyocardium. These locations are used to search iteratively for the ellipsoid that best represents the midmyocardial surface.[30] A refined estimate of midmyocardial points is found by searching for the myocardial perfusion count profile that best fits a Gaussian function across directions normal to the surface of the fitted ellipse. Cost functions are used to ensure that midmyocardial locations do not deviate unrealistically from their nearest neighbors.

Once this procedure is finished for the summed tomogram, the Gaussian fit is used along directions normal to the same basic ellipsoidal surface to find midmyocardial location estimates for each set of unsummed short-axis slices per each time interval throughout the cardiac cycle. The valve plane is computed as the 25% contrast threshold of myocardial counts of the summed tomogram. Epicardial and endocardial surfaces are generated starting from the estimated midmyocardial locations by further asymmetric Gaussian fits, and myocardial wall thickness between surfaces is adjusted throughout the cardiac cycle to guarantee that computed myocardial mass is the same as end-diastole and end-systole. As originally used, this method was fully automated, given a precomputed set of gated SPECT short-axis slices.[31]

Count-based models

In contrast to the constraint that the Gaussian midmyocardial detection model imposes on epicardial and endocardial surfaces to provide constant computed myocardial mass, count-based models use observed changes in myocardial perfusion counts between end diastole and end systole to measure the percentage of myocardial thickening.[5,78] The most striking distinction between gated SPECT myocardial perfusion images and those from other imaging methods is that myocardial counts seem to brighten as the ventricle contracts. This is attributed to partial volume effects, which were originally recognized in positron imaging,[41] and were subsequently used to derive myocardial wall thickening and motion indices from gated positron emission tomography (PET) studies.[89,90] Counts from structures smaller than the minimum resolvable volume incorrectly seem to be redistributed to uniformly occupy the minimum volume. Thus, two objects of different thicknesses that have the same count concentration will falsely register in a transaxial images as having two different count densities. Phantom exper-

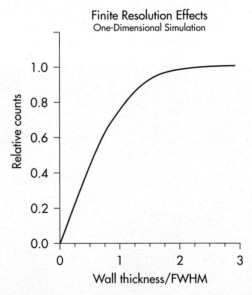

Finite Resolution Effects
One-Dimensional Simulation

Fig. 14-6. Percentage of relative counts are plotted against simulated myocardial wall thickness in units of full width at half maximum *(FWHM)* of an Anger camera. In this simulation, all myocardial walls have the same absolute count concentration. (From Galt JR, Garcia EV, Robbins WL: Effects of myocardial wall thickness of SPECT quantification, *IEEE Trans Med Imaging* 9:144-150, 1990. By permission of the IEEE.)

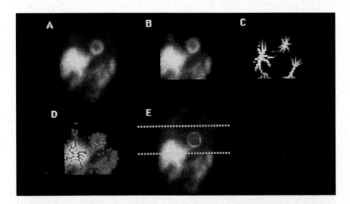

Fig. 14-5. Cluster analysis before Gaussian myocardial wall detection is demonstrated. The left anterior oblique summed tomogram *(A)* is masked *(B)*, then convolved with a two-dimensional Gaussian function *(C)*. Circles identifying local clusters *(C)* are compared with clusters of local maxima *(D)* to identify the single region that most likely represents myocardium *(E)*. (From Germano G, et al: Operator-less processing of myocardial perfusion SPECT studies, *J Nucl Med* 36:2127-2132, 1995. By permission of the Journal of Nuclear Medicine.)

iments have shown that as long as structures are smaller than the effective full width at half maximum (FWHM) of the point spread function, the percentage of observed counts is linearly related to the object size[27] (Fig. 14-6). If the myocardium maintains a constant concentration of tracer throughout the R-R interval and at its thickest is never as large as the FWHM, percentage count changes should be linearly related to wall thickening. This premise has been combined with midmyocardial location estimates to compute endocardial surfaces and, thereby gated SPECT ejection fraction.[8] Because isolated neighborhoods of gated myocardial perfusion scans may have "high noise-to-signal" ratios per individual time interval, one technique first forms the polar perfusion maps for all sets of short-axis time intervals individually,[83] then performs a first-order Fourier fit to counts within each pixel (Fig. 14-7).

This approach has the advantage of being able to construct polar thickening amplitude and phase maps with the same spatial relations as the original summed polar perfusion map.[28] Thus, territories that are abnormal on the polar perfusion map may be checked for abnormally decreased amplitudes or for phase anomalies that may indicate true or false aneurysms.

A potential disadvantage of the technique is that it assumes the myocardium to be uniformly 1 cm thick from apex to base for each patient, although this is known to not be the case.[71] Magnetic resonance imaging studies support the premise that the average myocardial thickness is 1 cm in humans,[44] and direct point-by-point comparisons of MRI short-axis images fused with endocardial borders by this technique have demonstrated excellent correlation.[22] It should be noted that related gated SPECT ejection fraction methods that only identify mid-

myocardial points and make no attempt to correct for nonzero myocardial wall thickness nevertheless yield left ventricular ejection fraction computations that agree well with gated equilibrium blood-pool left ventricular ejection fraction.[20,36] This observation has been bolstered by computer simulations and multimodality studies[5,78] demonstrating that gated SPECT models that use systolic thickening are insensitive to errors in the assumption of uniformly thick myocardium.[23]

Hybrid models

The technique described above may be considered a hybrid model, combining aspects of geometrical and count-based schema. In fact, none of the gated SPECT ejection fraction methods described above is purely geometric or count-based. At first glance, it may seem that the Dodge–Sandler and Simpson rule analogs are purely geometric. However, partial volume effects influence endocardial borders drawn according to fixed contrast thresholds (34%). This is because if apical myocardium is thinner than the midventricular myocardium, its maximum count is reduced. Consequently, the apical endocardial border will be drawn appropriately closer to the apical midmyocardial point than is the offset of the midventricular endocardial border to the midventricular midmyocardial point. Likewise, results of Gaussian midmyocardial detection are influenced by partial volume effects through use of a fixed percentage of standard deviation of Gaussian fitting parameters because the Gaussian standard deviations will be larger as the count rate increases for systolic frames.[31] Research on the optimal schema for identifying endocardial wall location from scintigraphic images remains active for gated SPECT and PET.[4,6,26,63]

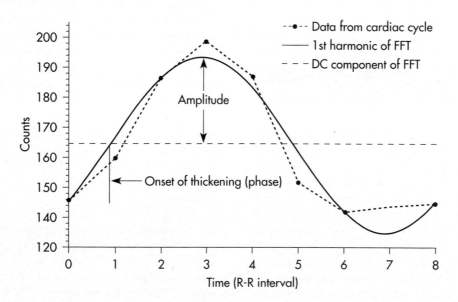

Fig. 14-7. Maximum counts of a short-axis tomogram are plotted against the time interval of a 2-methoxyisobutyl isonitrile study gated at 8 frames per cardiac cycle. Also shown *(solid line)* is the first harmonic of the Fourier fit to this data. (From Cooke CD, et al: Determining the accuracy of calculating systolic wall thickening using a fast Fourier transform approximation: A simulation study based on canine and patient data, *J Nucl Med* 35:1185-1192, 1994. By permission of the Journal of Nuclear Medicine.)

Automation

As with any imaging technique, the advantages of automation of gated SPECT ejection fraction processing are improvement in data processing reproducibility, accelerated learning of new techniques, and portability of methods from one institution to another. Although a high degree of interobserver agreement is achievable with practice, it may take new observers as many as 50 to 70 patient studies before a plateau of the learning curve is reached.[59]

Several of the methods described above have been automated, retaining the possibility for manual intervention or correction. Endocardial border generation by Dodge–Sandler analog methods are semiautomated,[70] relying on use of software designed to find the endocardial borders of contrast angiograms. The Simpson rule method is totally automated[59] from the point of using midventricular vertical long-axis and horizontal long-axis cine input, with the ability to change left ventricular center locations, end-diastolic and end-systolic frame numbers, and endocardial borders if necessary. The relaxation labeling technique requires manual identification of left ventricular symmetry axes and centers[25] but is automatic beyond that point. The Gaussian midmyocardial detection model is totally automatic,[31] but manual alterations to left ventricular are allowed limits in the event of incorrect inclusion of noncardiac counts.[1,32] Correction of midventricular endocardial and epicardial borders is also allowed. Finally, some uses of count-based models suggest automatically the apex-to-base limits for construction of polar perfusion maps for each of the time intervals,[8] but these may be changed manually as needed.

Enhancements

Enhancements to gated SPECT ejection fraction methods include compensation for the effects of the gamma camera's line-spread function on individual patient studies so that computed volumes are absolute, not relative, values.[4,13,45,64] Most gated SPECT quantitative methods produce absolute volumes, allowing direct comparisons of ventricular volume methods with those from other imaging methods, as described below. Considerable progress has also been made in the quantitation of regional wall thickening.[28,78]

Recent advances include regional image-contrast modification designed to enhance myocardial territories even in severe regional hypoperfusion. Currently, such data require that the observer manually alter the brightness and contrast of computer displays to verify the success of endocardial border generation or to alter borders. This simple technique has the advantages of optimally and automatically altering contrast, thereby providing edge detection algorithms with more consistent input data and assisting the observer verification process[61] (Fig. 14-8). This technique has enabled observers to perceive regional wall motion in agreement with echo measurements for hypoperfused patients[65] similar to results found previously for normal patient populations.

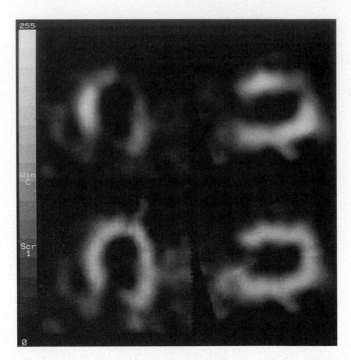

Fig. 14-8. Severely hypoperfused end-diastole midventricular sections *(top)* can be transformed by local contrast enhancement to produce images that reveal a uniform appearance of the myocardium *(bottom)*. This can result in improved endocardial border identification and aid in the verification of automated edges.

Limitations

One limitation of gated SPECT imaging is that acquisition of more than 8 to 16 frames per R-R interval becomes futile because too few counts are acquired beyond that limit. The most common acquisition mode is only 8 frames per cardiac cycle. Although phantom and clinical studies have shown that this mode underestimates ejection fraction, it depresses the ejection fraction by only 3% to 4% and produces a constant decrease in ejection fraction regardless of absolute ejection fraction values.[31,40] Therefore, this drawback is not serious. Linear regression analysis has demonstrated a correlation coefficient of 0.99 ($n = 65$) of gated SPECT ejection fractions for patient data acquired at 16 frames per R-R interval and reanalyzed as 8-frame cines.[31] The small number of frames and wide beat acceptance window used in gated SPECT require thorough gating quality assurance.[66,67]

Another concern arises from assumptions made by count-based methods, particularly those that rely on Fourier analysis.[8,37] Systolic count changes influence gated SPECT computations; this is demonstrated by the fact that myocardial mass estimates differ when they are derived from end-diastolic instead of end-systolic tomograms.[85] If partial volume effects linking count changes to myocardial thickening were truly linear,[27,41] the phenomenon would help in schema to relocate the computed endocardial border away from midmyocardial points within a cinematic frame.[13,78,86] However, recent studies called this assumption into question,[63] especially for abnormal cases for which noise artifacts resulting from severely hypoperfused myocardia may confound count-based algorithms.[37,87] Consequently, this area of investigation remains active.[4,87]

Several reasons could account for possible nonlinearity, including the assumption that all patients have myocardial wall thickness well below the tomographic resolution of the camera. A recent study demonstrated patients' myocardia to be thinner than most Anger cameras' resolution limit.[63] Technology has improved to the point that for some cameras, ^{99m}Tc tomographic resolution at 10 cm of depth is reported to be less than 9 mm,[55] in which case some patients may have thickened myocardia that exceed the 2-FWHM limit at end systole.[63] Nonlinearity could also be caused by inconstancy of myocardial count density, possibly due to changes of myocardial vascular compartments during cardiac contraction.[26]

Validations

Clinical validations of gated SPECT left ventricular functional parameter measurements that used simple manual techniques,[13,70] relaxation labeling combined with wall thickening,[8,21] and Gaussian midmyocardial detection[20,31] have been reported. Gated SPECT ejection fractions are accurate compared with those obtained by gated blood equilibrium ($r = 0.91$, $n = 23$),[5] ($r = 0.94$, $n = 40$), ($r = 0.87$, $n = 77$)[68] Anger camera gated first-pass ($r = 0.87$, $n = 67$)[68] and ($r = 0.87$, $n = 38$)[88] multicrystal camera first-pass ($r = 0.91$, $n = 65$)[31] and ($r = 0.73$, $n = 47$),[84] echocardiography ($r = 0.79$, $n = 33$),[47] MRI ($r = 0.82$, $n = 10$),[22] ($r = 0.89$, $n = 18$),[56] and radiographic contrast ventriculography ($r = 0.85$, $n = 75$)[70] ($r = 0.83$, $n = 54$),[88] $r = 0.84$, $n = 18$,[82] and $r = 0.83$, $n = 25$[56] ($r = 0.86$, $n = 58$).[64] Good agreement was also found for gated SPECT regional wall motion assessment compared with echocardiography.[45,65]

Left ventricular end diastolic volumes from gated SPECT methods have also been compared with those from biplane Anger camera gated first-pass ($r = 0.92$, $n = 40$)[60] multicrystal camera first-pass ($r = 0.85$, $n = 47$),[84] echocardiography ($r = .79$, $n = 49$),[54] ($r = .87$, $n = 52$)[10] ($r = 0.90$, $n = 33$),[47] MRI ($r = 0.92$, $n = 10$) ($r = 81$, $n = 17$)[39] and ($r = 0.94$, $n = 18$),[56] and radiographic ventriculography ($r = 0.65$, $n = 11$)[45] and ($r = 0.92$, $n = 25$)[56] ($r = 0.87$, $n = 58$)[64] ($r = 0.74$-0.90, $n = 27$).[33] Excellent data processing reproducibility of gated SPECT measurements has been reported for repeated measurements by one observer,[1,31,59,88] among observers at the same institution,[59,88] and among observers at different institutions.[59] Excellent reproducibility ($r = 0.92$; $n = 77$) of gated SPECT ejection fraction for serial data acquisitions for nonischemic patients has also been reported.[62]

CLINICAL APPLICATIONS

Gated SPECT myocardial perfusion imaging has several clinically relevant applications.

Myocardial infarction

In patients with myocardial infarction, both the size and severity of the perfusion defect as well as regional and global ventricular function can be assessed. The value of myocardial perfusion imaging in patients with myocardial infarction is well established.[35,42,49,77] Patient prognosis is inversely related to the extent and severity of the resting perfusion defect. Stress perfusion imaging is of even greater value in risk stratifying of patients with previous myocardial infarction for future cardiac events. In patients without stress-induced ischemia, the risk for future events is relatively low (approximately 5%), whereas in those with demonstrated ischemia, the event rate is significantly higher (approximately 33%).

In addition to the rest and stress myocardial perfusion characteristics, left ventricular function has been shown to have important prognostic value. In the Thrombolysis in Myocardial Infarction Trial, in which 2989 patients were enrolled, cardiac event-free survival was directly proportional to resting left ventricular ejection fraction after myocardial infarction.[91] In the Multicenter Post-Infarction Trial, in which 799 patients were followed, an even more striking relation between ejection fraction and event-free survival was demonstrated.[58] Essentially, cardiac events increased logarithmically as ejection fraction decreased to below 50%. For instance, in a patient with an ejection fraction of 60% after infarction, the cardiac event rate was approximately 15, whereas in a patient with an ejection fraction of 30%, the cardiac event rate was approximately 15%. Therefore, gated myocardial perfusion SPECT provides information about infarct size, stress-induced ischemia, and resting left ventricular function, all of which are important diagnostic and prognostic variables. It is not yet known whether the functional data have incremental prognostic value compared with the perfusion data alone. An example of a gated SPECT perfusion scan in a patient with myocardial infarction is shown in Fig. 14-9.

First-pass radionuclide ventriculography can also be used to evaluate ventricular function in conjunction with injection of a ^{99m}Tc-labeled myocardial perfusion tracer (see Chapter 13). First-pass radionuclide ventriculography is the only method to date that has been validated to assess stress ventricular function in conjunction with perfusion imaging. The prognostic value of exercise left ventricular function measured by upright bicycle radionuclide ventriculography in patients with previous myocardial infarction has been well documented.[46] In addition, exercise radionuclide ventriculography seems to increase sensitivity in the detection of multivessel coronary artery disease compared with ^{99m}Tc sestamibi SPECT perfusion imaging alone.[69] Gated perfusion SPECT does not provide similar information about stress ventricular function. However, Talierico et al[80] reported that stress and rest ventricular function measured with equilibrium radionuclide ventriculography provided equivalent prognostic information with regard to cardiac event-free survival. Thus, it is has not been demonstrated that the potential incremental value of stress versus rest ventricular function is worth the investment of the extra camera and personnel time and the technical demands of first-pass radionuclide ventriculography compared with gated SPECT, which provides resting functional data with only minimal additional time and effort.

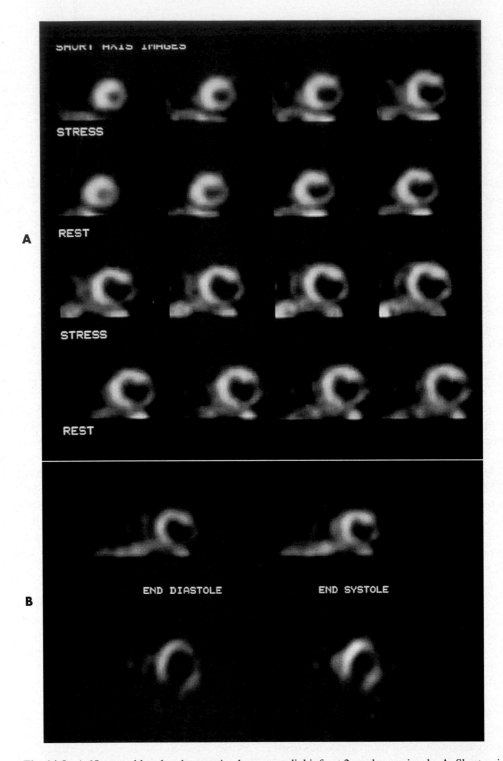

Fig. 14-9. A 65-year-old male who sustained a myocardial infarct 2 weeks previously. **A,** Short-axis tomograms demonstrate a marked and extensive fixed inferoposterior perfusion defect. **B,** Gated short-axis *(top)* and horizontal long-axis *(bottom)* tomograms show marked hypokinesis and decreased thickening of the distal two thirds of the inferoposterior wall. Left ventricular ejection fraction was 30%.

Primary left ventricular functional abnormalities

Many patients who are referred for myocardial perfusion imaging to evaluate chest pain or exertional fatigue or dyspnea, which are possible symptoms of coronary artery disease, may have known or occult left ventricular dysfunction; this condition may in part or totally account for their clinical presentation. Abnormalities of left ventricular function may be greater than perfusion defects in patients with valvular heart disease, cardiomyopathy, and small-vessel disease. Evaluation of both perfusion and function is particularly useful in patients in whom these conditions coexist with coronary artery disease.

For example, many patients referred for myocardial perfusion imaging have a history of hypertension, a well-recognized risk factor for coronary disease. Gated myocardial perfusion SPECT accurately detects regional ischemia in these patients and evaluates systolic left ventricular function. Unfortunately, the temporal resolution of gated perfusion SPECT is currently insufficient to evaluate diastolic ventricular dysfunction, which of course may affect patients with hypertensive cardiomyopathy. Rozanski et al[73] reported a series of 197 patients with normal stress and rest sestamibi perfusion distribution, 101 of whom had hypertension. Twenty-five of the 101 hypertensive patients had electrocardiographic evidence of left ventricular hypertrophy and 76 did not. These investigators found lower left ventricular ejection fractions (57.4% ± 14.0% vs 63.2% ± 9.9%) and greater end systolic volume indices (50.8% ± 35.9% vs 41.0% ± 14.7%) (p values 0.02 and 0.04, respectively) in the hypertensive patients with evidence of left ventricular hypertrophy compared with nonhypertensive patients and patients with hypertension but no evidence of left ventricular hypertrophy. An example of a patient with normal myocardial perfusion and clinically unsuspected left ventricular systolic dysfunction secondary to hypertension and left ventricular hypertrophy is shown in Fig. 14-10.

In patients with cardiomyopathy due to hypertension or other causes, left ventricular ejection fraction is an important prognostic variable. Gradman et al[38] demonstrated that in patients with cardiomyopathy and left ventricular ejection fraction less than 20%, the cardiac event–free survival rate was 27% at 16 months, whereas in patients with an ejection fraction 30% greater, it was 7%. By multiple logistic regression analysis, left ventricular ejection fraction was identified as the variable most closely associated with mortality. Therefore, gated perfusion SPECT may be of value in such patients in assessing function; the presence of coexistent coronary ischemia as a correctable cause of left ventricular dysfunction; and, possibly, myocardial viability (see below).

Another group of patients frequently encountered in the nuclear cardiology laboratory are abusers of substances that include alcohol and, increasingly cocaine. Like hypertensive patients, although patients who abuse substances may have coronary disease, their symptoms may be explained in part or totally by left ventricular dysfunction secondary to cardiomyopathy.

Although echocardiography is currently the noninvasive imaging method of choice to evaluate patients with valvular heart disease, such patients are sometimes also referred for stress myocardial perfusion imaging to assess the presence of coexistent coronary artery disease. Gated perfusion SPECT provides no information about the presence or severity of valvular disease per se, but the resting functional consequences (that is, ventricular volumes and ejection fraction) can be readily assessed. Figure 14-11 shows two sequential studies done 1 year apart in a patient with aortic and mitral insufficiency referred for perfusion imaging to evaluate recurrent atypical chest pain. A progressive increase in ventricular volume and decrease in ejection fraction are clearly visible, consistent with worsening valvular insufficiency that was subsequently confirmed by echocardiography. No stress or rest perfusion abnormalities were found to explain atypical chest pain symptoms.

Preoperative risk assessment

Another clinical circumstance in which both myocardial perfusion and left ventricular function provide valuable prognostic information is the assessment of the risk for perioperative cardiac events in patients undergoing major surgical procedures, particularly peripheral vascular surgery. Patients with scintigraphic evidence of stress-induced ischemia have a substantially higher incidence of perioperative cardiac events, including death.[3,9,48] However, it has been clearly demonstrated that poor left ventricular function places patients in increased jeopardy for perioperative events.[18,51] Before the introduction of gated perfusion SPECT with ^{99m}Tc agents, left ventricular dysfunction could only be assessed indirectly from perfusion scans in such patients. Emlein et al[19] reported that 335 vascular surgery patients with left ventricular cavity dilatation and homogenous tracer distribution present on ^{201}Tl SPECT had an increased incidence of perioperative cardiac events compared with patients without left ventricular dilatation ($p < 0.0005$).[19] Recently, by using ^{99m}Tc sestamibi gated SPECT, Ghesani et al[34] reported that in 100 patients undergoing major surgery, the presence of fixed perfusion defects, a history of congestive heart failure, and a left ventricular ejection fraction less than 50% (measured quantitatively from the gated perfusion images) were more important prognostic indicators of perioperative cardiac events than reversible perfusion defects alone present on the stress/rest SPECT images.[34]

Differentiation of artifact from scar

Simultaneous evaluation of myocardial perfusion and function can differentiate myocardial scarring from artifact in patients with fixed defects. Artifacts or normal variation, such as apical thinning, diaphragmatic attenuation, and breast attenuation, often appear as fixed defects that mimic myocardial scarring and thus decrease test specificity for coronary artery disease. If a fixed defect is observed to move and thicken normally, it is probably an artifact. In contrast, areas of infarction are more likely to demonstrate decreased wall motion and wall thickening. In a series of 551 patients, DePuey et al[15] demonstrated a decrease in false-positive results for myocardial scar (and, thus, for coronary disease) from 16% to 3% when ^{99m}Tc

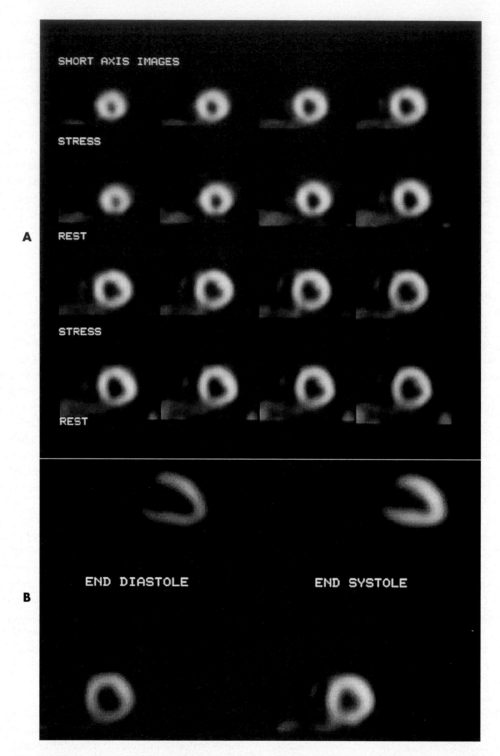

Fig. 14-10. A 55-year-old hypertensive man with atypical chest pain. **A,** Short-axis tomograms demonstrate normal stress and rest perfusion distribution. **B,** Gated vertical long-axis *(top)* and short-axis *(bottom)* tomograms demonstrate moderate, diffuse left ventricular hypokinesis.

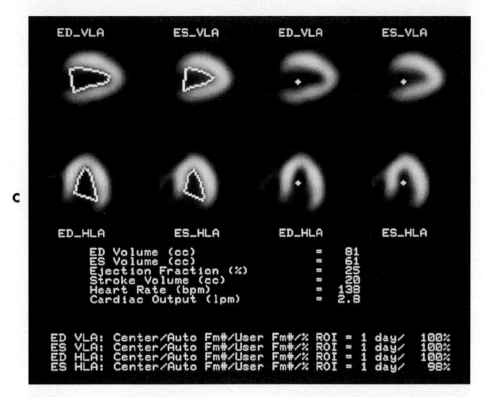

Fig. 14-10, cont'd. C, By quantitative analysis, left ventricular ejection fraction was 25%.

sestamibi perfusion tomograms were interpreted with a gated approach rather than a static or ungated approach.[15] The greatest benefit of gating was observed in women with large breasts and apparent fixed anterior perfusion defects and in men with fixed inferior defects presumably caused by diaphragmatic attenuation. More recently, in a series of 120 women who were either volunteers with a very low likelihood of coronary disease or patients undergoing coronary angiography, Taillefer et al[79] demonstrated an increase in [99mTc] sestamibi test specificity from 86% to 92% with the use of gated SPECT. Thus, because of its ability to substantially increase test specificity in patients referred for myocardial perfusion imaging in whom attenuation artifacts are commonly encountered, many laboratories now perform gated SPECT routinely in all patients. Examples of gated perfusion SPECT studies in which fixed defects are identified as attenuation artifacts rather than scars are shown in Fig. 14-12 and Fig. 14-13.

It should be emphasized that gated SPECT is useful only to differentiate fixed defects as scar versus artifact. In contrast, a stress perfusion defect that demonstrates normal wall motion and wall thickening but is reversible in separate resting images may represent either an artifact unique to the stress image or a reversible ischemic defect. These artifacts, which may affect only stress images, include patient motion and technical artifacts, such as flood-field nonuniformity, incorrect center of rotation, and tomographic reconstruction errors.

Myocardial viability

The simultaneous evaluation of exercise perfusion and resting function may potentially serve as an additional method of assessing myocardial viability. Although it is well known that areas of stunned or hibernating myocardium are frequently akinetic, the demonstration of preserved ventricular function in the distribution of a fixed perfusion defect may indicate viable, salvageable myocardium in many patients in whom revascularization is being considered. Logically, if an area of myocardium moves and thickens, it should be viable. However, if no motion or thickening is present, viability cannot be excluded, because areas of stunned or hibernating myocardium may be akinetic or dyskinetic, with no evidence of thickening but the ability to recover function after successful revascularization. DePuey et al[14] reported only a moderate correlation between [201Tl] uptake 3 hours after a resting injection and quantitative wall thickening in regions that demonstrated a fixed defect on stress/rest [99mTc] sestamibi SPECT.

There are several technical reasons why gated perfusion SPECT may overestimate viability, manifested by apparently preserved thickening and motion. Both normal and scarred, nonviable myocardium may be encompassed by the same minimum resolvable volume so that normally contracting myocardium will contribute to an increase in intensity of the scarred region during systole. A greater problem is the fact that the

Text continued on p. 232

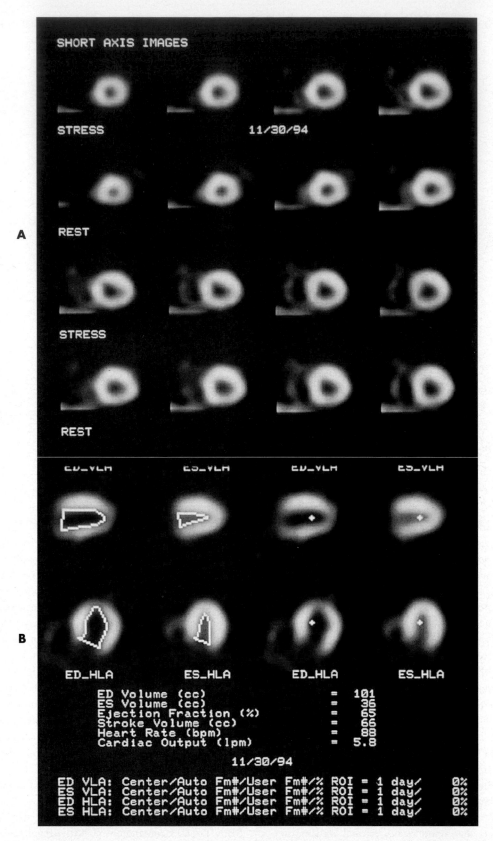

Fig. 14-11. A 50-year-old man with known aortic and mitral valve disease was referred for atypical chest pain. **A,** Short-axis tomograms demonstrate normal stress and rest perfusion distribution. **B,** Quantitative analysis of gated tomograms demonstrates borderline left ventricular dilatation (end-diastolic volume, 101 cc; end-systolic volume, 35 cc) and normal left ventricular ejection fraction (65%).

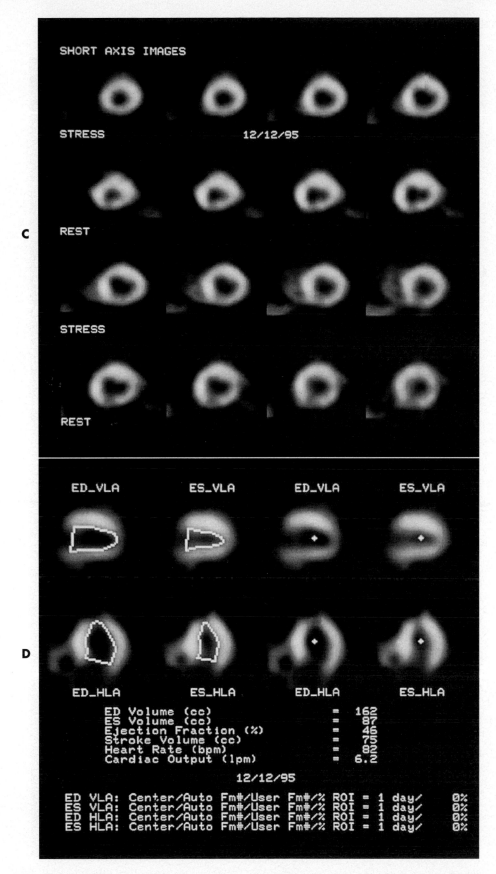

Fig. 14-11 cont'd. C, A follow-up study 1 year later demonstrates normal stress and rest perfusion distribution. **D,** Follow-up analysis demonstrates that left ventricular volume increased (end-diastolic volume, 162 cc; end-systolic volume, 87 cc) and systolic function worsened (left ventricular ejection fraction, 46%).

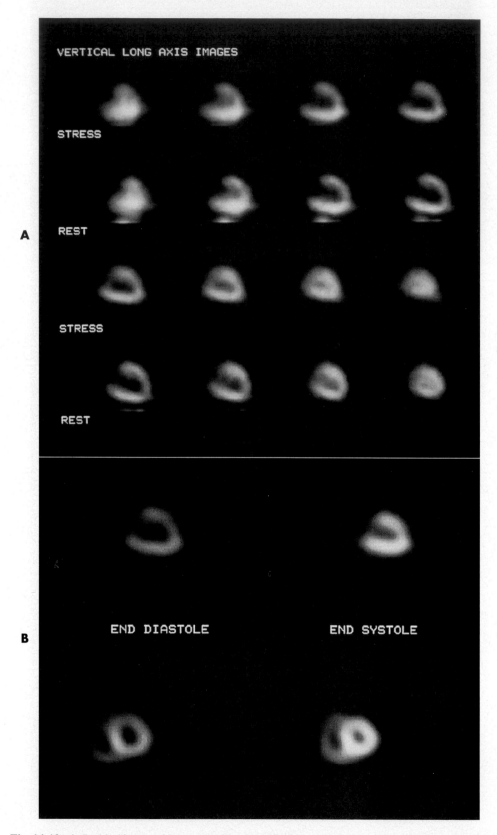

Fig. 14-12. A, In this 40-year-old woman with a low likelihood of coronary disease and a large chest circumference (bra cup, 44D), stress and rest vertical long-axis perfusion tomograms demonstrate an apparent fixed anterior wall defect. **B,** Vertical long-axis *(top)* and short-axis *(bottom)* gated tomograms demonstrate normal anterior wall motion and thickening consistent with a breast attenuation artifact rather than anterior scarring.

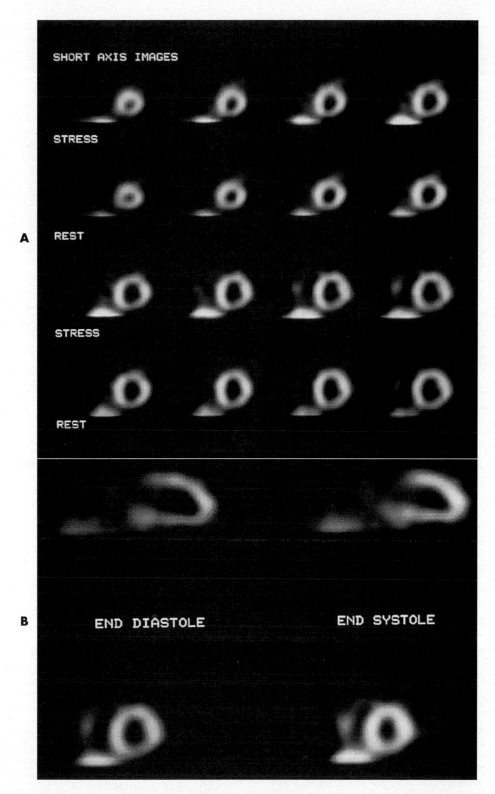

Fig. 14-13. A, In this 45-year-old hypertensive man, short-axis stress and rest perfusion tomograms demonstrate an apparent moderate fixed inferior perfusion defect. **B,** Gated vertical long-axis *(top)* and short-axis *(bottom)* tomograms demonstrate mild left ventricular dilatation and moderate, diffuse hypokinesis, consistent with cardiomyopathy. There is relative preservation of inferior wall motion and thickening, favoring a diaphragmatic attenuation artifact rather than inferior scar as the cause of the fixed inferior defect.

heart rotates and translates during the cardiac cycle. Therefore, if a region of normal myocardium at end systole displaces a region of scar present at end-diastole, the viability of the scar will be overestimated. It is hoped that gated SPECT reconstruction algorithms which compensate for cardiac motion will obviate this problem.

It is also not currently known what degree of wall thickening (that is, increase in myocardial intensity during systole) is necessary to predict recoverability of regional function after revascularization. Moreover, it is not known whether the systolic increase in count density of a fixed defect relative to normal myocardium or the baseline count density in the defect itself is a more reliable predictor of viability. Therefore, although gated perfusion SPECT may be an attractive potential technique to assess myocardial viability, several important technical and clinical questions must be resolved.

In summary, electrocardiographic gating is a relatively simple and clinically useful adjunct to SPECT myocardial perfusion imaging performed using ^{99m}Tc radiopharmaceuticals. Gating serves to further broaden its specificity and clinical utility.

REFERENCES

1. Achtert AD, King MA, Dahlberg ST, et al: An investigation of the estimation of ejection fractions and cardiac volumes by a quantitative gated SPECT software package in simulated gated SPECT images, *J Nucl Cardiol* 5:144–152, 1998.
2. Berman D, Salel A, DeNardo G, et al: Clinical assessment of left ventricular regional contraction patterns and ejection fraction by high-resolution gated scintigraphy, *J Nucl Med* 16:865–874, 1974.
3. Boucher CA, Brewster DC, Darling RC, et al: Determination of cardiac risk by dipyridamole-thallium imaging before peripheral vascular surgery, *N Engl J Med* 312:389–394, 1985.
4. Buvat I, Bartlett ML, Kitsiou AN, et al: A "hybrid" method for measuring myocardial wall thickening from gated PET/SPECT images, *J Nucl Med* 38:324–329, 1997.
5. Calnon DA, Kastner RJ, Smith WH, et al: Validation of a new counts-based gated single photon emission computed tomography method for quantifying left ventricular systolic function: Comparison with equilibrium radionuclide angiography, *J Nucl Cardiol* 4:464–471, 1997.
6. Case JA, Cullom SJ, Bateman TM, et al: Overestimation of LVEF by gated MIBI myocardial perfusion SPECT in patients with small hearts, *J Am Coll Cardiol* 31(2):43A, 1998 (abstract).
7. Chua T, Kiat H, Germano G, et al: Gated technetium-99m sestamibi for simultaneous assessment of stress myocardial perfusion, postexercise regional ventricular function and myocardial viability. Correlation with echocardiography and rest thallium-201 scintigraphy, *J Am Coll Cardiol* 23:1107–1114, 1994.
8. Cooke CD, Garcia EV, Cullom SJ, et al: Determining the accuracy of calculating systolic wall thickening using a fast Fourier transform approximation: a simulation study based on canine and patient data, *J Nucl Med* 35:1185–1192, 1994.
9. Cutler BS, Leppo JA: Dipyridamole thallium 201 scintigraphy to detect coronary artery disease before abdominal aortic surgery, *J Vasc Surg* 5:91–100, 1987.
10. Cwajg E, Cwajg J, He ZX, et al: Comparison between gated-SPECT and echocardiography for the analysis of global and regional left ventricular function and volumes, *J Am Coll Cardiol* 31(2):440A, 1998 (abstract).
11. DePuey EG, Grant C, Nichols K, et al: Can resting Tc-99m sestamibi SPECT be performed 15 minutes post-injection? *J Nucl Med* 37:48P, 1996 (abstract).
12. DePuey EG, Nichols KN, Dobrinsky C: Left ventricular ejection fraction from gated technetium-99m-sestamibi SPECT, *J Nucl Med* 34:1871–1876, 1993.
13. DePuey EG, Nichols K, Dobrinsky C, et al: Left ventricular ejection fraction from gated Tc-99m-sestamibi SPECT, *J Nucl Med* 33:927, 1992 (abstract).
14. DePuey EG, Nichols K, Salensky H, et al: Gated technetium-99m-sestamibi correlates of myocardial viability assessed with rest/delayed Tl-201 SPECT, *J Nucl Med* 36:56P, 1995 (abstract).
15. DePuey EG, Rozanski A: Using gated technetium-99m-sestamibi SPECT to characterize fixed myocardial defects as infarct or artifact, *J Nucl Med* 36:952–955, 1995.
16. Dodge HT, Sandler H, Ballew DW, et al: Use of biplane angiocardiography for the measurement of left ventricular volume in man, *Am Heart J* 60:762–776, 1960.
17. Dulce MC, Mostbeck GH, Friese KK, et al: Quantification of the left ventricular volumes and function with cine MR imaging: comparison of geometric models with three-dimensional data, *Radiology* 188: 371–376, 1993.
18. Eagle EA, Singer DE, Brewster DC, et al: Dipyridamole-thallium scanning in patients undergoing vascular surgery. Optimizing preoperative evaluation of cardiac risk, *JAMA* 257:2185–2189, 1987.
19. Emlein G, Villegas B, Dahlberg S, et al: Left ventricular cavity size determined by preoperative dipyridamole thallium scintigraphy as a predictor of late cardiac events in vascular surgery patients, *Am Heart J* 131:907–914, 1996.
20. Everaert H, Bossayt A, Franken PR, et al: Left ventricular ejection fraction and volumes from gated single photon emission tomographic myocardial perfusion studies: Comparison between two algorithms working in three-dimensional space, *J Nucl Cardiol* 4:472–476, 1997.
21. Faber TL, Akers MS, Peshock RM, et al: Three-dimensional motion and perfusion quantification in gated single-photon emission computed tomograms, *J Nucl Med* 32:2311–2317, 1991.
22. Faber TL, Cooke CD, Pettigrew RI, et al: Left ventricular volumes and mass from gated perfusion tomograms using a standard processing package, *J Nucl Med* 36:12P, 1995 (abstract).
23. Faber TL, Cooke CD, Vansant JP, et al: Sensitivity of an automated ejection fraction calculation from gated perfusion tomograms to modeling assumptions, *J Nucl Med* 37:213P, 1996 (abstract).
24. Faber TL, Stokely EM: Feature detection in 3-D medical images using shape information, *IEEE Trans Med Imaging* MI-6:8–13, 1987.
25. Faber TL, Stokely EM, Peshock RM, et al: A model-based four-dimensional left ventricular surface detector, *IEEE Trans Med Imaging* 10:321–392, 1991.
26. Fukuchi K, Uehara T, Morozumi T, et al: Quantification of systolic count increase in technetium-99m-MIBI gated myocardial SPECT, *J Nucl Med* 38:1067–1073, 1997.
27. Galt JR, Garcia EV, Robbins WL: Effects of myocardial wall thickness on SPECT quantification, *IEEE Trans Med Imaging* 9:144–150, 1990.
28. Germano G, Erel J, Lewin H, et al: Automatic quantitation of regional myocardial wall motion and thickening from gated technetium-99m sestamibi myocardial perfusion single-photon emission computed tomography, *J Am Coll Cardiol* 30:1360–1367, 1997.
29. Germano G, Kavanaugh PB, Chen J, et al: Operator-less processing of myocardial perfusion SPECT studies, *J Nucl Med* 36:2127–2132, 1995.
30. Germano G, Kavanaugh PB, Su HT, et al: Automatic reorientation of three-dimensional, transaxial myocardial perfusion SPECT images, *J Nucl Med* 36:1107–1114, 1995.
31. Germano G, Kiat H, Kavanaugh PB, et al: Automatic quantification of ejection fraction from gated myocardial perfusion SPECT, *J Nucl Med* 36:2138–2147, 1995.
32. Germano G, Kavanaugh PB, Berman DS: An automatic approach to the analysis, quantitation and review of perfusion and function from myocardial perfusion SPECT images. *International Journal of Cardiac Imaging* 13:337–346, 1994.

33. Germano G, Vandecker W, Mintz R, et al: Validation of left ventricular volumes automatically measured with gated myocardial perfusion SPECT, *J Am Coll Cardiol* 31(2):43A, 1998 (abstract).

34. Ghesani M, DePuey EG, Nichols K, et al: Risk stratification of patients for peri-operative cardiac events using gated Tc-99m sestamibi SPECT, *J Nucl Med* 37:116P, 1996 (abstract).

35. Gibson RS, Watson DD, Craddock GB, et al: Prediction of cardiac events after uncomplicated myocardial infarction: a prospective study comparing predischarge exercise thallium-201 scintigraphy and coronary angiography, *Circulation* 68:321–336, 1983.

36. Goris ML, Thompson C, Malone L, et al: Modeling the integration of myocardial regional perfusion and function. *Nucl Med Commun* 15:9–20, 1994.

37. Gradel C, Staib LH, Heller EN, et al: Limitations of ECG-gated SPECT for assessment of regional thickening: Experimental comparison with ECG-gated MRI, *J Am Coll Cardiol* 27:241A, 1996 (abstract).

38. Gradman A, Deedwania P, Cody R, et al: Predictors of total mortality and sudden death in mild to moderate heart failure, Captopril-Digoxin Study Group, *J Am Coll Cardiol* 14:564–570, 1989.

39. He ZX, Vick GW, Vaduganathan P, et al: Comparison of left ventricular volumes and ejection fraction measured by gated SPECT and by cine magnetic resonance imaging, *J Am Coll Cardiol* 31(2):44A, 1998 (abstract).

40. Hillel PG, Hastings DL: A three-dimensional second-derivative surface-detection algorithm for volume determination on SPECT images, *Phys Med Biol* 38:583–600, 1993.

41. Hoffman EJ, Huang SC, Phelps ME: Quantitation in positron emission computed tomography: 1. Effect of object size, *J Comput Assist Tomogr* 5:299–308, 1979.

42. Hung J, Goris ML, Nash E, et al: Comparative value of maximal treadmill testing, exercise thallium myocardial perfusion scintigraphy and exercise radionuclide ventriculography for distinguishing high- and low-risk patients soon after acute myocardial infarction, *Am J Cardiol* 53:1221–1227, 1984.

43. Johnson LL, Verdesca SA, Aude WY, et al: Postischemic stunning can affect left ventricular ejection fraction and regional wall motion on post-stress gated sestamibi tomograms, *J Am Coll Cardiol* 30:1641–1648, 1997.

44. Kaul S, Wismer GL, Brady TJ, et al: Measurement of normal left heart dimensions using optimally oriented MR images, *AJR Am J Roentgenol* 146:75–79, 1986.

45. Klodas E, Rogers PJ, Sinak LJ, et al: Quantitation of regional ejection fractions using gated tomographic imaging with Tc-99m-sestamibi, *J Am Coll Cardiol* 27:215A, 1996 (abstract).

46. Lee KL, Pryor DB, Pieper KS, et al: Prognostic value of radionuclide angiography in medically treated patients with coronary artery disease. A comparison with clinical and catheterization variables, *Circulation* 82:1705–1717, 1990.

47. Lefkowitz D, Nichols K, Rozanski A, et al: Echocardiographic validation of left ventricular volume measurements by Tc-99m sestamibi gated SPECT, *J Am Coll Cardiol* 27:241A, 1996 (abstract).

48. Leppo J, Plaja J, Gionet M, et al: Noninvasive evaluation of cardiac risk before elective vascular surgery, *J Am Coll Cardiol* 9:269–276, 1987.

49. Leppo JA, O'Brien J, Rothendler JA, et al: Dipyridamole-thallium-201 scintigraphy in the prediction of future cardiac events after acute myocardial infarction, *N Engl J Med* 310:1014–1018, 1984.

50. Lilly P, Jenkins J, Bourdillon P: Automatic contour definition of left ventriculograms by image evidence and a multiple template-based model, *IEEE Trans Med Imaging* 8:173–185, 1989.

51. L'Italien G, Hendel PS, Leppo J, et al: Development and validation of a Bayesian model for perioperative cardiac risk assessment in a cohort of 1,081 vascular surgical candidates. *J Am Coll Cardiol* 27:779–786, 1996.

52. Marcassa C, Marzullo P, Parodi O, et al: Anew method for noninvasive quantitation of segmental myocardial wall thickening using technetium-99m-2 methoxy-isobutyl-isonitrile scintigraphy—results in normal subjects, *J Nucl Med* 31:173–177, 1990.

53. Massie BM, Kramer BL, Gertz EW, et al: Radionuclide measurement of left ventricular volume: comparison of geometric and counts-based methods, *Circulation* 65:725–730, 1982.

54. Mathew D, Zabrodina Y, Manting F: Volumetric and functional analysis of left ventricle by gated SPECT: A comparison with echocardiographic measurements, *J Am Coll Cardiol* 31(2):44A, 1998 (abstract).

55. Fakhri GE, Burat I, Pelegrini H, et al: Quantitative accuracy in cardiac SPECT: What are the respective roles of attenuation, collimator response and scatter corrections? *J Nucl Med* 39:179P, 1998.

56. Mochizuki T, Murase K, Tanake H, et al: Assessment of left ventricular volume utilizing ECG-gated SPECT with technetium-99m-MIBI and technetium-99m tetrofosmin, *J Nucl Med* 38:53–57, 1997.

57. Mullick R, Ezquerra NF: Automatic determination of LV orientation from SPECT data, *IEEE Trans Med Imaging* 14:58–90, 1995.

58. Risk stratification and survival after myocardial infarction. *N Engl J Med* 309:331–336, 1983.

59. Nichols K, DePuey EG, Rozanski A: Automation of gated tomographic left ventricular ejection fraction, *J Nucl Cardiol* 3:475–482, 1996.

60. Nichols K, DePuey EG, Salensky H, et al: Ventricular volume measured from sestamibi gated tomograms, *J Nucl Med* 35:70P, 1994 (abstract).

61. Nichols K, DePuey EG, Salensky H, et al: Image enhancement of severely hypoperfused myocardia for computation of tomographic ejection fraction, *J Nucl Med* 37:105P, 1996 (abstract).

62. Nichols K, DePuey EG, Salensky H, et al: Reproducibility of ejection fractions from stress versus rest gated perfusion SPECT, *J Nucl Med* 37:115P, 1996 (abstract).

63. Nichols K, DePuey EG, Friedman MI, et al: Do patient data ever exceed the partial volume limit in gated SPECT studies? *J Nucl Cardiol* [in press for 1998; accepted for publication on 1/19/98].

64. Nichols K, Tamis J, DePuey EG, et al: Relationship of gated SPECT ventricular function parameters to angiographic measurements, *J Nucl Cardiol* [in press for 1998; accepted for publication on 10/27/97].

65. Nichols K, DePuey EG, Krasnow N, et al: Reliability of enhanced gated SPECT in assessing wall motion of severely hypoperfused myocardia: An echocardiographic validation. *J Nucl Cardiol* [in press for 1998; accepted for publication on 1/26/98].

66. Nichols K, Dorbala S, Yao SS, et al: Influence of gating errors on SPECT myocardial perfusion quantitative parameters, *J Nucl Med* 39:45P, 1998 (abstract).

67. Nichols K, DePuey EG, Dorbala S, et al: Prevalence of gating errors in myocardial perfusion SPECT data, *J Nucl Med* 39:45P, 1998 (abstract).

68. Nichols K, Rozanski A, Salensky H, et al: Accuracy and reproducibility of automated tomographic ventricular function measurements, *J Am Coll Cardiol* 27:215A, 1996 (abstract).

69. Palmas W, Friedman JD, Diamond GA, et al: Incremental value of simultaneous assessment of myocardial function and perfusion with technetium-99m sestamibi for prediction of extent of coronary artery disease, *J Am Coll Cardiol* 25:1024–1031, 1995.

70. Piriz JM, Kiernan FJ, Eldin A, et al: Correlation of left ventricular ejection fraction by gated SPECT Tc-99m sestamibi imaging with contrast ventriculography at subsequent cardiac catheterization, *J Nucl Med* 37:105P, 1996 (abstract).

71. Prigent F, Bellil D, Maddahi J, et al: Quantification of % hypoperfusion by thallium-201 SPECT: development of an algorithm for correction for variation in myocardial slice mass in man, *J Nucl Med* 30:750, 1989 (abstract).

72. Rosenfeld A, Kak AC: Segmentation in Digital Picture Processing, vol 2, Academic Press, New York, NY, pp. 57–190, 1982.

73. Rozanski A, Nichols K, Malhotra S, et al: Functional abnormalities in hypertensive patients with normal myocardial perfusion demonstrated by gated SPECT, *J Nucl Med* 37:115P, 1996 (abstract).

74. Sandler H, Dodge HT: The use of single plane angiocardiograms for the calculation of left ventricular volume in man, *Am Heart J* 75:325–334, 1968.

75. Seldin DW, Esser PD, Nichols AB, et al: Left ventricular volume determined from scintigraphy and digital angiography by a semi-automated geometric method, *Radiology* 149:809–813, 1983.

76. Slomka PJ, Hurwitz GA, Stephenson J, et al: Automated alignment and sizing of myocardial stress and rest scans to three-dimensional normal templates using an image registration algorithm, *J Nucl Med* 36:1115–1122, 1995.

77. Smeets JP, Rigo P, Legrand V, et al: Prognostic value of thallium-201 stress myocardial scintigraphy with exercise ECG after myocardial infarction, *Cardiology* 68 (Suppl 2):67, 1981 (abstract).

78. Smith WH, Kastner RJ, Calnon DA, et al: Quantitative gated single photon emission computed tomography imaging: A counts-based method for display and measurement of regional and global ventricular systolic function, *J Nucl Cardiol* 4:451–463, 1997.

79. Taillefer R, DePuey EG, Udelson JE, et al: Comparative diagnostic accuracy of Tl-201 and Tc-99m sestamibi SPECT imaging (perfusion and ECG-gated SPECT) in detecting coronary artery disease in women, *J Am Coll Cardiol* 29:69–77, 1997.

80. Taliercio CP, Clements IP, Zinsmerster AR, et al: Prognostic value and limitations of exercise radionuclide angiography in medically treated coronary artery disease, *Mayo Clin Proc* 63:573–582, 1988.

81. Tortoledo FA, Quinones MA, Fernandez GC, et al: Quantification of left ventricular volumes by two-dimensional echocardiography: a simplified and accurate approach, *Circulation* 67:579–584, 1983.

82. Trujillo NP, Quaife RA, Adiseshan P, et al: A new automated method for assessment of left ventricular function and myocardial perfusion using gated Tc-99m sestamibi imaging: comparison with cardiac catheterization, *J Nucl Med* 37:179P, 1996 (abstract).

83. Van Train KF, Areeda J, Garcia EV, et al: Quantitative same-day rest-stress technetium-99m-sestamibi SPECT: definition and validation of stress normal limits and criteria for abnormality, *J Nucl Med* 34:1494–1502, 1993.

84. Vansant JP, Faber TL, Folks RD, et al: Resting left ventricular volumes and ejection fraction from gated SPECT: correlation to first pass, *Circulation* 92:I–11, 1995 (abstract).

85. Williams KA, Lang RM, Reba RC, et al: Comparison of technetium-99m sestamibi-gated tomographic perfusion imaging with echocardiography and electrocardiography for determination of left ventricular mass, *Am J Cardiol* 77:750–755, 1996.

86. Williams KA, Taillon LA: Reversible ischemia in severe stress technetium 99m-labeled sestamibi perfusion defects assessed from gated single-photon emission computed tomographic polar map Fourier analysis, *J Nucl Cardiol* 2:199–206, 1995.

87. Williams KA, Taillon LA: Five methods for evaluation of left ventricular function with technetium-99m-sestamibi: a comparison with contrast ventriculography, *J Nucl Med* 37:104P, 1996 (abstract).

88. Williams KA, Taillon LA: Left ventricular function in patients with coronary artery disease assessed by gated tomographic myocardial perfusion images. Comparison with assessment by contrast ventriculography and first-pass radionuclide angiography, *J Am Coll Cardiol* 27:173–181, 1996.

89. Yamashita K, Tamaki N, Yonekura Y, et al: Quantitative analysis of regional wall motion by gated myocardial positron emission tomography: validation and comparison with left ventriculography, *J Nucl Med* 30:1775–1786, 1989.

90. Yamashita K, Tamaki N, Yonekura Y, et al: Regional wall thickening of left ventricle evaluated by gated positron emission tomography in relation to myocardial perfusion and glucose metabolism, *J Nucl Med* 32:679–685, 1991.

91. Zaret BL, Wackers FJ, Terrin M, et al: Value of radionuclide rest and exercise left ventricular ejection fraction in assessing survival of patient after thrombolytic therapy for acute myocardial infarction: Result of thrombolysis in myocardial infarction (CTIMI) Phase II Study, *J Am Coll Cardiol* 26:73–79, 1995.

PERFUSION IMAGING IN CHRONIC CORONARY DISEASE

Chapter 15

State of the art for coronary artery disease detection: thallium-201

John J. Mahmarian

Thallium-201 (^{201}Tl) myocardial perfusion scintigraphy is well recognized as a useful technique in the evaluation and management of patients with coronary artery disease. Advances in computer technology and the development of multidetector camera systems prompted the transition from planar to single-photon emission computed tomography (SPECT). Not only is SPECT more accurate than planar imaging for detection of individual coronary artery stenosis, it allows accurate quantification of the extent of hypoperfused myocardium. The latter feature is critically important when one is stratifying patient risk for subsequent cardiac events. The introduction of pharmacologic stressors greatly expanded the applicability of nuclear cardiac imaging to the general population of patients with suspected or known coronary artery disease. The role of ^{201}Tl scintigraphy for evaluating patients with coronary artery disease will be discussed in relation to the various advances that have been made over the past decade.

PROTOCOLS FOR PERFORMING THALLIUM-201 SCINTIGRAPHY

Thallium-201 SPECT can be performed after treadmill exercise or pharmacologic stress. The typical dose of ^{201}Tl for a 70-kg person is 3 mCi, adjusted for patient weight. Technetium (Tc)-based radiopharmaceuticals are recommended in patients who weigh more than 200 pounds because of the greater potential for soft-tissue photon attenuation in this patient population.

Exercise stress imaging

When performing exercise scintigraphy, ^{201}Tl is injected at peak exercise, and the patient continues to exercise on the treadmill for an additional 1 to 2 minutes to maintain maximal hyperemia until the isotope has cleared from the systemic circulation. Clearance of ^{201}Tl from the blood is approximately 90% within several minutes of intravenous injection[6] (Fig. 15-1). Imaging should commence 5 to 10 minutes after termination of exercise because ^{201}Tl clearance from the myocardium begins shortly after its initial uptake. Of note, myocardial clearance is slower with pharmacologic stressors than with exercise.[96] When performing SPECT, the images are generally acquired on a 64 × 64 matrix with 32 projections at 40 seconds

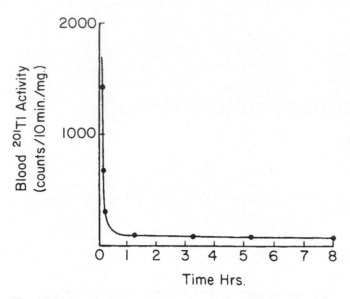

Fig. 15-1. Blood clearance curve for thallium-201 after intravenous injection in a dog. A nadir in counts occurs within 20 minutes of administration. It then reaches a plateau over several hours. (Reproduced with permission from Beller GA, Watson DD, Achell P, et al: Time course of thallium-201 redistribution after transient myocardial ischemia, *Circulation* 61:791-797, 1980.)

per projection. The total acquisition time is approximately 22 minutes. Repeat imaging at rest is performed approximately 4 hours later by using the same acquisition specifications as those used in the stress study.

Dipyridamole stress imaging

The recommended protocol for intravenous dosing of dipyridamole is 0.14 mg/kg/min over 4 minutes (0.56 mg/kg).[58] Because the peak effect of dipyridamole occurs within 3 to 7 minutes of administration, ^{201}Tl is usually injected 3 minutes after completing the 4-minute infusion.[119,133] Because maximal pharmacologic vasodilation may not occur in all patients at the dose of 0.56 mg/kg, some investigators have advocated administering doses of 0.84 mg/kg. This is particularly important for echocardiography, in which higher dipyridamole doses may be needed to escalate heterogeneity in coronary flow to frank ischemia in order to detect transient regional wall-motion abnormalities in a greater percentage of patients.[21] Theophylline competes with adenosine for its receptors; therefore, this medication should not be given for 24 hours before performing the test, and caffeine-containing beverages should be withheld for at least 12 hours before giving dipyridamole.

Adenosine stress imaging

The protocol for adenosine administration requires a continuous infusion system for maximizing and maintaining hyperemia. In patients with relative contraindications to adenosine, the infusion should be incremental, starting at 50 μg/kg/min and increasing to 75, 100, and 140 μg/kg/min at 1-minute intervals (Table 15-1). In all other patients, adenosine can be infused at a dose of 140 μg/kg/min for 6 minutes, with injection

Table 15-1. Contraindications to pharmacologic vasodilators (adenosine and dipyridamole)

Absolute contraindications
Known reactive airway disease or wheezing on physical examination (chronic obstructive pulmonary disease or asthma)
Sick sinus syndrome (without pacemaker)
Second- or third-degree atrioventricular block (without pacemaker)
Hypotension (systolic blood pressure <90 mm Hg)
Ongoing treatment with theophylline or dipyridamole

Relative contraindications
Chronic obstructive pulmonary disease without wheezing
Unstable angina pectoris
Recent (<1 week) myocardial infarction

of ^{201}Tl at minute 3. The rationale for a 6-minute infusion is based on hemodynamic data showing that maximal hyperemia occurs within 84±46 seconds (range, 23 to 125 seconds) of adenosine administration, with return to baseline values within 145±67 seconds (range, 54 to 310 seconds) of terminating the infusion.[187]

Dobutamine stress imaging

Dobutamine is administered as an intravenous infusion, starting at 5 μg/kg/min and increasing to 10, 20, 30, and up to 40 μg/kg/min at 3-minute intervals. Thallium-201 is injected 1 minute into infusion of the maximally tolerated dobutamine dose, and the infusion is continued for an additional 2 minutes after ^{201}Tl injection. The half-life of dobutamine is approximately 2 minutes. Atropine (0.5 to 1 mg) can be administered if the heart rate remains submaximal at the highest tolerated dobutamine dose. Dobutamine is reserved primarily for patients who cannot perform an adequate exercise test but have an absolute contraindication to the pharmacologic vasodilators adenosine and dipyridamole (Table 15-1).

Redistribution imaging

The purpose of the 4-hour rest image is to assess the extent of ^{201}Tl redistribution in initially hypoperfused regions. Redistribution results from slower clearance of ^{201}Tl from hypoperfused regions than from normal regions[7] and is considered evidence of potentially ischemic but viable myocardium.[91] Conversely, incomplete ^{201}Tl redistribution in initially hypoperfused regions does not necessarily imply scar, because this can occur in patients without previous myocardial infarction.[24] In patients with severe coronary stenosis or occluded coronary arteries supplied by collaterals, ^{201}Tl redistribution may take longer than the expected 4 hours.[156,176] Furthermore, low blood levels of ^{201}Tl may delay redistribution of this isotope into underperfused regions that are still viable.[19] In patients who demonstrate incomplete redistribution at 4 hours, 24-hour to 72-hour imaging has been advocated to allow greater time for ^{201}Tl redistribution to occur.[88,91] Although delayed imaging en-

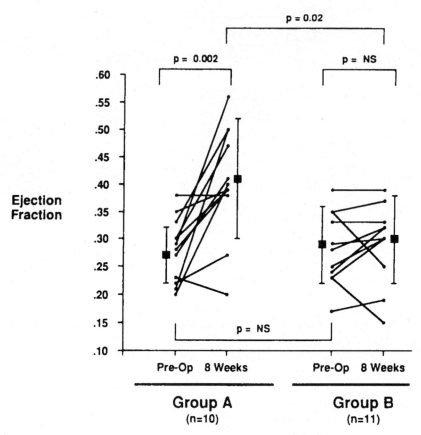

Fig. 15-2. Changes in global left ventricular ejection fraction *(LVEF)* based on preoperative rest-redistribution thallium-201 scintigraphy. The mean resting LVEF for all patients was 27% ± 5%. Patients who had more than seven viable segments by thallium-201 scintigraphy *(Group A)* had a significant improvement in global LVEF following coronary artery bypass surgery. Patients with less than seven viable segments *(Group B)* had no significant change in left ventricular ejection fraction with coronary revascularization. (Reproduced with permission from Ragosta M, Beller GA, Watson DD, et al: Quantitative planar rest-redistribution Tl-201 imaging in detection of myocardial viability and prediction of improvement in left ventricular function after coronary bypass surgery in patients with severely depressed left ventricular function, *Circulation* 87:1630–1641, 1993.)

hances the detection of viable myocardium, image quality is generally poor because of low myocardial counts. If delayed imaging is performed with SPECT, the time per projection should be increased to 60 seconds, thereby increasing the total acquisition time to approximately 32 minutes.

In patients without previous infarction, lack of complete redistribution has little clinical significance, because it can be assumed that the entire stress-induced perfusion defect represents viable myocardium. This may explain why the size alone of the stress-induced perfusion defect can accurately stratify risk in patients with chronic coronary artery disease.[64,81]

In patients with previous infarction, the detection of ischemic, potentially viable myocardium, is of critical importance. This is particularly true among patients with coronary artery disease who have global left ventricular dysfunction, because only approximately 20% of these patients will have improvement in left ventricular ejection fraction after coronary artery bypass surgery.[115] Rest-redistribution imaging and reinjection of ^{201}Tl following stress–rest imaging can be used to help identify viable myocardium in this subset of patients.

Thallium-201 rest-redistribution imaging

This imaging protocol is performed in a manner similar to that of stress-redistribution imaging. Three millicuries of ^{201}Tl are injected at rest, and imaging commences approximately 15 minutes later. After a minimum of 3 hours, imaging is repeated to determine whether initially hypoperfused regions show tracer uptake. The presence and extent of ^{201}Tl redistribution predicts improvement in regional and global left ventricular function after coronary artery bypass surgery[153] (Fig. 15-2). Patients with depressed left ventricular function and myocardial viability on scintigraphy seem to have improved long-term survival after bypass surgery.[37]

Imaging after reinjection of thallium-201

Reinjection of 1 to 1.5 mCi of ^{201}Tl after stress-redistribution imaging improves detection of viable myocardium[35,76,141] and predicts improvement in regional wall motion after coronary revascularization.[35,76,141] However, 20% to 30% of nonreversible perfusion defects may still show metabolic activity on positron emission tomography.[10,36,174] In view of this, we have

Fig. 15-3. Changes in the extent of defect reversibility from 4-hour redistribution to reinjection imaging among patients with and without collaterals based on nitroglycerin use. Defect reversibility was greatly enhanced when nitroglycerin was administered before thallium-201 reinjection, but only in patients who had coronary artery collaterals. SEM = standard error of the mean. (Adapted with permission from He ZX, Medrano R, Hays JT, et al: Nitroglycerin-augmented Tl-201 reinjection enhances detection of reversible myocardial hypoperfusion: A randomized, double-blind, parallel, placebo-controlled trial, *Circulation* 95:1799-1805, 1997.)

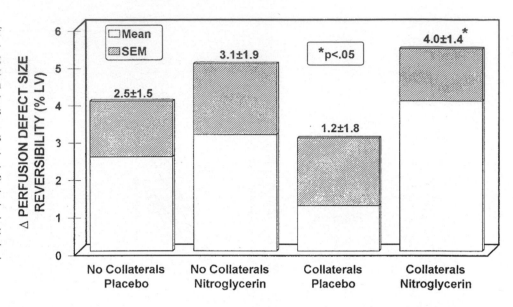

advocated administering 0.8 mg of sublingual nitroglycerin before reinjection.[66-68] Nitrates have important effects on preload[1,60] and afterload,[38,89] which may improve subendocardial blood flow at rest. They are also potent epicardial coronary[14,15] and collateral vasodilators.[3,125] In a recent study, 96 patients with persistent perfusion defects at 4 hours were randomized in a double-blind manner to receive an additional 1 mCi of ^{201}Tl after placebo or 0.8 mg of sublingual nitroglycerin.[67] In the overall population, a similar percentage of patients who received nitroglycerin and patients who received placebo showed additional defect reversibility (45% and 33%, respectively). However, in patients with predominantly fixed defects at 4 hours, only 33% of those who received placebo showed further reversibility compared with 50% of those who received nitroglycerin before ^{201}Tl reinjection ($p < 0.05$). This enhancement in defect reversibility was particularly striking among patients with coronary collaterals who received nitroglycerin (Fig. 15-3). On the basis of this study[67] and others,[66,68,164] it seems appropriate to recommend nitrate-augmented ^{201}Tl reinjection imaging in patients who have persistent defects on 4-hour redistribution imaging to best identify the presence of viable myocardium.

QUALITY CONTROL ISSUES WITH THALLIUM-201 SPECT

When performing ^{201}Tl SPECT, numerous technical and patient-related issues must be addressed to avoid study misinterpretation. The technical problems are generally avoidable, especially if proper testing of camera uniformity and image resolution and linearity are performed with daily cobalt-57 floods and weekly bar phantoms, respectively. Center-of-rotation analysis should be performed daily to avoid errors in back-projection resulting from differences in spatial alignment between the electronic matrix of the detector and the mechanical center of rotation. This becomes important in image interpretation, because failure to correct for center of rotation will result in misregistration of pixels during reconstruction. When the misalignment is greater than 2 pixels in a 64 × 64 matrix, artifactual perfusion defects occur. Cardiac motion during image acquisition will also cause improper back-projection during SPECT reconstruction that may result in spurious perfusion defects. Cardiac motion is most commonly caused by patient motion during image acquisition or diaphragmatic movement that occurs during heavy breathing after termination of exercise.

Cardiac motion due to diaphragmatic excursion is of particular concern when performing exercise ^{201}Tl SPECT, because imaging with this isotope must begin within minutes of terminating exercise.[50] With ^{99m}Tc sestamibi, imaging is usually not performed for at least half an hour after injection depending on the stressor used; thus, the likelihood of significant diaphragmatic excursion is minimized. Furthermore, if patient motion occurs during a sestamibi acquisition, imaging can be readily repeated because this isotope displays little, if any, myocardial redistribution.[104,144,168]

Before interpreting all ^{201}Tl SPECT images, the raw projection data sets must be reviewed for possible patient motion artifacts. Review of the raw image data can also identify other potential sources of artifact. High count activity in extracardiac structures (such as liver or bowel) can cause a relative diminution in cardiac activity that is perceived as a perfusion defect. Overlying bowel may also mask inferior and inferolateral perfusion defects. Furthermore, soft-tissue photon attenuation, which is commonly seen when using ^{201}Tl, can produce artifacts in the inferior and anterior myocardial regions.

Recently, several manufacturers developed attenuation correction devices to minimize these errors in interpretation. Attenuation correction can be done with triple-headed camera systems using a solitary point source and fan-beam collimation.[44] Dual-headed camera systems use scanning line sources (such as gadolinium-153) with simultaneous acquisition of emission and transmission data.[71] Attenuation correction has been attempted with ^{201}Tl and ^{99m}Tc sestamibi.[44-46,71] At the time of this writing, most of the validation studies have been

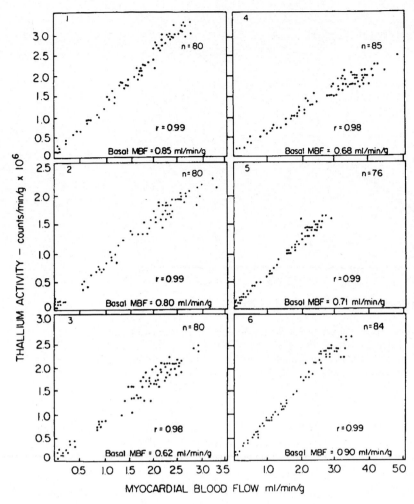

Fig. 15-4. Relation between thallium-201 activity and myocardial blood flow *(MBF)* in six dogs during exercise. A linear relation is noted except at the highest blood flows, where counts begin to reach a plateau. (Reproduced with permission from Nielsen AP, Morris KG, Murdock R, et al: Linear relationship between the distribution of thallium-201 and blood flow in ischemic and nonischemic myocardium during exercise, *Circulation* 61:797, 1980.)

performed with ^{99m}Tc,[46,71] although algorithms for correcting soft-tissue artifacts with ^{201}Tl are in progress. Preliminary results have demonstrated improved specificity at the expense of sensitivity.[71] This may be due in part to the restraints associated with visual interpretation of the corrected images. Quantification of the corrected images, with development of appropriate normal data files for both ^{201}Tl and Tc radiopharmaceuticals, may improve overall accuracy.[46]

DETECTION OF CORONARY STENOSIS BY THALLIUM-201: RELATION TO CORONARY FLOW RESERVE

Coronary blood flow is primarily regulated at the arteriolar level; minimal resistance to flow is observed in normal epicardial arteries.[120] Thus, during times of increasing myocardial oxygen demands (as in dynamic exercise) arteriolar vasodilation allows blood flow to increase twofold to threefold.[69,149,187] This ability to dramatically increase flow from basal resting levels is termed the *intrinsic coronary flow reserve* of a vascular bed. In patients with coronary artery disease many factors increase epicardial resistance, including the severity and length of stenosis,[41,58,59] the presence of sequential arterial lesions,[31] and intrinsic epicardial vasomotion.[52,161] Regardless of the

mechanisms responsible for altering vascular resistance, resting myocardial perfusion is generally maintained even when focal obstructions occlude 80% to 90% of the arterial cross-sectional area.[59] This is achieved through progressive distal arteriolar vasodilation with worsening stenosis. However, as coronary reserve is spent, there is less capability for further hyperemia with exercise or pharmacologic stressors.

The development of myocardial perfusion defects with exercise or pharmacologic stressors depends on induction of heterogeneous blood flow. During exercise[69] and particularly with pharmacologic stress,[187] coronary blood flow to the vascular bed of a normal artery will dramatically increase, whereas perfusion through a stenosed artery may change minimally despite a maximal hyperemic response. The initial uptake of [201]Tl (Fig. 15-4) and Tc-based radiopharmaceuticals (Fig. 15-5) is flow dependent within physiologic ranges,[100,121] although the extraction fraction of ^{201}Tl is higher than that observed for ^{99m}Tc sestamibi (0.85, 0.40, respectively).[33] In this regard, at higher myocardial blood flows, peak ^{201}Tl count activity should continue to increase and only reach a plateau at the highest levels. This clearly occurs, because myocardial ^{201}Tl counts are higher when maximal hyperemia is induced with pharmacologic vasodilators compared with exercise stress.[96] Regardless of the stressor used,

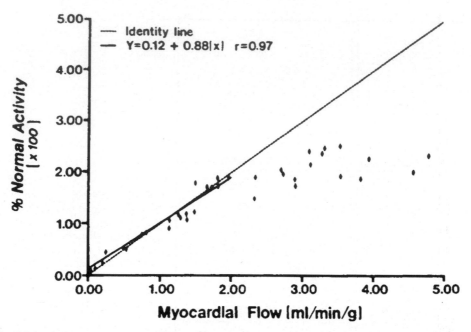

Fig. 15-5. Relation between technetium-99m sestamibi myocardial count activity and myocardial blood flow determined by microspheres. Technetium-99m count activity is linearly related to flow only up to 2.0 ml/min/gram, after which the former underestimates flow. (Reproduced with permission from Glover DK, Okada RD: Myocardial kinetics of Tc-MIBI in canine myocardium after dipyridamole, *Circulation* 81:628, 1990.)

the relative myocardial radionuclide concentration will be greater in vascular beds supplied by a normal coronary artery compared with those perfused by an artery with a severe obstruction. To detect a perfusion abnormality with scintigraphy, two-fold difference in relative count activity is required.[58] This is clinically important when assessing the functional significance of a coronary stenosis, because many moderate lesions (50% to 70%) may cause severe relative flow abnormalities, whereas others of similar angiographic severity may induce relatively minor regional differences and go undetected.[34,130,185,188]

During exercise stress, ischemia will occur in most patients when myocardial oxygen demands exceed increments in coronary flow, whereas with pharmacologic vasodilators (adenosine or dipyridamole) ischemia is infrequently induced.[80,137] However, although induction of ischemia with exercise stress may occur simultaneously with changes in regional myocardial blood flow, the latter is responsible for creating perfusion defects with ^{201}Tl scintigraphy. Dobutamine, unlike pharmacologic vasodilators, more commonly induces ischemia in patients with severe coronary lesions by markedly increasing myocardial contractility, heart rate, and blood pressure. Dobutamine also creates heterogeneous coronary blood flow, but to a lesser extent than that created by dipyridamole.[51]

DETECTION OF CORONARY ARTERY DISEASE: EXERCISE THALLIUM-201 SCINTIGRAPHY

Extensive data are published on several thousand patients that demonstrate the high sensitivity of both ^{201}Tl planar and SPECT imaging for detecting coronary artery disease. The sensitivity and specificity of qualitative planar imaging reported in the literature in more than 4000 patients are 82% (range, 74% to 96%) and 88% (range, 63% to 100%), respectively.[108] Sensitivity varies with the extent of coronary artery disease* (Fig. 15-6). When quantitative analysis is applied to the planar images sensitivity increases to 89% but at the expense of specificity.[8,86,106,179]

Pooled data from the largest series evaluating SPECT also indicate a high sensitivity of more than 90% (range, 82% to 98%) (Table 15-2).† Most patients with single-vessel disease (83%) and almost all patients with double- (93%) and triple-vessel disease (95%) will have an abnormal result on ^{201}Tl SPECT. The overall sensitivity is high for detecting patients without a history of myocardial infarction (85%) and patients with significant (>50%) single-vessel (75%), double-vessel (89%), and triple-vessel (96%) stenosis. Although comparative studies are few, SPECT seems to be superior to planar imaging, particularly for detecting individual coronary artery stenoses on the basis of localization of stress-induced perfusion defects.[47]

Detection of individual coronary artery stenosis by exercise SPECT

Two of the major advances from planar imaging to SPECT is the ability to detect individual coronary artery stenoses with greater accuracy and to quantify the extent of hypoperfused myocardium specific to an individual vascular bed. The overall

*References 4, 13, 39, 97, 123, 124, 127, 157, 177, 181.
†References 31, 78, 107, 109, 173, 179, 180.

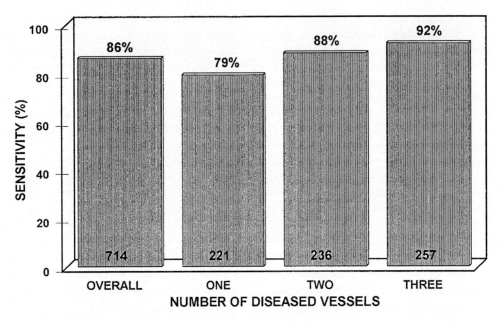

Fig. 15-6. Sensitivity of exercise planar thallium-201 scintigraphy for detecting coronary artery disease on the basis of the number of arteries with stenosis greater than 50%. (Adapted with permission from Maddahi J, Rodrigues E, Berman DS, et al: State-of-the-art myocardial perfusion imaging, *Cardiol Clin* 12:199-222, 1994.)

Table 15-2. Sensitivity and specificity of exercise thallium-201 SPECT*

Study (number of patients)	Patients with MI (%)	Sensitivity						Specificity	Normalcy rate
		Overall	MI	No MI	SVD	DVD	TVD		
		(%)							
Tamaki et al[171] (n = 104)	39	80/82 (98)	32/32 (100)	48/50 (96)	–	–	–	20/22 (91)	–
DePasquale et al[31] (n = 210)	26	170/179 (95)	47/47 (100)	123/134 (92)	85/93 (91)	72/73 (99)	13/13 (100)	23/31 (74)	–
Iskandrian et al[78] (n = 461)	18	224/272 (82)	49/50 (98)	174/222 (78)	45/70 (64)	93/107 (87)	86/95 (91)	35/58 (60)	123/131 (94)
Maddahi et al[107] (n = 138)	47	87/92 (95)	43/43 (100)	44/49 (90)	15/18 (83)	32/33 (97)	40/41 (98)	10/18 (56)	24/28 (86)
Mahmarian et al[109] (n = 360)	33	192/221 (87)	73/74 (99)	68/86 (79)	119/142 (84)	60/66 (91)	13/13 (100)	65/75 (87)	–
VanTrain et al[178] (n = 318)	40	185/196 (94)	78/78 (100)	106/118 (90)	56/64 (88)	69/72 (96)	60/60 (100)	15/35 (43)	62/76 (82)
Total	31% of all patients with MI	938/1042 (90)	322/324 (99)†	563/659 (85)	320/387 (83)	326/351 (93)‡	212/222 (95)‡	168/239 (70)	209/235 (89)

*DVD = double-vessel disease; MI = myocardial infarction; SPECT = single-photon emission computed tomography; SVD = single-vessel disease; TVD = triple-vessel disease.
†$p = 0.0001$ compared with no MI.
‡$p = 0.0001$ compared with SVD.
Modified with permission from Mahmarian JJ, Verani MS: Exercise thallium-201 perfusion scintigraphy in the assessment of ischemic heart disease, *Am J Cardiol* 67:2D-11D, 1991.

sensitivity and specificity of planar imaging for identifying significant (>50%) stenosis in individual vascular beds are 59% and 91%, respectively* (Fig. 15-7). In contrast, pooled data from the largest patient series using exercise SPECT demonstrate an overall 79% sensitivity for detecting individual vessel stenosis, which includes 80% of left anterior descending artery stenoses, 83% of right artery stenoses, and 72% of circumflex artery stenoses (Table 15-3).[78,107,109,173,180]

The lower detection rate of individual stenoses compared with patients with coronary artery disease may result from several potential factors. First, since the presence of a perfusion defect is determined by relative differences in regional myocardial ^{201}Tl uptake, it is conceivable that a vascular territory with a mild decrease in tracer uptake might be overshadowed by a territory with a perfusion defect of relatively greater severity. The region with only a mild count reduction would appear normal on scintigraphy. Second, the assignment of myocardial regions to specific coronary arteries is imperfect because of the great heterogeneity in the size and location of vascular beds supplied by a specific coronary artery in any given patient.[30,77,110] For example, a large perfusion defect caused by proximal stenosis of a left anterior descending artery might extend into the lateral wall and mask a smaller hypoperfused area in the territory of a stenosed obtuse marginal artery. Thus, although coronary angiography demonstrates double-vessel disease, the scintigraphic pattern may only appear as that seen with single-vessel stenosis. Third, in a patient with multivessel disease who is performing treadmill exercise, the development

* References 39, 97, 123, 128, 155, 157.

of ischemia within the vascular territory of a severe coronary artery stenosis may lead to termination of exercise before the development of maximal hyperemia, thus limiting the detection of additional coronary stenoses. Fourth, to a variable extent, collaterals may prevent ischemia within vascular beds supplied by arteries with severe stenoses. Fifth, antiischemic medications may reduce heterogeneity in coronary flow during exercise and thereby decrease the size of a perfusion defect or limit the defect to one vascular bed.[103,112,169,199] Finally, many moderate coronary artery stenoses identified as significant by angiography will not alter coronary blood flow during stress and will therefore go undetected.[34,130,185,188]

Despite these potential limitations, the sensitivity for detecting individual vessel stenosis with SPECT is reasonably high, even in patients without previous myocardial infarction (Table 15-4). In a study by Mahmarian et al.[109] of patients with severe stenosis (≥70%) and no previous myocardial infarction, sensitivities for individual vessel detection were 89% for the left anterior descending artery, 77% for the right artery, and 87% for the circumflex coronary artery, with an overall detection rate of 82%.

Detection of coronary artery bypass graft stenosis

Several studies have addressed whether ^{201}Tl planar scintigraphy can detect coronary artery bypass graft stenosis.[152,154] Rasmussen et al[154] studied 41 patients 6 months after bypass surgery and reported a 71% sensitivity and a 94% specificity for detecting graft closure. Pfisterer et al[152] reported similar findings in 55 patients. Although the overall sensitivity was 80% for detecting graft closure, the problem graft could be lo-

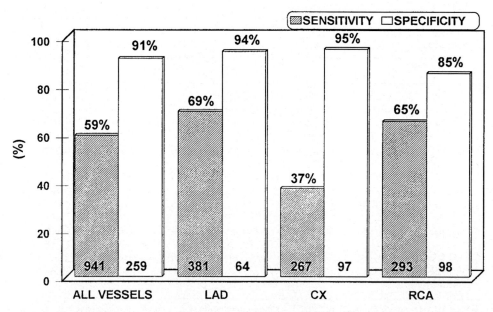

Fig. 15-7. Sensitivity and specificity of exercise planar thallium-201 scintigraphy for individual coronary artery disease detection (>50% stenosis). CX = circumflex coronary artery; LAD = left anterior descending; RCA = right coronary artery. (Adapted with permission from Maddahi J, Rodrigues E, Berman DS, et al: State-of-the-art myocardial perfusion imaging, *Cardiol Clin* 12:199-222, 1994.)

calized in only 61% of patients. The result is consistent with the known limitations of planar imaging for identifying individual coronary artery stenosis.[152] Lakkis et al[94] studied 50 patients without previous myocardial infarction who were referred for exercise ^{201}Tl SPECT to evaluate typical (60%) and atypical (40%) chest pain symptoms that recurred late (51 ± 47 months) after coronary artery bypass surgery. All patients had coronary angiography within 3 months of SPECT. Exercise SPECT had greater sensitivity for detecting patients with graft stenosis (80%) compared with stress electrocardiography (31%) (Fig. 15-8) regardless of whether patients presented with typical (84% vs 24%; $p<0.0001$) or atypical (70% vs 50%; $p<0.01$) chest pain symptoms. Thallium-201 SPECT detected most of the 48 grafts with more than 50% stenosis (83%) and accurately

localized graft stenoses to the proper vascular bed (Table 15-5). Similar results were reported for adenosine SPECT.[90] These data support the use of ^{201}Tl SPECT for evaluating patients after coronary bypass surgery. Whether SPECT can define patient risk for subsequent cardiac events following bypass surgery awaits further study.[147]

Effect of stenosis severity on results of scintigraphy

Although the extent of coronary artery disease predicts an abnormal scan result, the severity of stenosis is probably a more critical factor. Patients with multivessel disease have abnormal scan results more often because they commonly have at least one stenosis of high-grade severity. In our series, most patients (79%) who had a false-negative result on exercise SPECT were

Table 15-3. Exercise thallium-201 SPECT: individual vessel analysis (>50% stenosis)*

Study	Left anterior descending coronary artery		Right coronary artery		Circumflex artery		Overall	
	Sensitivity	Specificity	Sensitivity	Specificity	Sensitivity	Specificity	Sensitivity	Specificity
				n/n (%)				
Tamaki[171]	55/63 (87)	40/41 (98)	45/49 (92)	51/55 (93)	25/32 (78)	69/72 (96)	125/144 (87)	160/168 (95)
DePasquale[31]	75/96 (78)	95/114 (83)	93/104 (89)	92/106 (87)	51/78 (65)	125/132 (95)	219/278 (79)	312/352 (89)
Maddahi[107]	60/77 (78)	28/33 (85)	56/68 (82)	30/42 (71)	49/62 (79)	29/48 (60)	165/207 (80)	87/123 (71)
Mahmarian[109]	79/98 (81)	130/142 (92)	103/137 (75)	145/147 (99)	60/78 (77)	178/196 (91)	242/313 (77)	453/485 (93)
Van Train[178]	115/148 (78)	59/94 (63)	118/141 (84)	63/101 (62)	66/97 (68)	98/145 (68)	299/386 (77)	220/340 (65)
Total	384/482 (80)†	352/424 (83)	415/499 (83)‡	381/451 (84)	251/347 (72)	499/593 (84)	1050/1328 (79)	1232/1468 (84)

*SPECT = single-photon emission computed tomography.
†$p = 0.01$ compared with circumflex artery.
‡$p = 0.005$ compared with circumflex artery.
Reprinted with permission from Mahmarian JJ, Verani MS: Exercise thallium-201 perfusion scintigraphy in the assessment of ischemic heart disease, *Am J Cardiol* 67:2D-11D, 1991.

Table 15-4. Exercise thallium-201 SPECT: individual vessel detection (>50% stenosis) excluding patients with myocardial infarction*

Study	Left anterior descending coronary artery	Right coronary artery	Circumflex artery	Overall
		(%)		
Tamaki, et al[171]	32/38 (84)	28/31 (90)	14/19 (74)	74/88 (84)
DePasquale, et al[31]	83/103 (81)	89/99 (90)	37/58 (64)	209/260 (80)
Maddahi, et al[107]	27/40 (68)	24/32 (75)	29/38 (76)	80/110 (73)
Mahmarian, et al[109]	24/34 (71)	33/52 (63)	23/29 (79)	80/115 (70)
Van Train, et al[178]	62/86 (72)	65/83 (78)	42/63 (67)	169/232 (73)
Total	228/301 (76)	239/297 (80)	145/207 (70)	612/805 (76)

*SPECT = single-photon emission computed tomography.
Reprinted with permission from Mahmarian JJ, Verani MS: Exercise thallium-201 perfusion scintigraphy in the assessment of ischemic heart disease, *Am J Cardiol* 67:2D-11D, 1991.

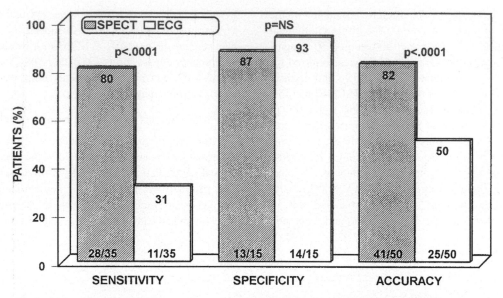

Fig. 15-8. Sensitivity, specificity, and overall accuracy of exercise thallium-201 single photon emission computed tomography and exercise electrocardiography (*ECG*) for detecting graft stenosis (>50%) in patients after coronary artery bypass surgery. SPECT = single-photon emission computed tomography. (Adapted with permission from Lakkis NM, Mahmarian JJ, Verani MS: Exercise thallium-201 single photon emission computed tomography for evaluation of coronary artery bypass graft patency, *Am J Cardiol* 76:107-111, 1995, with permission from Excerpta Medica, Inc.)

Table 15-5. Exercise thallium-201 SPECT: localizing bypass graft stenosis*

Graft	Sensitivity	Specificity	Positive predictive value	Negative predictive value
			%	
Left anterior descending coronary artery (*n* = 28)	82	90	85	88
Right coronary artery (*n* = 12)	92	91	85	95
Circumflex artery (*n* = 8)	75	75	60	86

*SPECT = single-photon emission tomography.
Reproduced from Lakkis NM, Mahmarian JJ, Verani MS: Exercise thallium-201 single photon emission computed tomography for evaluation of coronary artery bypass graft patency, *Am J Cardiol* 76:107–111, 1995, with permission from Excerpta Medica, Inc.

those with single-vessel disease, of whom 91% had only moderate coronary stenosis.[109] In fact, most of the patients with double-vessel disease and a false-negative result (67%) also had stenoses of only moderate severity. In a recent analysis from the Asymptomatic Cardiac Ischemia Pilot (ACIP) study, univariate predictors of an abnormal perfusion scan were the extent and severity of coronary stenosis.[116] However, on multivariate analysis, stenosis severity was the most important determinant of an abnormal scan ($p<0.001$), followed by impaired treadmill exercise duration ($p=0.016$) and older age ($p<0.05$). Pooled data from the literature substantiate that individual vessel detection substantially increases with stenosis severity[31,109,173,180] (Fig. 15-9). In the ACIP SPECT substudy, only 42% of patients with moderate stenosis were detected compared with 84% of those with severe stenosis.[116]

The seemingly variable and unpredictable detection of moderate stenosis with ^{201}Tl scintigraphy is due in part to the im-

precise gold standard used to assess the severity of coronary artery disease—coronary angiography. It is well established, particularly with moderate stenoses, that impairment in coronary flow reserve cannot be predicted from angiographic findings.[34,130,185,186] This has been confirmed by using noninvasive nitrogen-13 ammonia positron emission tomography[34] as well as coronary artery Doppler flow wires in the cardiac catheterization laboratory.[130] In the recent study by Miller et al,[130] only 47% of moderate stenoses (50% to 69%) had impaired coronary flow reserve defined as a twofold or lesser increase in myocardial blood flow velocity after intracoronary adenosine.[130] However, in the study by Miller et al[130] and that of Di Carli et al,[34] coronary flow reserve was abnormal in most arteries with stenosis of 70% or more (Fig. 15-10). In addition, Miller et al[130] demonstrated a high concordance (90%) for normalcy and abnormalcy between ^{99m}Tc sestamibi SPECT and Doppler flow measurements during adenosine-induced hyper-

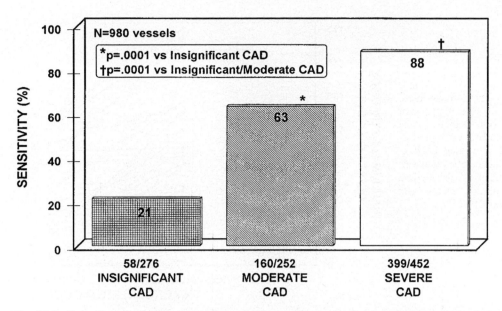

Fig. 15-9. Detection of coronary artery disease with exercise single-photon emission computed tomography in individual vessels based on stenosis severity. Insignificant coronary artery disease *(CAD)* = <50% stenosis; moderate CAD = 51 to 70% stenosis; severe CAD = ≥70% stenosis. Sensitivity increased significantly with severity of CAD stenosis.

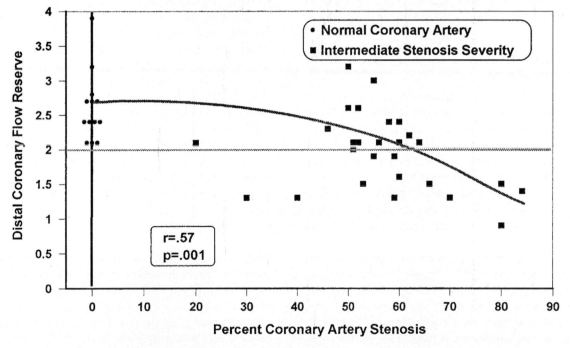

Fig. 15-10. Distal coronary flow reserve compared with coronary artery stenosis severity. Although flow reserve during adenosine-induced hyperemia is abnormal (≤ 2) *(horizontal line)* in most patients with stenosis >70%, the results are highly variable among arteries of lesser severity. (Adapted with permission from Miller DD, Gersh BJ, Christian TF, et al: Correlation of pharmacological Tc-99m-sestamibi myocardial perfusion imaging with poststenotic coronary flow reserve in patients with angiographically intermediate coronary artery stenoses, *Circulation* 89:2150-2160, 1994.)

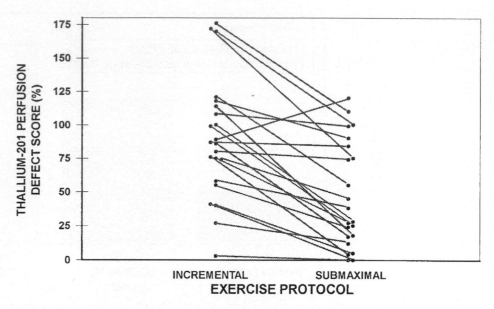

Fig. 15-11. Influence of exercise intensity on the extent of quantified planar thallium-201 perfusion defects in the same patients. (Adapted with permission from Heller GV, Ahmed I, Tilkemeier PL, et al: Influence of exercise intensity on the presence, distribution, and size of thallium-201 defects, *Am Heart J* 123:909-916, 1992.)

emia. On the basis of these data, the sensitivity for detecting severe coronary stenosis ($\geq$70%) is expected to be high and predictable. However, these studies emphasize that true flow-limiting moderate stenoses are also readily detected with perfusion imaging.

Influence of exercise performance on the detection of coronary artery disease

Few studies in the literature have evaluated sensitivity of perfusion scintigraphy with respect to treadmill exercise intensity. Iskandrian et al[78] reported their results in 272 patients with coronary artery disease. The patient population consisted of those who had a positive result on exercise electrocardiography for ischemia and/or achieved more than 85% of their predicted target heart rate (Group 1) or those who performed submaximal exercise (<85% of predicted target heart rate) and did not have a positive result on stress electrocardiography (Group 2). Compared with Group 2, Group 1 achieved a greater exercise workload (7.5 ± 0.2 vs 6.1 ± 0.3 metabolic equivalents; p<0.001), heart rate (136 ± 2 vs 111 ± 2 beats/minute, p<0.001), and systolic blood pressure (177 ± 2 vs 166 ± 3 mm Hg, p<0.001). Conversely, Group 2 patients were more frequently receiving antiischemic medications in the form of nitrates (65% vs 46%; p<0.01) and calcium antagonists (72% vs 59%; p<0.04) compared with Group 1 patients. The overall sensitivity of SPECT was significantly higher (p<0.002) in Group 1 than in Group 2 (88% vs 73%; p<0.002) as well as in the subset patients without previous myocardial infarction (86% vs 67%, respectively). These data imply that an abnormal result on SPECT is related to exercise intensity. However, confounding variables in this study were the substantially higher use of antiischemic medications among Group 2 patients and the inclusion in Group 1 of patients who performed submaximal exercise but had ischemia on electrocardiography.

We reported the effects of exercise intensity on SPECT results in 221 patients with coronary artery disease who performed symptom-limited treadmill exercise.[109] In contrast to the study by Iskandrian et al,[78] the sensitivity for detecting coronary artery disease was high (87%), regardless of exercise intensity. Similar findings were also reported by Esquivel et al[42] in a study of 290 patients with coronary artery disease who had exercise ^{201}Tl quantitative planar scintigraphy. Eighty-six percent of patients who performed maximal exercise and 89% who performed submaximal exercise had an abnormal result. This was also true in patients without previous myocardial infarction (maximal 89% vs submaximal 85%, respectively). As in our study, patients who performed submaximal compared with maximal exercise had a substantially higher incidence of multivessel coronary artery disease, which may have biased the results.

No definitive conclusions can be drawn from the results of the above trials because the patients studied clearly differed in many respects beyond the intensity of their exercise performance. To assess the effects of exercise effort on ^{201}Tl scintigraphy, two separate tests at different intensities would need to be performed in the same patients. Heller et al[70] reported the results of using such a protocol in 22 patients with coronary artery disease who underwent planar ^{201}Tl scintigraphy on separate days following maximal and submaximal (70% of predicted heart rate) exercise.[70] With maximal exercise, all patients had a reversible perfusion defect. However, so did 20 of 22 patients (91%) after submaximal exercise. Although scan abnormalcy was similar regardless of exercise intensity, the extent of the ^{201}Tl perfusion defect was much smaller with submaximal exercise compared with maximal exercise (Fig. 15-11). In support of this finding, Nishimura et al[139] demonstrated that the quantified SPECT perfusion defect size is smaller when the same patients undergo submaximal exercise

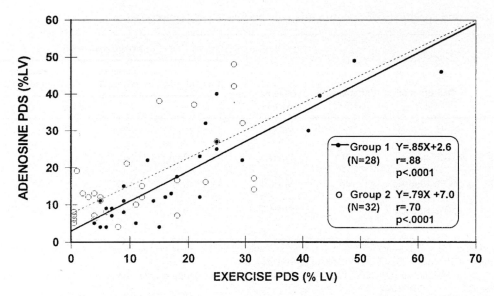

Fig. 15-12. Relation between exercise and adenosine-induced single-photon emission computed tomography perfusion defect sizes in the same patients as assessed by linear regression analysis. Patients who performed maximal exercise (≥85% of the predicted heart rate) *(Group 1)* had a similar defect size during adenosine stress (*r* = 0.88). However, in patients who performed submaximal exercise *(Group 2)*, the size of the perfusion defect was underestimated compared with that observed with adenosine stress. LV = left ventricle; PDS = perfusion defect size.

compared with maximal hyperemia with adenosine stress (11 ± 10% vs 15 ± 12%, respectively; *p* = 0.09). However, similar perfusion defect sizes were observed with adenosine and maximal exercise (19 ± 13% vs 18 ± 15%; *p* value not significant (Fig. 15-12).

These data indicate that in patients who prematurely terminate exercise because of a noncardiac reason, the perfusion abnormality may be substantially underestimated owing to an inability to maximize heterogeneity in coronary blood flow. Because the total size of perfusion defect is of prognostic importance, its underestimation may result in imprecise risk assessment. Patients who can perform only submaximal exercise because of a cardiac limitation will generally have more extensive coronary artery disease and an abnormal result on scintigraphy. However, in patients who cannot perform maximal exercise because of a noncardiac reason, pharmacologic stress testing is preferred.

PHARMACOLOGIC STRESS TESTING FOR DETECTING CORONARY ARTERY DISEASE

The introduction of pharmacologic stressors as a substitute for exercise has clearly broadened the clinical availability of perfusion scintigraphy, because 25% to 30% of patients referred for imaging cannot perform adequate exercise stress testing. The pharmacologic stressors currently available in clinical practice are the coronary vasodilators (such as adenosine and dipyridamole) and the β-agonist dobutamine. Adenosine, when administered as an intravenous infusion, binds with specific receptors at the coronary arteriolar level to induce vasodilation.[9] Dipyridamole is an indirect coronary artery vasodilator that in-

creases the extracellular concentration of adenosine by blocking its cellular reuptake and metabolism.[48,92] Because dipyridamole works indirectly through adenosine, the maximal hyperemic response is less predictable and may not occur in 20% to 30% of patients.[159] This may limit detection of coronary artery disease and underestimate the extent of hypoperfused myocardium in the same manner as submaximal exercise. Dobutamine is a β-agonist with direct chronotropic and inotropic effects that indirectly induce arteriolar coronary vasodilation by markedly increasing myocardial oxygen demands. Dobutamine is less potent than dipyridamole or adenosine for maximizing coronary artery blood flow.[51]

Dipyridamole

Intravenous and oral dipyridamole have been extensively studied for the detection of coronary artery disease with planar ^{201}Tl scintigraphy* and, more recently, SPECT† (Tables 15-6 and 15-7). As with exercise scintigraphy, coronary artery disease can be diagnosed with greater sensitivity in patients with more extensive and severe disease than in those with single-vessel involvement. In a series of 100 consecutive patients that combined oral dipyridamole (300 mg) with SPECT,[117] the detection of patients with single-, double-, and triple-vessel disease was 85%, 90%, and 100%, respectively. Furthermore, 82% of vessels with stenosis of 70% or more were identified compared with 67% of those with moderate stenosis (51% to 69%). The specificity for normal vessels was 90%. Similar re-

*References 2, 49, 74, 93, 95, 98, 129, 142, 174.
†References 5, 11, 32, 49, 73, 75, 129.

Table 15-6. Sensitivity and specificity of oral dipyridamole perfusion scintigraphy*

Study (number of patients)	Definition of CAD	Patients with MI (%)	Imaging method	Overall	Patients with MI	Patients without MI	Specificity
				Sensitivity			
						(%)	
Homma et al[74] (n = 53)	>50% stenosis	0	Planar	42/43 (91)	NA	42/43 (91)	8/10 (80)
Taillefer et al[169] (n = 50)	≥70% stenosis	NA	Planar	29/39 (74)†	NA	NA	11/11 (100)
Beer et al[5] (n = 65)	>50% stenosis	45	SPECT	41/48 (85)	NA	NA	11/17 (65)
Borges-Neto et al[11] (n = 100)	>50% stenosis	30	SPECT	77/84 (92)	29/30 (97)	48/54 (89)	14/16 (88)

CAD = coronary artery disease; MI = myocardial infarction; NA = not available; SPECT = single-photon emission computed tomography.
†Sensitivity 65% (200 mg of dipyridamole) and 84% (400 mg of dipyridamole).
Reprinted with permission from Mahmarian JJ, Verani MS: Myocardial perfusion imaging during pharmacologic stress testing. In Crawford ME (ed.), Nuclear Cardiology, *Cardiol Clin* 12:223-245, 1994.

Table 15-7. Sensitivity and specificity of intravenous dipyridamole perfusion scintigraphy*

Study (number of patients)	Definition of CAD	Patients with MI (%)	Imaging method	Overall	Patients with MI	Patients without MI	Specificity
				Sensitivity			
						(%)	
Albro et al[2] (n = 62)	≥50% stenosis	NA	Planar	34/51 (67)	NA	NA	10/11 (91)
Leppo et al[98] (n = 56)	>50% stenosis	29	Planar	37/40 (93)	16/16 (100)	21/24 (88)	16/20 (80)
Okada et al[142] (n = 30)	≥50% stenosis	30	Planar	21/23 (91)	12/13 (92)	9/10 (90)	7/7 (100)
Taillefer et al[169] (n = 50)	≥70% stenosis	NA	Planar	32/39 (82)	NA	NA	10/11 (91)
Lam et al[95] (n = 141)	≥70% stenosis	15	Planar	93/110 (85)	NA	NA	22/31 (71)
Kong et al[93] (n = 114)	>50% stenosis	7	Planar	86/94 (91)	NA	NA	12/20 (60)
Mendelson et al[129] (n = 79)	≥70% stenosis	70	Planar	51/76 (67)	41/55 (75)	11/22 (50)	NA
			SPECT	68/76 (89)	51/55 (93)	18/22 (82)	NA
Francisco et al[49] (n = 86)	≥70% stenosis	29	Planar	41/51 (80)	24/25 (96)	17/26 (65)	16/24 (67)
			SPECT (visual)	39/51 (76)	23/25 (92)	16/26 (62)	16/24 (67)
			SPECT (quantitative)	47/51 (92)	25/25 (100)	21/26 (81)	23/24 (96)
Huikuri et al[75] (n = 93)	≥70% stenosis	27	SPECT	78/81 (96)	NA	NA	9/12 (75)
DePuey et al[32] (n = 76)	>50% stenosis	NA	SPECT	45/51 (89)	NA	NA	7/15 (47)
Ho et al[73] (n = 54)	≥50% stenosis	NA	SPECT	42/43 (98)	NA	NA	NA
Total planar				395/484 (82)	93/109 (85)	58/82 (71)	93/124 (75)
Total visual SPECT				272/302 (90)	74/80 (93)	34/48 (71)	32/47 (68)

*CAD = coronary artery disease; MI = myocardial infarction; NA = not available; SPECT = single-photon emission computed tomography.
Modified with permission from Mahmarian JJ, Verani MS: Myocardial perfusion imaging during pharmacologic stress testing. In Crawford ME (ed.), Nuclear Cardiology, *Cardiol Clin* 12:223-245, 1994.

Table 15-8. Sensitivity and specificity of adenosine thallium-201 SPECT*

Study (number of patients)	Definition of CAD	Patients with MI (%)	Sensitivity						Specificity
			Overall	Patients with single-vessel disease	Patients with double-vessel disease	Patients with triple-vessel disease	Patients with MI	Patients without MI	
			(%)						
Iskandrian et al[80] (n = 148)	≥50% stenosis	25	121/132 (92)	47/54 (87)	34/37 (92)	40/41 (98)	35/37 (95)	86/95 (91)	14/16 (88)
Ngyuen et al[134] (n = 60)	≥50% stenosis	37	49/53 (92)	NA	NA	NA	NA	NA	7/7 (100)
Nishimura et al[135] (n = 101)	>50% stenosis	25	61/70 (87)	26/32 (81)	20/22 (91)	15/16 (94)	24/25 (96)	37/45 (82)	28/31 (90)
Verani et al[180] (n = 45)	>50% stenosis	25	24/29 (83)	11/15 (73)	9/10 (90)	4/4 (100)	NA	NA	15/16 (94)
Total			255/284 (90)	84/101 (83)	63/69 (91)	59/61 (97)	59/62 (95)	123/140 (88)	64/70 (91)

*CAD = coronary artery disease; MI = myocardial infarction; NA = not available; SPECT = single-photon emission computed tomography.
Adapted with permission from Mahmarian JJ, Verani MS: Myocardial perfusion imaging during pharmacologic stress testing. In Crawford ME (ed.), Nuclear Cardiology, *Cardiol Clin* 12:223-245, 1994.

sults were reported when intravenous dipyridamole was combined with SPECT.[32,49,73,75,129] In the series by Mendelson et al,[129] [201]Tl SPECT was shown to be superior to planar dipyridamole imaging for overall detection of coronary artery disease (89% vs 67%; *p*<0.001) and on identification of patients with moderate (83% vs 58%; *p*<0.05) and severe (90% vs 69%; *p*<0.01) stenosis.

Numerous studies have directly compared dipyridamole with exercise scintigraphy,[61,75,83,186] and found both stressors to be similar. However, dipyridamole seems to be superior to exercise stress testing for evaluating patients with left bundle-branch block,[20,84,158,178] who commonly have false-positive results for septal perfusion defects.

Adenosine

Adenosine SPECT has a reported overall sensitivity and specificity for detecting coronary artery disease of 90% and 91%, respectively (Table 15-8).* Detection of disease in individual vessels (≥70% stenosis) is equally high (91%), and specificity is retained (93%).[135] As with dipyridamole, adenosine has been directly compared to exercise stress.[25,62,136] Nishimura et al[136] reported the results of a multicenter study comparing adenosine with symptom-limited exercise SPECT in 175 patients who had both tests within 1 month.[136] Agreement between the two stressors for normalcy and abnormalcy was 83% by visual analysis and 86% by quantitative analysis. A concordance of 72% was observed on the type of defect (reversible or fixed). Close agreement was also found for the presence or absence of perfusion abnormalities within specific vascular beds (range, 82.7% to 90.0%) by using quantitative SPECT. Gupta et al[62] and Coyne et al[25] published the results of two separate multicenter

*References 25, 62, 80, 134, 135, 182.

trials comparing exercise and adenosine SPECT with coronary angiography. The sensitivity and specificity of the stressors were similar (Table 15-9). Adenosine stress is an acceptable alternative to exercise stress in patients who cannot adequately exercise or have left bundle-branch block.[145,146,178]

Dipyridamole and adenosine have only been directly compared in two recent but small patient series in which the scintigraphic results with both stressors were similar.[132,172] In the study by Taillefer et al,[172] the sensitivities of adenosine and dipyridamole when combined with planar scintigraphy were similar (91% vs 87%, respectively), although adenosine tended to detect more ischemic segments (170 vs 135, respectively). Patients preferred adenosine over dipyridamole mainly because of the short duration of side effects with the former agent.

Dobutamine

Mason et al[122] in 1984 were first to report the feasibility of dobutamine ^{201}Tl scintigraphy (at doses up to 20 µg/kg/min) for detecting coronary artery disease in patients without previous infarction.[122] The sensitivity and specificity of the test were 94% and 87%, respectively. Subsequent reports have confirmed these results[65,150,151] (Table 15-10). In the series by Hays et al,[65] the sensitivity and specificity of dobutamine SPECT were 86% and 90%, respectively, with reasonable individual vessel detection (78%) when stenosis severity was 70% or more.[65] Cid, Verani, and Mahmarian[23] reported an overall sensitivity of 81% with dobu-tamine SPECT in a larger cohort of 198 patients. In patients without a history of myocardial infarction, the sensitivity for detecting coronary artery disease was 76%. Overall, individual vessel detection (>50% stenosis) was only 57% and was particularly low in arteries with moderate stenosis (51% to 69%) (33% of arteries) compared with severe stenosis (≥70%) (66% of arteries). These data suggest that dobutamine may not be as ef-

Table 15-9. Adenosine versus exercise SPECT: diagnostic accuracy*

Variable	Coyne et al[25] (n = 100)		Gupta et al[62] (n = 144)	
	Exercise SPECT	Adenosine SPECT	Exercise SPECT	Adenosine SPECT
Sensitivity, %	81	83	82	83
Specificity, %	74	75	80	87
Normalcy rate, %	80	80	–	–
Positive predictive value, %	73	75	90	93
Negative predictive value, %	81	83	67	70
Overall accuracy, %	77	79	81	84

*SPECT = single-photon emission computed tomography.
Adapted with permission from Mahmarian JJ, Verani MS: Myocardial perfusion imaging during pharmacologic stress testing. In Crawford ME (ed.), Nuclear Cardiology, *Cardiol Clin* 12:223-245, 1994.

Table 15-10. Detection of coronary artery disease with dobutamine scintigraphy*

Author	Patients (n)	Patients with MI (%)	Dobutamine dose (μg/kg/min)	Imaging technique	Sensitivity			Specificity
					Overall	Patients with MI	Patients without MI	
					(%)			
Mason et al[122]	24	0	20	Planar	15/16 (94)	–	15/16 (94)	7/8 (87)
Pennell et al[149]	50	30	20	SPECT	39/40 (97)	15/15 (100)	24/25 (96)	8/10 (80)
Hays et al[65]	84	15	40	SPECT	49/57 (86)	13/13 (100)	26/34 (76)	9/10 (90)
Pennell et al[150]	20	0	40	SPECT	10/11 (91)	–	10/11 (91)	7/9 (78)
Total	178	–	–	–	113/124 (91)	28/28 (100)	75/86 (87)	31/37 (84)

*MI = myocardial infarction; SPECT = single-photon emission computed tomography.
Modified with permission from Mahmarian JJ, Verani MS: Myocardial perfusion imaging during pharmacologic stress testing. In Crawford ME (ed.), Nuclear Cardiology, *Cardiol Clin* 12:223-245, 1994.

fective as the pharmacologic vasodilators for detecting patients or individual arteries with significant coronary artery disease.

INCREASED LUNG UPTAKE DURING THALLIUM-201 SCINTIGRAPHY

Increased lung uptake during exercise results from high pulmonary capillary wedge pressures and is best observed in the anterior projection of planar and SPECT images. High lung uptake occurs in patients who have decreased left ventricular compliance caused by extensive coronary artery disease[102] but is also seen in other conditions that increase left ventricular end-diastolic pressure (such as valvular heart disease and cardiomyopathy). Although increased pulmonary uptake is a nonspecific finding, it portends a poor prognosis.[56,87,140]

Increased lung uptake is observed with dipyridamole scintigraphy in 20% to 35% of patients and occurs mostly in those who also exhibit ^{201}Tl redistribution and left ventricular cavity dilation.[143,183] Similar findings were reported for adenosine stress.[79,138] In a recent study from our laboratory, patients with single vessel and, particularly, multivessel coronary artery disease had a substantially greater lung-to-heart ratio than did normal volunteers or patients with normal coronary arteries.[138] Conversely, patients with increased lung uptake had a higher

frequency of previous myocardial infarction, a lower left ventricular ejection fraction, a larger initial perfusion defect, and more extensive ^{201}Tl redistribution. The sensitivity for detecting coronary artery disease on the basis of high lung uptake was only 30% but was similar to that previously reported with exercise stress.[56,87,140] At the present time, the prognostic significance of increased lung uptake of pharmacologic stressors is not known.

TRANSIENT LEFT VENTRICULAR DILATION

Transient left ventricular cavity dilation is best observed by comparing postexercise and 4-hour redistribution ^{201}Tl images. This scintigraphic pattern usually results from transient left ventricular systolic dysfunction in global myocardial ischemia and extensive coronary artery disease.[170,184] The sensitivity and specificity of this finding for identifying patients with critical multivessel disease were reported to be 60% and 95%, respectively.[184]

Transient left ventricular cavity dilation with dipyridamole occurs in approximately 22% of patients. As in exercise stress, this effect is indicative of severe triple-vessel disease, presence of coronary collateral vessels, and defect reversibility.[22] Lette et al[101] reported that patients with transient left ventricular di-

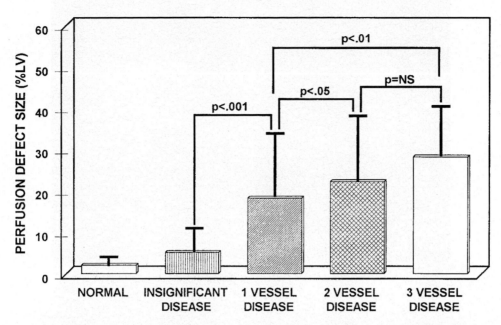

Fig. 15-13. Perfusion defect sizes observed in patients undergoing exercise single-photon emission computed tomography based on the extent of coronary artery disease. Normal = ≤25% stenosis; insignificant disease = 26 to 50% stenosis; 1,2,3, vessel disease = number of arteries with >50% stenosis. (Reprinted with permission from the American College of Cardiology. Modified from Mahmarian JJ, Boyce TM, Goldberg RK, et al: Quantitative exercise thallium-201 single-photon emission computed tomography for the enhanced diagnosis of ischemic heart disease, *J Am Coll Cardiol* 15:318-329, 1990.)

lation had severe coronary artery disease and an unusually high (64%) 1-year cardiac event rate, with most events occurring within 4 months of scintigraphy. Furthermore, in a subgroup of patients who had noncardiac surgery, postoperative event rates were 2% in 101 patients with normal scans or fixed defects, 9% in those with ^{201}Tl redistribution, and 58% in the 12 patients with transient cavity dilation.

Iskandrian et al[79] reported the importance of left ventricular dilation with adenosine in patients with coronary artery disease compared with normal persons. Cavity dilation was indicative of extensive coronary artery involvement and probably predicts as poor a prognosis as that predicted by dipyridamole and exercise stress.

ASSESSING THE EXTENT OF JEOPARDIZED MYOCARDIUM WITH THALLIUM-201 SPECT

Quantitative analysis of ^{201}Tl SPECT allows accurate estimation of the extent of stress-induced hypoperfusion and the percentage of scar and ischemia on the basis of relative changes in count activity from stress to redistribution imaging.[111] Many factors are known to influence left ventricular hypoperfusion beyond the intensity of exercise stress. The angiographic extent, location, and severity of coronary artery disease are important in defining the resultant perfusion defect size. In general, size of the perfusion defect increases with more extensive coronary artery disease (Fig. 15-13), but this effect is highly variable in any given patient.[109] Likewise, patients with moder-

ate coronary artery disease stenosis (51% to 69%) compared with those with severe stenosis (≥70%) have smaller perfusion defects regardless of the coronary artery involved.[110] However, the correlation between stenosis severity and perfusion defect size is modest at best ($r = 0.48$; $p = 0.004$).[110] The presence of coronary artery collaterals may dramatically affect defect size regardless if they are angiographically visible (Fig. 15-14).

The location of stenosis is a major determinant of the exercise-induced perfusion defect size. We addressed this issue by studying 158 patients who had single-vessel coronary artery disease by performing coronary angiography.[110] Stenosis-induced perfusion defects in the proximal left anterior descending artery are approximately twice as large as those observed for the right and circumflex coronary arteries (Fig. 15-15). These findings are consistent with reports demonstrating a greater reduction in left ventricular ejection fraction after anterior infarction than after inferior or lateral infarction.[163,165] Furthermore, proximal stenosis of the left anterior descending coronary artery was associated with substantially larger perfusion defects than stenoses in the midvessel or distal vessel (Fig. 15-16). One striking finding was the marked heterogeneity in myocardial perfusion defect sizes among individual patients with stenoses of similar anatomic severity and location. Angiographic findings did not predict the size of the vascular bed supplied by a given coronary artery. In this regard, the ^{201}Tl perfusion results can be used to clarify the functional significance of anatomic lesions identified at the time of coronary angiography.

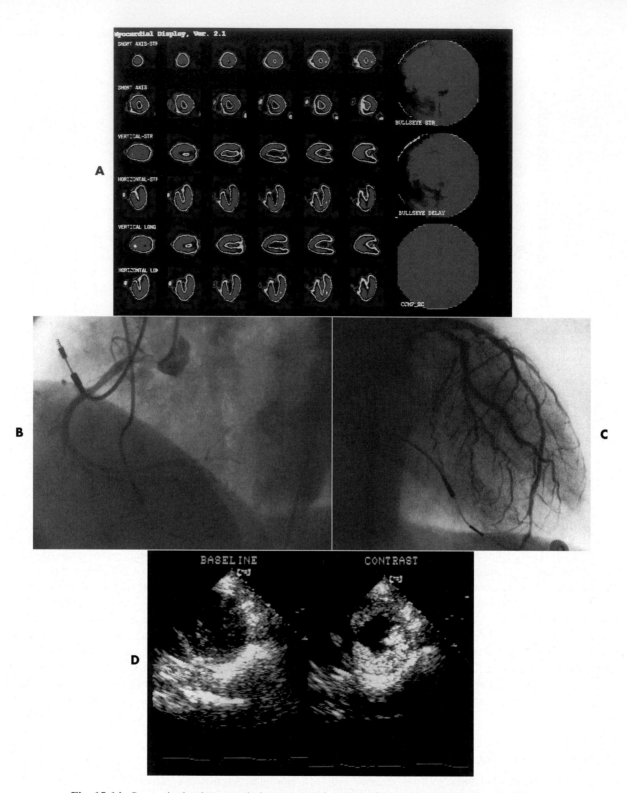

Fig. 15-14. Stress single-photon emission computed tomography reoriented and polar plot images. **A,** Right coronary artery arteriogram; **B,** left anterior descending coronary artery arteriogram; **C,** circumflex coronary arteriogram; and the short-axis two-dimensional echocardiographic images **(D)** at baseline *(left)* and after contrast injection down the LAD coronary artery *(right)*. Although this patient had a normal dobutamine thallium-201 SPECT with no discernible perfusion defect after comparison to the normal databank *(COMPSC)* **(A),** the right coronary artery is noted to have a subtotal ostial stenosis **(B).** No collaterals are observed to the right coronary artery after left main contrast injection **(C).** However, on echocardiography **(D),** intense contrast enhancement is noted in the inferior wall after injection of sonicated microbubbles down the LAD, verifying the presence of coronary collaterals to the right coronary artery. Despite a severe right coronary artery stenosis, this patient did not develop a stress perfusion defect because of the well-developed collateral circulation, which was apparent on echocardiography but not arteriography.

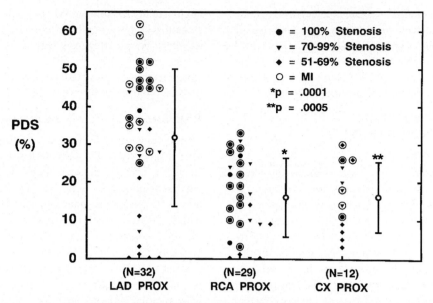

Fig. 15-15. Quantified mean *(solid bar)* and individual left ventricular perfusion defect size *(PDS)* in patients with proximal *(PROX)* stenoses of the left anterior descending *(LAD)*, right *(RCA)*, or circumflex *(CX)* coronary arteries. Although proximal LAD stenosis resulted in a significantly larger mean PDS than did RCA or CX stenosis, the anatomic information was imprecise in predicting the extent of jeopardized myocardium in any given artery. MI = myocardial infarction. (Reprinted with permission from the American College of Cardiology. From Mahmarian JJ, Pratt CM, Boyce TM, et al: The variable extent of jeopardized myocardium in patients with single vessel coronary artery disease: Quantification by thallium-201 single-photon emission computed tomography, *J Am Coll Cardiol* 17:355-362, 1991.)

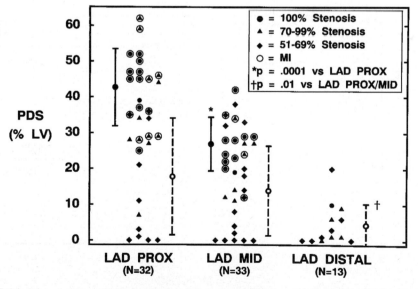

Fig. 15-16. Mean left ventricular perfusion defect size *(PDS)* in patients with *(solid bar)* and without *(broken bar)* myocardial infarction *(MI)* for the left anterior descending *(LAD)* coronary artery with proximal stenosis *(PROX)*, mid-stenosis, or distal stenosis. Proximal LAD stenosis generally led to a larger PDS than did mid or distal vessel stenosis, but there was significant individual vessel heterogeneity. (Reprinted from the American College of Cardiology. From Mahmarian JJ, Pratt CM, Boyce TM, et al: The variable extent of jeopardized myocardium in patients with single vessel coronary artery disease: Quantification by thallium-201 single-photon emission computed tomography, *J Am Coll Cardiol* 17:355-362, 1991.)

The size of the stress-induced perfusion defect assessed by ^{201}Tl SPECT is known to accurately predict patients at risk for subsequent cardiac events. The complementary data obtained by combining the scintigraphic and angiographic results would therefore be expected to improve the precision of clinical decision making when contemplating therapeutic options.

RISK STRATIFICATION WITH THALLIUM-201 SCINTIGRAPHY

Stable coronary artery disease

Thallium-201 scintigraphy can be used to assess risk across a broad spectrum of patients with coronary artery disease. Patients referred for perfusion imaging who have normal results have an exceedingly low (<1%) annual cardiac event rate.[16] The importance of quantifying perfusion defects has only recently become apparent.[81,105] One study compared the relative prognostic value of the exercise stress test results by using the Duke scoring system with results of SPECT and coronary angiography in 316 patients with coronary artery disease.[81] Over 28 ± 15 months of follow-up, 35 patients died or had nonfatal myocardial infarction. Although the treadmill exercise score and the extent of coronary artery disease did not define a high-risk or low-risk population for cardiac events, the size of exercise-induced perfusion defect size was a strong predictor. Patients with a small (<15%) left ventricular perfusion defect had an annual cardiac event rate of less than 1% compared with a 20% annual event rate over 4 years in patients with larger (≥15%) defects (Fig. 15-17). Of note, the scintigraphic results greatly improved risk assessment over clinical, stress test, and

angiographic variables alone (Fig. 15-18). These data demonstrate that both a normal or minimally abnormal scan confer an excellent overall prognosis regardless of the coronary angiographic findings. The importance of the total size of the perfusion defect in assessing risk has also been demonstrated among patients referred for adenosine SPECT (Fig. 15-19).[85]

Risk assessment after acute myocardial infarction

The value of ^{201}Tl perfusion scintigraphy for defining risk after acute myocardial infarction was reported with exercise stress[17,54,55,189] and pharmacologic stress.[18,57,99,114,188] Patients without scintigraphic ischemia have a very low cardiac event rate (<5%), whereas approximately 40% to 50% of patients with ischemia develop cardiac events (Table 15-11). Some of the most compelling initial data with scintigraphy were reported by Gibson et al.[54] In this study, 36% of 140 seemingly low risk patients had a subsequent cardiac event over 15 ± 12 months. The presence of scintigraphic ischemia, particularly when multiple vascular territories were involved, was the most powerful prognosticator. Fifty-nine percent of patients with ^{201}Tl redistribution and 86% of those with redistribution in multiple vascular beds had a subsequent cardiac event (Fig. 15-20). These data were the first to imply that patients with the largest ischemic burden were also at highest risk.

Similar findings were reported with dipyridamole perfusion scintigraphy. In the series by Leppo et al.[99] the presence of ^{201}Tl redistribution was the only significant predictor of cardiac death or recurrent myocardial infarction. Brown et al[18] performed dipyridamole imaging in 50 stable patients very

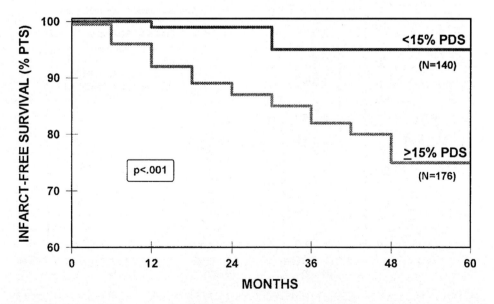

Fig. 15-17. Kaplan–Meier curves depicting infarct-free survival on the basis of the exercise-induced perfusion defect size *(PDS)* in 316 patients with coronary artery disease. The PDS dichotomized at 15% accurately predicted a low- and high-risk group for subsequent cardiac events. (Reprinted with permission from the American College of Cardiology. Adapted with permission from Iskandrian AS, Chae SC, Heo JT, et al: Independent and incremental prognostic value of exercise single-photon emission computed tomographic (SPECT) thallium imaging in coronary artery disease, *J Am Coll Cardiol* 22:665-670, 1993.)

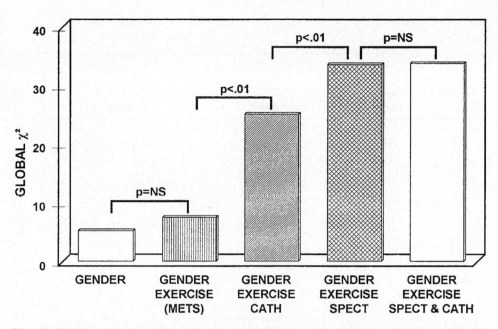

Fig. 15-18. Independent and incremental prognostic power of patient sex, exercise workload in metabolic equivalents *(METS)*, cardiac catheterization *(CATH)* variables, and thallium-201 tomographic imaging *(SPECT)* variables. Data shown represent the chi-square statistics for several combinations of variables. SPECT significantly added prognostic power to the model that combined sex, exercise, and CATH variables. However, the CATH information did not improve the chi-square statistic when SPECT was already included. (Reprinted with permission from the American College of Cardiology. Adapted with permission from Iskandrian AS, Chae SC, Heo JT, et al: Independent and incremental prognostic value of exercise single-photon emission computed tomographic (SPECT) thallium imaging in coronary artery disease, *J Am Coll Cardiol* 22:665-670, 1993.)

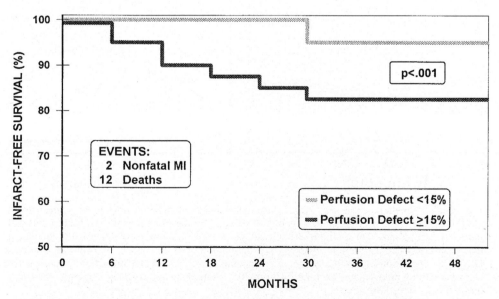

Fig. 15-19. Kaplan–Meier curves illustrating infarct-free survival based on the adenosine-induced perfusion defect size in 177 patients with coronary artery disease. Patients with large perfusion defects (≥15%) had a significantly worse prognosis than those with smaller defects. MI = myocardial infarction. (Adapted with permission from Kamal AM, Fattah AA, Pancholy S, et al: Prognostic value of adenosine single-photon emission computed tomographic thallium imaging in medically treated patients with angiographic evidence of coronary artery disease, *J Nucl Cardiol* 1:254, 1994.)

Table 15-11. Comparison of exercise and pharmacologic coronary vasodilators for risk assessment after myocardial infarction*

Method of vasodilation	Patients (n)	Follow-up (mo)	Type of events	Predictor	Positive predictive accuracy (%)	Negative predictive accuracy (%)
Exercise						
Wilson et al[187]	97	39	Death, MI, unstable angina	Infarct zone redistribution	42	77
Brown et al[17]	59	37	Death, MI, unstable angina	Infarct zone redistribution	28	100
Gibson et al[54]	140	15	Death, MI, unstable angina	Redistribution	59	94
Gibson et al[55]	241	27	Death, MI	Infarct zone redistribution	31	97
Overall	537				40	93
Dipyridamole						
Gimple et al[57]	36	6	Death, MI, unstable angina	Non–infarct zone redistribution	26 (42)	88
Younis et al[188]	68	12	Death, MI	Redistribution	22	94
Leppo et al[99]	51	19	Death, MI	Redistribution	33	94
Brown et al[118]	50	12	Death, MI, unstable angina	Redistribution	45	100
Overall	205				30	94
Adenosine						
Mahmarian et al[114]	92	15	Death, MI, unstable angina, congestive heart failure	Redistribution (5% left ventricle)	50	97

*MI = myocardial infarction.
Reprinted with permission from Mahmarian et al: *Cardiol Clin* 12:223-245, 1994.

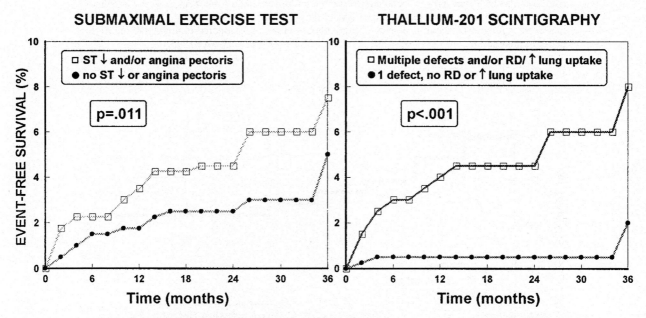

Fig. 15-20. Cumulative cardiac event rates in 140 stable patients who survived acute myocardial infarction on the basis of presence of ischemia as assessed by the submaximal exercise test and thallium-201 scintigraphy. The thallium-201 scintigraphic results best predicted risk for subsequent cardiac events. RD = redistribution. (Adapted with permission from Gibson RS, Watson DD, Craddock GB, et al: Prediction of cardiac events after uncomplicated myocardial infarction: A prospective study comparing predischarge exercise thallium-201 scintigraphy and coronary angiography, *Circulation* 68:321-336, 1983.)

early (mean of 62 ± 121 hours) after infarction. No patient had a complication from the test. When scintigraphic, clinical, and angiographic variables were compared, the only significant predictor of in-hospital cardiac events was the presence of infarct-zone ^{201}Tl redistribution. Events occurred in 45% of patients with redistribution but in none of the 30 patients without redistribution. Of note, patients without scintigraphic ischemia remained event-free over 1 year of follow-up, whereas 3 additional patients with ^{201}Tl redistribution had a cardiac event.

We recently reported the utility of quantitative adenosine ^{201}Tl SPECT for predicting risk in 92 stable patients after acute infarction.[114] Thirty patients (33%) had a cardiac event over 16 ± 5 months of follow-up. Univariate predictors of events were size of quantified perfusion defect, absolute extent of left ventricular ischemia, and left ventricular ejection fraction (Fig. 15-21). Measurement of these variables greatly improved risk assessment beyond the clinical and angiographic information (Fig. 15-22) and were the only risk predictors according to multivariate analysis.

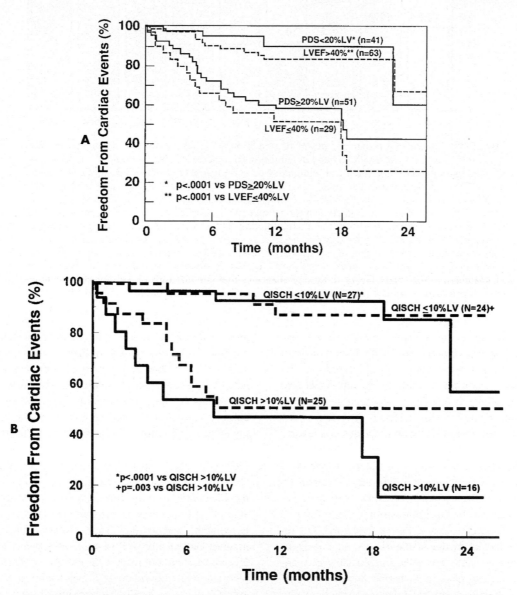

Fig. 15-21. Kaplan–Meier curves depicting freedom from cardiac events on the basis of (**A**) left ventricular *(LV)* perfusion defect size *(PDS)* and ejection fraction *(EF)* and (**B**) quantified extent of left ventricular ischemia *(QISCH)*. The total PDS and global LVEF were inversely related and provided similar prognostic information. The QISCH was the best univariate predictor of risk and did so regardless of initial therapy during acute infarction. Solid lines in **B** = early reperfusion therapy; dashed lines = no early reperfusion therapy. (Reprinted with permission from the American College of Cardiology. Reproduced from Mahmarian JJ, Mahmarian AC, Marks GF, et al: Role of adenosine thallium-201 tomography for defining long-term risk in patients after acute myocardial infarction, *J Am Coll Cardiol* 25:1333-1340, 1995.)

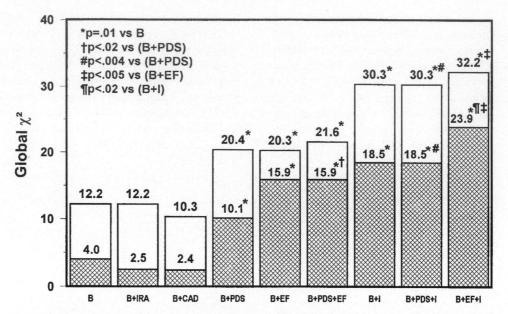

Fig. 15-22. Incremental prognostic power of scintigraphic variables and left ventricular ejection fraction *(LVEF)* compared with that of a baseline clinical model *(B)* for predicting all events *(crosshatched and open bars)* or death and reinfarction *(cross-hatched bar)*. The LVEF, perfusion defect size *(PDS)*, and, particularly, the extent of scintigraphic ischemia *(I)* predicted risk significantly better than did the baseline clinical model *(B)*. Furthermore, extent of ischemia improved the predictive power of the combined baseline clinical model and PDS *(B+PDS)* or baseline model and LVEF *(B+LVEF)* for all events and for death and reinfarction. The LVEF added to the combined baseline model and PDS *(B+PDS)* or the baseline model and extent of ischemia *(B+I)* for predicting death and reinfarction. CAD = extent of coronary artery disease; IRA = infarct artery patency, χ^2 = chi-square analysis. (Reprinted from the American College of Cardiology. Reproduced from Mahmarian JJ, Mahmarian AC, Marks GF, et al: Role of adenosine thallium-201 tomography for defining long-term risk in patients after acute myocardial infarction, *J Am Coll Cardiol* 25:1333-1340, 1995.)

To further validate these retrospective results, we prospectively studied 133 stable survivors of acute infarction with adenosine ^{201}Tl SPECT within several days of infarction.[28] Patients were stratified according to initial perfusion defect size and extent of scintigraphic ischemia. As observed in our initial series, patients with small perfusion defects (<20%) had a relatively low cardiac event rate (17%) with no deaths and few reinfarctions (7%) over 11 ± 5 months. In contrast, patients with large perfusion defects (≥20%) had a significantly higher overall event rate (50%; p<0.001), which was further influenced by the extent of scintigraphic ischemia. Patients with large reversible perfusion defects had a significantly higher event rate than those with scintigraphic scar (78% vs 29%; p<0.001, respectively). These data imply that stable patients after acute infarction who had small perfusion defects can usually be managed conservatively; aggressive antiischemic therapy can be reserved for those with large reversible defects who are known to be at high risk for subsequent cardiac events.

Risk assessment following thrombolytic therapy after acute myocardial infarction

The important prognostic information obtained with ^{201}Tl myocardial perfusion scintigraphy has recently been challenged in patients after thrombolysis. At present, however, al-

most no data suggest that perfusion imaging should be any less predictive of cardiac events in patients receiving thrombolytic agents.[63,131,175] One recent report from Tilkemeier et al[173] evaluated submaximal planar ^{201}Tl scintigraphy in 171 patients who did or did not have interventions (percutanious transluminal coronary angioplasty or thrombolytic therapy) during acute myocardial infarction. The positive predictive value of exercise-induced scintigraphic ischemia was similar in both groups (36% vs 33%, respectively). Furthermore, the presence of scintigraphic ischemia identified 80% (4 out of 5) of patients in the intervention group who died or had recurrent infarction. Within the limitations of this study (submaximal exercise, planar imaging, and no quantification of ischemia), ^{201}Tl perfusion imaging did equally well in predicting events in patients who received and did not receive thrombolysis. Similar findings are reported with dipyridamole[18] and adenosine[114] in heterogeneous populations in which approximately half received thrombolytic therapy during the acute phase of infarction.

In a recent series of 71 patients from our laboratory (all of whom received reperfusion therapy),[26] the exercise-induced total (p = 0.002) and ischemic (p<0.0005) SPECT perfusion defect sizes as well as the left ventricular ejection fraction (p<0.0005) were all strong univariate predictors of subsequent cardiac events over 26 ± 18 months of follow-up (Fig. 15-23).

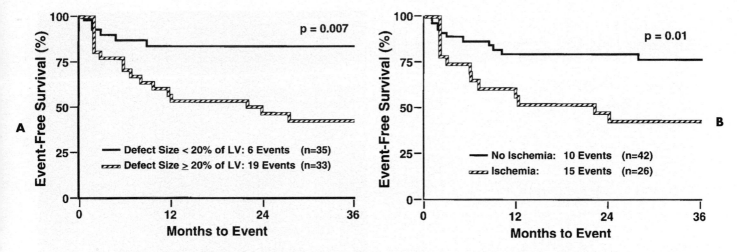

Fig. 15-23. Kaplan–Meier curves showing event-free survival as a function of perfusion defect size (**A**) and presence of myocardial ischemia (**B**). Events were defined as cardiac death, myocardial re-infarction, unstable angina, or congestive heart failure. LV = left ventricle. (Reproduced from Dakik HA, Mahmarian JJ, Kimball KT, et al: Prognostic value of exercise thallium-201 tomography in patients treated with thrombolytic therapy during acute myocardial infarction, *Circulation* 94:2735-2742, 1996.)

As in a previous study using adenosine SPECT after infarction,[114] only the left ventricular ejection fraction and the ischemic defect size predicted risk by multivariate analysis. Furthermore, the ejection fraction and scintigraphic variables contributed substantially to predicting risk beyond the clinical variables alone; no additional information was gained from the angiographic variables.

Patients without ischemia after thrombolysis as assessed by noninvasive testing have an excellent prognosis. This is apparent whether SPECT is combined with adenosine[114] or exercise stress testing.[26] Ellis et al[40] studied 87 patients with residual high-grade stenosis of the infarct-related artery but no objective ischemia by noninvasive testing (48% by ^{201}Tl scintigraphy). These patients were randomly allocated to medical therapy or coronary angioplasty. The 1-year mortality rate for the total group was 0%, with only 5 recurrent infarctions (4 in the angioplasty group). The infarct-free 1-year survival was 98% in the medically treated patients. Absence of ischemia in these patients conferred an excellent prognosis after infarction that did not improve with coronary revascularization. These data are consistent with reports from the prethrombolytic era but await confirmation.

THALLIUM-201 SPECT FOR ASSESSING THE RESULTS OF ANTIISCHEMIC THERAPY

An emerging new area of investigation is the evaluation of antiischemic therapy with sequential ^{201}Tl perfusion scintigraphy. It has long been appreciated that the antiischemic effects of coronary revascularization can be assessed by comparing pre- and postintervention stress ^{201}Tl scintigraphy.* Recently,

*References 24, 72, 82, 118, 159, 162.

the antiischemic effects of various medical therapies have been explored with sequential ^{201}Tl SPECT.

Exercise scintigraphy

Improvements in myocardial perfusion after antiischemic medical therapy can be defined in patients with coronary artery spasm (Fig. 15-24)[53] and in those who have fixed obstructive coronary artery disease.[103,112] We recently conducted a prospective, randomized, double-blind, placebo-controlled trial to assess the antiischemic effects of transdermal nitroglycerin patches in patients with significant coronary artery disease (>50%) who had scintigraphic ischemia on baseline exercise SPECT.[112] Following the baseline study, patients were randomly allocated to receive placebo or intermittent (12 hours on and 12 hours off) active nitroglycerin patch therapy that delivered 0.4 mg/h. Exercise SPECT was repeated a mean of 6.1 ± 1.8 days after randomization. A significant reduction in the total ($-8.9\% \pm 11.1\%$) and ischemic ($-8.5\% \pm 10.4\%$) perfusion defect size was observed in patients randomly allocated to active drug therapy compared with those receiving placebo ($p<0.04$). A ≥9% reduction of 9% or more in the total defect size defines the 95% confidence limit for a significant change in defect size beyond that attributable to technique variability.[113] Significantly more patients decreased their total defect size with active patch therapy (33%) than with placebo (5%; $p = 0.002$) (Fig. 15-25). By multivariate analysis, the only two variables that predicted a reduction in perfusion defect size were the initial size of the perfusion defect and random allocation to active nitroglycerin patch therapy. Figure 15-26 illustrates the sequential polar plots of a patient who received active nitroglycerin patch therapy. A similar recent study by Lewin et al[103] demonstrated efficacy with isosorbide mononitrate as assessed by sequential exercise ^{201}Tl scintigraphy.

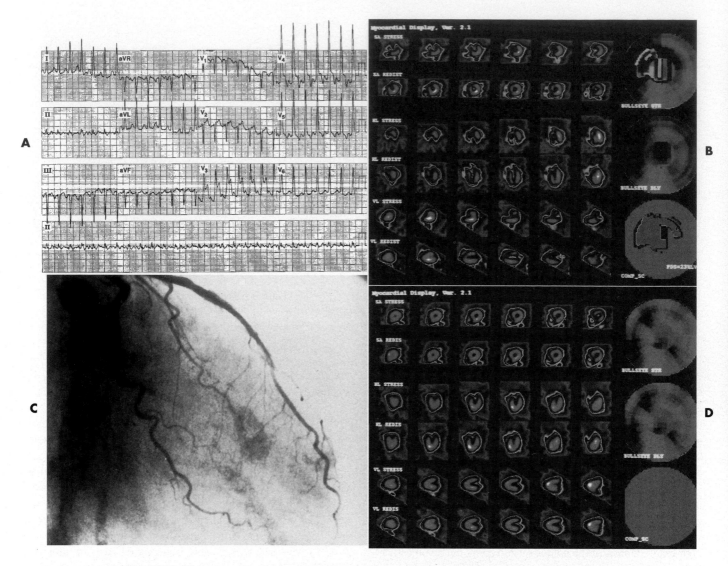

Fig. 15-24. This patient has coronary artery spasm that responded favorably to calcium-channel antagonist therapy. During the initial exercise single-photon emission computed tomography (SPECT) study, the patient developed chest pain and significant ST-segment elevation on 12-lead electrocardiography (**A**). The corresponding SPECT images (**B**) show an anterior exercise (stress)–induced perfusion defect that normalizes on 4-hour redistribution *(REDIST)* imaging. The polar maps *(right)* show a 23% total perfusion defect after comparison with a normal databank (COMPSC). The patient underwent coronary angiography and was found to have normal coronary arteries (**C**). After starting antiischemic medical therapy, a repeat exercise SPECT was performed several weeks later (**D**) that was now entirely normal. Medical therapy eliminated exercise-induced ischemia in this patient as assessed by sequential SPECT imaging. Black = scar; DLY = delay; HL = horizontal long axis; PDS = perfusion defect size; SA = short axis; STR = stress; VL = vertical long axis.

Exercise ^{201}Tl SPECT can also assess the effects of other factors on myocardial ischemia. Mahmarian et al.[117] reported the results of a study designed to evaluate the safety of transdermal nicotine patches as an aid to smoking cessation in patients with known (>50%) coronary artery stenosis. As in the previous nitrate patch study by those authors, all patients were required to have a perfusion defect greater than 5% on baseline SPECT. After the baseline study, patients were given 14-mg nicotine patches and were encouraged to stop smoking. Repeat SPECT imaging was performed after approximately 1 week of

14-mg and then 21-mg nicotine patch therapy. Levels of exhaled carbon monoxide and nicotine and plasma blood levels of cotinine were assessed before each exercise test. Despite a statistically significant rise in nicotine levels over the course of the study, the size of the exercise-induced perfusion defect significantly decreased ($p<.001$). Consistent with the overall results, 31% of patients significantly decreased their total defect size by 9% or more (Fig. 15-27). The reduction in defect size paralleled decreases in exhaled carbon monoxide levels as patients reduced their cigarette smoking by approximately 75% (Fig.

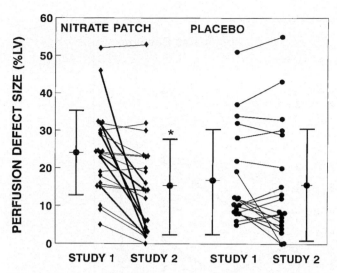

Fig. 15-25. Mean and individual patient changes in exercise-induced left ventricular *(LV)* perfusion defects from study 1 (baseline placebo patch) to study 2 (active nitrate compared with placebo patch). Nitroglycerin patch therapy significantly reduced the mean perfusion defect size compared with placebo therapy (*p = 0.04). Bold lines indicate the seven patients receiving active patch therapy who reduced their perfusion defect size by 9% or more (absolute). (Reproduced from Mahmarian JJ, Ferrimore NL, Marks GF, et al: Transdermal nitroglycerin patch therapy reduces the extent of exercise-induced myocardial ischemia: Results of a double-blind, placebo-controlled trial using quantitative thallium-201 tomography, *J Am Coll Cardiol* 24:25-32, 1994.)

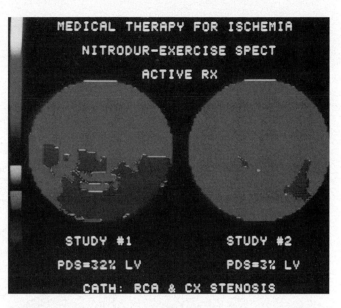

Fig. 15-26. Polar maps in a patient with angiographic stenosis of the right *(RCA)* and circumflex *(CX)* coronary arteries before *(left)* and after *(right)* nitrate patch therapy. The polar map on the left demonstrates a 32% ischemic perfusion defect following symptom-limited treadmill exercise. The patient underwent a second exercise test 6 days after starting nitrate patch therapy. The polar map after therapy *(right)* showed almost complete resolution of scintigraphic ischemia. PDS = perfusion defect size. (Reproduced from Mahmarian JJ, Verani MS: Use of radionuclide imaging in assessing medical therapy. In Iskandrian AS (ed.), Myocardial Perfusion Imaging, Part II: Acute Coronary Syndromes and Interventions, *Am J Cardiol* CME Series, 19, 1993.)

15-28). This study inferred that the extent of exercise-induced myocardial ischemia can be dramatically reduced when patients stop smoking with the aid of nicotine patches (Fig. 15-29), and it supports further the clinical utility of exercise ^{201}Tl SPECT for assessing dynamic changes in myocardial ischemia.

Pharmacologic stressors

Whether the results observed with exercise Tl-201 SPECT can be extended to pharmacologic stressors remains an important area of investigation. Despite the lack of supportive evidence, the current belief is that antiischemic medications should not alter the presence or extent of perfusion defects induced by pharmacologic stressors because these agents create heterogeneity in coronary flow without substantially altering myocardial oxygen demands or causing ischemia. However, even with exercise stress, perfusion defects result primarily from heterogeneity in coronary flow and not necessarily the accompanying myocardial ischemia. Several recent studies suggest that myocardial perfusion results can be altered with pharmacologic stressors. Cid et al[23] investigated which factors most affect the diagnostic accuracy of dobutamine Tl-201 SPECT. As anticipated, the severity of coronary artery stenosis was an important predictor of an abnormal scan result. An unexpected finding from this analysis was that the use of antiischemic medications greatly altered the perfusion results. Patients who took

at least 1 antiischemic medication had approximately one seventh the likelihood of an abnormal scan result compared with those who did not take medications. The overall sensitivity for detecting coronary artery disease increased from 67% for patients taking antiischemic medications to 90% for patients not taking antianginal agents. Of note, the angiographic extent, location, or severity of coronary artery disease did not differ significantly between the two groups. Shehata et al also demonstrated significant reductions in total and ischemic defect sizes when propranolol was administered to patients undergoing sequential dobutamine Tc-99m sestamibi SPECT imaging (Fig. 15-30).[167]

Similar preliminary results were found for pharmacologic vasodilators.[29,165] Dakik et al[29] reported the effects of antiischemic medications on adenosine-induced perfusion defects in 22 patients who survived acute myocardial infarction.[29] After a baseline adenosine SPECT study, patients received combination therapy with nitrates, β-blockers, and calcium antagonists. On repeat adenosine SPECT after therapy, significant reductions in the quantified total (38 ± 13% to 26 ± 16%; p<0.001) and ischemic (22 ± 12% to 10 ± 10%; p<0.001) perfusion defect sizes were observed. Sharir et al[167] studied the effects of antiischemic medications on perfusion defect size in 26 patients with coronary artery disease undergoing dipyridamole SPECT combined with submaximal exercise testing. Baseline SPECT

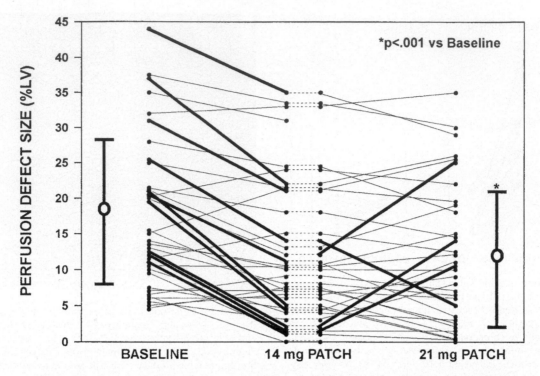

Fig. 15-27. Mean and individual patient changes in exercise-induced left ventricular *(LV)* perfusion defects from baseline to 14-mg and 21-mg nicotine patch therapy. Bold lines represents patients whose perfusion defect size changed by 9% or more (beyond technique variability). (Reprinted with permission from the American College of Cardiology. Reproduced from Mahmarian JJ, Moye LA, Nasser GA, et al: Nicotine patch therapy in smoking cessation reduces the extent of exercise-induced myocardial ischemia, *J Am Coll Cardiol* 30:125-130, 1997.)

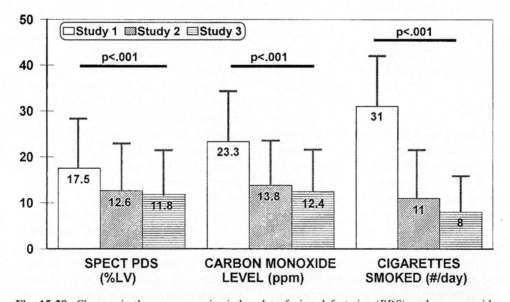

Fig. 15-28. Changes in the mean exercise-induced perfusion defect size *(PDS)*, carbon monoxide level, and number of cigarettes smoked from single-photon emission computed tomography (SPECT) study 1 *(baseline)* to SPECT study 2 (14-mg nicotine patches) and SPECT study 3 (21-mg nicotine patches). The significant reduction in PDS over the course of the study was associated with significant reductions in both exhaled carbon monoxide levels and number of cigarettes smoked. LV = left ventricle.

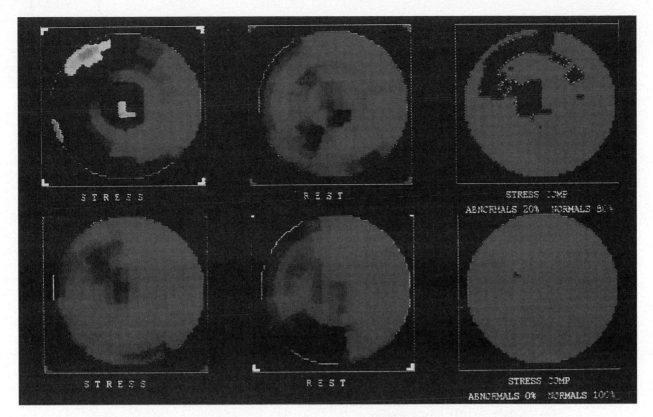

Fig. 15-29. The raw data and statistical polar maps of a patient at baseline (study 1) *(upper panel)* and while receiving 21-mg nicotine patches (study 3) *(lower panel)* are displayed. The improvement in myocardial perfusion on the raw data stress polar map at study 3 compared with baseline is evident. The quantified 20% exercise-induced perfusion defect at baseline *(STRESS COMP)* is virtually eliminated at study 3 despite severe stenosis of the proximal left anterior descending coronary artery. This patient stopped smoking while receiving nicotine patch therapy and had a dramatic reduction in exhaled carbon monoxide levels (from 13 ppm to 3 ppm). Plasma nicotine levels increased from 13.8 ng/ml at baseline to 39.6 ng/ml while the patient was receiving 21-mg patch therapy.

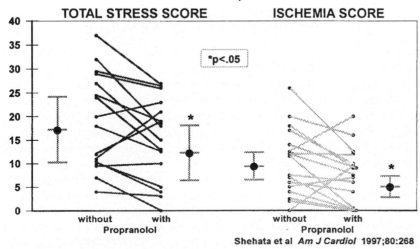

Fig. 15-30. The change in total and ischemia scores from baseline dobutamine SPECT (without propranolol) to dobutamine SPECT after pretreatment with propranolol. (Modified with permission from Shehata AR, Gillam LD, Mascitelli VA, et al: Impact of acute propranolol administration on dobutamine-induced myocardial ischemia as evaluated by myocardial perfusion imaging and echocardiography, *Am J Cardiol* 80:268–272, 1997.) βB Rx = beta-blocker therapy; SPECT = single-photon emission computed tomography.

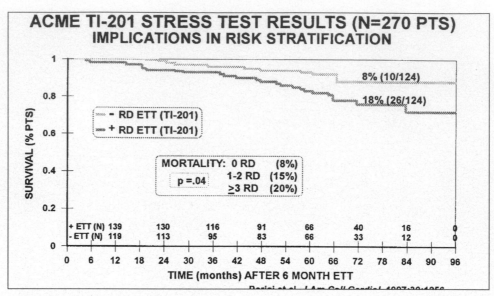

Fig. 15-31. Kaplan-Meier survival curves for patients having exercise thallium planar scintigraphy 6 months after randomization to antiischemic medical therapy or coronary angioplasty. Patients who normalized their perfusion scans (−RD ETT) had a significant improvement in survival as compared to those who continued to have ischemia (+RD ETT). Mortality increased with the number of RD segments. (Modified with permission from Parisi AF, Hartigan PM, Folland ED, et al: Evaluation of exercise thallium scintigraphy versus exercise electrocardiography in predicting survival outcomes and morbid cardiac events in patients with single- and double-vessel disease. Findings from the Angioplasty Compared to Medicine (ACME) study. *J Am Coll Cardiol* 30:1256-1263, 1997.) ETT = exercise treadmill test; RD = redistribution.

was performed while the patients were not taking antiischemic medications and was repeated after administration of calcium antagonists (21 patients), nitrates (19 patients), and β-blockers (8 patients). No significant changes in heart rate or blood pressure were observed from the first SPECT study to the second SPECT study. However, the size of the total left ventricular perfusion defect was significantly reduced from 33 ± 13% to 24 ± 13% with the use of antiischemic medications.

Although the mechanisms underlying the effects of antiischemic medications on pharmacologically induced perfusion defects are currently unknown, the above studies support the existence of this phenomenon. The most likely explanation may lie in the effects of medications on resting coronary flow reserve. Nitrates have clearly been shown to improve resting myocardial blood flow in patients with coronary artery disease as assessed by positron emission tomography.[43] The improved detection of tissue viability in underperfused myocardium after nitroglycerin-augmented ^{201}Tl reinjection imaging further supports this finding.[66-68] Likewise, β-blockers reduce resting myocardial oxygen demands in normal persons and thereby increase coronary flow reserve after dipyridamole-induced hyperemia.[12] This may result primarily from the effects of those agents on resting heart rate.[126] On the basis of these data, it is hypothesized that antiischemic medications allow less utiliza-

tion of coronary flow reserve at rest by reducing resting myocardial oxygen demands, thereby increasing coronary blood flow during pharmacologically induced hyperemia. This may reduce the heterogeneity in coronary flow during pharmacologic stress between vascular beds supplied by normal and stenosed arteries, resulting in smaller discrepancies in count activity and, therefore, smaller perfusion defects. Further studies are warranted to confirm these initial results.

DOES A REDUCTION IN PERFUSION DEFECT SIZE CONFER IMPROVED OUTCOME?

An important remaining question is whether the reduction in perfusion defect size observed with various antiischemic therapies is simply cosmetic or confers an actual reduction in risk for subsequent cardiac events. In the arena of coronary revascularization, initial reports indicate that patients without residual ischemia after anatomically successful coronary angioplasty are at low risk for developing recurrent angina and coronary restenosis.[82,162]

Studies assessing the effects of antiischemic therapies with sequential imaging were not available. Therefore, Dakik et al[27] addressed this issue in 42 stable high-risk survivors of acute myocardial infarction. For inclusion in the study, all patients were required to have both large total (≥20%) and ischemic

(≥10%) perfusion defects as assessed by adenosine ^{201}Tl SPECT. After initial SPECT, patients were randomized to receive aggressive antiischemic medical therapy or coronary revascularization. Repeat imaging was performed in all patients at 42 ± 26 days. Over 11 months of follow-up, 7 of the 42 patients had a subsequent cardiac event. The risk for subsequent cardiac events was strongly influenced by temporal changes in perfusion defect size. The respective reductions in total and ischemic perfusion defect size were significantly greater in the 35 patients without a subsequent cardiac event (–15% and –14%) than in the 7 with (–6% and –5%) a subsequent event. In fact, 96% of patients who had a significant reduction (≥9%) in defect size were event-free at follow-up, whereas 35% of patients in whom the size of the defect could not be reduced had a subsequent cardiac event ($p<0.007$). These preliminary data indicate that ^{201}Tl scintigraphy can not only assess initial risk but also track subsequent risk by evaluating the efficacy of various therapies on myocardial ischemia. The recently published Angioplasty Compared to Medicine (ACME) Study likewise demonstrated that patients who normalized a previously ischemic planar thallium-201 perfusion scan, with either medical therapy or coronary angioplasty, have a significantly higher survival rate (92%) as compared to those who continued to have exercise-induced ischemia (82%, $p=.02$) (Fig. 15-31).[148]

CONCLUSIONS

Thallium-201 scintigraphy is a versatile and clinically invaluable tool for the diagnosis and evaluation of patients with coronary artery disease. Although much has been written about the high diagnostic accuracy of ^{201}Tl scintigraphy for detecting coronary stenosis, its other applications seem to have far greater clinical importance. Specifically, the ability to quantify perfusion defects with ^{201}Tl SPECT has greatly enhanced risk stratification across a wide spectrum of patients with coronary artery disease. Newer applications of ^{201}Tl scintigraphy for assessing dynamic changes in myocardial perfusion after antiischemic therapy will further enhance the attractiveness of this technique as a cost-effective method for guiding patient management.

REFERENCES

1. Abrams J: Hemodynamic effects of nitroglycerin and long-acting nitrates, *Am Heart J* 110(1pt2):216–224, 1985.
2. Albro PC, Gould KL, Westcott RJ, et al: Noninvasive assessment of coronary stenoses by myocardial imaging during pharmacologic coronary vasodilatation. III. Clinical trial, *Am J Cardiol* 42:751–760, 1978.
3. Aoki M, Sakai K, Koyanagi S, et al: Effect of nitroglycerin on coronary collateral function during exercise evaluated by quantitative analysis of thallium-201 single photon emission computed tomography, *Am Heart J* 121:1361–1366, 1991.
4. Bailey IK, Giffith LS, Rouleau J, et al: Thallium-201 myocardial perfusion imaging at rest and during exercise. Comparative sensitivity to electrocardiography in coronary artery disease, *Circulation* 55:79–87, 1977.
5. Beer SG, Heo J, Kong B, et al: Use of oral dipyridamole SPECT thallium-201 imaging in detection of coronary artery disease, *Am Heart J* 118(5pt1):1022–1027, 1989.
6. Beller GA, Watson DD, Ackell P, et al: Time course of thallium-201 redistribution after transient myocardial ischemia, *Circulation* 61:791–797, 1980.
7. Beller GA, Pohost GM: Mechanism for thallium-201 redistribution after transient myocardial ischemia, *Circulation* 56(Suppl III):III-141, 1977 (abstract).
8. Berger BC, Watson DD, Taylor GJ, et al: Quantitative thallium-201 exercise scintigraphy for detection of coronary artery disease, *J Nucl Med* 22:585–593, 1981.
9. Berne RM: The role of adenosine in the regulation of coronary blood flow, *Circ Res* 47:807–813, 1980.
10. Bonow RO, Dilsizian V, Cuscolo A, et al: Identification of viable myocardium in patients with chronic coronary artery disease and left ventricular dysfunction. Comparison of thallium scintigraphy with reinjection and PET imaging with ^{18}F-fluorodeoxyglucose, *Circulation* 83:26–37, 1991.
11. Borges-Neto S, Mahmarian JJ, Jain A, et al: Quantitative thallium-201 single photon emission computed tomography after oral dipyridamole for assessing the presence, anatomic location and severity of coronary artery disease, *J Am Coll Cardiol* 11:962–969, 1988.
12. Bottcher M, Czernin J, Sun K, et al: Effect of β1 adrenergic receptor blockade on myocardial blood flow and vasodilatory capacity, *J Nucl Med* 38:442–446, 1997.
13. Botvinick EH, Taradash MR, Shames DM, et al: Thallium-201 myocardial perfusion scintigraphy for the clinical clarification of normal, abnormal and equivocal electrocardiographic stress tests. *Am J Cardiol* 41:43–51, 1978.
14. Brown BG: Response of normal and diseased epicardial coronary arteries to vasoactive drugs: quantitative arteriographic studies, *Am J Cardiol* 56:23E–29E, 1985.
15. Brown BG, et al: The mechanisms of nitroglycerin action: stenosis vasodilation as a major component of the drug response, *Circulation* 64:1089–1097, 1981.
16. Brown KA: Prognostic value of thallium-201 myocardial perfusion imaging. A diagnostic tool comes of age, *Circulation* 83:363–381, 1991.
17. Brown KA, Weiss RM, Clements JP, et al: Usefulness of residual ischemic myocardium within prior infarct zone for identifying patients at high risk late after acute myocardial infarction, *Am J Cardiol* 60:15–19, 1987.
18. Brown KA, O'Meara J, Chambers CE, et al: Ability of dipyridamole-thallium-201 imaging one to four days after acute myocardial infarction to predict in-hospital and late recurrent myocardial ischemic events, *Am J Cardiol* 65:160–167, 1990.
19. Budinger TF, Pohost GM, Bischoff P: Thallium-201 integral blood concentration over 2 hours explains persistent defects in patients with no evidence of MI by ECG, *Circulation* 76(Suppl IV):IV-64, 1987 (abstract).
20. Burns RJ, Galligan L, Wright LM, et al: Improved specificity of myocardial thallium-201 single-photon emission computed tomography in patients with left bundle branch block by dipyridamole, *Am J Cardiol* 68:504–508, 1991.
21. Casanova R, Patronici A, Guidalotti PL, et al: Dose and test for dipyridamole infusion and cardiac imaging early after uncomplicated acute myocardial infarction, *Am J Cardiol* 70:1402–1406, 1992.
22. Chouraqui P, Rodrigues EA, Berman DS, et al: Significance of dipyridamole-induced transient dilation of the left ventricle during thallium-201 scintigraphy in suspected coronary artery disease, *Am J Cardiol* 66:689–694, 1990.
23. Cid E, Verani MS, Mahmarian JJ: Factors affecting the diagnostic accuracy of quantitative single photon tomography combined with dobutamine stress: Importance of anti-ischemic medications, *J Nucl Med* 37:58P, 1996 (abstract).
24. Cloninger KG, DePuey EG, Garcia EV, et al: Incomplete redistribution in delayed thallium-201 single photon emission computed tomographic (SPECT) images: an overestimation of myocardial scarring, *J Am Coll Cardiol* 12:955–963, 1988.

25. Coyne EP, Belvedere DA, Vande Streer PR, et al: Thallium-201 scintigraphy after intravenous infusion of adenosine compared with exercise thallium testing in the diagnosis of coronary artery disease, *J Am Coll Cardiol* 17:1289–1294, 1991.

26. Dakik HA, Mahmarian JJ, Kimball KT, et al: Prognostic value of exercise ^{201}Tl tomography in patients treated with thrombolytic therapy during acute myocardial infarction, *Circulation* 94:2735–2742, 1996.

27. Dakik HA, Verani MS, He Z-X, et al: Adenosine SPECT to assess anti-ischemic drug therapy vs coronary revascularization following acute myocardial infarction: A prospective randomized trial, *J Nucl Cardiol* 4:S44, 1997 (abstract).

28. Dakik HA, Farmer JA, He Z-X, et al: Quantitative adenosine thallium-201 single photon tomography accurately predicts risk following acute myocardial infarction: the results of a prospective trial, *J Am Coll Cardiol* 29(Suppl A):228A, 1997 (abstract).

29. Dakik HA, Farmer JA, Kleiman NS, et al: A strategy of aggressive anti-ischemic drug therapy versus coronary revascularization in high risk patients after myocardial infarction: Results of a prospective, randomized trial, *J Am Coll Cardiol* 29(Suppl A):53A, 1997 (abstract).

30. DePace NL, Iskandrian AS, Nadell R, et al: Variation in the size of jeopardized myocardium in patients with isolated left anterior descending coronary artery disease, *Circulation* 67:988–994, 1983.

31. DePasquale EE, Nody AC, DePuey EG et al: Quantitative rotational thallium-201 tomography for identifying and localizing coronary artery disease, *Circulation* 77:316–327, 1988.

32. DePuey EG, Guertler-Krawczynska E, D'Amato PH, et al: Thallium-201 single-photon emission computed tomography with intravenous dipyridamole to diagnose coronary artery disease, *Coron Heart Dis* 1:75–85, 1990.

33. DePuey EG, Berman DS, Garcia EV: *Cardiac SPECT imaging*, Philadelphia, 1996, Lippincott–Raven.

34. Di Carli M, Czernin J, Hohek, et al: Relation among stenosis severity, myocardial blood flow, and flow reserve in patients with coronary artery disease, *Circulation* 91:1944–1951, 1995.

35. Dilsizian V, Rocco TP, Freedman NM, et al: Enhanced detection of ischemic but viable myocardium by the reinjection of thallium after stress-redistribution imaging, *N Engl J Med* 323:141–146, 1990.

36. Dilsizian V, Arrishi JA, Diodati JG, et al: Myocardial viability in patients with chronic coronary artery disease. Comparison of ^{99m}Tc-sestamibi with thallium reinjection and [^{18}F]fluorodeoxyglucose, *Circulation* 89:578–587, 1994.

37. Dreyfus GD, Duboc D, Blasco A, et al: Myocardial viability assessment in ischemic cardiomyopathy: benefits of coronary revascularization, *Ann Thorac Surg* 57:1402–1407, 1994.

38. Duchier J, Iannoscoli F, Safar M: Antihypertensive effect of sustained-release isosorbide dinitrate for isolated systolic systemic hypertension in the elderly, *Am J Cardiol* 60:99–102, 1987.

39. Elkayam U, Weinstein M, Berman D, et al: Stress thallium-201 myocardial scintigraphy and exercise technetium ventriculography in the detection and location of chronic coronary artery disease: comparison of sensitivity and specificity of these noninvasive tests alone and in combination, *Am Heart J* 101:657–666, 1981.

40. Ellis SG, Mooney MR, George BS, et al: Randomized trial of late elective angioplasty versus conservative management for patients with residual stenoses after thrombolytic treatment of myocardial infarction. Treatment of Post Thrombolytic Stenoses (TOPS) Study Group, *Circulation* 86:1400–1406, 1992.

41. Epstein SE, Talbot TL: Dynamic coronary tone in precipitation, exacerbation and relief of angina pectoris, *Am J Cardiol* 48:797–803, 1981.

42. Esquivel L, Pullock SG, Beller GA, et al: Effect of the degree of effort on the sensitivity of the exercise thallium-201 stress test in symptomatic coronary artery disease, *Am J Cardiol* 63:160–165, 1989.

43. Fallen EL, Nahmias C, Scheffel A, et al: Redistribution of myocardial blood flow with topical nitroglycerin in patients with coronary artery disease, *Circulation* 91:1381–1388, 1995.

44. Ficaro EP, Fessler JA, Rogers WL, et al: Comparison of americium-241 and technetium-99m as transmission sources for the attenuation correction of thallium-201 SPECT imaging of the heart, *J Nucl Med* 35:652–663, 1994.

45. Ficaro EP, Fessler JA, Ackermann RJ, et al: Simultaneous transmission-emission thallium-201 cardiac SPECT: effect of attenuation correction on myocardial tracer distribution, *J Nucl Med* 36:921–931, 1995.

46. Ficaro EP, Fessler JA, Shreve PD, et al: Simultaneous transmission/emission myocardial perfusion tomography. Diagnostic accuracy of attenuation-corrected ^{99m}Tc-sestamibi single-photon emission computed tomography, *Circulation* 93:463–473, 1996.

47. Fintel DJ, Links JM, Brinker JA, et al: Improved diagnostic performance of exercise thallium-201 single photon emission computed tomography over planar imaging in the diagnosis of coronary artery disease: a receiver operating characteristic analysis, *J Am Coll Cardiol* 13:600–612, 1989.

48. FitzGerald GA: Dipyridamole, *N Engl J Med* 316:1247–1257, 1987.

49. Francisco DA, Collins SM, Go RT, et al: Tomographic thallium-201 myocardial perfusion scintigrams after maximal coronary artery vasodilation with intravenous dipyridamole. Comparison of qualitative and quantitative approaches, *Circulation* 66:370–379, 1982.

50. Friedman J, Van Train K, Maddahi J, et al: "Upward creep" of the heart: a frequent source of false-positive reversible defects during thallium-201 stress-redistribution SPECT, *J Nucl Med* 30:1718–1722, 1989.

51. Fung AY, Gallagher KP, Buda AJ: The physiologic basis of dobutamine as compared with dipyridamole stress interventions in the assessment of critical coronary stenosis, *Circulation* 76:943–951, 1987.

52. Gage JE, Hesso M, Murakami T, et al: Vasoconstriction of stenotic coronary arteries during dynamic exercise in patients with classic angina pectoris: reversibility by nitroglycerin, *Circulation* 73:865–876, 1986.

53. Gallik DM, Bucay M, Mahonarian JJ, et al: Thallium-201 tomography in the management of exercise-induced coronary spasm, *Am Heart J* 124:1078–1081, 1992.

54. Gibson RS, Watson DD, Craddock GB, et al: Prediction of cardiac events after uncomplicated myocardial infarction: a prospective study comparing predischarge exercise thallium-201 scintigraphy and coronary angiography, *Circulation* 68:321–336, 1983.

55. Gibson RS, Beller GA, Gheorghiade M, et al: The prevalence and clinical significance of residual myocardial ischemia 2 weeks after uncomplicated non-Q wave infarction: a prospective natural history study, *Circulation* 73:1186–1198, 1986.

56. Gill JB, Ruddy TD, Finkelstein DM, et al: Prognostic importance of thallium uptake by the lungs during exercise in coronary artery disease, *N Engl J Med* 317:1486–1489, 1987.

57. Gimple LW, Hutter AM Jr, Guiney TE, et al: Prognostic utility of predischarge dipyridamole-thallium imaging compared to predischarge submaximal exercise electrocardiography and maximal exercise thallium imaging after uncomplicated acute myocardial infarction, *Am J Cardiol* 64:1243–1248, 1989.

58. Gould KL: Noninvasive assessment of coronary stenoses by myocardial perfusion imaging during pharmacologic coronary vasodilatation: I. Physiologic basis and experimental validation, *Am J Cardiol* 41:267–278, 1978.

59. Gould KL, Lipscomb K: Effects of coronary stenosis on coronary flow reserve and resistance, *Am J Cardiol* 34:48–55, 1974.

60. Greenberg H, Dwyer EM Jr, Jameson AG, et al: Effects of nitroglycerin on the major determinants of myocardial oxygen consumption. An angiographic and hemodynamic assessment, *Am J Cardiol* 36:426–432, 1975.

61. Gunalp B, Dokumaci B, Uyan C, et al: Value of dobutamine technetium-99m-sestamibi SPECT and echocardiography in the detection of coronary artery disease compared with coronary angiography, *J Nucl Med* 34:889–894, 1993.

62. Gupta NC, Esterbrooks DJ, Hilleman DE, et al: Comparison of adenosine and exercise thallium-201 single-photon emission computed tomography (SPECT) myocardial perfusion imaging. The GE SPECT Multicenter Adenosine study group, *J Am Coll Cardiol* 19:248–257, 1992.

63. Haber HL, Beller GA, Watson DD, et al: Exercise thallium-201 scintigraphy after thrombolytic therapy with or without angioplasty for acute myocardial infarction, *Am J Cardiol* 71:1257–1261, 1993.

64. Hachamovitch R, Berman DS, Kiat H, et al: Exercise myocardial perfusion SPECT in patients without known coronary artery disease: incremental prognostic value and use in risk stratification, *Circulation* 93:905–914, 1996.

65. Hays JT, Mahmarian JJ, Cochran AJ, et al: Dobutamine thallium-201 tomography for evaluating patients with suspected coronary artery disease unable to undergo exercise or pharmacologic stress testing, *J Am Coll Cardiol* 21:1583–1590, 1993.

66. He ZX, Darcourt J, Guignier A, et al: Nitrates improve detection of ischemic but viable myocardium by thallium-201 reinjection SPECT, *J Nucl Med* 34:1472–1477, 1993.

67. He ZX, Medrano R, Hays JT, et al: Nitroglycerin-augmented ^{201}Tl reinjection enhances detection of reversible myocardial hypoperfusion. A randomized, double-blind, parallel, placebo-controlled trial, *Circulation* 95:1799–1805, 1997.

68. He ZX, Verani MS, Liu XJ: Nitrate-augmented myocardial imaging for assessment of myocardial viability, *J Nucl Cardiol* 2:352–357, 1995.

69. Heiss HW, Barmeyer J, Wink K, et al: Studies on the regulation of myocardial blood flow in man. I.: Training effects on blood flow and metabolism of the healthy heart at rest and during standardized heavy exercise, *Basic Res Cardiol* 71:658–675, 1976.

70. Heller GV, Ahmed I, Tilkemeier PL, et al: Influence of exercise intensity on the presence, distribution, and size of thallium-201 defects, *Am Heart J* 123:909–916, 1992.

71. Hendel RC, Berman DS, Follansbee WP, et al: Effects of attenuation corrected SPECT myocardial perfusion imaging on diagnostic accuracy: Results of a multicenter trial, *Circulation* 94(Suppl I):I-303, 1996 (abstract).

72. Hirzel HO, Nuesch K, Gwentzig AR, et al: Short- and long-term changes in myocardial perfusion after percutaneous transluminal coronary angioplasty assessed by thallium-201 exercise scintigraphy, *Circulation* 63:1001–1007, 1981.

73. Ho F-M, Huang PJ, Liau CS, et al: Dobutamine stress echocardiography compared with dipyridamole thallium-201 single-photon emission computed tomography in detecting coronary artery disease, *Eur Heart J* 16:570–575, 1995.

74. Homma S, Callahan RJ, Ameer B, et al: Usefulness of oral dipyridamole suspension for stress thallium imaging without exercise in the detection of coronary artery disease, *Am J Cardiol* 57:503–508, 1986.

75. Huikuri HV, Karhonen UR, Airaksimen J, et al: Comparison of dipyridamole-handgrip test and bicycle exercise test for thallium tomographic imaging, *Am J Cardiol* 61:264–268, 1988.

76. Inglese E, Brambilla M, Dondi M, et al: Assessment of myocardial viability after thallium-201 reinjection or rest-redistribution imaging: a multicenter study. The Italian Group of Nuclear Cardiology, *J Nucl Med* 36:555–563, 1995.

77. Iskandrian AS, Lichtenberg R, Segal BL, et al: Assessment of jeopardized myocardium in patients with one-vessel disease, *Circulation* 65:242–247, 1982.

78. Iskandrian AS, Heo J, Kong B, et al: Effect of exercise level on the ability of thallium-201 tomographic imaging in detecting coronary artery disease: analysis of 461 patients, *J Am Coll Cardiol* 14:1477–1486, 1989.

79. Iskandrian AS, Heo J, Nguyen T, et al: Left ventricular dilatation and pulmonary thallium uptake after single-photon emission computed tomography using thallium-201 during adenosine-induced coronary hyperemia, *Am J Cardiol* 66:807–811, 1990.

80. Iskandrian AS, Heo J, Nguyen T, et al: Assessment of coronary artery disease using single-photon emission computed tomography with thallium-201 during adenosine-induced coronary hyperemia, *Am J Cardiol* 67:1190–1194, 1991.

81. Iskandrian AS, Chae SC, Heo J, et al: Independent and incremental prognostic value of exercise single-photon emission computed tomographic (SPECT) thallium imaging in coronary artery disease, *J Am Coll Cardiol* 22:665–670, 1993.

82. Jain A, Mahmarian JJ, Boyes-Neto S, et al: Clinical significance of perfusion defects by thallium-201 single photon emission tomography following oral dipyridamole early after coronary angioplasty, *J Am Coll Cardiol* 11:970–976, 1988.

83. Josephson MA, Brown BG, Hecht HS, et al: Noninvasive detection and localization of coronary stenoses in patients: comparison of resting dipyridamole and exercise thallium-201 myocardial perfusion imaging, *Am Heart J* 103:1008–1018, 1982.

84. Jukema JW, Vander Wall EE, vander Vis-Melsen MJ, et al: Dipyridamole thallium-201 scintigraphy for improved detection of left anterior descending coronary artery stenosis in patients with left bundle branch block, *Eur Heart J* 14:53–56, 1993.

85. Kamal AM, Fattah AA, Pancholy S, et al: Prognostic value of adenosine single-photon emission computed tomographic thallium imaging in medically treated patients with angiographic evidence of coronary artery disease, *J Nucl Cardiol* 1:254–261, 1994.

86. Kaul S, Boucher CA, Newell JB, et al: Determination of the quantitative thallium imaging variables that optimize detection of coronary artery disease, *J Am Coll Cardiol* 7:527–537, 1986.

87. Kaul S, Finkelstein DM, Homma S, et al: Superiority of quantitative exercise thallium-201 variables in determining long-term prognosis in ambulatory patients with chest pain: a comparison with cardiac catheterization, *J Am Coll Cardiol* 12:25–34, 1988.

88. Kayden DS, Sigal S, Soufer R, et al: Thallium-201 for assessment of myocardial viability: quantitative comparison of 24-hour redistribution imaging with imaging after reinjection at rest, *J Am Coll Cardiol* 18:1480–1486, 1991.

89. Kelly RP, Gibbs HH, O'Rourke MF, et al: Nitroglycerin has more favourable effects on left ventricular afterload than apparent from measurements of pressure in a peripheral artery, *Eur Heart J* 11:138–144, 1990.

90. Khoury AF, Rivera JM, Mahmarian JJ, et al: Adenosine thallium-201 tomography in evaluation of graft patency late after coronary artery bypass graft surgery, *J Am Coll Cardiol* 29:1290–1295, 1997.

91. Kiat H, Berman DS, Maddahi J, et al: Late reversibility of tomographic myocardial thallium-201 defects: an accurate marker of myocardial viability, *J Am Coll Cardiol* 12:1456–1463, 1988.

92. Knabb RM, Gidday JM, Ely SW, et al: Effects of dipyridamole on myocardial adenosine and active hyperemia, *Am J Physiol* 247(5Pt2):H804–H810, 1984.

93. Kong BA, Shaw L, Miller DD, et al: Comparison of accuracy for detecting coronary artery disease and side-effect profile of dipyridamole thallium-201 myocardial perfusion imaging in women versus men, *Am J Cardiol* 70:168–173, 1992.

94. Lakkis NM, Mahmarian JJ, Verani MS: Exercise thallium-201 single photon emission computed tomography for evaluation of coronary artery bypass graft patency, *Am J Cardiol* 76:107–111, 1995.

95. Lam JY, Chaitman BR, Glaenzer M, et al: Safety and diagnostic accuracy of dipyridamole-thallium imaging in the elderly, *J Am Coll Cardiol* 11:585–589, 1988.

96. Lee J, Chae JC, Lee K, et al: Biokinetics of thallium-201 in normal subjects: comparison between adenosine, dipyridamole, dobutamine and exercise, *J Nucl Med* 35:535–541, 1994.

97. Lenaers A, Block P, Thiel EV, et al: Segmental analysis of T1-201 stress myocardial scintigraphy, *J Nucl Med* 18:509–516, 1977.

98. Leppo J, Boucher CA, Okada RD, et al: Serial thallium-201 myocardial imaging after dipyridamole infusion: diagnostic utility in detect-

ing coronary stenoses and relationship to regional wall motion, *Circulation* 66:649–657, 1982.

99. Leppo JA, O'Brien J, Rothendler JA, et al: Dipyridamole-thallium-201 scintigraphy in the prediction of future cardiac events after acute myocardial infarction, *N Engl J Med* 310:1014–1018, 1984.

100. Leppo JA, Meerdink DJ: Comparison of the myocardial uptake of a technetium-labeled isonitrile analogue and thallium, *Circ Res* 65:632–639, 1989.

101. Lette J, Lapointe J, Watus D, et al: Transient left ventricular cavitary dilation during dipyridamole-thallium imaging as an indicator of severe coronary artery disease, *Am J Cardiol* 66:1163–1170, 1990.

102. Levy R, Rosanski A, Berman DS, et al: Analysis of the degree of pulmonary thallium washout after exercise in patients with coronary artery disease, *J Am Coll Cardiol* 2:719–728, 1983.

103. Lewin HC, Williams C, Tecson J et al: Sustained quantitative reduction of reversible defect extent by exercise Tc-99m sestamibi/rest thallium-201 myocardial perfusion SPECT with isosorbide mononitrate (IMDUR), *Circulation* 94:I-302, 1996 (abstract).

104. Liu P, Houle J, Mills L, et al: Kinetics of Tc-99m MIBI in clearance in ischemia-reperfusion: comparison with Tl-201, *Circulation* 76(Suppl IV):IV-216, 1987 (abstract).

105. Machecourt J, Longere P, Fagret D, et al: Prognostic value of thallium-201 single-photon emission computed tomographic myocardial perfusion imaging according to extent of myocardial defect. Study in 1,926 patients with follow-up at 33 months. *J Am Coll Cardiol* 23:1096–1106, 1994.

106. Maddahi J, Garcia EV, Berman DS, et al: Improved noninvasive assessment of coronary artery disease by quantitative analysis of regional stress myocardial distribution and washout of thallium-201, *Circulation* 64:924–935, 1981.

107. Maddahi J, Van Train K, Prigent F, et al: Quantitative single photon emission computed thallium-201 tomography for detection and localization of coronary artery disease: optimization and prospective validation of a new technique, *J Am Coll Cardiol* 14:1689–1699, 1989.

108. Maddahi J, Rodrigues E, Berman DS, et al: State-of-the-art myocardial perfusion imaging, *Cardiol Clin* 12:199–222, 1994.

109. Mahmarian JJ, Boyce TM, Goldberg RK, et al: Quantitative exercise thallium-201 single photon emission computed tomography for the enhanced diagnosis of ischemic heart disease, *J Am Coll Cardiol* 15:318–329, 1990.

110. Mahmarian JJ, Pratt CM, Boyce TM, et al: The variable extent of jeopardized myocardium in patients with single vessel coronary artery disease: quantification by thallium-201 single-photon emission computed tomography, *J Am Coll Cardiol* 17:355–362, 1991.

111. Mahmarian JJ, Pratt CM, Nishimura S, et al: Quantitative adenosine ²⁰¹Tl single-photon emission computed tomography for the early assessment of patients surviving acute myocardial infarction, *Circulation* 87:1197–1210, 1993.

112. Mahmarian JJ, Fenimore NL, Mark GF, et al: Transdermal nitroglycerin patch therapy reduces the extent of exercise-induced myocardial ischemia: results of a double-blind, placebo-controlled trial using quantitative thallium-201 tomography, *J Am Coll Cardiol* 24:25–32, 1994.

113. Mahmarian JJ, Moye LA, Verani MS, et al: High reproducibility of myocardial perfusion defects in patients undergoing serial exercise thallium-201 tomography, *Am J Cardiol* 75:1116–1119, 1995.

114. Mahmarian JJ, Mahmarian AC, Marks GF, et al: Role of adenosine thallium-201 tomography for defining long-term risk in patients after acute myocardial infarction, *J Am Coll Cardiol* 25:1333–1340, 1995.

115. Mahmarian JJ, Taillefer R, Pippin JJ, et al: Improvement in left ventricular ejection fraction and cardiac volumes following coronary artery bypass surgery in patients with depressed left ventricular function: a prospective study *J Nucl Med* 37:93P, 1996 (abstract).

116. Mahmarian JJ, et al: Relation between ambulatory electrocardiographic monitoring and myocardial perfusion imaging to detect coronary artery disease and myocardial ischemia: an ACIP ancillary study.

The Asymptomatic Cardiac Ischemia Pilot (ACIP) Investigations, *J Am Coll Cardiol* 29:764–769, 1997.

117. Mahmarian JJ, Moye LA, Nasser GA, et al: Nicotine patch therapy in smoking cessation reduces the extent of exercise-induced myocardial ischemia, *J Am Coll Cardiol* 30:125–130, 1997.

118. Manyari DE, Knudtson M, Kloiber R, et al: Sequential thallium-201 myocardial perfusion studies after successful percutaneous transluminal coronary artery angioplasty: delayed resolution of exercise-induced scintigraphic abnormalities, *Circulation* 77:86–95, 1988.

119. Marchant E, Pichard A, Rodriguez JA, et al: Acute effects of systemic versus intracoronary dipyridamole on coronary circulation, *Am J Cardiol* 57:1401–1404, 1986.

120. Marcus ML, Chilian WM, Kanatsuka H, et al: Understanding the coronary circulation through studies at the microvascular level, *Circulation* 82:1–7, 1990.

121. Marshall RC, Leidholdt EM Jr, Zhang DY, et al: Technetium-99m hexakis 2-methoxy-2-isobutyl isonitrile and thallium-201 extraction, washout, and retention at varying coronary flow rates in rabbit heart, *Circulation* 82:998–1007, 1990.

122. Mason JR, Palac RT, Freeman ML, et al: Thallium scintigraphy during dobutamine infusion: nonexercise-dependent screening test for coronary disease, *Am Heart J* 107:481–485, 1984.

123. Massie BM, Botvinick EH, Brundage BH: Correlation of thallium-201 scintigrams with coronary anatomy: factors affecting region by region sensitivity, *Am J Cardiol* 44:616–622, 1979.

124. McCarthy DM, Blood DK, Sciacca RR, et al: Single dose myocardial perfusion imaging with thallium-201: application in patients with nondiagnostic electrocardiographic stress tests, *Am J Cardiol* 43:899–906, 1979.

125. McFadden EP, Clarke JG, Davies GJ, et al: Effect of intracoronary serotonin on coronary vessels in patients with stable angina and patients with variant angina, *N Engl J Med* 324:648–654, 1991.

126. McGinn AL, White CW, Wilson RF: Interstudy variability of coronary flow reserve. Influence of heart rate, arterial pressure, and ventricular preload, *Circulation* 81:1319–1330, 1990.

127. McKillop JH, Murray RJ, Turner JG, et al: Can the extent of coronary artery disease be predicted from thallium-201 myocardial images? *J Nucl Med* 20:714–719, 1979.

128. McLaughlin PR, Martin RP, Doherty P, et al: Reproducibility of thallium-201 myocardial imaging. *Circulation* 55:497–503, 1977.

129. Mendelson MA, Spies SM, Spies WG, et al: Usefulness of single-photon emission computed tomography of thallium-201 uptake after dipyridamole infusion for detection of coronary artery disease, *Am J Cardiol* 69:1150–1155, 1992.

130. Miller DD, Donohue TJ, Yourus LT, et al: Correlation of pharmacological 99mTc-sestamibi myocardial perfusion imaging with post-stenotic coronary flow reserve in patients with angiographically intermediate coronary artery stenoses, *Circulation* 89:2150–2160, 1994.

131. Miller TD, Gersh BJ, Christian TF, et al: Limited prognostic value of thallium-201 exercise treadmill testing early after myocardial infarction in patients treated with thrombolysis, *Am Heart J* 130:259–266, 1995.

132. Mohiuddin SM, Gupta NC, Esterbooks DJ, et al: Thallium-201 myocardial imaging in patients with coronary artery disease: comparison of intravenous adenosine and oral dipyridamole, *Ann Pharmacother* 26:1352–1357, 1992.

133. Moser GH, Schrader J, Deussen A: Turnover of adenosine in plasma of human and dog blood, *Am J Physiol* 256(4 Pt 1):C799–C806, 1989.

134. Nguyen T, Heo J, Ogilby JD, et al: Single photon emission computed tomography with thallium-201 during adenosine-induced coronary hyperemia: correlation with coronary arteriography, exercise thallium imaging and two-dimensional echocardiography, *J Am Coll Cardiol* 16:1375–1383, 1990.

135. Nishimura S, Mahmarian JJ, Boyce TM, et al: Quantitative thallium-201 single-photon emission computed tomography during maximal

pharmacologic coronary vasodilation with adenosine for assessing coronary artery disease, *J Am Coll Cardiol* 18:736–745, 1991.

136. Nishimura S, Mahmarian JJ, Boyce TM, et al: Equivalence between adenosine and exercise thallium-201 myocardial tomography: a multicenter, prospective, crossover trial, *J Am Coll Cardiol* 20:265–275, 1992.

137. Nishimura S, Kimball KT, Mahmarian JJ, et al: Angiographic and hemodynamic determinants of myocardial ischemia during adenosine thallium-201 scintigraphy in coronary artery disease, *Circulation* 87:1211–1219, 1993.

138. Nishimura S, Mahmarian JJ, Verani MS: Significance of increased lung thallium uptake during adenosine thallium-201 scintigraphy, *J Nucl Med* 33:1600–1607, 1992.

139. Nishimura S, Mahmarian JJ, Verani MS: Effect of exercise level on equivalence between adenosine and exercise thallium-201 myocardial tomography in coronary artery disease, *J Nucl Med* 34:95P, 1993 (abstract).

140. Nygaard TW, Gibson RS, Ryan JM, et al: Prevalence of high-risk thallium-201 scintigraphic findings in left main coronary artery stenosis: comparison with patients with multiple- and single-vessel coronary artery disease, *Am J Cardiol* 53:462–469, 1984.

141. Ohtani H, Tamaki N, Yonakura Y, et al: Value of thallium-201 reinjection after delayed SPECT imaging for predicting reversible ischemia after coronary artery bypass grafting, *Am J Cardiol* 66:394–399, 1990.

142. Okada RD, Lim YL, Rothendler J, et al: Split dose thallium-201 dipyridamole imaging: a new technique for obtaining thallium images before and immediately after an intervention, *J Am Coll Cardiol* 1:1302–1310, 1983.

143. Okada RD, Dai YH, Boucher CA, et al: Significance of increased lung thallium-201 activity on serial cardiac images after dipyridamole treatment in coronary heart disease, *Am J Cardiol* 53:470–475, 1984.

144. Okada RD, Glover D, Geoffrey T, et al: Myocardial kinetics of technetium-99m-hexakis-2-methoxy-2-methylpropyl-isonitrile, *Circulation* 77:491–498, 1988.

145. O'Keefe JH Jr, Bateman TM, Silvestri R, et al: Safety and diagnostic accuracy of adenosine thallium-201 scintigraphy in patients unable to exercise and those with left bundle branch block, *Am Heart J* 124:614–621, 1992.

146. O'Keefe JH Jr, Bateman TM, Barnhart CS: Adenosine thallium-201 is superior to exercise thallium-201 for detecting coronary artery disease in patients with left bundle branch block, *J Am Coll Cardiol* 21:1332–1338, 1993.

147. Palmas W, Bingham S, Diamond GA, et al: Incremental prognostic value of exercise thallium-201 myocardial single-photon emission computed tomography late after coronary artery bypass surgery, *J Am Coll Cardiol* 25:403–409, 1995.

148. Parisi AF, Hartigan PM, Folland ED for the ACME Investigators. Evaluation of exercise thallium scintigraphy versus exercise electrocardiography in predicting survival outcomes and morbid cardiac events in patients with single- and double-vessel disease. Findings from the Angioplasty Compared to Medicine (ACME) Study. *J Am Coll Cardiol* 30:1256–1263, 1997.

149. Parker JO, West RO, Di Giorgi S: The effect of nitroglycerin on coronary blood flow and the hemodynamic response to exercise in coronary artery disease. *Am J Cardiol* 27:59–65, 1971.

150. Pennell DJ, Underwood SR, Swanton RH, et al: Dobutamine thallium myocardial perfusion tomography, *J Am Coll Cardiol* 18:1471–1479, 1991.

151. Pennell DJ, Underwood SR, Ell PJ: Safety of dobutamine stress for thallium-201 myocardial perfusion tomography in patients with asthma, *Am J Cardiol* 71:1346–1350, 1993.

152. Pfisterer M, Emmenegger H, Schmitt HE, et al: Accuracy of serial myocardial perfusion scintigraphy with thallium-201 for prediction of graft patency early and late after coronary artery bypass surgery. A controlled prospective study, *Circulation* 66:1017–1024, 1982.

153. Ragosta M, Beller GA, Watson DD, et al: Quantitative planar rest-redistribution ^{201}Tl imaging in detection of myocardial viability and prediction of improvement in left ventricular function after coronary bypass surgery in patients with severely depressed left ventricular function, *Circulation* 87:1630–1641, 1993.

154. Rasmussen SL, Nielsen SL, Amtoys O, et al: 201-Thallium imaging as an indicator of graft patency after coronary artery bypass surgery, *Eur Heart J* 5:494–499, 1984.

155. Rehn T, Griffith LS, Achroff JC, et al: Exercise thallium-201 myocardial imaging in left main coronary artery disease: sensitive but not specific, *Am J Cardiol* 48:217–223, 1981.

156. Rigo P, Becker LC, Griffith LS, et al: Influence of coronary collateral vessels on the results of thallium-201 myocardial stress imaging, *Am J Cardiol* 44:452–458, 1979.

157. Rigo P, Bailey IK, Griffith LS, et al: Value and limitations of segmental analysis of stress thallium myocardial imaging for localization of coronary artery disease, *Circulation* 61:973–981, 1980.

158. Rockett JF, Wood WC, Moinuddin M, et al: Intravenous dipyridamole thallium-201 SPECT imaging in patients with left bundle branch block, *Clin Nucl Med* 15:401–407, 1990.

159. Rosing DR, Van Raden MJ, Mincemoyer RM, et al: Exercise, electrocardiographic and functional responses after percutaneous transluminal coronary angioplasty, *Am J Cardiol* 53:36C–41C, 1984.

160. Rossen JD, Quillen JE, Lopez AG, et al: Comparison of coronary vasodilation with intravenous dipyridamole and adenosine, *J Am Coll Cardiol* 18:485–491, 1991.

161. Santamore WP, Walinsky P: Altered coronary flow responses to vasoactive drugs in the presence of coronary arterial stenosis in the dog, *Am J Cardiol* 45:276–285, 1980.

162. Scholl JM, et al: Exercise electrocardiography and myocardial scintigraphy in the serial evaluation of the results of percutaneous transluminal coronary angioplasty, *Circulation* 66:380–390, 1982.

163. Seals AA, Pratt CM, Mahmarian JJ, et al: Relation of left ventricular dilation during acute myocardial infarction to systolic performance, diastolic dysfunction, infarct size and location, *Am J Cardiol* 61:224–229, 1988.

164. Senior R, et al: Dobutamine echocardiography and thallium-201 imaging predict functional improvement after revascularization in severe ischaemic left ventricular dysfunction, *Br Heart J* 74:358–364, 1995.

165. Shah PK, Pichler M, Berman DS, et al: Left ventricular ejection fraction determined by radionuclide ventriculography in early stages of first transmural myocardial infarction. Relation to short-term prognosis, *Am J Cardiol* 45:542–546, 1980.

166. Sharir T, Rabinowitz B, Livschitz S, et al: Underestimation of extent and severity of coronary artery disease by dipyridamole stress thallium-201 single-photon emission computed tomographic myocardial perfusion imaging in patients taking antianginal drugs, *J Am Coll Cardiol* 31:1540–1546, 1998.

167. Shehata AR, Gillam LD, Mascitelli VA, et al: Impact of acute propranolol administration of dobutamine-induced myocardial ischemia as evaluated by myocardial perfusion imaging and echocardiography. *Am J Cardiol* 80:268–272, 1997.

168. Sinusas AJ, Trautman KA, Bergin JD, et al: Quantification of area at risk during coronary occlusion and degree of myocardial salvage after reperfusion with technetium-99m methoxyisobutyl isonitrile, *Circulation* 82:1424–1437, 1990.

169. Stegaru B, Loose R, Keller H, et al: Effects of long-term treatment with 120 mg of sustained-release isosorbide dinitrate and 60 mg of sustained-release nifedipine on myocardial perfusion, *Am J Cardiol* 61:74E–77E, 1988.

170. Stolzenberg J: Dilatation of the left ventricular cavity on stress thallium scan as an indicator of ischemic disease, *Clin Nucl Med* 5:289–291, 1980.

171. Taillefer R, Lette J, Phaneuf DC, et al: Thallium-201 myocardial imaging during pharmacologic coronary vasodilation: comparison of

oral and intravenous administration of dipyridamole, *J Am Coll Cardiol* 8:76–83, 1986.

172. Taillefer R, Amyot R, Turpin S, et al: Comparison between dipyridamole and adenosine as pharmacologic coronary vasodilators in detection of coronary artery disease with thallium 201 imaging, *J Nucl Cardiol* 3:204–211, 1996.

173. Tamaki N, Yonekura Y, Mukai T, et al: Stress thallium-201 transaxial emission computed tomography: quantitative versus qualitative analysis for evaluation of coronary artery disease, *J Am Coll Cardiol* 4:1213–1221, 1984.

174. Tamaki N, Ohtani H, Yamashita K, et al: Metabolic activity in the areas of new fill-in after thallium-201 reinjection: comparison with positron emission tomography using fluorine-18-deoxyglucose, *J Nucl Med* 32:673–678, 1991.

175. Tilkemeier PL, Guiney TE, LaRaia PJ, et al: Prognostic value of pre-discharge low-level exercise thallium testing after thrombolytic treatment of acute myocardial infarction, *Am J Cardiol* 66:1203–1207, 1990.

176. Tubau JF, Chaitman BR, Bouressa MG, et al: Importance of coronary collateral circulation in interpreting exercise test results, *Am J Cardiol* 47:27–32, 1981.

177. Uhl GS, Kay TN, Hickman JR Jr: Computer-enhanced thallium scintigrams in asymptomatic men with abnormal exercise tests, *Am J Cardiol* 48:1037–1043, 1981.

178. Vaduganathan P, He ZX, Raghavan C, et al: Detection of left anterior descending coronary artery stenosis in patients with left bundle branch block: exercise, adenosine or dobutamine imaging? *J Am Coll Cardiol* 28:543–550, 1996.

179. Van Train KF, Berman DS, Garcia EV, et al: Quantitative analysis of stress thallium-201 myocardial scintigrams: a multicenter trial, *J Nucl Med* 27:17–25, 1986.

180. Van Train KF, Maddahi J, Berman DS et al: Quantitative analysis of tomographic stress thallium-201 myocardial scintigrams: a multicenter trial, *J Nucl Med* 31:1168–1179, 1990.

181. Verani MS, Marcus ML, Razzak MA, et al: Sensitivity and specificity of thallium-201 perfusion scintigrams under exercise in the diagnosis of coronary artery disease, *J Nucl Med* 19:773–782, 1978.

182. Verani MS, Mahmarian JJ, Hixson JB, et al: Diagnosis of coronary artery disease by controlled coronary vasodilation with adenosine and thallium-201 scintigraphy in patients unable to exercise, *Circulation* 82:80–87, 1990.

183. Villanueva FS, Kaul S, Smith WH, et al: Prevalence and correlates of increased lung/heart ratio of thallium-201 during dipyridamole stress imaging for suspected coronary artery disease, *Am J Cardiol* 66:1324–1328, 1990.

184. Weiss AT, Berman DS, Law AS, et al: Transient ischemic dilation of the left ventricle on stress thallium-201 scintigraphy: a marker of severe and extensive coronary artery disease, *J Am Coll Cardiol* 9:752–759, 1987.

185. White CW, Wright CB, Doty DB, et al: Does visual interpretation of the coronary arteriogram predict the physiologic importance of a coronary stenosis? *N Engl J Med* 310:819–824, 1984.

186. Wilde P, Walker P, Watt I, et al: Thallium myocardial imaging: recent experience using a coronary vasodilator, *Clin Radiol* 33:43–50, 1982.

187. Wilson RF, Wyche K, Christensen BV, et al: Effects of adenosine on human coronary arterial circulation, *Circulation* 82:1595–1606, 1990.

188. Wilson RF, Marcus ML, White CW: Prediction of the physiologic significance of coronary arterial lesions by quantitative lesion geometry in patients with limited coronary artery disease, *Circulation* 75:723–732, 1987.

189. Wilson WW, Gibson RS, Nygaard TW, et al: Acute myocardial infarction associated with single vessel coronary artery disease: an analysis of clinical outcome and the prognostic importance of vessel patency and residual ischemic myocardium, *J Am Coll Cardiol* 11:223–234, 1988.

190. Younis LT, Byers S, Shaw L, et al: Prognostic value of intravenous dipyridamole thallium scintigraphy after an acute myocardial ischemic event, *Am J Cardiol* 64:161–166, 1989.

191. Zacca NM, Verani MS, Chalrine RA, et al: Effect of nifedipine on exercise-induced left ventricular dysfunction and myocardial hypoperfusion in stable angina, *Am J Cardiol* 50:689–695, 1982.

Chapter 16

State of the art in coronary artery disease detection: technetium-99m–labeled myocardial perfusion imaging agents

Frans J. Th. Wackers

For almost 15 years, thallium-201 (^{201}Tl) has been the cornerstone of myocardial perfusion imaging and clinical nuclear cardiology. The widespread use and acceptance of ^{201}Tl imaging in clinical cardiology is rooted in a plethora of published data documenting the value of radionuclide myocardial perfusion imaging for the detection of coronary artery disease and for risk stratification of patients with known coronary artery disease. Nevertheless, it was well recognized that ^{201}Tl has significant limitations as an imaging agent. Planar ^{201}Tl images were usually of good diagnostic quality, but single-photon emission computed tomography (SPECT) ^{201}Tl images were often of inconsistent and, at times, suboptimal quality.

The emergence of technetium-99m (^{99m}Tc)–labeled myocardial perfusion imaging agents in the late 1980s changed markedly the clinical practice of myocardial perfusion imaging.[18,42] The ^{99m}Tc label of these radiopharmaceuticals allows administration of a substantially higher radioisotope dose than was feasible with ^{201}Tl. This higher dose, along with concurrent important technical advances in gamma-camera technology, resulted in spectacular improvement of quality of SPECT images in the 1990s (Fig. 16-1). When identical imaging protocol and equipment are used, the count density of images is approximately 3 to 5 times higher with ^{99m}Tc-labeled agents than with ^{201}Tl. This is of clinical relevance because higher count density translates into better image quality, which in turn results in greater confidence in and greater accuracy of the interpretation of images. The relatively high dose also allows simultaneous assessment of left ventricular function, either by a first-pass technique[16] or by electrocardiographically gated SPECT imaging.[2] Another important difference between ^{99m}Tc-labeled agents and ^{201}Tl is that the former lacks substantial myocardial redistribution.[36] This characteristic has the disadvantage that two separate injections of radiopharmaceutical are necessary for evaluation of myocardial perfusion at rest and exercise; on the other hand, it has the advantage that regional myocardial perfusion at the time of radionuclide administration is more or less frozen over time and can be imaged conveniently during subsequent hours.[41] An important difference between ^{99m}Tc and ^{201}Tl is the substantial subdiaphragmatic accumulation of ^{99m}Tc-labeled agents, especially after injection at rest and after pharmacologic intervention. This extracardiac accumulation presents a great problem for planar imaging in particular. Because subdiaphragmatic radioactivity is superimposed on radioactivity in the left ventricle, planar imaging with Tc-labeled agents is not an attractive imaging method. In contrast, because radioactivity in the heart is spatially separated from that in other organs by three-dimensional reconstruction, SPECT is the imaging method of choice with these agents. Accordingly, the following discussion of imaging with ^{99m}Tc-labeled agents is largely limited to the SPECT technique.

Five ^{99m}Tc-labeled radiopharmaceuticals have been introduced in recent years: ^{99m}Tc-teboroxime,[32] ^{99m}Tc-sestamibi,[42] ^{99m}Tc-tetrofosmin,[43] ^{99m}Tc-furifosmin,[11] and ^{99m}Tc-bis(N-ethoxy, N-ethyl dithiocarbamato nitrido (NOET).[5] Only the first three agents have been approved by the U.S. Food and Drug Administration. At the time of this writing, only ^{99m}Tc sestamibi and ^{99m}Tc tetrofosmin have found widespread clinical use. Imaging with ^{99m}Tc-teboroxime, which clears from the myocardium within a few minutes, proved to be too demanding for practical clinical imaging.

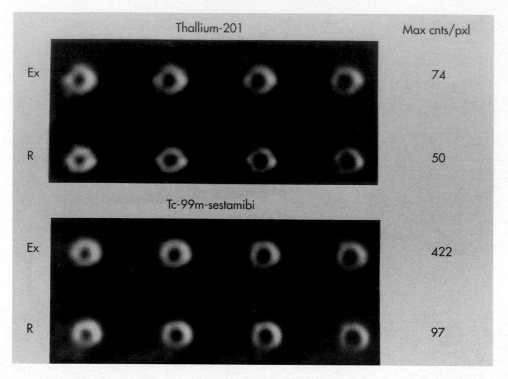

Fig. 16-1. Exercise *(Ex)*–rest *(R)* thallium-201 single-photon emission computed tomography (SPECT) *(top)* and technetium-99m sestamibi SPECT *(bottom)* images acquired in the same patient by using identical imaging protocols. Maximal count density per pixel *(Max cnts/pxl)* is substantially higher with technetium-99m sestamibi than with thallium-201, which is reflected in the better image quality of technetium-99m sestamibi images.

IMAGING PROTOCOLS

As mentioned above, stress and rest myocardial perfusion imaging with ^{99m}Tc-labeled agents requires two separate injections of radiopharmaceutical.[39] On the basis of dosimetry, whole-body exposure, and target organ exposure, the maximal allowable patient dose of ^{99m}Tc-labeled agents is 30 mCi per day. For optimal imaging and, in particular, for optimal SPECT imaging, adequate count density in the heart is a first requirement. Consequently, consistently good results are insured by using an imaging protocol that involves two 30-mCi injections of ^{99m}Tc on two different days, one at peak stress and one at rest. This is known as the two-day imaging protocol.

Two-day protocol

The two-day protocol may be inconvenient especially for outpatients.[39] However, for hospitalized patients, it is feasible to schedule rest images a few days before the expected day of predischarge stress testing. The various imaging protocols for ^{99m}Tc sestamibi and ^{99m}Tc tetrofosmin are schematically shown in Fig. 16-2 and Fig. 16-3. Technetium-99m sestamibi and ^{99m}Tc tetrofosmin clear through the biliary system and accumulate in the gall bladder and gastrointestinal tract.[14,42] Because liver clearance is relatively rapid after exercise injection, a favorable heart-to-liver ratio for imaging occurs early: Imaging can generally be started approximately 15 to 30 minutes after injection. A longer delay can be disadvantageous because ra-

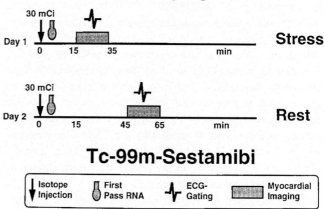

Fig. 16-2. Schematic representation of a two-day technetium-99m sestamibi single-photon emission computed tomography (SPECT) myocardial perfusion imaging protocol combined with first-pass radionuclide angiography and gated SPECT acquisition.

dioactivity travels through the intestines and reaches the bowel loops adjacent to the inferior wall of the left ventricle in 45 to 60 minutes, where it may interfere substantially with visualization of the left ventricle. After injection at rest, ^{99m}Tc sestamibi and ^{99m}Tc tetrofosmin differ substantially. Resting ^{99m}Tc sestamibi imaging should be delayed for at least 45 to 60 minutes

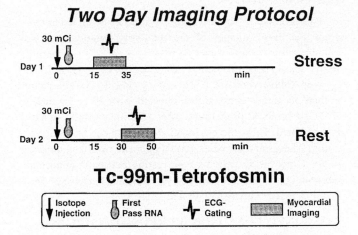

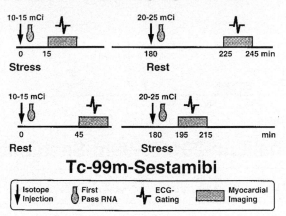

Fig. 16-3. Schematic representation of a two-day technetium-99m tetrofosmin single-photon emission computed tomography (SPECT) myocardial perfusion imaging protocol combined with first-pass radionuclide angiography and gated SPECT acquisition.

Fig. 16-4. Schematic representation of a same-day technetium-99m sestamibi single-photon emission computed tomography (SPECT) myocardial perfusion imaging protocol combined with first-pass radionuclide angiography and gated SPECT acquisition.

to achieve adequate clearance from the liver. In contrast, ^{99m}Tc tetrofosmin clears considerably faster from the liver after rest injection than does ^{99m}Tc sestamibi. Resting ^{99m}Tc tetrofosmin images can therefore can be obtained 15 to 30 minutes after resting injection. Ingestion of milk or a greasy meal has been advocated as a means to enhance liver and gall bladder clearance. However, in our experience, this does not noticeably improve the quality of rest images.

Same-day protocol

Although the two-day protocol is optimal from a technical point of view, a same-day protocol is currently used in most laboratories because it is more convenient (Fig. 16-4 and Fig. 16-5).[39] For this imaging protocol, the first dose usually consists of 10 to 15 mCi of the ^{99m}Tc-labeled agent. After approximately 3 to 4 hours, a second, larger dose (20 to 25 mCi) is injected for the second study. Because of the faster clearance of ^{99m}Tc tetrofosmin from the liver, the total time involved in stress–rest ^{99m}Tc tetrofosmin imaging can be somewhat shorter than that with ^{99m}Tc sestamibi. Using the same-day protocol, the second dose of radiopharmaceutical should be approximately three times larger than the first dose. During the usual interval of approximately 3 hours, the radioisotope decays by one quarter and approximately 25% of the imaging agent clears from the heart. This results in a favorable ratio between radioactivity from the first and second doses.

Using the same-day imaging protocol, either the exercise image or the rest image can be acquired first. The rest–stress sequence is the preferred protocol. The stress–rest sequence has the following potential limitations:

1. If the exercise image is abnormal, it may create an inhomogenous background for the resting image. Because of shine-through of the exercise defect on the rest image, particularly when the interval between the two injections

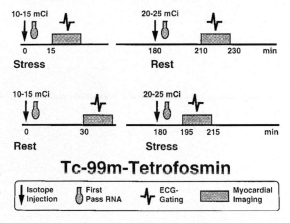

Fig. 16-5. Schematic representation of a same-day technetium-99m tetrofosmin single-photon emission computed tomography (SPECT) myocardial perfusion imaging protocol combined with first-pass radionuclide angiography and gated SPECT acquisition.

is too short or when the second dose is relatively low, defect reversibility may be underestimated (Fig. 16-6).[37]

2. Because the first image (the stress image) is acquired with a lower dose, the quality of the exercise image is jeopardized. In particular, electrocardiographically gated SPECT images may be of suboptimal quality. In addition, the lower dose may result in suboptimal images in obese patients. Nevertheless, the stress–rest sequence may, for practical reasons, be preferred in selected patients. For instance, in patients with an intermediate or low likelihood of coronary artery disease, the likelihood of obtaining normal exercise images is high. If the exercise images are normal, the patient usually does not need additional rest imaging. Thus, time and money can be saved by omitting the rest image.

Dual Isotope Imaging Protocol

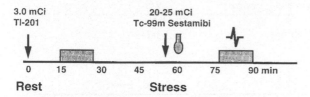

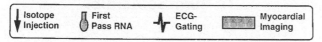

Thallium-201/Tc-99m-Sestamibi

Fig. 16-6. Schematic representation of a dual-isotope thallium-201 rest–technetium-99m sestamibi stress single-photon emission computed tomography (SPECT) myocardial perfusion imaging protocol combined with first-pass radionuclide angiography and gated SPECT acquisition.

Dual-isotope protocol

This protocol is a hybrid imaging protocol designed to overcome the disadvantages of the relatively lengthy same-day imaging protocol that uses two injections of ^{99m}Tc-sestamibi.[1] In the dual-isotope protocol, a rest injection of [201]Tl (3.5 mCi) is given, followed by rest ^{201}Tl imaging (Fig. 16-7). The patient is then put under stress and is injected with 25 to 30 mCi of ^{99m}Tc sestamibi at peak stress; after 15 minutes stress imaging is performed. This efficient imaging protocol can be completed within 2 hours and provides good diagnostic results in most patients. However, in patients with resting perfusion abnormalities, defect reversibility may be overestimated because of physical differences between ^{201}Tl and [99m]Tc.[35]

COMBINED FUNCTION–PERFUSION IMAGING

The high photon flux of ^{99m}Tc-labeled agents allows assessment of left ventricular function in conjunction with myocardial perfusion imaging in two ways: The injections at rest and exercise can be used for first-pass radionuclide angiocardiography,[16] and SPECT images can be acquired with electrocardiographically synchronized gating.[2] First-pass radionuclide angiocardiography requires a gamma camera with high count sensitivity-particularly during exercise. Traditionally, exercise

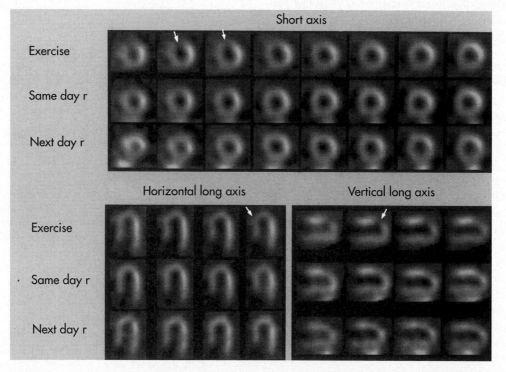

Fig. 16-7. Example of underestimation of exercise defect size reversibility due to early rest imaging after exercise. The patient experienced exercise-induced chest pain and ischemic electrocardiographic changes. Exercise single-photon emission computed tomography was performed after injection of 15 mCi of ^{99m}Tc tetrofosmin. Immediately after completion of exercise imaging, 25 mCi of ^{99m}Tc tetrofosmin was injected at rest, and imaging was started after 30 minutes *(Same-Day Rest)*. The following day, the patient had a repeat 25-mCi injection of ^{99m}Tc tetrofosmin at rest *(Next-Day Rest)*. The reversible anteroseptal exercise defect seems less reversible on the same-day rest study than on the next-day rest study because of shine-through of the exercise defect in the same-day rest study.

first-pass studies are acquired by using upright bicycle exercise.[15] However, some investigators have shown that it is feasible to perform first-pass angiography during treadmill exercise by using sophisticated motion-correction software.[7] The results obtained by exercise–rest first-pass angiography and exercise–rest SPECT myocardial perfusion imaging complement each other and provide incremental diagnostic and prognostic information. In patients with concordant function–perfusion results, the confidence of interpretation is strengthened. For instance, if myocardial perfusion abnormalities are equivocal, the results of exercise first-pass radionuclide angiocardiography may be helpful to reach a definitive decision (normal or abnormal). Several investigators have demonstrated that the combined information derived from first-pass left ventricular ejection fraction and myocardial perfusion imaging may allow better stratification of patients according to the extent of coronary artery disease.[28] Peak exercise left ventricular ejection fraction has long been valued as a powerful predictor of future cardiac events. Resting left ventricular ejection fraction has also been shown to be a prognostic predictor in patients with coronary artery disease.[24,44] Because the heart rate is lower at rest, first-pass angiography can be acquired with longer frame rates than images acquired during exercise; thus, adequate count statistics are more easily achieved. When first-pass angiography equipment is not available, resting first-pass studies of adequate quality can be acquired by using state-of-the-art single crystal cameras.[26] In our laboratory, we routinely acquire resting first-pass studies with rest injection of ^{99m}Tc-labeled agents. In addition to providing prognostic information, evaluation of resting wall motion may identify artifacts on myocardial perfusion images caused by breast tissue or diaphragmatic attenuation.[4,33] Normal regional wall motion in an area with a rest defect suggests attenuation artifact. The potential to distinguish between artifact and true defect is limited. If the patient has a severe myocardial perfusion defect and severely abnormal wall motion in the same area, a transmural myocardial infarction is most likely present. However, if the perfusion defect is mild and regional function is preserved, it is not always possible to differentiate between a small transmural infarction, a nontransmural myocardial infarction, and subdiaphragmatic attenuation.

Electrocardiographically gated SPECT has received substantial attention in recent years. Although the acquisition of gated SPECT is now routine in most laboratories, the criteria for its interpretation are not standardized. A major limitation of gated SPECT imaging is the subjective nature of the interpretation of wall motion and wall thickening images. Nevertheless, in selected patients, gated SPECT images may be useful to identify artifacts. Preliminary results in our laboratory with software used to quantify regional wall thickening on gated SPECT perfusion images have been encouraging in overcoming the limitations of visual analysis.[34] Recently, software to calculate resting left ventricular ejection fraction from ECG gated SPECT images became commercially available (Fig. 16-8).[3,9] This method has been shown to be highly reproducible and to correlate well with resting left ventricular ejection frac-

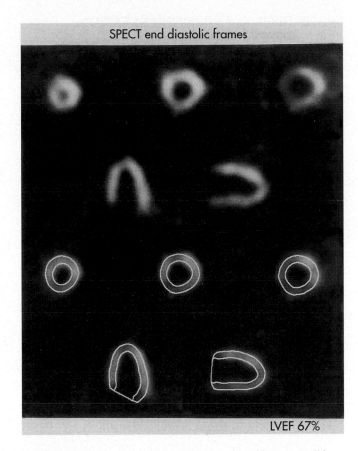

Fig. 16-8. End-diastolic frames of technetium-99m sestamibi reconstructed single-photon emission computed tomography slices *(top two rows)*. The bottom two rows show automatically derived edges used for automatic quantification of left ventricular ejection fraction *(LVEF)*.

tion derived from conventional methods to determine left ventricular ejection fraction.

ADMINISTRATION OF NITROGLYCERIN

Because ^{99m}Tc-labeled agents do not redistribute substantially in the myocardium after initial accumulation, myo-cardial uptake of the radiopharmaceutical is predominantly determined by regional myocardial blood flow at the time of injection. There has been considerable concern that because of this, myocardial viability is underestimated by ^{99m}Tc-labeled agents when resting hypoperfusion exists. Resting defects have occasionally been noted in patients without apparent infarction. Some data suggest that in such patients it may be beneficial to administer nitroglycerin sublingually, orally, or as an intravenous infusion before a resting injection of ^{99m}Tc-labeled agents.[10,31] Although improvement of resting uptake has been demonstrated in selected patients, in most patients, myocardial uptake after rest injection reflects accurately the regional distribution of viable myocardium. Several recent studies indicate that regional myocardial uptake of ^{99m}Tc sestamibi at rest correlates well with histologic regional distribution of viable and scarred myocardium.[22]

IMAGE DISPLAY AND INTERPRETATION

On ^{201}Tl images, particularly those obtained after exercise, uptake of ^{201}Tl is most intense in the heart. Little ^{201}Tl accumulates in adjacent organs. In contrast, on ^{99m}Tc-labeled images, intense radioactivity is almost invariably present outside the heart in the gall bladder, intestines, or liver. Because most computers display images relative to the hottest pixel within the field of view, in the presence of intense extracardiac activity, the image of the heart is displayed in the low end of the gray scale, and the left ventricle is only faintly visible (Fig. 16-9). This faulty normalization may render visual interpretation of ^{99m}Tc-labeled images difficult. Thus, it is important to normalize such images to the hottest pixel within the heart and use the full gray scale for imaging of the heart.[38] Display of myocardial perfusion images is best performed by using a linear gray scale. If color is used, a monochromatic color scale is preferred. Multichrome color scales are preferred for the display of gated SPECT images to appreciate wall thickening and for the display of polar maps but not for the display of reconstructed tomographic slices.

Imaging with ^{99m}Tc-labeled agents has, without doubt, advanced the field of myocardial perfusion imaging to a higher level of quality. Consistently good, diagnostic quality SPECT images are now routinely obtained. As in planar imaging, normal variations in regional myocardial uptake of radiotracer occur in normal SPECT images. It is at times difficult to differentiate normal regional variations from mild, true myocardial perfusion abnormalities by using subjective visual analysis. We advocate strongly quantification of myocardial perfusion images.[19,23,40] Quantification of regional tracer uptake can be done by using circumferential count profile display or polar map display. In circumferential count profile display, regional myocardial distribution of radiopharmaceutical is displayed as a graph normalized to the area with maximal uptake. This normalized display is particularly useful when substantial extra cardiac activity is present. Circumferential count profiles can be displayed simultaneously with a curve indicating the lower limit of normal radiotracer uptake. The polar map display (or bull's-eye display) is based on a similar principle. Regional myocardial tracer uptake is normalized to the area of maximal uptake and is displayed relative to normal data files. The use of normal data files provides a means of quantifying the degree of a myocardial perfusion abnormality.[25,40] Extensive literature provides evidence that the quantified degree of myocardial perfusion abnormalities has important prognostic significance.[12,17,20,21,29]

When ^{99m}Tc-labeled radiopharmaceuticals were introduced, it was expected that attenuation artifacts, which plagued ^{201}Tl imaging for years, would be less troublesome with these new imaging agents. Unfortunately, this expectation was unrealistic. Attenuation of the 140 keV photons of ^{99m}Tc is only a factor of 0.7 less than that of the 80 keV photons of ^{201}Tl. However, ^{201}Tl images are degraded to a much greater extent by low-energy Compton scatter than are images acquired with ^{99m}Tc-labeled agents. Several gamma camera manufacturers have developed attenuation correction hardware, software, and acquisition protocols. The basic principle is to generate a transmission attenuation map that allows mathematical correction of soft-tissue photon absorption. It is now clear that in addition to attenuation correction, scatter correction and resolution compensation are required. At the time of this writing, most commercially developed attenuation–scatter correction packages are still investigational. However, it seems to be only a matter of time before attenuation artifacts can be corrected adequately and routinely in clinical imaging.[6] This will be a major advance in clinical SPECT.

In summary, imaging with ^{99m}Tc-labeled agents can provide consistently high quality myocardial perfusion images. This requires state-of-the-art equipment, such as the multiheaded system, adherence to standardized and optimized imaging protocols,[8,39] and simultaneous assessment of ventricular function and perfusion. Attenuation correction is an important advance, still on the horizon, that can be expected to compensate for tissue attenuation artifacts, one of the most important limitations of SPECT imaging. Once attenuation correction has been perfected, absolute image quantification may be possible. Radionuclide evaluation of coronary artery disease is an exciting and dynamic area of invesigation that continues to develop.

Even after more than two decades, myocardial perfusion imaging is in a state of evolution. None of the existing imaging agents is ideal. It is anticipated that in the near future, metabolic

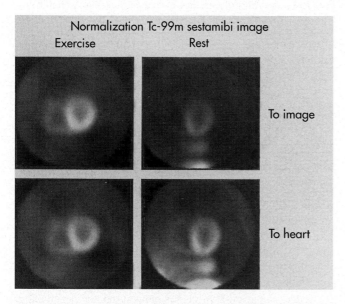

Fig. 16-9. Normalization of exercise–rest technetium-99m sestamibi images. Intense subdiaphragmatic activity *(arrow)* may cause problems with adequate display of the image of the heart. Radionuclide images are usually normalized to the hottest area in the field of view. On the exercise sestamibi images, the heart is the hottest organ. However, on the rest image, the gastrointestinal tract is the hottest area *(arrow)*. Consequently, when the rest image is normalized to subdiaphragmatic activity, the heart is visualized only faintly *(top)*. Using technetium-99m-labeled myocardial perfusion imaging agents, images should be normalized to the heart *(bottom)* for adequate visualization of the heart.

agents will be developed for SPECT.[13,27] Positron-emitting agents may be routinely imaged with standard SPECT cameras.[30]

REFERENCES

1. Berman DS, Kiat H, Friedman JD, et al: Separate acquisition rest thallium-201/stress technetium-99m sestamibi dual-isotope myocardial perfusion single-photon emission computed tomography: a clinical validation study, *J Am Coll Cardiol* 22:1455–1464, 1993.

2. Chua T, Kiat H, Germano G, et al: Gated technetium-99m sestamibi for simultaneous assessment of stress myocardial perfusion, postexercise regional ventricular function and myocardial viability. Correlation with echocardiography and rest thallium-201 scintigraphy, *J Am Coll Cardiol* 23:1107–1114, 1994.

3. DePuey EG, Nichols K, Dobrinsky C: Left ventricular ejection fraction assessed from gated technetium-99m-sestamibi SPECT, *J Nucl Med* 34:1871–1876, 1993.

4. DePuey G, Rozanski A: Using gated technetium-99m-sestamibi SPECT to characterize fixed myocardial defects as an infarct or artifact, *J Nucl Med* 36:952–955, 1995.

5. Fagret D, Marie PY, Brunotte F, et al: Myocardial perfusion imaging with technetium-99m-Tc NOET: comparison with thallium-201 and coronary angiography, *J Nucl Med* 36:936–943, 1995.

6. Ficaro EP, Fessler JA, Shreve PD, et al: Simultaneous transmission/emission myocardial perfusion tomography. Diagnostic accuracy of attenuation-corrected ^{99m}Tc-sestamibi single-photon emission computed tomography, *Circulation* 93:463–473, 1996.

7. Friedman JD, Berman DS, Kiat H, et al: Rest and treadmill exercise first-pass radionuclide ventriculography: validation of left ventricular ejection fraction measurements, *J Nucl Cardiol* 1:382–388, 1994.

8. Garcia EV: Imaging guidelines for nuclear cardiology procedures. Part 1, *J Nucl Cardiol* 3:G1–G646, 1996.

9. Germano G, Kiat H, Kavanaugh PB, et al: Automatic quantification of ejection fraction from gated myocardial perfusion SPECT, *J Nucl Med* 36:2138–2147, 1995.

10. He ZX, Verani MS, Liu XJ: Nitrate-augmented myocardial imaging for assessment of myocardial viability, *J Nucl Cardiol* 2:352–357, 1995.

11. Hendel RC, Verani MS, Miller DD, et al: Diagnostic utility of tomographic myocardial perfusion imaging with technetium 99m furifosmin (Q12) compared with thallium 201: results of a phase III multicenter trial, *J Nucl Cardiol* 3:291–300, 1996.

12. Iskandrian AS, Chae SC, Heo J, et al: Independent and incremental prognostic value of exercise single-photon emission computed tomographic (SPECT) thallium imaging in coronary artery disease, *J Am Coll Cardiol* 22:665–670, 1993.

13. Iskandrian AS, Powers J, Cave V, et al: Assessment of myocardial viability by dynamic tomographic iodine 123 iodophenylpentadecanoic acid imaging: comparison with rest-redistribution thallium 201 imaging, *J Nucl Cardiol* 2(2 Pt 1):101–109, 1995.

14. Jain D, Wackers FJ, Mattera J, et al: Biokinetics of technetium-99m-tetrofosmin: myocardial perfusion imaging agent: implications for a one-day imaging protocol, *J Nucl Med* 34:1254–1259, 1993.

15. Jones RH, McEwan P, Newman GE, et al: Accuracy of diagnosis of coronary artery disease by radionuclide measurement of left ventricular function during rest and exercise, *Circulation* 64:586–601, 1981.

16. Jones RH, Borges-Neto S, Potts JM: Simultaneous measurement of myocardial perfusion and ventricular function during exercise from a single injection of technetium-99m sestamibi in coronary artery disease, *Am J Cardiol* 66:68E–71E, 1990.

17. Kamal AM, Fattah AA, Pancholy S, et al: Prognostic value of adenosine single-photon emission computed tomographic thallium imaging in medically treated patients with angiographic evidence of coronary artery disease, *J Nucl Cardiol* 1:254–261, 1994.

18. Kiat H, Maddali J, Roy LT, et al: Comparison of technetium 99m methoxy isobutyl isonitrile and thallium 201 for evaluation of coronary artery disease by planar and tomographic methods, *Am Heart J* 117:1–11, 1989.

19. Klein JL, Garcia EV, DePuey EG, et al: Reversibility bulls-eye: a new polar bull's-eye map to quantify reversibility of stress-induced SPECT thallium-201 myocardial perfusion defects, *J Nucl Med* 31:1240–1246, 1990.

20. Machecourt J, Longere P, Fagret D, et al: Prognostic value of thallium-201 single-photon emission computed tomographic myocardial perfusion imaging according to extent of myocardial defect. Study in 1,926 patients with follow-up at 33 months, *J Am Coll Cardiol* 23:1096–1106, 1994.

21. Marie PY, Danchin N, Durand JF, et al: Long-term prediction of major ischemic events by exercise thallium-201 single-photon emission computed tomography. Incremental prognostic value compared with clinical, exercise testing, catheterization and radionuclide angiographic data, *J Am Coll Cardiol* 26:879–886, 1995.

22. Medrano R, Lowry RW, Young JB, et al: Assessment of myocardial viability with ^{99m}Tc sestamibi in patients undergoing cardiac transplantation. A scintigraphic/pathological study, *Circulation* 94:1010–1017, 1996.

23. Mortelmans L, Nuyts J, Scheys I, et al: A new quantitative method for the analysis of cardiac perfusion tomography (SPET): validation in post-infarction patients treated with thrombolytic therapy, *Eur J Nucl Med* 20:1193–1200, 1993.

24. Risk stratification and survival after myocardial infarction, *N Engl J Med* 309:331–336, 1983.

25. Naruse H, Daher E, Sinusas A, et al: Quantitative comparison of planar and SPECT normal data files of thallium-201, technetium-99m-sestamibi, technetium-99m-tetrofosmin, and technetium-99m furifosmin, *J Nucl Med* 37:1783–1788, 1996.

26. Nichols K, DePuey EG, Gooneratne N, et al: First-pass ventricular ejection fraction using a single-crystal nuclear camera, *J Nucl Med* 35:1292–1300, 1994.

27. Nishimura T, Uchara T, Shimonagata T, et al: Clinical results with b-methyl-p (^{123}I) iodophenylpentadecanoic acid, single-photon emission computed tomography in cardiac disease, *J Nucl Cardiol* 1(2 Pt 2):S65–S71, 1994.

28. Palmas W, Friedman JD, Diamond GA, et al: Incremental value of simultaneous assessment of myocardial function and perfusion with technetium-99m sestamibi for prediction of extent of coronary artery disease, *J Am Coll Cardiol* 25:1024–1031, 1995.

29. Petretta M, Cuocola A, Carpimelli A, et al: Prognostic value of myocardial hypoperfusion indexes in patients with suspected or known coronary artery disease, *J Nucl Cardiol* 1:325–337, 1994.

30. Sandler MP, Videlefsky S, Delbeke D, et al: Evaluation of myocardial ischemia using a rest metabolism/stress perfusion protocol with fluorine-18 deoxyglucose/technetium-99m MIBI and dual-isotope simultaneous-acquisition single-photon emission computed tomography, *J Am Coll Cardiol* 26:870–878, 1995.

31. Sciagra R, Bisi G, Santoro GM, et al: Influence of the assessment of defect severity and intravenous nitrate administration during tracer injection on the detection of viable hibernating myocardium with data-based quantitative technetium 99m-labeled sestamibi single-photon emission computed tomography, *J Nucl Cardiol* 3:221–230, 1996.

32. Seldin DW, Johnson U, Blood DK, et al: Myocardial perfusion imaging with technetium-99m SQ30217: comparison with thallium-201 and coronary anatomy, *J Nucl Med* 30:312–319, 1989.

33. Shen MYH, et al: Quantitative analysis of SPECT imaging in combination of first-pass radionuclide angiography permits identification of interior wall attenuation from scar, *J Nucl Med* 37:81P, 1996.

34. Shen MYH, et al: A new method for quantification of regional and temporal wall thickening on gated SPECT, *J Nucl Cardiol* 4:S102, 1997.

35. Siebelink HMJ, Natale D, Sinusas AJ, et al: Quantitative comparison of single-isotope and dual-isotope stress-rest single-photon emission computed tomographic imaging for reversibility of defects. *J Nucl Cardiol* 3(6 Pt 1):483–493, 1996.

36. Sinusas AJ, Bergin JD, Edwards NC, et al: Redistribution of ^{99m}Tc-sestamibi and ^{201}Tl in the presence of a severe coronary artery stenosis, *Circulation* 89:2332–2341, 1994.

37. Taillefer R, Gagnon A, LaFlamme L, et al: Same day injections of Tc-99m methoxy isobutyl isonitrile (hexamibi) for myocardial tomographic imaging: comparison between rest-stress and stress-rest injection sequences, *J Nucl Med* 15:113–117, 1989.

38. Wackers FJTh: Artifacts in planar and SPECT myocardial perfusion imaging, *Am J Cardiac Imaging* 6:42–58, 1992.

39. Wackers FJTh: The maze of myocardial perfusion imaging protocols in 1994, *J Nucl Cardiol* 1(2 Pt 1):180–188, 1994.

40. Wackers FJTh: Science, art and artifacts: how important is quantification for the practicing physician interpreting myocardial perfusion studies? *J Nucl Cardiol* 1(5 Pt 2):S109–S117, 1994.

41. Wackers FJTh, Gibbons RJ, Verani MS, et al: Serial quantitative planar technetium-99m isonitrile imaging in acute myocardial infarction: efficacy for noninvasive assessment of thrombolytic therapy, *J Am Coll Cardiol* 14:861–873, 1989.

42. Wackers FJTh, Berman DS, Maddahi J, et al: Technetium-99m hexakis 2-methoxyisobutyl isonitrile: human biodistribution, dosimetry, safety, and preliminary comparison to thallium-201 for myocardial perfusion imaging, *J Nucl Med* 30:301–311, 1989.

43. Zaret BL, Rigo P, Wackers FJ, et al: Myocardial perfusion imaging with ^{99m}Tc tetrofosmin. Comparison to ^{201}Tl imaging and coronary angiography in a phase III multicenter trial. Tetrofosmin International Trial Study Group, *Circulation* 91:313–319, 1995.

44. Zaret BL, Wackers FJ, Terrin ML, et al: Value of radionuclide rest and exercise left ventricular ejection fraction in assessing survival of patients after thrombolytic therapy for acute myocardial infarction: results of thrombolysis in Myocardial (TIMI) phase II study. The TIMI Study Group, *J Am Coll Cardiol* 26:73–79, 1995.

Chapter 17

Dual-isotope myocardial perfusion SPECT with rest thallium-201 and stress technetium-99m sestamibi

Daniel S. Berman, Aman M. Amanullah, Sean Hayes, John D. Friedman,
Rory Hachamovitch, Xingping Kang, Howard C. Lewin, Hosen Kiat, Kenneth F. Van Train,
Sanjay Dahr, and **Guido Germano**

The commercial availability of technetium-99m (^{99m}Tc)–labeled myocardial perfusion agents has added choices in the noninvasive clinical assessment of coronary artery disease. Several studies have suggested that rest–stress technetium-99m sestamibi single-photon emission computed tomography (SPECT) has a sensitivity and specificity similar to that of thallium-201 (^{201}Tl) SPECT for the detection of coronary artery disease.[26, 27, 34] Preferential use of ^{99m}Tc sestamibi has been advocated for stress imaging, principally because of improved image quality and flexibility, which results from the combined physical and biological characteristics of this agent.[10,12,13] However, rest–stress ^{99m}Tc sestamibi studies, which require two injections using same-day or two-day protocols, have drawbacks.[14] Two-day protocols are not ideal for patients because they require two visits to the imaging laboratory. Same-day rest–stress protocols are more convenient but involve the superimposition of a resting perfusion pattern on a stress SPECT pattern, thereby potentially reducing defect contrast. In addition, same-day rest–stress studies lack ideal efficiency because a 1-hour delay is needed after rest injection before imaging to allow for hepatobiliary clearance. With respect to the assessment of myocardial viability, rest–stress sestamibi imaging has theoretical constraints in separating hibernating myocardium from infarction that do not apply to ^{201}Tl because of its redistribution properties.

Given these limitations of standard ^{99m}Tc sestamibi protocols, our group decided to investigate another approach to ^{99m}Tc sestamibi SPECT—dual-isotope rest–stress myocardial perfusion SPECT, which takes advantage of the Anger camera's ability to collect data in different energy windows. For the dual-isotope approach, separate radiopharmaceuticals are used for the rest injection and the stress injection.

PROTOCOLS

The two fundamental types of procedures are simultaneous[16,31] or separate acquisition dual-isotope SPECT.[10] With either approach, considerations of radiation dosimetry from standard ^{201}Tl or ^{99m}Tc protocols are relevant because two radiopharmaceuticals are used. Table 17-1 illustrates the comparative doses used in ^{201}Tl protocols with and without reinjection, dual-isotope approaches, and rest–stress ^{99m}Tc sestamibi techniques. Because of differences in the critical organs involved with ^{201}Tl and ^{99m}Tc sestamibi, the dual-isotope procedures result in essentially the same radiation dose to both the critical organ and the whole body as that observed in ^{201}Tl stress reinjection protocols.

Simultaneous acquisition

The protocol for the simultaneous dual-isotope study is illustrated in Fig. 17-1. After resting administration of ^{201}Tl, SPECT imaging is not performed. Instead, the patient immediately undergoes treadmill exercise with administration of ^{99m}Tc sestamibi at the peak of stress. Fifteen minutes thereafter, dual-isotope myocardial perfusion SPECT is performed. The entire procedure is completed in less than 1 hour, and only one SPECT acquisition of approximately 20 minutes' duration is required. In principle, this simultaneous acquisition of a rest ^{201}Tl and a stress sestamibi study would have many advantages compared with the conventional stress and rest protocols. It would halve camera utilization time and substantially abbreviate overall study time. Furthermore, the inherent registration of stress and rest image sets would reduce the frequency of unrecognized artifacts associated with separate stress and rest image acquisitions.

This protocol, however, rests on unproven assumptions. Because no rest SPECT is performed before exercise, the simultaneous dual-isotope approach assumes that the resting ^{201}Tl distribution does not change during exercise. We have preliminary data suggesting that this assumption is correct.[32] More importantly, this approach also assumes that the effects of cross-scatter of gamma rays between the two energy windows are insignificant or can be accounted for. Kiat et al[31] demonstrated in a report of patient studies that ^{99m}Tc sestamibi cross-talk (downscatter) into the lower energy ^{201}Tl window causes substantial reduction in ^{201}Tl defect contrast (20%) leading to an overestimation of defect reversibility. Thus, although simultaneous dual-isotope SPECT is an appealing protocol, the contribution of ^{99m}Tc in the ^{201}Tl window is substantial with this approach. For optimal clinical application, this approach requires correction for downscatter to assess defect reversibility. The correction for ^{99m}Tc downscatter is not trivial, however. The contribution of downscatter to the lower energy image is not simply a scaled portion of the activity distribution of the higher energy image and, as such, cannot be corrected for by simple subtraction.[42,51] Several laboratories, including our own, are currently working on this important problem. At present, we do not recommend general clinical use of this simultaneous dual-isotope protocol.

Separate acquisition

After extensive consideration of various approaches, we elected to develop separate rest ^{201}Tl–stress ^{99m}Tc sestamibi dual-isotope SPECT[10] for clinical use. Because of the negligible contribution of ^{201}Tl in the ^{99m}Tc window (2.9%),[31] the separate acquisition approach using rest ^{201}Tl and exercise ^{99m}Tc sestamibi provides an alternative that does not require correction for cross-contamination between the two isotopes. In phantom and clinical studies, Kiat et al[31] reported that the concurrent presence of ^{201}Tl causes an imperceptible reduction in defect contrast in ^{99m}Tc sestamibi images. Our current routine clinical protocol is shown in Fig. 17-2. For the separate acquisition study, a standard dose of 3 mCi of ^{201}Tl is injected intravenously at rest; the exact dose depends on patient weight. Rest ^{201}Tl SPECT is begun 10 minutes after

Table 17-1. Comparison of radiation dosimetry

| | Thallium-201 protocol | | | |
| | Stress | Reinjection | Dual-isotope | Same-day |
Site	3.5 mCi	1 mCi	Thallium, 3.0 mCi and technetium, 25 mCi	Technetium, 8 mCi and 22 mCi
Whole body	0.7	1.0	1.1	0.5
Kidneys	4.2	5.4	5.3	2.0
Large intestine	0.9	1.1	5.2	5.4

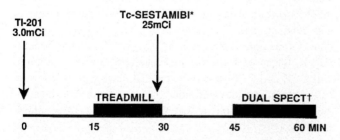

Fig. 17-1. Simultaneous rest thallium-201–stress technetium-99m sestamibi dual-isotope myocardial perfusion study protocol. Until background subtraction techniques are developed, this protocol is not recommended. * = Peak exercise first-pass study is optional.

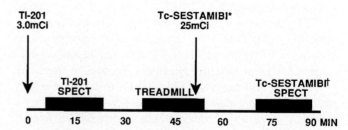

Fig. 17-2. Separate acquisition rest thallium-201–stress technetium-99m sestamibi dual-isotope myocardial perfusion study protocol. TM = treadmill. * = Peak exercise first-pass study is optional; † = gated single-photon emission computed tomography is optional.

injection. Immediately following ^{201}Tl SPECT, the patient is prepared for treadmill exercise. At near-maximal exercise, a standard dose of 25 mCi of ^{99m}Tc sestamibi is injected; the dose is again based on the patient weight. For patients weighing more than 70 kg, the rest ^{201}Tl dose is 0.043 mCi/kg, and the exercise ^{99m}Tc sestamibi dose is 0.36 mCi/kg. Technetium-99m sestamibi SPECT is begun 15 minutes after injection.

Both the rest ^{201}Tl and stress ^{99m}Tc sestamibi studies use a high-resolution collimator, use 180-degree acquisition over 64 projections, and take 20 seconds per projection. In ^{201}Tl imaging, two energy windows are used. Our previous protocol used a 15% window centered on the 68- to 80-keV peak and a 10% window centered on the 167-keV peak. On the basis of work performed at Emory University by Garcia et al, we adopted a 30% symmetric window for the 68- to 80-keV peak and a 20% window for the 167-keV ^{201}Tl photopeak for the rest ^{201}Tl SPECT. The new windows for ^{201}Tl acquisition provide an increase of approximately 40% in counts compared with the previous protocol without a loss in resolution. For ^{99m}Tc sestamibi SPECT, a 15% window centered on the 140-keV peak is used. This window is narrower than that used with other ^{99m}Tc ses-

tamibi protocols to reduce scatter from ^{201}Tl. With the separate acquisition dual-isotope protocol, completion of the entire procedure is possible in less than 2 hours.

Preprocessing for ^{201}Tl uses a Butterworth filter of order 5 with a cut-off frequency of 50% Nyquist. For ^{99m}Tc sestamibi images, a Butterworth filter of order 2.5 with a cut-off frequency of 66% Nyquist is used. A ramp filter is used to reconstruct the transaxial tomograms of 6.4-mm slices that make up the entire heart. Short-axis, vertical, and horizontal long-axis tomograms of the left ventricle are extracted from the reconstructed transaxial tomograms by performing coordinate transformation with appropriate interpolation. No attenuation or scatter correction is used. All of the filters are identical to those used for the rest–stress same-day ^{99m}Tc sestamibi–only protocol.[13] Image interpretation is performed in the same way as with ^{99m}Tc sestamibi.[13] The only difference is that visual compensation is made for the slightly smaller cavity size and slightly thicker myocardial walls observed with a normal ^{201}Tl resting study compared with a normal ^{99m}Tc sestamibi rest study. Example of a normal study is shown in Fig. 17-3. A study demonstrating a reversible defect is shown in Fig. 17-4.

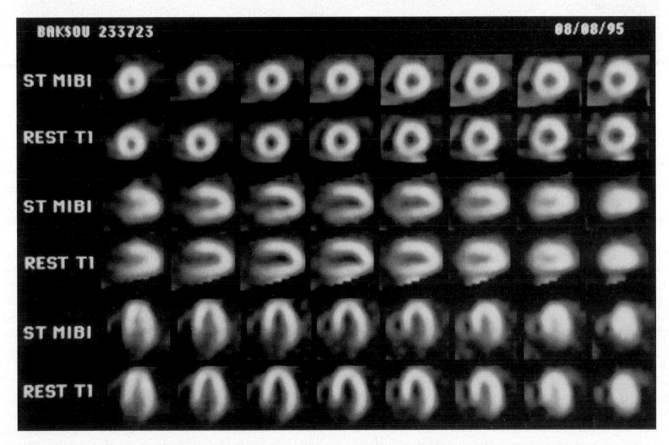

Fig. 17-3. A normal case example of a separate acquisition rest thallium-201 *(bottom row)*–stress technetium-99m sestamibi *(top row)* dual-isotope single-photon emission computed tomography. ST mibi = stress technetium sestamibi; Tl = thallium-201.

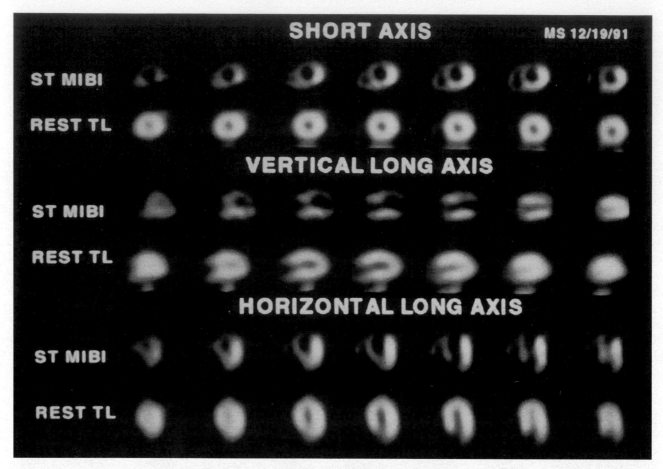

Fig. 17-4. A case example of a reversible defect on separate acquisition dual-isotope single-photon emission computed tomography. Rows 1, 3, and 5 show the stress technetium sestamibi images, and rows 2, 4, and 6 show the rest thallium-201 images. A clear large reversible defect is noted throughout the left anterior descending coronary artery territory.

RECENT PROTOCOL MODIFICATIONS

Prone imaging

Image acquisition of ^{201}Tl and ^{99m}Tc sestamibi SPECT has traditionally been performed with the patient in the supine position. Unfortunately, acquisition in the supine position frequently results in diaphragmatic attenuation of inferior wall counts. This artifact decreases the specificity of the study due to a higher false positive rate for inferior wall ischemia. SPECT acquisition of ^{201}Tl with the patient in the prone position decreases diaphragmatic attenuation by lowering the diaphragm and allowing the heart to move closer to the chest wall and results in an increase in inferior and septal wall counts.[33,41a] Using prone imaging for stress-redistribution ^{201}Tl SPECT, Kiat et al. demonstrated specificities of 94%, 71%, and 94% for the detection of coronary artery disease (≥50% stenosis) in the right, left circumflex, and left anterior descending coronary arteries, respectively; the sensitivities were 88%, 89%, and 78%.[33] The prone position is also associated with reduced patient motion; in the study of Kiat et al, mild and severe patient motion occurred in 12% and 4% of the supine studies, respectively, but in only 3.5% and 0% of the prone studies. With ^{99m}Tc sestamibi,

our laboratory has recently reported preliminary results that patients with inferior wall defects on supine SPECT imaging but normal prone SPECT imaging have the same low event rate as patients with normal supine SPECT.[25] Therefore, because prone imaging decreases false positive results as well as patient motion, we now routinely perform combined prone and supine imaging on all patients. Prone imaging alone is not recommended because of frequent anteroseptal defects which mimic left anterior descending coronary artery disease.[38a,41a] Supine and prone imaging is also not recommended for general stress ^{201}Tl imaging because rapid redistribution occurs in approximately 20% of cases, complicating the interpretation of supine thallium defects which disappear on prone imaging.[18]

Adenosine walk

Many patients are unable to perform adequate treadmill exercise, which has led to the increasing use of pharmacologic stress imaging protocols. Matzer et al have validated separate acquisition rest ^{201}Tl/adenosine or dipyridamole stress ^{99m}Tc sestamibi SPECT with a sensitivity of 97% and specificity of 81% for the detection of coronary artery disease (stenosis

Table 17-2. Sensitivity, specificity, and normalcy rate by rest thallium-201–treadmill stress technetium-99m sestamibi separate acquisition dual-isotope SPECT*

Variable	Overall CAD	Left anterior descending CAD	Right anterior descending CAD	Left circumflex artery CAD
≥50% CAD				
Sensitivity, n/n (%)	50/55 (91)	22/36 (61)	33/34 (97)	15/27 (56)
Specificity, n/n (%)	6/8 (75)	25/27 (93)	25/29 (86)	35/36 (97)
≥70% CAD				
Sensitivity, n/n (%)	50/52 (96)	22/27 (81)	30/31 (97)	15/24 (63)
Specificity, n/n (%)	9/11 (82)	34/36 (94)	25/32 (78)	40/41 (98)
Normalcy rate, n/n (%)	102/117 (95)			

*CAD = coronary artery disease; SPECT = single-photon emission computed tomography. Adapted from Berman DS, Kiat H, Friedman JD, et al: Separate acquisition rest thallium-201/stress technetium 99m sestamibi dual-isotope myocardial perfusion SPECT: A clinical validation study, *J Am Coll Cardiol* 22:1455-1464, 1993. With permission from American College of Cardiology.

≥70%).[37] Subsequently our laboratory reported high sensitivity, specificity, and normalcy rate in women with adenosine ^{99m}Tc sestamibi SPECT.[6] We have recently reported preliminary confirmation of an approach combining adenosine stress and treadmill exercise as initially described by Pennell et al.[39] The addition of low level treadmill exercise reduces the noncardiac side effects of simultaneous adenosine infusion and allows for early post-stress imaging, thereby shortening study time.[38a] We have therefore modified our separate acquisition adenosine protocol to include simultaneous low level treadmill exercise (modified Bruce protocol, stage I, 1.7 mph, 0% grade) for the duration of the six minute infusion of adenosine (140 μg/kg/min intravenously). At the end of the three minutes of adenosine infusion with treadmill exercise, 25 mCi of sestamibi is injected. Hayes et al have recently demonstrated the incremental value of adding first-pass radionuclide angiography obtained using a Scinticor SIM-400 camera to adenosine low level treadmill exercise dual-isotope SPECT for detecting multivessel coronary artery disease.[24] We now routinely add low level treadmill exercise with first-pass radionuclide angiography to all adenosine SPECT studies except for patients who cannot walk on a treadmill or who have a left bundle branch block or paced rhythm on baseline ECG.

CLINICAL VALIDATION

Detection of coronary artery disease

The dual-isotope separate acquisition method has been validated at Cedars-Sinai Medical Center where it is the standard clinical routine and has been used in approximately 16,000 patients as of December 1996. Our initial validation was described in a report[10] of the results of the dual-isotope procedure in 63 patients without previous myocardial infarction undergoing coronary angiography to evaluate sensitivity and specificity for coronary artery disease and in 107 patients with a low likelihood of coronary artery disease to evaluate the normalcy rate. To validate defect reversibility, the dual-isotope SPECT study was also compared with stress–rest ^{99m}Tc sestamibi SPECT studies in a separate group of 31 patients with documented previous myocardial infarction who underwent a rest ^{99m}Tc sestamibi study in addition to the dual-isotope SPECT study.[10]

The angiographic correlations are shown in Table 17-2. Dual-isotope SPECT demonstrated high sensitivity for detecting patients with 50% or greater coronary artery stenosis (91%, n = 55) and 70% or greater stenosis (96%, n = 52). Although high values for specificity were found in this study (75% for <50% stenosis and 82% for <70% stenosis), little significance was attributed to this finding because of the small number of patients (n = 11) with normal coronary arteriograms. A referral bias that overestimates test sensitivity[40,41] and underestimates test specificity was operative in this study. In our clinical study, patients were more likely to be catheterized when scintigraphic findings were positive than when they were negative. However, this referral bias has been present in several recent studies from our institution[34,47,49] correlating myocardial perfusion SPECT and angiographic results. In those studies, sensitivities similar to those observed in the present study were reported. Therefore, findings suggest that the sensitivity of separate acquisition dual-isotope SPECT is similar to that of SPECT studies using ^{201}Tl or ^{99m}Tc sestamibi alone.

We advocate the use of the normalcy rate of a scintigraphic test as a proxy for specificity when referral bias is operative.[40,49] A very high normalcy rate of 95% was found in a large population of patients with a low likelihood of coronary artery disease evaluated in this study. With ^{201}Tl SPECT, the normalcy rate has been reported to be between 82% and 89%.[47,49] No large study of ^{201}Tl has suggested a SPECT normalcy rate as high as that observed in this study. The high normalcy rate observed in this examination most likely represents a true characteristic of ^{99m}Tc sestamibi SPECT studies. It is related to improved counts and less attenuation and scatter, and may be one of the most important reasons for considering the clinical use of any ^{99m}Tc sestamibi protocol.[12-14] The high normalcy rate is also related to the ability to repeat imaging when artifact is suspected; thus, when motion or diaphragmatic attenuation is observed, imaging can be repeated in the prone position[31] (Fig. 17-5).

In this study, the sensitivity and specificity for detecting individual coronary artery stenoses were also similar to those found previously with ^{201}Tl SPECT[35,49] and ^{99m}Tc sestamibi SPECT.[13,26,27,33,47] Compared with angiography, dual-isotope SPECT had a tendency to underestimate the number of

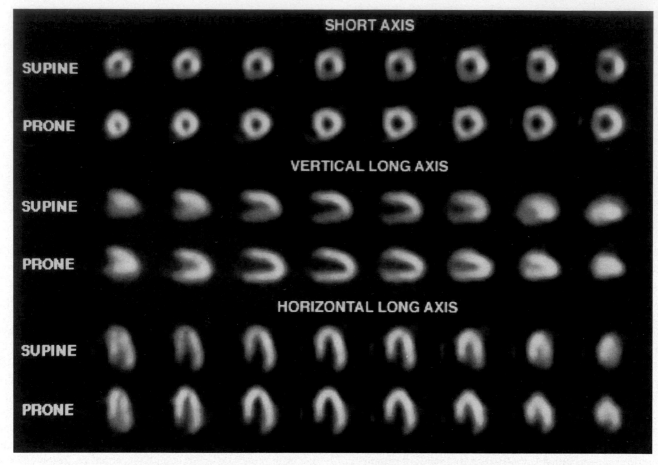

Fig. 17-5. A normal case example of a separate acquisition dual-isotope study showing inferior wall defect on supine stress images due to diaphragmatic attenuation. This defect resolved completely on prone images.

stenosed vessels. In this respect, dual-isotope myocardial perfusion SPECT seems to be similar to single-isotope SPECT.

The separate acquisition dual-isotope protocol is effective with pharmacologic stress using adenosine, dipyridamole, or dobutamine. The pharmacologic stress dual-isotope protocol is illustrated in Fig. 17-6. In a study of 132 patients undergoing adenosine (*n* = 82) or dipyridamole (*n* = 50) dual-isotope protocol, Matzer et al.[37] have shown a high sensitivity (92% and 97% for ≥50% and ≥70% stenosis, respectively) and specificity (85% and 81% for ≥50% and ≥70% stenosis, respectively). Recently, Amanullah et al[2] demonstrated a similar a high sensitivity, specificity, and accuracy of 93%, 73%, and 88%, respectively, in a consecutive series of 222 patients undergoing adenosine dual-isotope study. In another recent study of a large consecutive series of women, adenosine dual-isotope protocol had a high sensitivity and specificity for detection of coronary artery disease in women regardless of presenting symptoms or pretest likelihood of coronary disease (Table 17-3).[6] In this study, the normalcy rate in 71 women with a low pretest likelihood of coronary artery disease was 93%. The protocol has also been validated in patients with left ventricular hypertrophy[7] and in very elderly persons (age ≥80 years).[50]

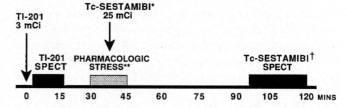

Fig. 17-6. Injection and acquisition protocol for a pharmacologic dual-isotope protocol. * = Peak stress first-pass study is optional; †gated single-photon emission computed tomography is optional; † = adenosine, dipyridamole, or dobutamine (duration of stress varies with stress agent).

The dual-isotope myocardial perfusion SPECT protocol would be expected to work well with ^{99m}Tc agents other than sestamibi. ^{99m}Tc tetrofosmin is a new lipophilic diphosphine cationic radiopharmaceutical used for myocardial perfusion SPECT. As with ^{99m}Tc sestamibi, the high count statistics of ^{99m}Tc tetrofosmin allow for acquisition of exercise wall motion via first-pass radionuclide angiography during the bolus injection as well as post-stress resting wall motion via gated SPECT. Takahashi et al have demonstrated the feasibility of stress ^{99m}Tc

Table 17-3. The sensitivity, specificity, predictive accuracy, and normalcy rate of adenosine technetium-99m sestamibi SPECT*

| Patient category | Stenosis of 50% or more | | | Stenosis of 70% or more | | | Normalcy rate |
| | Sensitivity | Specificity | Predictive accuracy | Sensitivity | Specificity | Predictive accuracy | |
	% (n/n)			% (n/n)			% (n/n)
Low likelihood of CAD (<10%; n = 71)							93 (66/71)
Catheterized patients							
All patients (n = 130)	93 (87/94)	78 (28/36)	88 (115/130)	95 (79/83)	66 (31/47)	85 (110/130)	
Patients without previous MI (n = 103)	91 (61/67)	78 (28/36)	86 (89/103)	95 (54/57)	67 (31/46)	83 (85/103)	
Patients with angina (n = 74)	92 (47/51)	83 (19/23)	89 (66/74)	96 (44/46)	75 (21/28)	88 (65/74)	
Patients without angina (n = 56)	93 (40/43)	69 (9/13)	88 (49/56)	95 (35/37)	53 (10/19)	80 (45/56)	
Relatively low likelihood of CAD (<25%; n = 22)	82 (9/11)	82 (9/11)	82 (18/22)	88 (7/8)	71 (10/14)	77 (17/22)	
Intermediate likelihood of CAD (25% to 75%; n = 68)	93 (43/46)	73 (16/22)	87 (59/68)	97 (38/39)	62 (18/29)	82 (56/68)	
High likelihood of CAD (>75%; n = 40)	95 (35/37)	100 (3/3)	95 (38/40)	94 (34/36)	75 (3/4)	93 (37/40)	

*CAD = coronary artery disease; MI = myocardial infarction; SPECT = single-photon emission computed tomography. Adapted from Amanullah AM, Kiat H, Friedman JD, et al: Adenosine technetium-99m sestamibi myocardial perfusion SPECT in women: diagnostic efficacy in detection of coronary artery disease, *J Am Coll Cardiol* 27:803-809, 1996. With permission from American College of Cardiology.

tetrofosmin with first-pass radionuclide angiography for combined myocardial perfusion and function assessment.[46] We await the publication of studies validating the diagnostic and prognostic accuracy of dual-isotope rest ^{201}Tl/stress ^{99m}Tc tetrofosmin SPECT.

Assessment of defect reversibility

With respect to defect reversibility, our initial validation compared the dual-isotope procedure with rest–stress ^{99m}Tc sestamibi SPECT.[10] The κ-statistic and its standard error were used for agreement analysis; a value of 1 denoted perfect agreement and a value of 0 indicated no agreement beyond chance. In general, κ-values of 0.6 or greater are considered to indicate good agreement. In the patient group assessed for defect reversibility, segmental agreement for defect type between rest ^{201}Tl and rest ^{99m}Tc sestamibi studies was 97% (κ = 0.79; p<0.001) in zones with no previous myocardial infarction. In myocardial infarct zones, segmental agreement for defect type was 98% (κ = 0.93; p<0.001).[10] The agreement for defect reversibility pattern (normal, reversible, or nonreversible) between first and second readings was 95% (κ = 0.89; p<0.001).[10] The agreements for exact segmental score (range, 0 to 4) were 86% (κ = 0.67; p<0.001) and 84% (κ = 0.71, p<0.001) for rest ^{201}Tl and rest–stress ^{99m}Tc sestamibi, respectively.[10] An example of a patient with an extensive nonreversible defect on rest ^{201}Tl and stress ^{99m}Tc sestamibi SPECT is shown in Fig. 17-7.

One of the principal advantages of the dual-isotope approach over standard rest–stress sestamibi approaches relates to the use of ^{201}Tl for the evaluation of defect reversibility. This advantage derives from the greater redistribution of ^{201}Tl into areas of ischemic but viable myocardium than is observed with ^{99m}Tc sestamibi. Thus, in patients with resting ^{201}Tl defects, assessment of myocardial viability can be enhanced with the dual-isotope approach over rest–stress ^{99m}Tc sestamibi imaging by the use of redistribution ^{201}Tl imaging.[10,30] Patients can be brought back for 24-hour imaging the next day, or a rest-redistribution study can be completed before the ^{99m}Tc stress sestamibi injection. In 24-hour imaging, because of the 6-hour half-life of ^{99m}Tc, only one sixteenth of the injected ^{99m}Tc sestamibi dose would remain because of physical decay, whereas a much higher proportion of ^{201}Tl remains because of its 73-hour half-life. Unpublished observations from our laboratory show that the amount of ^{99m}Tc contributing to the ^{201}Tl peak at 24 hours is less than 10%.

Incorporation of 24-hour rest-redistribution ^{201}Tl scintigraphy into the dual-isotope protocol provides the detection of an additional 8% to 15% of reversible segments, which would go undetected by rest scintigraphy alone.[30] The protocol for the late redistribution imaging is illustrated in Fig. 17-8, and a patient with late reversibility with this protocol is shown in Fig. 17-9. The approach potentially provides more information about myocardial viability than does rest–stress ^{99m}Tc sestamibi studies, because rest-redistribution ^{201}Tl studies can be

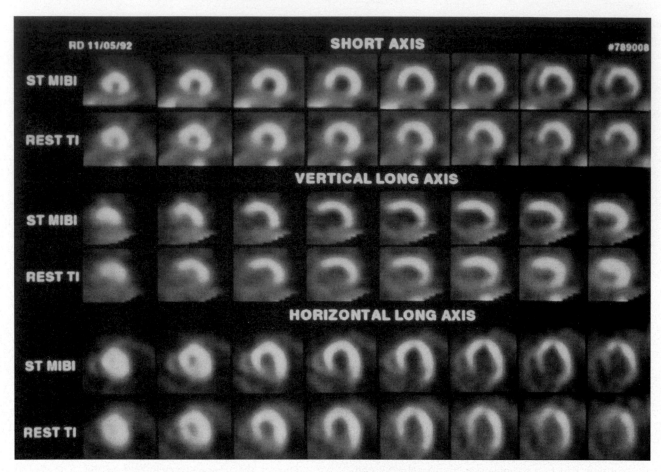

Fig. 17-7. A case example of a nonreversible defect on separate acquisition dual-isotope single-photon emission computed tomography. A severe nonreversible defect can be seen in the inferoseptal and inferior left ventricular walls.

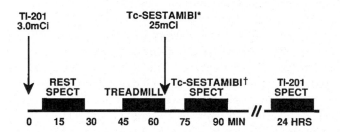

Fig. 17-8. Late-redistribution protocol for separate acquisition dual-isotope myocardial perfusion single-photon emission computed tomography (SPECT). This protocol is used if the rest thallium-201 study demonstrates a defect. * = Peak stress first-pass study is optional; † = gated SPECT is optional.

performed before or after the dual-isotope procedure, capturing additional information about hibernating myocardium from the redistribution phase of the Tl study.

As a practical routine, we inject inpatients with ^{201}Tl the night before stress studies. The next day, we begin imaging with a 12-hour postinjection redistribution Tl study, followed immediately by stress ^{99m}Tc sestamibi SPECT (Fig. 17-10). With this approach, 24-hour imaging after the stress study is not necessary. Thus, when the patient who has had myocardial

infarction is considered ready for predischarge stress testing (usually pharmacologic), the redistribution ^{201}Tl–stress ^{99m}Tc sestamibi dual-isotope protocol can be accomplished faster than standard ^{201}Tc protocols. The protocol is faster because the late redistribution ^{201}Tl image frequently needed in these patients can be obtained on the day of the stress study rather than the following day, thereby potentially decreasing the length of hospitalization by 1 day.

Quantitative analysis

Because of the minimal contribution of the rest ^{201}Tl study to the ^{99m}Tc stress sestamibi SPECT images, the stress normal limits that have been developed for rest–stress ^{99m}Tc sestamibi imaging[48] are directly applicable without modification to the dual-isotope procedure. However, separate normal limits for the dual-isotope procedure are required for assessment of defect reversibility. Commercially available normal limits (Cedars–Emory quantitative analysis) for assessment of defect reversibility for rest ^{201}Tl–stress ^{99m}Tc sestamibi dual-isotope SPECT have recently been developed.[8,28] To determine whether quantitative same-day rest–stress sestamibi SPECT is applicable to dual-isotope myocardial perfusion SPECT, Kiat et

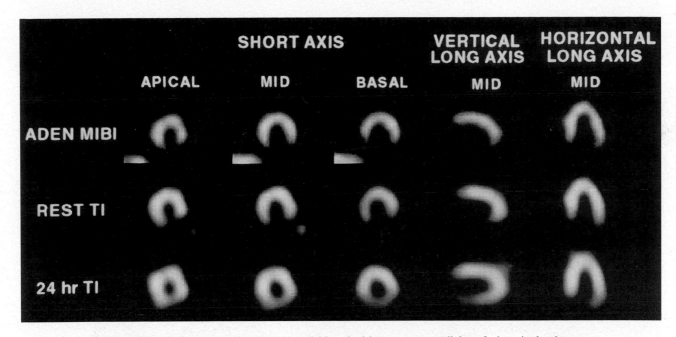

Fig. 17-9. Case example of separate acquisition dual-isotope myocardial perfusion single-photon emission computed tomography showing adenosine sestamibi stress studies *(top row)*, rest thallium-201 studies *(middle row)*, and 24-hour redistribution thallium-201 studies following a rest injection *(bottom row)*. The stress–rest studies alone demonstrated a nonreversible defect in the inferior left ventricular wall. On 24-hour redistribution imaging, however, the inferior wall defect was seen to be clearly reversible. ADEN = adenosine.

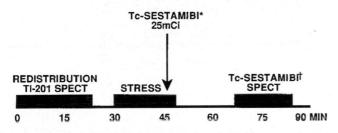

Fig. 17-10. Injection of thallium-201 the night before stress protocol for separate acquisition dual-isotope myocardial perfusion single-photon emission computed tomography (SPECT) that is used in patients after myocardial infarction. * = Peak stress first-pass study is optional; † = gated SPECT is optional.

al[29] studied 60 male patients using sex-specific normal limits for rest–stress sestamibi and dual-isotope myocardial perfusion SPECT[27] (Fig. 17-11, *A, B, C*). Quantitative rest–stress sestamibi significantly and systematically overestimated defect reversibility. The differences in assessment of stress defect extent and severity, however, were minimal. In a series of 67 patients undergoing quantitative dual-isotope myocardial perfusion SPECT, Kiat et al.[28] preliminarily validated these limits by demonstrating high correlations of the quantitative assessment of the extent, severity, and reversibility of the stress defect with expert visual analysis. Dual-isotope images acquired separately from a patient with combined reversible and nonreversible defects and results of quantitative analysis using the standard rest–stress ^{99m}Tc sestamibi limits and special dual-isotope normal limits are shown in Fig. 17-12, *A, B, C*. By using the

rest–stress ^{99m}Tc sestamibi limits for quantitative analysis of the dual-isotope studies, a defect reversibility is systematically overestimated.

Image quality

A study of 170 patients[10] showed that image quality tends to be good to excellent in most dual-isotope studies. The images were considered to be poor in only 2% of studies, all of which were rest ^{201}Tl images. The minor differences in image quality noted between ^{99m}Tc sestamibi and ^{201}Tl studies with dual-isotope SPECT have not been proven to be clinically significant, providing adequate doses and acquisition times are used.

Although differences in image quality between stress ^{99m}Tc sestamibi and rest ^{201}Tl SPECT could be a source of criticism of the dual-isotope technique, several factors reduce the importance of this difference. The difference in image resolution with the two radionuclides is minimized by the use of high-resolution collimation for both ^{99m}Tc sestamibi and ^{201}Tl SPECT acquisitions. The total myocardial counts in the rest ^{201}Tl SPECT studies are similar to those seen in the rest segment of low-dose–high-dose same-day ^{99m}Tc sestamibi SPECT.[48] Furthermore, the use of different isotopes to evaluate different myocardial characteristics is common and is not limited to the comparison of ^{99m}Tc sestamibi with ^{201}Tl. In myocardial positron emission tomography (PET), for example, perfusion studies are sometimes performed using rubidium-82 (maximum positron energy, 3.35 MeV; range, 2.6 mm full width half maximum [FWHM]), whereas viability studies use fluorine-18 fluorodeoxyglucose (maximum positron energy, 0.63 MeV; range,

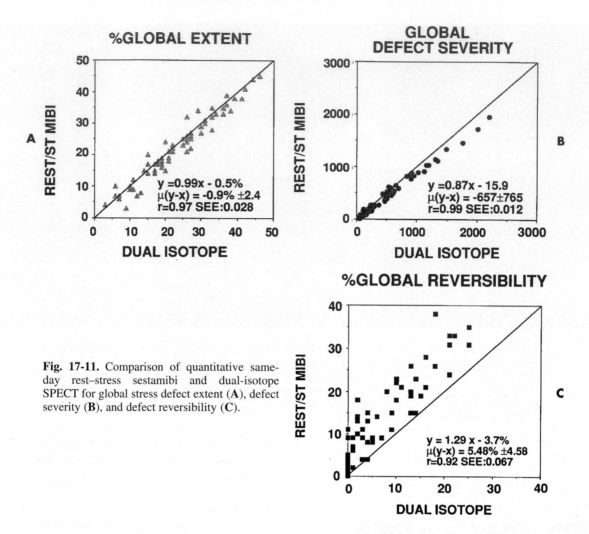

Fig. 17-11. Comparison of quantitative same-day rest–stress sestamibi and dual-isotope SPECT for global stress defect extent (**A**), defect severity (**B**), and defect reversibility (**C**).

0.22 mm FWHM). Images acquired by using these two agents show strikingly different resolution, more so than ^{99m}Tc and ^{201}Tl images; however, even in an inherently quantitative environment, such as PET, no attempt is made to equalize reconstructed resolution of the perfusion and viability image sets. The use of separate acquisition dual-isotope protocols to assess different physiologic processes is ubiquitous in nuclear medicine. For example, ventilation–perfusion imaging with xenon-133 gas and ^{99m}Tc-labeled particles is one of the most commonly performed procedures. Even in laboratories that use sestamibi rest stress studies as a routine, follow-up ^{201}Tl studies are often done when viability remains a question. This application necessitates the comparison of different radionuclides for assessment of a given myocardial region.

ASSESSMENT OF PROGNOSIS

Recently, the prognostic implications of dual-isotope SPECT have been extensively validated. To optimally determine the level of patient risk from the extent and severity of perfusion abnormalities, a series of combined variables were derived by using a 5-point scoring system (0 = normal, 1 = equivocal, 2 = moderate, 3 = severe reduction of isotope uptake, and 4 = absence of detectable tracer uptake in a segment) and a 20-segment model (Fig. 17-13). The summed stress score reflects the extent and severity of stress perfusion defects. Stress–rest differences indicate the degree of reversibility which is measured by the *summed difference score*.[10] The results of nuclear testing are divided into four categories on the basis of the summed stress score: normal (0 to 3), mildly abnormal (4 to 8), moderately abnormal (9 to 13), and severely abnormal (>13) scans. By using the dual-isotope protocol, Berman et al.[9] found that in patients with normal scans, the cardiac event rate (nonfatal myocardial infarction or cardiac death) over a 20-month follow-up period was low (<1% per year) regardless of the prescan likelihood of coronary disease. In addition, patients with a low and intermediate prescan risk were significantly stratified by the results of perfusion scanning in a cost-efficient manner.

Sex-related differences in prognosis with this protocol were evaluated by Hachamovitch et al.[20] The combination of clinical, exercise, and nuclear variables yielded incremental prognostic information both in women and men. Of interest, nuclear

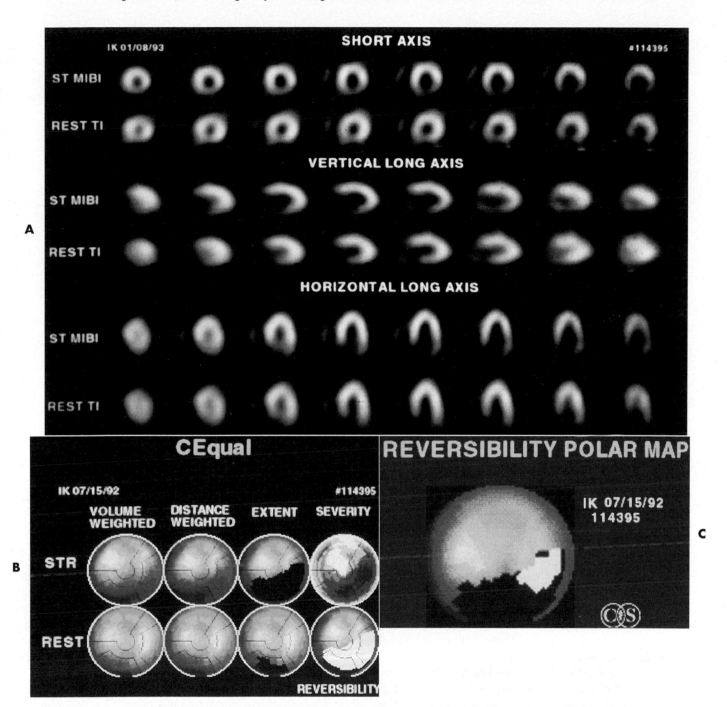

Fig. 17-12. A, A case example of separate acquisition dual-isotope myocardial perfusion single-photon emission computed tomography demonstrating a small reversible defect in the inferolateral wall and a nonreversible defect in the inferior left ventricular wall. **B,** Cedars–Emory quantitative analysis *(CEqual)* quantitation using the standard normal limits of same-day rest–stress technetium-99m sestamibi demonstrates close correspondence to the visual abnormalities with respect to the extent of the stress defect but a lack of correspondence in defect reversibility. **C,** The reversibility in polar map using special dual-isotope normal limits is shown. This map shows the small reversible component and the larger nonreversible component, which accurately represents the visual findings in this patient.

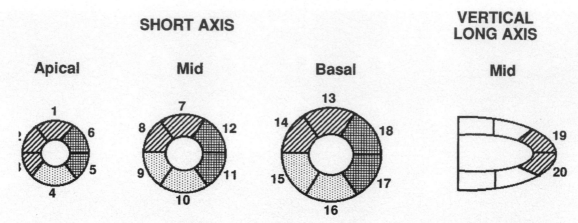

Fig. 17-13. Assignment of myocardial regions for scoring of single-photon emission computed tomographic images. Usually, scans with multiple segments scored as having stress–rest scores of 0 or 1 or a single segment with a stress score of 2 were classified as equivocal. Scans with 2 segments assigned stress scores of 2 were classified as probably abnormal, and scans containing 2 or more stress segments assigned scores of 2 or scans with one or more segments assigned scores of 3 were classified as definitely abnormal. Assignment of segmental scores took into account knowledge of normal segment variation. Reversibility of segmental scores influenced the interpretation toward abnormal. When fixed defects on the stress study were considered to be secondary to attenuation, their score was decreased to 1. If apparent apical defects were considered likely to represent normal apical thinning or if defects were considered to be secondary to breast attenuation, they were assigned a score of 1. On the basis of these scoring guidelines, the observers judged each patient's study as normal, probably normal, equivocal, probably abnormal, or definitely abnormal in a reading blinded to the patients' clinical, historical, and exercise treadmill information. The observers were then made aware of the patients' other relevant nonnuclear information and formed a final interpretation of the study (scan result), which by agreement among observers could not vary by more than 1 grade from the initial interpretation.

information added substantially more information in women than in men, the first demonstration of the superiority of a non-invasive test in women compared with men. Furthermore, the study showed that women were risk stratified more efficiently than men, suggesting the potential for a more cost-efficient strategy in women using dual-isotope SPECT.

Our group also evaluated this protocol in a large series of patients without known coronary artery disease.[4,22] Dual-isotope SPECT significantly stratified this population and added substantial incremental prognostic value over clinical, historical, and exercise treadmill data alone.[22] Of more clinical importance, dual-isotope myocardial perfusion SPECT significantly stratified patients who had low-intermediate and high Duke treadmill scores (Fig. 17-14). Patients with a low Duke treadmill score had a hard event rate of less than 1%; those with intermediate scores had an event rate of 2.5%; and those with high scores had an event rate of 7.7%. Patients with an intermediate Duke treadmill score constituted more than half of our study population; because 70% of this group had normal results on nuclear testing, they were considered to be at low risk and do not need further intervention. The remaining patients with moderate or severely abnormal myocardial perfusion scans were at greatly increased risk for adverse events. Thus, the nuclear tests were able to stratify patients who could not be differentiated according to risk by Duke treadmill score alone. This study also documented that a dual-isotope scan result con-

tributed 95% of the information about referral to catheterization. Importantly, of these 1624 patients (74%) in this study with normal scan results, only 23 (1%) were referred to early catheterization (less than 60 days after testing).

A recent large patient series (more than 5000 patients) revealed that the scan threshold for abnormality may vary with the prognostic end point used. Confirming the work of Berman et al[11] patients with normal scan results were at low risk for subsequent myocardial infarction and cardiac death. Also, as demonstrated before, patients with moderately and severely abnormal scans were at intermediate risk for both cardiac death and myocardial infarction. The new finding was that patients with mildly abnormal results on their scans were at intermediate risk for myocardial infarction (2.7% risk for myocardial infarction per 1 year of follow-up) but were at low risk for subsequent cardiac mortality (0.8% cardiac death rate per 1 year of follow-up). On the basis of these data, it would appear that it may be possible in the future to treat patients with normal and mildly abnormal scans with medical therapy alone, a method previously shown to reduce the risk of myocardial infarction (for example, lipid lowering agents, aspirin, angiotensin-converting enzyme inhibitors, and β-blockers) instead of referring them directly to catheterization and possible subsequent revascularization.

Substantial preliminary data using this protocol suggest that the prognostic results obtained in general patient populations

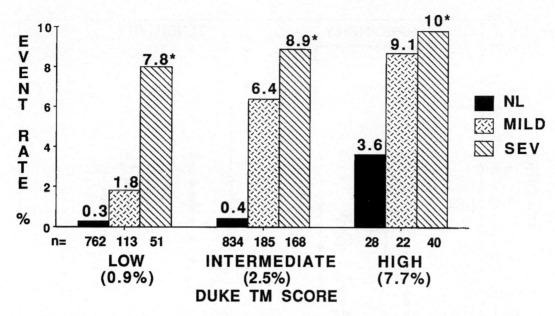

Fig. 17-14. Duke treadmill *(TM)* score category and scan results compared with the hard event rate (myocardial infarction or cardiac death). Rates of hard events over the follow-up period are given for patients in low, intermediate, and high Duke treadmill score categories with normal *(NL)*, mildly abnormal *(MILD)*, and severely abnormal *(SEV)* scans. The figures in parentheses under Duke Treadmill subgroups show hard event rate in these groups. * = $p<0.05$ across scan results.

(detailed above) are also present when specific patient subgroups are examined. The prognostic implications of this protocol have been assessed in women,[5,20] patients with left ventricular hypertrophy,[1] patients with previous coronary artery bypass surgery,[21] elderly patients,[3,23] and patients without known coronary artery disease.[4,22]

ADVANTAGES OF THE SEPARATE DUAL-ISOTOPE APPROACH

Standard ^{201}Tl redistribution and same-day or two-day rest–stress ^{99m}Tc sestamibi protocols are time-consuming. The separate dual-isotope acquisition protocol is briefer than the standard ^{201}Tl or ^{99m}Tc sestamibi protocols; it can be completed in approximately 2 hours. The protocol also permits the performance of more patient studies per camera or computer system per day. More rapid completion of studies is appreciated as an advantage by patients, technologists, interpreting and referring physicians, nurses, and hospital administration personnel. Because of resting background radioactivity, same-day rest–stress ^{99m}Tc protocols have a disadvantage compared with 2-day sestamibi protocols of potential reduction of defect severity. The separate acquisition dual-isotope SPECT procedure described minimizes this contrast reduction. Because of the low abundance of high-energy ^{201}Tl photons, which scatter into the ^{99m}Tc window, the contribution of ^{201}Tl scatter to the ^{99m}Tc sestamibi images at the doses used is only 2.9%.[31] Perhaps most important, because ^{201}Tl redistributes more than ^{99m}Tc sestamibi, the dual-isotope approach may be more effective for assessment of myocardial viability than pure sestamibi studies through the use of ^{201}Tl redistribution imaging,

either before the ^{99m}Tc sestamibi injection or 24 to 48 hours later.

Myocardial perfusion imaging is also of use in some patients with unstable angina. Whereas high risk patients should undergo coronary angiography, low to intermediate risk patients can undergo stress myocardial perfusion imaging after medical stabilization with no recurrent chest pain for 48 hours.[15] Predischarge stress ^{99m}Tc sestamibi SPECT provides additional risk stratification as well as quantification of the amount of myocardium at risk.[43,44] The advantage of the separate acquisition dual-isotope rest ^{201}Tl–stress ^{99m}Tc sestamibi SPECT protocol compared to a stress–rest protocol is that the rest ^{201}Tl image can be evaluated prior to performing the stress test. When the rest ^{201}Tl SPECT image shows an unexpected defect in a patient with no history of myocardial infarction and no Q waves on ECG, unnecessary stress imaging can be avoided, and rest–redistribution ^{201}Tl imaging can be performed instead to evaluate defect reversibility.

Another clinically useful application of rest ^{201}Tl–stress ^{99m}Tc sestamibi dual-isotope SPECT occurs in patients with acute chest pain being evaluated for possible acute ischemic syndrome. Ziffer et al. have reported high accuracy as well as cost effectiveness of a protocol which substitutes ^{201}Tl at rest for ^{99m}Tc sestamibi in patients whose acute chest pain has resolved by the time of injection.[52,53] If a perfusion defect is present in a patient with no prior myocardial infarction, an acute ischemic syndrome is likely as it would be with ^{99m}Tc sestamibi imaging. Redistribution imaging may be useful in this setting. In patients in whom no perfusion defect is noted on the rest thallium injected following resolution of chest pain, stress

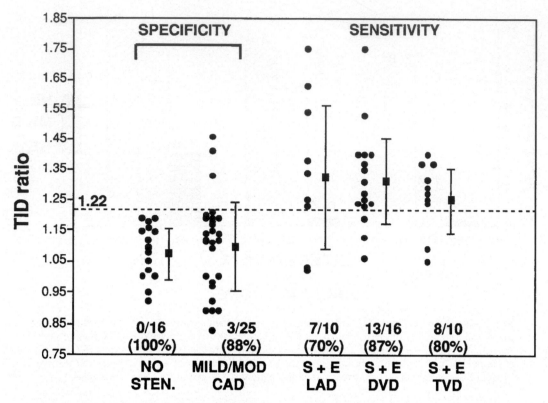

Fig. 17-15. Relation between the transient ischemic dilation ratio and presence, extent, and severity of coronary artery disease. TID = transient ischemic dilation; STEN = stenosis; MILD/MOD = mild/moderate disease; CAD = coronary artery disease; S + E = severe and extensive disease; DVD = double-vessel disease; TVD = triple-vessel disease. (Adapted from Kiat H, Biasio Y, Wong FP, et al: Frequency of reversible resting hypoperfusion in patients undergoing rest T1-201/stress Tc-sestamibi separate acquisition on dual-isotope myocardial perfusion SPECT, *J Am Coll Cardiol* 21:222A, 1993. With permission of the American College of Cardiology.)

^{99m}Tc sestamibi imaging can be immediately performed to virtually exclude coronary disease as a source of the patient's acute chest pain.

ASSESSMENT OF PERFUSION AND FUNCTION

As with any high-dose sestamibi studies, gated SPECT or first-pass radionuclide angiography can be added to the dual-isotope procedure (Fig. 17-2 and Fig. 17-6). Gated SPECT can easily be performed in this protocol and facilitates the identification of attenuation artifacts as a region with fixed defect that moves and thickens normally. In addition, post-stress resting left ventricular ejection fraction can be assessed in this protocol by using automatic computer software.[17] This assessment of ejection fraction may add prognostic value to perfusion SPECT in certain patient subsets.[36] The processing of quantitative left ventricular volumes can also be applied to standard (nongated) rest and stress SPECT images, and volume estimates can be extracted for computation of the transient ischemic dilation ratio. Mazzanti et al,[38] using the dual-isotope protocol, showed that this ratio is moderately sensitive and highly specific for identifying patients with severe and extensive coronary artery disease[38] (Fig. 17-15). A case example of a patient with severe proximal left anterior descending coronary artery stenosis and

transient ischemic dilatation of the left ventricle is shown in Fig. 17-16. Use of ^{99m}Tc sestamibi also allows performance of an exercise first-pass study of ventricular function. This information has been shown to add incremental prognostic value over that provided by dual-isotope SPECT alone.[19] This study also showed that a normal first-pass study may be prognostically equivalent to a normal SPECT study.

COST CONSIDERATIONS

Given the current need for cost containment in medicine, the potential of increased cost due to the use of two radiopharmaceuticals merits discussion. If only supply costs and current prices of these agents are considered, pure ^{201}Tl protocols provide the least expensive approach. If ^{99m}Tc sestamibi is used, it is purchased from the manufacturer or a radiopharmacy. The comparative costs of the radiopharmaceuticals for rest–stress ^{99m}Tc sestamibi and dual-isotope studies are illustrated in Table 17-4. The manufacturer currently charges $300 per vial or a minimum of $50 per dose of ^{99m}Tc sestamibi. Thallium-201 is available at a cost of approximately $50 to $80 per 3-mCi dose, depending on the volume used by the laboratory. In laboratories performing six or more studies a day, therefore, the supply cost for the dual-isotope

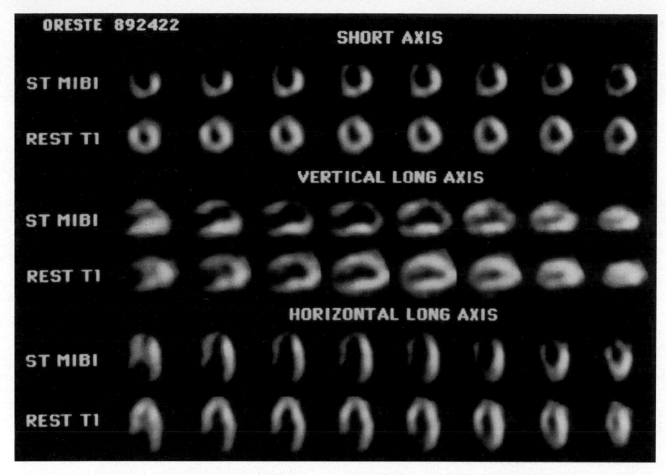

Fig. 17-16. Case example of an abnormal separate acquisition dual-isotope stress study demonstrating a reversible defect in the anterior septal and apical regions. The findings are consistent with severe proximal left anterior descending coronary artery disease. Note the transient dilatation of the left ventricle during stress. ST MIBI = Stress technetium-99m sestamibi; Tl = thallium-201.

Table 17-4. Comparative radiopharmaceutical costs for technetium-99m sestamibi and dual-isotope procedures

Type of procedure	Manufacturer's pricing by number of patients studied per day*					Radiopharmacy pricing by number of patients studied per day†				
	2	3	4	5	6	2	3	4	5	6
	$/patient study					*$/patient study*				
Rest–stress ^{99m}Tc sestamibi	150	100	100	100	100	180	170	160	145	135
Rest ^{201}Tl–stress ^{99m}Tc sestamibi (A)	200	150	125	110	100	155	155	155	150	145
Rest ^{201}Tl–stress ^{99m}Tc sestamibi (B)	230	180	155	140	130	170	170	170	165	160

*DuPont Pharma, April 1993: technetium-99m sestamibi = $300 per vial or $50 per dose if more than 6 doses per vial; thallium-201 = $50 per 3 mCi (A); $80 per 3 mCi (B).
†Syncor, April 1993

Sliding scale	
Doses per month	**Cost per dose, $**
0–90	90
90–125	85
126–175	80
176–240	72.50
>240	67.50

Thallium-201: $65 per 3 mCi (A), $80 per 3 mCi (B)

procedure approach equals that for the rest–stress ^{99m}Tc sestamibi study if the lower ^{201}Tl price is available. Smaller numbers of patient studies or incremental increases in ^{201}Tl pricing would increase the supply cost per procedure. When using a radiopharmacy distributor, the supply costs for the dual-isotope approach are similar to those for the rest–stress ^{99m}Tc sestamibi technique, even at low volumes.

In assessing the impact of using the dual-isotope procedure on the economics of health care, more than radiopharmaceutical costs must be considered. In view of the increased efficiency and throughput of the procedure, modest increases in radiopharmaceutical cost can be balanced by increased productivity; more efficient utilization of equipment and physical plant; and, potentially, a decrease in overtime costs. Furthermore, in assessing overall benefits, the additional value provided by higher quality images, the potential for adding first-pass or gated SPECT studies of ventricular function, and improved viability information should be considered.

CLINICAL IMPLICATIONS

Separate acquisition dual-isotope SPECT with rest ^{201}Tl and stress ^{99m}Tc sestamibi represents a simple, efficient technique. Because of the ease of implementation, the practical advantages provided by its use, and its potential superiority in assessing myocardial viability, we currently consider separate acquisition rest ^{201}Tl–stress ^{99m}Tc sestamibi dual-isotope myocardial perfusion SPECT to be one of the protocols of choice for ^{99m}Tc sestamibi SPECT when combined assessment of stress myocardial perfusion and myocardial viability is desired.

REFERENCES

1. Amanullah AM, Berman DS, Friedman JD, et al: Enhanced prognostic stratification of patients with left ventricular hypertrophy using myocardial perfusion imaging, *Circulation* 94:I-445, 1996 (abstract).
2. Amanullah AM, Berman DS, Kiat H, et al: Usefulness of hemodynamic changes during adenosine infusion in predicting the diagnostic accuracy of adenosine ^{99m}Tc sestamibi SPECT, *Am J Cardiol* 79:1319–1322, 1997.
3. Amanullah AM, Hachamovitch R, Erel J, et al: Prognostic value of exercise and adenosine myocardial perfusion SPECT in the very elderly, *J Am Coll Cardiol* 29:228A, 1997 (abstract).
4. Amanullah AM, Hachamovitch R, Friedman JD, et al: Adenosine SPECT in patients without known coronary artery disease: prediction of cardiac events and test utilization, *J Am Coll Cardiol* 29:362A, 1997 (abstract).
5. Amanullah AM, Berman DS, Erel J, et al: Incremental prognostic value of adenosine myocardial perfusion imaging in women, *Am J Cardiol* 1998 (abstract).
6. Amanullah AM, Kiat H, Friedman JD, et al: Adenosine technetium-99m sestamibi myocardial perfusion SPECT in women: diagnostic efficacy in detection of coronary artery disease, *J Am Coll Cardiol* 27:803–809, 1996.
7. Amanullah AM, Kiat H, Raina A, et al: Exercise Tc-99m sestamibi SPECT for detection and localization of coexistent coronary artery disease in patients with left ventricular hypertrophy, *J Nucl Med* 37:182P, 1996.
8. Areeda J, Van Train K, Kiat H, et al: Quantitative assessment of reversibility for rest Tl-201-stress Tc-99m sestamibi separate acquisition dual-isotope myocardial perfusion SPECT: development and prospective validation, *J Nucl Med* 34:64P, 1993.
9. Berman DS, Hachamovitch R, Kiat H, et al: Incremental value of prognostic testing in patients with known or suspected ischemic heart disease: a basis for optimal utilization of exercise technetium-99m sestamibi myocardial perfusion single-photon emission computed tomography, *J Am Coll Cardiol* 26:639–647, 1995.
10. Berman DS, Kiat H, Friedman JD, et al: Separate acquisition rest thallium-201/stress technetium-99m sestamibi dual-isotope myocardial perfusion single-photon emission computed tomography: a clinical validation study, *J Am Coll Cardiol* 22:1455–1464, 1993.
11. Berman DS, Kiat H, Hachamovitch R, et al: Prediction of cardiac mortality in 5125 patients using stress technetium-99m myocardial perfusion SPECT, *J Am Coll Cardiol* 27:285A, 1996.
12. Berman DS, Kiat H, Maddahi J: The new ^{99m}Tc myocardial perfusion imaging agents: ^{99m}Tc-sestamibi and ^{99m}Tc-teboroxime, *Circulation* 84:I17–I21, 1991.
13. Berman DS, Kiat H, Van Train K, et al: Technetium 99m sestamibi in the assessment of chronic coronary artery disease, *Semin Nucl Med* 21:190–212, 1991.
14. Berman DS, Kiat HS, Van Train KF, et al: Myocardial perfusion imaging with technetium-99m-sestamibi: comparative analysis of available protocols, *J Nucl Med* 35:681–688, 1994.
15. Braunwald E, Mark DB, Jones RH, et al: Unstable angina: diagnosis and management, Clinical Practice Guidelines Number 10, AHCPR Publication 94-0602, Rockville, Md. 1994.
16. Friedman J, Van Train K, Kiat H, et al: Simultaneous dual-isotope rest/stress myocardial perfusion scintigraphy: a feasibility study, *J Am Coll Cardiol* 17:390A, 1991.
17. Germano G, Kiat H, Kavanagh PB, et al: Automatic quantification of ejection fraction from gated myocardial perfusion SPECT, *J Nucl Med* 36:2138–2147, 1995.
18. Gutman J, Berman DS, Freeman M, et al: Time to completed redistribution of thallium-201 in exercise myocardial scintigraphy: relationship to the degree of coronary artery stenosis, *Am Heart J* 106:989–995, 1983.
19. Hachamovitch R, Benari B, Kiat H, et al: Exercise first pass adds additional prognostic information in patients with abnormal Tc-99m myocardial perfusion SPECT, *Circulation* 90:I–10, 1994 (abstract).
20. Hachamovitch R, Berman DS, Kiat H, et al: Gender-related differences in clinical management after exercise nuclear testing, *J Am Coll Cardiol* 26:1457–1464, 1995.
21. Hachamovitch R, Berman DS, Kiat H, et al: The evaluation of patients more than five years after coronary bypass surgery: potential cost savings of a nuclear exercise testing approach, *J Nucl Med* 36:13P, 1995.
22. Hachamovitch R, Berman DS, Kiat H, et al: Exercise myocardial perfusion SPECT in patients without known coronary artery disease: incremental prognostic value and use in risk stratification, *Circulation* 93:905–914, 1996.
23. Hachamovitch R, Diamond GA, Kiat H, et al: Noninvasive risk stratification of the elderly patient: use of nuclear testing to identify high-risk patient populations, *Circulation* 90:I–102, 1994 (abstract).
24. Hayes SW, Dhar SC, Cordero H, et al: First-pass radionuclide angiography adds incremental value to adenosine low level treadmill exercise Tc-99m sestamibi SPECT for detecting multivessel coronary artery disease, *J Nucl Med* 39:102P, 1998.
25. Hayes SW, Dhar SC, Hsu P, et al: Improved prognostic discrimination by prone imaging in patients with inferior wall defects on supine SPECT imaging, *J Nucl Med* 39:154P, 1998.
26. Iskandrian AS, Heo J, Kong B. et al: Use of technetium-99m isonitrile (RP-30A) in assessing left ventricular perfusion and function at rest and during exercise in coronary artery disease, and comparison with coronary arteriography and exercise thallium-201 SPECT imaging, *Am J Cardiol* 64:270–275, 1989.
27. Kahn JK, McGhie I, Akers MS, et al: Quantitative rotational tomog-

raphy with ^{201}Tl and [99m]Tc 2-methoxy-isobutyl-isonitrile. A direct comparison in normal individuals and patients with coronary artery disease, *Circulation* 79:1282–1293, 1989.

28. Kiat H, Areeda J, Van Train K, et al: Quantitative assessment of stress defect extent and reversibility on rest Tl-201/stress Tc-99m sestamibi dual-isotope myocardial perfusion SPECT: a prospective validation, *Circulation* 88:I–440, 1993 (abstract).

29. Kiat H, Areeda J, Van Train K, et al: Applicability of quantitative same-day rest/stress Tc-99m sestamibi limits to separate acquisition dual isotope myocardial perfusion SPECT, *J Nucl Med* 35:103P, 1994.

30. Kiat H, Biasio Y, Wong FP, et al: Frequency of reversible resting hypoperfusion in patients undergoing rest Tl-201/stress Tc-sestamibi separate acquisition dual-isotope myocardial perfusion SPECT, *J Am Coll Cardiol* 21:222A, 1993.

31. Kiat H, Germano G, Friedman JD, et al: Comparative feasibility of separate or simultaneous rest thallium-201/stress technetium-99m-sestamibi dual isotope myocardial perfusion SPECT, *J Nucl Med* 35:542–548, 1994.

32. Kiat H, Germano G, William C, et al: Comparison of rest Tl-201 myocardial perfusion patterns before and after exercise: a prelude to the validation of simultaneous rest Tl-201/stress Tc-99m sestamibi dual isotope SPECT, *J Nucl Cardiol* 2:P03–070, 1995.

33. Kiat H, Van Train KF, Friedman JD, et al: Quantitative stress-redistribution thallium-201 SPECT using prone imaging: methodologic development and validation, *J Nucl Med* 33:1509–1515, 1992.

34. Kiat H, Van Train K, Maddahi J, et al: Development and prospective application of quantitative 2-day stress-rest Tc-99m methoxy isobutyl isonitrile SPECT for the diagnosis of coronary artery disease, *Am Heart J* 120:1255–1266, 1990.

35. Maddahi J, Rodrigues E, Berman DS: *Assessment of myocardial perfusion by single-photon agents.* In: Pohost GM, O'Rourke RA, eds, *Principles and practices of cardiovascular imaging,* Boston 1991, Little, Brown.

36. Mahmarian JJ, Mahmarian AC, Marks GF, et al: Role of adenosine thallium-201 tomography for defining long-term risk in patients after acute myocardial infarction, *J Am Coll Cardiol* 25:1333–1340, 1995.

37. Matzer L, Kiat H, Wang FP, et al: Pharmacologic stress dual-isotope myocardial perfusion single-photon emission computed tomography, *Am Heart J* 128:1067–1076, 1994.

38. Mazzanti M, Germano G, Kiat H, et al: Identification of severe and extensive coronary artery disease by automatic measurement of transient ischemic dilatation of the left ventricle in dual-isotope myocardial perfusion SPECT, *J Am Coll Cardiol* 27:1612–1620, 1996.

38a. Parikh A, Kiat H, Kang X, et al: Addition of low-level treadmill exercise to adenosine stress Tc-99m sestamibi myocardial perfusion SPECT allows for early post-stress imaging, *J Nucl Med* 37:59P, 1996.

39. Pennell DJ, Mavrogeni SI, Forbat SM, et al: Adenosoine combined with dynamic exercise for myocardial perfusion imaging, *J Am Coll Cardiol* 25:1300–1309, 1995.

40. Rozanski A, Berman DS: The efficacy of cardiovascular nuclear medicine exercise studies, *Semin Nucl Med* 17:104–120, 1987.

41. Rozanski A, Diamond GA, Berman DS, et al: The declining specificity of exercise radionuclide ventriculography, *N Engl J Med* 309:518–522, 1983.

41a. Segall GM, Davis MJ: Prone versus supine thallium myocardial SPECT: A method to decrease artifactual inferior wall defects, *J Nucl Med* 30:548–555, 1998.

42. Smith WH, Watson DD: Technical aspects of myocardial planar imaging with technetium-99m sestamibi, *Am J Cardiol* 66:16E–22E, 1990.

43. Stratmann HG, Tamesis BR, Younis LT, et al: Prognostic value of predischarge dipyridamole technetium 99m sestamibi myocardial tomography in medically treated patients with unstable angina. *Am Heart J* 130:734–740, 1995.

44. Stratmann HG, Younis LT, Wittry MD, et al: Exercise technetium-99m myocardial tomography for the risk stratification of medically treated patients with unstable angina pectoris. *Am J Cardiol* 76:236–240, 1995.

45. Taillefer R, Primeau M, Costi P, et al: Technetium-99m-sestamibi myo-cardial perfusion imaging in detection of coronary artery disease: comparison between initial (1-hour) and delayed (3-hour) postexercise images, *J Nucl Med* 32:1961–1965, 1991.

46. Takahashi N, Tamaki N, Tadamura E, et al: Combined assessment of regional perfusion and wall motion in patients with coronary artery disease with technetium 99m tetrofosmin, *J Nucl Cardiol* 1:29–38, 1994.

47. Van Train KF, Areeda J, Garcia EV, et al: Quantitation of same-day technetium-99m-sestamibi myocardial SPECT: multicenter trial validation, *J Nucl Med* 33:876, 1992 (abstract).

48. Van Train KF, Areeda J, Garcia EV, et al: Quantitative same-day rest-stress technetium-99m-sestamibi SPECT: definition and validation of normal limits and criteria for abnormality, *J Nucl Med* 34:1494–1502, 1993.

49. Van Train KF, Maddahi J, Berman DS, et al: Quantitative analysis of tomographic stress thallium-201 myocardial scintigrams: a multicenter trial, *J Nucl Med* 31:1168–1179, 1990.

50. Wang FP, Amanullah AM, Kiat H, et al: Diagnostic efficacy of stress technetium 99m-labeled sestamibi myocardial perfusion single-photon emission computed tomography in detection of coronary artery disease among patients over age 80, *J Nucl Cardiol* 2:380–388, 1995.

51. Watson DD, Smith WH, Glover DK, et al: Dual-isotope SPECT imaging of Tc-99m sestamibi and Tl201: comparing myocardial defect magnitudes. *Circulation* 84:II–314, 1991 (abstract).

52. Ziffer JA, Nateman DR, Janowitz WR, et al: Improved patient outcomes and cost effectiveness of utilizing nuclear cardiology protocols in an emergency department chest pain center: two year results in 6,548 patients, *J Nucl Med* 39:139P, 1998.

53. Ziffer JA, Nateman DR, Janowitz WR, et al: The role of stress imaging subsequent to rest imaging in patients presenting to an emergency department with resolved, acute chest pain, *J Nucl Med* 39:140P, 1998.

Chapter 18

Detection of coronary artery disease in women

Gary V. Heller and **Andrea T. Fossati**

THE SIGNIFICANCE OF HEART DISEASE IN WOMEN

Cardiovascular disease is recognized as the leading cause of death in men and women in the United States, with similar morbidity and mortality in both sexes. The published mortality data support this observation: Deaths in women accounted for 52% of all cardiovascular deaths, or a total of almost 480,000 women in 1992.[2] Each year more women die of cardiovascular disease than of all cancers combined (Fig. 18-1). Coronary artery disease remains the primary cause of death among women in the United States, resulting in over 250,000 deaths per year (roughly 28% of all deaths).[26] Despite the similarities in mortality in both sexes, a substantial number of gender-related differences in cardiac disease present unique challenges to the detection of heart disease in women.

The profile of women with heart disease

Several classic studies detailed the differences in the presentation of heart disease between women and men. The Framingham Study data revealed that women present with their first anginal symptoms 10 years later and sustain their first myocardial infarction 20 years later than their male counterparts.[32] Castelli[5] demonstrated an age-related increase in the incidence of coronary artery disease in women, with a similar incidence in postmenopausal women and in men[5] (Fig. 18-2). This increase is gradual and does not change abruptly at the onset of menopause. By the age of 75, the rates for coronary morbidity and mortality are similar in men and women.[37]

Women and men share the major cardiac risk factors of hypertension, diabetes, high cholesterol levels, smoking, and family history; however, their risk factor profiles differ. In women, the risk of hypertension is lower at an early age, but by age 55, the prevalence is essentially the same as that of men, and by age 75, the prevalence is higher than that in men.[2] Diabetes is more prevalent in women at all ages, and several studies have found that it imparts a twofold higher risk of heart disease in women compared with men.[46,59] The lipid profiles of women generally remain favorable before menopause; however, after menopause levels of both low-density and total cholesterol are higher than those in men in a similar age group.[59] Obesity and physical inactivity have each been independently associated with an increased risk for heart disease in women.[13,46] In general, women have more risk factors and comorbid conditions associated with the initial presentation of heart disease.

Estrogen plays cardioprotective role in women in the prevention of coronary artery disease. Recent nonrandomized trials[13] have shown risk reduction of 50% in postmenopausal women receiving estrogen replacement therapy. The beneficial effect of estrogen on lipid profiles have been described, as have several other theories about the possible mechanisms by which estrogen imparts a cardioprotective effect.[13] The gradual age-related increase in coronary disease without an abrupt change at menopause may be viewed as support of estrogen's protective role, because menopause represents the result of a gradual

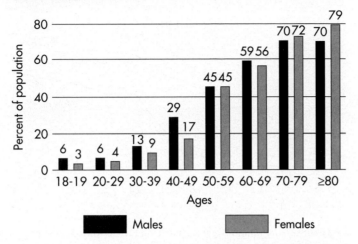

Estimated Prevalence of Cardiovascular Diseases by Age and Sex
United States: 1988–91

Source: Unpublished data from the National Health and Nutrition
Examination Survey III (NHANES III), 1988–91, National Center
for Health Statistics and the American Heart Association.

Fig. 18-1. Leading causes of death for men and women in the United States: 1995 Mortality Final Data. (From National Center for Health Statistics and the American Heart Association.)

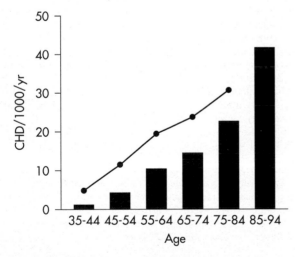

Fig. 18-2. Annual rate of coronary heart disease (CHD) in men (line) and women (bars) from the Framingham Heart Study. (From Castelli WP: *Am J Obstet Gynecol* 158:1553-1560, 1988.)

rather than an abrupt loss of ovarian function over many years.[46] Despite the late appearance of coronary artery disease in women, the risk for disease in premenopausal women remains substantial and should not be disregarded, especially given an appropriate index of suspicion.

Gender-related differences in the outcomes of coronary artery disease

The Framingham Study was the first to demonstrate important gender differences in the rates of coronary events and their complications. Nonfatal myocardial infarction was a more common initial cardiac event in men than in women, although women were clearly shown to have a worse prognosis and higher mortality rate after infarction.[33,37] Women were found to have an early mortality rate (within 30 days post infarction) of 28% compared with 16% for men; this rate increased to 47% and 38% in women and men, respectively; if sudden cardiac death was included in the analysis.[33] The 1-year mortality rate after myocardial infarction was higher in women than men.[33]

Women have been found to have a higher rate of reinfarction within the first 5 years after myocardial infarction (39%) compared with men (13%), which contributes to the higher 1-year mortality rate in women.[33] This outcome may be related to the higher rate of non–Q-wave myocardial infarction found in women.[53] The Framingham Study also determined that a large portion of all infarctions in women were silent (34% compared with 27% in men).[37] Both men and women who sustained silent infarctions were found to have increased risk for subsequent cardiac failure, stroke, and death.[37] Heart failure after infarction has been found to occur more commonly in women than men despite better preservation of the systolic function in women, a

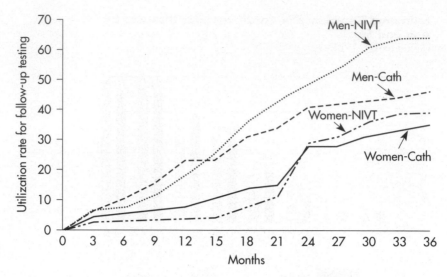

Fig. 18-3. A gender-based comparison of noninvasive test use rates over time. A greater percentage of men than women received follow-up noninvasive testing (NIVT) ($p < 0.001$). Similarly, a comparison of use of coronary arteriography during the 2-year follow-up period showed that a greater percentage of men than women subsequently had catheterization (Cath) ($p < 0.001$). (From Shaw LJ, Miller DD, Romeis JC, et al: *Ann Intern Med* 120:559-566, 1994.)

result that has been attributed to a higher incidence of diastolic dysfunction.[53] Overall, studies have concluded that the consequences of myocardial infarction are clinically more profound in women than in men.

Several studies demonstrated striking differences in the evaluation and management of suspected coronary artery disease in women and men. A retrospective analysis of patients enrolled in the Survival and Ventricular Enlargement (SAVE) Study showed a lower rate of referral for coronary catheterization in women (15%) than in men (27%), despite the greater functional limitations caused by anginal symptoms in women.[51] Women were referred later in the course of disease for catheterization and revascularization, although after cardiac catheterization, no sex difference in referral for surgical intervention was found. A lower rate of referral for diagnostic testing has been demonstrated in women with suspected coronary disease, despite positive results on exercise tests and dipyridamole thallium imaging similar to those in men[48] (Fig. 18-3). These findings were associated with a lower rate of revascularization and a higher rate of adverse outcomes in women than in men (Table 18-1). Although such data have determined that women are underserved in diagnostic studies, these findings have been challenged by more recent studies that found similar rates of referral in men and women after radionuclear stress imaging.[23,36,54]

Various gender-related differences have been demonstrated in the morbidity and mortality associated with revascularization. Women have been found to be older and to have more cardiovascular complications than men referred for revascularization.[60] Despite the lower incidence of previous myocardial infarction and multivessel coronary disease and better preservation of systolic function in women compared with men, stud-

Table 18–1. Cardiac death, nonfatal myocardial infarction, unstable angina, or revascularization procedure rates in patients referred for noninvasive testing*

Variable	Women (*n* = 391)	Men (*n* = 449)	*P* value
Cardiac death or myocardial infarction, *n (%)*	27 (3.5)	11 (1.2)	0.002
Cardiac death	9 (1.1)	3 (0.3)	0.05
Myocardial infarction	18 (2.3)	8 (0.9)	0.02
Total death, *n (%)*	18 (4.7)	14 (3.1)	0.26
Unstable angina, *n (%)*	8 (1.0)	4 (0.4)	0.16
Revascularization procedures, *n (%)*	8 (1.0)	22 (2.5)	0.03
PTCA	3 (0.4)	10 (1.1)	
CABS	5 (0.6)	12 (1.3)	

*Percentages represent annual cardiac event rates. CABS = coronary artery bypass surgery; total death = noncardiac and cardiac death; PTCA = percutaneous transluminal coronary angioplasty. Adapted from Shaw LJ, Miller DD, Romeis JC, et al: Gender differences in the noninvasive evaluation and management of patients with suspected coronary artery disease, *Ann Intern Med* 120:559-566, 1994.

ies have demonstrated a higher incidence of adverse outcomes related to coronary artery bypass surgery in women. This includes higher rates of perioperative mortality and congestive heart failure, although 5- and 10-year survival rates have been found to be similar in men and women.[60]

DIAGNOSING HEART DISEASE IN WOMEN

Several challenges exist in the detection of coronary artery disease in women. The diagnostic workup of women may be limited by physician and patient misperceptions about the risk

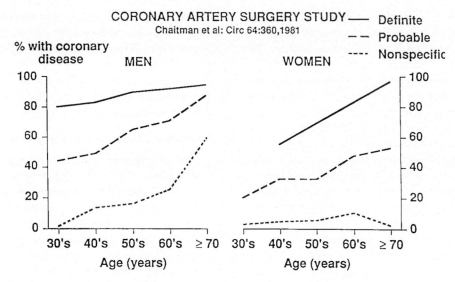

Fig. 18-4. Prevalence of coronary disease according to age, sex, and symptoms. (Adapted by D. Waters, MD, from Coronary Artery Surgery Study (CASS) data in Chaitman BR, Bowassa MG, Davis K, et al: *Circulation* 64:360–367, 1981.)

for coronary artery disease in women. The symptomatology of women with suspected coronary disease often differs from that of men and may result in a lower rate of referral for diagnostic evaluation. In addition, women are evaluated with diagnostic testing standards that are based on data in men.

The diagnostic value of clinical history

The complexity of chest pain syndromes observed in women makes the detection of coronary disease in women challenging. The Framingham Study was the first to characterize the diagnostic value of chest pain in men and women. Although a larger proportion of the women enrolled in the study presented with angina (65% compared with 37% of men), they sustained fewer myocardial infarctions during 5 years of follow-up (14% compared with 25% in men).[32,60] Initially, these data suggested that the course of coronary disease was less aggressive in women and that the presence of angina was associated with a better prognosis in women compared with men. Although this conclusion was challenged by later studies that correlated the clinical presentation of patients with angiographic findings, it contributed to longstanding misperceptions about the risk of coronary disease in women.

The largest randomized angiographic study, the Coronary Artery Surgery Study (CASS), found that 50% of the 2810 women compared with 17% of the men referred for coronary catheterization for evaluation of chest pain had no significant coronary obstruction.[35,60] In women classified as having definite angina, the prevalence of coronary disease (stenosis ≥70%) was 72% compared with 93% in similar men, suggesting a lack of specificity for anginal symptoms in women.[7] The prevalence of coronary disease in this relatively high-risk group of women increased from 56% in those who were 40 years of age to 96% in those who were 70 years of age and older; this finding sup-

ports studies in which a higher prevalence of obstructive disease was found in postmenopausal women.[7] The prevalence of heart disease was proportionally lower in patients classified with probable angina and nonspecific chest pain. In each group, the prevalence of coronary disease in premenopausal women remained lower than that in age-matched men (Fig. 18-4).[7]

The CASS and similar studies have demonstrated a high prevalence of noncardiac chest pain in premenopausal women,[7,30,58] reinforcing the view that the presence of anginal symptoms alone is not a valuable predictor of heart disease in women. Our inability to accurately predict coronary disease in women by history coupled with predisposition of women for adverse outcomes from cardiac events emphasizes the need for early, accurate diagnosis of heart disease in women at risk.

Role of exercise testing in women

Exercise tolerance testing is the most commonly used noninvasive method for the evaluation of patients with suspected coronary artery disease, although it has been shown to be a less sensitive predictor of coronary disease in women than in men. Several studies have detailed the lack of diagnostic value of exercise testing in women[4,11,15,20,21,30,49,57] (Table 18-2). In a classic study, Sketch et al[49] determined that a positive exercise stress test was a useful predictor of angiographically significant coronary disease in men (stenosis ≥75%) but was not useful in women because of the high rate of false-positive responses.[49] The trend towards false-positive test results in women has been supported by several studies,[4,11,57] including Weiner et al[57] (Fig. 18-5). A negative result on an exercise tolerence test has been found to be a valuable measure in the exclusion of coronary disease (stenosis ≥75%) in women.[49]

Possible causes for gender-related differences in the diagnostic value of exercise testing have been extensively studied.

The classic electrocardiographic criteria for a positive study are based on data obtained in men, which may account in part for the diminished diagnostic value of the test in women. The lower prevalence of heart disease in premenopausal women contributes to a lower pretest probability of disease and a decreased predictive value of exercise testing.[4,17,57] Women present with heart disease at a later age, with an altered exercise capacity and a greater number of concurrent disease processes. Although a decrease in exercise capacity may be compensated for by the use of pharmacologic stress testing, baseline gender-related differences exist in the normal physiologic response to exercise. Those differences include lower ejection fraction, peak work load, and oxygen consumption in women than in similarly conditioned men.[18] Such physiologic differences during stress may affect the exercise test variable measured.

Differences in the severity of the type of coronary disease most prevalent in men and women may affect the value of exercise testing. Single-vessel disease is more common in women, and multivessel and left main disease are more common in men.[7,58] Exercise stress testing has a higher sensitivity in detecting multivessel disease compared with single-vessel disease, and patients with more severe disease were found to have a higher incidence of abnormal test results.[29,30] Microvascular angina, a nonobstructive cause of cardiac chest pain, is also more prevalent in women than in men of the same age and may account for some of the gender-related differences in the reliability of exercise testing.

To identify factors that affect the sensitivity and specificity of exercise testing, Hlatky et al[29] analyzed the results of exercise tests performed in patients undergoing coronary angiography over a 12-year period. A total of 3094 patients were studied, and multivariate logistic regression analysis was performed to identify these factors. The five variables that were found to independently affect the sensitivity of exercise testing were maximal heart rate achieved, number of diseased vessels, presence of typical angina, patient age, and patient gender. The only variable found to independently affect test specificity was maximal exercise heart rate. The study demonstrated a decreased sensitivity of exercise testing in women compared to men, which was independent of the variables studied.[29]

Because exercise testing lacks sensitivity in women, many investigators have attempted to identify alternate stress test criteria to improve the diagnostic value of the test,[8,44,47] although these criteria have yet to be adopted for general use. The results of exercise stress testing in women remain inconsistent because the current test variables are affected by numerous factors other than the presence of coronary disease.

Noninvasive alternatives to stress testing

Several noninvasive methods have been studied with regard to their role in the detection of heart disease in women.[30] One of the most important noninvasive methods for the diagnosis of coronary artery disease is radionuclide perfusion imaging. Combined with an exercise or pharmacologic stress test, this method has demonstrated increased diagnostic value in the detection of coronary disease that is most notable in women. It is highly accurate in assessing viability and ventricular function and in identifying regions of myocardium at risk.

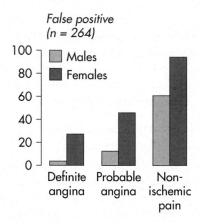

Fig. 18-5. Percentage of false-positive results in men and women undergoing exercise testing. (From Weiner DA, Ryan TJ, et al: Exercise Stress Testing: Correlations among History of Angina, ST-Segment Response and Prevalence of Coronary-Artery Disease in the Coronary Artery Surgery Study (CASS), *N Engl J Med* 301:230-235. Copyright © 1979 Massachusetts Medical Society. Adapted with permission. All rights reserved.)

Table 18-2. Value of exercise electrocardiographic testing*

Study, year	Women	Men	Angiographic endpoint (degree of stenosis)	Sensitivity	Specificity
	n			%	
Detry et al, 1979†	47	231	≥50	80 in women/87 in men	63 in women/74 in men
Weiner et al, 1979	580	1465	≥70 or ≥50% LM	76 in women/80 in men	64 in women/74 in men
Barolsky et al, 1979	92	85	≥75	60 in women/65 in men	68 in women/89 in men
Friedman et al, 1982	60	NA	≥70	32	41
Guiteras et al, 1982	112	NA	≥70	79	66
Hung et al, 1984	92	NA	≥70 or 50% LM	73	59

*NA = not applicable; LM = left main coronary stenosis.
†Included patients with and without history of myocardial infarction. All other studies cited excluded patients with history of myocardial infarction.

RADIONUCLIDE STRESS IMAGING IN WOMEN: DIAGNOSTIC ACCURACY

Exercise radionuclide imaging

Improved sensitivity and specificity in the detection of coronary disease have been described with the use of radionuclide stress imaging compared with exercise testing.[3] Early studies reported an overall sensitivity of 82% and specificity of 91% for exercise thallium imaging in predominantly male patient populations.[43] More recent studies of exercise thallium imaging in women demonstrated a similar diagnostic benefit compared with exercise testing.[15,19,30,41] Planar imaging was found to have a sensitivity of 71% to 75% and a notable specificity of 91% to 97% in women with no history of heart disease[19] (Table 18-3). Positive studies were based on exercise-induced perfusion defects, and a loss of specificity occurred when fixed defects were also considered abnormal.[15,30] In a study of 92 symptomatic women, Hung et al[30] found a high specificity of exercise thallium planar imaging, which was especially useful in the identification of women with false-positive results on exercise tests. The highest sensitivity for imaging was found in women with multivessel disease; 93% of these women were found to have one or more exercise-induced perfusion defects compared with 54% of women with single-vessel disease. This finding is similar to the results of other studies.[30]

Exercise SPECT has been found to be more sensitive than planar imaging in the overall diagnosis of coronary artery disease, as illustrated by the paired receiver-operating characteristic (ROC) curves in Fig. 18-6.[14] Although the sensitivity of SPECT imaging would thus be expected to be higher than that of planar imaging in women, few studies are available to confirm this assumption. Chae et al[6] retrospectively studied 243 women with known or suspected coronary disease who underwent exercise thallium SPECT within 3 months of coronary angiography. The study demonstrated a sensitivity of 71% and a specificity of 65% for exercise thallium SPECT in 243 women. This method was not compared with planar imaging.[6] These results may have been influenced by the submaximal exercise response in 104 of the women, with subsequent underestimation

Table 18-3. Diagnostic value of exercise thallium planar imaging in women

Study, year	Women	Angiographic endpoint (degree of stenosis)	Sensitivity	Specificity
	n		*%*	
Friedman et al, 1982	60	≥70	75	97
Hung et al, 1984	92	≥70 or ≥50 LM	75	91
Melin et al, 1985	93	≥50	71	91

of the presence and extent of coronary disease in these patients. The use of pharmacologic stress to achieve target heart rate responses, as well as the use of technetium-based imaging agents, has improved reported diagnostic values for SPECT imaging in women.[1,52]

Pharmacologic radionuclide imaging

An important adjunct to noninvasive testing in women is the use of pharmacologic stress. Early studies that examined the exercise response of women during stress testing described varying abilities of women to achieve target exercise levels. This may be because women present with heart disease at a later age, have more associated risk factors and disease states than their male counterparts, and have decreased exercise capacity in general. Pharmacologic myocardial perfusion imaging presents an alternative to exercise imaging studies in women who are limited by these conditions.

The diagnostic value of pharmacologic radionuclide imaging has been demonstrated by numerous studies but has been largely based on data obtained in men. In a review of these studies, Mahmarian and Verani[40] reported an overall sensitivity of 89% and a specificity of 78% for dipyridamole radionuclide SPECT; this result is similar to the overall sensitivity and specificity of 90% and 91%, respectively, demonstrated by studies of adenosine thallium SPECT. Both methods of pharmacologic

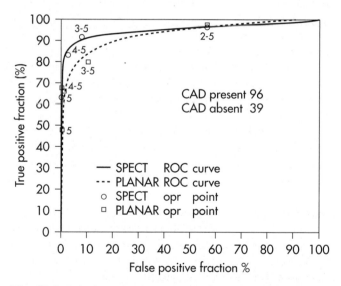

Fig. 18-6. Paired receiver-operating characteristic (ROC) curves for the overall diagnosis of coronary artery disease (CAD). The solid line indicates single-photon emission computed tomography (SPECT) ROC curve; the dotted line indicates planar ROC curve. Individual operating points (circle = tomography, square = planar) were obtained by using varying decision thresholds for a positive and negative test. The SPECT ROC curve is shifted upward and leftward of the planar ROC curve, implying improved diagnostic performance at each diagnostic threshold. Numbers on the curves indicate criteria for a positive scan. opr point = operating point. (Reprinted with permission from the American College of Cardiology. From Fintel DJ, Links JM, Brinker JA, et al: *J Am Coll Cardiol* 13:600-612, 1989.)

stress were found to be comparable to exercise imaging.[40] A recent study by Stein et al[50] suggested an improved diagnostic yield (on the basis of increased extent and severity of ischemia on imaging) with the addition of symptom-limited arm exercise in a group of 49 patients undergoing dipyridamole–thallium SPECT. In a prospective study of 144 patients (25% women) undergoing both adenosine and exercise stress thallium SPECT, Gupta et al[22] demonstrated similar efficacies for adenosine and exercise imaging and reported a concordance of 90% to 95% between those two methods in the detection of individual coronary lesions (>50% stenosis).[22] A review of studies involving dobutamine imaging (planar and SPECT) revealed a slightly lower overall sensitivity and specificity of 82% and 73%, respectively, with this agent.[40]

In total, these studies demonstrated a similar diagnostic accuracy of pharmacologic testing and exercise testing. These data suggest that pharmacologic imaging should be particularly useful for women with diminished exercise capacity. However, fewer data are available on the application of these techniques in women.

Amanullah et al[1] prospectively studied 201 consecutive women who underwent adenosine SPECT imaging using a rest thallium-201 (^{201}Tl)–stress-technetium-99m (^{99m}Tc) sestamibi separate aquisition protocol. The group was divided into 130 women with suspected heart disease who underwent coronary angiography within 2 months of imaging and 71 women with a low prescan likelihood (<10%) of disease who did not undergo catheterization. Evidence of previous myocardial infarction was found in 21% of patients in the catheterized group. In this study, adenosine SPECT imaging was found to have high accuracy and excellent sensitivity, specificity, and normalcy rates for the detection of coronary disease in women. For detection of stenosis of 70% or more, the sensitivity, specificity, and accuracy were 95%, 66%, and 85%, respectively and the normalcy rate was 93%.[1] Of particular importance, these results were similar for all patients regardless of presenting symptoms, history of myocardial infarction, or pretest probability of coronary disease.[1]

Myocardial perfusion imaging has been found to provide valuable diagnostic information in the evaluation of women suspected of having coronary disease and is superior to exercise testing alone. Although this approach compensates for many of the inaccuracies of exercise testing in women, it also introduces diagnostic challenges that are intrinsic to radionuclide imaging in women.

DIAGNOSTIC CHALLENGES OF RADIONUCLIDE STUDIES IN WOMEN

Factors that affect the accuracy of radionuclide imaging in both men and women have been reviewed in detail.[9,12,55,56] These include such technical aspects as suboptimal count densities, degree of energy scatter by distance, patient motion, and various potential artifacts. The patient's condition is also a factor: The severity of disease, presence of myocardial scarring, and inability to attain target exercise levels have been found to affect test accuracy. Two factors that have demonstrated a predominant effect on image accuracy in women are breast attenuation, with 8% to 30% of female patients displaying breast attenuation defects in several studies,[12,15,19,30] and a higher prevalence of single-vessel compared with multivessel coronary artery disease in women than in men. The smaller left ventricular chamber size found in women has also been shown to affect the accuracy of SPECT.[25]

Breast attenuation

Breast attenuation on planar imaging produces several characteristic perfusion defects, the extent of which depend on the size and density of the breast and its position in relation to the heart. For positions in which the left breast completely covers the heart, no perfusion defects are detected, because attenuation is uniform. In patients in whom the left breast incompletely obscures the heart, nonuniform attenuation perfusion defects that are characteristic for each planar view have been described. An important way to distinguish breast artifact from a true positive test result is the fact that the defect should remain fixed during stress and rest (delayed) imaging. However, the breast position may shift during the two acquisitions in the same patient, creating a partially (or, less often, totally) reversible defect. These shifts create even greater challenges for the interpreting physician.

Several factors related to breast artifacts may further complicate planar imaging in women. Wackers[56] has described small angle scatter, which may occur along the breast margin and produces linear photon densities that often extend beyond the cardiac image.[56] In addition, false-positive increased lung uptake has been demonstrated with thallium imaging. This results from breast attenuation that occurs to a greater extent over the heart compared with the upper lung fields, creating what appears to be increased lung uptake.[56]

Breast attenuation artifacts on SPECT imaging often appear less extensive and more localized than those on planar imaging. This may be partially attributed to the large number of projections obtained and the computerized processing used in tomographic imaging. This process averages attenuation artifacts, producing a more subtle defect that may closely mimic true perfusion defects. The SPECT images most commonly demonstrate anteroseptal breast attenuation defects, although this location may vary depending on the position of the breast in individual patients. Image defects often present in more than one view, particularly the short axis and vertical long axis.

Several methods have been proposed to minimize breast attenuation defects in radionuclide imaging. DePuey and Garcia[9] recommended a review of patient characteristics during scan interpretation, including sex, weight, chest circumference, bra cup size, history of mastectomy or breast implants, and any other pertinent information about the habitus. Planar imaging has been shown to have improved diagnostic accuracy with such positioning techniques as obtaining left lateral images with patients lying on their right side rather than supine.[31] This technique, developed to decrease diaphragmatic attenuation through cardiac repositioning, has been used in women to reduce breast attenuation artifacts.[56] Improved recognition of breast artifacts in planar imaging has been observed with the use of breast markers. It has also been suggested that the contour of the breast may be identified in certain patients as a negative or positive linear density extending beyond the cardiac image.[56]

To improve the diagnostic accuracy of SPECT image interpretation, it is recommended that unprocessed photon images be reviewed for breast shadows. The use of technetium-based imaging agents has been found to increase image quality because of the increased energy windows and higher count rates that result in decreased attenuation and lower energy scatter.[56] The higher energy of technetium also allows the acquisition of enough counts for gated imaging, which improves identification of attenuation defects.[56] The enhanced accuracy of technetium and echocardiographic gating for the detection of coronary disease in women were recently supported in a study by Taillefer et al[52] and will be detailed later in this chapter.

Single-vessel vs multivessel disease

Premenopausal women have been found to have a higher proportion of single-vessel disease compared to multivessel disease in age-matched men and postmenopausal women.[7,58] Although radionuclide imaging has been found to have a higher sensitivity than exercise stress testing for the detection of single-vessel disease.[34] Its superior diagnostic accuracy in detecting multivessel compared with single-vessel disease has also been detailed by several studies.

In a study described earlier in this chapter, Hung et al demonstrated a higher sensitivity for the detection of multivessel disease than for single-vessel disease in a group of women who underwent exercise thallium planar imaging. The presence of a positive scan increased the posttest probability of coronary disease in a woman with typical angina from 44% to 77%; this likelihood increased to 100% when two or more vascular segments were abnormal.[30] Chae et al[6] also found an increased sensitivity for the detection of multivessel disease than for single-vessel disease in women (82% and 52%, respectively).

Women in that study were further grouped according to the presence of no disease, single-vessel disease, or double-vessel disease and those with left main or triple-vessel disease. Independent variables associated with the group of women with left main or triple-vessel disease included a high incidence of abnormal thallium images, reversible perfusion defects, and left ventricular cavity dilatation; a greater number of abnormal vascular segments on imaging; and more extensive perfusion abnormalities[6] (Table 18-4).

Amanullah et al[1] found similar results in a prospective study of 201 women with a known or suspected history of coronary disease by using adenosine stress and ^{99m}Tc sestamibi SPECT imaging. The study groups were composed of 130 women who underwent cardiac angiography and 71 women with a low likelihood (<10%) of coronary disease. Sensitivities for the detection of stenosis 50% or more were 84%, 93%, and 100% for single-vessel, double-vessel, and triple-vessel disease, respectively. These sensitivities increased to 91%, 96%, and 100% for the detection of stenosis 70% or greater. This result was better than the data reported for planar ^{201}Tl imaging.

These studies confirm that the diagnostic accuracy of radionuclide imaging is higher in patients with multivessel disease than in those with single-vessel disease, a finding that may have a greater impact on the detection of coronary artery disease in premenopausal women because of their higher prevalence of single-vessel disease. They also emphasize the superior diagnostic accuracy of radionuclide imaging compared with alternative approaches in detecting single-vessel disease, a factor that should be strongly considered in the choice of noninvasive diagnostic testing for women.

Left ventricular chamber size

Hansen et al[25] recently evaluated the effect of left ventricular chamber size on the accuracy of ^{201}Tl SPECT myocardial perfusion imaging in men and women. A total of 323 patients were prospectively studied: 127 women and 196 men were grouped as normal patients (<5% probability of coronary artery disease) or as patients who underwent coronary angiography within 60 days of stress testing. Left ventricular size

Table 18-4. Results of exercise tomographic thallium imaging in patients with left main or triple-vessel coronary disease (group 1) and those with no single-vessel or double-vessel disease (group 2)

Result	Group 1 (n = 58)	Group 2 (n = 185)	P value
Abnormal thallium imaging, n (%)	49 (84)	94 (51)	0.0001
Reversible perfusion defects, n (%)	44 (76)	64 (35)	0.0001
Increased lung/heart ratio, n (%)	18 (31)	20 (11)	0.0002
Left ventricular cavity dilation, n (%)	14 (24)	11 (6)	0.0002
Mean segments with perfusion defects ±SD, n	8.2 ± 5.7	3.8 ± 4.9	0.0001
Mean segments with reversible defects ±SD, n	6.3 ± 5.1	2.6 ± 4.3	0.0001
Extent of perfusion abnormality, %	25 ± 9	15 ± 12	0.0001
Multivessel thallium abnormality, n (%)	32 (55)	37 (20)	0.0001

From Chae SC, Heo J, Iskandrian AS, et al: Identification of extensive coronary artery disease in women by exercise single-photon emission computed tomographic (SPECT) thallium imaging, *J Am Coll Cardiol* 21:1305-1311, 1993.

was graded as large or small, and 67% of women and 20% of men were found to have small chamber sizes. The ROC curve areas were used to compare the accuracy of SPECT between groups and showed greater accuracy of imaging in men than in women (0.93 and 0.82; $p<0.05$), without associated differences between severity of disease or coronary flow measurements during exercise. There was no difference by gender in ROC curve areas for patients with large chamber size.[25] These results introduce smaller left ventricular chamber size as a factor affecting the accuracy of ^{201}Tl SPECT in women. Whether the same phenomenon occurs with ^{99m}Tc-based imaging is not known.

NUCLEAR MYOCARDIAL PERFUSION IMAGING TECHNIQUES

Technetium imaging agents

The use of technetium-based imaging agents in radionuclide imaging has improved count densities, image quality, and the diagnostic value of imaging with the addition of gated SPECT. Studies of sensitivity, specificity, and normalcy rates for thallium and technetium have reported similar results for both agents,[39] although it is generally agreed that improved accuracy occurs with the use of technetium-based imaging agents in obese patients.

To examine the comparative diagnostic value of these agents in the detection of heart disease in women, Taillefer et al[52] prospectively studied 115 women who underwent ^{201}Tl and ^{99m}Tc sestamibi SPECT perfusion imaging with and without gating during a 2-day protocol. Eighty-five women referred for evaluation of suspected coronary artery disease underwent coronary angiography, and 30 women with a low likelihood of coronary disease (<5%) did not undergo catheterization. The study demonstrated sensitivities of 84.3% and 80.4% (p value not significant) for the detection of coronary disease (stenosis ≥70%) with thallium and technetium SPECT, respectively. The use of technetium resulted in a significantly higher specificity compared with thallium (84.4% and 67.2%; $p = 0.02$)[52] (Fig. 18-7).

Gated single-photon emission computed tomography

The higher count densities obtained with technetium-based agents have made the use of gated SPECT possible. Gated SPECT allows myocardial perfusion and function to be assessed in the same patient. For gating, the patient is electrocardiographically monitored, and data are separated into eight frames during aquisition. Because of this additional splitting of data, technetium-based imaging agents are required for gating studies. By this procedure, the viewer is able to observe resting

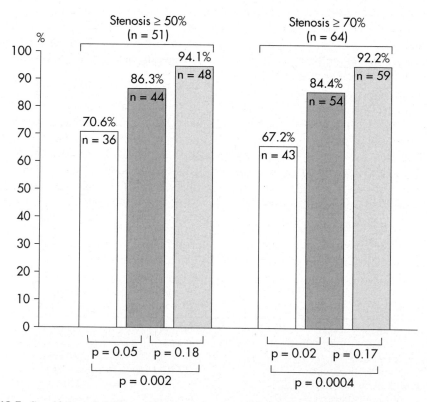

Fig. 18-7. Specificity of thallium-201 (open bars), technetium-99m sestamibi perfusion (striped bars), and technetium-99m sestamibi perfusion and gated SPECT (speckled bars) studies for patients with coronary artery disease and the group of normal volunteers. (Reprinted with permission from the American College of Cardiology. From Taillefer R, DePuey EG, Udelson JE, et al: *J Am Coll Cardiol* 29:69-77, 1997.)

ventricular function and evaluate function in the area of a perfusion defect.

Gated SPECT may be particularly useful in the evaluation of women. As stated previously, most breast attenuation artifacts appear as fixed defects. If a gated SPECT study shows normal ventricular function in the area of a defect, the defect is assumed to be artifactual. A recent study by DePuey and Rozanski[10] corroborated this finding by showing a decrease in the potential false-positive rate of images confirmed in women with the addition of gating.[10] In the study by Taillefer et al,[52] a higher specificity was found with the use of technetium compared with thallium in women. The addition of gating to ^{99m}Tc SPECT imaging further increased the specificity from 67.2% to 92.2% compared with ^{201}Tl imaging ($p = 0.0004$)[52] (Fig. 18-7). Thus, gated SPECT techniques can be successfully used in women for improved specificity without a loss of sensitivity.

OUTCOMES OF RADIONUCLIDE IMAGING IN WOMEN

Prognostic value of radionuclide imaging

Myocardial perfusion imaging has contributed to the noninvasive assessment of patients with known or suspected coronary disease by its ability to provide prognostic information. Studies over the past 15 years have clearly shown that patients with normal scans have a very good prognosis for future cardiac events, whereas those with abnormal scans (particularly those with multivessel ischemia) have a much worse prognosis.[27] Physicians have used these findings to assist in decision-making in various circumstances, including preoperative and postmyocardial evaluation. In a recent prospective study of 732 patients (519 men and 213 women) with stable coronary disease, Pattillo et al[45] concluded that the quantitative measurement of exercise induced perfusion defects on SPECT was the most important predictor of future cardiac events (myocardial infarction or cardiac death), superior to quantitative data obtained from coronary angiography or exercise stress testing.[45] This study, however, did not compare the prognostic value of SPECT imaging in men and women. Similarly, most previous studies have examined prognostic data from predominantly male populations. Prognostic studies of radionuclide imaging in women are only now beginning to emerge.

A retrospective study of 4136 patients by Hachamovitch et al[24] demonstrated the prognostic value of rest thallium–exercise technetium SPECT in 2742 men and 1394 women who were followed for a mean of 20 months for the recurrence of myocardial infarction or cardiac death. Radionuclide imaging was found to identify a greater proportion of women at high risk than men, and a more effective risk stratification was demonstrated in women by odds ratios analysis (Fig. 18-8).

The predictive value of SPECT was confirmed by Travin et al[54] in a prospective study of 2377 patients. The study included 1226 men and 1151 women with known or suspected coronary disease who underwent exercise or dipyridamole technetium SPECT. Abnormal images were present in 70% of men and 39% of women. Patients were followed for a mean of 15 months for cardiac events. A decreased cardiac event–free survival rate was found in both men and women with abnormal scans (Fig. 18-9). Similar event rates were found for men and women, with a higher rate of unstable angina and congestive heart failure in women and a higher rate of myocardial infarction and death in men[54] (Fig. 18-10).

Several investigations have studied the prognostic value of pharmacologic radionuclide imaging. Lette et al[38] evaluated the predictive value of clinical variables and dipyridamole–^{201}Tl planar imaging in the risk stratification of patients for future events. The final study population consisted of 395 men and 293 women referred for evaluation of known or suspected coronary disease who were unable to achieve target exercise levels because of physical inability or β-blocker therapy. Patients were followed for a mean of 16 months for the occurrence of myocardial infarction or cardiac death; those who underwent revascularization during follow-up were excluded from the study. Patients with normal stress thallium scans were found to have very low risk for future cardiac events (2.7% in 296 patients) regardless of their pretest likelihood of coronary disease.[38] Figure 18-11 illustrates the stratification of patients into low-risk, intermediate-risk, and high-risk groups on the basis of the results of dipyridamole thallium SPECT.

To confirm the prognostic value of a normal result on dobutamine–atropine stress sestamibi SPECT imaging in women, Geleijnse et al[16] studied a group of 80 women with various pretest probabilities of coronary disease (9 with low probability, 43 with intermediate probability, and 28 with high probability) who were found to have normal scans. Patients were followed for 23 ± 13 months for subsequent cardiac events. Over this period, two patients in the high probability group underwent revascularization, whereas no patient had a cardiac event, such as cardiac death and myocardial infarction. This correlated

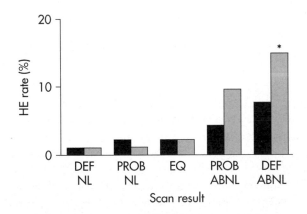

Fig. 18-8. Event rates in men (solid bars) and women (hatched bars) as a function of scan result. The event rate in women with definitely abnormal (DEF ABNL) scan results was significantly greater than that in men (*$p < 0.001$). EQ = equivalent; DEF NL = definitely normal; HE rate = hard event rate over the follow-up period; PROB ABNL = probably abnormal; PROB NL = probably normal. (Reprinted with permission from the American College of Cardiology. From Hachamovitch R, Berman DS, Kiat H, et al: *J Am Coll Cardiol* 28:34-44, 1996.)

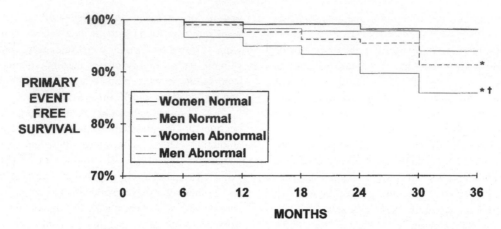

Fig. 18-9. Event free survival. Kaplan–Meier curves showing lack of nonfatal myocardial infarction or cardiac death (MI/CD) in relation to sex and SPECT image results. *$p < 0.01$ compared with normal images for same sex; $p < 0.05$ compared with normal women (From Travin MI, et al: *Am Heart J* 134:73-82, 1997.)

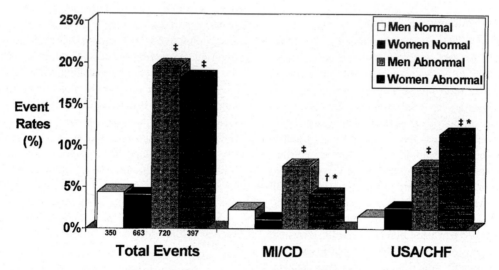

Fig. 18-10. Cardiac events in relation to SPECT results. Numbers below columns are numbers of patients in each group. *$p < 0.05$ compared with men; †$p < 0.01$ compared with normal images for same sex; ‡$p < 0.001$ compared with normal images for same sex. CD = cardiac death; CHF = congestive heart failure; MI = myocardial infarction; USA = unstable angina. (From Travin MI, et al: *Am Heart J* 134:73-82, 1997.)

with an event rate of 1.3% per year in the study group; therefore, the study concluded that the prognosis of women with a normal dobutamine–atropine stress sestamibi scan was excellent, even for patients with a high pretest likelihood of disease.[16]

The high predictive value of normal and abnormal radionuclide images has been clearly demonstrated by studies in both men and women. In response to earlier studies that found sex-related differences in referral for diagnostic testing and revascularization,[48] numerous studies have also explored the outcomes of men and women with positive scan results.

Clinical management of women after imaging

In a retrospective study of 3211 patients (2137 men and 1074 women), Hachamovitch et al[23] examined sex-related dif-

ferences in referral patterns of men and women for catheterization in relation to the severity of perfusion abnormalities on dual-isotope SPECT. The investigators hypothesized that differences in the prevalence and extent of coronary disease in men and women referred for imaging would result in differences in the extent of perfusion abnormalities on imaging and would account for previously reported discrepancies in subsequent referral for catheterization. Study patients with various cardiac histories underwent rest thallium–stress technetium SPECT and were followed for referral to cardiac catheterization or revascularization within 60 days of imaging. The study showed that men had a higher incidence of infarction and ischemia on imaging; however, this may have been due to the higher levels of exercise that they attained. Although the overall rate of catheterization was greater in men, on stratification

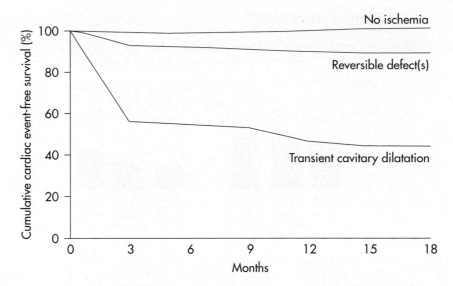

Fig. 18-11. Proportion of patients remaining free of cardiac events who had normal scans or fixed defects, reversible perfusion defects, or transient dipyridamole-induced left ventricular cavitary dilation. Patients with normal scans were at low risk. Patients with reversible defects were at increased risk but clearly cannot be considered together as "high risk" with others. (From Lette J, Bertrand C, Gossard D, et al: *Am Heart J* 129:880–886, 1995.)

by quantitative analysis of their perfusion abnormalities, men and women did not differ for catheterization or revascularization referral rates. In both men and women, catheterization referral increased with the amount of reversibility seen on scan.[23]

A prospective study by Lauer et al[36] evaluated the referral rates for coronary angiography within 90 days of exercise thallium SPECT in 2351 men and 1318 women with no history of catheterization or revascularization. The study determined that fewer women than men underwent follow-up catheterization (6% and 14%, respectively); however, this correlated with a lower percentage of abnormal thallium scans in women compared with men (8% and 29%, respectively; *P*<0.001). Logistic regression analysis used to adjust for patient age and degree of thallium scan abnormality revealed no significant differences in referral patterns for men and women.[36] In the study by Travin et al[54] of 1226 men and 1151 women evaluated by exercise or dipyridamole ^{99m}Tc sestamibi SPECT imaging, similar effects were observed with comparable rates of catheterization (24.3% for men and 22.3% for women) and revascularization (14.7% of men and 12.7% of women).[54]

These data suggest that the presence of abnormal myocardial perfusion images greatly affects subsequent management of patients, regardless of sex. These findings are probably caused by the high degree of accuracy of various methods of radionuclide imaging combined with the high prognostic value of these studies, which have affirmed radionuclide imaging as reliable means of noninvasive testing in women.

The cost-effectiveness of evaluating women with chest pain syndromes by coronary catheterization compared with perfusion imaging was recently studied by Miller et al.[42] Data were obtained in 4638 women who underwent either direct coronary angiography or stress radionuclide imaging with subsequent

angiography in the presence of reversible perfusion defects. During follow-up, patients with invasive approaches and noninvasive approaches did not differ for cardiac death rates. However, analysis of the total cost of diagnostic testing and follow-up care for each approach found substantially lower costs with the initial use of noninvasive screening compared with catheterization for each subgroup regardless of the pretest probability of coronary disease[42] (Fig. 18-12).

CONCLUSIONS

The detection of coronary artery disease represents an important aspect of health care in women, given our current knowledge of the morbidity and mortality associated with the disease. A higher rate of silent and non–Q wave myocardial infarction has been described in women, and women have been found to have higher mortality rates and rates of reinfarction compared with men after their first myocardial infarction. Previous studies have demonstrated that the consequences of revascularization are associated with poorer outcomes in women than in men, a finding that may be attributed to the later or less comprehensive workup of suspected coronary artery disease in women.

The diagnostic value of radionuclide imaging in the detection of coronary disease in women has been firmly established, with similar results reported for exercise and pharmacologic stress myocardial perfusion imaging. These methods are superior to the use of clinical variables or exercise stress testing alone. In addition, studies investigating the prognostic value of myocardial perfusion scans in women have begun to emerge, and a strong correlation was found between abnormal images and increased risk for cardiac events. Normal images have similarly been correlated with a very low risk for future cardiac events. These stud-

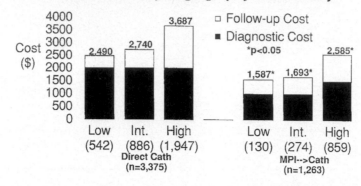

Fig. 18-12. Cost of screening with myocardial perfusion imaging compared with direct coronary angiography: economics of noninvasive diagnosis (END) study. (Reprinted with permission from the Society of Nuclear Medicine. From Miller DD, et al: *J Nucl Med* 264:69D, 1996 (abstract).

ies in women have primarily examined exercise radionuclide imaging, although a few studies have confirmed the predictive value of imaging with pharmacologic stress.

Technetium-99m–based imaging agents may be superior to ^{201}Tl for the detection of coronary disease in women. Gated SPECT seems to play an important role in increasing the accuracy and predictive value of radionuclide imaging in women, although this presumption needs to be further demonstrated. In particular, the use of gated SPECT for improvement of the detection of soft-tissue attenuation defects in women and the effect of this improvement on prognosis should be studied. Likewise, the role of attenuation correction in reducing artifact in women has not yet been evaluated.

Finally, although the clinical management of women has recently been demonstrated to be similar to that of men after radionuclide imaging, the results of subsequent intervention in these women have not been well established. Although some preliminary data exist, controversy remains about the outcomes of revascularization and the role of post-interventional myocardial perfusion imaging in women. Studies on the effects of pharmacologic interventions (for example, estrogen agents) and their impact on the results of myocardial perfusion imaging are ongoing and may provide additional important information about the use of these agents for the treatment of coronary disease in women.

REFERENCES

1. Amanullah AM, Kiat H, Friedman JD, et al: Adenosine technetium-99m sestamibi myocardial perfusion SPECT in women: diagnostic efficacy in detection of coronary artery disease, *J Am Coll Cardiol* 27:803–809, 1996.
2. American Heart Association: *Heart and stroke facts: 1996 statistical supplement,* Dallas, 1996, American Heart Association.
3. Bailey IK, Griffith LS, Rouleau J, et al: Thallium-201 myocardial perfusion imaging at rest and during exercise. Comparative sensitivity to electrocardiography in coronary artery disease, *Circulation* 55:79–87, 1977.
4. Barolsky SM, Gilbert CA, Faruqui A, et al: Differences in electrocardiographic response to exercise of women and men: a non-Bayesian factor, *Circulation* 60:1021–1027, 1979.
5. Castelli WP: Cardiovascular disease in women, *Am J Obstet Gynecol* 158(6 Pt 2):1553–1560, 1988.
6. Chae SC, Hes J, Iskandrian AS, et al: Identification of extensive coronary artery disease in women by exercise single-photon emission computed tomographic (SPECT) thallium imaging, *J Am Coll Cardiol* 21:1305–1311, 1993.
7. Chaitman BR, Bourassa MG, Davis K, et al: Angiographic prevalence of high-risk coronary artery disease in patient subsets (CASS), *Circulation* 64:360–367, 1981.
8. Deckers JW, Rensing BJ, Simons ML, et al: Diagnostic merits of exercise testing in females, *Eur Heart J* 10:543–550, 1989.
9. DePuey EG, Garcia EV: Optimal specificity of thallium-201 SPECT through recognition of imaging artifacts, *J Nucl Med* 30:441–449, 1989.
10. DePuey EG, Rozanski A: Using gated technetium-99m-sestamibi SPECT to characterize fixed myocardial defects as infarct or artifact, *J Nucl Med* 36:952–955, 1995.
11. Detry JM, Kapita BM, Cosyms J, et al: Diagnostic value of history and maximal exercise electrocardiography in men and women suspected of coronary heart disease, *Circulation* 56:756–761, 1977.
12. Dunn RF, Wolff L, Wagner S, et al: The inconsistent pattern of thallium defects: a clue to the false positive perfusion scintigram, *Am J Cardiol* 48:224–232, 1981.
13. Eaker ED, Chesebro JH, Sacks FM, et al: Cardiovascular disease in women, *Circulation* 88:1999–2009, 1993.
14. Fintel DJ, Linles JM, et al: Improved diagnostic performance of exercise thallium-201 single photon emission computed tomography over planar imaging in the diagnosis of coronary artery disease: a receiver operating characteristic analysis, *J Am Coll Cardiol* 13:600–612, 1989.
15. Friedman TD, Greene AC, Iskandrian AS, et al: Exercise thallium-201 myocardial scintigraphy in women: correlation with coronary arteriography, *Am J Cardiol* 49:1632–1637, 1982.
16. Geleijnse ML, Elhendy A, van Domberg RT, et al: Prognostic significance of normal dobutamine-atropine stress sestamibi scintigraphy in women with chest pain, *Am J Cardiol* 77:1057–1061, 1996.
17. Gibbons RJ: *Exercise ECG testing with and without radionuclide studies.* In Wenger NK, Speroff L, Packard B, eds: *Cardiovascular health and disease in women,* Greenwich, 1993, Lejaq Communications.
18. Gibbons RJ, Lee KL, Cobb F, et al: Ejection fraction response to exer-

cise in patients with chest pain and normal coronary arteriograms, *Circulation* 64:952–957, 1981.

19. Goodgold HM, et al: Improved interpretation of exercise Tl-201 myocardial perfusion scintigraphy in women: characterization of breast attenuation artifacts, *Radiology* 165:361–366, 1987.

20. Gordon EE: Noninvasive diagnosis of coronary artery disease in women, *Cardio* December 1992: pp. 29–32, 37–39, 58.

21. Guiteras P, Chaitman BR, Waters DD, et al: Diagnostic accuracy of exercise ECG lead systems in clinical subsets of women, *Circulation* 65:1465–1474, 1982.

22. Gupta NC, Esterbrooks DJ, Hilleman DE, et al: Comparison of adenosine and exercise thallium-201 single-photon emission computed tomography (SPECT) myocardial perfusion imaging. The GE SPECT Multicenter Adenosine Study Group, *J Am Coll Cardiol* 19:248–257, 1992.

23. Hachamovitch R, Berman DS, Kiat H, et al: Gender-related differences in clinical management after exercise nuclear testing, *J Am Coll Cardiol* 26:1457–1464, 1995.

24. Hachamovitch R, Berman DS, Kiat H, et al: Effective risk stratification using exercise myocardial perfusion SPECT in women: gender-related differences in prognostic nuclear testing, *J Am Coll Cardiol* 28:34–44, 1996.

25. Hansen CL, Crabbe D, Rubin S: Lower diagnostic accuracy of thallium-201 SPECT myocardial perfusion imaging in women: an effect of smaller chamber size, *J Am Coll Cardiol* 28:1214–1219, 1996.

26. Harvard Medical School: Coronary heart disease, *Women's Health Watch* 1:6, 1994.

27. Heller GV, Brown KA: Prognosis of acute and chronic coronary artery disease by myocardial perfusion imaging, *Cardiol Clin* 12:271–287, 1994.

28. Higginbotham MB, Morris KG, Coleman RE, et al: Sex-related differences in the normal cardiac response to upright exercise, *Circulation* 70:357–366, 1984.

29. Hlatky MA, Pryor DB, Harrell FE Jr, et al: Factors affecting sensitivity and specificity of exercise electrocardiography. Multivariable analysis, *Am J Med* 77:64–71, 1984.

30. Hung J, Chaitman BR, Lam J, et al: Noninvasive diagnostic test choices for the evaluation of coronary artery disease in women: a multivariate comparison of cardiac fluoroscopy, exercise electrocardiography and exercise thallium myocardial perfusion scintigraphy, *J Am Coll Cardiol* 4:8–16, 1984.

31. Johnstone DE, et al: Effect of patient positioning on left lateral thallium-201 myocardial images, *J Nucl Med* 20:183–188, 1979.

32. Kannel WB, Feinleib M: Natural history of angina pectoris in the Framingham Study. Prognosis and survival, *Am J Cardiol* 29:154–163, 1972.

33. Kannel WB, Sorlie P, McNamara PM: Prognosis after initial myocardial infarction: the Framingham Study, *Am J Cardiol* 44:53–59, 1979.

34. Kaul S, Kiess M, Liu P, et al: Comparison of exercise electrocardiography and quantitative thallium imaging for one-vessel coronary artery disease, *Am J Cardiol* 56:257–261, 1985.

35. Kennedy JW, Killip T, Fisher LD, et al: The clinical spectrum of coronary artery disease and its surgical and medical management, 1974–1979. The Coronary Artery Surgery Study, *Circulation* 66(5 Pt 2):16–23, 1982.

36. Lauer MS, Pashkow FJ, Snader CE, et al: Gender and referral for coronary angiography after treadmill thallium testing, *Am J Cardiol* 78:278–283, 1996.

37. Lerner DJ, Kannel WB: Patterns of coronary heart disease morbidity and mortality in the sexes: a 26-year follow-up of the Framingham population, *Am Heart J* 111:383–390, 1986.

38. Lette J, Bertrand C, Gossard D, et al: Long-term risk stratification with dipyridamole imaging, *Am Heart J* 129:880–886, 1995.

39. Maddahi J, et al: *Technetium-99m-sestamibi myocardial perfusion imaging for evaluation of coronary artery disease.* In Zaret BL, Beller G, eds: *Nuclear cardiology: state of the art and future directions,* ed 1, St. Louis, 1993, Mosby.

40. Mahmarian JJ, Verani MS: Myocardial perfusion imaging during pharmacologic stress testing, *Cardiol Clin* 12:223–245, 1994.

41. Melin JA, Wijns W, Vanbutsele RJ, et al: Alternative diagnostic strategies for coronary artery disease in women: demonstration of the usefulness and efficiency of probability analysis, *Circulation* 71:535–542, 1985.

42. Miller DD, et al: Cost analysis of stress myocardial perfusion imaging in 4,638 women with stable angina: comparison to a strategy of direct coronary angiography, *J Nucl Med* 37:68P, 1996 (abstract).

43. Okada RD, Boucher CA, Strauss HW, et al: Exercise radioniclide imaging approaches to coronary artery disease, *Am J Cardiol* 46:1188–1204, 1980.

44. Okin PM, Kligfield P: Gender-specific criteria and performance of the exercise electrocardiogram, *Circulation* 92:1209–1216, 1995.

45. Pattillo RW, Fuchs S, Johnson J, et al: Predictors of prognosis by quantitative assessment of coronary angiography, single photon emission computed tomography thallium imaging, and treadmill exercise testing, *Am Heart J* 131:582–590, 1996.

46. Rich-Edwards JW, Manson JE, Hennekens CH, et al: The primary prevention of coronary heart disease in women, *N Engl J Med* 332:1758–1766, 1995.

47. Robert AR, Melin JA, Detry JM: Logistic discriminant analysis improves diagnostic accuracy of exercise testing for coronary artery disease in women, *Circulation* 83:1202–1209, 1991.

48. Shaw LJ, Miller DD, Romeis JC, et al: Gender differences in the noninvasive evaluation and management of patients with suspected coronary artery disease, *Ann Intern Med* 120:559–566, 1994.

49. Sketch MH, Mohiuddin SM, Lynch JD, et al: Significant sex differences in the correlation of electrocardiographic exercise testing and coronary arteriograms, *Am J Cardiol* 36:169–173, 1975.

50. Stein L, Burt R, Oppenheim B, et al: Symptom-limited arm exercise increases detection of ischemia during dipyridamole tomographic thallium stress testing in patients with coronary artery disease, *Am J Cardiol* 75:568–572, 1995.

51. Steingart RM, Packer M, Hamm P, et al: Sex differences in the management of coronary artery disease. Survival and Ventricular Enlargement Investigators, *N Engl J Med* 325:226–230, 1991.

52. Taillefer R, DePuey EG, Udelson JE, et al: Comparative diagnostic accuracy of Tl-201 and Tc-99m sestamibi SPECT imaging (perfusion and ECG-gated SPECT) in detecting coronary artery disease in women, *J Am Coll Cardiol* 29:69–77, 1997.

53. Tofler GH, Stone PH, Muller JE, et al: Effects of gender and race on prognosis after myocardial infarction: adverse prognosis for women, particularly black women, *J Am Coll Cardiol* 9:473–482, 1987.

54. Travin MI, et al: Relationship of gender to physician use of test results and to the prognostic value of stress technetium 99m sestamibi myocardial single-photon emission computed tomography scintigraphy, *Am Heart J* 134:73–82, 1997.

55. Wackers FJTh: Artifacts in planar SPECT myocardial perfusion imaging. *Am J Card Imaging* 6:42–58, 1992.

56. Wackers FJTh: Diagnostic pitfalls of myocardial perfusion imaging in women, *J Myocardial Ischemia* 4:23–37, 1992.

57. Weiner DA, Ryan TA, McCabe CH, et al: Exercise stress testing. Correlations among history of angina, ST-segment response and prevalence of coronary artery-disease in the Coronary Artery Surgery Study (CASS), *N Engl J Med* 301:230–235, 1979.

58. Welch CC, Proudfit WL, Sheldon WC: Coronary arteriographic findings in 1,000 women under age 50, *Am J Cardiol* 35:211–215, 1975.

59. Wenger NK: *Coronary heart disease: diagnostic decision making.* In Douglas P, ed: *Cardiovascular health and disease in women,* Philadelphia, 1993, WB Saunders Company.

60. Wenger NK: Coronary heart disease in women: an overview (myths, misperceptions, and missed opportunities), *Cardiovascular Review and Reports* 14:24–41, 1993.

Chapter 19

State of the art for pharmacologic stress imaging

Ami E. Iskandrian

In many tertiary referral medical centers, pharmacologic stress testing constitutes roughly 30% of all stress tests performed for the detection of coronary artery disease (CAD) and for risk assessment.* The ideal candidates are patients who cannot exercise or can perform only limited exercise (Box 19-1). Iskandrian et al[56] reported that submaximal exercise single-photon emission computed tomography (SPECT) perfusion imaging is significantly less sensitive than maximal exercise in detecting

*References 7, 9, 10, 54, 55, 60, 61, 79, 121.

any coronary artery disease and in correctly identifying patients with multivessel coronary artery disease; thus, even when the test result is positive, extent of disease and ischemic myocardium is underestimated. Methods of detecting coronary artery disease with pharmacologic stress testing are shown in Box 19-2. The stress agents can be divided into vasodilators and inotropes/chronotropes (Box 19-3). The U.S. Food and Drug Administration has approved the use of dipyridamole (1992), adenosine (1995), and arbutamine (1997) for stress testing. Stress agents that are used to provoke coronary spasm, such as ergonovine and acetylcholine, are not discussed in this chapter.

PHARMACOLOGY

Adenosine

Adenosine is a small heterocyclic compound with a molecular weight of 267.25. It is made of a purine base and the sugar ribose. The chemical structure is 6-amino-9-B-D-ribofuranosyl-9H-purine. It is available for use in myocardial perfusion imaging as a 20 or 30 mL vial containing 60 or 90 mg of adenosine (Adenoscan). When infused intravenously, adenosine has a very short half-life (less than 2 seconds).[60] Endogenous adenosine is produced intracellularly through two pathways: the adenosine triphosphate (ATP) pathway and S-adenosyl methionine (SAM) pathways. Endogenous adenosine crosses the cellular membrane and interacts with special purine cell surface receptors (Fig. 19-1). Activation of A_2 receptors causes coronary vasodilation through the production of adenylate cyclase and cyclic adenosine monophosphate stimulation of potassium channels; decreased intracellular calcium uptake also occurs.[8] A_{2a} receptors are predominantly found in the coronary vasculature, and A_{2b} receptors are found in the systemic circulation. The density and distribution of these receptors are species-specific, suggesting the need for caution in extrapolating results from animal experiments to humans. Stimulation of A_1 receptors causes atrioventricular conduction delay, which explains why adenosine is the treatment of choice for supraventricular tachycardia. Other types of receptors (A_3 and A_4) are probably

---

Box 19-1 Contraindications to exercise stress testing

Peripheral arteriosclerotic vascular disease
Disabling arthritis
History of stroke
Orthopedic problems (such as low back pain)
Chronic pulmonary disease
Extremity amputation
Poor motivation to exercise
Poor exercise capacity due to noncardiac endpoints (such as fatigue)
β-Blocking drugs that limit heart rate response
Left bundle-branch block (false-positive result on exercise perfusion scans)
Soon after myocardial infarction (<5 days)

Reproduced with permission from Beller GA, ed: *Pharmacologic stress imaging in clinical nuclear cardiology*, Philadelphia, 1995, WB Saunders Company.

Box 19-2 Methods of detecting coronary artery disease with a pharmacologic stress test

Electrocardiography
Perfusion imaging
Radionuclide angiography
Two-dimensional echocardiography
Positron emission tomography
Magnetic resonance imaging

Box 19-3 Types of pharmacologic stress agents

Coronary vasodilator

Adenosine
Dipyridamole
Adenosine triphosphate
Others agents, such as a selective A_2 agonist

Inotropes/chronotropes

Dubotamine
Arbutamine

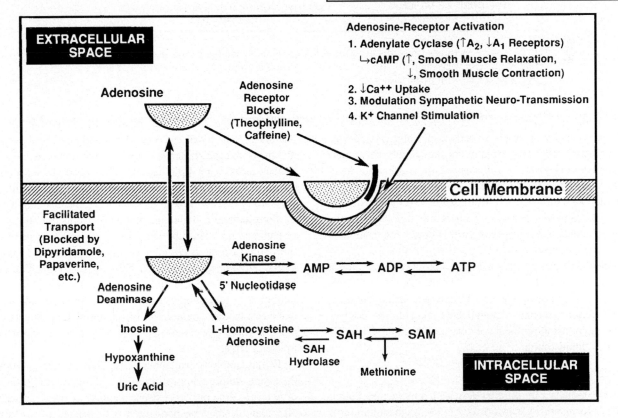

Fig. 19-1. Synthesis and site of action of endogenous adenosine. (From Verani MS: Adenosine thallium 201 myocardial perfusion scintigraphy, *Am Heart J* 122:269-278, 1991. Reproduced with permission.)

in the mast cells and other organs of the body and may have a relation to bronchospasm in susceptible persons.[8,60] Theophylline and caffeine are nonselective competitive blockers of adenosine receptors and thus antagonize the effects of adenosine (Fig. 19-2).

After activation of adenosine receptors, adenosine reenters the intracellular compartment through a facilitated transport mechanism by an unknown substance. Once adenosine is inside the cell, it is converted to ATP and SAM or is deaminated to inosine (which eventually is metabolized to uric acid) by the en-

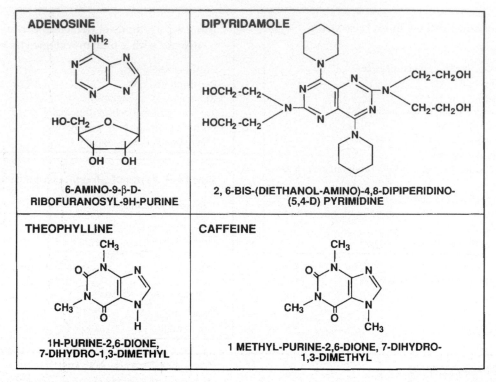

Fig. 19-2. The chemical structures of adenosine, dipyridamole, caffeine, and theophylline. (From Verani MS: Adenosine thallium 201 myocardial perfusion scintigraphy, *Am Heart J* 122:269-278, 1991. Reproduced with permission.)

zyme adenosine deaminase.[122] Exogenously administered adenosine is rapidly taken up by cells, especially erythrocytes and endothelial cells; this explains its remarkably short half-life. Adenosine is given at a dosage of 140 μg/kg/min for 6 minutes by using an infusion pump. The radiotracer is best administered into a different vein from that used for adenosine infusion. It is, however, possible to inject the radiotracer in the same intravenous line, provided that it is done with caution so as not to produce a bolus effect.

In Japan, ATP was recently used as a coronary vasodilator in conjunction with perfusion imaging. The mechanism of vasodilation is probably conversion of ATP into adenosine, but a direct vasodilator mechanism cannot be excluded. The dose of ATP and the infusion protocol are very similar to those used in adenosine administration.[123]

Dipyridamole

Dipyridamole is a pyrimidine base with a molecular weight of 504.62. Its chemical structure is 2,6-bis-(diethanol-amino)-4,8-dipiperidino-(5,4-D)pyrimidine. Most if not all of the vasodilatory effects of dipyridamole are secondary to elevation of interstitial levels of adenosine. At high doses, dipyridamole is also a phosphodiesterase inhibitor, but it is unclear whether this property contributes to the vasodilatory effects in the doses used in humans.* Dipyridamole blocks the transport of adeno-

*References 9, 10, 60, 68, 76, 113, 115.

sine into the cells, thereby raising the interstitial levels of adenosine, which causes coronary vasodilation. McLaughlin et al[85] measured the coronary sinus level of adenosine after intravenous infusion of dipyridamole. They observed an increased adenosine level in both normal persons and patients with coronary artery disease; this suggests that the mechanism of action of dipyridamole is the augmentation of the local concentration of endogenous adenosine (Fig. 19-3). After intravenous injection, dipyridamole is completely distributed within 15 minutes and is eliminated. Its plasma half-life is 20 to 30 minutes. Dipyridamole also has antiplatelet actions, probably because of inhibition of phosphodiesterase, increase in adenosine triphosphate levels, and potentiation of the antiplatelet effects of aspirin. It should be noted that adenosine also has a direct antiplatelet effect.

Dipyridamole is available in 2-ml vials containing 10 mg of the agent. Before administration, it is diluted with 20 to 50 ml of normal saline or 5% dextrose solution in water. Infusion of dipyridamole may be performed with the aid of an infusion pump or through a slow intravenous push over 4 minutes. The recommended dose in the United States is 142 μg/kg/min for 4 minutes. In Europe, a 50% higher dose is often used with echocardiography.

Dobutamine

Dobutamine is a powerful inotropic agent that is often used in the treatment of heart failure. Dobutamine hydrochloride is a

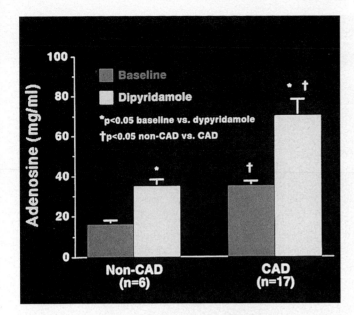

Fig. 19-3. Changes in the coronary sinus level of adenosine in response to intravenous administration of dipyridamole in normal patients and in patients with coronary artery disease *(CAD)*. An increase is seen in both groups. (From McLaughlin DP, Beller GA, Linden J, et al: Hemodynamic and metabolic correlates of dipyridamole-induced myocardial thallium-201 perfusion abnormalities in multivessel coronary artery disease, *Am J Cardiol* 74:1159-1164, 1994. Reproduced with permission from Excerpta Medica, Inc.)

Table 19-1. The actions of dobutamine and related compounds

| | Adrenergic receptor activity | | |
Agent	Peripheral (A)	Cardiac (β_1)	Peripheral (β_2)
Norepinephrine	+ + + +	+ + + +	0
Epinephrine	+ + + +	+ + + +	+ +
Dopamine	+ + + +	+ + + +	+ +
Isoproterenol	0	+ + + +	+ + + +
Dobutamine	+	+ + + +	+ +
Methoxamine	+ + + +	0	0
Arbutamine	+	+ + + +	+ +

+ Mild effect
+ + + + Strong effect
0 No effect

synthetic catecholamine; chemically, it is the ($\pm$)-4-[-2-[[3-(*p*-hydroxyphenyl)-1-methylpropyl]amino]ethyl] procatechol hydrochloride, with a molecular weight of 337.85. It is available in 20 mL-vials containing 20 mg of dobutamine hydrochloride and a small amount of sodium bisulfide.

The onset of action of dobutamine occurs 1 or 2 minutes after starting the intravenous infusion, but the peak effect is achieved several minutes later.[10,33,36,45] The plasma half-life of dobutamine is about 2 minutes, and the drug is metabolized through methylation of the catechol group (by the enzyme catechol *o* methyltransferase) and conjugation. The commercially available dobutamine preparation contains levorotatory isomer, which produces α_1 stimulation and dextrorotatory isomer, which produces β_1- and β_2-receptor stimulation (Table 19-1). Dobutamine is given as intravenous infusion by using an infusion pump in incremental doses starting at 5 to 10 μg/kg/min to a maximum of 40 μg/kg/min.[60,83,98,120,124]

Arbutamine

Arbutamine is a synthetic catecholamine that is structurally similar to dobutamine. It has a mixed β_1- and β_2-adrenoreceptor agonist activity and a mild affinity for α receptors. Its chemical structure is R(-1)-1(3,4-dihydroxyphenyl)-2-[(4-hydroxyphenyl) butylamino]-ethanol hydrochloride. Compared with dipyridamole, arbutamine has a similar degree of inotropic and chronotropic activity, but it has less vasodilator activity than isoproterenol and less inotropic activity than dobutamine. Its plasma half life is approximately 8 minutes.[65] Arbutamine was developed in conjunction with a closed-loop delivery device that uses the patient's heart rate response (heart rate feedback) to modulate the rate of administration within prespecified heart rate and blood pressure limits. The delivery system stops the arbutamine infusion when a total dose of 10 μg/kg per body weight is administered or when there is no further increase in heart rate at the maximum infusion rate of 0.8 μg/kg/min, roughly 1/50th of the dose of dobutamine. The closed-loop system automatically monitors the heart rate at 5-second intervals and blood pressure at 2-minute intervals throughout the infusion period. It provides audible and visible messages in response to potentially important changes in heart rate or blood pressure and automatically interrupts the arbutamine infusion if the heart rate or blood pressure changes exceed the programmed limits. At the end of the test, the results are summarized on a printout, and complete data are stored on magnetic media by using a laptop computer linked to the system (Fig. 19-4).

CHANGES IN CORONARY BLOOD FLOW

Resting myocardial blood flow is dependent on myocardial oxygen demand. The peak flow represents the flow at the maximum effect of an intervention, such as the effect of intracoronary injection of papaverine, which has been used as the gold standard to measure maximum coronary hyperemia. The absolute coronary flow reserve ratio represents the ratio of the peak flow to the baseline flow. The relative coronary flow reserve ratio represents the ratio of the peak flow in a diseased coronary artery to the peak flow in a normal coronary artery. Unlike the absolute flow reserve, this ratio is independent of changes in heart rate, blood pressure, and baseline flow and is more meaningful to the understanding of results of perfusion imaging. Both nitric oxide and adenosine produce vasodilation and decrease coronary vascular resistance, but the interaction between these two endogenous substances is not clear.[75,100,107,111] Lefroy et al[75] showed that acetylcholine-induced dilation of epicardial arteries is mediated by nitric oxide because synthesis of the latter substance is inhibited

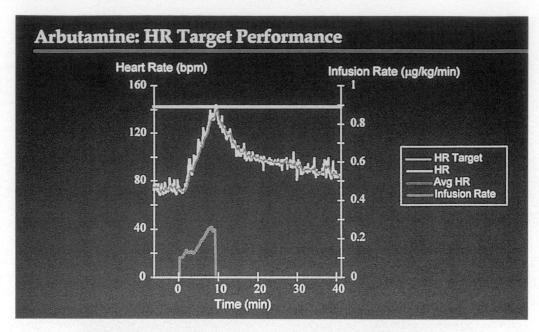

Fig. 19-4. The response of the heart rate to arbutamine infusion. A gradual increase is seen.

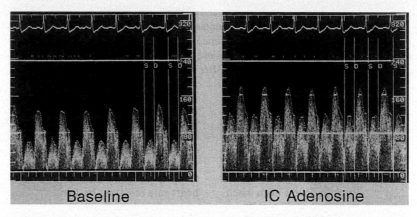

Fig. 19-5. Measurements of coronary flow velocity by Doppler wire at baseline and in response to adenosine. An increase is seen with adenosine. (From Iskandrian AS, Verani MS, Heu J: Pharmacologic stress testing: mechanisms of action, hemodynamic responses, and results in detection of coronary artery disease, *J Nucl Cardiol* 1:94-111, 1994. Reproduced with permission.)

by N-monomethyl-L-arginine [L-NMMA], whereas acetyl choline–induced dilation of resistance vessels (and, hence, degree of coronary hyperemia) is not mediated in this manner. Using the Doppler flow wire method, Shiode et al[109] showed that the coronary flow reserve ratio was 4.0 before and 3.4 after L-NMMA administration in normal subjects (*p* value not significant). It is possible that nitric oxide and adenosine act at different levels of the coronary microvasculature; nitric oxide may act proximally and adenosine may act distally. In vessels with normally functioning endothelium, nitric oxide maintains dilation of the proximal segments, which exposes the distal sites to a high perfusion pressure, leading to vasoconstriction. Under these circumstances, adenosine could produce maximal vasodilation and hyperemia. In the presence of low levels of nitric oxide due to endothelial dysfunction, the proximal segments are

vasoconstricted, leading to a lower distal pressure and partial vasodilation at distal sites. In this situation, adenosine produces less-than-maximal hyperemia.

NORMAL PATIENTS

The coronary vasodilatory properties of adenosine have been recognized since the report by Drury and Szent-Gyorgyi in 1929.[32] Using Doppler flow wire, Wilson et al[125] demonstrated an average 4.4-fold increase in coronary blood flow velocity in normal human coronary arteries at an adenosine dosage of 140 μg/kg/min given intravenously (Fig. 19-5). The response was similar to that achieved with intercoronary papaverine. At a dosage of 70 μg/kg/min of adenosine, maximal vasodilation was achieved in 84% of normal patients, whereas at a dose of 140 μg/kg/min, maximal hyperemia occurred in 92% of the patients. Of note, at a dosage of adenosine less than 140 µg/kg/min, there was fluctuation in the coronary flow response that was abolished at the dosage of 140 µg/kg/min. These fluctuations may have reflected transient changes in blood adenosine concentrations. Rossen et al[102,103] observed a slightly higher absolute coronary flow velocity reserve ratio with papaverine than with adenosine or dipyridamole (3.9, 3.4, and 3.1, respectively). The maximum coronary flow velocity was reached earlier after adenosine administration than after dipyridamole administration (55 compared with 287 seconds). Chan et al,[20] using positron emission tomography to measure absolute myocardial blood flow (with nitrogen-(^{13}N)–labeled ammonia), observed an absolute coronary flow reserve ratio of 4.3 with adenosine and 4.0 with dipyridamole. Brown et al[13] observed a 2.4-fold increase in coronary flow (measured by the coronary sinus thermodilution technique) with dipyridamole, which increased further by the addition of hand-grip exercise. Rossen et al[103] and Czernin et al,[27] however, could not demonstrate an advantage of combining hand-grip exercise with dipyridamole to further augment coronary blood flow. Although the standard dosage of dipyridamole (142 µg/kg/min for 4 minutes) can induce maximum or near-maximum coronary vasodilation in most patients, a submaximal response is noted in as many as 20% to 25% of normal patients. Furthermore a 50% higher dose of dipyridamole did not result in further augmentation of the myocardial blood flow above the level achieved with the standard dosage, but these studies did not address specifically the subgroup of patients with submaximal response. It is conceivable that the combination of submaximal exercise and a higher dose of dipyridamole may result in further increase in the hyperemic response in some patients.[60,102,103] Krivokapich et al,[70] using ^{13}N-labeled ammonia, observed a threefold increase in myocardial blood flow (range, 2 to 4.8) in response to dobutamine in normal patients. Myocardial flow correlated significantly with the heart rate, systolic blood pressure, and rate-pressure product, suggesting that high-dose dobutamine infusion (40 µg/kg/min) can increase coronary flow to the same level that is achieved with exercise (Fig. 19-6).

Recent data also reveal that the absolute coronary flow reserve decreases with age and smoking (Fig. 19-7).[8,12,28,110,118] In both of these conditions, the decrease is caused by an increase in baseline flow secondary to increase in blood pressure in elderly persons and blood pressure and heart rate with smoking. In addition, caffeine decreases the coronary flow reserve by decreasing the peak hyperemic response; the latter seems to be dose dependent, because it is a competitive inhibitor. These observations are important in the interpretation of perfusion test results because a history of recent smoking or caffeine intake is often not volunteered by the patients. Although no sex-related

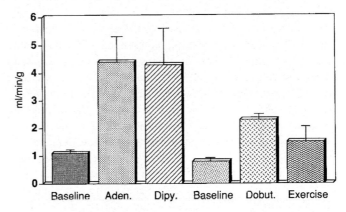

Fig. 19-6. Coronary blood flow reserve ratio in response to adenosine, dipyridamole, dobutamine, and exercise stress. (From Iskandrian AS, Verani MS, Heu J: Pharmacologic stress testing: mechanism of action, hemodynamic responses, and results in detection of coronary artery disease, *J Nucl Cardiol* 1:94-111, 1994. Reproduced with permission.)

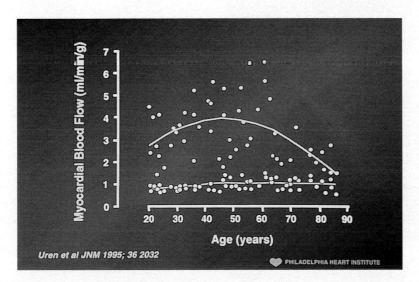

Fig. 19-7. Coronary blood flow reserve ratio in relation to age. A decrease is seen with aging. (From Uren NG, Camici PG, Melin JA, et al: Effect of aging on myocardial perfusion reserve, *J Nucl Med* 36:2032-2036, 1995. Reproduced with permission.)

differences have been observed in coronary flow responses, on average, women develop coronary artery disease a decade later than men; therefore, age-related differences may be especially important in women. Abnormal flow reserve has been observed in diabetic patients, especially those with autonomic neuropathy in the absence of epicardial coronary disease.

PATIENTS WITH CORONARY ARTERY DISEASE

In the presence of coronary stenosis, the ability to augment the myocardial blood flow with pharmacologic stimulation is reduced with an inverse relation to the severity of stenosis (Fig. 19-8). The smaller increase in flow is explained by dilation of microvasculature at baseline as a compensatory mechanism to maintain resting flow. Therefore, the administration of a coronary vasodilator will result in no or minimal additional dilation (exhaustion of reserve mechanism).* In a series of landmark experiments by Gould et al,[40-42] it was shown that coronary flow reserve begins to decrease when the coronary diameter stenosis is roughly 45% to 50%, representing a 75% reduction in the cross-sectional area. In contrast, the resting myocardial blood flow remains basically within normal limits, at least until the luminal diameter is decreased by 90%. The heterogeneity in myocardial blood flow during coronary vasodilation in territories of normal and diseased coronary arteries underscores the mechanism of production of perfusion defects in many patients with coronary artery disease. Voudris et al[123] recently used dual Doppler flow wires, one in a normal vessel and another in a diseased artery, and documented differences in coronary flow reserves in these two vessels in response to dipyr-

*References 13, 20, 27, 40–42, 70, 87, 119, 123, 125.

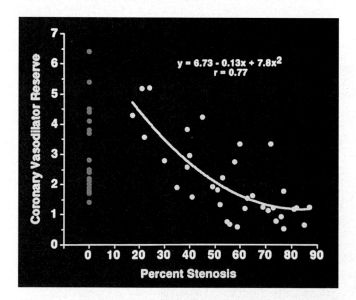

Fig. 19-8. The relation between coronary flow reserve ratio and degree of coronary stenosis. An inverse curvilinear relation is seen. (From Uren NG, Melin JA, DeBruyne B, et al: Relation between myocardial blood flow and the severity of coronary artery stenosis, *N Engl J Med* 330:1782-1788, 1994. Reproduced with permission.)

idamole (2.6 and 1.1, respectively). On a separate day, these patients had demonstrated perfusion defects on dipyridamole SPECT perfusion imaging in the territory of the diseased artery. Strauss and Pitt[105] first demonstrated perfusion defects by the use of ethyladenosine in dogs with experimental coronary stenosis of the left circumflex artery. Later, Gould et al[40] and Leppo et al[76] confirmed the observations that perfusion defects can be demonstrated in the presence of coronary stenosis (Fig. 19-9). The greater increase in myocardial blood flow in normal coronary arteries compared with diseased coronary arteries would create a difference in tracer concentration in the territories of these vessels. In addition, because the increase in coronary flow is greater than the increase in cardiac output with adenosine and dipyridamole, the myocardial tracer concentration is considerably higher, provided that the injected dose and the extraction fraction are kept constant according to the Sapirstein principle. However, for most tracers, the first-pass extraction fraction decreases at high flow rates (roll-off), which means that the myocardial tracer concentration underestimates the flow.*

The mechanism underlying this decrease in extraction is not totally clear, but it may be related to excessive blood flow velocity in the presence of normal or mildly increased myocardial oxygen demand. This roll-off differs from one tracer to another; for example, it is greater with technetium-99m (^{99m}Tc) sestamibi, ^{99m}Tc tetrofosmin, and ^{99m}Tc furifosmin than with thallium and is less with ^{99m}Tc teboroxime or ^{99m}Tc NOET, (bis[N-ethoxy, N-ethyl dithiocarbamate]nitrids), suggesting a rationale for using different tracers to identify mild to moderate coronary stenosis (Fig. 19-10). Heller et al[50] compared the results of adenosine thallium imaging with stenosis severity assessed by angiography and with coronary flow reserve in patients with moderate stenosis.[50] They found that most lesions with coronary flow reserve ratio less than 1.7 were associated with perfusion defects. Ideally, the detection of mild to moderate stenosis requires the production of maximum hyperemia in the normal zone and administration of a radiotracer that has a linear extraction fraction at high flow.

It is often asked whether the detection of mild to moderate coronary stenosis is important. The answer may not be straightforward, because one can argue that detection may lead to unnecessary cardiac catheterizations and interventions. This reasoning assumes that any abnormal perfusion result is a prelude to catheterization, which it should not be. An alternative viewpoint is that the detection of early atherosclerosis is vitally important because medical management strategies, such as control of hyperlipidemia, are most effective in the early stage of the disease. In the presence of more severe stenosis, it is likely that all tracers will yield similar results; therefore, the choice among tracers will depend on other factors, such as physical characteristics, imaging characteristics, or cost, rather than physiologic differences.

*References 16, 35, 38, 47, 51, 73, 105.

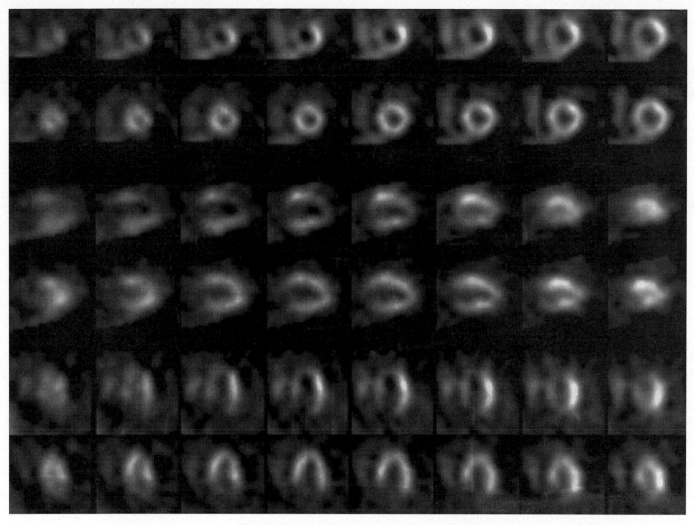

Fig. 19-9. Adenosine–redistribution single-photon emission computed tomography thallium images showing a large reversible anteroseptal abnormality.

Fig. 19-10. The relation between myocardial concentration of sestamibi and thallium and flow in an animal model. The roll-off of sestamibi is greater than that of thallium. (From Glover DK, Ruiz M, Edwards C, et al: Comparison between thallium-201 and Tc-99m sestamibi uptake during adenosine-induced vasodilation as a function of coronary stenosis severity, *Circulation* 91:813-820, 1995. Reproduced with permission.)

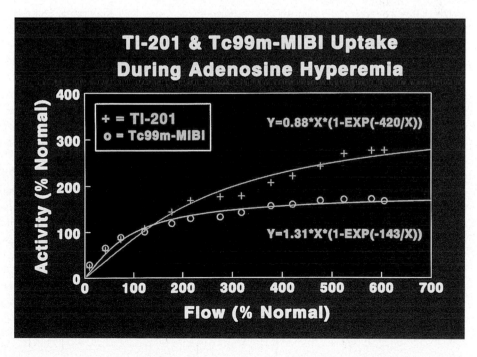

As with exercise, the increase in myocardial blood flow with dobutamine is secondary to increased myocardial oxygen demand (secondary vasodilation).

CORONARY STEAL DURING PHARMACOLOGIC VASODILATION

Coronary steal represents an absolute decrease in flow distal to coronary stenosis in response to coronary vasodilation. It can be intercoronary or intracoronary in type.[6,10,52,60,96] Intercoronary steal occurs when the coronary bed distal to high-grade stenosis is perfused by collateral vessels originating from a different coronary artery. During maximal vasodilation, the coronary resistance decreases in the normal donor artery, leading to an increase in flow in the normal area and a decrease in collateral flow in the stenotic artery. This type of steal most often occurs when mild and noncritical stenosis is present in the donor artery but may occur in the absence of such stenosis. Intracoronary steal (also called subendocardial or transmural steal) denotes a shift of blood flow from the endocardial layer into the subepicardial layer in a vascular territory perfused by a stenotic artery. This type of steal occurs because the subepicardial vessels retain residual vasodilator reserve that is greater than the reserve in the subendocardial layer (Fig. 19-11). This degree of steal is considerably smaller in quantitative terms than intercoronary steal. Branch steal denotes shift of flow from one region of myocardium to another in the same vascular territory. Seilen et al, using intracoronary Doppler flow velocity measurements, concluded that coronary steal occurs in 10% of patients with a wide range of coronary collaterals to the vascular area from which blood flow is redistributed.[107]

Factors other than steal may contribute to myocardial ischemia during pharmacologic vasodilation. These include a decrease in distal coronary perfusion pressure; an increase in myocardial oxygen demand (because of reflex tachycardia); and, possibly, collapse at the stenosis site because of a decrease in coronary pressure. We could not confirm the presence of collapse in humans by using quantitative coronary angiography during adenosine infusion.[93] If myocardial ischemia occurs because of steal, it may lead to regional wall-motion abnormality, ST-segment depression, metabolic abnormality, and lactate production. Fung et al[36] observed a decrease in regional left ventricular contraction in few of their experimental animals in response to dipyridamole, suggesting that methods that rely on heterogeneity of blood flow (such as perfusion imaging) are superior to methods that rely on the demonstration of wall-motion abnormality (such as echocardiography) during vasodilator stress testing. These observations have been confirmed clinically. Vatner and Baig[120] observed augmentation of coronary blood flow in normal or moderately stenosed arteries but not in severely ischemic zones in response to dobutamine administration in experimental animals.[120] They also observed that the degree of tachycardia affected the endocardial-to-epicardial blood flow ratio in severely ischemic zones. In the presence of coronary artery disease, the increase in coronary blood flow with dobutamine is blunted, and the heterogeneity in flow between

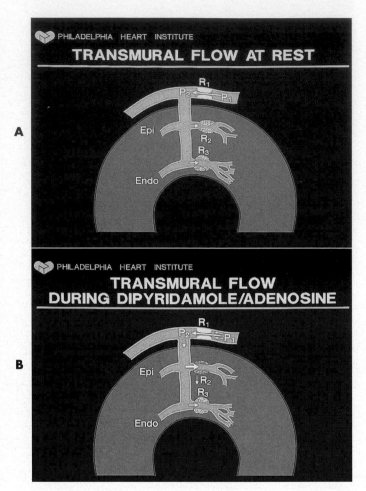

Fig. 19-11. Transmural steal during coronary vasodilation with redistribution of flow from endocardial to epicardial layer. **(A)** At baseline, **(B)** during adenosine infusion.

the normal and diseased arteries is the mechanism for the detection of perfusion defects. Unlike with coronary vasodilators, however, the territory of the diseased artery may become ischemic because of the increase in myocardial oxygen demand. Therefore, with both vasodilators and inotropes/chronotropes, perfusion defects are caused by heterogeneity in flow, which may reflect true ischemia with dobutamine and arbutamine but reflect mere flow differences with adenosine and dipyridamole (unless ischemia is also produced by coronary steal).

HEMODYNAMIC EFFECTS

The hemodynamic effects of adenosine appear almost immediately after infusion is started and disappear very rapidly after termination of infusion. The hemodynamic effects of dipyridamole peak at approximately the seventh minute after the start of infusion and may last 30 to 45 minutes after the infusion is completed.*

Both adenosine and dipyridamole produce a slight increase in heart rate (adenosine more so than dipyridamole) and a slight

*References 34, 46, 49, 62, 66, 67, 85, 92, 93.

decrease in systemic arterial pressure (adenosine more so than dipyridamole). A slight increase in the double product (heart rate multiplied by systolic blood pressure) is observed with both agents. Cardiac output increases slightly (average, 50% with adenosine and 35% with dipyridamole).[93] Adenosine causes a small increase in pulmonary capillary wedge pressure that is greater in patients with coronary artery disease than in normal patients. The changes in pulmonary capillary wedge pressure are minimal with dipyridamole. The causes of this increase in pulmonary capillary pressure are shown in Box 19-4. Increased left ventricular stiffness may be caused by increased myocardial blood volume. In support of that hypothesis, we have seen a slight but significant increase in myocardial thickness during the effect of adenosine. The greater increase in left ventricular filling pressure in patients with coronary artery disease may suggest an additional effect of ischemia. This ischemia, however, may produce diastolic rather than systolic dysfunction because of its mild nature. Diastolic dysfunction alters left ventricular stiffness by shifting the pressure–volume relation. Ogilby et al[93] did not observe substantial changes in left ventricular end-diastolic volume and ejection fraction. Others, however, have measured a slight increase in end-diastolic volume and have suggested that the increase in the filling pressure is caused by increased preload.[92] This increase in preload is thought to result from venoconstriction. In our opinion, the slight change in end-diastolic volume could not account for the observed change in filling pressure without simultaneous changes in stiffness.

With dobutamine and arbutamine, the increase in heart rate is greater than that achieved by adenosine or dipyridamole but is less than that achieved with maximal exercise. The mean heart rate at a dosage of 40 μg/kg/min of dobutamine or 0.8 μkg/min of arbutamine is 120 to 125 beats per minute in normal patients. The stroke volume, cardiac output, and systolic blood pressure also increase, although hypotension may occur even in normal patients (especially at high infusion rates). This most likely results from the stimulation of β2 adrenoreceptors, causing peripheral vasodilation. Dynamic obstruction of left ventricular outflow tract may also cause hypotension.

It has been suggested that adenosine has a negative indirect inotropic effect or antiadrenergic effect: that is, it depresses contractility when there is baseline adrenergic stimulation. However, this effect has not been documented in humans.

Box 19-4 Mechanisms of increased pulmonary capillary wedge pressure during adenosine infusion

Increased left ventricular stiffness
Cardiodepressant effect and direct coronary steal
  Direct
  Indirect because of coronary steal → ischemia
Negative lusitropic effect
Increased preload

Adenosine is an important vasodilator in all arteriolar beds except for the preglomerular arterioles in the kidneys, where it produces vasoconstriction.[67] The hypotensive effect of adenosine has been used during intracranial vascular operations[49,62] and in the treatment of pulmonary hypertension.[46] Other effects of adenosine include myocardial protection during ischemic preconditioning and thrombolytic therapy in acute myocardial infarction and during coronary artery bypass surgery.

PERFUSION IMAGING

The earliest work with perfusion imaging with adenosine was done by Strauss and Pitt.[115] Gould et al[40] first investigated dipyridamole, and dobutamine was first researched by Mason et al.[83] Since then, extensive clinical experience has been reported, especially with dipyridamole and adenosine, and both agents are approved by the U.S. Food and Drug Administration for use with perfusion imaging. Although dobutamine has been used for this purpose, it has not been approved for this indication, and arbutamine is awaiting approval. The paradigm most commonly adopted is that in patients who have exercise limitations, coronary vasodilators are the first choice, and in those who have contraindications to coronary vasodilators, dobutamine is used. These agents have been used with thallium-201 (^{201}Tl), ^{99m}Tc sestamibi, ^{99m}Tc teboroxime, and ^{99m}Tc tetrofosmin. Because of the short half-life of adenosine the radiotracer is injected during the infusion; in contrast, dipyridamole is injected 3 minutes after the completion of the infusion. With dobutamine and arbutamine, the radiotracer is injected at the peak effect. The imaging protocols are shown in Fig. 19-12. In some laboratories, hand-grip exercise or submaximal treadmill exercise is combined with dipyridamole. This combination helps to decrease subdiaphragmatic activity and improve target-to-background ratio and may decrease side effects secondary to hypotension. Some have suggested the use of exercise in combination with adenosine, possibly for the same reasons, but the justification and the logistics for this combination seem to be more difficult to defend. A high dose of dipyridamole (0.84 mg/kg) is used in Europe, especially with echocardiography; this dose has not been approved by the U.S. Food and Drug Administration. Atropine may be combined with dobutamine in patients with indaquate heart rate response to the maximum dose. The thallium protocol is stress–4-hour redistribution (or reinjection, or both). The protocol with the technetium-labeled tracers can be same-day stress–rest or rest–stress or separate-day stress–rest. Gated imaging and attenuation/scatter compensation may be used as with exercise, although the functional data (ejection fraction by gating or first-pass radionuclide angiography) are less helpful with adenosine and dipyridamole than with exercise.[10,60]

RESULTS

The results of stress perfusion imaging depend on patient selection, extent of coronary artery disease, severity of stenosis, presence of previous myocardial infarction, and the experience of the observer. The average sensitivity from multiple studies is

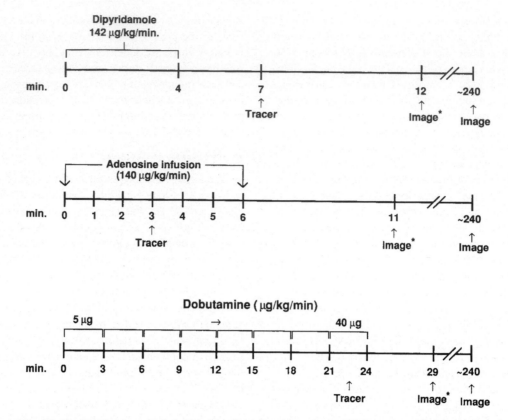

Fig. 19-12. Imaging protocols with adenosine, dipyridamole, and dobutamine. (From Iskandrian AS, Verani MS, Heo J: Pharmacologic stress testing: Mechanism of action, hemodynamic responses, and results in detection of coronary artery disease, *J Nucl Cardiol* 1:94-111, 1994. Reproduced with permission.)

Table 19-2. Summary results of pharmacologic single-photon emission computed tomography perfusion imaging

Variable	Dipyridamole	Adenosine	Dobutamine	Arbutamine
Sensitivity, %	89	90	82	87
Specificity, %	78	91	73	90*

*Normalcy rate.

80% to 90% and the specificity is 80% to 90% (Table 19-2).* In our experience, the results of SPECT perfusion imaging are better in patients with multivessel disease than in those with single-vessel disease and are better in men than in women (Fig. 19-13). Investigators from Cedars-Sinai Medical Center[3] showed a high sensitivity in detecting coronary artery disease in women by using adenosine dual-isotope imaging (rest thallium adenosine ^{99m}Tc sestamibi). Using stepwise discriminate analysis Iskandian et al[57] showed that the most important predictors of extensive coronary artery disease (left main or triple-vessel disease) are the presence of perfusion abnormality in more than one vascular territory, increased lung thallium uptake, and ST-segment depression. These variables were also the most important variables during exercise testing.[60] The tech-

netium-labeled tracers provide results similar to those of thallium because most patients included in these studies have severe coronary artery disease.

As discussed earlier, no comparative data exist for patients with mild to moderate stenosis. A phase III trial comparing adenosine teboroxime infusion with adenosine sestamibi infusion in patients with mild to moderate stenosis by angiography is under way. The results of perfusion imaging with adenosine and dipyridamole, unlike those with dobutamine, are not related to the degree of systemic hemodynamic changes (heart rate or blood pressure) or symptoms. On the basis of tracer kinetics, we prefer thallium in patients with average body weight (<200 lb in men and <175 lb in women). In obese patients, we use technetium-labeled tracers (^{99m}Tc sestamibi or ^{99m}Tc tetrofosmin) with adenosine or dipyridamole. The image quality with thallium in such patients is very good because of marked increase in myocardial blood flow.

* References 25, 31, 32, 43, 53, 57, 58, 63, 68, 76, 88, 90, 91, 95, 113, 115, 117, 122.

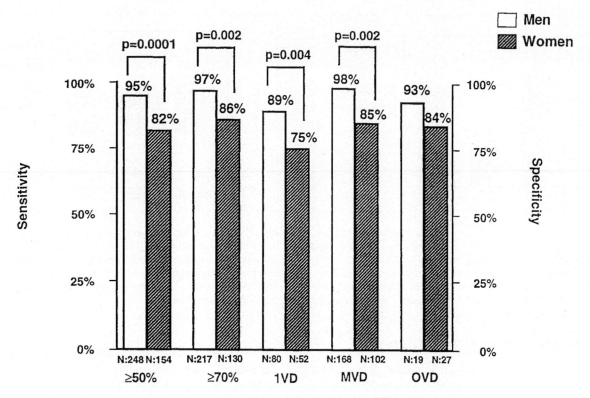

Fig. 19-13. Results of adenosine single-photon emission computed tomography thallium imaging in relation to extent of coronary artery disease in men and women (From Iskandrian AS: *Perfusion imaging for the diagnosis and risk assessment of CAD in women.* In Marwick T, ed: *Cardiac stress testing and imaging,* New York, 1996, Churchill Livingstone Company. Reproduced with permission.)

Taillefer et al[113] compared the results of dipyridamole and adenosine thallium imaging in 54 patients with coronary artery disease, by using quantitative planar imaging. Dipyridamole thallium images were abnormal in 47 patients, and adenosine images were abnormal in 49 patients (difference not significant).[113] All 6 patients who received adenosine and 8 patients who received dipyridamole who had normal images had single-vessel coronary artery disease. There were 35 more reversible defects with adenosine than with dipyridamole; most of these defects were in territories of vessels with 50% to 70% stenosis. The ischemic-to-normal thallium ratio was lower with adenosine than with dipyridamole (0.78 and 0.83; p <0.001), suggesting a higher flow in the normal zone. The same authors also observed more reversible defects with high-dose dipyridamole thallium than with the standard dose.[71] The difference between administration of a high dose and standard dose could not be shown when ^{99m}Tc sestamibi was used by Casanova et al,[16] probably because of differences in tracer kinetics. The results with arbutamine (Table 19-2) were from a U.S. multicenter study that included 122 patients with coronary artery disease on angiography and 62 patients with a low likelihood of coronary artery disease. In 69 patients, both arbutamine and exercise tests were done on separate days, and 92% agreement in the presence of perfusion defects was found (κ = 0.80; p <0.001).[65] Recently, Sharir et al reported that continued use of antianginal drugs before dipyridamole plus low level exercise SPECT thallium imaging reduced the extent and severity of perfusion defects resulting in underestimation of CAD.[108]

LEFT VENTRICULAR DILATION

Transient left ventricular dilation may occur during adenosine or dipyridamole infusion which most likely reflects a decrease (relative or absolute) in subendocardial flow. This finding is more common in patients with extensive CAD and multiple perfusion defects, and therefore, is a marker of high risk. Transient dilation could also be observed with dobutamine.[10,22,59,60]

LUNG THALLIUM UPTAKE

Increased lung thallium uptake (measured qualitatively or by a lung-to-heart ratio >50%) during infusion of adenosine, dipyridamole, or dobutamine is more common in patients with multivessel disease and in patients with multiple perfusion defects. It is unclear whether increased lung thallium uptake is associated with transient left ventricular dilation.[10,59,60] It is thought that increased lung thallium uptake is secondary to elevation of left ventricular filling pressure, a mechanism similar to that observed during exercise testing; however, this hypothesis could not be proven in one study.

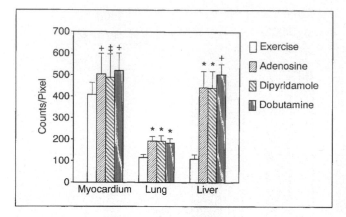

Fig. 19-14. The concentration of thallium in the myocardium, liver, and lungs during exercise, adenosine, dipyridamole, and dobutamine testing in normal volunteers. (From Lee J, Chae SC, Lee K, et al: Biokinetics of thallium-201 in normal subjects: Comparison between adenosine, dipyridamole, dobutamine, and exercise, *J Nucl Med* 35:535-541, 1994. Reproduced with permission from the Society of Nuclear Medicine.)

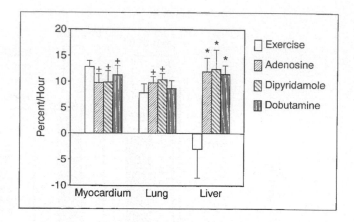

Fig. 19-15. Thallium wash-out from the myocardium, liver, and lungs in normal volunteers. (From Lee J, Chae SC, Lee K, et al: Biokinetics of thallium-201 in normal subjects: comparison between adenosine, dipyridamole, dobutamine, and exercise, *J Nucl Med* 35:535-541, 1994. Reproduced with permission from the Society of Nuclear Medicine.)

SUBDIAPHRAGMATIC TRACER ACTIVITY

Unlike in exercise testing, little, if any, redistribution of the cardiac output occurs in adenosine or dipyridamole infusion; therefore, prominent hepatic activity is seen.[60] This is true with thallium and, especially, with technetium-labeled perfusion tracers. With SPECT imaging this activity generally does not interfere with image interpretation. Bowel activity may be more of problem than liver activity. Nonetheless, it has been suggested that imaging with technetium-labeled agents should be performed 30 to 60 minutes after injection of the tracer rather than 15 to 30 minutes after infusion, as is recommended with exercise.

THALLIUM WASH-OUT (CLEARANCE)

The thallium concentration in the myocardium, lung, and liver with adenosine, dipyridamole, dobutamine, and exercise testing in normal volunteers are shown in Fig. 19-14 and Fig. 19-15.[73] Myocardial activity was higher with pharmacologic stress tests than with exercise, but myocardial wash-out was slower. Slower wash-out is probably due to a higher blood concentration of thallium as a result of thallium reentering the blood pool from the liver and other noncardiac tissues. Therefore, despite higher myocardial uptake with thallium than with exercise, wash-out is slower. The myocardial uptake of ^{99m}Tc sestamibi in another study was similar with adenosine, dipyridamole, and exercise, probably because the extraction fraction of ^{99m}Tc sestamibi is lower than that of thallium.[105]

PATIENTS WITH LEFT BUNDLE-BRANCH BLOCK

Twenty percent to 50% of patients with left bundle-branch block may have transient defects in the septum during exercise perfusion imaging in the absence of disease of the left anterior descending coronary artery. These patients are therefore candidates for pharmacologic stimulation with adenosine or dipyridamole (with no supplemental exercise).* The septal perfusion defect is related to tachycardia; for this reason, dobutamine is not a suitable choice in these patients. On the basis of measurement of blood flow and metabolism in dogs during right ventricular pacing, Ono et al[95] concluded that these defects represent a decrease in diastolic flow in the left anterior descending artery because a decrease in myocardial tension with no evidence of true ischemia occurred.[95] Matzer et al[84] observed that involvement of the apex could separate true abnormality caused by left anterior descending artery stenosis from bundle-branch–related defect.[84] We do not believe that this scintigraphic finding is reliable. Conduction defects of other types are not associated with specific patterns of perfusion.

ST-SEGMENT DEPRESSION

ST-segment depression is more common with dobutamine than with adenosine and dipyridamole and is less prominent with dobutamine than with exercise testing. With dobutamine, it reflects the presence of myocardial ischemia due to increased demand; with dipyridamole and adenosine, it reflects myocardial ischemia due to coronary steal.[19,60,89] The presence of coronary collateral vessels on angiography has been shown to be an important predictor of ST-segment depression with adenosine or dipyridamole; this result supports the idea of coronary steal as an underlying mechanism. In nonselected patients, ST-segment depression occurs in 5% to 10% of patients undergoing adenosine or dipyridamole testing, but in patients with coronary artery disease, the incidence may be 20% to 30%, depending on the extent and severity of disease and the presence or absence of collaterals. Occasionally, ST-segment depression

*References 14, 23, 29, 72, 84, 94.

may occur in the absence of coronary artery disease (10% of patients with ST-segment depression). ST-segment elevation may also be observed but is very rare in the absence of Q-wave myocardial infarctions.

CONTRAINDICATIONS

Contraindications to adenosine or dipyridamole include bronchospasm, baseline hypotension (systolic blood pressure <90 mm Hg), acute myocardial infarction (within 24 hours), acute coronary syndromes, second-degree or higher atrioventricular block in the absence of a functioning pacemaker, and hypersensitivity reaction.[7,9,10,60] Oral dipyridamole should be discontinued for 24 hours, and compounds that contain caffeine and xanthine should not be taken for 12 hours. Contraindications to dobutamine stress testing include severe hypotension or hypertension, uncontrolled atrial flutter or fibrillation, recurrent ventricular tachycardia, severe left ventricular outflow obstruction, recent acute myocardial infarction, acute coronary syndromes, large aortic aneurysms, and decompensated heart failure. Therapy with β-blockers and calcium-channel antagonists should be discontinued for 24 to 48 hours.

SIDE EFFECTS

Roughly 70% to 80% of patients receiving adenosine have one or more side effects. In general, these effect are short-lived and mild, and rarely require treatment or discontinuation of the infusion (Table 19-3). Side effects include chest pains, flushing, shortness of breath, dyspnea, gastrointestinal discomfort, headaches, lightheadedness, and ST changes.* Chest pains are caused by adenosine A_1 receptor stimulation and may be observed in patients with normal coronary angiograms.[26] Dyspnea is caused by adenosine-induced hyperventilation acting through stimulation of the carotid chemoreceptor; therefore, it is not a sign of heart failure. First-degree atrioventricular block occurs in about 10% of patients but is hemodynamically unimportant.[60,74] Second-degree atrioventricular block occurs in 4% of patients and is well tolerated. Third-degree atrioventricular block occurs in less than 1% of patients and requires either decrease of the infusion rate or discontinuation of the infusion,

depending on the heart rate and blood pressure responses and symptoms. It rarely requires reversal with aminophylline. Atropine is not effective in reversing atrioventricular block caused by adenosine. Atrioventricular block generally occurs in the first 2 minutes of infusion and may be intermittent. Ironically, ST-segment depression is considered a side effect of dipyridamole or adenosine infusion but not of exercise testing. Aminophylline is used to treat side effects of adenosine or dipyridamole.

The safety of adenosine and dipyridamole has been confirmed in numerous studies, and serious side effects, such as death, myocardial infarction, or serious arrhythmias, are extremely unusual. Both agents are also safe in patients with carotid disease, but care should be taken in patients with hypotension and recent transient ischemic attacks.[77] Of interest, adenosine produces an increase in cerebral blood flow. Side effects of dipyridamole occur in 50% of patients and include chest pain, headache, dizziness, ST changes, hypotension, flushing, dyspnea, and gastrointestinal symptoms. These side effects tend to last longer and require reversal with aminophylline. Routine use of aminophylline in the absence of side effects is not recommended.

Side effects of dobutamine occur in about 75% of patients and include chest pain, palpitations, headaches, flushing, dyspnea, paresthesias, nausea, and dizziness. In the study by Hays et al,[45] dobutamine infusion had to be discontinued in 26% of patients because of severe side effects. The most troublesome side effect is ventricular and atrial arrhythmias. Most patients prefer adenosine or dipyridamole over dobutamine.[45] Secknus et al[106] observed few serious side effects in nearly 3000 studies. Side effects of dobutamine are treated with short-acting β-blockers.

RISK ASSESSMENT

Pharmacologic stress testing has been used in risk assessment of patients with stable symptoms, after stabilization of patients with unstable angina, after acute myocardial infarction, and before major vascular surgery. These topics will be discussed in Chapters 20, 21, and 26.

*References 18, 69, 77, 78, 86, 97, 101.

Table 19-3. Common side effects (%)

Side effect	Adenosine	Dipyridamole	Dobutamine	Arbutamine
Flushing	37	43	14	10
Dyspnea	35	3	14	21
Chest pain	35	20	31	51
Headaches	14	12	14	11
Lightheadedness	12	7	4	5
Atrioventricular block	8	0	0	0
ST-T changes	6	8	30	50
Arrhythmias	2	5	50	53
Hypotension	5	3	0	8
Any	79	47	75	53

PHARMACOLOGIC TESTING WITH RADIONUCLIDE ANGIOGRAPHY

Adenosine and dipyridamole infusion may precipitate regional and global left ventricular dysfunction in some patients with coronary artery disease.[17,44,112] These abnormal responses are less frequent than perfusion abnormalities. Harris et al[44] found a sensitivity of 13% for dipyridamole radionuclide angiography compared with 88% with thallium. Sochor et al[112] found that only 31% of patients with perfusion defect had regional wall-motion abnormality. Better results were obtained by Cates et al[17] (67%) and Klein et al[66] (66%). Even with dobutamine, perfusion defects are more common than wall-motion abnormalities. An increase in left ventricular ejection fraction has been reported with dobutamine, even in patients with coronary artery disease.[5,24]

PHARMACOLOGIC STRESS TESTING WITH TWO-DIMENSIONAL ECHOCARDIOGRAPHY

Adenosine, dipyridamole, and dobutamine have been used with two-dimensional echocardiography; most experience, however, has been with dobutamine echocardiography.[48,64,80-82,99,127] When dipyridamole is used, a high dose rather than a standard dose is often used. The results depend on observer experience and patient selection. Marwick et al[82] compared ^{99m}Tc sestamibi SPECT with echocardiography during adenosine or dobutamine infusion.[83] Dobutamine sestamibi SPECT had a sensitivity of 80% and a specificity of 74% compared with a sensitivity of 86% and a specificity of 71% for adenosine sestamibi SPECT. Dobutamine echocardiography had a sensitivity of 85% and a specificity of 82%, and adenosine echocardiography had a sensitivity of 58% and a specificity of 87%. In another study by the same group, sensitivity was 76% for ^{99m}Tc sestamibi SPECT and 72% for dobutamine echocardiography, the specificity was 67% and 83%, respectively.[81] Most false-positive SPECT results were in patients with left ventricular hypertrophy. The sensitivity on echocardiography was lower in patients who were unable to complete the test because of side effects; in these patients, the sensitivity of ^{99m}Tc sestamibi SPECT was higher than that of echocardiography (71% and 59%). In patients with a negative result on submaximal dobutamine echocardiography (31 of 142 patients), SPECT had a sensitivity of 80%. In a recent multicenter study, dobutamine atropine echocardiography had a sensitivity of 82% and specificity of 94% (p value not significant). Santoro et al[104] examined 60 patients, 33 with and 27 without coronary artery disease on angiography.[104] In these patients, the sensitivity and specificity of dipyridamole echocardiography were 55% and 96%; on dobutamine echocardiography, they were 61% and 96%; on dipyridamole sestamibi infusion, 97% and 89%; and on dobutamine sestamibi infusion, 91% and 81% ($p <$ 0.005 on nuclear imaging vs echocardiography). Furthermore, of the 62 stenotic coronary arteries, dipyridamole echocardiography identified 32%, dobutamine echocardiography identified 39%, dipyridamole sestamibi identified 77%, and dobutamine sestamibi identified 73%. The sensitivity for correctly predict-ing multivessel disease was as follows: dipyridamole echocardiography, 14%; dobutamine echocardiography, 29%; dipyridamole sestamibi, 48%; and dobutamine sestamibi, 57%. Dibello et al[30] also found that the sensitivity of dobutamine sestamibi was higher than that of dobutamine echocardiography (87% and 76%), although the specificity of both techniques was similar (86% for each). Recent data suggest that for any given blood flow, the ratio of sestamibi counts in the abnormal to those in the normal areas of the myocardium is substantially smaller with dobutamine than with adenosine, suggesting that dobutamine may underestimate the degree and extent of ischemia in mild to moderate stenosis.[15] The precise reason for this observation is not clear but may be related to the effect of dobutamine on mitochondrial potential and, hence, on extraction, retention, or washout of ^{99m}Tc sestamibi.

Bach et al.[4] reported the results of the International Arbutamine Study Group in Europe. The sensitivity of arbutamine echocardiography was 71%, and its specificity was 67%. These results are in agreement with the results bound by Santoro et al.[104] using dobutamine echocardiography.

As mentioned earlier, when evaluating comparative data, the choice of the tracer and the stress agent in relation to the patient mix is important. For example, it is conceivable that thallium is better than ^{99m}Tc sestamibi in patients with moderate stenosis or that adenosine or dipyridamole is preferred over dobutamine with pharmacologic perfusion testing. In addition, the specificity with SPECT imaging is a complex issue and is largely dependent on the experience of the observer, the imaging technique used, and the incorporation of additional imaging methods, such as attenuation and scatter compensation and gating. These methods were not used in the previously cited studies.

POSITRON EMISSION TOMOGRAPHY WITH PHARMACOLOGIC STRESS TESTING

Most studies of positron emission tomography for the detection of coronary artery disease are done using rubidium -82 or ^{13}N-labeled ammonia during pharmacologic stimulation with adenosine or dipyridamole.[21,54] The results are dependent on qualitative assessment of perfusion pattern. In general, the results are similar to or slightly better than those obtained with SPECT perfusion imaging. A major advantage of positron emission tomography is the ability to compensate for attenuation. With attenuation and scatter compensation, SPECT results may also improve. Quantitative measurement of absolute myocardial blood flow is not routinely used for detection of coronary artery disease, probably because of considerable interperson variability. However, quantitative measurements are very useful for serial measurements (such as evaluation of effects of lipid lowering therapy or cardiac rehabilitation) because of small intraindividual variability.

MAGNETIC RESONANCE IMAGING

The experience with magnetic resonance imaging is limited, but it should be possible to quantitatively assess regional and global left ventricular function. The use of dipyridamole may be preferred in these circumstances because of its longer duration of pharmacologic effects.

NEW AGENTS

A selective adenosine A_2 receptor agonist, WCR-470, produces coronary vasodilation and hyperemia of similar magnitude to that produced by adenosine.[11,53] This agent is a selective A_{2a} agonist, suggesting that the decrease in coronary vascular resistance is far greater than the decrease in systemic vascular resistance. In animal studies, the ischemic-to-normal tracer ratio obtained with WCR-470 was similar to that obtained with adenosine. Because WCR-470 is a selective A_2 agonist, the side effects of A_1 receptor stimulation, such as atrioventricular block, are not encountered. Because chest pain during adenosine stimulation are due to A_1 stimulation, their occurrence with WCR-470 suggests that they may be used as markers of true ischemia.

A short-lived selective adenosine A_1 receptor agonist also exists. This agent may be combined with adenosine to counteract the undesirable effects of A_1 stimulation (chest pains and atrioventricular block).[11,39] As mentioned earlier, however, the side effects of adenosine are mild and short-lived; therefore, the combination of adenosine with A_1 receptor agonists, even if given as a bolus, would be rarely required for routine clinical use.

COMPARISON WITH EXERCISE

The sensitivity of vasodilator pharmacologic SPECT perfusion imaging is similar to that of maximal exercise testing and is better than that of submaximal exercise testing. Its specificity is also better than that of exercise. Mild side effects are more frequent with pharmacologic testing, but serious serous side effects are rare with either type of stress. ST depression is less frequent with pharmacologic testing. Antianginal medications affect the results of exercise, dobutamine, and arbutamine tests but not of adenosine and dipyridamole tests. Caffeine and xanthine compounds affect the results of adenosine and dipyridamole tests but not of exercise, dobutamine, and arbutamine tests. Pharmacologic stress testing can be used in patients with exercise limitations and may be better for serial studies and for the detection of mild stenosis, although the latter two issues have not been studied adequately.[60]

REFERENCES

1. Abreu A, Mahmarian JJ, Nishimura S, et al: Tolerance and safety of pharmacologic coronary vasodilation with adenosine in association with thallium-201 scintigraphy in patients with suspected coronary artery disease, *J Am Coll Cardiol* 18:730–735, 1991.
2. Allman KC, Berry T, Sucharski LA, et al: Determination of extent and location of coronary artery disease in patients without prior myocardial infarction by thallium-201 tomography with pharmacologic stress, *J Nucl Med* 33:2067–2073, 1992.
3. Amanullah AM, Kiat H, Friedman JD, et al: Adenosine technetium-99m sestamibi myocardial perfusion SPECT in women: diagnostic efficacy in detection of coronary artery disease, *J Am Coll Cardiol* 27:803–809, 1996.
4. Bach DS, Cohen JL, Fioretti PM, et al: Safety and efficacy of closed-loop arbutamine stress echocardiography detection of coronary artery disease. International Arbutamine Study Group, *Am J Cardiol* 81:32–35, 1998.
5. Bartunek J, Marwick JH, Rodrigues ACT, et al: Dobutamine-induced wall motion abnormalities: correlations with myocardial fractional flow reserve and quantitative coronary angiography, *J Am Coll Cardiol* 27:1429–1436, 1996.
6. Becker LC: Conditions for vasodilator-induced coronary steal in experimental myocardial ischemia, *Circulation* 57:1103–1110, 1978.
7. Beer SG, Heo J, Iskandrian AS: Dipyridamole thallium imaging, *Am J Cardiol* 67:18D–26D, 1991.
8. Belardinelli L, Linden J, Berne RM: The cardiac effects of adenosine, *Prog Cardiovasc Dis* 32:73–97, 1989.
9. Beller GA: Pharmacologic stress imaging, *JAMA* 265:633–638, 1991.
10. Beller GA, ed: *Pharmacologic stress imaging. In clinical nuclear cardiology,* Philadelphia, 1995, WB Saunders Company.
11. Bertolet BD, Belardinelli L, Franco EA, et al: Selective attenuation by N-0861 (N^6-endonorboran-2-yl-9-methyladenine) of cardiac A_1 adenosine receptor-mediated effects in humans, *Circulation* 93:1871–1876, 1996.
12. Böttcher M, Czernin J, Sun KT, et al: Effect of caffeine on myocardial blood flow at rest and during pharmacologic vasodilation, *J Nucl Med* 36:2016–2021, 1995.
13. Brown BG, Josephson MA, Peterson RB, et al: Intravenous dipyridamole combined with isometric handgrip for near maximal acute increase in coronary flow in patients with coronary artery disease, *Am J Cardiol* 48:1077–1085, 1981.
14. Burns RJ, Balligan L, Wright LM, et al: Improved specificity of myocardial thallium-201 single-photon emission computed tomography in patients with left bundle branch block by dipyridamole, *Am J Cardiol* 68:504–508, 1991.
15. Calnon DA, Glover DK, Beller GA, et al: Effects of dobutamine stress on myocardial blood flow, ^{99m}Tc sestamibi uptake, and systolic wall thickening in the presence of coronary artery disease: implications for dobutamine stress testing, *Circulation* 96:2353–2360, 1997.
16. Casanova R, Patroncini A, Guidalotti PL, et al: Dose and test for dipyridamole infusion and cardiac imaging early after uncomplicated acute myocardial infarction, *Am J Cardiol* 70:1402–1406, 1992.
17. Cates CU, Kronenberg MW, Collins HW, et al: Dipyridamole radionuclide ventriculography: a test with high specificity for severe coronary artery disease. *J Am Coll Cardiol* 13:841–851, 1989.
18. Cerqueira MD, Verani MS, Schwaiger M, et al: Safety profile of adenosine stress perfusion imaging: results from the Adenoscan Multicenter Trial Registry, *J Am Coll Cardiol* 23:384–389, 1994.
19. Chambers CE, Brown KA: Dipyridamole-induced ST segment depression during thallium-201 imaging in patients with coronary artery disease: angiographic and hemodynamic determinants, *J Am Coll Cardiol* 12:37–41, 1988.
20. Chan SY, Brunken RC, Czernin J, et al: Comparison of maximal myocardial blood flow during adenosine infusion with that of intravenous dipyridamole in normal men, *J Am Coll Cardiol* 20:979–985, 1992.
21. Chan SY, Kobashigawa J, Stevenson LW, et al: Myocardial blood flow at rest and during pharmacological vasodilation in cardiac transplants during and after successful treatment of rejection, *Circulation* 90:204–212, 1994.
22. Chouraqui P, Rodrigues EA, Berman DS, et al: Significance of dipyridamole-induced transient dilation of the left ventricle during thallium-201 scintigraphy in suspected coronary artery disease, *Am J Cardiol* 66:689–694, 1990.
23. Civelek AC, Gozukara I, Durski K, et al: Detection of left anterior descending coronary artery disease in patients with left bundle branch block, *Am J Cardiol* 70:1565–1570, 1992.
24. Coma-Canella I, Gomez Martinez MV, Rodrigo F, et al: The dobutamine stress test with thallium-201 single-photon emission computed tomography and radionuclide angiography: postinfarction study, *J Am Coll Cardiol* 22:399–406, 1993.

25. Coyne EP, Belvedere DA, Vande Streek PR, et al: Thallium-201 scintigraphy after intravenous infusion of adenosine compared with exercise thallium testing in the diagnosis of coronary artery disease, *J Am Coll Cardiol* 17:1289–1294, 1991.

26. Crea F, Pupita G, Galassi AR, et al: Role of adenosine in pathogenesis of anginal pain, *Circulation* 81:164–172, 1990.

27. Czernin J, Auerbach M, Sun KT, et al: Effects of modified pharmacologic stress approaches on hyperemic myocardial blood flow, *J Nucl Med* 36:575–580, 1995.

28. Czernin J, Müller P, Chan S, et al: Influence of age and hemodynamics on myocardial blood flow and flow reserve, *Circulation* 88:62–69, 1993.

29. DePuey EG, Guertler-Krawczynska E, Robbins WL: Thallium-201 SPECT in coronary disease patients with left bundle branch block, *J Nucl Med* 29:1479–1485, 1988.

30. Di Bello V, Bellina CR, Gori E, et al: Incremental diagnostic value of dobutamine stress echocardiography and dobutamine scintigraphy (technetium 99m-labeled sestamibi single-photon emission computed tomography) for assessment of presence and extent of coronary artery disease, *J Nucl Cardiol* 3:212–220, 1996.

31. Donohue TJ, Miller DD, Bach RG, et al: Correlation of poststenotic hyperemic coronary flow velocity and pressure with abnormal stress myocardial perfusion imaging in coronary artery disease, *Am J Cardiol* 77:948–954, 1996.

32. Drury AN, Szent-Gyorgyi A: The physiological activity of adenine compounds with special reference to their action upon the mammalian heart, *J Physiol* 68:213–219, 1929.

33. Elliot BM, Robinson JG, Zellner JL, et al: Dobutamine-201Tl imaging. Assessing cardiac risks associated with vascular surgery, *Circulation* 84(5 Suppl):III54–III60, 1991.

34. Feldman RL, Nichols WW, Pepine CJ, et al: Acute effect of intravenous dipyridamole on regional coronary hemodynamics and metabolism, *Circulation* 64:333–344, 1981.

35. Flamen P, Bossuyt A, Franken PR: Technetium-99m-tetrofosmin in dipyridamole-stress myocardial SPECT imaging: intraindividual comparison with technetium-99m-sestamibi, *J Nucl Med* 36:2009–2015, 1995.

36. Fung AY, Gallagher KP, Buda AJ: The physiologic basis of dobutamine as compared with dipyridamole stress interventions in the assessment of critical coronary stenosis, *Circulation* 76:943–951, 1987.

37. Ghods M, Mangal R, Iskandrian AS, et al: Importance of intraluminal pressure on hemodynamics and vasoconstriction response of stenotic arteries, *Circulation* 85:708–716, 1992.

38. Glover DK, Ruiz M, Edwards NC, et al: Comparison between ^{201}Tl and ^{99m}Tc sestamibi uptake during adenosine-induced vasodilation as a function of coronary stenosis severity, *Circulation* 91:813–820, 1995.

39. Glover DK, Ruiz M, Sansoy V, et al: Effect of N-0861, a selective A_1 receptor antagonist, on pharmacologic stress imaging with adenosine, *J Nucl Med* 36:270–275, 1995.

40. Gould KL: Noninvasive assessment of coronary stenoses by myocardial perfusion imaging during pharmacologic coronary vasodilation. I. Physiologic basis and experimental validation, *Am J Cardiol* 41:267–278, 1978.

41. Gould KL, Lipscomb K, Hamilton GW: Physiologic basis for assessing critical coronary stenosis. Instantaneous flow response and regional distribution during coronary hyperemia as measures of coronary flow reserve, *Am J Cardiol* 33:87–94, 1974.

42. Gould KL, Westcott RJ, Albro PC, et al: Noninvasive assessment of coronary stenoses by myocardial imaging during pharmacologic coronary vasodilation. II. Clinical methodology and feasibility, *Am J Cardiol* 41:279–287, 1978.

43. Gupta NC, Esterbrooks DJ, Hilleman DE, et al: Comparison of adenosine and exercise thallium-201 single-photon emission computed tomography (SPECT) myocardial perfusion imaging. The GE SPECT Multicenter Adenosine Study Group, *J Am Coll Cardiol* 19:248–257, 1992.

44. Harris D, Taylor D, Condon B, et al: Myocardial imaging with dipyridamole: comparison of sensitivity and specificity of ^{201}Tl versus MUGA. *Eur J Nucl Med* 7:1–5, 1982.

45. Hays JT, Mahmarian JJ, Cochran AJ, et al: Dobutamine thallium-201 tomography for evaluating patients with suspected coronary artery disease unable to undergo exercise or vasodilator pharmacologic stress testing, *J Am Coll Cardiol* 21:1583–1590, 1993.

46. Haywood GA, Sneddon JF, Bashir Y, et al: Adenosine infusion for the reversal of pulmonary vasoconstriction in biventricular failure. A good test but a poor therapy, *Circulation* 86:896–902, 1992.

47. He ZX, Iskandrian AS, Gupta NC, et al: Assessing coronary artery disease with dipyridamole technetium-99m-tetrofosmin SPECT: a multicenter trial, *J Nucl Med* 38:44–48, 1997.

48. Heinle S, Hanson M, Gracey L, et al: Correlation of adenosine echocardiography and thallium scintigraphy, *Am Heart J* 125:1606–1613, 1993.

49. Heistad DD, Marcus ML, Gourley JK, et al: Effect of adenosine and dipyridamole on cerebral blood flow, *Am J Physiol* 240:H775–H780, 1981.

50. Heller LI, Cates C, Pompa J, et al: Intracoronary Doppler assessment of moderate coronary artery disease: comparison with ^{201}Tl imaging and coronary angiography. FACTS Study Group. *Circulation* 96:484–490, 1997.

51. Iskandrian AS: What is the optimum dose of dipyridamole for cardiac imaging? *Am J Cardiol* 70:1485–1486, 1992.

52. Iskandrian AS: Myocardial ischemia during pharmacological stress testing, *Circulation* 87:1415–1417, 1993.

53. Iskandrian AS: Are the differences between adenosine and dipyridamole clinically relevant? *J Nucl Cardiol* 3:281–283, 1996.

54. Iskandrian AS, Heo J: *Pharmacologic stress testing*. In Zaret BL, Beller GA, eds: *Nuclear cardiology: state of the art and future directions,* St. Louis, 1992, Mosby–Year Book.

55. Iskandrian AS, Heo J, Askenase A, et al: Dipyridamole cardiac imaging, *Am Heart J* 115:432–443, 1988.

56. Iskandrian AS, Heo J, Kong B, et al: Effect of exercise level on the ability of thallium-201 tomographic imaging in detecting coronary artery disease: analysis of 461 patients, *J Am Coll Cardiol* 14:1477–1486, 1989.

57. Iskandrian AS, Heo J, Lemlek J, et al: Identification of high-risk patients with left main and three-vessel coronary artery disease by adenosine-single photon emission computed tomographic thallium imaging, *Am Heart J* 125:1130–1135, 1993.

58. Iskandrian AS, Heo J, Nguyen T, et al: Assessment of coronary artery disease using single-photon emission computed tomography with thallium-201 during adenosine-induced coronary hyperemia, *Am J Cardiol* 67:1190–1194, 1991.

59. Iskandrian AS, Heo J, Nguyen T, et al: Left ventricular dilatation and pulmonary thallium uptake after single-photon emission computed tomography using thallium-201 during adenosine-induced coronary hyperemia, *Am J Cardiol* 66:807–811, 1990.

60. Iskandrian AS, Verani MS, eds: *Pharmacologic stress testing and other alternative techniques in the diagnosis of coronary artery disease in nuclear cardiac imaging: principles and applications,* ed 2, Philadelphia, 1995, FA Davis Company.

61. Iskandrian AS, Verani MS, Heo J: Pharmacologic stress testing: mechanism of action, hemodynamic responses, and results in detection of coronary artery disease, *J Nucl Cardiol* 1:94–111, 1994.

62. Kassell NF, Boarini DJ, Olin JJ, et al: Cerebral and systemic circulatory effects of arterial hypotension induced by adenosine, *J Neurosurg* 58:69–76, 1983.

63. Kern MJ, Deligonul U, Tatineni S, et al: Intravenous adenosine: continuous infusion and low dose bolus administration for determination of coronary vasodilator reserve in patients with and without coronary artery disease, *J Am Coll Cardiol* 18:718–729, 1991.

64. Khattar RS, Senior R, Joseph D, et al: Comparison of arbutamine stress ^{99m}Tc-labeled sestamibi single-photon emission computed to-

mographic imaging and echocardiography for detection of the extent and severity of coronary artery disease and inducible ischemia, *J Nucl Cardiol* 4:211–216, 1997.

65. Kiat H, Iskandrian AS, Villegas BJ, et al: Arbutamine stress thallium-201 single-photon emission computed tomography using a computerized closed-loop delivery system. Multicenter trial for evaluation of safety and diagnostic accuracy. The International Arbutamine Study Group, *J Am Coll Cardiol* 26:1159–1167, 1995.

66. Klein HO, Ninio R, Eliyahu S, et al: Effects of the dipyridamole test on left ventricular function in coronary artery disease, *Am J Cardiol* 69:482–488, 1992.

67. Koglin J, Böhm M, von Scheidt W, et al: Antiadrenergic effect of carbachol but not of adenosine on contractility in the intact human ventricle in vivo, *J Am Coll Cardiol* 23:678–683, 1994.

68. Kong BA, Shaw L, Miller DD, et al: Comparison of accuracy for detecting coronary artery disease and side-effect profile of dipyridamole thallium-201 myocardial perfusion imaging in women versus men, *Am J Cardiol* 70:168–173, 1992.

69. Korkmaz ME, Mahmarian JJ, Guidry GW, et al: Safety of single-site adenosine thallium-201 scintigraphy, *Am J Cardiol* 73:200–204, 1994.

70. Krivokapich J, Smith GT, Huang SC, et al: 13N ammonia myocardial imaging at rest and with exercise in normal volunteers. Quantification of absolute myocardial perfusion with dynamic positron emission tomography, *Circulation* 80:1328–1337, 1989.

71. Lalonde D, Taillefer R, Lambert R, et al: Thallium-201-dipyridamole imaging: comparison between a standard dose and a high dose of dipyridamole in the detection of coronary artery disease, *J Nucl Med* 35:1245–1253, 1994.

72. Larcos G, Brown ML, Gibbons RJ: Role of dipyridamole thallium-201 imaging in left bundle branch block, *Am J Cardiol* 68:1097–1098, 1991.

73. Lee J, Chae SC, Lee K, et al: Biokinetics of thallium-201 in normal subjects: comparison between adenosine, dipyridamole, dobutamine and exercise, *J Nucl Med* 35:535–541, 1994.

74. Lee J, Heo J, Ogilby JD, et al: Atrioventricular block during adenosine thallium imaging, *Am Heart J* 123:1569–1574, 1992.

75. Lefroy DC, Crake T, Uren NG, et al: Effect of inhibition of nitric oxide synthesis on epicardial coronary artery caliber and coronary blood flow in humans, *Circulation* 88:43–54, 1993.

76. Leppo JA, Boucher CA, Okada RD, et al: Serial thallium-201 myocardial imaging after dipyridamole infusion: diagnostic utility in detecting coronary stenoses and relationship to regional wall motion, *Circulation* 66:649–657, 1982.

77. Lette J, Carini G, Tatum JL, et al: Safety of dipyridamole testing in patients with cerebrovascular disease, *Am J Cardiol* 75:535–537, 1995.

78. Lette J, Tatum JL, Fraser S, et al: Safety of dipyridamole testing in 73,806 patients: the Multicenter Dipyridamole Safety Study, *J Nucl Cardiol* 2:3–17, 1995.

79. Mahmarian JJ, Verani MS: Myocardial perfusion imaging during pharmacologic stress testing, *Cardiol Clin* 12:223–245, 1994.

80. Martin TW, Seaworth JF, Johns JP, et al: Comparison of adenosine, dipyridamole, and dobutamine in stress echocardiography, *Ann Intern Med* 116:190–196, 1992.

81. Marwick T, D'Hondt AM, Baudhuin T, et al: Optimal use of dobutamine stress for the detection and evaluation of coronary artery disease: combination with echocardiography or scintigraphy, or both? *J Am Coll Cardiol* 22:159–167, 1993.

82. Marwick T, Willemart B, D'Hondt AM, et al: Selection of the optimal nonexercise stress for the evaluation of ischemic regional myocardial dysfunction and malperfusion. Comparison of dobutamine and adenosine using echocardiography and ^{99m}Tc-MIBI single photon emission computed tomography, *Circulation* 87:345–354, 1993.

83. Mason JR, Palac RT, Freeman ML, et al: Thallium scintigraphy during dobutamine infusion: nonexercise-dependent screening test for coronary disease, *Am Heart J* 107:481–485, 1984.

84. Matzer LA, Kiat H, Friedman JD, et al: A new approach to the assessment of tomographic thallium-201 scintigraphy in patients with left bundle branch block, *J Am Coll Cardiol* 17:1309–1317, 1991.

85. McLaughlin DP, Beller GA, Linden J, et al: Hemodynamic and metabolic correlates of dipyridamole-induced myocardial thallium-201 perfusion abnormalities in multivessel coronary artery disease, *Am J Cardiol* 74:1159–1164, 1994.

86. Mertes H, Sawada SG, Ryan T, et al: Symptoms, adverse effects, and complications associated with dobutamine stress echocardiography. Experience in 1118 patients, *Circulation* 88:15–19, 1993.

87. Muller P, Czernin J, Choi Y, et al: Effect of exercise supplementation during adenosine infusion on hyperemic blood flow and flow reserve, *Am Heart J* 128:52–60, 1994.

88. Miyagawa M, Kumano S, Sekiya M, et al: Thallium-201 myocardial tomography with intravenous infusion of adenosine triphosphate in diagnosis of coronary artery disease, *J Am Coll Cardiol* 26:1196–1201, 1995.

89. Nishimura S, Kimball KT, Mahmarian JJ, et al: Angiographic and hemodynamic determinants of myocardial ischemia during adenosine thallium-201 scintigraphy intercoronary artery disease, *Circulation* 87:1211–1219, 1993.

90. Nishimura S, Mahmarian JJ, Boyce TM, et al: Quantitative thallium-201 single-photon emission computed tomography during maximal pharmacologic coronary vasodilation with adenosine for assessing coronary artery disease, *J Am Coll Cardiol* 18:736–745, 1991.

91. Nguyen T, Heo J, Ogilby JD, et al: Single photon emission computed tomography with thallium-201 during adenosine-induced coronary hyperemia: correlation with coronary arteriography, exercise thallium imaging and two-dimensional echocardiography, *J Am Coll Cardiol* 16:1375–1383, 1990.

92. Nussbacher A, Arie S, Kalil R, et al: Mechanism of adenosine-induced elevation of pulmonary capillary wedge pressure in humans, *Circulation* 92:371–379, 1995.

93. Ogilby JD, Iskandrian AS, Untereker WJ, et al: Effect of intravenous adenosine infusion on myocardial perfusion and function. Hemodynamic angiographic and scintigraphy study, *Circulation* 86:887–895, 1992.

94. O'Keefe JH Jr, Bateman TM, Barnhart CS: Adenosine thallium-201 is superior to exercise thallium-201 for detecting coronary artery disease in patients with left bundle branch block, *J Am Coll Cardiol* 21:1332–1338, 1993.

95. Ono S, Nohara R, Kambara H, et al: Regional myocardial perfusion and glucose metabolism in experimental left bundle branch block, *Circulation* 85:1125–1131, 1992.

96. Patterson RE, Kirk ES: Coronary steal mechanisms in dogs with one-vessel occlusion and other arteries normal, *Circulation* 67:1009–1015, 1983.

97. Pennell DJ, Underwood SR, Ell PJ: Safety of dobutamine stress for thallium-201 myocardial perfusion tomography in patients with asthma, *Am J Cardiol* 71:1346–1350, 1993.

98. Pennell DJ, Underwood SR, Swanton RH, et al: Dobutamine thallium myocardial perfusion tomography, *J Am Coll Cardiol* 18:1471–1479, 1991.

99. Pingitore A, Picano E, Colosso MQ, et al: The atropine factor in pharmacologic stress echocardiography. Echo Persatine (EPIC) and Echo Dobutamine International Cooperative (EDIC) Study Groups, *J Am Coll Cardiol* 27:1164–1170, 1996.

100. Quyyumi AA, Dakak N, Andrews NP, et al: Contribution of nitric oxide to metabolic coronary vasodilation in the human heart, *Circulation* 92:320–326, 1995.

101. Ranhosky A, Kempthorne-Rawson J: The safety of intravenous dipyridamole thallium myocardial perfusion imaging. Intravenous Dipyridamole Thallium Imaging Study Group, *Circulation* 81:1205–1209, 1990.

102. Rossen JD, Quillen JE, Lopez AG, et al: Comparison of coronary va-

sodilation with intravenous dipyridamole and adenosine, *J Am Coll Cardiol* 18:485–491, 1991.

103. Rossen JD, Simonetti I, Marcus ML, et al: Coronary dilation with standard dose dipyridamole and dipyridamole combined with handgrip, *Circulation* 79:566–572, 1989.

104. Santoro GM, Sciagra R, Buonamici P, et al: Head-to-head comparison of exercise stress testing, pharmacologic stress echocardiography, and perfusion tomography as first-line examination for chest pain in patients without history of coronary artery disease, *J Nucl Cardiol* 5:19–27, 1998.

105. Santos-Ocampo CD, Herman SD, Travin MI, et al: Comparison of exercise, dipyridamole, and adenosine by use of technetium 99m sestamibi tomographic imaging, *J Nucl Cardiol* 1:57–64, 1994.

106. Secknus MA, Marwick TH: Evolution of dobutamine echocardiography protocols and indications: safety and side effects in 3,011 studies over 5 years, *J Am Coll Cardiol* 29:1234–1240, 1996.

107. Seiler C, Fleish M, Meier B: Direct intracoronary evidence of collateral steal in humans, *Circulation* 96:4261–4267, 1997.

108. Sharir J, Rabinowitz B, Livschitz S, et al: Underestimation of extent and severity of coronary artery disease by dipyridamole stress thallium-201 single photon emission computed tomographic myocardial perfusion imaging in patients taking antianginal drugs, *J Am Coll Cardiol* 31:1540–1546, 1998.

109. Shiode N, Nakayama K, Morishima N, et al: Nitric oxide production by coronary conductance and resistance vessels in hypercholesterolemia patients, *Am Heart J* 131:1051–1057, 1996.

110. Smits P, Aengevaeren WR, Corstens FH, et al: Caffeine reduces dipyridamole-induced myocardial ischemia, *J Nucl Med* 30:1723–1726, 1989.

111. Smits P, Williams SB, Lipson DE, et al: Endothelial release of nitric oxide contributes to the vasodilator effect of adenosine in humans, *Circulation* 92:2135–2141, 1995.

112. Sochor H, Pachinger O, Ogris E, et al: Radionuclide imaging after coronary vasodilation: myocardial scintigraphy with thallium-201 and radionuclide angiography after administration of dipyridamole, *Eur Heart J* 5:500–509, 1984.

113. Stern S, Greenberg ID, Corne RA: Quantification of walking exercise required for improvement of dipyridamole thallium-201 image quality, *J Nucl Med* 33:2061–2066, 1992.

114. Stevens MJ, Dayanikli F, Raffel DM, et al: Scintigraphic assessment of regionalized defects in myocardial sympathetic innervation and blood flow regulation in diabetic patients with autonomic neuropathy, *J Am Coll Cardiol* 31:1575–1584, 1998.

115. Strauss HW, Pitt B: Noninvasive detection of subcritical coronary arterial narrowing with a coronary vasodilator and myocardial perfusion imaging, *Am J Cardiol* 39:403–406, 1977.

116. Taillefer R, Amyot R, Turpin S, et al: Comparison between dipyridamole and adenosine as pharmacologic coronary vasodilators in detection of coronary artery disease with thallium 201 imaging, *J Nucl Cardiol* 3:204–211, 1996.

117. Takeishi Y, Chiba J, Abe S, et al: Adenosine-induced heterogenous perfusion accompanies myocardial ischemia in the presence of advanced coronary artery disease, *Am Heart J* 127:1262–1268, 1994.

118. Uren NG, Camici PG, Melin JA, et al: Effect of aging on myocardial perfusion reserve, *J Nucl Med* 36:2032–2036, 1995.

119. Uren NG, Melin JA, DeBruyne B, et al: Relation between myocardial blood flow and the severity of coronary artery stenosis, *N Engl J Med* 330:1782–1788, 1994.

120. Vatner SF, Baig H: Importance of heart rate in determining the effects of sympathomimetic amines on regional myocardial function and blood flow in conscious dogs with acute myocardial ischemia, *Circ Res* 45:793–803, 1979.

121. Verani MS, Mahmarian JJ: Myocardial perfusion scintigraphy during maximal coronary artery vasodilation with adenosine, *Am J Cardiol* 67:12D–17D, 1991.

122. Verani MS, Mahmarian JJ, Hixson JB, et al: Diagnosis of coronary artery disease by controlled coronary vasodilation with adenosine and thallium-201 scintigraphy in patients unable to exercise, *Circulation* 82:80–87, 1990.

123. Voudris V, Manginas A, Vassilikos V, et al: Coronary flow velocity changes after intravenous dipyridamole infusion: measurements using intravascular Doppler guide wire. A documentation of flow inhomogeneity, *J Am Coll Cardiol* 27:1148–1155, 1996.

124. Willerson JT, Hutton I, Watson JT, et al: Influence of dobutamine on regional myocardial blood flow and ventricular performance during acute and chronic myocardial ischemia in dogs, *Circulation* 53:828–833, 1976.

125. Wilson RF, Wyche K, Christensen BV, et al: Effects of adenosine on human coronary arterial circulation, *Circulation* 82:1595–1606, 1990.

126. Yamada H, Azuma A, Hirasaki S, et al: Intracoronary adenosine 5′-triphosphate as an alternative to papaverine for measuring coronary flow reserve, *Am J Cardiol* 74:940–941, 1994.

127. Zoghbi WA, Cheirif J, Kleiman NS, et al: Diagnosis of ischemic heart disease with adenosine echocardiography, *J Am Coll Cardiol* 18:1271–1279, 1991.

Chapter 20

Prognosis in stable coronary artery disease

Kenneth A. Brown

The prognostic value of myocardial perfusion imaging for patients with stable coronary artery disease is well established. The ability of this technique to identify patients at high risk and low risk for cardiac events has played an important role in directing patient management decisions. As emphasis on cost control and managed care increases, a tool such as myocardial perfusion imaging will have increasing value; this procedure can act as a "gatekeeper" by distinguishing patients who are most and least likely to benefit from additional, more costly procedures. However, scrutiny of all technologic procedures will increase. It is therefore important to examine the established data supporting the use of myocardial perfusion imaging for risk stratification of patients with stable coronary artery disease and to evaluate new developments and future directions.

ESTABLISHED DATA AND PRINCIPLES

Jeopardized viable myocardium

Perhaps the most consistent observation in the literature concerning the prognostic value of myocardial perfusion imaging is that the presence and extent of transient myocardial perfusion imaging defects, a marker of jeopardized viable myocardium, predict important future cardiac events.[10,12] A direct relation between the presence and extent of jeopardized viable myocardium determined by exercise thallium-201 (^{201}Tl) myocardial imaging and cardiac risk was first reported in 1983 by Brown et al.[14] When results of ^{201}Tl imaging were compared with clinical, exercise electrocardiographic, and angiographic data in patients without known previous myocardial infarction who presented for evaluation of chest pain, the best predictor of cardiac death or nonfatal myocardial infarction was the number of myocardial segments with transient defects on ^{201}Tl imaging (Fig. 20-1). Of note, although angiographic data had significant univariate predictive value, they added no significant prognostic value to the noninvasive marker of the extent of jeopardized viable myocardium. Many studies have confirmed and expanded this observation. In a larger group of patients presenting with suspected coronary disease, Ladenheim et al.[47] found that among clinical and scintigraphic variables, the number of reversible defects on ^{201}Tl imaging was the best predictor of future cardiac events.[47] Many other studies have since documented a significant relation between the presence and extent of myocardium at risk (reflected in transient myocardial perfusion imaging defects) and the probability of future important cardiac events.[10,12] These data established an important principle: Although the presence of jeopardized viable myocardium identifies patients at increased risk for cardiac events, more importantly cardiac risk is directly related to the *extent* of jeopardized viable myocardium.

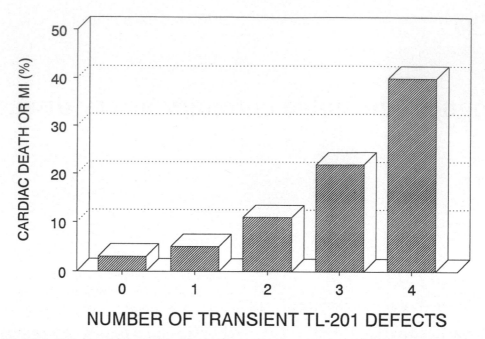

Fig. 20-1. Risk for cardiac death or myocardial infarction as a function of the number of transient defects on exercise thallium-201 imaging. (From Brown KA, Boucher CA, Oleada RD, et al: Prognostic value of exercise thallium-201 imaging in patients presenting for evaluation of chest pain, *J Am Coll Cardiol* 1:994-1001, 1983. Reprinted with permission from the American College of Cardiology.)

Scintigraphic indices of left ventricular dysfunction and prognosis

Increased lung uptake on exercise ^{201}Tl imaging has been shown to reflect resting left ventricular dysfunction, exercise-induced left ventricular dysfunction, and extent of angiographic coronary artery disease.* Not surprisingly, increased lung uptake of ^{201}Tl has been associated with an increased risk of cardiac events. Kaul et al.[40] found that increased lung uptake of ^{201}Tl was the overall best predictor of cardiac events.[40] In addition, Gill et al.[32] reported that increased lung uptake of ^{201}Tl on exercise studies was the best predictor of cardiac events in a series of patients with suspected coronary artery disease. Although the presence and extent of transient defects was also a powerful univariant predictor of cardiac events, these variables did not add any significant prognostic value to increased ^{201}Tl uptake.[32]

Left ventricular dilation determined from myocardial perfusion imaging studies has also been shown to be a marker of extensive coronary artery disease and left ventricular dysfunction.[52,76] Lette et al.[52] found that transient left ventricular dilation during dipyridamole infusion was associated with an increased risk of perioperative and long-term cardiac events.[52] More recently, Krawczynska et al.[42] reported the outcome of 291 patients with large perfusion defects in the left anterior descending coronary artery as a function of the presence or absence of left ventricular dilation. They found that patients with substantial left ventricular dilation at stress images had a reduced 3-year survival rate compared to patients with nondilated

left ventricles. Because left ventricular dilation is related to left ventricular function, these data are consistent with previous studies that showed an inverse relation between resting ejection fraction and prognosis.[60] An association between transient, exercise-induced left ventricular dilation seen on stress myocardial perfusion imaging compared with rest images and the presence of extensive coronary artery disease has also been described.[81] Although it may be reasonable to infer that such a marker of extensive underlying coronary disease would have important adverse prognostic implications, confirmation of this idea awaits additional data.

Vasodilator myocardial perfusion imaging

It is now established that myocardial perfusion imaging performed with dipyridamole, a coronary vasodilator, has prognostic value similar to exercise imaging.[10,12,37,73,84] Consistent with exercise imaging data, transient defects on ^{201}Tl imaging have significant predictive value for cardiac events and have been shown to be superior to clinical or angiographic data.[84] A similar prognostic value of transient defects has also been reported for patients undergoing atrial pacing stress.[49,77]

Normal myocardial perfusion imaging

It is well established that a normal result on myocardial perfusion imaging predicts a benign outcome. Many clinical studies have consistently demonstrated that patients with normal myocardial perfusion images have a very low cardiac event rate (<1% per year for death or myocardial infarction). This rate approaches that seen in the general population.[10,12,63,80]

---

*References 4, 9, 15, 31, 45, 55.

NEW DEVELOPMENTS

Normal myocardial perfusion imaging

Discordance between myocardial perfusion imaging results and other data. Recent studies suggest that even in patients with exercise electrocardiographic (ST-segment depression) or angiographic (multivessel disease) markers of poor outcome, the prognosis remains benign when myocardial perfusion imaging is normal.* Fagan et al[27] reported an annual cardiac event rate of 0.7% in 70 patients with positive results on exercise electrocardiography and normal results on ^{201}Tl imaging.[27] Prognosis seems to be benign when myocardial perfusion imaging is normal, even when marked ST-segment depression is seen on exercise electrocardiography. Schalet et al.[72] reported no death or myocardial infarction over a mean follow-up of 34 ± 17 months among 154 patients with ST-segment depression of 2 mm or more on exercise electrocardiography but normal results on stress ^{201}Tl imaging.[72] Similarly, in a group of 32 patients without reversible defects on ^{201}Tl exercise myocardial perfusion imaging and ST-segment depression of more than 2 mm on stress electrocardiography, no cardiac events were observed over a mean follow-up of 38 months.[43]

When myocardial perfusion imaging is normal in patients with documented angiographic coronary artery disease, the clinician is faced with a dilemma. The physician must decide whether the result of myocardial perfusion imaging is a false negative and underestimates cardiac risk or whether it is a true physiologic negative result, indicating that the angiographic disease is not hemodynamically significant and risk for cardiac events is low. Several studies confirm the latter scenario. Brown and Rowen[19] compared the outcome of 75 patients with angiographic coronary disease (including 36 with multivessel disease) who had normal results on exercise ^{201}Tl imaging to 101 patients with normal results on thallium studies who had no evidence of coronary disease on the basis of angiographic, clinical, and stress electrocardiographic data.[49] Over a mean follow-up of 2 years, the event rate for cardiac death or nonfatal myocardial infarction was equally low in both groups: 0.7% per year in patients with angiographic coronary disease and 1.0% per year in patients without coronary disease. These observations have been confirmed by Abdel-Fattah et al,[1] who reported the outcome of 97 patients with angiographic coronary disease (including 45 with multivessel disease) who had normal results on exercise single-photon emission computed tomography (SPECT) ^{201}Tl imaging. Over a mean follow-up of 32 months, only 3 cardiac deaths or nonfatal myocardial infarctions occurred, for an annual cardiac event rate of 1% per year. Likewise, in a preliminary report, Doat et al[24] described the mean 5-year outcome of patients who underwent exercise ^{201}Tl imaging and coronary angiography. When significant disease on angiography was present but results of thallium-201 imaging were normal, the annual rate of cardiac death or nonfatal myocardial infarction was 0.7%; this rate did not differ from that in patients with normal results on ^{201}Tl studies and no substantial

disease on angiography (0.6%). In contrast, among patients with disease on angiography and ischemia on ^{201}Tl myocardial perfusion imaging, the annual rate of cardiac death or myocardial infarction was 6.5%.

Table 20-1 presents the results of studies evaluating the annual cardiac event rate in patients with normal results on myocardial perfusion imaging and angiographically significant coronary artery disease. The summary of the data is based on the studies described above and smaller cohorts of patients derived from earlier reports. The overall annual rate of cardiac death or nonfatal myocardial infarction rate is less than 1% per year, similar to the event rate in patients with normal study results independent of angiographic coronary disease. These findings may have a major clinical impact. They strongly imply that patients with coronary disease on angiography but normal results on stress myocardial perfusion imaging will not benefit from coronary revascularization procedures because their outcome is very benign. Myocardial perfusion imaging can therefore play an important role in reducing medical costs by eliminating more expensive coronary revascularization procedures in patients who are unlikely to derive a clinical benefit but for whom coronary revascularization may be recommended on the basis of anatomic criteria.

Impact of antianginal medications and level of stress. It is possible that the low risk implied by normal results on exercise myocardial perfusion imaging may not apply when patients are taking antianginal medications or when the level of exercise achieved is low. In these patients, it is possible that antianginal medication or poor level of stress could result in a normal myocardial perfusion imaging study that underestimates the extent of coronary disease and, therefore, the risk of future cardiac events. However, insight into this issue provided by Brown and Rowen[18] suggests that this concern is not warranted. They reported the outcome of 261 patients with normal results on exercise ^{201}Tl studies followed for approximately 2 years as a function of antianginal medication usage and level of stress achieved. The overall rate of cardiac death or nonfatal

Table 20-1. Outcome of patients with coronary artery disease and normal results on myocardial perfusion imaging

Study	Patients	Events	Annual rate of cardiac events*
	n	n	%
Brown and Rosen[19]	75	1	0.75
Abdel-Fattah et al.[1]	97	3	1.1
Doat et al.[24]	52	2	0.7
Wahl, Hakki, and Iskandrian[80]	8	0	0
Pamelia et al.[63]	22	2	3.2
Younis et al.[84]	36	0	0
Summary	290	8	0.9

*Cardiac death or nonfatal myocardial infarction.

---

*References 1, 19, 24, 27, 43, 72.

myocardial infarction was 1.2% per year, similar to previous data. They found that use of antianginal medications, including β-blockers, and level of stress (defined by a peak heart rate or final Bruce treadmill stage) did not affect the low risk seen in patients with normal results on ^{201}Tl imaging (Table 20-2).

Technetium-99m sestamibi myocardial perfusion imaging. Given the similar sensitivity for the detection of coronary artery disease, it would be anticipated that normal Tc-99m sestamibi imaging would predict a benign prognosis comparable to normal thallium-201 imaging. Recent data have confirmed this expectation. Brown and colleagues reported the outcome of 234 patients undergoing exercise or dipyridamole Tc-99m sestamibi myocardial perfusion imaging.[13] Cardiac death or nonfatal myocardial infarction occurred in only 1 patient, resulting in an annualized cardiac event rate of 0.5% per year. Similar to thallium-201 imaging data described above, the prognosis remained benign even among patients who had exercise- or dipyridamole-induced ST segment depression. These observations have been confirmed by several studies. Raiker and colleagues found that only 1 of 208 patients with normal stress ^{99m}Tc sestamibi myocardial perfusion imaging developed cardiac death or nonfatal myocardial infarction, resulting in an annualized cardiac event rate of 0.5%.[69] More recently, in a large series of 1702 patients, Berman found that exercise ^{99m}Tc sestamibi studies were associated with a benign prognosis (<0.5% death/myocardial infarction rate) even when the likelihood of coronary artery disease was high.[3]

Long-term follow up. The observational follow up period for studies evaluating the outcome of patients with normal myocardial perfusion imaging have generally been in the 2-4 year range. Since coronary disease can clearly progress over this time frame, the event rate in patients with a normal study may increase as time progresses. However, recent data suggest that the benign prognosis indicated by a normal result on myocardial perfusion imaging is maintained even over a very long follow-up period. Steinberg et al.[74] described the outcome of 309 patients with normal results on stress ^{201}Tl imaging who were followed for an average of 10 years. In this cohort, the annual cardiac event rate remained very low: 0.1% for cardiac death and 0.6% for nonfatal myocardial infarction. However, it is not known whether such a long-term low cardiac event rate would be maintained in patients with known angiographic disease, in whom the potential for substantial progression over time is greater. Additional studies are needed to address this issue.

In summary, a large body of data has established that normal result on myocardial perfusion imaging identifies patients with a very low risk for future cardiac death or nonfatal myo-cardial infarction. Recent studies suggest that even when the result of stress electrocardiography is markedly positive or when angiographically significant coronary artery disease is present, the prognosis remains very benign. Furthermore, concurrent use of antianginal medications and a low peak level of stress do not seem to result in an underestimation of cardiac risk when the result of myocardial perfusion imaging is normal. The important clinical implication derived from these studies is that patients can be identified who are at such low risk for cardiac events that the expense and risk of further intervention (such as coronary angiography or coronary revascularization) are not justified, because these interventions are very unlikely to improve prognosis.

Myocardial perfusion imaging with technetium-99m–based imaging agents

With the growing use of myocardial perfusion imaging for risk stratification, it will be important to establish the prognostic value of scintigraphy using new imaging agents as they become available. Given the similar sensitivity and specificity of imaging agents for the detection of coronary artery disease, it

Table 20-2. Annual rate of cardiac death or nonfatal myocardial infarction as a function of antianginal therapy or stress indices in patients with a normal result on myocardial perfusion imaging*

Variable	Patients with cardiac death or nonfatal myocardial infarction	Annual event rate	P value
	n/n	%	
Antianginal therapy	3/133	1.2	n.s. (≥0.6)
No antianginal therapy	3/128	1.2	
β-Blocker use	2/77	1.4	n.s. (≥0.6)
No β-blocker use	4/184	1.1	
Peak heart rate			
≥85% maximal predicted heart rate	4/178	1.2	n.s. (≥0.6)
<85% maximal predicted heart rate	2/83	1.2	
≥60% maximal predicted heart rate	6/249	1.3	
<60% maximal predicted heart rate	0/12	0.0	
Final Bruce stage			
≥3	3/152	1.0	n.s. (≥0.6)
≤2	3/109	1.4	
≤1	0/39	0.0	

*n.s. = not significant.

would be expected that the prognostic value of new imaging agents will be similar to that of ^{201}Tl imaging. Accumulating data seem to confirm these expectations. As described above, several studies show that a normal result on technetium-99m (^{99m}Tc) sestamibi imaging indicates a benign prognosis similar to that indicated by a normal result on ^{201}Tl imaging.[3,13,69] Recently, Stratmann et al.[79] described the predictive value of exercise ^{99m}Tc sestamibi myocardial perfusion imaging in 548 patients with stable angina. Consistent with previous studies, cardiac events (cardiac death or nonfatal myocardial infarction) occurred in only 0.5% of patients with normal results on ^{99m}Tc sestamibi imaging compared to 8% of patients with reversible defects (p < 0.01) and 11% of patients with reversible defects in more than one coronary territory. The presence of reversible defects and myocardial perfusion abnormalities had significant independent predictive value for cardiac events when multivariate analysis was performed. These investigators have reported similar observations when using dipyridamole vasodilator stress with ^{99m}Tc sestamibi imaging.[78] An abnormal scan or the presence of reversible defects had the greatest value for predicting cardiac death or nonfatal myocardial infarction in a multivariate analysis that compared scintigraphic, clinical, electrocardiographic, and angiographic data. Cardiac events occurred in 17% of patients with reversible defects compared

with only 1.7% of patients with normal results over a mean follow-up of 13 months. More recently, Heller et al.[36] confirmed the prognostic value of dipyridamole ^{99m}Tc sestamibi myocardial perfusion imaging and, of more importance, showed that just as with ^{201}Tl imaging the risk for cardiac events was directly related to the extent of myocardium at risk demonstrated by myocardial perfusion imaging. Among 512 patients, those with reversible defects had the highest rate of cardiac death or nonfatal myocardial infarction (12.3% at 18 months) compared with patients who had normal results (1.7%; p < 0.01) (Fig. 20-2). These investigators also examined the relation between outcome and size of perfusion defects. They found that cardiac events, as well as need for future hospitalization, were directly related to the size of the perfusion defect (Fig. 20-3), a finding similar to that described for ^{201}Tl imaging.

Recently, the benign outcome of ^{99m}Tc sestamibi imaging was reported when this type of imaging is performed in conjunction with dobutamine atropine stress.[29] Geleijnse et al.[24] observed no cardiac events over a mean 23 month follow-up among 80 women with chest pain who had a normal result on dobutamine atropine ^{99m}Tc sestamibi imaging. Of note, 89% of patients had an intermediate or high probability of having coronary artery disease; nonetheless, the prognosis remained benign.

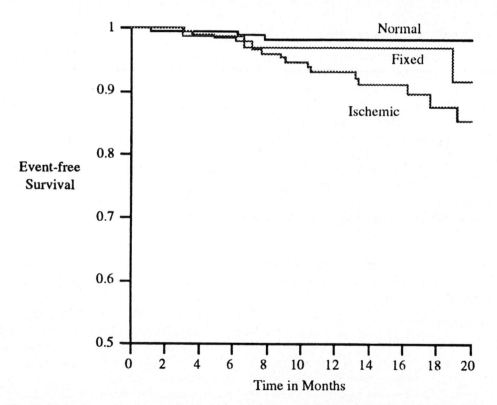

Fig. 20-2. Cardiac event–free survival in patients with normal results on dipyridamole technetium-99m sestamibi imaging or with fixed or transient (ischemia) defects. Event-free survival was reduced in patients with transient defects compared with those with normal results (p < 0.01). (From Heller GV, Herman SD, Travin MI, et al: Independent prognostic value of intravenous dipyridamole with technetium-99m sestamibi tomographic imaging in predicting cardiac events and cardiac-related hospital admissions, *J Am Coll Cardiol* 26:1202-1208, 1995. Reprinted with permission from the American College of Cardiology.)

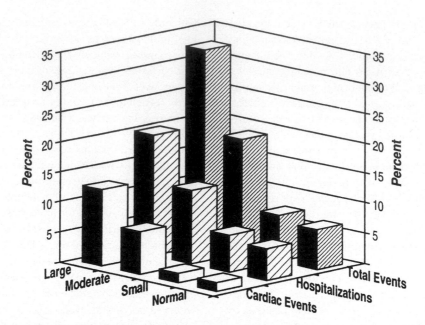

Fig. 20-3. Annual rate of cardiac death or nonfatal myocardial infarction and cardiac-related hospitalizations as a function of myocardial perfusion defect size. Cardiac events and hospitalizations increase progressively with increasing size of defects. (From Heller GV, Herman SD, Travin MI, et al: Independent prognostic value of intravenous dipyridamole with technetium-99m sestamibi tomographic imaging in predicting cardiac events and cardiac-related hospital admissions, *J Am Coll Cardiol* 26:1202-1208, 1995. Reprinted with permission from the American College of Cardiology.)

Single-photon emission computed tomography

The prognostic value of myocardial perfusion imaging was established by studies that used planar imaging.[10] Because of its greater sensitivity and ability to distinguish coronary artery territories, SPECT would have be expected to have a prognostic value at least as good as that of planar imaging. A growing number of studies has substantiated this expectation. Machecourt et al.[57] recently described the outcome of 1926 patients undergoing stress SPECT ^{201}Tl imaging. The extent of initial perfusion defect was the best prognostic imaging variable and added significant predictive value to clinical variables and exercise electrocardiography. Furthermore, the cardiac event rate in patients with normal results on SPECT ^{201}Tl imaging was 0.4% per year, a result similar to those of the planar imaging studies described above. In addition, other already cited studies that have shown significant prognostic value have used SPECT myocardial perfusion imaging.[43,69,72,78,79]

Fixed thallium-201 defects

A standard tenet for many years after the introduction of ^{201}Tl myocardial perfusion imaging was that reversible defects reflected jeopardized viable myocardium, whereas fixed defects reflected infarction or scar.[10] This idea was supported by a very consistent observation that in contrast to reversible defects, defects that are fixed on standard 2- to 4-hour delayed images generally do not predict future cardiac events.* Recent data

*References 6, 8, 10, 12, 16, 21, 25, 26, 30, 32, 33, 37, 41, 48, 50, 51, 53, 54, 65, 71, 77, 82, 85.

have supported these earlier observations. In a study of 896 patients with known coronary artery disease undergoing stress ^{201}Tl imaging, the cardiac event rate in 217 patients with defects that were fixed on standard delayed imaging was very low and was identical to that of 310 patients with normal results on imaging (death rate < 1%), whereas in 369 patients with reversible defects, death was substantially increased (5%; $p < 0.001$) (Fig. 20-4).[5]

It is now evident, however, that some defects that do not show redistribution in 2 to 4 hours probably do not represent infarction or scar, particularly in the absence of electrocardiographic Q waves or in the presence of normal regional wall motion.[7,22,23,56,83] As a result, various imaging protocols have been developed, including reinjection imaging and delayed imaging, to maximize the detection of viable myocardium in segments that appear to be fixed on standard stress delayed imaging. However, given the remarkably consistent lack of prognostic value for defects that are fixed on standard delayed imaging, the clinical implications of defects that are made reversible with reinjection or late imaging remain unclear. Brown, Rowen, and Altland[20] recently provided some insight into this issue when they reported the outcome of 100 patients without previous myocardial infarction who had isolated fixed defects on standard ^{201}Tl stress 2- to 4-hour delayed imaging. Because the fixed defects in these patients do not represent scar, these patients represent a cohort that is very likely to show reversibility with reinjection or delayed imaging. Over a mean follow-up of 2 years, only 1 patient developed nonfatal myocardial infarction and no patient developed cardiac death, yielding an annual car-

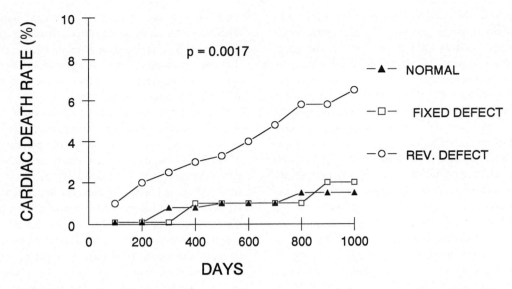

Fig. 20-4. Cardiac death rate as a function of result of exercise thallium-201 imaging. Patients with reversible *(REV)* defects had a significantly higher death rate than patients with fixed defects or normal results on studies. (Adapted from Bodenheimer MM, Wackers FJTh, Schwartz, RG, et al: Prognostic significance of a fixed thallium defect one to six months after onset of acute myocardial infarction or unstable angina, *Am J Cardiol* 74:1196-1200, 1994. Reprinted with permission from Excerpta Medica Inc.)

diac event rate of 0.5%. Thus, even in patients in whom fixed defects probably do not represent scar or infarction and who would be expected to show reversibility with reinjection or delayed imaging, the prognosis remained benign, just as in patients with a normal result on ^{201}Tl imaging. Furthermore, a recent preliminary report suggests that fixed defects that become reversible after reinjection are not associated with an increased risk for cardiac events.[64] Thus, although reinjection or delayed imaging may result in new reversibility in defects that are fixed on standard delayed imaging, such defects seem unlikely to have the same clinical importance as those that show reversibility on standard delayed imaging. Substitution of a reinjection image for the standard 2- to 4-hour delayed redistribution image has been advocated by some laboratories. Although this technique may be advantageous when the principal aim is detection of viable myocardium, caution should be used in changing standard imaging protocols when the goal is risk stratification until the prognostic significance of this phenomenon is demonstrated. Because previous reinjection studies have shown that some defects that would otherwise be reversible on standard delayed imaging will appear to be fixed with reinjection,[23] substituting a reinjection image for delayed imaging could result in underestimation of cardiac risk.

Relation between location of perfusion defect and site of subsequent myocardial infarction

Although the presence and extent of perfusion defects, especially transient defects, predict future cardiac events (including myocardial infarction), few data were published on the relation of the location of jeopardized myocardium to the site of future infarction. Two recent studies now shed some light on the sub-

ject. Miller and colleagues[59] examined 25 patients with acute myocardial infarction following stress ^{99m}Tc sestamibi myocardial perfusion imaging. Perfusion defects corresponding to the coronary territories of subsequent infarction were observed in 17 (68%) patients; 14 defects were reversible, and 3 were fixed. Galvin and Brown[28] reported findings in 34 patients with acute myocardial infarction who had a previous stress myocardial perfusion imaging study showing transient defects. They found that the duration of time between myocardial perfusion imaging study and subsequent infarction (which could confound the results because of disease progression during the interval) greatly influenced the relation between site of transient defect and infarction. Among patients with a transient defect and less than 2 years between infarction and imaging, 11 of 14 (79%) had an infarction in the same coronary territory as the previous transient defect *(p < 0.0005)*. This association decreased to only 5 of 20 patients (25%) when the interval was 2 years or more. In a subgroup of patients with angiographic data, no relation was seen between the most severe coronary lesion and site of subsequent infarction, regardless of the interval between the two events. These studies suggest that a direct regional relation exists between demonstration of jeopardized viable myocardium and risk for subsequent myocardial infarction, although this relation is not absolute. Thus, it seems that the hemodynamic significance of a coronary lesion is an important factor in the pathophysiology of acute myocardial infarction. However, undefined factors also may play a causative role.

Incremental value of myocardial perfusion imaging

Although the prognostic value of myocardial perfusion imaging is clearly established, increasing scrutiny of health care costs has made it important to demonstrate that such testing adds substantially to the prognostic value of data that is less expensive to obtain, such as clinical information and stress electrocardiograms. Likewise, it is important to ask what more invasive and expensive procedures, such as coronary angiography, add to the prognostic value of less expensive, noninvasive tests, such as myocardial perfusion imaging. An early report by Ladenheim et al[46] examined the incremental prognostic value of exercise ^{201}Tl imaging in a series of 1659 patients with suspected coronary artery disease. They found that ^{201}Tl data provided the greatest additive predictive power in patients with abnormal results on resting electrocardiography or with an intermediate to high preexercise probability of coronary disease. Subsequently, Pollock et al[67] determined the additive incremental prognostic information obtained in hierarchical order from clinical data, exercise electrocardiography, ^{201}Tl imaging, and coronary angiography in a series of patients presenting with suspected coronary artery disease who were originally described by Kaul et al[41] The global chi-square value derived from the Cox proportional hazards regression model was used as a index of the relative predictive value. The authors demonstrated that stress electrocardiography data added significantly to the prognostic value of clinical information alone (Fig. 20-5). However, the addition of ^{201}Tl data (presence of transient defects) almost doubled the ability to predict cardiac events when this test was added to stress electrocardiography (Fig. 20-5). Of note, the incremental improvement with ^{201}Tl data

was similar to that observed with cardiac catheterization data. Therefore, this study demonstrated that although it is more expensive, ^{201}Tl imaging data greatly increase the ability to predict cardiac events compared with stress electrocardiographic and clinical data and provide incremental prognostic value similar to that of angiographic data.

This principle has now been confirmed by several other investigators. Iskandrian et al[38] examined the prognostic value of clinical data, exercise electrocardiography, exercise ^{201}Tl SPECT, and cardiac catheterization in patients with known coronary artery disease. Among all variables, myocardial perfusion imaging had the greatest predictive value. More importantly, when testing methods were evaluated in a hierarchical incremental model, exercise testing did not add significant prognostic value to clinical variables, but myocardial perfusion imaging data improved the ability to predict cardiac events by a factor of more than 4 (Fig. 20-6). The increment in prognostic value with myocardial perfusion imaging data was greater than with cardiac catherization data (Fig. 20-6), which did not add any significant prognostic value to ^{201}Tl imaging. Thus, not only did myocardial perfusion imaging data greatly improve the prognostic value of the less expensive stress electrocardiography, the more expensive cardiac catherization data did not improve the predictive value of myocardial perfusion imaging.

More recently, Palmas et al[62] found that the extent of jeopardized viable myocardium reflected in a ^{201}Tl SPECT summed reversibility score, significantly improved the prognostic infor-

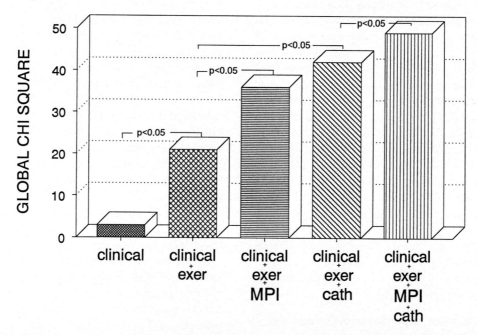

Fig. 20-5. The relative predictive value of clinical data, exercise electrocardiography *(exer)*, myocardial perfusion imaging *(MPI)*, and cardiac catheterization *(CATH)*. The addition of MPI data had substantial and statistically significant incremental prognostic value when added to clinical and exercise data; this result was similar to the additive value of CATH data. (From Pollock SG, Abbott RD, Boucher CA, et al: Independent and incremental prognostic value of tests performed in hierarchial order to evaluate patients with suspected coronary artery disease, *Circulation* 85:237-248, 1992.)

mation available from clinical and exercise data in patients who had undergone previous coronary bypass surgery, doubling the predictive model chi-square value. A similar finding was reported by Marie et al.,[58] who examined the incremental prognostic value of exercise ^{201}Tl SPECT over a long-term follow-up of approximately 6 years compared with clinical data, exercise testing, catheterization, and radionuclide angiography. They observed that ^{201}Tl imaging variables were the best predictors of cardiac death or myocardial infarction and that ^{201}Tl imaging data added substantially to the predictive value of clinical data, exercise testing, and cardiac catheterization. The extent of reversible defects seen in ^{201}Tl perfusion imaging provided additional prognostic information even when clinical data and results of exercise and cardiac catheterization data were all added. Furthermore, the testing extent of reversible defects provided additional predictive value compared with the extent of nonreversible defects and was the sole ^{201}Tl imaging variable that provided additional prognostic information compared with left ventricular ejection fraction by radionuclide imaging.

Hachamovitch et al.[35] took this approach one step further. In a series of 2200 patients without known coronary disease who underwent exercise myocardial SPECT, these researchers confirmed that nuclear testing added incremental predictive value to the best clinical and exercise variables, resulting in a doubling of prognostic information.[35] Of note, they also found that rates of referral for early catheterization and revascularization were strongly influenced by the results of myocardial perfusion

imaging. Referral rates were very low in patients with normal scan results even when stress test results and clinical data suggested the presence of coronary disease. Significant increases in referral rates were seen as scan results worsened (Fig. 20-7). Thus, not only did myocardial perfusion SPECT add incremental prognostic value in risk-stratified patients even after clinical and exercise information was known, it was apparent that referring physicians used this test in an appropriate manner in selecting patients for referral for cardiac catheterization or coronary revascularization. In another study, these investigators demonstrated that after controlling for differences in perfusion scan abnormalities, no sex-related difference exists for referral for cardiac catheterization.[34] In the setting of severe ischemia seen on myocardial perfusion imaging, women were referred for cardiac catheterization more frequently than men. However, this higher rate seemed to be clinically appropriate because the cardiac event rate was higher in women with severely abnormal scan results than in men (Fig. 20-8). This greater risk in women may have been underappreciated because the increased rate of cardiac death or myocardial infarction in women with severely abnormal scan results was disproportionate to the smaller increase in the rate of referral for cardiac catheterization. The authors suggested that this high-risk subgroup of women was underreferred for cardiac catheterization relative to men and called for a need to better identify women at high risk for cardiac events.

In summary, compelling data show that myocardial perfu-

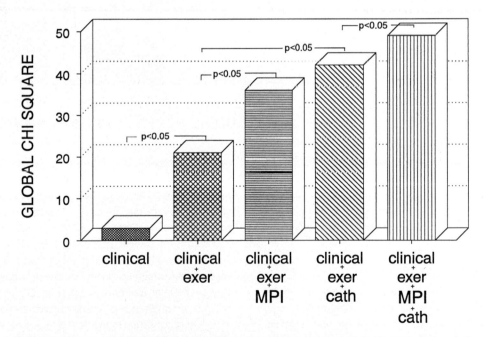

Fig. 20-6. Incremental hierarchical prognostic value of clinical data *(clin)*, exercise electrocardiography *(exer)*, myocardial perfusion imaging *(MPI)*, and cardiac catheterization (CATH). When added to clinical and exercise data, myocardial perfusion imaging data increased the predictive power to a much greater degree than angiographic data did. Furthermore, catheterization did not add predictive value to myocardial perfusion imaging data. (From Iskandrian AS, Chae SC, Heo J, et al: Independent and incremental prognostic value of exercise single-photon emission computed tomographic (SPECT) thallium imaging in coronary artery disease, *J Am Coll Cardiol* 22:665-670, 1993. Reprinted with permission from the American College of Cardiology.)

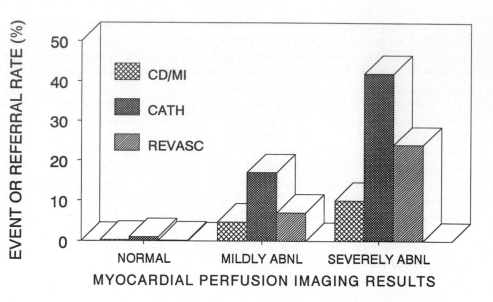

Fig. 20-7. Rates of cardiac death *(CD)* and myocardial infarction *(MI)*, cardiac catheterization *(CATH)*, or coronary revascularization *(REVASC)* as a function of myocardial perfusion imaging results. Referral rates for catheterization and revascularization paralleled cardiac event rates in all scan categories: they were very low in patients with normal results and increased significantly as imaging abnormalities *(ABNL)* increased. (From Hachamovitch R, Berman DS, Kiat H, et al: Exercise myocardial perfusion (SPECT) in patients with known coronary artery disease: incremental prognostic value and use in risk stratification, *Circulation* 93:905-914, 1996.)

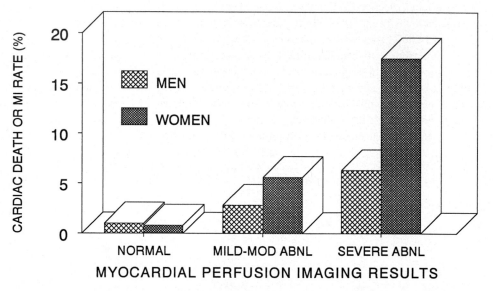

Fig. 20-8. Rate of cardiac death or myocardial infarction *(MI)* rate as a function of sex and results of myocardial perfusion imaging. Cardiac events increased as imaging results worsened for both men and women. However, the event rate was higher in women than in men (*p* < 0.05) when imaging results were severely abnormal *(ABNL)*. (Adapted from Hachamovitch R, Berman DS, Kiat H, et al: Gender-related differences in clinical management after exercise nuclear testing, *J Am Coll Cardiol* 26:1457-1464, 1995. Reprinted with permission from the American College of Cardiology.)

sion imaging adds statistically significant and substantial prognostic value to more easily obtained and less expensive clinical and exercise testing data. Equally important, more expensive cardiac catheterization and angiographic data do not seem to add significant incremental prognostic value to myocardial perfusion imaging.

Outcomes research

Because of its established diagnostic and prognostic significance, stress myocardial perfusion imaging could play a major role as a "gatekeeper" for more costly invasive and interventional procedures. The emerging health care environment, which places increasing emphasis on cost containment, may result in the integration of myocardial perfusion imaging into standardized practice guidelines, mandating that certain tests be done before more expensive procedures. In the meantime, there seems to be widespread appreciation of the clinical implications of myocardial perfusion imaging that affect the use of car-

diac catheterization and coronary revascularization. As described above, Hachamovitch et al[34,35] showed that clinicians used stress myocardial perfusion imaging results to make decisions about referrals for cardiac catheterization and coronary revascularization. Only a small percentage of patients with normal results on nuclear studies are referred for cardiac catheterization, even when they have a high likelihood of coronary disease as determined by stress electrocardiography (Fig. 20-9, *A*) or a high Duke treadmill score (Fig. 20-10, *B*).[35] Even fewer patients are referred for coronary revascularization (Fig. 2-9, *B*). This low referral rate is justified by a very low event rate (Figs. 20-9, *A* and 20-10, *A*). In contrast, positive scan results (particularly when they are severely abnormal) result in a high referral rate for cardiac catherization and coronary revascularization (Figs. 20-9, *B* and *C* and 20-10, *B*).

Other investigators have described similar observations. In a series of 4162 patients who underwent stress ^{201}Tl imaging, only 3.5% of patients without reversible defects were referred

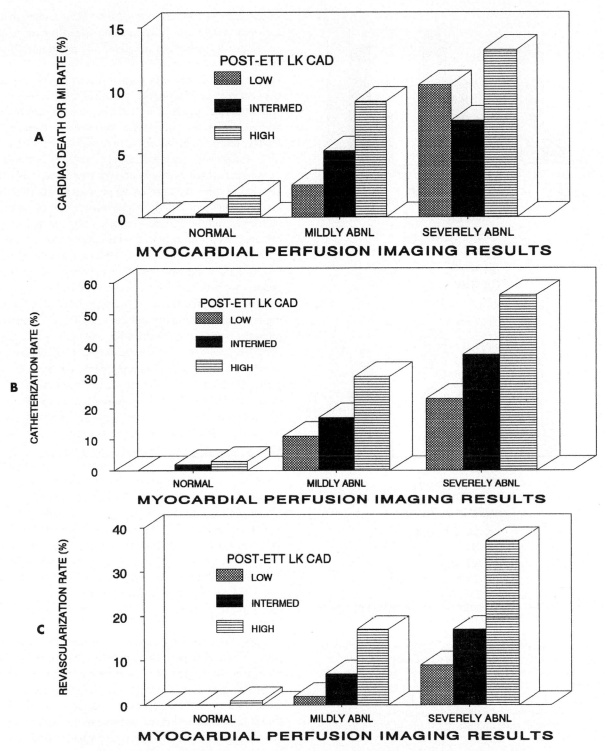

Fig. 20-9. A, Rate of cardiac death or myocardial infarction *(MI)* as a function of myocardial perfusion imaging results and postexercise treadmill test *(ETT)* likelihood of coronary artery disease *(LK CAD)*. **B,** Rate of cardiac catheterization and **C,** rate of coronary revascularization as a function of the same variables. Catheterization and revascularization rates were very low when imaging results were normal even if the likelihood of coronary artery disease was high, reflecting the low event rate seen in this group. Utilization rates of catheterization and revascularization increased as the degree of abnormality of imaging results increased, reflecting the corresponding higher event rates in these groups. (From Hachamovitch R, Berman DS, Kiat H, et al: Exercise myocardial perfusion (SPECT) in patients with known coronary artery disease: incremental prognostic value and use in risk stratification, *Circulation* 93:905-914, 1996.)

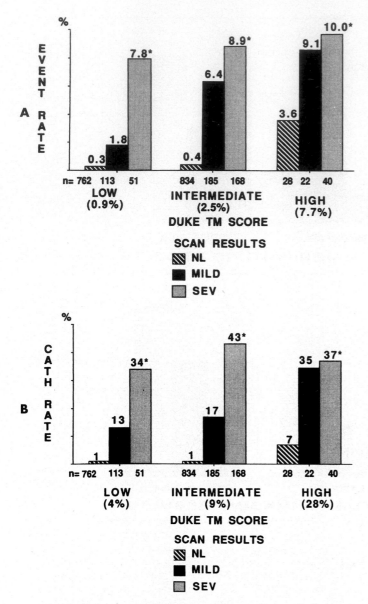

Fig. 20-10. A, Cardiac death or myocardial infarction as a function of Duke treadmill *(TM)* score and myocardial perfusion imaging results (nl = normal; mild = mildly abnormal; sev = severely abnormal). For each Duke TM category, the event rate was related to imaging results ($p < 0.05$). **B,** Cardiac catheterization rate as a function of the same variables. Catheterization rates were directly related to imaging results across treadmill scores ($p < 0.05$). (From Hachamovitch R, Berman DS, Kiat H, et al: Exercise myocardial perfusion (SPECT) in patients with known coronary artery disease: incremental prognostic value and use in risk stratification, *Circulation* 93:905-914, 1996.)

for cardiac catheterization compared with 32% of patients with reversible defects.[2] Furthermore, consistent with previous observations, clinicians seemed to respond to the details of imaging results: Among patients with reversible defects, 60% with high-risk imaging result (multiple coronary territories, left anterior descending artery territory, or increased lung uptake) were referred for cardiac catheterization compared with only 9% of patients without these findings. Of the total cohort, approxi-

mately 80% of patients referred for cardiac catheterization had high-risk results on ^{201}Tl imaging. Nallamothu et al.[61] also found that the results of exercise ^{201}Tl imaging influenced referrals for cardiac catheterization in a cohort of 2700 patients. Only 3% of patients with normal results on ^{201}Tl imaging underwent coronary angiography compared with 36% of patients with abnormal results. Furthermore, among patients with abnormal results, the referral rate for cardiac catheterization was directly related to the extent of myocardial perfusion abnormalities. Previously, Steingart et al.[75] used a questionnaire to demonstrate that the results of exercise nuclear studies greatly affected likelihood that referring physicians would recommend coronary angiography. The perceived need for coronary angiography was significantly reduced after performance of a nuclear exercise test for all patient groups encompassing a low to high probability of coronary disease. The impact of the nuclear stress test for influencing decisions about cardiac catheterization was greatest for patients with known coronary artery disease.

In summary, the results of stress myocardial perfusion imaging seem to substantially influence clinicians' decisions about referral for cardiac catheterization and coronary revascularization. Clinicians seem to recommend these procedures after stress myocardial perfusion imaging on the basis of an appropriate understanding of the prognostic implications of imaging results. Patients at low risk for future cardiac events (as defined by a normal result on a nuclear study) are generally not referred for cardiac catheterization or coronary revascularization, even when their probability of having angiographic coronary disease is high on the basis of clinical data and the results of stress electrocardiography. Cardiac catheterization and coronary revascularization seem to be reserved for patients who are identified as having high risk for future cardiac events on the basis of stress myocardial perfusion imaging results. Therefore, stress nuclear techniques seem to currently play an important role in limiting health care costs by controlling access to more expensive procedures and interventions. Such use is likely to have growing value in the foreseeable health care environment.

FUTURE DIRECTIONS

Earlier studies firmly established the prognostic value of stress myocardial perfusion imaging, and new developments have clearly extended these observations and have brought additional insight to the field. It is gratifying that many of the topics defined as future directions in the previous edition of this book[11] have been addressed over the past several years. Nevertheless, areas in which additional information is needed remain, providing an impetus for future study.

New myocardial perfusion agents

New imaging agents are generally released on the basis of documentation of their sensitivity for detection of coronary artery disease. Although initial uptake during stress is usually similar to that of the gold standard of ^{201}Tl and yields a comparable sensitivity and specificity for coronary disease, the kinetics of new tracers are often quite different. Differences in kinetics exist even among technetium-based agents. As a result, the prognostic implications of transient defects compared with fixed defects must be established for these new tracers. In addition to the recently released ^{99m}Tc tetrofosmin, several agents are now on the horizon for evaluation, including ^{99m}Tc furifosmin, ^{99m}Tc NOET, and iodine-123–labeled fatty acids (such as IPPA and BMIPP). In addition, use of iodine-123 MIBG, which has been shown to provide functional assessment of cardiac sympathetic activity, may have important prognostic implications. Data must be obtained, and this will clearly be a fruitful area for new investigation.

Cost-effectiveness

Although many studies have established that stress myocardial perfusion imaging can greatly affect clinician decisions about referral for cardiac catheterization and coronary revascularization,[2,34,35,61,75] additional data are needed on the cost-effectiveness of various strategies using clinical data, stress electrocardiography, and stress radionuclide imaging for controlling global health care costs and maximizing patient benefit.

Impact of coronary revascularization

Data are needed on the impact of coronary revascularization in patients identified by stress myocardial perfusion imaging as having high risk. While stress myocardial perfusion imaging can clearly identify patients at high risk for cardiac events resulting in referral for cardiac catheterization and revascularization, it is important to establish that such a management approach has a beneficial clinical outcome.

Comparison with stress echocardiography

Stress echocardiography has seen growing use as an alternative to stress myocardial perfusion imaging in the clinical management of patients with coronary artery disease. Initial data suggest that stress echocardiography may be substantially less sensitive than stress myocardial perfusion imaging for detecting patients with coronary artery disease who are at risk for cardiac events, resulting in an unacceptably high event rate in patients with negative results on imaging studies. Several studies have reported annual rates of death or myocardial infarction of 5% to 7% in patients with negative results on stress echocardiography who have known coronary artery disease.[39,44,66,68,70] As discussed above, this cardiac event rate is much higher than that observed with stress myocardial perfusion imaging.[1,10,12,19,24] In addition to the obvious undesirability of failing to detect patients at risk for serious cardiac events, these findings have important medicoeconomic implications. As discussed previously, rates of cardiac catheterization and coronary revascularization utilization after stress myocardial perfusion imaging reflect perceived and established cardiac risk associated with imaging results.[2,34,35,61,75] Consequently, referral rates following a negative result on stress myocardial perfusion imaging study are very low (1% to 3%). Such rates may not be as low after stress echocardiography because of this technique's seemingly lower sensitivity for detecting patients at risk. Comparative studies of global costs associated with myocardial perfusion imaging compared with stress echocardiography may have important value.

CONCLUSIONS

Use of stress myocardial perfusion imaging to establish cardiac risk and to identify patients who are most and least likely to benefit from additional, more costly procedures is likely to remain a growth area in nuclear cardiology. An increasing number of studies have consistently demonstrated the statistically significant and substantial incremental value that stress myocardial perfusion imaging adds to prognostic information derived from less expensively obtained clinical data and stress testing. It is likely that the prognostic value of stress myocardial perfusion imaging will continue to play an important role in patient management, allowing clinicians to make rational decisions about referral for cardiac catheterization and coronary revascularization and serving a justifiable "gatekeeper" function for more expensive procedures, thereby helping to control global health care costs.

REFERENCES

1. Abdel-Fattah A, Kamal AM, Pancholy S, et al: Prognostic implications of normal exercise tomographic thallium images in patients with angiographic evidence of significant coronary artery disease, *Am J Cardiol* 74:769–771, 1994.
2. Bateman TM, O'Keefe JH Jr, Dong VM, et al: Coronary angiographic rates after stress single-photon emission computed tomographic scintigraphy, *J Nucl Cardiol* 2:217–223, 1995.
3. Berman DS, Hachamovitch R, Kiat H, et al: Incremental value of prognostic testing in patients with known or suspected ischemic heart disease: a basis for optimal utilization of exercise technetium-99m sestamibi myocardial perfusion single-photon emission computed tomography, *J Am Coll Cardiol* 26:639–647, 1995.
4. Bingham JB, McKusick KA, Strauss HW, et al: Influence of coronary artery disease on pulmonary uptake of thallium-201, *Am J Cardiol* 46:821–826, 1980.
5. Bodenheimer MM, Wackers FJTh, Schwartz RG, et al: Prognostic significance of a fixed thallium defect one to six months after onset of acute myocardial infarction or unstable angina. Multicenter Myocardial Ischemia Research Group, *Am J Cardiol* 74:1196–1200, 1994.
6. Bosch X, March R, Magrina J, et al: Prediction of in-hospital cardiac events using dipyridamole perfusion scintigraphy after myocardial infarction, *Circulation* 80(suppl II):II–307, 1989 (abstract).
7. Botvinick EH: Late reversibility: a viability issue, *J Am Coll Cardiol* 15:341–344, 1990.
8. Boucher CA, Brewster DC, Darling RC, et al: Determination of cardiac risk by dipyridamole-thallium imaging before peripheral vascular surgery, *N Engl J Med* 312:389–394, 1985.
9. Boucher CA, Zir LM, Beller GA, et al: Increased lung uptake of thallium-201 during exercise myocardial imaging: clinical, hemodynamic and angiographic implications in patients with coronary artery disease, *Am J Cardiol* 46:189–196, 1980.
10. Brown KA: Prognostic value of thallium-201 myocardial perfusion imaging. A diagnostic tool comes of age, *Circulation* 83:363–381, 1991.
11. Brown KA: *Critical assessment of prognostic applications of thallium-201 myocardial perfusion imaging. In Zaret BL, Beller GA, eds: Nuclear cardiology: state of the art and future directions,* St. Louis, 1993, Mosby–Year Book.
12. Brown KA: Prognostic value of myocardial perfusion imaging: state of the art and new developments, *J Nucl Cardiol* 3(6P+1):516–537, 1996.

13. Brown KA, Altland E, Rowen M: Prognostic value of normal technetium-99m-sestamibi cardiac imaging, *J Nucl Med* 35:554–557, 1994.

14. Brown KA, Boucher CA, Okada RD, et al: Prognostic value of exercise thallium-201 imaging in patients presenting for evaluation of chest pain, *J Am Coll Cardiol* 1:994–1001, 1983.

15. Brown KA, Boucher CA, Okada RD, et al: Quantification of pulmonary thallium-201 activity after upright exercise in normal persons: importance of peak heart rate and propranolol usage in defining normal values, *Am J Cardiol* 53:1678–1682, 1984.

16. Brown KA, O'Meara J, Chambers CE, et al: Ability of dipyridamole-thallium-201 imaging one to four hours after myocardial infarction to predict in-hospital and later recurrent myocardial ischemic events, *Am J Cardiol* 65:160–167, 1990.

17. Brown KA, Rimmer J, Haisch C: Noninvasive cardiac risk stratifications of diabetic and nondiabetic uremic renal allograft candidates using dipyridamole-thallium-201 imaging and radionuclide ventriculography, *Am J Cardiol* 64:1017–1021, 1989.

18. Brown K, Rowen M: Impact of antianginal medications, peak heart rate and stress level on the prognostic value of a normal exercise myocardial perfusion imaging study, *J Nucl Med* 34:1467–1471, 1993.

19. Brown KA, Rowen M: Prognostic value of a normal exercise myocardial perfusion imaging study in patients with angiographically significant coronary artery disease, *Am J Cardiol* 71:865–867, 1993.

20. Brown KA, Rowen M, Altland E: Prognosis of patients with an isolated fixed thallium-201 defect and no prior myocardial infarction, *Am J Cardiol* 72:1199–1201, 1993.

21. Brown KA, Weiss RM, Clements JP, et al: Usefulness of residual ischemic myocardium within prior infarct zone for identifying patients at high risk late after acute myocardial infarction, *Am J Cardiol* 60:15–19, 1987.

22. Brunken R, Schwaiger M, Grover-McKay M, et al: Positron emission tomography detects tissue metabolic activity in myocardial segments with persistent thallium perfusion defects, *J Am Coll Cardiol* 10:557–567, 1987.

23. Dilsizian V, Rocco TP, Freedman NMT, et al: Enhanced detection of ischemic but viable myocardium by the reinjection of thallium after stress-redistribution imaging, *N Engl J Med* 323:141–146, 1990.

24. Doat M, Podio V, Pavin D, et al: Long term prognostic significance of normal or abnormal exercise Tl-201 myocardial scintigraphy in patients with or without significant coronary stenosis, *J Am Coll Cardiol* 158A, 1994 (abstract).

25. Eagle KA, Coley CM, Newell JB, et al: Combining clinical and thallium data optimizes preoperative assessment of cardiac risk before major vascular surgery, *Ann Intern Med* 110:859–866, 1989.

26. Eagle KA, Singer DE, Brewster DC, et al: Dipyridamole-thallium scanning in patients undergoing vascular surgery. Optimizing preoperative evaluation of cardiac risk, *JAMA* 257:2185–2189, 1987.

27. Fagan LF Jr, Shaw L, Kong BA, et al: Prognostic value of exercise thallium scintigraphy in patients with good exercise tolerance and a normal or abnormal exercise electrocardiogram and suspected or confirmed coronary artery disease, *Am J Cardiol* 69:607–611, 1992.

28. Galvin GM, Brown KA: The site of acute myocardial infarction is related to the coronary territory of transient defects on prior myocardial perfusion imaging, *J Nucl Cardiol.*

29. Geleijnse ML, Elhendy A, van Domburg RT, et al: Prognostic value of dobutamine-atropine stress technetium-99m sestamibi perfusion scintigraphy in patients with chest pain, *J Am Coll Cardiol* 28:447–454, 1996.

30. Gibson RS, Beller GA, Gheorghiade M, et al: The prevalence and clinical significance of residual myocardial ischemia 2 weeks after uncomplicated non-Q-wave myocardial infarction: a prospective natural history study, *Circulation* 73:1186–1198, 1986.

31. Gibson RS, Watson DD, Carabello BA, et al: Clinical implications of increased lung uptake of thallium-201 during exercise scintigraphy 2 weeks after myocardial infarction, *Am J Cardiol* 49:1586–1593, 1982.

32. Gill JB, Ruddy TD, Newell JB, et al: Prognostic importance of thallium uptake by the lungs during exercise in coronary artery disease, *N Engl J Med* 317:1486–1489, 1987.

33. Gimple LW, Hutter AM Jr, Guiney TE, et al: Prognostic utility of predischarge dipyridamole-thallium imaging compared to predischarge submaximal exercise electrocardiography and maximal exercise imaging after uncomplicated acute myocardial infarction, *Am J Cardiol* 64:1243–1248, 1989.

34. Hachamovitch R, Berman DS, Kiat H, et al: Gender-related differences in clinical management after exercise nuclear testing, *J Am Coll Cardiol* 26:1457–1464, 1995.

35. Hachamovitch R, Berman DS, Kiat H, et al: Exercise myocardial perfusion SPECT in patients with known coronary artery disease: incremental prognostic value and use in risk stratification, *Circulation* 93:905–914, 1996.

36. Heller GV, Herman SD, Travin MI, et al: Independent prognostic value of intravenous dipyridamole with technetium-99m sestamibi tomographic imaging in predicting cardiac events and cardiac-related hospital admissions, *J Am Coll Cardiol* 26:1202–1208, 1995.

37. Hendel RC, Layden JJ, Leppo JA: Prognostic value of dipyridamole thallium scintigraphy for evaluation of ischemic heart disease, *J Am Coll Cardiol* 15:109–116, 1990.

38. Iskandrian AS, Chae SC, Heo J, et al: Independent and incremental prognostic value of exercise single-photon emission computed tomographic (SPECT) thallium imaging in coronary artery disease, *J Am Coll Cardiol* 22:665–670, 1993.

39. Kamaran M, Teague SM, Finkelhor RS, et al: Prognostic value of dobutamine stress echocardiography in patients referred because of suspected coronary artery disease, *Am J Cardiol* 76:887–891, 1995.

40. Kaul S, Finkelstein DM, Homma S, et al: Superiority of quantitative exercise thallium-201 variables in determining long-term prognosis in ambulatory patients with chest pain: a comparison with cardiac catheterization, *J Am Coll Cardiol* 12:25–34, 1988.

41. Kaul S, Lilly DR, Gasho JA, et al: Prognostic utility of the exercise thallium-201 test in ambulatory patients with chest pain: comparison with cardiac catheterization, *Circulation* 77:745–758, 1988.

42. Krawczynska EG, Weintraub WS, Garcia EV, et al: Left ventricular dilatation and multivessel coronary artery disease on thallium-201 SPECT are important prognostic indicators in patients with large defects in the left anterior descending distribution, *Am J Cardiol* 74:1233–1239, 1994.

43. Krishnan R, Lu J, Dae MW, et al: Does myocardial perfusion scintigraphy demonstrate clinical usefulness in patients with markedly positive exercise tests? An assessment of the method in a high-risk subset, *Am Heart J* 127(4 pt 1):804–816, 1994.

44. Krivokapich J, Child JS, Gerber RS, et al: Prognostic usefulness of positive or negative exercise stress echocardiography for predicting coronary events in ensuing twelve months, *Am J Cardiol* 71:646–651, 1993.

45. Kushner FG, Okada RD, Kirshenbaum HD, et al: Lung thallium-201 uptake after stress testing in patients with coronary artery disease, *Circulation* 63:341–347, 1981.

46. Ladenheim ML, Kotler TS, Pollock BH, et al: Incremental prognostic power of clinical history, exercise electrocardiography and myocardial perfusion scintigraphy in suspected coronary artery disease, *Am J Cardiol* 59:270–277, 1987.

47. Ladenheim ML, Pollock BH, Rozanski A, et al: Extent and severity of myocardial hypoperfusion as predictors of prognosis in patients with suspected coronary artery disease, *J Am Coll Cardiol* 7:464–471, 1986.

48. Lane SE, Lewis SM, Pippin JJ, et al: Predictive value of quantitative dipyridamole-thallium scintigraphy in assessing cardiovascular risk after vascular surgery in diabetes mellitus, *Am J Cardiol* 64:1275–1279, 1989.

49. Le Feuvre C, Vacheron A, Metzger JP, et al: Prognostic value of thallium-201 myocardial scintigraphy after atrial transesophageal pacing in patients with suspected coronary artery disease, *Eur Heart J* 14:1195–1199, 1993.

50. Leppo J, Plaja J, Gionet M, et al: Noninvasive evaluation of cardiac risk before elective vascular surgery, *J Am Coll Cardiol* 9:269–276, 1987.

51. Leppo JA, O'Brien J, Rothendler JA, et al: Dipyridamole-thallium-201 scintigraphy in the prediction of future cardiac events after acute myocardial infarction, *N Engl J Med* 310:1014–1018, 1984.

52. Lette J, Lapointe J, Waters D, et al: Transient left ventricular cavity dilation during dipyridamole-thallium imaging as an indicator of severe coronary artery disease, *Am J Cardiol* 66:1163–1170, 1990.

53. Lette J, Waters D, Lapointe J, et al: Usefulness of the severity and extent of reversible perfusion defects during thallium-dipyridamole imaging for cardiac risk assessment before noncardiac surgery, *Am J Cardiol* 64:276–281, 1989.

54. Lette J, Waters D, Lassonde J, et al: Postoperative myocardial infarction and cardiac death. Predictive value of dipyridamole-thallium imaging and five clinical scoring systems based on multifactorial analysis, *Ann Surg* 211:84–90, 1990.

55. Liu P, Kiess M, Okada RD, et al: Increased thallium lung uptake after exercise in isolated left anterior descending coronary artery disease, *Am J Cardiol* 55:(13 pt 1)1469–1473, 1985.

56. Liu P, Kiess MC, Okada RD: The persistent defect on exercise thallium imaging and its fate after myocardial revascularization: does it represent scar or ischemia? *Am Heart J* 110:996–1001, 1985.

57. Machecourt J, Longere P, Fagret D, et al: Prognostic value of thallium-201 single-photon emission computed tomographic myocardial perfusion imaging according to extent of myocardial defect. Study in 1,926 patients with follow-up at 33 months, *J Am Coll Cardiol* 23:1096–1106, 1994.

58. Marie PY, Danchin N, Durand JF, et al: Long-term prediction of major ischemic events by exercise thallium-201 single-photon emission computed tomography. Incremental prognostic value compared with clinical, exercise testing, catheterization and radionuclide angiographic data, *J Am Coll Cardiol* 26:879–886, 1995.

59. Miller GL, Herman SD, Heller GV, et al: Relation between perfusion defects on stress technetium-99m sestamibi SPECT scintigraphy and the location of a subsequent acute myocardial infarction, *Am J Cardiol* 78:26–30, 1996.

60. Risk stratification and survival after myocardial infarction, *N Engl J Med* 309:331–336, 1983.

61. Nallamothu N, Pancholy SB, Lee KR, et al: Impact on exercise single-photon emission computed tomographic thallium imaging on patient management and outcome, *J Nucl Cardiol* 2:334–338, 1995.

62. Palmas W, Bingham S, Diamond GA, et al: Incremental prognostic value of exercise thallium-201 myocardial single-photon emission computed tomography late after coronary artery bypass surgery, *J Am Coll Cardiol* 25:403–409, 1995.

63. Pamelia FX, Gibson RS, Watson DD, et al: Prognosis with chest pain and normal thallium-201 exercise scintigrams, *Am J Cardiol* 55:920–926, 1985.

64. Pieri PL, Tisselli A, Moscatelli G, et al: Prognostic value of Tl-201 reinjection (RI) in patients with chronic myocardial infarction, *J Nucl Cardiol* 2:S89, 1995 (abstract).

65. Pirelli S, Inglese E, Suppa M, et al: Dipyridamole-thallium-201 scintigraphy in the early post-infarction period, (Safety and accuracy in predicting the extent of coronary disease and future recurrence of angina in patients suffering from their first myocardial infarction), *Eur Heart J* 9:1324–1331, 1988.

66. Poldermans D, Fioretti PM, Boersma E, et al: Dobutamine-atropine stress echocardiography and clinical data for predicting late cardiac events with suspected coronary artery disease, *Am J Med* 97:119–125, 1994.

67. Pollock SG, Abbott RD, Boucher CA, et al: Independent and incremental prognostic value of tests performed in hierarchial order to evaluate patients with suspected coronary artery disease. Validation of models based on these tests, *Circulation* 85:237–248, 1992.

68. Quintana M, Lindvall K, Ryden L, et al: Prognostic value of predischarge exercise stress echocardiography after acute myocardial infarction, *Am J Cardiol* 76:1115–1121, 1995.

69. Raiker K, Sinusas AJ, Wackers FJTh, et al: One-year prognosis of patients with normal planar or single-photon emission computed tomographic technetium-99m-labeled sestamibi exercise imaging, *J Nucl Cardiol* 1(5 Pt 1):449–456, 1994.

70. Ryan T, Armstrong WF, O'Donnell JA, et al: Risk stratification after acute myocardial infarction by means of exercise two-dimensional echocardiography, *Am Heart J* 114:1305–1316, 1987.

71. Sachs RN, Tellier P, Larmignat P, et al: Assessment by dipyridamole-thallium-201 myocardial scintigraphy of coronary risk before peripheral vascular surgery, *Surgery* 103:584–587, 1988.

72. Schalet BD, Kegel JG, Heo J, et al: Prognostic implications of normal exercise SPECT thallium images in patients with strongly positive exercise electrocardiograms, *Am J Cardiol* 72:1201–1203, 1993.

73. Shaw L, Chaitman BR, Hilton TC, et al: Prognostic value of dipyridamole thallium-201 imaging in elderly patients, *J Am Coll Cardiol* 19:1390–1398, 1992.

74. Steinberg EH, Koss JH, Lee M, et al: Prognostic significance from 10-year follow-up of a qualitatively normal planar exercise thallium test in suspected coronary artery disease, *Am J Cardiol* 71:1270–1273, 1993.

75. Steingart RM, Wassertheil-Smoller S, Tobin JN, et al: Nuclear exercise testing and the management of coronary artery disease, *J Nucl Med* 32:753–758, 1991.

76. Stolzenberg J: Dilatation of left ventricular cavity on stress thallium scan as an indicator of ischemic disease, *Clin Nucl Med* 5:289–291, 1980.

77. Stratmann HG, Mark AL, Walter KE, et al: Prognostic value of atrial pacing and thallium-201 scintigraphy in patients with stable chest pain, *Am J Cardiol* 64:985–990, 1989.

78. Stratmann HG, Tamesis BR, Younis LT, et al: Prognostic value of dipyridamole technetium-99m sestamibi myocardial tomography in patients with stable chest pain who are unable to exercise, *Am J Cardiol* 73:647–652, 1994.

79. Stratmann HG, Williams GA, Wittry MD, et al: Exercise technetium-99m sestamibi tomography for cardiac risk stratification of patients with stable chest pain, *Circulation* 89:615–622, 1994.

80. Wahl JM, Hakki AH, Iskandrian AS: Prognostic implications of normal exercise thallium 201 images, *Arch Intern Med* 145:253–256, 1985.

81. Weiss AT, Berman DS, Lew AS, et al: Transient ischemic dilation of the left ventricle on stress thallium-201 scintigraphy: a marker of severe and extensive coronary artery disease, *J Am Coll Cardiol* 9:752–759, 1987.

82. Wilson WW, Gibson RS, Nygaard TW, et al: Acute myocardial infarction associated with single vessel coronary artery disease: an analysis of clinical outcome and the prognostic importance of vessel patency and residual ischemic myocardium, *J Am Coll Cardiol* 11:223–234, 1988.

83. Yang LD, Berman DS, Kiat H, et al: The frequency of late reversibility in SPECT thallium-201 stress-redistribution studies, *J Am Coll Cardiol* 15:334–340, 1990.

84. Younis LT, Byers S, Shaw L, et al: Prognostic importance of silent myocardial ischemia detected by intravenous dipyridamole thallium myocardial imaging in asymptomatic patients with coronary artery disease, *J Am Coll Cardiol* 14:1635–1641, 1989.

85. Younis LT, Byers S, Shaw L, et al: Prognostic value of intravenous dipyridamole thallium scintigraphy after an acute myocardial ischemic event, *Am J Cardiol* 64:161–166, 1989.

Chapter 21

Preoperative risk stratification: an overview

Mylan C. Cohen and **Kim A. Eagle**

"Just say something appropriate, like "cleared for the O.R.""

SURGICAL INTERN REQUESTING A PREOPERATIVE
CARDIOLOGY CONSULTATION

Because of the aging population, the prevalence of coronary artery disease, and constantly improving surgical and anesthetic techniques, many patients at risk for cardiac complications undergo noncardiac surgery each year. Cardiologists are frequently asked to evaluate patients to estimate cardiovascular risk associated with noncardiac surgical procedures and to assist in the management of postoperative cardiac complications. However, when requesting a preoperative cardiac evaluation, the surgical intern may not realize that the purpose of the interaction between the patient and the cardiology service may not be merely to get the patient through surgery. The preoperative cardiovascular evaluation represents an opportunity to identify cardiovascular conditions that may cause long-term illness and death and to manage the patient's overall cardiovascular health. This chapter reviews the epidemiology of postoperative cardiac complications, methods for risk assessment, a stepwise approach to preoperative cardiac evaluation and management, and future directions in the field, with a focus on the identification and management of coronary artery disease.

EPIDEMIOLOGY

More than 25 million patients undergo noncardiac surgery in the United States each year. Of these patients, 1 million have diagnosed coronary artery disease, 2 to 3 million have multiple risk factors for coronary disease, and 4 million are older than 65 years of age.[95] These patients account for approximately 80% of the 1 million persons in whom surgery is complicated by perioperative cardiac morbidity and mortality; the accompanying in-hospital costs exceed $12 billion annually.[102] Perhaps partially because of the lack of results of clinical trials to guide decision making, practice related to risk stratification varies widely.[11] The process of risk assessment is costly, having been estimated at $3.7 billion annually,[11] and most patients who undergo risk assessment will not die or sustain postoperative myocardial infarction.

Over the past 30 years, the risk for postoperative myocardial infarction has remained low (<1%).[134,140] A history of myocardial infarction increases the risk for postoperative myocardial infarction, especially when surgery is performed soon after an index infarction.[61,134,140,146] The peak risk for myocardial infarction occurs within the first 3 days after surgery.[7,73,123,140,146] Most postoperative myocardial infarctions are non–Q-wave in type and are detected within the first 24 hours after surgery, likely because of increased surveillance with frequent electrocardiography and cardiac enzyme evaluation.[18,19,127] Because of the residual effects of anesthesia and the effects of narcotics and sedatives, the presentation of postoperative myocardial infarction is often silent or subtle. Nonspecific symptoms, such as new or worsening congestive heart failure, hypotension, nausea, altered mental status, or arrhythmias, may be the only clinical indications of infarction.[7,62] For these reasons and because the average mortality rate associated with postoperative myocardial infarction can be as high as 50%,[7,61,134,140,146] close perioperative surveillance with prompt initiation of therapy if infarction is suspected is warranted.

Cardiac surgical risk is a function of patient-specific, surgical procedure–specific, and institution-specific factors. Emergency, intrathoracic, and intraperitoneal procedures are associated with higher risk for perioperative cardiac complications. Orthopedic and vascular surgery are also associated with higher rates of postoperative cardiac morbidity and mortality.[61,134,140] The high association between peripheral vascular disease and coronary artery disease is already well recognized.[66] Other procedures have higher risk because of associated blood loss; higher risk for hypotension; intravascular and extravascular fluid shifts; or the tendency for older, debilitated patients to require the procedure. Conversely, procedures performed under local anesthesia are usually associated with very low risk. For example, ophthalmologic procedures and herniorrhaphies have been safely performed soon after infarction.[5,103]

CLINICAL PREDICTION

Several investigators have sought to stratify risk on the basis of clinical criteria. One of the first attempts was made by Dripps et al[35] on the basis of their surgical experience in more than 33,000 patients over 10 years (1947–1957). Patients were assigned to a physical status class before receiving anesthesia. No deaths occurred in 16,000 "physically fit" patients. However, in "moribund" patients, 1 in 16 patients given spinal anesthesia and 1 in 10 patients given general anesthesia died. Although Dripps's modification of the index of physical status is still used today by the American Society of Anesthesiologists (Table 21-1)[3] and has been validated in a large cohort of patients,[145] it is subjective and may be less predictive in some subsets of patients, such as elderly persons, obese persons, and persons with previous myocardial infarction or mild systemic disease.[117]

In part because of the limitations of the Dripps–ASA Index, Goldman et al[61,62] developed a multifactorial index to assess the cardiac risk of noncardiac surgery in 1001 consecutive general surgery patients 40 years of age and older.[61,62] There were 19 postoperative cardiac deaths, 18 perioperative myocardial infarctions, 36 episodes of pulmonary edema, and 12 cases of ventricular tachycardia. The overall nonfatal cardiac event rate was 3.9%. Using multivariate analysis to evaluate 39 variables, nine independent, statistically significant predictors of periop-

erative cardiac events were identified. Each predictor was assigned a discriminate function coefficient reflecting its relative weight in the logistic regression equation. The coefficients were used to assign a point value to each variable. From the point scores, a preoperative cardiac risk index composed of four classes was created (Table 21-2). Patients in risk class I (0 to 5 points) of the Goldman multifactorial index had a 0.9% incidence of life-threatening cardiac complications or cardiac death. Complications increased incrementally by class, with class IV patients (>26 points) having a complication rate of 78%. Class IV included 18 high-risk patients who accounted for more than half of cardiac deaths (10 of 19).

Although the Goldman risk index has been prospectively validated,[152] its applicability for more specific patient subsets and types of surgery has been questioned. For example, Gerson et al[57] evaluated the predictive value of patient history, physical examination, and rest and exercise radionuclide ventriculography to risk-stratify 155 geriatric patients presenting for nonemergency abdominal, thoracic, or aortic surgery. Dripps–ASA and Goldman risk indices were calculated for each patient. Inability to bicycle 2.0 minutes to a heart rate greater than 99 beats per minute was the only significant pre-

Table 21-1. Dripps's modification of the index of physical status, American Society of Anesthesiologists

1. A normal healthy patient
2. A patient with mild systemic disease
3. A patient with a severe systemic disease that limits activity but is not incapacitating
4. A patient with an incapacitating systemic disease that is a constant threat to life
5. A moribund patient who is not expected to survive 24 hours with or without operation

In the event of emergency operation, precede the number with an E.

Reprinted with permission from American Society of Anesthesiologists. New classification of physical status, *Anesthesiology* 24:111, 1963.

Table 21-2. The Goldman Multifactorial Cardiac Risk Index

Criterion	Points, n
History	
Age > 70 years	5
Myocardial infarction in previous 6 months	10
Physical examination	
S_3 gallop or jugular venous distention	11
Important valvular aortic stenosis	3
Electrocardiography results	
Rhythm other than sinus or premature atrial contractions on last preoperative electrocardiography	7
> 5 premature ventricular contractions per minute documented at any time before surgery	7
General status	
P_{O_2} < 60 mm Hg or P_{CO_2} > 50 mm Hg, potassium level < 3.0 mEq/L or bicarbonate level < 20 mEq/L, blood urea nitrogen concentration > 50 mg/dL or creatinine concentration > 3.0 mg/dL, abnormal serum glutamic-oxaloacetic transaminase, signs of chronic liver disease, or bedridden from noncardiac causes	3
Surgery	
Intraperitoneal, intrathoracic, or aortic surgery	3
Emergency surgery	4
Total	**53**

Reprinted with permission from Goldman L, Caldera DL, Nussbaum SR, et al: Multifactorial index of cardiac risk in noncardiac surgical procedures, *N Engl J Med* 297:845-850, 1977.

dictor of a cardiac event. No clinical predictor, including the Dripps–ASA and Goldman indices, provided any additional independent predictive information.

To adjust risk estimates for a specific planned surgical procedure, Detsky et al[32] developed a modified index of perioperative cardiac risk.[32] They altered several features of Goldman's original index on the basis of their clinical experiences (Table 21-3). Detsky's modified multifactorial index included categories describing the severity of coronary artery disease as reflected by Canadian Heart Association angina class, a more precise definition of congestive heart failure, and consideration of the proximity of the episode of heart failure to the surgical procedure. The scoring system was also simplified by using multiples of five. Finally, the type of surgery was considered in the pretest probability of postoperative cardiac complications. Detsky et al determined the pretest probability of postoperative cardiac events for each type of surgery at the first author's institution. The risk scores for the entire group were used to generate likelihood ratios (the proportion of patients with and without cardiac complications for any given risk score). The individual patient information contained in the risk score was used

Table 21-3. The Modified Multifactorial Cardiac Risk Index

Criterion	Points, n
Coronary artery disease	
MI within 6 months	10
MI more than 6 months	5
Canadian Heart Association angina	
Class 3	10
Class 4	20
Unstable angina within 3 mos.	10
Alveolar pulmonary edema	
Within 1 week	10
Ever	5
Valvular disease	
Suspected critical aortic stenosis	20
Arrhythmias	
Sinus plus atrial premature beats or rhythm other than sinus on last preoperative electrocardiogram	5
> 5 ventricular premature depolarization at any time before surgery	5
Poor general medical status*	5
Age older than 70 years	5
Emergency surgery	10

$PO_2 < 60$ mm Hg; $PCO_2 > 50$ mm Hg; serum potassium level < 3.0 mmol/L; serum bicarbonate level < 20 mmol/L; blood urea nitrogen concentration ≥ 18 mmol/L; serum creatinine concentration > 260 mmol/L; abnormal aspartate aminotransferase level; signs of chronic liver disease; or bedridden because of noncardiac causes.
Reprinted with permission from Detsky AS, Abrams HB, McLaughlin JR, et al: Predicting cardiac complications in patients undergoing non-cardiac surgery, *J Gen Intern Med* 1:211-219, 1986.

to convert the pretest probability of a cardiac complication (the average risk for all patients undergoing a similar procedure) to a posttest probability (the average risk for patients with similar index scores) via the likelihood ratio associated with that particular risk score. These investigators prospectively evaluated 455 consecutive patients who were referred for preoperative consultation for cardiac risk assessment before noncardiac surgery. Receiver-operating characteristic curves showed that cardiac risk was progressively greater for increasing modified risk index scores and for surgical procedures associated with higher complication rates.[32,33]

Several factors may limit the predictive value of these clinical indices. To our knowledge, the modified risk index has never been validated externally, and the pretest probabilities and likelihood ratios are likely to vary by institution and patient population. Furthermore, confounding clinical problems and events not considered in the risk index may influence the management of individual patients. When estimating surgical risk, relevant patient-specific, institution-specific, and procedure-specific factors must be considered. Since these risk indices were introduced, there has been increased appreciation of the value of screening patients before surgery. Many patients who may have had surgery previously may cancel surgery. Thus, indices may lose predictive value in current patient populations who continue on to surgery after evaluation. These considerations, as well as the desire to increase predictive precision, have stimulated investigations of noninvasive tests to determine whether it is possible to more accurately identify patients at major risk.

STRESS TESTING AND ASSESSMENT OF LEFT VENTRICULAR FUNCTION

Because poor functional capacity in patients who have coronary artery disease or have sustained myocardial infarction is associated with an increased incidence of subsequent cardiac events,[113] it is not surprising that one of the first noninvasive technologies to be evaluated for use in preoperative cardiac risk stratification was exercise treadmill testing. Cutler et al[30] reviewed the results of preoperative exercise treadmill test in 130 patients with substantial peripheral vascular disease who subsequently underwent peripheral vascular surgery.[30] The investigators correlated the results of preoperative exercise treadmill testing with the development of postoperative cardiac complications (myocardial infarction or ischemia and congestive heart failure). Patients who achieved greater than 75% of their predicted maximal heart rate without an ischemic electrocardiographic response were at lowest risk (0 events in 35 patients). In contrast, patients who had myocardial ischemia at a low level of exercise (peak heart rate less than 75% of the predicted maximum) were at the highest perioperative cardiac risk (10 postoperative cardiac complications, including 7 myocardial infarctions [5 fatal] in 26 patients). Patients who had an ischemic electrocardiographic response to exercise at a heart rate greater than 75% of the predicted maximum were at intermediate risk (6 of 23 patients had postoperative cardiac complications, but 0 died).[30]

Carliner et al[17] prospectively evaluated preoperative exercise testing in 200 consecutive patients older than 40 years of age (mean age, 59 years) scheduled for major noncardiac surgical procedures (52% abdominal, 34% vascular, and 14% thoracic). Three postoperative deaths and three myocardial infarctions occurred. Twenty-seven patients developed postoperative myocardial ischemia or injury (manifested by postoperative electrocardiographic changes without elevation of the creatine phosphokinase-MB fraction or an elevated creatine phosphokinase-MB fraction without accompanying diagnostic electrocardiographic changes). An abnormal result on preoperative electrocardiography was the only statistically significant predictor of risk in multivariate analysis, and only one of the six patients who had myocardial infarction died or had a positive ST- segment response to exercise. However, five of the six had a maximal exercise capacity of less than 5 metabolic equivalents (MET).[17]

The importance of exercise capacity as an important predictor of cardiac outcome after noncardiac surgery was further demonstrated by McPhail et al,[109] who performed preoperative exercise testing in 101 consecutive patients with clinical evidence of coronary artery disease before peripheral vascular surgery. Sixty-one patients underwent exercise treadmill testing according to the standard Bruce protocol, and 40 underwent arm ergometry. Patients who achieved greater than 85% of the predicted maximal heart rate during exercise testing had a cardiac complication rate (cardiac death, myocardial infarction, congestive heart failure, or malignant ventricular ectopic activity) of 6%; whereas those who achieved less than 85% of the predicted maximal heart rate had a complication rate of 24%. Although the degree of ST-segment depression during exercise testing was not an independent predictor of cardiac complications, patients who attained less than 85% of the predicted maximal heart rate and had a positive result on a stress test (ST depression >1.0 mm) had the highest complication rate (7 of 21 [33%]).[109]

In addition, supine bicycle ergometry has been performed in patients who are unable to exercise on a treadmill. Gerson et al[56] showed that the inability to perform 2 minutes of supine bicycle exercise to raise the heart rate above 99 bpm was a good predictor of perioperative pulmonary, cardiac, and combined cardiopulmonary complications.[56]

These studies and others (Table 21-4) suggest that the inability to perform even modest levels of exercise identifies patients who are at higher risk. Furthermore, poor exercise capac-

Table 21-4. Preoperative exercise testing before major noncardiac surgery*

Study, year	Patients with abnormal test result n (%)	Criteria for abnormal test	Events	Predictive value of positive test result	Predictive value of negative test result	Event	Comments
				% (n/n)			
Peripheral vascular surgery or abdominal aortic aneurysm repair							
McCabe et al, 1981[104]†	314(36)	STD, CP, or A	38(15/39)	81(13/16)	91(21/23)	D,M,I,II,A	
Cutler et al, 1981[30]	130(39)	STD	7(9/130)	16(8/50)	99(79/80)	D,M	< 75% MPHR increased risk
Arous, Baum, and Cutler, 1984[4]†	808(17)	STD	NR	21(19/89)	NR	D,M	
Laughlin et al, 1985[92]†	86(48)	STD	11(2/19)	11(1/9)	90(9/10)	D,M	
von Knorring and Lepantals, 1986[147]	105(25)	STD, A, or CP	3(3/105)	8(2/26)	99(78/79)	D,M	
Leppo et al, 1987[87]‡	60(28)	STD	12(7/60)	25(3/12)	92(44/48)	D,M	Exercise test results used to refer patients for revascularization
Hanson et al, 1988[64]†	74(57)	STD	3(1/37)	5(1/19)	100(18/18)	D,M	Arm ergometry
McPhail et al, 1988[109]‡	100(70)	<85% MPHR	19(19/100)	24(17/70)	93(28/30)	D,M,A,F	<85% MPHR; $p = 0.04$; STD; NS
Urbinati et al, 1994[143]	121(23)	STD	0	0(0/28)	100(93/93)	D,M	Carotid endarterectomy patients; STD predicted late death
Peripheral vascular surgery or major noncardiac surgery							
Carliner et al, 1985[17]	200(16)	STD	32(16/200)	16(5/32)	93(157/168)	D,M	5 METs (NS)

*STD = exercise-induced electrocardiographic ischemia; CP, chest pain; A, cardiac arrhythmia; D, death; M, myocardial infarction; I, myocardial ischemia; H, hypotension; MPHR = maximum predicted heart rate; NR, not reported; F, failure; NS, not significant; MET, metabolic equivalent.

†Studies with prospective collection of postoperative electrocardiography and cardiac enzyme tests.

‡The total number of patients undergoing peripheral vascular surgery was less than the total number tested.

Modified from Eagle KA, Brundage BH, Chaitman BR, et al: Guidelines for perioperative cardiovascular evaluation for noncardiac surgery. Report of the American College of Cardiology/American Heart Association Task Force on Practice Guidelines (Committee on Perioperative Cardiovascular Evaluation for Noncardiac Surgery), *J Am Coll Cardiol* 27:910-948, 1996.

ity, along with electrocardiographic changes that are diagnostic for myocardial ischemia, are associated with a particularly high risk. The frequency of an abnormal result on exercise electrocardiography is related to the patient's clinical history and increases with a history of myocardial infarction or an abnormal result in resting electrocardiography.

In an attempt to find alternative methods for identifying patients with significant coronary artery disease, some investigators turned to radionuclide ventriculography to assess resting and exercise left ventricular function. Pasternack et al performed resting radionuclide ventriculography in 50 patients undergoing elective aortic aneurysm repair[122] and 100 patients before elective lower extremity revascularization.[123] No perioperative myocardial infarctions occurred in any patient with a normal left ventricular ejection fraction, even though 20% of these patients had a history of angina or infarction. Of the patients with left ventricular ejection fraction of 36% to 55%, 20% experienced perioperative non–Q wave myocardial infarction and 75% with a left ventricular ejection fraction of <35% or less experienced a perioperative non–Q wave myocardial infarction. All of the high-risk patients had a history of myocardial infarction or angina. Although there were few high-risk patients in each study, a resting left ventricular ejection fraction of <35% or less was a better predictor of perioperative myocardial infarction than any other clinical variable. In a later study of 200 patients referred for all types of vascular surgery, Pasternack et al[120] reported similar results.

These findings were confirmed in several other cohorts, including 73 patients scheduled to undergo carotid endarterectomy,[76] 41 patients referred for aortic surgery,[114] 72 patients undergoing aortic surgery,[49] 20 patients referred for aortic surgery,[43] and 94 patients undergoing noncardiac surgery.[86] However, subsequent studies by Kazmers, Cerqueira, and Zierler;[74,75] Franco et al;[51] McCann and Clements;[105] and McEnroe et al[108] failed to show a statistically significant relation between resting left ventricular ejection fraction and development of perioperative adverse cardiac events. Thus, taken together, the data indicate that resting left ventricular ejection fraction is a relatively insensitive and nonspecific marker for postoperative myocardial infarction and cardiac death. However, poor left ventricular systolic or diastolic dysfunction may predict postoperative congestive heart failure and undoubtedly correlates with long-term mortality. Because of this shortcoming, left ventricular ejection fraction determined by radionuclide ventriculography was evaluated.

Jain et al[72] examined exercise first-pass radionuclide ventriculography in 78 patients referred for peripheral vascular surgery. Surgery was canceled so that coronary angiography could be performed, along with other cardiac interventions (if warranted), in suitable patients if the resting left ventricular ejection fraction was less than 50% with wall-motion abnormalities or if the exercise left ventricular ejection fraction increased less than 5%. Of 53 patients with abnormal results, 27 patients underwent coronary angiography, 6 underwent coronary artery bypass graft (CABG) surgery, 11 had a modified

surgical procedure, and five had anesthesia changed from general to local. No deaths or myocardial infarctions were noted in patients who had normal results. Other studies, however, have not shown that exercise radionuclide ventriculography–determined left ventricular ejection fraction is predictive of postoperative myocardial infarction or cardiac death. However, these studies did confirm the importance of good functional capacity in avoiding postoperative cardiac events.[72] Gerson et al[57] evaluated rest and exercise radionuclide ventriculography in patients 65 years of age or older who were scheduled to undergo elective abdominal or noncardiac thoracic surgery. The investigators used bicycle ergometry starting at 50 rpm and a workload of 25 watts, which was increased by 12.5 watts every minute until the patients developed fatigue, dyspnea, or chest pain. At peak exercise, a 2-minute acquisition was obtained in the left anterior oblique position. In a preliminary investigation in 100 patients, 13 had 22 perioperative cardiac complications, including six deaths. Multivariate analysis identified the inability to exercise for 2 minutes with a heart rate less than 99 bpm and regional wall-motion abnormalities on resting radionuclide ventriculography as statistically significant predictors of adverse perioperative cardiac events. The investigators then tested these results in 55 consecutive patients 65 years of age or older. In this cohort, 10 patients had 12 cardiac complications, including two deaths. The only significant predictor of a perioperative cardiac complication was the inability to bicycle for 2 minutes and achieve a heart rate of more than 99 bpm.[57] In another cohort of 148 patients undergoing bicycle ergometry before peripheral vascular surgery, cardiac events did not correlate with left ventricular ejection fraction, wall-motion abnormalities, or exercise-induced myocardial ischemia. All 11 perioperative adverse cardiac events (five deaths, five myocardial infarctions, and one cardiac arrest) occurred in patients who were unable to achieve 4.5 METs.[52] Thus, these studies indicate that resting left ventricular ejection fraction and exercise-induced wall-motion abnormalities are insensitive predictors of postoperative myocardial infarction and cardiac death. However, poor functional capacity was confirmed as being of prognostic benefit (Table 21-4).

PERFUSION IMAGING

Thallium-201 myocardial scintigraphy

Functional capacity seems to be a strong determinant of overall prognosis and a significant predictor of perioperative cardiac risk; but many patients are limited in their ability to exercise. Thus, exercise testing has limited prognostic value[53,71,111] in some elderly, deconditioned, or obese patients, as well as in many patients scheduled to undergo peripheral vascular, orthopedic, or neurosurgical procedures. Alternative methods of preoperative cardiac risk assessment are necessary in these patient populations, and pharmacologic stress imaging represents a major advance. The most common forms of pharmacologic stress imaging used for preoperative cardiac risk assessment are dobutamine stress echocardiography and intravenous dipyridamole myocardial perfusion scintigraphy, although other agents and combinations of imaging methods have been investigated.

Boucher et al[9] first demonstrated the utility of dipyridamole thallium scanning for preoperative cardiac risk assessment in patients who are unable to exercise. They evaluated 54 stable patients with suspected coronary artery disease (on the basis of an abnormal result on resting electrocardiography or a history of chest pain or myocardial infarction) before vascular surgery. Of the 48 patients (89%) who underwent vascular surgery without coronary angiography, 16 patients had thallium redistribution on preoperative dipyridamole thallium scintigraphy. Eight perioperative ischemic cardiac events occurred (unstable angina, myocardial infarction, or cardiac death). All eight events occurred in the group of 16 patients who had preoperative thallium redistribution. No adverse postoperative cardiac events occurred in the 20 patients with a normal result on dipyridamole thallium scanning or in the 12 patients with only persistent defects on thallium imaging. All six patients who underwent coronary angiography before surgery had multivessel coronary disease; four patients underwent CABG surgery followed by peripheral vascular surgery without postoperative cardiac ischemic events.

Leppo et al[87] performed dipyridamole thallium imaging in 100 consecutive patients, 69 of whom also underwent exercise stress testing, before elective abdominal aortic or peripheral vascular surgery. Noninvasive test results were not blinded; thus, 11 patients were referred for coronary angiography before surgery. The remaining 89 patients underwent vascular surgery without further intervention; among these patients, 15 postoperative myocardial infarctions occurred. The presence of either an abnormal result on thallium imaging or thallium redistribution was a significant predictor of postoperative myocardial infarction. Of interest, no events occurred in the 12 patients who were able to perform more than 9 minutes of treadmill exercise (reaching stage IV of the Bruce protocol), even though 4 patients had thallium redistribution and 2 patients had both ST depression and redistribution. The presence of thallium redistribution was the most significant prognostic indicator of adverse postoperative outcome in a multivariate analysis to identify independent clinical predictors of postoperative myocardial infarction or death. Only the presence of ST depression during dipyridamole infusion and a history of diabetes had significant prognostic value in addition to thallium redistribution. Total exercise time and ST depression with exercise were borderline predictors of postoperative cardiac events, but neither added prognostic power once thallium redistribution was entered into the model. Among the 11 patients who underwent coronary angiography, 4 patients died, 1 after CABG and 1 after peripheral vascular surgery that was not preceded by CABG. In addition, two deaths occurred in the interval between cardiac catheterization and planned coronary intervention. Finally, one patient had a cerebrovascular accident 24 hours after coronary angiography and one had a non–Q wave myocardial infarction after combined CABG and abdominal aortic aneurysm resection.

The studies discussed above used a purely qualitative approach to image interpretation and classified scans as normal or abnormal. Defects were further classified as either having or not having reversibility. Several investigators hypothesized that the predictive power of preoperative dipyridamole thallium imaging could be improved by using a more quantitative approach to image interpretation. Lette et al[89] performed dipyridamole thallium scintigraphy in 66 consecutive patients referred for testing before major general surgery (18 patients) or vascular surgery (48 patients). The authors defined semiquantitative indices of the extent and severity of reversible thallium abnormalities. A strong correlation was seen between the indices of severity and extent of thallium redistribution and postoperative cardiac death or myocardial infarction. Cardiac complications occurred in 9 of 21 patients (43%) with thallium redistribution, whereas no events occurred in 30 patients with normal results or in 9 patients with fixed defects. Only 1 of 11 patients classified as intermediate risk (limited extent of thallium redistribution) had a postoperative event. However, 8 of 10 patients classified as high risk (extensive thallium redistribution) had a postoperative cardiac event (seven cardiac deaths and one myocardial infarction). Reversible left ventricular cavity dilation was also a significant predictor of postoperative cardiac complications.

Likewise, Levinson et al[90] retrospectively analyzed clinical and scintigraphic predictors of perioperative cardiac complications in 62 patients with redistribution on preoperative dipyridamole thallium scintigraphy. In these 62 patients, there were 17 ischemic cardiac events, including 7 myocardial infarctions or deaths. The authors hypothesized that a semiquantitative analysis of the number of segments, views, or coronary arterial territories demonstrating thallium redistribution would improve the specificity and predictive value of dipyridamole thallium scintigraphy for perioperative ischemic events. Patients with redistribution in four or more myocardial segments were more likely than patients with three or fewer such segments to experience a perioperative ischemic cardiac event (38% compared with 12%; $p = 0.03$). Postoperative cardiac complications in patients with three or fewer segments showing redistribution were ischemic pulmonary edema (one patient), unstable angina (one patient), and myocardial infarction (one patient); no patients died. Patients with redistribution in two or three views were significantly more likely than patients with such redistribution in only one view to have a perioperative ischemic event (36% compared with 0%; $p = 0.005$). No patient with redistribution in only one view had any cardiac complication after vascular surgery, regardless of the number of abnormal segments in that view. Finally, patients with dipyridamole thallium redistribution in two or three coronary artery territories were significantly more likely than patients with redistribution in only one coronary artery territory to have a perioperative cardiac complication (43% compared with 13%; $p = 0.007$). Patients with redistribution in only one coronary territory had ischemic pulmonary edema (three patients) and unstable angina (one patient); no myocardial infarctions or deaths recurred. Dipyridamole-induced chest pain or ischemic electrocardiographic changes, fixed or reversible left ventricular cavity dilation, and increased lung uptake were not significant independent predictors of perioperative ischemic cardiac events. Multivariate analysis identified thallium redistribution in more than one view ($p<0.001$) as the strongest predictor of perioperative cardiac complications. After controlling for redistribution in multiple views, redistribution in more than one coronary territory remained significant.

Lane et al[84] also evaluated preoperative dipyridamole thallium scintigraphy quantitatively in 101 patients with diabetes mellitus who underwent peripheral vascular surgery. Thallium scans were analyzed visually and by using computer quantification. The overall cardiac event rate was 11% (3 deaths, 6 nonfatal myocardial infarctions, 3 episodes of unstable angina [2 of which were associated with subsequent infarction], and 5 episodes of congestive heart failure [3 of which ccurred in patients who eventually died]). At least one scintigraphic abnormality was found in more than 80% of these patients. Thallium abnormalities were present in 59% of patients without clinically evident coronary disease. The perioperative event rate in patients with thallium redistribution was 14% (10 of 71 patients) compared with 3.3% (1 of 30 patients) in patients without redistribution. The demonstration of two or more myocardial segments with thallium redistribution was sensitive (82%) but not specific (56%) for predicting perioperative ischemic events. Subgroups of patients at particularly high risk for adverse postoperative cardiac events included 9 patients who had five or more segments of thallium redistribution, 4 of whom (44%) had events, and 27 patients who had redistribution in the left anterior descending territory, 7 of whom (27%) had postoperative ischemic events. Patients at low risk were identified by an absence of angina pectoris (3.7% event rate) and no more than one segment with thallium redistribution (3.8% event rate).

Although it seems that thallium redistribution is sensitive for predicting postoperative ischemic cardiac events, its specificity is low. Specificity could be improved by applying the test in a higher risk cohort and not performing the test in low-risk subsets. Stratification of patients into groups who should and should not have further noninvasive cardiac assessment was the focus of two studies by Eagle et al.[38,39] In the first study, the authors evaluated the predictive value of dipyridamole thallium imaging for postoperative cardiac events in 61 patients referred for elective aortic surgery (resection of abdominal aortic aneurysm[39] or aortoiliac reconstruction). Thallium redistribution predicted postoperative ischemic events (unstable angina, ischemic pulmonary edema, myocardial infarction, or cardiac death). Several clinical variables, including Q waves on electrocardiography; history of congestive heart failure; and, possibly, diabetes, also had predictive value. The absence of these variables was considered, along with the history of myocardial infarction or angina, in an attempt to identify a clinically low-risk subset of patients who could proceed directly to vascular surgery without further noninvasive testing. Only 1 of 29 low-risk patients (3.4%), defined by absence of all five clinical

markers, experienced a perioperative ischemic event (unstable angina), whereas 7 (22%) higher-risk patients (patients with one or more of the five clinical markers) had a perioperative ischemic event. The stratification instrument was then prospectively validated in 50 patients undergoing vascular procedures. No ischemic events occurred in 23 low-risk patients. Among the 27 patients with one or more clinical markers, the event rate was 37%, including 3 cardiac deaths. Each patient who died had thallium redistribution on preoperative dipyridamole thallium scintigraphy.

These investigators later extended their observations by retrospectively analyzing 200 consecutive patients referred for vascular surgery (aortoiliac or aortofemoral bypass graft in 67 patients; abdominal aortic aneurysm resection in 71 patients; and peripheral vascular procedures, such as femoral popliteal bypass or carotid endarterectomy, in 62 patients).[38] Postoperative cardiac events occurred in 30 patients (15%) (six cardiac deaths [3%], nine acute nonfatal myocardial infarctions [4.5%], nine cases of acute ischemic pulmonary edema [4.5%], and 19 cases of unstable angina pectoris [8.5%]). In multivariate analysis, Q waves on preoperative electrocardiography, history of angina, history of ventricular ectopic activity requiring treatment, diabetes requiring pharmacologic therapy, and age older than 70 years were independent clinical predictors of postoperative ischemic events. The two independent dipyridamole thallium scan predictors of ischemic events were thallium redistribution and ischemic electrocardiographic changes during or after dipyridamole infusion ($p<0.01$). Three logistic regression models were created to predict postoperative cardiac ischemic events: 1) clinical variables alone, 2) dipyridamole thallium test results alone, and 3) both clinical and dipyridamole thallium test variables. The sensitivities and specificities of these three models were compared.

Thallium redistribution was the most sensitive predictor, but it was less specific than several of the clinical variables, particularly Q waves on preoperative electrocardiography. The model that used both clinical markers and dipyridamole thallium test results achieved a significantly higher specificity at equivalent sensitivity levels than models using either clinical variables alone or dipyridamole thallium test results alone (Fig. 21-1). Of 64 patients with none of the five clinical variables, only 2 patients (3.1% [95% confidence interval (CI), 0% to 8%]) experienced postoperative cardiac ischemic events compared with 10 of 20 patients (50% [95% CI, 29% to 71%]) with three or more clinical markers. Patients with either one or two clinical variables had an intermediate risk, with 18 ischemic events in 116 patients (15.5% [95% CI, 7% to 21%]). The presence or absence of thallium redistribution further delineated the intermediate-risk group into low-risk and high-risk categories; only 2 of the 62 patients (3.2% [95% CI, 0% to 8%]) in the intermediate-risk subgroup without thallium redistribution had events compared with 16 events in the 54 patients with thallium redistribution (29.6% [95% CI, 16% to 44%]).

Taken together, these studies indicate that the specificity of preoperative dipyridamole thallium scintigraphy can be im-

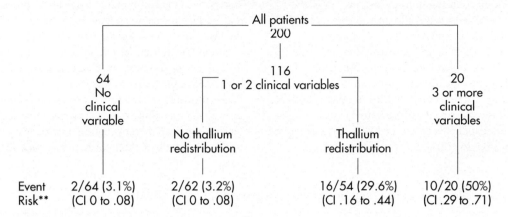

Fig. 21-1. Clinical markers of risk and thallium redistribution. (Reprinted with permission from Eagle KA, Coley CM, Newell JB, et al: Combining clinical and thallium data optimizes preoperative assessment of cardiac risk before major vascular surgery, *Ann Intern Med* 110:859-866, 1989.)

proved by considering clinical variables. Low-risk and high-risk subsets of vascular surgery patients can be identified clinically. Dipyridamole thallium imaging may be most useful to risk-stratify vascular surgery patients who are determined by clinical criteria to be at intermediate risk.

Further support for selective use of preoperative dipyridamole thallium scanning comes from a study by Baron et al.[6] They prospectively evaluated 457 consecutive patients undergoing elective surgery for abdominal aortic aneurysm with dipyridamole thallium single-photon emission computed tomography (SPECT) and radionuclide ventriculography. The cardiac event rate was 19% (prolonged myocardial ischemia in 61 patients, myocardial infarction in 22, congestive heart failure in 20, severe ventricular tachyarrhythmia in 2, and death from any cause in 20). Clinical evidence of coronary artery disease (odds ratio (OR), 2.6 [95% CI, 1.6 to 4.3]) and age greater than 65 years (OR, 2.3; 95% CI, 1.4 to 3.6) were better predictors of adverse outcome than thallium redistribution (OR, 1.1 [95% CI, 0.6 to 2.0]). Left ventricular ejection fraction assessed by radionuclide ventriculopathy only predicted postoperative congestive heart failure. Age older than 65 years was the only predictor of death (OR, 26.4 [95% CI, 3.5 to 200.0]). The authors concluded that the routine use of dipyridamole thallium SPECT and radionuclide ventriculography for preoperative cardiac risk assessment before abdominal aortic surgery may not be justified. Mangano et al[98] also questioned the utility of routine preoperative thallium scanning when they found that thallium redistribution had a positive predictive value of 14% (2 myocardial infarctions and 1 cardiac death among 22 patients with thallium redistribution) for hard end points. In both of these studies, treating physicians were blinded to test results.

In a multicenter study that sought to develop and validate a Bayesian risk prediction model for vascular surgery candidates, L'Italien et al[91] developed a prediction model in 567 patients from two centers on the basis of clinical variables (age >70 years, angina, history of myocardial infarction, diabetes mellitus, history of congestive heart failure, and prior coronary revascularization). A second model was developed from dipyridamole thallium scan results (perfusion abnormalities and ST-segment changes). Model performance, alone and in combination, was evaluated with receiver-operating curve (ROC) analysis. The models were then validated in a separate cohort of 514 patients from three centers. The observed and predicted cardiac event rates were similar for both patient sets. The addition of dipyridamole thallium scan data reclassified more than 80% of intermediate-risk patients into low-risk (3% event rate) and high-risk (19% event rate) categories (*p*<0.0001) but provided no stratification for patients classified as low risk or high risk by the clinical model. The authors concluded that clinical markers, weighted according to prognostic impact, will reliably stratify risk in patients who are candidates for dipyridamole thallium scintigraphy, thus obviating the need for more expensive testing.[91]

Because of the association of coronary artery disease with peripheral vascular disease and a higher event rate in this population of patients with peripheral vascular disease, most investigations have evaluated noninvasive testing in patients requiring vascular surgery. However, preoperative noninvasive cardiac risk assessment has been evaluated in patients undergoing other noncardiac surgery. Brown et al[14] assessed dipyridamole thallium scintigraphy and radionuclide ventriculography in renal transplantation on the basis of candidates. In a cohort of 65 patients, 4 patients did not undergo transplantation on the basis of test results (3 with thallium redistribution and 1 with left ventricular ejection fraction <30%), and 35 of the 61 remaining patients received a renal allograft. Although none of the 35 patients had thallium redistribution or experienced postoperative cardiac events, thallium redistribution and reduced left ventricular ejection fraction were strong predictors of future adverse cardiac outcomes in the entire group. Similar results were obtained by Camp et al.[16] Studies in other groups of patients have demonstrated a positive predictive value for myocardial infarction or death between 8% and 27% and a negative predictive value of 98% to 100%.[23,70,132,139,149]

Recently, a joint task force of the American College of Cardiology (ACC) and the American Heart Association (AHA) summarized the current knowledge about preoperative myocardial perfusion imaging methods (Table 21-5).[37] The report of the task force noted that the predictive value of thallium redistribution for myocardial infarction or death ranged from 4% to 20% in selected reports that included more than 100 patients. The positive predictive value has decreased over time, an effect that is probably related to use of thallium information for therapeutic interventions, such as coronary revascularization or intensive medical therapy before noncardiac surgery. Furthermore, the results of thallium scanning may lead to the perfor-

Table 21-5. Dipyridamole thallium imaging for preoperative assessment of cardiac risk*

Study, year	Patients who underwent surgery	Patients with ischemia by thallium redistribution	Myocardial infarction on death
	n	*n(%)*	*n(%)*
Vascular surgery			
Boucher et al, 1985[9]	48	16(33)	3(6)
Cutler and Leppo, 1987[29]	116	54(47)	11(10)
Fletcher et al, 1988[48]	67	15(22)	3(4)
Sachs et al, 1988[130]	46	14(31)	2(4)
Eagle et al, 1989[38]	200	82(41)	15(8)
McEnroe et al, 1990[108]	95	34(36)	7(7)
Younis et al, 1990[150]	111	40(36)	8(7)
Mangano et al, 1991[98]	60	22(37)	3(5)
Strawn and Guernsey, 1991[138]	68	N/A	4(6)
Watters et al, 1991[148]	26	15(58)	3(12)
Hendel et al, 1992[65]	327	167(51)	28(9)
Lette et al, 1992[88]	355	161(45)	30(8)
Madsen et al, 1992[93]	65	45(69)	5(8)
Brown and Rosen, 1993[14]	231	77(33)	12(5)
Kresowik et al, 1993[80]	170	67(39)	5(3)
Baron et al, 1994[6]	457	160(35)	22(5)
Bry et al, 1994[15]	237	110(46)	17(7)
Nonvascular surgery†			
Camp et al, 1990[16]	40	9(23)	6(15)
Iqbal et al, 1991[70]	31	11(41)	3(11)
Coley et al, 1992[23]	100	36(36)	4(4)
Shaw et al, 1992[132]	60	28(47)	6(10)
Takase et al, 1993[139]	53	15(28)	6(11)
Younis et al, 1994[149]	161	50(31)	15(9)

N/A = not available.

*All studies except those by Coley et al[23] and Shaw et al[132] acquired patient information prospectively. Only in reports by Mangano et al[98] and Baron et al[6] were attending physicians blinded to scan results.

†Patients with fixed defects were omitted from calculations of positive and negative predictive value.

Reprinted from Eagle KA, Brundage BH, Chaitman BR, et al: Guidelines for perioperative cardiovascular evaluation for noncardiac surgery. Report of the American College of Cardiology/American Heart Association Task Force on Practice Guidelines (Committee on Perioperative Cardiovascular Evaluation for Noncardiac Surgery), *J Am Coll Cardiol* 27:910-948, 1996.

mance of less extensive procedures or cancellation of surgery. Nevertheless, the negative predictive value has remained high (approximately 99%), and the prognosis associated with a normal result on scanning is excellent.[37]

Dipyridamole technetium-99m sestamibi myocardial scintigraphy

There is limited experience with ^{99m}Tc sestamibi myocardial scintigraphy for preoperative risk assessment. Bry et al[15] retrospectively evaluated their experience over 6 years in 237 patients who underwent dipyridamole myocardial scintigraphy with either thallium or ^{99m}Tc sestamibi before vascular

surgery. Of 110 patients with at least one reversible defect, 51 underwent preoperative coronary angiography, 6 underwent coronary artery bypass surgery, and 3 underwent coronary angioplasty. Only congestive heart failure and two or more reversible defects on myocardial perfusion scintigraphy predicted adverse cardiac outcomes in multiple logistic regression analysis.

Stratmann et al reported on the prognostic value of dipyridamole ^{99m}Tc sestamibi scintigraphy in 229 consecutive patients being considered for vascular surgery[137] and 285 consecutive patients being considered for major and minor nonvascular surgery.[136] In the first study, vascular surgery was performed

Perioperative events		
Scan with thallium redistribution positive predictive value†	Normal scan negative predictive value†	Comments
%(n/n)		
19(3/16)	100(32/32)	First study to define risk of thallium redistribution
20(11/54)	100(60/60)	Only aortic surgery
20(3/15)	100(56/56)	
14(2/14)	100(24/24)	
16(13/82)	98(61/62)	Defined clinical risk
9(3/34)	96(44/46)	Fixed defects predict events
15(6/40)	100(51/51)	Includes long-term follow-up
5(1/22)	95(19/20)	Managing physicians blinded to scan result
N/A	100(21/21)	
20(3/15)	100(11/11)	Includes transesophageal echocardiography
14(23/167)	99(97/98)	Included long-term follow-up
17(28/161)	99(160/162)	Used quantitative scan index
11(5/45)	100(20/20)	
13(10/77)	99(120/121)	Prognostic utility enhanced by combined scan and clinical factors
4(3/67)	98(64/65)	Did not analyze for cardiac death; no independent value of scan
4(7/160)	96(195/203) (nonfatal only)	Cost-effectiveness data included
11(12/110)	100(97/97)	
67(6/9)	100(23/23)	Diabetes mellitus, renal transplant
27(3/11)	100(20/20)	86% of patients had exercise imaging instead of dipyridamole, diabetes mellitus, pancreas transplant
8(3/36)	98(63/64)	Define clinical risk factors in patients with known or suspected coronary artery disease
21(6/28)	100(19/19)	Used adenosine
27(4/15)	100(32/32)	Patients with documented or suspected coronary artery disease include rest echocardiography
18(9/50)	98(87/89)	Intermediate- to high-risk coronary artery disease

within 3 months of testing in 197 patients. Cardiac death, non-fatal myocardial infarction, unstable angina, or ischemic pulmonary edema occurred in 9 (5%) patients (3% in patients with normal results on ^{99m}Tc sestamibi imaging, 5% in those with abnormal results, and 6% in patients with ischemia). The occurrence of perioperative cardiac events in patients with abnormal results on ^{99m}Tc sestamibi imaging who had coronary revascularization or an increase in antiischemic medical therapy did not significantly differ from that in those who did not have these results or undergo these procedures.[137] In the second study, 140 major and 89 minor procedures were performed within 4 months of ^{99m}Tc sestamibi scanning. Unstable angina, acute ischemic pulmonary edema, nonfatal myocardial infarction, or cardiac death occurred in 11 patients (8%) undergoing major nonvascular surgery and 1 patient (1%) undergoing a minor procedure. Goldman class II or higher, an abnormal result on ^{99m}Tc sestamibi imaging, and a fixed perfusion defect were associated with increased risk. In the 60 patients whose Goldman class was II or higher, only an abnormal result on ^{99m}Tc sestamibi and a fixed perfusion defect were associated with incremental risk for perioperative cardiac events. Perioperative cardiac events occurred in 4% of patients with a normal result on ^{99m}Tc sestamibi scanning, 27% with an abnormal result ($p <0.05$), 24% with ischemia (p = 0.45), and 37% with a fixed defect ($p<0.01$).[136]

Late cardiac events

Dipyridamole thallium or ^{99m}Tc sestamibi myocardial scintigraphy performed before peripheral vascular surgery has long-term prognostic value as well. Hendel et al[65] evaluated 360 patients, of whom 327 underwent vascular surgery. Operative death and nonfatal myocardial infarction occurred in 4.9% and 6.7% of patients, respectively. A cardiac event (nonfatal myocardial infarction or cardiac death) occurred in 14.4% of patients with a transient thallium defect and in 1% of patients with a normal result ($p<0.001$). Multivariate analysis revealed that the best predictor of perioperative events was the presence of a reversible thallium defect. Late cardiac events occurred in 53 (15.2%) survivors of surgery or nonsurgically treated patients who were followed for a mean of 31 months. The late event rate was 24% in patients with a fixed perfusion abnormality compared with 4.9% in those with a normal dipyridamole thallium study result ($p<0.01$). Cox regression analysis showed that a fixed thallium defect was the most powerful predictor of late events and increased the relative risk by almost fivefold. A history of congestive heart failure was the only significant clinical variable that contributed additional value to that of a fixed defect alone. Life-table analysis confirmed the strong relationship between fixed defects and cardiac event–free survival ($p<0.0001$).

Younis et al[150] also evaluated late outcomes in 131 patients scheduled for peripheral vascular surgery. The actuarial event-free survival rate for patients with thallium redistribution was approximately 50% at 2 years. Urbinati et al[144] evaluated early and late cardiac events in 106 patients with neither a history nor

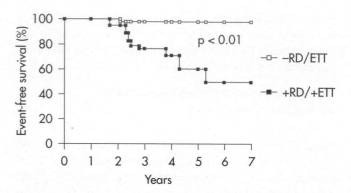

Fig. 21-2. Long-term prognostic value of exercise thallium imaging before carotid endarterectomy. Event-free survival rate was significantly lower in patients with reversible thallium defects *(RD)* and positive results on stress electrocardiography *(ETT)* compared with patients without such results. (Reprinted with permission from Goldman L, Caldera DL, et al: Multifactorial index of cardiac risk in non-cardiac surgical procedures, *N Engl J Med* 297:845-850, copyright 1997 Massachusetts Medical Society. All rights reserved.)

symptoms of coronary artery disease who underwent exercise thallium myocardial perfusion imaging before carotid endarterectomy. No cardiac deaths or myocardial infarctions occurred within 30 days of surgery. However, actuarial survival without coronary events was 51% in patients with a positive stress scan and thallium redistribution compared with 98% in patients without such results ($p<0.01$) by 7 years (Fig. 21-2).

In 172 patients who were followed for a mean of 21±14 months after elective vascular surgery, event-free survival was significantly lower in patients with abnormal ^{99m}Tc sestamibi scan results compared with those with normal scan results (74% and 96%; $p<0.0001$). After controlling for other clinical factors by using Cox proportional-hazards models, an abnormal ^{99m}Tc sestamibi study (relative risk, 3.7 [95% CI, 1.2 to 11.4]) and ^{99m}Tc sestamibi–detected ischemia (relative risk, 2.7 [95% CI, 1.2 to 6.1]) remained significant predictors of increased risk of late cardiac events.[137]

ALTERNATIVE METHODS OF RISK STRATIFICATION

Several reports have evaluated the accuracy of pharmacologic stress echocardiography to identify patients at risk for postoperative cardiac events* (Table 21-6). Most studies used dobutamine, although dipyridamole has also been used. The populations examined have been predominantly patients undergoing vascular surgery. Only one study blinded clinicians to the results of echocardiography.[126] In the other studies, results affected patient management, including the decision to perform preoperative coronary angiography and coronary revascularization. Among the studies of preoperative dobutamine echocardiography, the positive predictive value for myocardial infarction and death ranged from 7% to 23%. The negative predictive

*References 31, 40, 81, 83, 85, 125, 126, 141.

Table 21-6. Studies examining the value of dobutamine stress echocardiography for preoperative risk assessment*

Author	Patients with ischemia who underwent surgery	Events (death or myocardial infarction)		Criteria for abnormal test result	Predictive value†		Comments
					Positive	Negative	
Lane et al, 1991[83]	38	50	3(8)	New WMA	16(3/19)	100(19/19)	Vascular and general surgery
Lalka et al, 1992[81]	60	50	9(15)	New or worsening WMA	23(7/30)	93(28/30)	Multivariate analysis
Eichelberger et al, 1993[40]	75	36	2(3)	New or worsening WMA	7(2/27)	100(48/48)	Managing physicians blinded to DSE results
Langan et al, 1993[85]	74	24	3(4)	New WMA or electrocardiographic changes	17(3/18)	100(56/56)	
Poldermans et al, 1993[126]	131	27	5(4)	New or worsening	14(5/35)	100(96/96)	Multivariate analysis; managing physicians blinded to DSE results
Davila-Roman et al, 1993[31]	88	23	2(2)	New or worsening WMA	10(2/20)	100(68/68)	Included long-term follow-up

*DSE, dobutamine stress echocardigraphy; WMA, wall motion abnormality.
Table reprinted from Eagle KA, Brundage BH, Chaitman BR, et al: Guidelines for perioperative cardiovascular evaluation for noncardiac surgery. Report of the American College of Cardiology/American Heart Association Task Force on Practice Guidelines (Committee on Perioperative Cardiovascular Evaluation for Noncardiac Surgery), *J Am Coll Cardiol* 27:910-948, 1996.

value was 100% in all but one study. The severity of wall-motion changes with low-dose dobutamine infusion may be especially important. Furthermore, Poldermans et al[124] showed that stress-induced ischemia on dobutamine echocardiography is predictive of late cardiac events after vascular surgery. Therefore, although the published experience with stress echocardiography is not as extensive as that with exercise testing or radionuclide perfusion imaging, the literature suggests that dobutamine stress echocardiography is a valuable risk stratification method.

The predictive value of preoperative ambulatory echocardiographic monitoring for 24 to 48 hours was myocardial infarction and death has been reported by several investigators in patients undergoing vascular and other types of noncardiac surgery.* Although some of these reports have suggested favorable utility, preoperative ST-segment monitoring has several important limitations including variation in study protocols that affects predictive value, low predictive value compared with other risk stratification modalities, inability to perform screening in large numbers of patients because of baseline electrocardiographic abnormalities, a binary outcome that does not quantify the amount of myocardium at risk (which is useful in making a decision about performing coronary angiography), and inability to perform and interpret the test in a limited time for urgent surgical cases. However, im-

provements in technology, such as real-time identification of ischemic ST changes, may increase the utility of the method for postoperative surveillance and identify patients who may benefit from intensified medical regimens.

Finally, other imaging methods may have limited utility. Coronary calcification on computed tomographic scans obtained before noncardiac thoracic surgery has been shown to be predictive of postoperative cardiac morbidity.[112] Stress magnetic resonance imaging or ultrafast cine computed tomography in theory should identify patients at risk. However, less expensive and more widely available technologies exist.

STUDIES USING DECISION ANALYTIC AND COST-EFFECTIVENESS METHODOLOGIES

Investigations using decision analytic and cost-effectiveness methodologies have primarily evaluated management strategies involving myocardial perfusion imaging and coronary angiography in patients undergoing vascular surgery.[15,22,47,101,131] These studies indicate that selective screening should only be performed in patients with intermediate risk for coronary artery disease when the expected risk for surgical death is greater than about 5%.[22,47,101] In addition, the expected risk for death related to coronary revascularization should be low (less than approximately 2% to 3%).[101] With a selective approach to screening and coronary revascularization, the marginal cost per year of life saved is approximately $20,000.[22] Although this is a favorable amount, constantly improving surgical and anesthetic

*References 45, 46, 78, 79, 96, 110, 120, 127.

techniques are decreasing the cost-effectiveness of preoperative coronary artery disease screening and treatment.[15,31] Further evaluation is required to determine the cost-effectiveness of screening and treatment strategies over longer periods of follow-up.

RISK REDUCTION

Once a patient with intermediate to high cardiovascular risk for noncardiac surgery has been identified, what measures can be taken to reduce risk? Clinicians caring for the patient must consider the necessity and urgency of the proposed surgical procedure. If the procedure is elective or nonurgent, surgery might be canceled. Alternatively, a less extensive procedure involving shorter duration of anesthesia; less potential blood loss; or a percutaneous approach, such as peripheral angioplasty for treatment of vascular disease, might be contemplated. Evidence suggests that optimization of preoperative hemodynamics may be beneficial,[8] and careful perioperative hemodynamic monitoring may decrease cardiac morbidity.[128] However, the routine use of pulmonary arterial catheters in the initial care of critically ill patients has recently been questioned,[24] and there are no data from controlled clinical trials to guide the operative or postoperative use of pulmonary arterial catheters.

Several studies suggest that β-blockade may be beneficial perioperatively and long-term in patients who have undergone noncardiac surgery (Table 21-7).[97,119,121,135] Perioperative administration of nitroglycerin may decrease the incidence of intraoperative myocardial ischemia[26]; however, reduction in the incidence of myocardial infarction or cardiac death has not been demonstrated.[26,34] One small study evaluated the efficacy of intravenous diltiazem in patients undergoing vascular surgery. Less myocardial ischemia was noted in patients receiving diltiazem, but the study was too small to draw conclusions about myocardial infarction or death.[58] Presumably, these interventions may prevent postoperative adverse cardiac events that are preceded by tachycardia and electrocardiographic evi-

Table 21-7. Perioperative prophylactic antiischemic medications and cardiac morbidity

Study, year	Surgical procedure	Number of patients	Type of control
Nitroglycerin			
Coriat et al, 1984[26]	Carotid endarterectomy	45	Nitroglycerin, 0.5 μg/kg/min
Dodds et al, 1993[34]	Noncardiac	45	Placebo
Calcium-channel blockers			
Godet et al, 1987[58]	Vascular	30	Placebo
β-adrenergic blockers			
Pasternack et al, 1987[121]	Abdominal aortic aneurysmorrhaphy	83	Case–control
Pasternack et al, 1989[119]	Vascular	200	Unblinded
Stone et al, 1988[135]	Noncardiac	128	Placebo
Mangano et al, 1996[87]	Noncardiac	200	Placebo

*$p < .05$ for drug group versus control group.
†$p = 0.019$ for two-year mortality.
Reprinted with modifications from Eagle KA, Brundage BH, Chaitman BR, et al: Guidelines for perioperative cardiovascular evaluation for noncardiac surgery. Repoprt of the American College of Cardiology/American Heart Association Task Force on Practice Guidelines (Committee on Perioperative Cardiovascular Evaluation for Noncardiac Surgery), *J Am Coll Cardiol* 27:910-948, 1996.

dence of ischemia.* Furthermore, interventions aimed at increasing oxygen supply through increased oxygen delivery[10] or improved blood flow through intraaortic balloon counterpulsation may reduce postoperative cardiac morbidity and mortality.[55,133]

Studies by Golden et al[59] and Younis et al[149] suggest that coronary intervention in patients identified as high risk by myocardial perfusion scintigraphy may improve cardiac outcomes. These investigators reported no perioperative death or myocardial infarction in high-risk patients in whom revascularization was performed. In addition, adjustment of medication dosages and intraoperative hemodynamic monitoring may have contributed to a significant reduction in all perioperative cardiac events (from 47% to 8%; $p<0.001$) in the study by Younis et al.[149]

Other retrospective studies of percutaneous transluminal coronary angioplasty[2,41,54,68] and coronary artery bypass

*References 44, 82, 99, 105, 116, 127.

surgery* have shown that patients who have had recent coronary revascularization before noncardiac surgery have postoperative cardiac morbidity and mortality rates that are similar to those in patients with no clinical evidence of coronary artery disease. Manske et al[100] performed a randomized trial in which patients with coronary disease who were scheduled to undergo renal transplantation were assigned to receive medical therapy or CABG surgery. Although a 57% reduction in cumulative probability of unstable angina, myocardial infarction, or death at 12 months was observed in revascularized patients compared with medically treated patients, the study was terminated early, and loss to follow-up and small size were limitations. No randomized trials have evaluated preoperative coronary angioplasty, and optimal timing of noncardiac surgery after angioplasty remains poorly defined. Because of the increased chance of acute reocclusion in the first 1 to 2 days and the risk for restenosis at 1 to 3 months, it seems appropriate to delay non-

*References 1, 27, 28, 66, 94, 107, 129.

Drug	Occurrence of myocardial ischemia		Occurrence of myocardial infarction	
	Control group	Drug group	Control group	Drug group
Nitroglycerin, 1.0 µg/kg/min intraoperatively	14/22	4/23	0/22	0/23
Nitroglycerin 0.9 µg/kg/min intraoperatively	7/22	7/23	1/22	0/23
Diltiazem, 3 µg/kg/min intraoperatively	11/15	6/15	0/15	0/15
Metoprolol, 50 mg by mouth			9/51 (17.6%)	1/32† (3.1%)*
Metoprolol, 50 mg by mouth preoperatively	0.8 + 1.6 episodes	1.8 + 3.2 episodes		
Labetalol, atenolol, and olprenolol by mouth preoperatively	11/39 (28%)	2/89 (2%)	0/39	0/89
Atenolol preoperatively and postoperatively			21/101 (21%)	9/99 (10%)†

cardiac surgery several days to no more than several weeks after percutaneous transluminal coronary angioplasty. Presumably, patients who have had intracoronary stent placement should also be at lower risk for coronary events after noncardiac surgery, although no study to date has confirmed this idea. Because of the current practice of administering antiplatelet agents after stent placement, surgery should be delayed until therapy with medications can be safely discontinued. In determining whether any preoperative revascularization should be performed, the clinician must balance the short-term risks and the long-term benefits.

A postoperative hypercoagulable state exists[118,142] with increased circulating catecholamines.[12] This milieu may predispose patients to plaque rupture with thrombosis, resulting in fatal transmural myocardial infarction. Thus, improved pain control and low-level anticoagulation (with low-dose heparin or aspirin) in conjunction with β-blockade may block the pathophysiologic substrate for fatal postoperative myocardial infarction. However, no results of randomized trials exist to support these hypotheses.

STEPWISE APPROACH TO PREOPERATIVE CARDIAC RISK ASSESSMENT

Preoperative cardiac testing assesses short-term and long-term risk. With current anesthetic, surgical, and medical care, it is rare for the clinician to encounter a patient in whom the noncardiac surgical risk exceeds that of coronary artery bypass surgery. Percutaneous transluminal coronary angioplasty is an intuitively sound alternative because the long-term outcomes are similar to those of bypass surgery.[63,69,77] However, the appropriate prospective studies have not been performed in patients scheduled to undergo noncardiac surgery. Therefore, strategies that are known to improve long-term outcomes[151] should guide decision making; in this regard, the preoperative setting represents the first opportunity for coronary evaluation for many patients. In addition, preoperative evaluation may have value other than the detection of significant coronary artery disease, including the identification of asymptomatic or minimally symptomatic valvular or myocardial disease that requires long-term management. Costs and quality of testing methods vary locally and regionally. The cost-effectiveness of alternative methods, such as preoperative stress echocardiography, has not yet been evaluated. The clinician must weigh these factors in determining a risk assessment strategy that is appropriate for a specific patient.

On the basis of current knowledge, the ACC and the AHA jointly produced guidelines for cardiac evaluation before noncardiac surgery. A general strategy for preoperative cardiac risk assessment is summarized in Fig. 21-3. A stepwise approach to risk stratification includes the following:[37]

1. Determine the urgency of noncardiac surgery. Postoperative risk stratification may be appropriate for patients who must undergo emergency surgery, precluding preoperative assessment.

2. Determine whether the patient has undergone coronary revascularization in the past 5 years. Previous coronary revascularization probably reduces cardiac risk of noncardiac surgery.[50,68]

3. Determine whether the patient has had an adequate, favorable cardiac evaluation in the past 2 years. If there have been no new intercurrent symptoms, costly repeated testing may not be necessary.

4. Determine whether the patient has an unstable coronary syndrome or a major clinical predictor of risk (such as decompensated heart failure, significant arrhythmias, or severe valvular disease), which usually leads to cancellation or delay of surgery until the problem has been diagnosed and treated.

5. Determine whether the patient has intermediate clinical predictors of risk (such as previous myocardial infarction by history or electrocardiography, angina pectoris, compensated or previous heart failure, or diabetes mellitus). Consider the patient's functional capacity and surgery-specific risk.

6. Patients without major but with intermediate predictors of clinical risk and at least moderate functional capacity can generally undergo intermediate-risk surgery with a low probability of perioperative myocardial infarction or death. Conversely, patients with poor functional capacity (inability to exercise 4 METs) or who have multiple markers of risk and who are undergoing higher risk surgery should undergo noninvasive evaluation to further stratify risk. If the anticipated risk of surgery is high and results of noninvasive testing show abnormalities suggesting significant coronary artery disease,[20] coronary angiography with the intention to perform coronary revascularization given suitable coronary anatomy should be considered.

7. Noncardiac surgery is generally safe for patients with neither major nor intermediate predictors of clinical risk and at least moderate functional capacity.

8. Use results of the preoperative evaluation, including noninvasive testing in selected patients, to determine further preoperative management. Use information gained during preoperative evaluation and careful postoperative surveillance to tailor long-term therapy and follow-up.

No large, prospective studies have examined preoperative cardiac risk reduction, in part because of the difficulties associated with designing and carrying out such investigations.[21] Because of the lack of sufficient sound evidence, the decision to perform coronary angiography based on preoperative noninvasive cardiac testing remains difficult, controversial, and costly. The ACC/AHA guidelines for perioperative cardiovascular evaluation before noncardiac surgery do not address whether to perform coronary angiography in response to specific test results.[37] Therefore, using a modification of the "Delphi method" (a term sometimes used to describe a reiterative process by

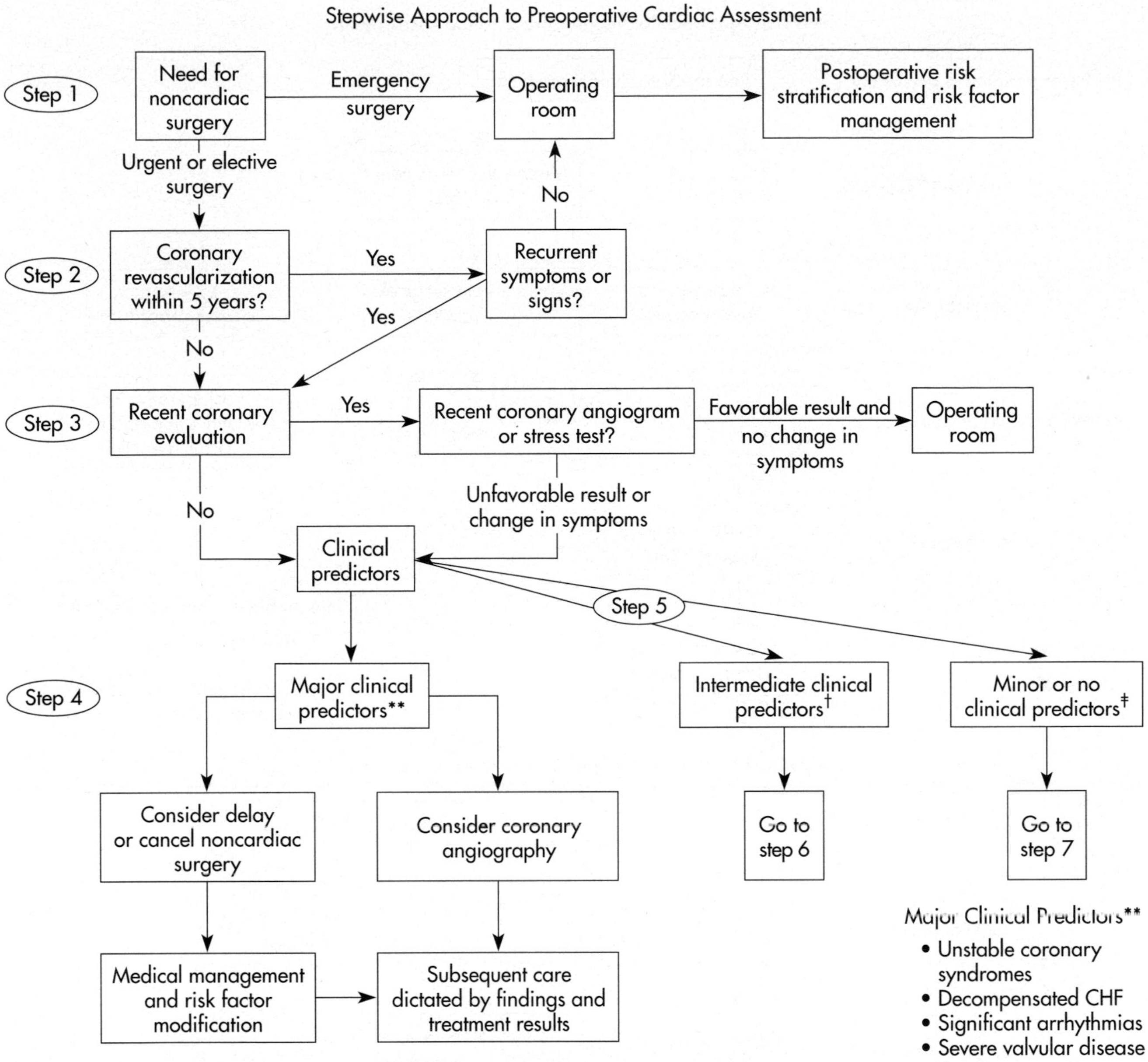

Stepwise Approach to Preoperative Cardiac Assessment

Fig. 21-3. A stepwise approach to preoperative cardiac assessment. Steps are discussed in text. * = Subsequent care may include cancellation or delay of surgery, coronary revascularization followed by noncardiac surgery, or intensified care. (Reprinted with permission from Eagle KA, Brundage BH, Chaitman BR, et al: Guidelines for perioperative cardiovascular evaluation for noncardiac surgery. Report of the American College of Cardiology/American Heart Association Task Force on Practice Guidelines [Committee on Perioperative Cardiovascular Evaluation for Noncardiac Surgery], *J Am Coll Cardiol* 27:910-948, 1996.)

Stepwise Approach to Preoperative Cardiac Assessment

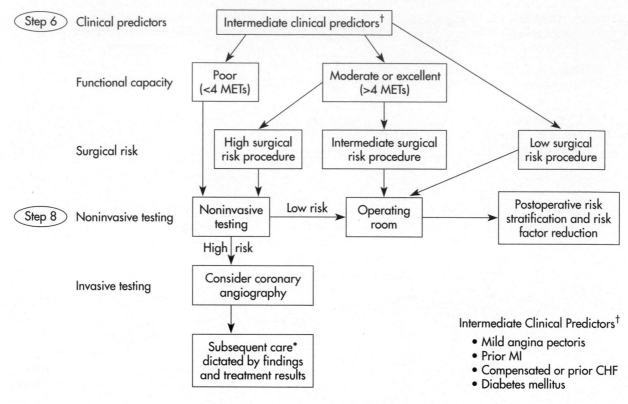

Stepwise Approach to Preoperative Cardiac Assessment

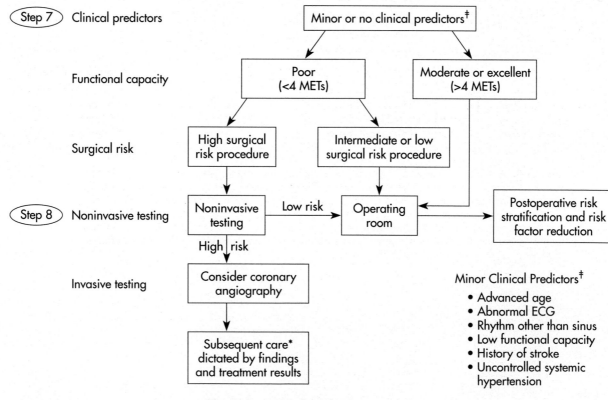

Fig. 21-3, cont'd. For legend see page 361.

which consensus panels make recommendations), we determined expert opinion regarding the indications for preoperative coronary angiography when results of noninvasive tests are known. It was agreed that catheterization should be performed for: 1) exercise electrocardiographic ischemia with a blood pressure decrease of more than 10 mm Hg, 2) stress perfusion scan reversibility in greater than or equal to one half of SPECT slices, and 3) stress echocardiographic ischemia in more than than five segments, more than two coronary artery zones, or four left anterior descending coronary artery segments. Therefore, in general, coronary angiography should be performed in the appropriate clinical context on the basis of noninvasive test results that indicate large zones of myocardial ischemia and should not be performed for limited ischemia without other significant clinical findings.[20]

Preoperative cardiac evaluation is frequently sought for a history of cardiovascular disease, hypertension, or chest pain; the presence of a murmur or arrhythmia; or an abnormal result on electrocardiography.[36,42,60] Congestive heart failure is an important harbinger of poor postoperative outcome.[25,33,61] Therefore, efforts should be made to identify and treat unsuspected heart failure by taking a careful history and doing a physical examination. The cause of congestive heart failure may have prognostic implications.[37]

Cardiac murmurs are common. The cardiology consultant must determine the cause of the murmur and distinguish important murmurs from those that are not clinically important. Severe aortic stenosis confers high risk[61] and may justify postponement or cancellation of surgery. Rarely, percutaneous balloon aortic valvuloplasty may be justified in a patient who is not a candidate for aortic valve replacement, the preferred treatment before noncardiac surgery.[37] Mild or moderate mitral stenosis requires monitoring to maintain reasonable control of heart rate to reduce the risk for pulmonary congestion associated with a decreased diastolic filling period. Patients with severe mitral stenosis may benefit from balloon mitral valvuloplasty or open surgical repair before high-risk noncardiac surgery.[37] Patients with regurgitant lesions may benefit from rate control, antibiotic prophylaxis, or afterload reduction, depending on cause and severity.[37] Patients with mechanical prosthetic valves may require a short course of heparin.

Cardiac arrhythmias and conduction disturbances are common in the perioperative period.[61,62,67] Although supraventricular and ventricular arrhythmias have been associated with increased risk for postoperative adverse cardiac events, they are probably markers for underlying cardiopulmonary disease that places a patient at higher risk. Most arrhythmias are not dangerous, but they may expose underlying disease that may endanger the patient (such as new atrial fibrillation with rapid ventricular response that precipitates ischemia and subsequent congestive heart failure). Patients with conduction disease and no history of high-grade block generally do well. However, high-grade atrioventricular block may require insertion of a temporary pacing wire. Transcutaneous pacing allows rapid response to sudden, hemodynamically significant heart block.[37]

CONCLUSIONS

Because of the aging population and the prevalence of coronary artery disease, many patients at risk for cardiac complications will undergo noncardiac surgery. Improvements in surgical and anesthetic technique have created a situation in which surgery may be considered one of the many potential triggers of cardiac morbidity and mortality[115] with which a person may come in contact during daily life. "Universal precautions," including intensified antiischemic drug regimens and close hemodynamic monitoring combined with constantly improving surgical and anesthetic techniques, may make preoperative cardiac risk assessment less cost-effective. However, the preoperative cardiac evaluation may increasingly represent an opportunity to initiate or modify cardiac care, including primary and secondary preventive measures that have long-term benefits beyond decreasing surgical morbidity and mortality. Future research may better define cost-effective strategies for risk assessment and reduction. Prospective studies may also better define subsets of patients that may benefit from certain management strategies. Although there is extensive experience with radionuclide methods, availability and expertise may vary from center to center. Nevertheless, radionuclide perfusion techniques are sensitive for detecting patients at risk for short-term and long-term postoperative cardiac events. Patient-related, institution-related, and test-related factors interact, and the clinician must consider all of these elements before deciding whether to test and which test to order. Once the results of testing are known, efforts to achieve risk reduction may be made in selected patients. These interventions should not only improve postoperative prognosis but also lead to improved long-term cardiovascular health.

REFERENCES

1. Akl BF, Talbot W, Neal JF, et al: Noncardiac operations after coronary revascularization, *West J Med* 136:91–94, 1982.
2. Allen JR, Helling TS, Hartzler GO: Operative procedures not involving the heart after percutaneous transluminal coronary angioplasty, *Surg Gynecol Obstet* 173:285–288, 1991.
3. American Society of Anesthesiologists I. New classification of physical status. *Anesthesiology* 24:111, 1963.
4. Arous EJ, Baum PL, Cutler BS: The ischemic exercise test in patients with peripheral vascular disease. Implications for management, *Arch Surg* 119:780–783, 1984.
5. Backer CL, Tinker JH, Robertson DM, et al: Myocardial reinfarction following local anesthesia for ophthalmic surgery, *Anesth Analg* 59:257–262, 1980.
6. Baron JF, Mundler O, Bertrand M, et al: Dipyridamole-thallium scintigraphy and gated radionuclide angiography to assess cardiac risk before abdominal aortic surgery, *N Engl J Med* 330:663–669, 1994.
7. Becker RC, Underwood DA: Myocardial infarction in patients undergoing noncardiac surgery, *Cleve Clin J Med* 54:25–28, 1987.
8. Berlauk JF, Abrams JH, Gilmour IJ, et al: Preoperative optimization of cardiovascular hemodynamics improves outcome in peripheral vascular surgery. A prospective, randomized clinical trial, *Ann Surg* 214:289–297, 1991.
9. Boucher CA, Brewster DC, Darling RC, et al: Determination of cardiac risk by dipyridamole-thallium imaging before peripheral vascular surgery, *N Engl J Med* 312:389–394, 1985.

10. Boyd O, Grounds RM, Bennett ED: A randomized clinical trial of the effect of deliberate perioperative increase of oxygen delivery on mortality in high-risk surgical patients, *JAMA* 270:2699–2707, 1993.

11. Brener S, Cohen MC, Talley JD, et al: Striking hospital to hospital variation in pre-operative cardiac work-up for patients referred for major non-cardiac surgery, *Circulation* 92:I-679, 1995 (abstract).

12. Breslow MJ, Jordan DA, Christopherson R, et al: Epidural morphine decreases postoperative hypertension by attenuating sympathetic nervous system hyperactivity, *JAMA* 261:3577–3581, 1989.

13. Brown KA: Prognostic value of myocardial perfusion imaging: state of the art and new developments, *J Nucl Cardiol* 3(6 Pt 1):516–537, 1996.

14. Brown KA, Rowen M: Extent of jeopardized viable myocardium determined by myocardial perfusion imaging best predicts perioperative cardiac events in patients undergoing noncardiac surgery, *J Am Coll Cardiol* 21:325–330, 1993.

15. Bry JD, Belkin M, O'Donnell TF Jr, et al: An assessment of the positive predictive value and cost-effectiveness of dipyridamole myocardial scintigraphy in patients undergoing vascular surgery, *J Vasc Surg* 19:112–121, 1994.

16. Camp AD, Garvin PJ, Hoff J, et al: Prognostic value of intravenous dipyridamole thallium imaging in patients with diabetes mellitus considered for renal transplantation, *Am J Cardiol* 65:1459–1463, 1990.

17. Carliner NH, Fisher ML, Plotnick GD, et al: Routine preoperative exercise testing in patients undergoing major noncardiac surgery, *Am J Cardiol* 56:51–58, 1985.

18. Charlson ME, MacKenzie CR, Ales KL, et al: Surveillance for postoperative myocardial infarction after noncardiac operations, *Surg Gynecol Obstet* 167:407–414, 1988.

19. Charlson ME, MacKenzie CR, Ales KL, et al: The post-operative electrocardiogram and creatine kinase: implications for diagnosis of myocardial infarction after non-cardiac surgery, *J Clin Epidemiol* 42:25–34, 1989.

20. Cohen MC, Eagle KA: Expert opinion regarding cardiac catheterization prior to noncardiac surgery, *Circulation* 92:I-602, 1995 (abstract).

21. Cohen MC, McKenna C, Lewis SM, et al: Requirements for controlled clinical trials of preoperative cardiovascular risk reduction, *Control Clin Trials* 16:89–95, 1995.

22. Coley CM, Eagle KA, Singer DE, et al: Decision analysis for preoperative cardiac risk evaluation before vascular surgery, *Clin Res* 35:342A, 1987 (abstract).

23. Coley CM, Field TS, Abraham SA, et al: Usefulness of dipyridamole-thallium scanning for preoperative evaluation of cardiac risk for nonvascular surgery, *Am J Cardiol* 69:1280–1285, 1992.

24. Connors AF Jr, Speroff T, Dawson NV, et al: The effectiveness of right heart catheterization in the initial care of critically ill patients. SUPPORT Investigators, *JAMA* 276:889–897, 1996.

25. Cooperman M, Pflug B, Martin EW Jr, Evans WE. Cardiovascular risk factors in patients with peripheral vascular disease, *Surgery* 84:505–509, 1978.

26. Coriat P, Daloz M, Bousseau D, et al: Prevention of intraoperative myocardial ischemia during noncardiac surgery with intravenous nitroglycerin, *Anesthesiology* 61:193–196, 1984.

27. Crawford ES, Morris GC Jr, Howell JF, et al: Operative risk in patients with previous coronary artery bypass, *Ann Thorac Surg* 26:215–221, 1978.

28. Cruchley PM, Kaplan JA, Hug CC Jr, et al: Non-cardiac surgery in patients with prior myocardial revascularization, *Can Anaesth Soc J* 30:629–634, 1983.

29. Cutler BS, Leppo JA: Dipyridamole thallium 201 scintigraphy to detect coronary artery disease before abdominal aortic surgery, *J Vasc Surg* 5:91–100, 1987.

30. Cutler BS, Wheeler HB, Paraskos JA, et al: Applicability and interpretation of electrocardiographic stress testing in patients with peripheral vascular disease, *Am J Surg* 141:501–506, 1981.

31. Davila-Roman VG, Waggoner AD, Sicard GA, et al: Dobutamine stress echocardiography predicts surgical outcome in patients with an aortic aneurysm and peripheral vascular disease, *J Am Coll Cardiol* 21:957–963, 1993.

32. Detsky AS, Abrams HB, Forbath N, et al: Cardiac assessment for patients undergoing noncardiac surgery. A multifactorial clinical risk index, *Arch Intern Med* 146:2131–2134, 1986.

33. Detsky AS, Abrams HB, McLaughlin JR, et al: Predicting cardiac complications in patients undergoing non-cardiac surgery, *J Gen Intern Med* 1:211–219, 1986.

34. Dodds TM, Stone JG, Coromilas J, et al: Prophylactic nitroglycerin infusion during noncardiac surgery does not reduce perioperative ischemia, *Anesth Analg* 76:705–713, 1993.

35. Dripps RD, Lamont A, Eckenhoff JE: The role of anesthesia in surgical mortality, *JAMA* 178:261–266, 1961.

36. Dudley JC, Brandenburg JA, Hartley LH, et al: Last-minute preoperative cardiology consultations: epidemiology and impact, *Am Heart J* 131:245–249, 1996.

37. Eagle KA, Brundage BH, Chaitman BR, et al: Guidelines for perioperative cardiovascular evaluation for noncardiac surgery. Report of the American College of Cardiology/American Heart Association Task Force on Practice Guidelines (Committee on Perioperative Cardiovascular Evaluation for Noncardiac Surgery), *J Am Coll Cardiol* 27:910–948, 1996.

38. Eagle KA, Coley CM, Newell JB, et al: Combining clinical and thallium data optimizes preoperative assessment of cardiac risk before major vascular surgery, *Ann Intern Med* 110:859–866, 1989.

39. Eagle KA, Singer DE, Brewster DC, et al: Dipyridamole-thallium scanning in patients undergoing vascular surgery. Optimizing preoperative evaluation of cardiac risk, *JAMA* 257:2185–2189, 1987.

40. Eichelberger JP, Schwarz KQ, Black ER, et al: Predictive value of dobutamine echocardiography just before noncardiac vascular surgery, *Am J Cardiol* 72:602–607, 1993.

41. Elmore JR, Hallett JW Jr, Gibbons RJ, et al: Myocardial revascularization before abdominal aortic aneurysmorrhaphy: effect of coronary angioplasty, *Mayo Clin Proc* 68:637–641, 1993.

42. Ferguson RP, Rubinstien E: Preoperative medical consultations in a community hospital, *J Gen Intern Med* 2:89–92, 1987.

43. Fiser WP, Thompson BW, Thompson AR, et al: Nuclear cardiac ejection fraction and cardiac index in abdominal aortic surgery, *Surgery* 94:736–739, 1983.

44. Fleisher LA, Nelson AH, Rosenbaum SH: Postoperative myocardial ischemia: etiology of cardiac morbidity or manifestation of underlying disease? *J Clin Anesth* 7:97–102, 1995.

45. Fleisher LA, Rosenbaum SH, Nelson AH, et al: The predictive value of preoperative silent ischemia for postoperative ischemic cardiac events in vascular and nonvascular surgery patients, *Am Heart J* 122:980–986, 1991.

46. Fleisher LA, Rosenbaum SH, Nelson AH, et al: Preoperative dipyridamole thallium imaging and ambulatory electrocardiographic monitoring as a predictor of perioperative cardiac events and long-term outcome, *Anesthesiology* 83:906–917, 1995.

47. Fleisher LA, Skolnick ED, Holroyd KJ, et al: Coronary artery revascularization before abdominal aortic aneurysm surgery: a decision analytic approach, *Anesth Analg* 79:661–669, 1994.

48. Fletcher JP, Antico VF, Gruenewald S, et al: Dipyridamole-thallium scan for screening of coronary artery disease prior to vascular surgery, *J Cardiovasc Surg* (Torino) 29:666–669, 1988.

49. Fletcher JP, Antico VF, Gruenewald S, et al: Risk of aortic aneurysm surgery as assessed by preoperative gated heart pool scan, *Br J Surg* 76:26–28, 1989.

50. Foster ED, Davis KB, Carpenter JA, et al: Risk of noncardiac operation in patients with defined coronary disease: The Coronary Artery Surgery Study (CASS) registry experience, *Ann Thorac Surg* 41:42–50, 1986.

51. Franco CD, Goldsmith J, Veith FJ, et al: Resting gated pool ejection

fraction: a poor predictor of perioperative myocardial infarction in patients undergoing vascular surgery for infrainguinal bypass grafting, *J Vasc Surg* 10:656–661, 1989.

52. Freeman WK, Gibbons RJ, Shub C: Preoperative assessment of cardiac patients undergoing noncardiac surgical procedures, *Mayo Clin Proc* 64:1105–1117, 1989.

53. Gage AA, Bhayana JN, Balu V, et al: Assessment of cardiac risk in surgical patients, *Arch Surg* 112:1488–1492, 1977.

54. Gagnon RM, Dumont G, Sestier F, et al: The role of coronary angioplasty in patients with associated noncardiac medical and surgical conditions, *Can J Cardiol* 6:287–292, 1990.

55. Georgeson S, Coombs AT, Eckman MH: Prophylactic use of the intra-aortic balloon pump in high-risk cardiac patients undergoing noncardiac surgery: a decision analytic view, *Am J Med* 92:665–678, 1992.

56. Gerson MC, Hurst JM, Hertzberg VS, et al: Prediction of cardiac and pulmonary complications related to elective abdominal and noncardiac thoracic surgery in geriatric patients, *Am J Med* 88:101–107, 1990.

57. Gerson MC, Hurst JM, Hertzberg VS, et al: Cardiac prognosis in noncardiac geriatric surgery, *Ann Intern Med* 103:832–837, 1985.

58. Godet G, Coriat P, Baron JF, et al: Prevention of intraoperative myocardial ischemia during noncardiac surgery with intravenous diltiazem: a randomized trial versus placebo, *Anesthesiology* 66:241–245, 1987.

59. Golden MA, Whittemore AD, Donaldson MC, et al: Selective evaluation and management of coronary artery disease in patients undergoing repair of abdominal aortic aneurysms. A 16-year experience, *Ann Surg* 212:415–20, 1990.

60. Golden WE, Lavender RC: Preoperative cardiac consultations in a teaching hospital, *South Med J* 82:292–295, 1989.

61. Goldman L, Caldera DL, Nussbaum SR, et al: Multifactorial index of cardiac risk in noncardiac surgical procedures, *N Engl J Med* 297:845–850, 1997.

62. Goldman L, Caldera DL, Southwick FS, et al: Cardiac risk factors and complications in non-cardiac surgery, *Medicine* (Baltimore) 57:357–370, 1978.

63. Hamm CW, Reimers J, Ischinger T, et al: A randomized study of coronary angioplasty compared with bypass surgery in patients with symptomatic multivessel coronary disease. German Angioplasty Bypass Surgery Investigation, *N Engl J Med* 331:1037–1043, 1994.

64. Hanson P, Pease M, Berkoff H, et al: Arm exercise testing for coronary artery disease in patients with peripheral vascular disease, *Clin Cardiol* 11:70–74, 1988.

65. Hendel RC, Whitfield SS, Villegas BJ, et al: Prediction of late cardiac events by dipyridamole thallium imaging in patients undergoing elective vascular surgery, *Am J Cardiol* 70:1243–1249, 1992.

66. Hertzer NR, Beven EG, Young JR, et al: Coronary artery disease in peripheral vascular patients. A classification of 1000 coronary angiograms and results of surgical management, *Ann Surg* 199:223–233, 1984.

67. Hollenberg M, Mangano DT, Browner WS, et al: Predictors of postoperative myocardial ischemia in patients undergoing noncardiac surgery. The Study of Perioperative Ischemia Research Group, *JAMA* 268:205–209, 1992.

68. Huber KC, Evans MA, Bresnahan JF, et al: Outcome of noncardiac operations in patients with severe coronary artery disease successfully treated preoperatively with coronary angioplasty, *Mayo Clin Proc* 67:15–21, 1992.

69. Hueb WA, Bellotti G, de Oliveira SA, et al: The Medicine, Angioplasty or Surgery Study (MASS): a prospective, randomized trial of medical therapy, balloon angioplasty or bypass surgery for single proximal left anterior descending artery stenoses, *J Am Coll Cardiol* 26:1600–1605, 1995.

70. Iqbal A, Gibbons RJ, McGoon MD, et al: Noninvasive assessment of cardiac risk in insulin-dependent diabetic patients being evaluated for pancreatic transplantation using thallium-201 myocardial perfusion scintigraphy, *Transplant Proc* 23(1 Pt 2):1690–1691, 1991.

71. Iskandrian AS, Heo J, Kong B, et al: Effect of exercise level on the ability of thallium-201 tomographic imaging in detecting coronary artery disease: analysis of 461 patients, *J Am Coll Cardiol* 14:1477–1486, 1989.

72. Jain KM, Patil KD, Doctor US, et al: Preoperative cardiac screening before peripheral vascular operations, *Am Surg* 51:77–79, 1985.

73. Jeffrey CC, Kunsman J, Cullen DJ, et al: A prospective evaluation of cardiac risk index, *Anesthesiology* 58:462–464, 1983.

74. Kazmers A, Cerqueira MD, Zierler RE: Perioperative and late outcome in patients with left ventricular ejection fraction of 35% or less who require major vascular surgery, *J Vasc Surg* 8:307–315, 1988.

75. Kazmers A, Cerqueira MD, Zierler RE: The role of preoperative radionuclide ejection fraction in direct abdominal aortic aneurysm repair, *J Vasc Surg* 8:128–136, 1988.

76. Kazmers A, Cerqueira MD, Zierler RE: The role of preoperative radionuclide left ventricular ejection fraction for risk assessment in carotid surgery, *Arch Surg* 123:416–419, 1988.

77. King SB 3rd, Lembo NJ, Weintraub WS, et al: A randomized trial comparing coronary angioplasty with coronary bypass surgery. Emory Angioplasty versus Surgery Trial (EAST), *N Engl J Med* 331:1044–1050, 1994.

78. Kirwin JD, Ascer E, Gennaro M, et al: Silent myocardial ischemia is not predictive of myocardial infarction in peripheral vascular surgery patients, *Ann Vasc Surg* 7:27–32, 1993.

79. Knight AA, Hollenberg M, London MJ, et al: Perioperative myocardial ischemia: importance of the preoperative ischemic pattern, *Anesthesiology* 68:681–688, 1988.

80. Kresowik TF, Bower TR, Garner SA, et al: Dipyridamole thallium imaging in patients being considered for vascular procedures, *Arch Surg* 128:299–302, 1993.

81. Lalka SG, Sawada SG, Dalsing MC, et al: Dobutamine stress echocardiography as a predictor of cardiac events associated with aortic surgery, *J Vasc Surg* 15:831–840, 1992.

82. Landesberg G, Luria MH, Cotev S, et al: Importance of long-duration postoperative ST-segment depression in cardiac morbidity after vascular surgery, *Lancet* 341:715–719, 1993.

83. Lane RT, Sawada SG, Segar DS, et al: Dobutamine stress echocardiography for assessment of cardiac risk before noncardiac surgery, *Am J Cardiol* 68:976–977, 1991.

84. Lane SE, Lewis SM, Pippin JJ, et al: Predictive value of quantitative dipyridamole-thallium scintigraphy in assessing cardiovascular risk after vascular surgery in diabetes mellitus, *Am J Cardiol* 64:1275–1279, 1989.

85. Langan EM 3rd, Youkey JR, Franklin DP, et al: Dobutamine stress echocardiography for cardiac risk assessment before aortic surgery, *J Vasc Surg* 18:905–911, 1993.

86. Lazor L, Russell JC, DaSilva J, et al: Use of the multiple uptake gated acquisition scan for the preoperative assessment of cardiac risk, *Surg Gynecol Obstet* 167:234–238, 1988.

87. Leppo J, Plaja J, Gionet M, et al: Noninvasive evaluation of cardiac risk before elective vascular surgery, *J Am Coll Cardiol* 9:269–276, 1987.

88. Lette J, Waters D, Cerino M, et al: Preoperative coronary artery disease risk stratification based on dipyridamole imaging and a simple three-step, three-segment model for patients undergoing noncardiac vascular surgery or major general surgery, *Am J Cardiol* 69:1553–1558, 1992.

89. Lette J, Waters D, Lapointe J, et al: Usefulness of the severity and extent of reversible perfusion defects during thallium-dipyridamole imaging for cardiac risk assessment before noncardiac surgery, *Am J Cardiol* 64:276–281, 1989.

90. Levinson JR, Boucher CA, Coley CM, et al: Usefulness of semiquantitative analysis of dipyridamole-thallium-201 redistribution for

improving risk stratification before vascular surgery, *Am J Cardiol* 66:406–410, 1990.

91. L'Italien GJ, Paul SD, Hendel RC, et al: Development and validation of a Bayesian model for perioperative cardiac risk assessment in a cohort of 1,081 vascular surgical candidates, *J Am Coll Cardiol* 27:779–786, 1996.

92. Loughlin V, Beniwal JS, Cassidy K, et al: Comparison of risk factor and left ventricular stroke work index as predictors of cardiac complications in vascular surgery, *Eur J Vasc Surg* 4:83–87, 1990.

93. Madsen PV, Vissing M, Munck O, et al: A comparison of dipyridamole thallium 201 scintigraphy and clinical examination in the determination of cardiac risk before arterial reconstruction, *Angiology* 43:306–311, 1992.

94. Mahar LJ, Steen PA, Tinker JH, et al: Perioperative myocardial infarction in patients with coronary artery disease with and without aorta–coronary artery bypass grafts, *J Thorac Cardiovasc Surg* 76:533–537, 1978.

95. Mangano DT: Perioperative cardiac morbidity, *Anesthesiology* 72:153–184, 1990.

96. Mangano DT, Browner WS, Hollenberg M, et al: Association of perioperative myocardial ischemia with cardiac morbidity and mortality in men undergoing noncardiac surgery. The Study of Perioperative Ischemia Research Group, *N Engl J Med* 323:1781–1788, 1990.

97. Mangano DT, Layug EL, Wallace A, et al: The Multicenter Study of Perioperative Ischemia Research Group. Effect of atenolol on mortality and cardiovascular morbidity after noncardiac surgery, *N Engl J Med* 335:1713–1720, 1996.

98. Mangano DT, London MJ, Tubau JF, et al: Dipyridamole thallium–201 scintigraphy as a preoperative screening test. A reexamination of its predictive potential. Study of Perioperative Ischemia Research Group, *Circulation* 84:493–502, 1991.

99. Mangano DT, Wong MG, London MJ, et al: Perioperative myocardial ischemia in patients undergoing noncardiac surgery—II: Incidence and severity during the 1st week after surgery. The Study of Perioperative Ischemia (SPI) Research Group, *J Am Coll Cardiol* 17:851–857, 1991.

100. Manske CL, Wang Y, Rector T, et al: Coronary revascularisation in insulin-dependent diabetic patients with chronic renal failure, *Lancet* 340:998–1002, 1992.

101. Mason JJ, Owens DK, Harris RA, et al: The role of coronary angiography and coronary revascularization before noncardiac vascular surgery, *JAMA* 273:1919–1925, 1995.

102. Massie BM, Mangano DT: Risk stratification for noncardiac surgery. How (and why)? *Circulation* 87:1752–1755, 1993.

103. McAuley CE, Watson CG: Elective inguinal herniorrhaphy after myocardial infarction, *Surg Gynecol Obstet* 159:36–38, 1984.

104. McCabe CJ, Reidy NC, Abbott WM, et al: The value of electrocardiogram monitoring during treadmill testing for peripheral vascular disease, *Surgery* 89:183–186, 1981.

105. McCann RL, Clements FM: Silent myocardial ischemia in patients undergoing peripheral vascular surgery: incidence and association with perioperative cardiac morbidity and mortality, *J Vasc Surg* 9:583–587, 1989.

106. McCann RL, Wolfe WG: Resection of abdominal aortic aneurysm in patients with low ejection fractions, *J Vasc Surg* 10:240–244, 1989.

107. McCollum CH, Garcia-Rinaldi R, Graham JM, et al: Myocardial revascularization prior to subsequent major surgery in patients with coronary artery disease, *Surgery* 81:302–304, 1977.

108. McEnroe CS, O'Donnell TF Jr, Yeager A, et al: Comparison of ejection fraction and Goldman risk factor analysis to dipyridamole-thallium 201 studies in the evaluation of cardiac morbidity after aortic aneurysm surgery, *J Vasc Surg* 11:497–504, 1990.

109. McPhail N, Calvin JE, Shariatmadar A, et al: The use of preoperative exercise testing to predict cardiac complications after arterial reconstruction. *J Vasc Surg* 7:60–68, 1988.

110. McPhail NV, Ruddy TD, Barber GG, et al: Cardiac risk stratification using dipyridamole myocardial perfusion imaging and ambulatory ECG monitoring prior to vascular surgery, *European J Vasc Surg* 7:151–155, 1993.

111. McPhail NV, Ruddy TD, Calvin JE, et al: A comparison of dipyridamole-thallium imaging and exercise testing in the prediction of postoperative cardiac complications in patients requiring arterial reconstruction, *J Vasc Surg* 10:51–55, 1989.

112. Moore EH, Greenberg RW, Merrick SH, et al: Coronary artery calcifications: significance of incidental detection on CT scans, *Radiology* 172:711–716, 1989.

113. Morris CK, Ueshima K, Kawaguchi T, et al: The prognostic value of exercise capacity: a review of the literature, *Am Heart J* 122:1423–1431, 1991.

114. Mosley JG, Clarke JM, Ell PJ, et al: Assessment of myocardial function before aortic surgery by radionuclide angiocardiography, *Br J Surg* 72:886–887, 1985.

115. Muller JE, Tofler GH, Stone PH: Circadian variation and triggers of onset of acute cardiovascular disease, *Circulation* 79:733–743, 1989.

116. Ouyang P, Gerstenblith G, Furman WR, et al: Frequency and significance of early postoperative silent myocardial ischemia in patients having peripheral vascular surgery, *Am J Cardiol* 64:1113–1116, 1989.

117. Owens WD, Felts JA, Spitznagel EL Jr: ASA physical status classifications: a study of consistency of ratings, *Anesthesiology* 49:239–243, 1978.

118. Paramo JA, Alfaro MJ, Rocha E: Postoperative changes in the plasmatic levels of tissue-type plasminogen activator and its fast-acting inhibitor—relationship to deep vein thrombosis and influence of prophylaxis, *Thromb Haemost* 54:713–716, 1985.

119. Pasternack PF, Grossi EA, Baumann FG, et al: Beta blockade to decrease silent myocardial ischemia during peripheral vascular surgery, *Am J Surg* 158:113–116, 1989.

120. Pasternack PF, Grossi EA, Baumann FG, et al: The value of silent myocardial ischemia monitoring in the prediction of perioperative myocardial infarction in patients undergoing peripheral vascular surgery, *J Vasc Surg* 10:617–625, 1989.

121. Pasternack PF, Imparato AM, Baumann FG, et al: The hemodynamics of beta-blockade in patients undergoing abdominal aortic aneurysm repair, *Circulation* 76:III1–III7, 1987.

122. Pasternack PF, Imparato AM, Bear G, et al: The value of radionuclide angiography as a predictor of perioperative myocardial infarction in patients undergoing abdominal aortic aneurysm resection, *J Vasc Surg* 1:320–325, 1984.

123. Pasternack PF, Imparato AM, Riles TS, et al: The value of the radionuclide angiogram in the prediction of perioperative myocardial infarction in patients undergoing lower extremity revascularization procedures, *Circulation* 72(3 Pt 2):II13–II17, 1985.

124. Poldermans D, Arnese M, Fioretti PM, et al: Sustained prognostic value of dobutamine stress echocardiography for late cardiac events after major noncardiac vascular surgery, *Circulation* 95:53–58, 1997.

125. Poldermans D, Arnese M, Fioretti PM, et al: Improved cardiac risk stratification in major vascular surgery with dobutamine-atropine stress echocardiography, *J Am Coll Cardiol* 26:648–653, 1995.

126. Poldermans D, Fioretti PM, Forster T, et al: Dobutamine stress echocardiography for assessment of perioperative cardiac risk in patients undergoing major vascular surgery, *Circulation* 87:1506–1512, 1993.

127. Raby KE, Goldman L, Creager MA, et al: Correlation between preoperative ischemia and major cardiac events after peripheral vascular surgery, *N Engl J Med* 321:1296–1300, 1989.

128. Rao TL, Jacobs KH, El-Etr AA: Reinfarction following anesthesia in patients with myocardial infarction, *Anesthesiology* 59:499–505, 1983.

129. Reul GJ Jr, Cooley DA, Duncan JM, et al: The effect of coronary by-

pass on the outcome of peripheral vascular operations in 1093 patients, *J Vasc Surg* 3:788–798, 1986.

130. Sachs RN, Tellier P, Larmignat P, et al: Assessment by dipyridamole-thallium-201 myocardial scintigraphy of coronary risk before peripheral vascular surgery, *Surgery* 103:584–587, 1988.

131. Shaw LJ, Miller DD: Cost-effectiveness analysis of preoperative pharmacologic stress myocardial imaging in 3,623 vascular surgery candidates, *Circulation* 92:I521–I522, 1995 (abstract).

132. Shaw L, Miller DD, Kong BA, et al: Determination of perioperative cardiac risk by adenosine thallium-201 myocardial imaging, *Am Heart J* 124:861–869, 1992.

133. Siu SC, Kowalchuk GJ, Welty FK, et al: Intra-aortic balloon counterpulsation support in the high-risk cardiac patient undergoing urgent noncardiac surgery, *Chest* 99:1342–1345, 1991.

134. Steen PA, Tinker JH, Tarhan S: Myocardial reinfarction after anesthesia and surgery, *JAMA* 239:2566–2570, 1978.

135. Stone JG, Foex P, Sear JW, et al: Myocardial ischemia in untreated hypertensive patients: effect of a single small oral dose of a beta-adrenergic blocking agent, *Anesthesiology* 68:495–500, 1988.

136. Stratmann HG, Younis LT, Wittry MD, et al: Dipyridamole technetium 99m sestamibi myocardial tomography for preoperative cardiac risk stratification before major or minor nonvascular surgery, *Am Heart J* 132:536–541, 1996.

137. Stratmann HG, Younis LT, Wittry MD, et al: Dipyridamole technetium-99m sestamibi myocardial tomography in patients evaluated for elective vascular surgery: prognostic value for perioperative and late cardiac events, *Am Heart J* 131:923–929, 1996.

138. Strawn DJ, Guernsey JM: Dipyridamole thallium scanning in the evaluation of coronary artery disease in elective abdominal aortic surgery, *Arch Surg* 126:880–884, 1991.

139. Takase B, Younis LT, Byers SL, et al: Comparative prognostic value of clinical risk indexes, resting two-dimensional echocardiography, and dipyridamole stress thallium-201 myocardial imaging for perioperative cardiac events in major nonvascular surgery patients, *Am Heart J* 126:1099–1106, 1993.

140. Tarhan S, Moffitt EA, Taylor WF, et al: Myocardial infarction after general anesthesia, *JAMA* 220:1451–1454, 1972.

141. Tischler MD, Lee TH, Hirsch AT, et al: Prediction of major cardiac events after peripheral vascular surgery using dipyridamole echocardiography, *Am J Cardiol* 68:593–597, 1991.

142. Tuman KJ, McCarthy RJ, March RJ, et al: Effects of epidural anesthesia and analgesia on coagulation and outcome after major vascular surgery, *Anesth Analg* 73:696–704, 1991.

143. Urbinati S, Di Pasquale G, Andreoli A, et al: Preoperative noninvasive coronary risk stratification in candidates for carotid endarterectomy, *Stroke* 25:2022–2027, 1994.

144. Urbinati S, Di Pasquale G, Andreoli A, et al: Frequency and prognostic significance of silent coronary artery disease in patients with cerebral ischemia undergoing carotid endarterectomy, *Am J Cardiol* 69:1166–1170, 1992.

145. Vacanti CJ, VanHouten RJ, Hill RC: A statistical analysis of the relationship of physical status to postoperative mortality in 68,388 cases, *Anesthesia & Analgesia* 49:564–566, 1970.

146. von Knorring J: Postoperative myocardial infarction: a prospective study in a risk group of surgical patients, *Surgery* 90:55–60, 1981.

147. von Knorring J, Lepantalo M: Prediction of perioperative cardiac complications by electrocardiographic monitoring during treadmill exercise testing before peripheral vascular surgery, *Surgery* 99:610–613, 1986.

148. Watters TA, Botvinick EH, Dae MW, et al: Comparison of the findings on preoperative dipyridamole perfusion scintigraphy and intraoperative transesophageal echocardiography: implications regarding the identification of myocardium at ischemic risk, *J Am Coll Cardiol* 18:93–100, 1991.

149. Younis L, Stratmann H, Takase B, et al: Preoperative clinical assessment and dipyridamole thallium-201 scintigraphy for prediction and prevention of cardiac events in patients having major noncardiovascular surgery and known or suspected coronary artery disease, *Am J Cardiol* 74:311–317, 1994.

150. Younis LT, Aguirre F, Byers S, et al: Perioperative and long-term prognostic value of intravenous dipyridamole thallium scintigraphy in patients with peripheral vascular disease, *Am Heart J* 119:1287–1292, 1990.

151. Yusuf S, Zucker D, Peduzzi P, et al: Effect of coronary artery bypass graft surgery on survival: overview of 10-year results from randomised trials by the Coronary Artery Bypass Graft Surgery Trialists Collaboration, *Lancet* 344:563–570, 1994.

152. Zeldin RA: Assessing cardiac risk in patients who undergo noncardiac surgical procedures, *Can J Surg* 27:402–404, 1984.

Chapter 22

Stress echocardiography versus nuclear imaging

Mario S. Verani

Both nuclear cardiac imaging and stress echocardiography are useful techniques to assess patients with suspected or documented coronary artery disease. Nuclear cardiac imaging has been incorporated into clinical practice in the past 20 years, whereas stress echocardiography, although initially examined in the late 1970s, has only recently gained popularity.

In 1997, approximately 3.7 million patients underwent myocardial perfusion scintigraphy, most during stress. It is not known how many patients underwent stress echocardiography, but it seems that a major increase in the use of this method can be traced to the use of dobutamine stress echocardiography, followed by use of exercise echocardiography.

According to unpublished industry data, use of nuclear cardiology procedures increased 20% between April 1995 and April 1996 in the United States. Presumably, most of this increase was in the area of stress perfusion imaging. It also seems likely that most of the recent increase in nuclear cardiology procedures can be explained by the growing interest of cardiologists in the practice of nuclear cardiology. At present, approx-

imately 50% of all Medicare charges for myocardial perfusion imaging are submitted by cardiologists; the remaining 50% are divided among radiologists, nuclear physicians, and internists.

PHYSIOLOGIC BASIS OF CARDIAC IMAGING DURING STRESS

It has long been appreciated that patients with even severe coronary artery disease may have normal myocardial perfusion and ventricular function, including normal left ventricular wall motion at rest. This is because as coronary stenosis progresses, compensatory adaptations occur in the coronary circulation, including arteriolar coronary vasodilation, that may maintain normal myocardial blood flow. As long as the myocardial supply–demand balance is maintained, perfusion and function remain normal. Only very severe coronary stenosis (>85% of the luminal diameter) is ordinarily (but not necessarily) associated with decreased coronary blood flow distal to the site of stenosis. When the myocardial blood flow decreases to 50% below the basal resting flow, the subtended myocardium begins to show abnormal thickening and abnormal wall motion.

Physiologic basis of stress myocardial perfusion imaging

The underlying mechanism of perfusion defects induced by any stress method is a differential increase in coronary blood flow, with a higher increase occurring in the normal arteries and a smaller increase or no increase (or, occasionally, a decrease) of blood flow toward the territory perfused by a coronary artery with significant stenosis.[27,20,41] The normal coronary flow reserve varies between fourfold and sixfold; that is, flow increases maximally fourfold to sixfold in the normal arteries. This maximal flow reserve, however, varies with the technique used to assess it. It is higher when measured by a flowmeter and is lower when measured by coronary sinus thermodilution positron emission tomography, or a coronary flow wire technique, with the tip of the wire placed distal to the stenosis. Transient coronary occlusion for a few seconds, followed by reperfusion, or intracoronary administration of adenosine or papaverine is capable of inducing maximal or near maximal coronary hyperemia. Both intravenous adenosine and intravenous dipyridamole have been shown to produce an average increase in myocardial blood flow of more than fourfold.[63,50] High-dose intravenous dobutamine (40 μg/kg/min) increases the coronary blood flow by about threefold.[30] Inotropic stimulation, such as exercise, produces an indirect increase in coronary blood flow that is secondary to the increased myocardial oxygen demands. Therefore, whereas the changes in heart rate and blood pressure or contractility are modest during pharmacologic vasodilation and do not correlate with the maximal increase in flow, the increase in coronary flow with dobutamine administration or exercise stress is directly related to the myocardial oxygen demands and depends on the relative increase in heart rate, systolic blood pressure, and contractility. A practical corollary of these observations is that a submaximal increase in heart rate, blood pressure, or systolic pressure–heart rate product during exercise stress or dobutamine administration will be associated with a submaximal increase in blood flow and therefore a lesser chance to create differential coronary flow between normal and abnormal arteries.

During exercise stress, the relation between flow and thallium uptake remains approximately linear up to a flow of about three times higher than the baseline values.[41] However, when the coronary flow is markedly elevated (especially during pharmacologic stress), the increase in tracer uptake lags behind the increase in flow. This "roll-off" threshold occurs at approximately 2.5 times the baseline flow values and is more severe for tracers that have lower myocardial extraction, such as technetium-99m (^{99m}Tc) sestamibi, ^{99m}Tc tetrofosmin, or ^{99m}Tc furofosmin, and is less severe for thallium, which has a higher extraction rate.[11,27,36]

A common misconception is that myocardial ischemia must be induced to produce a perfusion defect. In reality, myocardial ischemia or hypoxia decrease tracer uptake only slightly; thus, the predominant reason for a stress-induced perfusion defect is the differential increase in flow. Thus, although transient, stress-induced perfusion defects are commonly designated as ischemia, they do not strictly require the presence of physiologic ischemia. This explains why stress-induced defects occur much more frequently than electrocardiographic abnormalities or angina pectoris during stress.

Physiologic basis of stress echocardiography

The diagnosis of coronary artery disease by stress echocardiography depends on demonstrating deterioration of left ventricular wall thickening or wall motion, or both, during stress. Because stress-induced myocardial ischemia is secondary to a supply–demand imbalance, it follows that maximal stress is pivotal. Submaximal stress that is not sufficient to provoke myocardial ischemia may not allow the identification of coronary artery disease. Thus, although one strives for a maximal test under most circumstances, it is particularly critical during stress echocardiography.

It is also intuitive that coronary vasodilation may not be a very effective type of stress in combination with echocardiog-

raphy, because wall motion deterioration would only be expected to occur in patients who develop true myocardial ischemia during pharmacologic vasodilation. The available evidence[14,18] suggests that few such patients develop true myocardial ischemia, as evidenced by a low frequency of ischemic electrocardiographic changes and myocardial production of lactate.

To the best of my knowledge, there are no reports of animal laboratory experiments with exercise two-dimensional echocardiography. The same can be said of exercise radionuclide angiography by either first-pass or gated (MUGA) techniques, which have been used for more than 20 years for diagnosis and evaluation of patients with coronary artery disease. Thus, the demonstration by exercise two-dimensional echocardiography of deterioration of wall motion–induced myocardial ischemia was modeled after exercise radionuclide angiography. The principal difference between exercise radionuclide angiography and exercise echocardiography is that the former method solely assesses wall motion, whereas the latter assesses wall thickening and motion. With exercise radionuclide angiography a common criterion for abnormality is the response of the left ventricular ejection fraction during exercise, with an increase of less than 5% usually considered abnormal. Because of problems in measuring and reproducing ejection fraction measurements by two-dimensional echocardiography, this criterion is not ordinarily used during exercise two-dimensional echocardiography.

Several experimental studies in animals assessed the use of echocardiography during high-dose dobutamine administration.[16,22,55] Fung, Gallagher, and Buda[16] used an open-chest anesthetized dog model to compare dipyridamole with dobutamine echocardiography. They concluded that wall-motion deterioration occurs infrequently during infusion of standard dipyridamole dose (0.56 mg/kg) but is more frequent during dobutamine administration. In a more recent study, Hammond and McKinnan[22] concluded that dobutamine enhanced regional ventricular function in normal vascular territories and in those perfused by arteries with high-grade stenosis, despite a reduced endocardial to epicardial blood flow ratio in the latter areas during dobutamine infusion. Although both the vascular territory perfused by normal arteries and that perfused by a chronically occluded circumflex artery showed increased wall thickening with dobutamine, the increase was smaller in the latter region. Thus, had echocardiography been done at that time, it may have been possible to discern heterogeneous regional contraction, even though in reality both had increased function relative to the rest study. In this model, however, the resting percent of myocardial thickening was smaller in the abnormal vascular territories than in the normal ones.

Schulz et al[55] investigated the effect of dobutamine administration on regional myocardial blood flow and function in anesthetized swine. These investigators also found that intracoronary infusion of dobutamine led to enhancement of maximal work in the ischemic myocardium despite decreased subendocardial blood flow. The clinical counterpart of these observations may be the report by Movahed et al,[39] which showed that dobutamine enhanced the regional ventricular function in normal patients and those with coronary artery disease; it improved the wall motion in more than 80% of patients studied by radionuclide angiography.

MYOCARDIAL PERFUSION IMAGING

Advantages

In disease such as coronary artery disease, which primarily affects myocardial blood flow and secondarily (if at all) affects myocardial contraction, it seems reasonable that a technique that assesses myocardial blood flow may be more powerful than one that tracks regional ventricular contraction. Box 22-1 lists several of the advantages of stress myocardial perfusion imaging. With the advent of the ^{99m}Tc tracers (sestamibi and tetrofosmin), good images can be obtained in most patients, including those weighing almost 300 pounds. With any imaging technique, the importance of image quality cannot be overemphasized. High-quality interpretations can only be done with high-quality images. Not even the most highly skilled and experienced physician can accurately interpret images of suboptimal quality. In this regard, computer techniques have proven their utility in enhancing image display by color coding, data smoothing, contrast enhancement, and background subtraction. The current ability to combine perfusion and functional evaluation by assessing regional function on gated single-photon emission computed tomography (SPECT) images or by combining SPECT with first-pass radionuclide angiography is particularly powerful for risk-stratification of patients with coronary artery disease in whom perfusion assessment and left ventricular ejection fraction are important and complementary. The ability to perform computer quantification of nuclear perfusion images is a major asset that not only increases the accuracy of the method but decreases in part the variability of the interpretations. Of note, stress myocardial perfusion imaging is a time-proven technique with a solid diagnostic and prognostic track record.[8,27,31,32,43]

Disadvantages

Box 22-2 lists some disadvantages of stress myocardial perfusion imaging. Myocardial perfusion imaging by single-photon techniques (planar or SPECT) assesses relative myocardial blood flow, not absolute flow. Positron emission tomography, on the other hand, can measure absolute flow. It is thus theoretically possible that in a patient with a perfectly similar degree of stenosis in all three major coronary arteries, the resulting perfusion pattern may still appear to be homogeneous, although uniformly decreased. Fortunately, this occurs rarely. A more likely scenario is that severe coronary stenosis or complete occlusion will create such a severe defect that milder defects in the remaining areas may not be recognized.

One of the major hindrances of myocardial perfusion imaging is the attenuation encountered by the photons as they traverse different body tissues on their path from the heart to the gamma camera. Because this attenuation varies from patient to patient, artifacts may occur, especially in obese patients or patients with other physical characteristics that cause excessive attenuation (such as large breasts or breast implants). This, in fact, may be an important reason for the suboptimal specificity observed with stress perfusion imaging. It is likely that a large fraction of false-positive scans are caused by photon attenuation. Fortunately, attenuation correction is rapidly becoming a reality and should lead to enhanced specificity of stress perfusion imaging (Fig. 22-1).

The lack of standardization of processing, display, and computer analysis of images can lead to substantial interinstitutional variation as studies are done using gamma camera systems. Although many elements of recording images are standardized, such as the back-projection technique, spatial reconstruction, and filters, intersystem variation is sufficient to confound the field. Wackers et al[62] recently reported on the interobserver variability of myocardial perfusion images. When institutions were requested to interpret images by using a qualitative analysis on their particular display format, the agreement yielded a κ value of 0.53. However, when the same institutions were given uniformly processed images with a common image display format, the agreement increased substantially (κ = 0.70). Agreement improved further to a κ value of 0.80 when quantitative analysis was done. Thus, with a common display method, trained observers are very consistent with respect to interpretations of results of myocardial perfusion scintigraphy.

Finally, a perceived disadvantage of stress myocardial perfusion imaging is the relatively high cost of the gamma cameras, tracers, and chemical stressors. This cost, coupled with strict regulations by federal and state governments, represents a hindrance to nuclear cardiology. The charges for nuclear cardi-

---

Box 22-1. Advantages of stress perfusion imaging

1. Good images can be obtained in most patients by using technetium-99m
2. Amenable to computer quantification
3. Ability to combine perfusion and functional evaluation
4. Relatively easy to interpret
5. Less observer dependency
6. Can be done during treadmill exercise
7. Time proven
8. Solid diagnostic and prognostic data base

Box 22-2. Disadvantages of stress perfusion imaging

1. Assesses relative flow
2. Presence of photon attenuation and other artifacts
3. Low specificity
4. Lack of standardization
5. Tracer roll-off at high flows
6. Cost, availability, and regulatory issues

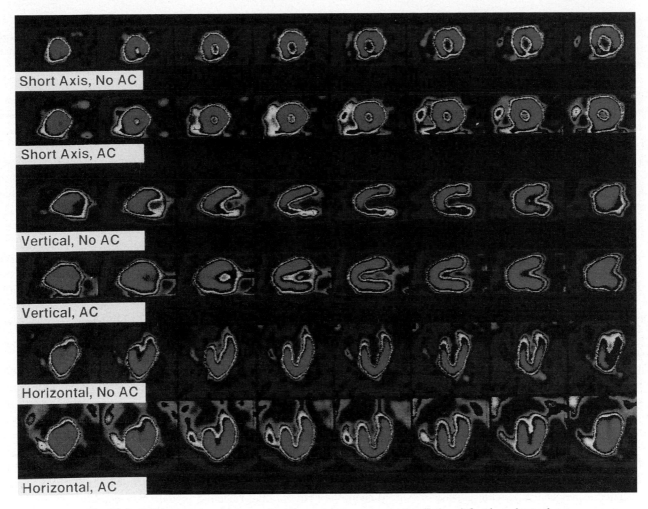

Fig. 22-1. Inferoposterior photon attenuation causing an apparent perfusion defect in a short, obese male patient. The apparent defect disappears after photon attenuation correction using gadolinium-153 line sources and a dual-headed SPECT system.

ology and echocardiographic procedures are being reevaluated in the context of managed care medicine; it is likely that the charges and the profit margins for these tests, as well as for many other tests in medicine, will decrease.

STRESS ECHOCARDIOGRAPHY

Advantages

Box 22-3 lists some of the advantages of stress echocardiography. The technique is truly noninvasive, insofar as administration of foreign substances is not required. Certainly, it does not require any exposure to radioactivity. Detection of deteriorating wall motion or wall thickening during stress is strong evidence of true, ongoing myocardial ischemia. The problem lies in being certain that wall motion deterioration has taken place.

Echocardiography is a comprehensive technique, allowing assessment of systolic and diastolic ventricular function, anatomic integrity, valvular structure and function and detection of pericardial effusion. The technique is well standardized, with similar views performed by virtually every laboratory. No sophisticated computers are required for posttest processing

> **Box 22-3. Advantages of stress echocardiography**
>
> 1. Totally noninvasive
> 2. Detects true ischemia
> 3. Comprehensive
> 4. Wide availability
> 5. Relatively low cost
> 6. Controlled by cardiologists

and storage. Doppler echocardiographic studies are clinically useful for the assessment of pulmonary arterial pressure, pulmonary arterial wedge pressure, and diastolic ventricular function. In addition, echocardiography is widely available and requires less space for storage and patient examination. An echocardiography machine costs considerably less than a sophisticated multihead, digital, highly computerized gamma camera (although single-headed gamma cameras may currently cost less than a state-of-the-art echocardiographer with multiple transducers, color-flow Doppler capability, and more).

In terms of competition with nuclear cardiology, echocardiography is in a privileged position because it is controlled by cardiologists (who also supply the patients), is readily available in hospitals and physician offices throughout the United States, and is rapidly becoming available throughout the world. With so many advantages, it is no wonder that echocardiography has become popular.

The truly tomographic nature of echocardiography is often cited as a major advantage of this technique. However, in most cases, echocardiographic cuts include sections of only one, two, or, at most, three different ventricular levels, unlike SPECT, in which the whole heart can be sectioned from top to bottom, side to side, and front to back.

Disadvantages

Box 22-4 lists some disadvantages of stress echocardiography. Suboptimal images are frequent with this technique. Although it is true that in many cases, a less-than-ideal image does not preclude diagnostic interpretation, it compromises the ability to visualize all myocardial segments and, hence, to identify every possible coronary stenosis. The predominant reason for suboptimal images is variable "echogenicity," which is particularly poor in older patients with hyperinflated lungs. The true incidence of poor images is difficult to ascertain, but it is likely that 10% of adult patients have poor echocardiographic windows. Evaluation of wall motion often depends on identifying the movement of the leading edge (the endocardium). Unfortunately, this leading edge is frequently indistinct and drops off at irregular intervals. This problem hinders the automatic quantification of wall motion; for example, for an automatic computerized technique that requires at least 75% of the endocardium to be discernible throughout the cardiac cycle, such quantification is only feasible in 59% of patients. Studies of poor technical quality occurred in 9.5% of patients in the multicenter report by Hoffmann et al;[24] in these patients, the agreement among different observers was only 43%, proving that what cannot be seen well cannot be evaluated well. Several regions of the left ventricle are difficult to evaluate precisely; these include but are not necessarily limited to the lateral wall, the apex, and the posterobasal segments. Thus, it is not surprising that the posterobasal segments have a particularly low interobserver reproducibility.[24]

Box 22-4. Disadvantages of stress echocardiography

1. Suboptimal images are common
2. Poor visualization of some regions
3. Computer quantification is difficult
4. Technical skill is pivotal
5. Loose criteria for normal response to stress
6. Difficult to do during exercise
7. Subjective interpretation
8. Difficult to identify ischemia superimposed on infarct

Another issue with echocardiography is the dependency on the skills of the technician or physician performing the study. For example, depending on the position of the transducer on the chest wall and its relative angulation, foreshortening or drop-off of cardiac walls can be a problem. In contrast, SPECT is done automatically, and image acquisition is controlled entirely by computer. Processing of SPECT requires some observer interaction, but the technical skills currently required are easily absorbed and well standardized.

The definition of a normal response during stress echocardiography is somewhat ambiguous. It is widely accepted that during inotropic stress, such as exercise or high-dose dobutamine, normally perfused cardiac walls contract more vigorously and, hence, have greater thickening and more dynamic wall motion.

Ginzton et al[19] reported on the variability of echocardiographic responses during maximal upright exercise in normal volunteers. They concluded that the variability among normal persons is so great that a mild abnormality, such as hypokinesis, may be a normal event. These investigators went on to suggest that only akinesis or dyskinesis should be considered abnormal during exercise.

A recent report by Borges et al[3] indicates that heterogeneity of left ventricular wall thickening may be induced or magnified by dobutamine infusion in normal persons. These investigators observed that the inferior wall often shows a lack of hyperkinesis or even relative hypokinesis when compared with the other myocardial regions. Moreover, Hammond et al,[22] using an experimental model of myocardial ischemia, reported that during dobutamine stimulation, not only the normally perfused but also the ischemic regions had increased rather than decreased wall thickening. The regions with normal perfusion had greater thickening than the regions with abnormal perfusion; nonetheless, if both the normal and abnormal regions improve with dobutamine, it may be difficult or impossible to discern deterioration of wall motion or thickening of the wall during dobutamine stress.

The issues discussed above pertaining to the technical and quality aspects of echocardiography are magnified during exercise stress because the increased respiratory rate and lung expansion further narrow the echocardiographic window. Moreover, in institutions where posttreadmill exercise echocardiography is used, the behavior of the left ventricle is not depicted during peak exercise because these studies are typically done immediately after rather than during exercise. In practice, this represents a delay of critical seconds during which myocardial ischemia may completely dissipate, especially in patients with single-vessel rather than multivessel coronary artery disease.

Upright and supine bicycle exercise stress testing are performed at some institutions. During upright bicycle exercise, only the subcostal or apical windows are usually accessible. Supine bicycle exercise can also be a challenging proposition, with a yield of only 70% to 80%.[12] Therefore, in many institutions, even when bicycle exercise is chosen, the images are frequently obtained after exercise. However, as demonstrated by Ryan et al,[52] the sensitivity of peak exercise testing is higher than that of the postexercise recording. A major problem with the bicycle exercise is that sedentary U.S. patients are often unable to reach a maximal heart rate, which is critical to achieve a high sensitivity. In the study by Ryan et al,[52] only 37% of patients reached their target heart rate during upright bicycle exercise echocardiography.

Perhaps the most important limitation of stress echocardiography is the subjective, solely visual analysis of the images. When this subjective element is combined with suboptimal images, incomplete delineation of the endocardium; and incomplete visualization of the lateral wall, posterolateral segments, and apex, considerable interobserver variability of the interpretation occurs. It is surprising that the reported results of stress echocardiography are not worse than they are. A recent multicenter study exposed a high interinstitutional variability of stress echocardiography.[24] In this study, five of the best echocardiographic laboratories in Europe were asked to select 30 stress echocardiograms each. All 150 studies were transferred to videotape and were interpreted at the five institutions. The results indicated that four of the five centers agreed in the designating the wall motion as normal or abnormal in only 73% of the patients. Among the 150 studies, the percentage of abnormal test interpretations ranged from as low as 25% to as high as 68%, depending on the institution interpreting the study. As expected, the lowest agreement was for evaluation of the basal inferior segments. The agreement was essentially perfect for the 9% of studies that had the highest quality images but was only 43% in the 9.5% of the studies with the lowest quality images. The agreement with respect to normal versus abnormal results in patients with single- or double-vessel disease was only 61% and 68%, respectively. This study clearly emphasizes that the subjective nature of the interpretation predictably leads to high interobserver variability.

Marwick et al[34] evaluated the confidence level of dobutamine and exercise echocardiographic interpretations. In this study, when the readers were asked to grade their own confidence levels, a high confidence level was given to only 17% of the dobutamine echocardiographic interpretations compared with 37% of exercise echocardiographic interpretations. In 55% of the patients during dobutamine echocardiography and 36% during exercise echocardiography, the interpretations were ranked as being of moderate confidence. In 27% and 28% of patients during dobutamine and exercise echocardiography, respectively, the confidence level of the interpretations was low.[34]

Finally, one of the most difficult areas in stress echocardiography is the evaluation of wall motion in regions with resting dysynergy. The decision of whether a given wall, particularly when it is akinetic or dyskinetic, is changing during stress is very difficult and is probably not very reproducible.[13,47,48]

CLINICAL RESULTS

Myocardial perfusion scintigraphy in the diagnosis of coronary artery disease

A meta-analysis of reports on exercise thallium-201 (^{201}Tl) planar scintigraphy that included a total of 52 publications and 5150 patients showed a sensitivity of 83% and a specificity of 88%.[10,60] For the most part, these studies were analyzed qualitatively. In the 16 studies that used quantification of ^{201}Tl planar imaging, the average sensitivity was 90% and specificity was 80%.[27,60]

In the past decade, SPECT has become the state-of-the-art of myocardial perfusion scintigraphy, and most studies are now performed using this tomographic technique. A recent meta-analysis[43] of 12 studies using exercise SPECT scintigraphy in a total of 2626 patients* showed an overall sensitivity of 90%, a specificity of 72%, and a normalcy rate of 89% (Fig. 22-2).

Pharmacologic perfusion imaging

Most of the reports on dipyridamole imaging have used ^{201}Tl planar scintigraphy. In 14 studies comprising 965 patients,

*References 4, 5, 8, 25, 28, 29, 31, 32, 56-59.

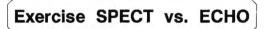

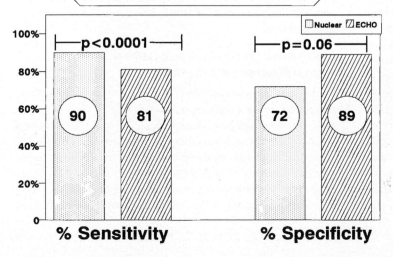

Fig. 22-2. Sensitivity and specificity of exercise SPECT and exercise echocardiography. (Adapted from O'Keefe JH Jr, Bateman TM, Silvestri R, et al: Safety and diagnostic accuracy of adenosine thallium-201 scintigraphy in patients unable to exercise and those with left bundle branch block, *Am Heart J* 124:614-621, 1992.)

the overall sensitivity was 87%, and the specificity was 75%. In four recent studies assessing dipyridamole SPECT imaging, the sensitivity was 90% and the specificity was 78%.[9,15,38,64] Adenosine SPECT scintigraphy also has a sensitivity and specificity comparable to that of exercise or dipyridamole imaging. In a recent review of 8 studies including 925 patients, the average sensitivity was 89% and the specificity was 83%.*

Dobutamine perfusion scintigraphy has recently seen wider use. A composite of three recent studies with dobutamine SPECT imaging with a total of 158 patients showed an average sensitivity of 91% and a specificity of 86%.[43]

Exercise stress echocardiography in coronary artery disease

A recent compilation of 12 studies using treadmill echocardiography in 913 patients yielded an average sensitivity of 81% and a specificity of 89%[43] (Fig. 22-2). These values are similar to those compiled in another review, which included some values of the earlier studies and studies performed during supine or upright bicycle exercise testing.[56] Although many problems are encountered when comparison of different cohorts of patients studied by either technique is attempted, this meta-analysis showed a statistically significant difference in favor of perfusion scintigraphy with respect to sensitivity and a borderline difference in favor of echocardiography with respect to specificity (Fig. 22-2). In the largest review thus far reported on exercise echocardiography, which included 3,679 patients, the sensitivity was 78% in men and 79% in women, with a specificity of 44% and 37%, respectively.[49]

Pharmacologic stress echocardiography

A recent composite evaluation of reported studies with dipyridamole, including standard and high-dose dipyridamole testing, showed an overall sensitivity of 63% and a specificity of 95%.[61] More recently, a large multicenter study compared the value of dipyridamole and dobutamine echocardiography with and without additional administration of atropine.[46] With dipyridamole, an overall sensitivity of 68% was found, which increased to 82% with concomitant atropine administration. The specificity with dipyridamole echocardiography was 94%. Dobutamine echocardiography had a sensitivity of 78%, which increased to 84% with atropine administration. The specificity of dobutamine echocardiography was 89%. The safety of dobutamine-atropine echocardiography was recently reported from a multicenter registry including 2799 patients.[45] In this series, 12% of patients could not complete the test because of side effects. Life-threatening complications or side effects requiring specific treatment and lasting more than 3 hours or necessitating a new hospital admission occurred in 1 of every 210 tests performed. This included two episodes of ventricular fibrillation, two instances of myocardial infarctions, three cases of sustained ventricular tachycardia, one case of prolonged ischemia, one instance of persistent and severe hypotension, and

five cases of central nervous system disturbances. Another study compared exercise, dipyridamole, and dobutamine echocardiography. In this study, the sensitivity was 76%, 72%, and 52% for exercise, dobutamine, and dipyridamole, respectively.[7]

Thus, dipyridamole and dobutamine echocardiography have a lower sensitivity than pharmacologic perfusion imaging with these agents or with adenosine. The sensitivity increases modestly with addition of atropine, but safety becomes more of a concern.

Correct identification of multivessel disease

One of the goals of stress cardiac imaging in addition to documentation or exclusion of the diagnosis of coronary artery disease is to ascertain the extent of coronary involvement. Several studies have reported on the detection of multivessel coronary artery disease by stress SPECT scintigraphy and stress echocardiography. Eight studies using stress echocardiography in 308 patients yielded an average sensitivity for correct identification of multivessel disease of 50%. On the other hand, five studies that reported on SPECT stress scintigraphy in 1020 patients showed an overall sensitivity for correct identification of multivessel disease of 72% ($p<0.001$)* (Fig. 22-3).

Correct localization of coronary artery stenosis

Several studies have addressed the issue of correct localization of individual coronary stenosis detected by exercise SPECT and exercise echocardiography. Together, these studies included 770 patients and 1328 stenotic coronary arteries.[43,61] The sensitivity was slightly higher with SPECT than with echocardiography for left anterior descending and right coronary artery stenoses but was markedly higher ($p<0.00001$) with SPECT than with exercise echocardiography for circumflex artery stenoses. Similar trends are seen with pharmacologic stress[43,61] (Fig. 22-4).

As compelling as all of the above numbers might be in demonstrating a higher sensitivity for stress SPECT imaging than for stress echocardiography, these data cannot be scientifically used to unquestionably demonstrate the superiority of one technique over another. Such an evaluation requires that patients be studied with the two techniques at the same time and with the same type of stress. Several recent studies have done just that.

Simultaneous perfusion scintigraphy and echocardiography during stress

A recent review compiled 11 studies comprising 808 patients who were simultaneously studied with perfusion imaging and echocardiography during exercise or pharmacologic stress.[43] The average sensitivity of these studies was slightly higher for perfusion scintigraphy than for stress echocardiography (83% compared with 78%; $p = 0.07$) (Fig. 22-5). In patients with single-vessel coronary artery disease the sensitivity was higher for stress SPECT than for stress echocardiography

---

*References 1, 6, 21, 26, 40, 42-44, 60.

*References 2, 8, 13, 17, 23, 25, 32, 33, 35, 37, 43, 51, 54, 57.

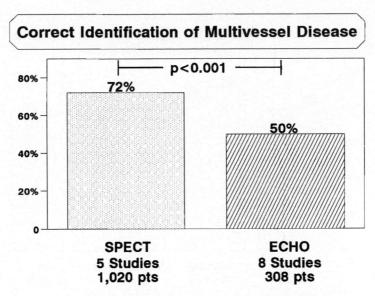

Fig. 22-3. Multivessel disease identification by SPECT and stress echocardiography. (Adapted from O'Keefe JH Jr, Bateman TM, Silvestri R, et al: Safety and diagnostic accuracy of adenosine thallium-201 scintigraphy in patients unable to exercise and those with left bundle branch block, *Am Heart J* 124:614-621, 1992.)

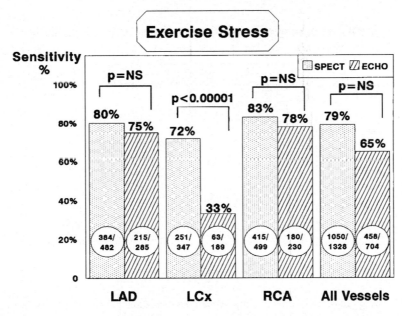

Fig. 22-4. Sensitivity of exercise SPECT and exercise echocardiography for individual coronary artery stenosis. (Adapted from O'Keefe JH Jr, Bateman TM, Silvestri R, et al: Safety and diagnostic accuracy of adenosine thallium-201 scintigraphy in patients unable to exercise and those with left bundle branch block, *Am Heart J* 124:614-621, 1992.)

(76% compared with 67%; $p < 0.05$) (Fig. 22-6). The specificity was slightly higher for echocardiography than for SPECT (86% compared with 77%), but this difference was not statistically significant. Santoro et al[53] recently compared the performance of exercise stress testing, dipyridamole echocardiography, dobutamine echocardiography, dipyridamole tomography, and dobutamine tomography in 60 patients. The sensitivities were 58%, 53%, 61%, 97%, and 91%, respectively. The specificities

were 67%, 96%, 89%, and 81%, respectively. The difference found in sensitivity found of tomography was statistically significant ($p < 0.005$).

THE FUTURE OF STRESS IMAGING

The field of stress cardiac imaging is very dynamic. Recent technological advances are gradually being incorporated into clinical practice. With respect to nuclear cardiology, the avail-

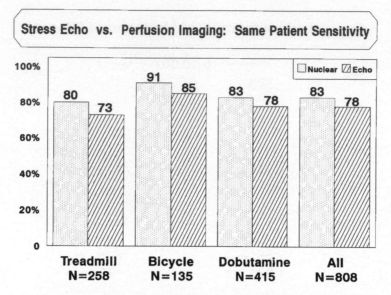

Fig. 22-5. Sensitivity of stress SPECT echocardiography in the same patients in Fig. 22-4. Although the sensitivity is slightly higher for every stressor used with SPECT, the differences are not statistically significant. (Adapted from O'Keefe JH Jr, Bateman TH, Silvestri R, et al: Safety and diagnostic accuracy of adenosine thallium-201 scintigraphy in patients unable to exercise and those with left bundle branch block, *Am Heart J* 124:614-621, 1992.)

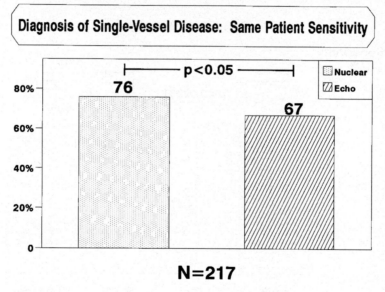

Fig. 22-6. Diagnosis of single-vessel disease. Same patient sensitivity.

ability of multidetector gamma cameras; improvement in computer technology, hardware, and software for correction of attenuation and scatter; and the ability to do gated SPECT of perfusion images by using 99mTc tracers have advanced the field. Other recent developments in hardware have provided the opportunity to perform myocardial metabolic studies with positron emitters (such as fluorine-18 fluorodeoxyglucose), by use of a standard gamma camera coupled with a high-energy collimator or by performance of coincidence imaging of positrons using modified gamma cameras without collimation.

Important advances have been made in echocardiography in the last several years, including digitization of images and stan-

dard format display. There is currently great interest in the potential of contrast echocardiography, and various contrast agents are being tested at several medical centers. Contrast echocardiography has not yet been tried during exercise or other types of stress, but the potential for this development exists.

Other stressors or imaging techniques have also been used, such as dobutamine in combination with magnetic resonance imaging and transesophageal echocardiography combined with atrial pacing. Although these variations of stress testing are feasible, they are not very practical and are therefore not used very often.

REFERENCES

1. Allman KC, Berry J, Sucharski LA, et al: Determination of extent and location of coronary artery disease in patients without prior myocardial infarction by thallium-201 tomography with pharmacologic stress, *J Nucl Med* 33:2067–2073, 1992.

2. Armstrong WF, O'Donnell J, Ryan T, et al: Effect of prior myocardial infarction and extent and location of coronary disease on accuracy of exercise echocardiography, *J Am Coll Cardiol* 10:531–538, 1987.

3. Borges AC, Pingitore A, Cordovil A, et al: Heterogeneity of left ventricular regional wall thickening following dobutamine infusion in normal human subjects, *Eur Heart J* 16:1726–1730, 1995.

4. Chouraqui P, Maddahi J, Ostrzega E: Quantitative exercise thallium-201 rotational tomography for evaluation of patients with prior myocardial infarction, *Am J Cardiol* 66:151–157, 1990.

5. Christian TF, Miller TD, Bailey KR, et al: Noninvasive identification of severe coronary artery disease using exercise tomographic thallium-201 imaging, *Am J Cardiol* 70:14–20, 1992.

6. Coyne EP, Belvedere DA, Vande Streek PR, et al: Thallium-201 scintigraphy after intravenous infusion of adenosine compared with exercise thallium testing in the diagnosis of coronary artery disease, *J Am Coll Cardiol* 17:1289–1294, 1991.

7. Dagianti A, Penco M, Agati L, et al: Stress echocardiography: comparison of exercise, dipyridamole and dobutamine in detecting and predicting the extent of coronary artery disease, *J Am Coll Cardiol* 26:18–25, 1995.

8. DePasquale EE, Nody AC, DePuey EG, et al: Quantitative rotational thallium-201 tomography for identifying and localizing coronary artery disease, *Circulation* 77:316–327, 1988.

9. DePuey EG, Gertler-Krawczynska E, D'Amato PH, et al: Thallium-201 single-photon emission computed tomography with intravenous dipyridamole to diagnose coronary artery disease, *Coron Artery Dis* 1:75–82, 1990.

10. Detrano R, Janosi A, Lyons KP, et al: Factors affecting sensitivity and specificity of a diagnostic test: the exercise thallium scintigram, *Am J Med* 84:699–710, 1988.

11. Di Rocco RJ, Rumsey WL, Kuczynski BL, et al: Measurement of myocardial blood flow using a co-injection technique for technetium-99m-teboroxime, technetium-96-sestamibi and thallium-201, *J Nucl Med* 33:1152–1159, 1992.

12. Feigenbaum H: *Echocardiography,* Philadelphia, 1986, Lea & Febiger.

13. Feigenbaum H: Evolution of stress testing, *Circulation* 85:1217–1218, 1992 (editorial).

14. Feldman RL, Nichols WW, Pepine CJ, et al: Acute effect of intravenous dipyridamole on regional coronary hemodynamics and metabolism, *Circulation* 64:333–344, 1981.

15. Francisco DA, Collins SM, Go RT, et al: Tomographic thallium-201 myocardial perfusion scintigrams after maximal coronary artery vasodilation with intravenous dipyridamole. Comparison of qualitative and quantitative approaches, *Circulation* 66:370–379, 1982.

16. Fung AY, Gallagher KP, Buda AJ: The physiologic basis of dobutamine as compared with dipyridamole stress interventions in the assessment of critical coronary stenosis, *Circulation* 76:943–951, 1987.

17. Galanti G, Sciagra R, Comeglio M, et al: Diagnostic accuracy of peak exercise echocardiography in coronary artery disease: comparison with thallium-201 myocardial scintigraphy, *Am Heart J* 122:1609–1616, 1991.

18. Gerwirtz H, Gross SL, Williams DO, et al: Contrasting effects of nifedipine and adenosine on regional myocardial flow distribution and metabolism distal to a severe coronary arterial stenosis: observations in sedated, closed-chest, domestic swine, *Circulation* 69:1048–1057, 1984.

19. Ginzton LE, Conant R, Brizendine M, et al: Quantitative analysis of segmental wall motion during maximal upright dynamic exercise: variability in normal adults, *Circulation* 73:268–275, 1986.

20. Gould KL: Noninvasive assessment of coronary stenoses by myocardial perfusion imaging during pharmacologic coronary vasodilatation:
I. Physiologic basis and experimental validation, *Am J Cardiol* 41:267–278, 1978.

21. Gupta NC, Esterbrooks DJ, Hilleman DE, et al: Comparison of adenosine and exercise thallium-201 single-photon emission computed tomography (SPECT) myocardial perfusion imaging. The GE SPECT Multicenter Adenosine Study Group, *J Am Coll Cardiol* 19:248–257, 1992.

22. Hammond HK, McKirnan MD: Effects of dobutamine and arbutamine on regional myocardial function in a porcine model of myocardial ischemia, *J Am Coll Cardiol* 23:475–482, 1994.

23. Hays JT, Mahmarian JJ, Cochran AJ, et al: Dobutamine thallium-201 tomography for evaluating patients with suspected coronary artery disease unable to undergo exercise or vasodilator pharmacologic stress testing, *J Am Coll Cardiol* 21:1583–1590, 1993.

24. Hoffmann R, Lethen H, Marwick T, et al: Analysis of interinstitutional observer agreement in interpretation of dobutamine stress echocardiograms, *J Am Coll Cardiol* 27:330–336, 1996.

25. Iskandrian AS, Heo J, Kong B, et al: Effect of exercise level on the ability of thallium-201 tomographic imaging in detecting coronary artery disease: analysis of 461 patients, *J Am Coll Cardiol* 14:1477–1486, 1989.

26. Iskandrian AS, Heo J, Lemlek J, et al: Identification of high-risk patients with left main and three-vessel coronary artery disease by adenosine-single photon emission computed tomographic thallium imaging, *Am Heart J* 125:1130–1135, 1993.

27. Iskandrian AS, Verani MS: *Nuclear Cardiac Imaging: Principles and Applications,* Philadelphia, 1996, F.A. Davis.

28. Kahn JK, McGhie I, Akers MS, et al: Quantitative rotational tomography with 201Tl and 99mTc-2-methoxy-isobutyl isonitrile. A direct comparison in normal individuals and patients with coronary artery disease, *Circulation* 79:1282–1293, 1989.

29. Kiat H, Maddahi J, Roy LT, et al: Comparison of technetium 99m methoxy isobutyl isonitrile and thallium 201 for evaluation of coronary artery disease by planar and tomographic methods, *Am Heart J* 117:1–11, 1989.

30. Krivokapich J, Huang SC, Schelbert HR: Assessment of the effects of dobutamine on myocardial blood flow and oxidative metabolism in normal human subjects using nitrogen-13 ammonia and carbon-11 acetate, *Am J Cardiol* 71:1351–1356, 1993.

31. Maddahi J, Van Train K, Prigent F, et al: Quantitative single photon emission computed thallium-201 tomography for detection and localization of coronary artery disease: optimization and prospective validation of a new technique, *J Am Coll Cardiol* 14:1689–1699, 1989.

32. Mahmarian JJ, Boyce TM, Goldberg RK, et al: Quantitative exercise thallium-201 single photon emission computed tomography for the enhanced diagnosis of ischemic heart disease, *J Am Coll Cardiol* 15:318–329, 1990.

33. Marwick T, Willemart B, D'Hondt AM, et al: Selection of the optimal nonexercise stress for the evaluation of ischemic regional myocardial dysfunction and malperfusion. Comparison of dobutamine and adenosine using echocardiography and 99mTc-MIBI single photon emission computed tomography, *Circulation* 87:345–354, 1993.

34. Marwick TH, D'Hondt AM, Mairesse GH, et al: Comparative ability of dobutamine and exercise stress in inducing myocardial ischaemia in active patients, *Br Heart J* 72:31–38, 1994.

35. Marwick TH, Nemec JJ, Stewart WJ, et al: Diagnosis of coronary artery disease using exercise echocardiography and positron emission tomography: comparison and analysis of discrepant results, *J Am Soc Echocardiogr* 5:231–238, 1992.

36. Mays AE Jr, Cobb FR: Relationship between regional myocardial blood flow and thallium-201 distribution in the presence of coronary artery stenosis and dipyridamole-induced vasodilation. *J Clin Invest* 73:1359–1366, 1984.

37. Mazeika PK, Nadazdin A, Oakley CM: Dobutamine stress echocardiography for detection and assessment of coronary artery disease, *J Am Coll Cardiol* 19:1203–1211, 1992.

38. Mendelson MA, Spies SM, Spies WG, et al: Usefulness of single-photon emission computed tomography of thallium-201 uptake after dipyridamole infusion for detection of coronary artery disease, *Am J Cardiol* 69:1150–1155, 1992.

39. Movahed A, Reeves WC, Rose GC, et al: Dobutamine and improvement of regional and global left ventricular function in coronary artery disease, *Am J Cardiol* 66:375–377, 1990.

40. Nguyen T, Heo J, Ogilby JD, et al: Single photon emission computed tomography with thallium-201 during adenosine-induced coronary hyperemia: correlation with coronary arteriography, exercise thallium and two-dimensional echocardiography. *J Am Coll Cardiol* 16:1375–1383, 1990.

41. Nielsen AP, Morris KG, Murdock R, et al: Linear relationship between the distribution of thallium-201 and blood flow in ischemic and non-ischemic myocardium during exercise, *Circulation* 61:797–801, 1980.

42. Nishimura S, Mahmarian JJ, Boyce TM, et al: Quantitative thallium-201 single photon emission computed tomography during maximal pharmacologic coronary vasodilation with adenosine for assessing coronary artery disease, *J Am Coll Cardiol* 18:736–745, 1991.

43. O'Keefe JH Jr, Barnhart CS, Bateman TM: Comparison of stress echocardiography and stress myocardial perfusion scintigraphy for diagnosing coronary artery disease and assessing its severity, *Am J Cardiol* 75:25D–34D, 1995.

44. O'Keefe JH Jr, Bateman TM, Silvestri R, et al: Safety and diagnostic accuracy of adenosine thallium-201 scintigraphy in patients unable to exercise and those with left bundle branch block, *Am Heart J* 124:614–621, 1992.

45. Picano E, Mathias W Jr, Pingitori A, et al: Safety and tolerability of dobutamine-atropine stress echocardiography: a prospective, multicentre study. Echo Dobutamine International Cooperative Study Group, *Lancet* 344:1190–1192, 1994.

46. Pingitore A, Picano E, Colosso MQ, et al: The atropine factor in pharmacologic stress echocardiography. Echo Persantine (EPIC) and Echo Dobutamine International Cooperative (EDIC) Study Groups, *J Am Coll Cardiol* 27:1164–1170, 1996.

47. Quinoñes MA: Clinical assessment of regional function: strengths and limitations, *Coron Artery Dis* 6:625–628, 1995.

48. Quiñones MA, Verani MS, Haichin RM, et al: Exercise echocardiography versus 201Tl single-photon emission computed tomography in evaluation of coronary artery disease. Analysis of 292 patients, *Circulation* 85:1026–1031, 1992.

49. Roger VL, Pellika PA, Bell MR, et al: Sex and test verification bias. Impact on the diagnostic value of exercise echocardiograph, *Circulation* 95:405–410, 1997.

50. Rossen JD, Quillen JE, Lopez AG, et al: Comparison of coronary vasodilation with intravenous dipyridamole and adenosine, *J Am Coll Cardiol* 18:485–491, 1991.

51. Ryan T, Segar DS, Sawada SG, et al: Detection of coronary artery disease with upright bicycle exercise echocardiography, *J Am Soc Echocardiogr* 6:186–197, 1993.

52. Ryan T, Vasey CG, Presti CF, et al: Exercise echocardiography: detection of coronary artery disease in patients with normal left ventricular wall motion at rest, *J Am Coll Cardiol* 11:993–999, 1988.

53. Santoro GM, Sciagrá R, Buonamici P, et al: Head-to-head comparison of exercise stress testing, pharmacologic stress echocardiography, and perfusion tomography as first-line examination for chest pain in patients without history of coronary artery disease, *J Nucl Cardiol* 5:19–27, 1998.

54. Sawada SG, Segar DS, Ryan T, et al: Echocardiographic detection of coronary artery disease during dobutamine infusion, *Circulation* 83:1605–1614, 1991.

55. Schulz R, Miyazaki S, Miller M, et al: Consequences of regional inotropic stimulation of ischemic myocardium on regional myocardial blood flow and function in anesthetized swine, *Circ Res* 64:1116–1126, 1989.

56. Svane B, Bone D, Holmgren A: Coronary angiography and thallium-201 single photon emission computed tomography in single vessel coronary artery disease, *Acta Radiol* 31:237–244, 1990.

57. Tamaki N, Yonekura Y, Mukai T, et al: Stress thallium-201 transaxial emission computed tomography: quantitative versus qualitative analysis for evaluation of coronary artery disease, *J Am Coll Cardiol* 4:1213–1221, 1984.

58. Van Train KF, Areeda J, Garcia EV, et al: Quantitative same-day rest-stress technetium-99m-sestamibi SPECT: definition and validation of stress normal limits and criteria for abnormality, *J Nucl Med* 34:1494–1502, 1993.

59. Van Train KF, Maddahi J, Berman DS, et al: Quantitative analysis of tomographic stress thallium-201 myocardial scintigrams: a multicenter trial, *J Nucl Med* 31:1168–1179, 1990.

60. Verani MS: Myocardial perfusion imaging versus two-dimensional echocardiography: comparative value in the diagnosis of coronary artery disease, *J Nucl Cardiol* 1:399–414, 1994.

61. Verani MS, Mahmarian JJ, Hixson JB, et al: Diagnosis of coronary artery disease by controlled coronary vasodilation with adenosine and thallium-201 scintigraphy in patients unable to exercise, *Circulation* 82:80–87, 1990.

62. Wackers FJTh, Bodenheimer M, Fleiss JL, et al: Factors affecting uniformity in interpretation of planar thallium-201 imaging in a multicenter trial. The Multicenter Study on Silent Myocardial Ischemia (MSSMI) Thallium-201 Investigators, *J Am Coll Cardiol* 21:1064–1074, 1993.

63. Wilson RF, Wyche K, Christensen BV, et al: Effects of adenosine on human coronary arterial circulation, *Circulation* 82:1595–1606, 1990.

64. Zhu YY, Chung WS, Botvinick EH, et al: Dipyridamole perfusion scintigraphy: the experience with its application in one hundred seventy patients with known or suspected unstable angina, *Am Heart J* 121(1Pt1):33–43, 1991.

Chapter 23

Myocardial perfusion imaging using nonnuclear tracers and detectors

Jonathan R. Lindner and **Sanjiv Kaul**

Although radionuclide imaging is currently the most widely used method for myocardial perfusion imaging in patients with known or suspected coronary artery disease, alternative techniques are emerging. These techniques include magnetic resonance imaging (MRI), ultrafast computed tomography (CT), and myocardial contrast echocardiography, all of which provide better spatial and temporal resolution than radionuclide imaging. In this chapter, we discuss the biophysical properties of contrast materials employed by these imaging modalities, as well as the principles used to assess myocardial perfusion. In addition, we comment on the properties of the detectors used for imaging. We do not discuss positron emission tomography because this topic is covered in another chapter.

BIOCHEMICAL AND KINETIC PROPERTIES OF TRACERS

Certain assumptions must be met for an exogenously administered tracer to be considered ideal for quantification of regional myocardial blood flow. It should be stable, mix rapidly and uniformly in blood, be negligible in volume compared with the myocardial blood volume, be hemodynamically inert, and not exhibit substantial recirculation.

Paramagnetic contrast agents

Assessment of myocardial perfusion with MRI relies on magnetic relaxivity and susceptibility changes in the local tissue environment produced by paramagnetic agents as they pass through the microcirculation. Most of the elements used to produce signal enhancement, such as gadolinium, manganese, or iron, have powerful proton-relaxing effects that can be attributed to the presence of unpaired electrons. As a result, they produce dose-dependent enhancement of the magnetic field and reduce the relaxation times of resonating atomic nuclei after a radiofrequency pulse.

Paramagnetic contrast agents can be classified by their predominant effects on either the T1 (relaxation agents) or T2 (susceptibility agents) relaxation times (Table 23-1). T1 reflects the rate at which the proton magnetic vector aligns longitudinally with the external magnetic field, whereas T2 reflects the rate at which the transverse vector decays after a 90° radiofrequency pulse. Although they may be characterized by their relative enhancement during T1- compared with T2-weighted imaging, all paramagnetic agents produce shortening of both relaxation times. The degree of shortening may vary depending on the concentration of the agents, the magnetic field strength, and the imaging technique.[67,80] Currently, most commercial preparations contain paramagnetic agents with a predominant effect on T1 relaxation at relatively low doses normally used.

Although chelation of paramagnetic agents considerably reduces their toxicity,[4,5] it also decreases their effectiveness as contrast agents because unpaired electrons are depleted in the process. However, the reduction in paramagnetism is more than compensated for by the ability to administer higher doses of less toxic formulations and, for some agents, by improved biodistribution. Currently, the most commonly employed formulation consists of gadolinium chelated with diethylenetriamine pentaacetic acid (Gd-DTPA). This complex is safe because of the very high binding affinity and specificity of DTPA for gadolinium. Although Gd-DTPA has a high osmolality (1960 mOsm/kg), its effects on hemodynamics and myocardial blood flow are minimal (Fig. 23-1) because the doses needed to produce myocardial signal enhancement are comparatively

Table 23-1. Characteristics of commonly used magnetic resonance contrast agents*

Agent	Intravascular kinetics	Predominant effects
Gadolinium-DTPA	Diffusible	T1
Gadolinium-DTPA-BMA	Diffusible	T1
Gadolinium-DOTA	Diffusible	T1
Gadolinium-DOTA	Diffusible	T1
Dysprosium-DTPA-BMA	Diffusible	T2
SPIO	Blood Pool	T1, T2
Gadolinium-DTPA-Albumin	Blood Pool	T1
Polylysine-Gadolinium-DTPA	Blood Pool	T1

*BMA = bis-methylamide; DOTA = tetraazacyclo-dodecanetetraacetic acid; DTPA = diethylenetriamine pentaacetic acid; SPIO = super-paramagnetic iron oxide.

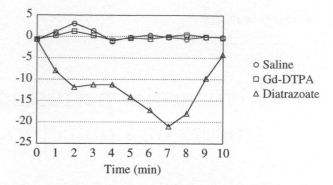

Fig. 23-1. Mean percent change in myocardial microvascular perfusion after administration of gadolinium-DTPA, 0.25 mmol/kg saline, and an iodinated radiographic contrast agent (diatrazoate) in 10 rats. (Adapted from Klopp R, Niemer W, Schippel W, et al: Changes in the microcirculation of the intact rat heart after iodinated and gadolinium-containing contrast media, *Invest Radiol* 30:69-74, 1995.)

small.[36,56] Similarly, myocardial blood volume changes little after injection of this agent.

Gadolinium-DTPA is highly soluble and mixes readily with blood. However, the application of tracer kinetic principles for the quantification of myocardial perfusion is complicated by the diffusion of this agent into the extracellular space.[31,38,71,82] Other paramagnetic relaxation agents, such as gadolinium tetraazacyclo-dodecanetetraacetic acid (Gd-DOTA), and susceptibility agents, such as dysprosium-DTPA-bis-methylamide, are also not retained strictly within the intravascular space. Flux of these diffusible agents into the myocardial extravascular space is dependent on the amount of microvascular flow, the volume of the interstitial space, and capillary permeability.[38,80] Under normal resting conditions, approximately 40% to 50% of Gd-DTPA diffuses from the vascular compartment to the interstitial space on initial capillary transit.[38,64,76,82] Diffusion of Gd-DTPA results in broadening of the time–intensity curve during the first pass of the agent through the myocardium, which complicates the evaluation of residue functions to determine transit rates unless only initial time points are considered (as shown in Fig. 23-2). Fitting a curve to time–signal intensity data in an ischemic region in which the peak intensity is low and its duration is long, is particularly difficult (Fig. 23-3). Moreover, the proportion of Gd-DTPA that diffuses into the extravascular space of the ischemic region is greater than that in normal regions because of an increased intravascular residence time[82] and, possibly, enhanced capillary permeability. Back-diffusion of these tracers also occurs, requiring correction for complex exchange kinetics between the intravascular, interstitial, and intracellular compartments to quantify myocardial blood flow.[47] The recirculation of paramagnetic agents may also complicate analysis of time–intensity data. Diffusion of the tracer into the interstitial space can preclude discrimination between first and second passes in the myocardium, especially in an ischemic region.

Although they are an impediment for absolute flow quantification, the diffusion characteristics of paramagnetic contrast agents have been successfully used to determine infarct size

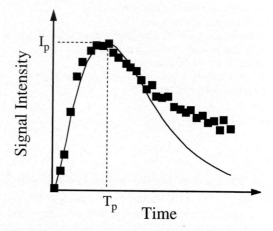

Fig. 23-2. Background-subtracted time versus signal intensity curve obtained from a normal myocardial region on magnetic resonance imaging after left atrial injection of gadolinium-DTPA, 0.05 mmol/kg. Diffusion of Gd-DTPA into the extravascular space resulted in artifactual widening of the curve and persistent myocardial enhancement. The γ-variate function must therefore be calculated from data points before signal intensity decreases to approximately 70% of peak intensity. I_p = peak intensity; T_p = time to peak intensity. (Adapted from Wilke N, Simm J, Zhang J, et al: Contrast-enhanced first pass myocardial perfusion imaging: correlation between myocardial blood flow in dogs at rest and during hyperemia, *Magn Reson Med* 29:485-497, 1993.)

and viability by MRI. Areas of edema and inflammation have greater accumulation and slower clearance of Gd-DTPA because of increased capillary permeability and expansion of the interstitial space after infarction.[4,47] The resulting enhanced myocardial contrast effect in the infarct bed forms the basis for determining infarct size and success of reperfusion with Gd-DTPA early after myocardial infarction (Fig. 23-4). Because washout of Gd-DTPA is more rapid in normal than in infarcted tissue, enhancement of an injured, reperfused region is maximal when imaging is delayed 10 to 30 minutes after administration.[68,79] In the chronic setting, Gd-DTPA diffusion into the

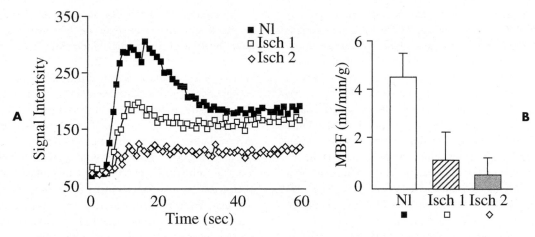

Fig. 23-3. A, Time–signal intensity curves during ultrafast magnetic resonance imaging (MRI) after left atrial injection of gadolinium (Gd)-DTPA in normal *(closed squares)* and two ischemic *(open squares and open triangles)* myocardial regions during hyperemia. **B,** Corresponding microsphere-derived regional myocardial blood flow measurements from these regions. (Adapted from Wilke N, Simm J, Zhang J, et al: Contrast-enhanced first pass myocardial perfusion imaging: correlation between myocardial blood flow in dogs at rest and during hyperemia, *Magn Reson Med* 29:485-497, 1993.)

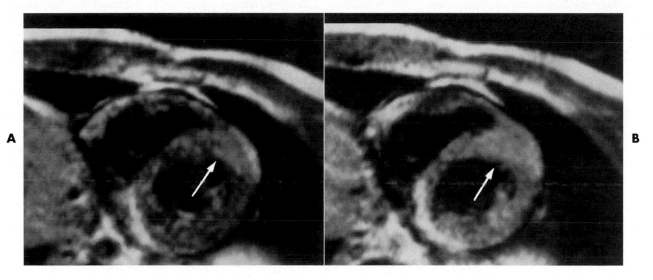

Fig. 23-4. Short-axis images obtained from a patient with a recent anteroseptal infarction by using magnetic resonance imaging before **(A)** and after **(B)** administration of gadolinium-DTPA. The infarct zone is defined by enhancement in the anteroseptal region after administration of contrast agent *(arrow).* (From van der Wall EE, Vliegen HW: In Iskandrian AS, van der Wall EE, eds: *Myocardial viability: detection and clinical relevance,* Dordrecht, the Netherlands, 1994, with kind permission from Kluwer Academic Publishers.)

infarct zone is absent because of the presence of poorly vascularized scar tissue.[49,69]

Like Gd-DTPA, manganese-bis-pyridoxal ethylenediamine diacetic acid (Mn-DPDP) can be used to define the spatial extent of an acute infarction because cytosolic swelling and loss of membrane integrity result in preferential retention of Mn-DPDP within the interstitial space.[57] A possible advantage of Mn-based compounds over Gd-DTPA is that their active cellular uptake by myocytes may allow detection of myocardial viability in the setting of chronic coronary artery disease.[15,50]

More ideal obligatory vascular MRI tracers have been developed by complexing paramagnetic elements with larger molecules. The biodistribution of these materials is determined by properties of the binding molecule rather than by the paramagnetic element. Because diffusion out of the intravascular space is greatly reduced by the increased molecular size of these agents, MRI first-pass and transit time analyses more closely reflect the relation of myocardial blood flow to myocardial volume. The greatest experience has been with poly-lysine-Gd-DTPA,[37,56,70,81] in which covalent linkage of Gd-DTPA to poly-L-lysine increases the molecular weight from approximately 600 to 50,000 D.[37] As a result, 97% to 98% of this agent is retained the blood pool 1 minute after intravenous injection.[37,81] Confinement within the vascular compartment, however, results in lower myocardial tissue concentrations and less signal enhancement of this agent compared with diffusible agents. Nonetheless, adequate myocardial enhancement is still achieved because of a relatively large myocardial blood volume in the heart (5–10% of total myocardial volume at rest).[9,45] The higher molecular weight of the compound also shortens the relaxation time of surrounding protons by several fold, causing a further increase in the signal.[81] Similar to polylysine-Gd-DTPA, the ability of Gd-DTPA to shorten T1 when covalently complexed to albumin[59] is also enhanced.

Even larger particulate intravascular MRI contrast agents are under investigation. Superparamagnetic iron oxide (SPIO) particles, which have strong effects on T1 and T2, are currently being evaluated. Contrast agents for MRI that incorporate SPIO particles are characterized by their large size (often several hundred nanometers in diameter) and their long intravascular half-life.[18] A hydrophilic outer coat surrounds the iron oxide core of these particles to ensure reliable biodistribution and to prevent extraction from the blood pool by the reticuloendothelial system.[80] Liposomal macroparticulate MRI contrast agents are even larger and are composed of phospholipid bilayers containing paramagnetic substances, such as manganese.[83] The high concentration of the paramagnetic agent within these particles results in strong effects on proton relaxation, which is further potentiated when manganese is incorporated into the microsphere membrane through alkylation.[66] These large microspheres (measured in micrometers) remain entirely within the intravascular space.

As alluded to earlier, the larger size of the intravascular agents described above may be advantageous for absolute quantification of myocardial blood flow, because there is less need to account for extravascular diffusion. Greater stability is also afforded because unlike diffusible agents, intravascular compounds are not readily excreted by the kidney. Once equilibrium distribution throughout the entire blood pool has been established, the concentration of intravascular agents within the myocardium compared with the blood pool should reflect the fractional myocardial blood volume. This estimate can be used to solve for myocardial blood flow quantification because data obtained from first-pass methods of analysis reflect the relation between myocardial blood flow and myocardial blood volume.[81,83] Fractional myocardial blood volume may also be estimated by the ratio of the areas under the enhancement curve for the myocardium and blood pool (Fig. 23-5).[81]

Contrast agents used for radiographic computed tomography

Intravascular injection of iodinated radiologic contrast agents is combined with tomographic imaging of the myocardium during ultrafast CT. Iodinated contrast agents increase the absorption of X-rays within the blood pool, which results in an increase in radiographic density (quantified as Hounsfield units). Similar to analyses performed with contrast-enhanced cardiac MRI, myocardial blood flow is assessed with CT by tissue residue or transfer functions[13,55,77] or first-pass indicator dilution (Stewart–Hamilton) analysis[23,84,85] from images obtained during the microvascular transit of the agent. Different contrast agent formulations are available for use, and all have the advantage of a relatively long shelf-life. They have been well characterized on the basis of their os-

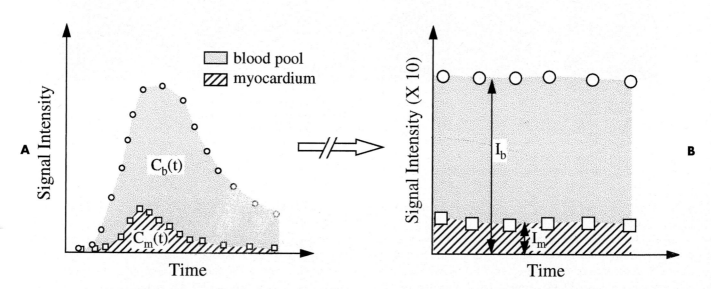

Fig. 23-5. Methods of determining myocardial blood volume after administration of a nondiffusible intravascular contrast agent. **A,** The area under the background-subtracted first-pass time versus signal intensity curves from the myocardium, $C_m(t)$, and from the blood pool, $C_b(t)$, may be compared. **B,** If the agent is stable, the ratio of signal intensities in the myocardium (I_m) and the blood pool (I_b) may be compared once equilibrium has been established.

molarity, calcium-chelating properties, and ionic composition (Table 23-2).

Agents used in CT have adverse effects on coronary hemodynamics and flow,[20,60,87] which worsen at higher doses. Intracoronary injection of sodium meglumine diatrizoate, an ionic compound with relatively high osmolarity, is followed by a triphasic coronary flow response (Fig. 23-6). An initial rapid decrease in myocardial blood flow is followed by a hyperemic response.[20,60] A gradual return to baseline flow is then seen. The nadir of flow reduction and the degree of hyperemia are related to the dose of contrast medium injected. In addition to the physiologic response to initial flow reduction, hyperemia also results from the hyperosmolarity[12] and calcium-chelating effects[32] of these agents and is less pronounced with isoosmolar agents and those containing disodium-calcium ethylenediamine tetraacetic acid.[11,16] Vagal responses,[87] histamine release,[2] direct effects on smooth muscle calcium channels,[32] and change in myocardial metabolic requirements[60] may also account for some of the hyperemia noted with CT-contrast agents. The dose of contrast required to enhance the myocardium by CT is small; consequently, the hemodynamic effects are not clinically important. Because they reduce hyperemia and do not expand the myocardial blood volume,[28] nonionic low osmolar agents are preferable for evaluation of myocardial perfusion using CT.

Diffusion of soluble iodinated contrast agents into the interstitial space may adversely influence flow measurements by CT,[8] particularly nonionic and low-molecular-weight compounds.[1,8] Fig. 23-7 shows background-subtracted myocardial CT time–intensity curves following aortic root injection of a conventional nonionic contrast agent (Ioversol) and a particu-

Table 23-2. Characteristics of commercially available iodinated radiographic contrast agents

Agent	Trade name	Iodine content mg/ml	Osmolarity mOsm/kg	Viscosity centipoise (CP) at 37°C	Ionic (mEq/L of sodium) or nonionic
Diatrazoate meglumine sodium	Hypaque-76	370	2016	9.0	Ionic (160)
Diatrazoate meglumine sodium	Renografin-76	370	1940	8.4	Ionic (190)
Diatrazoate meglumine sodium	Angiovist	370	2076	8.4	Ionic (160)
Ioxaglate meglumine	Hexabrix	320	600	7.5	Ionic (150)
Iopamidol	Isovue	370	796	9.4	Nonionic
Iohexol	Omnipaque-350	350	844	10.4	Nonionic
Ioversol	Optiray	320	702	5.8	Nonionic

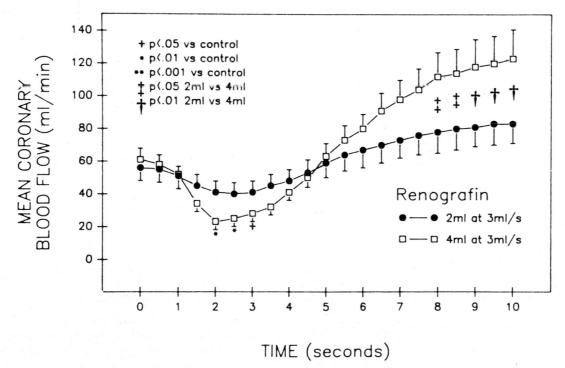

Fig. 23-6. Mean coronary blood flow (±SEM) after intracoronary injection of 2 and 4 ml of sodium meglumine diatrizoate (Renografin-76) at a constant rate. (Adapted from Friedman HZ, DeBee SF, McGillen MJ, et al: Immediate effects of graded ionic and nonionic contrast injections on coronary blood flow and myocardial function: Implications for digital coronary angiography, *Invest Radiol* 22:722-727, 1987.)

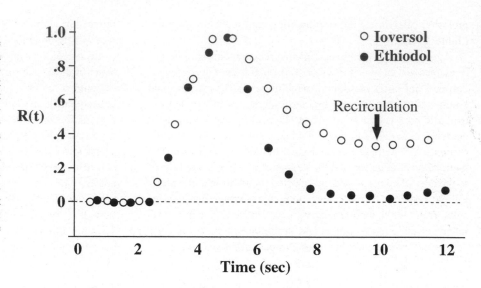

Fig. 23-7. Background-subtracted time versus intensity curves obtained from a normal myocardial region by using ultrafast computed tomography after aortic root injection of a diffusible nonionic contrast agent (ioversol) and an intravascular particulate emulsion (Ethiodol). Computed tomographic intensity values were plotted as a fraction of the peak intensity, *R(t)*. (Adapted from Canty JM, Judd RM, Brody AS, et al: First pass entry of nonionic contrast agent into the extravascular space: effect on radiographic estimates of transit time and blood volume, *Circulation* 84: 2071-2078, 1991. With permission of the American Heart Association.)

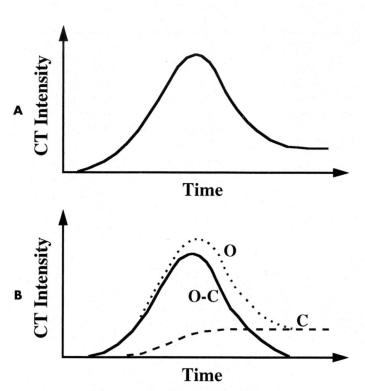

Fig. 23-8. Depiction of the method used to correct for extravascular diffusion of radiographic contrast agents. **A,** A typical time–intensity curve for computed tomography, obtained from the myocardium following aortic root injection of a diffusible radiographic contrast agent. **B,** The original curve *(O)* and the curve that describes the intensity attributable to contrast that has diffused extravascularly *(C)*, obtained by integrating and scaling the input obtained from a region of interest over the aortic root. Mathematical correction for diffusion results in a narrower time–intensity curve without residual myocardial contrast *(O-C)*. (Adapted from Wu X, Ewert DL, Liu YH, et al: In vivo relation of intramyocardial blood volume to myocardial perfusion: evidence supporting microvascular site for autoregulation, *Circulation* 85:730-737, 1992. With permission of the American Heart Association.)

late emulsion compound (Ethiodol). Compared with Ethiodol, which remains within the intravascular compartment and exhibits rapid myocardial washout, Ioversol diffuses into the extracellular space. This diffusion yields a wider time–intensity curve, and myocardial contrast enhancement persists at the time of recirculation *(arrow)*. First-pass entry of iodinated contrast agents into the extravascular compartment can be as great as 33% in normal beds and even higher in hypoperfused beds, in which the transit time of these agents is prolonged.[8]

Mathematical correction can be used to account for extravascular diffusion by deriving a curve that describes the myocardial enhancement attributable to the portion of contrast material that has diffused out of the vascular compartment (Fig. 23-8).[86] This sigmoid-shaped curve is generated by integrating the input curve from the aortic root. It is then rescaled so that the plateau at its terminal portion approximates the intensity at the terminal portion of the myocardial time–intensity curve. Correction for the diffusible properties of CT contrast agents is imperative for the estimation of myocardial blood flow in the setting of coronary artery disease, where regional differences in diffusion due to different vascular residence times and vascular permeability may be particularly confounding. Pure intravascular contrast agents, such as iodinated dextran polymer particles (with a molecular weight of approximately 30,000 d) are currently under investigation.[53] Their use may obviate the need for mathematical modeling to correct for diffusion.

Echocardiographic contrast agents

Myocardial contrast echocardiography is performed by combining cardiac ultrasound imaging with simultaneous intravascular injection of microbubbles that produce backscatter of ultrasound during their myocardial transit. Because the compressibility of a particle of a given size is the most important determinant of its ability to scatter ultrasound,[13] bubbles are the ideal ultrasound contrast agent. The ultrasonographic frequency required to produce backscatter for most microbubble agents used is within the range of frequencies routinely used for diagnostic ultrasonography.[13]

One of the earlier methods for standardizing microbubble size and concentration was sonication.[17] However, the lifespan of the bubbles produced using this technique was too short (seconds to minutes) to be useful in the clinical setting. Furthermore, the liquids in which the bubbles were prepared, such as dextrose solutions or iodinated radiopaque contrast agents, are not biologically inert. Thus, intracoronary injection of microbubbles produced in these media cause substantial (albeit transient) changes in coronary and systemic hemodynamics and in myocardial blood flow.[21,34,48] Of note, the hemodynamic effects are due to the toxic effects of the liquids themselves and not the microbubbles.[34,39,48]

When injected into the arterial system, air-filled albumin microbubbles, produced by sonication of 5% human serum albumin, are suitable for quantification of the relation of myocardial blood flow to myocardial blood volume. They produce almost no effect on systemic or coronary hemodynamics or on left ven-

tricular function (Fig. 23-9).[33,65] They are also stable, because heat generated by sonication leads to the formation of a shell, 15 nm thick, composed of insoluble denatured human albumin.[26] Encapsulation of air within this shell reduces outward diffusion of air in vitro, thereby prolonging the shelf-life. When injected intravenously, these microbubbles are removed from the blood pool by the reticuloendothelial system after their first pass, and 80% are cleared from the blood within 2 minutes.[72]

Sonicated albumin microbubbles possess a relatively narrow size distribution similar to that of erythrocytes, with a mean diameter of around 4 μm. Intravital studies using high-powered microscopy have demonstrated that the microvascular velocity profile and branch point flux of sonicated microbubbles are similar to those of erythrocytes (Fig. 23-10).[35] Figure 23-11 shows a time–intensity curve and a time–activity curve obtained from the myocardium after direct coronary injection of sonicated albumin microbubbles and ^{99m}Tc-labeled erythrocytes at the same coronary flow rate. The duration of injection (input function) was constant. A close correlation is found be-

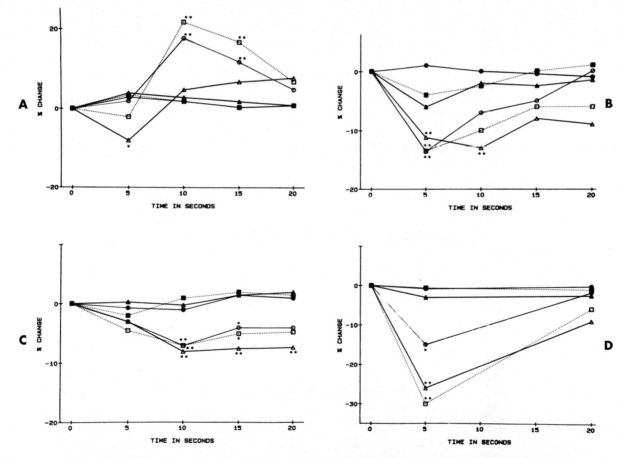

Fig. 23-9. Effect of sonicated and nonsonicated 5% human albumin and sodium meglumine diatrazoate (Renografin-76) on coronary blood flow **(A),** left ventricular dP/dt **(B),** mean arterial pressure **(C),** and **(D)** left ventricular wall thickening. Closed circles = control albumin; closed squares = 2.9-μm albumin bubbles; closed triangles = 5.5-μm albumin bubbles; open circles = control Renografin-76; open squares = sonicated Renografin-76; open triangles = hand-agitated Renografin-76. (From Keller MW, Glasheen WP, Teja K, et al: Myocardial contrast echocardiography without significant hemodynamic effects or reactive hyperemia: A major advantage in the imaging of myocardial perfusion, *J Am Coll Cardiol* 12:1039-1047, 1988. With permission of the American College of Cardiology.)

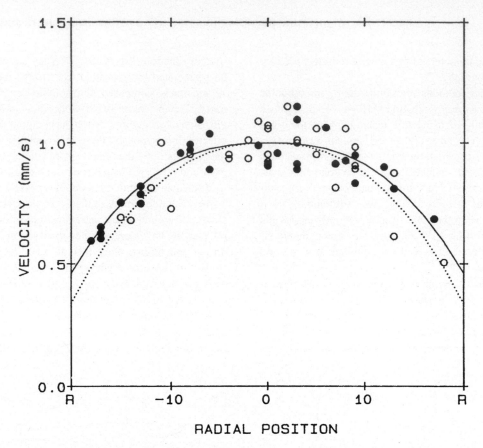

Fig. 23-10. Velocity profiles of microbubbles *(open circles)* and erythrocytes *(closed circles)* in an arteriole. The regression line describing the profile for microbubbles *(dashed line)* is similar to that obtained for erythrocytes *(solid line)*. (From Keller MW, Glasheen WP, Teja K, et al: Myocardial contrast echocardiography without significant hemodynamic effects or reactive hyperemia: A major advantage in the imaging of myocardial perfusion, *J Am Coll Cardiol* 12:1039-1047, 1988, with permission of the American College of Cardiology.)

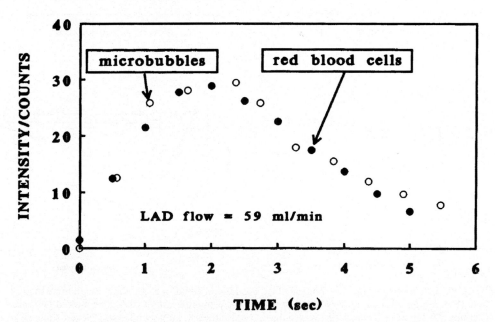

Fig. 23-11. A typical time–intensity and time–activity curve obtained from the myocardium after intracoronary injection of air-filled microbubbles and technetium-99m–labeled erythrocytes *(closed circles)* at the same flow rate in a dog. (From Jayaweera AR, Edwards N, Glasheen WP, et al: In vivo myocardial kinetics of air-filled albumin microbubbles during myocardial contrast echocardiography: comparison with radiolabeled red blood cells, *Circ Res* 74:1157-1165, 1994. With permission of the American Heart Association.)

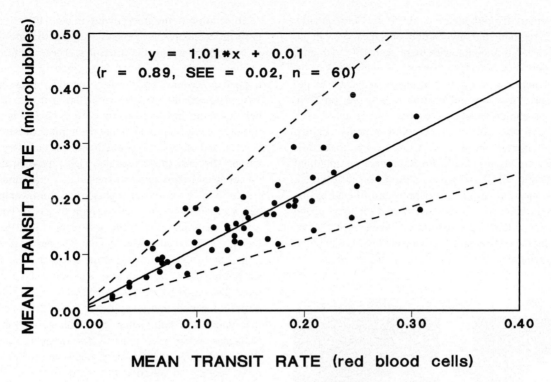

Fig. 23-12. Relation between mean transit rates (s^{-1}) of technetium-labeled erythrocytes and soni-cated albumin microbubbles after direct injection into the left anterior descending coronary artery at various flow rates. (From Jayaweera AR, Edwards N, Glasheen WP, et al: In vivo myocardial kinet-ics of air-filled albumin microbubbles during myocardial contrast echocardiography: comparison with radiolabeled red blood cells, *Circ Res* 74:1157-1165, 1994. With permission of the American Heart Association.)

Table 23-3. Characteristics of commercially produced echocardiographic contrast agents

Agent	Intravascular kinetics	Size μm	Shell concentration 10^{-9}	Shell composition	Gas
Albunex	Free flowing	4.3	0.5	Denatured albumin	Air
Optison	Free flowing	3.9	0.8	Denatured albumin	Perfluoropropane/air
DMP-115	Free flowing	2–2.5	1.0–1.5	Phospholipid/surfactant	Perfluoropropane/air
AFO150	Free flowing	5.0	0.5	Surfactant	Perfluorohexane
Sonovine	Free flowing	2.5	0.2	Phospholipid/surfactant	Sulfur hexafluoride/air
Levovist	Free flowing	2.0–4.0		Phospholipid/galactose	Air
Sonovist	Free flowing	1.0–2.0		Cyanoacrylate	Air
N100100	Free flowing				
Quantison	Free flowing	3.2	1.5	Denatured albumin	Air
AIP-201	Deposit	10.0	0.015	Denatured albumin	Air
Echogen	Deposit	3.0–10.0	3.0–5.0	No shell	Dodecafluoropentane
Sonogen	Deposit			No shell	Dodecafluoropentane

tween the mean myocardial transit rate of albumin microbub-bles and ^{99m}Tc-labeled erythrocytes through the beating heart in dogs[30] (Fig. 23-12) and in humans.[29]

Although air-filled albumin microbubbles possess many of the properties of an ideal tracer, the outward diffusion of air on exposure to blood diminishes their size. Because ultrasound backscatter is related to the sixth power of a bubble's radius, even a small decrease in its size results in a large decrease in acoustic signal.[13,14] This phenomenon limits the ability of son-

icated albumin microbubbles to produce myocardial opacifica-tion after venous injection. Left ventricular opacification after venous injection is poorer when cardiac output is reduced, be-cause time of exposure to blood before appearance in the left heart chambers is increased. In response to these limitations, second-generation microbubbles have been developed that con-tain high-molecular-weight gases with low solubility (Table 23-3). Microbubbles containing these gases have a longer half-life in blood and maintain their acoustic properties after transit through the venous and pulmonary circulations. Consequently, adequate and reproducible myocardial opacification can be achieved after venous injection with these agents.[19,40,46] Figure 23-13 shows perfusion defects in two patients with previous infarction following venous injection of one such agent. The defects correspond in intensity and location to those seen on ^{99m}Tc sestamibi single-photon emission computed tomography.

The hemodynamic effects of echocardiographic contrast agents depend largely on their size and composition. Microbubbles that are encapsulated with albumin or phospholipid shells are generally small and have a narrow size distribution. After venous injection, any larger bubbles are filtered by the pulmonary circulation so that entrapment and plugging of the coronary microvasculature are minimized.[61] As a result, venous injection produces no important alterations in myocardial blood flow or hemodynamics.[40,61]

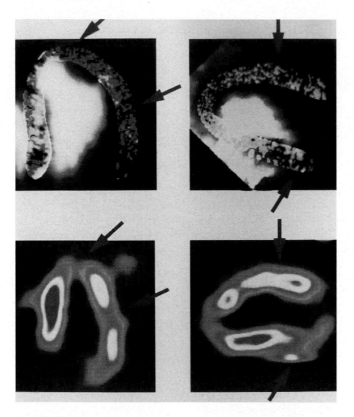

Fig. 23-13. Perfusion defects in two patients with previous myocardial infarction. The top panels show images obtained with intermittent harmonic myocardial contrast echocardiography; the bottom panels show images obtained using technetium-99m sestamibi. The first patient (*left,* four-chamber view) has a large anterolateral defect. The second patient (*right,* two-chamber view) has defects in two vascular territories: the anteroapical and the upper posterior walls. The contrast echocardiographic image from the apical two-chamber view in this patient is placed on its side to correspond to the vertical two-chamber view obtained using technetium sestamibi. (From Kaul S, Senior R, Dittrich H, et al: Detection of coronary artery disease with myocardial contrast echocardiography: comparison with 99mTc-sestamibi single-photon emission computed tomography, *Circulation* 96:785-792, 1997.)

In addition to the free-flowing tracers discussed above, deposit microbubbles have been developed that are large enough to be trapped within the arterioles. These preformed deposit bubbles cannot be injected intravenously, because they are trapped by the lungs and do not result in left heart opacification. When injected into the left atrium, left ventricle, or aorta, these bubbles result in excellent myocardial opacification and have no adverse effects provided that the number of bubbles injected is small and blocks only a fraction of the coronary microcirculation.[41] Because they have thick shells, these air-filled bubbles do not change their size on exposure to ultrasound.

One way to administer deposit tracers intravenously is to inject a liquid emulsion that converts to gas at body temperature.[24] The problem with this approach is that the size of the bubble cannot be controlled in vivo. The partial pressures of nitrogen and oxygen are higher in blood than in the bubbles. Therefore, these gases diffuse into the bubbles and enlarge them. The larger bubbles produced on initial exposure to blood obstruct the pulmonary capillaries, causing a decrease in cardiac output and pulmonary gas exchange and an increase in pulmonary artery pressures.[22,24] The smaller bubbles cross the lungs and enter the coronary microcirculation, where they grow, leading to microcirculatory obstruction.[3] Because the bubbles are large and persist in the myocardium, they produce striking myocardial opacification even after they have cleared the systemic circulation. Because of continued growth in bubble size within the myocardium, the myocardial contrast effect improves and left ventricular wall thickening and left ventricular and systemic pressures decline. Ex-vivo pre-activation of such substances may decrease some of these side effects, but the contrast enhancement is also decreased.[3]

CHARACTERISTICS OF IMAGING METHODS

To accurately quantify myocardial blood flow, the external detectors used during MRI, CT, and myocardial contrast echocardiography must fulfill certain physical prerequisites. A linear or other measurable, consistent relation must exist between the tissue concentration of the tracer and the signal intensity depicted by the imaging technique. The sensitivity of the system must allow determination of small differences in the tissue concentration of tracer. The spatial resolution must be sufficiently high to accurately assess regional and transmural differences in myocardial perfusion. The temporal resolution must also be high to assess cardiac cycle–related changes in myocardial perfusion. Finally, the availability, cost, and convenience of each imaging technique must be considered when determining its widespread clinical applicability.

Relation between tracer concentration and signal intensity

Alterations in the magnetic field produced by paramagnetic agents during MRI cause changes in the behavior of protons in their vicinity, resulting in variable signal enhancement during imaging. Effects on local magnetic moments are influenced not only by the local concentration of the paramagnetic compound but also by other imaging and tissue variables, complicating the relation between contrast concentration and MRI signal intensity.

The relative effects on T1 and T2 produced by gadolinium-containing MRI contrast agents are dependent on the dose used.[10,81] Figure 23-14 depicts MRI signal intensities obtained by using a spin-echo pulse sequence at various Gd-DTPA concentrations. At lower doses, the effect on T1 shortening predominates and causes a net increase in the MRI signal. Higher doses, which increase Gd-DTPA concentrations, result in a relatively greater effect on T2, producing a net decrease in MRI signal. Consequently, the most linear relation between Gd-DTPA concentration and T1 or T2 signal occurs at different tracer doses.

The shortening of T1 and T2 produced by MRI contrast agents is also influenced by the magnetic pulse sequences applied.[27,78] Rapid-gradient echo, produced by successive application of radiofrequency pulses, is the most commonly used sequence. It is characterized by very short repetition times (interval between radiofrequency pulses) and echo delay times (interval between initial radiofrequency pulse and signal acquisition).[25] Rapid-spin and gradient echo sequences have also been developed (echo planar imaging), in which a single radiofrequency pulse is followed by several sequential resonance signal acquisitions.[63] Different magnetic pulse sequences and signal acquisition methods encompassed by these techniques result in different relative effects on T1 and T2. The imaging method used affects the relation between the tissue concentration of the contrast agents and the degree of signal enhancement (Fig. 23-15).

The effects of paramagnetic agents on MRI relaxation times are also influenced by various local factors, such as the magnitude of myocardial blood flow[52] and the molecular environment unique to different biologic tissues.[6,10] For a given concentration of an agent, variation in proton density in different organs produces heterogeneity in the degree of signal enhancement during T1-weighted imaging (Fig. 23-16). Differences in the paramagnetic effects of MRI contrast agents may even exist among normal, ischemic, and infarcted regions of myocardium.[58] The complex relation between paramagnetic compound concentration and MRI signal described above is not prohibitive for the assessment of myocardial blood flow, provided that there is comprehensive understanding of the agents and the imaging techniques. The relation between tracer (iodine) concentration and radiographic intensity during CT is nonlinear, mostly because of imaging artifacts, such as beam hardening and photon scatter.[7,54,55] Because the transmitted X-ray beam encompasses a spectrum of energies, its mean energy at the region of interest increases or "hardens" as lower ener-

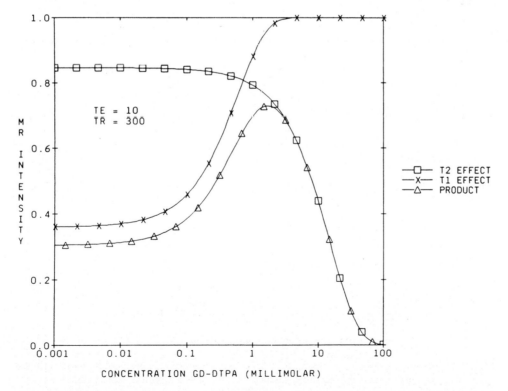

Fig. 23-14. Relative T1 and T2 effects for increasing concentration of gadolinium-DTPA. At low concentrations, T1 effects predominate, producing an increase in intensity; at higher concentrations, T2 effects are greater and lead to signal decline. The relation between tracer concentration and signal intensity *(triangles)* is therefore bimodal, with an initial increase followed by a decrease. TE = echo time; TR = sequence repetition time. (From Davis PL, Parker DL, Nelson JA, et al: Interactions of paramagnetic contrast agents and the spin echo pulse sequence, *Invest Radiol* 23:381-388, 1988.)

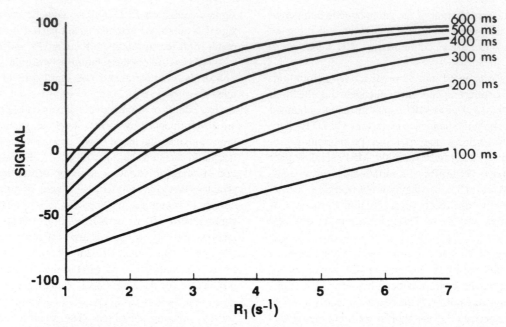

Fig. 23-15. Relation between the relaxation rate (R_1), which is proportional to gadolinium-DTPA concentration, and magnetic resonance signal intensity using a Turbo-FLASH sequence for different inversion times. (From Larsson HBW, Stubgaard M, Sondergaard L, et al: In vivo quantification of the unidirectional influx constant for Gd-DTPA diffusion across the myocardial capillaries with MR imaging, J Magn Reson Imaging 4:433-440, 1994, with permission from Elsevier Science.)

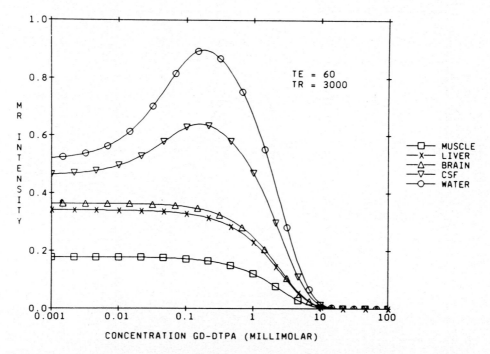

Fig. 23-16. Relation between gadolinium-DTPA and relative signal enhancement for various tissues using a T1-weighted spin-echo sequence. Tissues with the greatest proton density and, hence, the longest relaxation times are enhanced the most. TE = echo time; TR = sequence repetition time. (From Davis PL, Parker DL, Nelson JA, et al: Interactions of paramagnetic contrast agents and the spin echo pulse sequence, *Invest Radiol* 23:381-388, 1988.)

gies are attenuated by interposing tissue. This phenomenon results in a nonuniform relation between tracer concentration and CT intensity for different patients and even in various cardiac regions within the same patient.[43]

All imaging techniques that rely on radiographic energy are subject to artifacts caused by photon scatter, the degree of which depends on the geometry and energy of the beam and patient characteristics. Detection of radiographic energy from nonincident sources may introduce error in the actual degree of contrast enhancement. This limitation has been reduced but not eliminated by the use of parallel-hole collimators.

Beam hardening and photon scatter are particularly troublesome following venous injection of contrast agents when substantially higher concentrations of iodine accumulate in the left ventricular cavity compared with the myocardium.[7,54] As depicted in Fig. 23-17, artifacts caused by high concentration of iodine in the cavity adjacent to myocardial regions of interest may affect the intensity of various segments before myocardial appearance of the tracer and adversely affect estimations of myocardial tracer transit. Complex reconstruction algorithms

that correct for these artifacts are necessary for CT perfusion imaging to be clinically applicable.

Ultrasonographic systems used for routine echocardiography are not ideal for myocardial contrast echocardiography because of their limited dynamic range (the ratio of the highest to the lowest possible signal that can be measured). The number of bits on the analyze-to-digital converter for each channel determines this ratio and averages only 60 to 80 dB for most systems currently in use. Another variable that affects dynamic range is system noise, which is caused by leaks from the beam former, electrical connections, and the large number of interfaces within a system. To eliminate noise, most ultrasonographic systems have a threshold below which a signal is not registered, thus further decreasing the dynamic range of the system. The threshold that the microbubble concentration must exceed before contrast signal is detected in the tissue reduces the sensitivity of the system, particularly after venous injection of contrast, which is associated with a low myocardial concentration of microbubbles.[29]

The ultrasonographic signal threshold not only decreases the

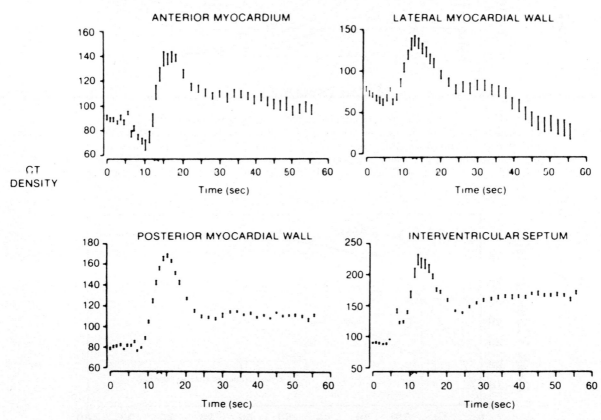

Fig. 23-17. Time–density curves for computed tomography, obtained simultaneously from four normal myocardial regions after intravenous injection of iohexol. The high concentration of iodine in the left ventricular cavity results in an artificial reduction in the myocardial intensity just before contrast appearance in the myocardium, which is most profound in the anterior segment *(arrow).* This artifact produces heterogeneity in the time–intensity curves from the various myocardial regions. (From Rumberger JA, Feiring AJ, Lipton MJ, et al: Use of ultrafast computed tomography to quantitate regional myocardial perfusion: A preliminary report, *J Am Coll Cardiol* 9:59-69, 1987. With permission of the American College of Cardiology.)

sensitivity of myocardial contrast echocardiography but may also adversely influence calculations of mean transit rate of microbubble tracers through the myocardium. As shown in Fig. 23-18, the threshold effect truncates the lower portion of the time–intensity curve and results in an artificial narrowing of the curve. As a result of this narrowing, the transit rate will overestimate myocardial blood flow, the extent of which varies depending on the dose of microbubbles used, the image postprocessing settings employed, and the ultrasonographic system used.[29,62]

The relation between microbubble concentration and video intensity is exponential; a linear range occurs only at lower concentrations (Fig. 23-19). The flat portion of the curve at higher concentrations is due in part to system saturation[30,62] and in part to the bubbles themselves. Because ultrasonographic backscatter must be displayed on a video screen with an even smaller dynamic range (30 to 40 dB) than the received signal (100 dB), some compression of the received signal must occur. When they reach a certain concentration, the bubbles scatter a large portion of the transmitted signal. Further increases in concentration result in decreases in video intensity because of attenuation of transmitted ultrasonographic energy.[30] To use video intensity as a surrogate of microbubble concentration, it is imperative that the number of bubbles injected be small enough to produce video intensities within the linear range of the curve describing the relation between the two elements.

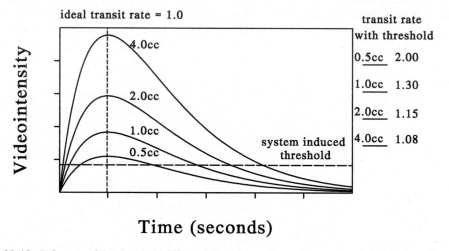

Fig. 23-18. Influence of the threshold effect of the echocardiographic system on estimation of mean microbubble transit rate. The ideal transit rate is $1.0\ s^{-1}$. Changes are apparent for different doses of microbubbles. (From Skyba DM, Jayaweera AR, Goodman NC, et al: Quantification of myocardial perfusion with myocardial contrast echocardiography during left atrial injection of contrast: implications for venous injection, *Circulation* 90:1513-1521, 1994. With permission of the American Heart Association.)

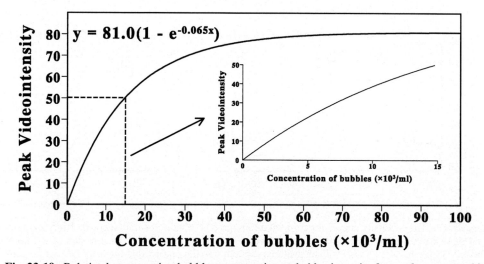

Fig. 23-19. Relation between microbubble concentration and video intensity for an ultrasonographic imaging system. (From Skyba DM, Jayaweera AR, Goodman NC, et al: Quantification of myocardial perfusion with myocardial contrast echocardiography during left atrial injection of contrast: implications for venous injection, *Circulation* 90:1513-1521, 1994. With permission of the American Heart Association.)

When exposed to ultrasound, microbubbles oscillate in a nonlinear fashion and are destroyed (Fig. 23-20).[5,13] In this process, they produce several acoustic frequencies in addition to the one at which they were insonified, which also include the harmonics of the insonification frequency. Because these harmonic signals emanate from the microbubbles and not from tissue, the signal-to-noise ratio is improved when receiving at the harmonic frequency.[40,75] Harmonic imaging results in a greater background-subtracted video intensity compared with fundamental (conventional) imaging, providing a means of detecting smaller myocardial concentrations of microbubbles.[40]

Temporal and spatial resolution

Use of MRI and CT for the evaluation of myocardial perfusion has until recently been limited by long acquisition times. Advances in imaging technology and computing power allow more rapid acquisition, thus improving temporal resolution and reducing motion artifacts and data misregistration.[55,73,77,85,86] Two rapid scanning methods have been developed for the assessment of myocardial blood flow by CT. In ultrafast CT scanning, the electron beam is successively directed to four tungsten targets that surround the patient and produce fans of radiography waves, which are received by a semicircular array of detectors. This form of imaging requires only 50 ms for digital acquisition and image reconstruction and may be gated to the electrocardiographic signal.[55,85] However, spatial resolution during ultrafast CT degraded compared with that of conventional CT, with final tomographic slice thicknesses of approximately 0.8 cm.[55] The second method uses the dynamic spatial reconstructor, which places a semicircular array of radiographic sources around the imaging subject that are activated at approximately 750-μs intervals, resulting in a single sweep that takes just over 10 ms.[42] Because of its complexity and cost, however, the dynamic spatial reconstructor is unlikely to be used clinically.

The reduction of acquisition times and sampling intervals has substantially diminished motion error with cardiac MRI and has permitted evaluation of myocardial tracer transit with adequate temporal resolution. Fast-gradient echo pulse sequences allow subsecond acquisitions of end-diastolic or end-systolic images.[44,82] Magnetic resonance imaging systems are now capable of gradient echo sequences and T1-weighted acquisition times as rapid as 100 to 200 ms. Echo planar imaging, which requires only a single radiofrequency pulse, has already achieved acquisition times of less than 100 ms. Image construction from the spectrum of received signals with all forms of cardiac MRI has also been improved by rapid Fourier analysis.

The temporal resolution of echocardiography is excellent (30 Hz using a 90° sector width with full depth). Because the speed of sound through tissue is constant, changing the size of the sector increases the sampling rate, although the use of parallel processing has increased the rate to 120 Hz without changing image size. The combination of high temporal resolution and the ability to destroy microbubbles with ultrasonography has led to the development of a novel method for quantification of myocardial perfusion after venous administration of microbubbles that does not require the application of classic indicator-dilution methods.[74] Microbubbles are delivered as a continuous infusion so that during steady state, their concentration in tissue is proportional to the myocardial blood volume fraction of tissue. The bubbles are then destroyed by an ultrasonographic pulse and their rate of replenishment in myocardial tissue is measured, providing an estimate of microbubble velocity which, in turn, reflects erythrocyte velocity.[30,35] Figure 23-21 illustrates this approach.

Consider the elevation (thickness) of an ultrasonographic beam to be E. After microbubbles are destroyed (A), the degree of beam replenishment will depend upon their velocity in tissue as well as the time between ultrasound pulses (pulsing inter-

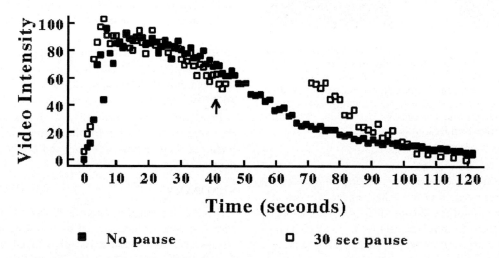

Fig. 23-20. Effect of pausing ultrasound on video intensity. (From Wei K, Skyba DM, Firschke C, et al: Interactions between microbubbles and ultrasound: in vitro and in vivo observations, *J Am Coll Cardiol* 29:1081-1088, 1997. With permission of the American College of Cardiology.)

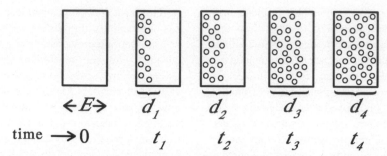

Fig. 23-21. Schematic diagram depicting microbubble replenishment of the ultrasonographic beam elevation *(E)* for different pulsing intervals. If all of the microbubbles in the elevation are destroyed by a single pulse of ultrasound at t_0, replenishment of the beam elevation (**B** to **E**) will depend on the velocity of microbubbles and the ultrasound pulsing interval t. (From Wei K, Jayaweera AR, Firoozan S, et al: Quantification of myocardial blood flow with ultrasound-induced destruction of microbubbles administered as a constant venous infusion, *Circulation* 97:473-483, 1998. With permission of the American Heart Association.)

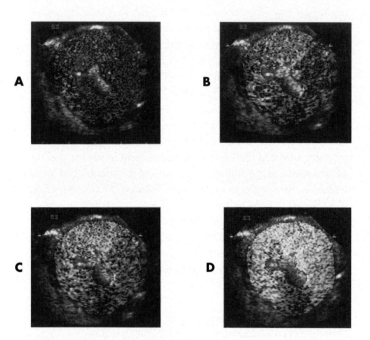

Fig. 23-22. End-systolic images obtained at a constant left anterior descending artery flow at four pulsing intervals (316, 536, 1608, and 5360 ms, respectively, in **A** to **D**). (From Wei K, Jayaweera AR, Firoozan S, et al: Quantification of myocardial blood flow with ultrasound-induced destruction of microbubbles administered as a constant venous infusion, *Circulation* 97:473-483, 1998. With permission of the American Heart Association.)

val). For the same microbubble velocity, as the pulsing interval is progressively increased *(B to D)*, enhancement of video intensity will be noted until the pulsing interval is long enough for the microbubbles to fill the entire beam *(E)*, after which prolongation of the pulsing interval will no longer result in an increase in video intensity.

Figure 23-22 illustrates four images obtained at end systole in a dog in which myocardial blood flow was altered mechani-

cally. The concentration and venous infusion rate of the microbubbles were constant, as was the flow in the left anterior descending coronary artery. The only difference between the images was the pulsing interval. When the pulsing interval was short, very little microbubble replenishment was seen *(A)*. As the pulsing interval increased, greater replenishment was noted *(B to D)* until a pulsing interval was reached *(D)* beyond which no further increase in video intensity was seen.[74]

When the pulsing interval versus video intensity data was plotted at different flows in a single dog, a faster rate constant was noted at higher flow rates (Fig. 23-23,*A*). The correlation between flow and the rate constant (signifying microbubble velocity) was also excellent (Fig. 23-23,*B*). Figure 23-24 illustrates data obtained from a model of coronary stenosis in which resting flow was normal. Flow disparities between the left anterior descending and left circumflex beds were induced by exogenous hyperemia. Flows in both beds were measured with radiolabeled microspheres and by the product of plateau video intensity (denoting the microbubble cross-sectional area) and microbubble velocity. An excellent relation was noted between the ratio of flows in the two beds derived by using both methods.[74] This method can also provide information regarding the transmural distribution of myocardial blood flow. This new myocardial contrast echocardiography method is being investigated clinically. In all likelihood, it will become the main approach for the quantification of myocardial perfusion (both capillary density and erythrocyte velocity) in humans.

SUMMARY

Each of the imaging methods discussed in this chapter has been historically characterized by excellent spatial resolution. Assessment of regional myocardial blood flow has become feasible with MRI and CT by improving the temporal resolution, which is excellent for myocardial contrast echocardiography. A unique approach independent of classic tracer

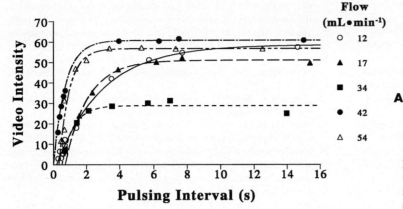

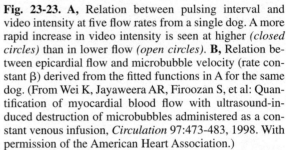

A

Fig. 23-23. A, Relation between pulsing interval and video intensity at five flow rates from a single dog. A more rapid increase in video intensity is seen at higher *(closed circles)* than in lower flow *(open circles)*. **B,** Relation between epicardial flow and microbubble velocity (rate constant β) derived from the fitted functions in A for the same dog. (From Wei K, Jayaweera AR, Firoozan S, et al: Quantification of myocardial blood flow with ultrasound-induced destruction of microbubbles administered as a constant venous infusion, *Circulation* 97:473-483, 1998. With permission of the American Heart Association.)

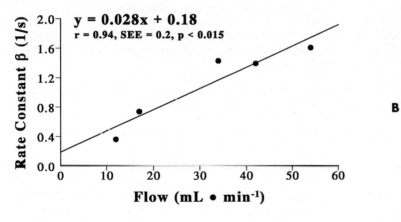

B

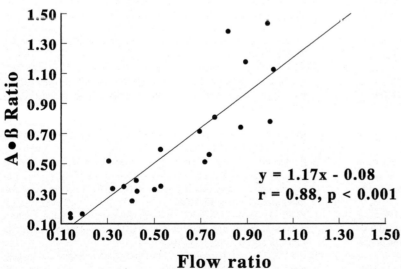

Fig. 23-24. Relation between the ratio of radiolabeled microsphere–derived myocardial blood flow from the stenosed and nonstenosed beds and the ratio derived by myocardial contrast echocardiography (using the product of microbubble velocity and plateau intensity). (From Wei K, Jayaweera AR, Firoozan S, et al: Quantification of myocardial blood flow with ultrasound-induced destruction of microbubbles administered as a constant venous infusion, *Circulation* 97: 473-483, 1998. With permission of the American Heart Association.)

kinetic models has been developed for myocardial contrast echocardiography, in which myocardial blood flow is calculated by the product of microbubble microvascular velocity and microvascular cross-sectional area at steady state. These techniques may provide an accurate assessment of myocar-

dial perfusion and, therefore, show great promise for providing valuable information in the routine clinical setting. Cost, ease of operation, and feasibility in the day-to-day practice of cardiology will determine which techniques will predominate.

REFERENCES

1. Almen T: Contrast media: the relation of chemical structure, animal toxicity and adverse clinical effects, *Am J Cardiol* 66:2F–8F, 1990.
2. Assem E, Bray K, Dawson P: The release of histamine from human basophils by radiological contrast agents, *Br J Radiol* 56:647–652, 1983.
3. Beppu S, Matsuda H, Shishido T, et al: Prolonged myocardial contrast echocardiography via peripheral venous administration of QW3600 injection (Echo-Gen): its efficacy and side effects, *J Am Soc Echocardiogr* 10:11–24, 1997.
4. Brasch RC, Weinmann H, Wesbey GE: Contrast-enhanced NMR imaging: animal studies using gadolinium-DTPA complex, *AJR Am J Roentgenol* 142:625–630, 1984.
5. Burns PN: Harmonic imaging with ultrasound contrast agents, *Clin Radiol* 51Suppl I:50–55, 1996.
6. Bydder GM, Young IR: Clinical use of the partial saturation and saturation recovery sequences in MR imaging, *J Comput Assist Tomogr* 9:1020–1032, 1985.
7. Canty JM Jr: Measurement of myocardial perfusion by fast computed tomography, *Am J Card Imaging* 7:309–316, 1993.
8. Canty JM Jr, Judd RM, Brody AS, et al: First-pass entry of nonionic contrast agent into the extravascular space. Effects on radiographic estimates of transit time and blood volume, *Circulation* 84:2071–2078, 1991.
9. Crystal GJ, Downey HF, Bashour FA: Small vessel and total coronary blood volume during intracoronary adenosine, *Am J Physiol* 241:H194–H201, 1981.
10. Davis PL, Parker DL, Nelson JA, et al: Interactions of paramagnetic contrast agents and the spin echo pulse sequence, *Invest Radiol* 23:381–388, 1988.
11. Dawson P: Chemotoxicity of contrast media and clinical adverse effects: a review, *Invest Radiol* 20(1 suppl):S81–S91, 1985.
12. Dawson P: Cardiovascular effects of contrast agents, *Am J Cardiol* 64:2E–9E, 1989.
13. de Jong N, ten Cate FJ, Lancee CT, et al: Principles and recent developments in ultrasound contrast agents, *Ultrasonics* 29:324–330, 1991.
14. de Jong N, Ten Cate FJ, Vletter WB, et al: Quantification of transpulmonary echo-contrast effects, *Ultrasound Med Biol* 19:279–288, 1993.
15. de Roos A, van der Wall EE: Evaluation of ischemic heart disease by magnetic resonance imaging and spectroscopy, *Radiol Clin North Am* 32:581–592, 1994.
16. Dundore RL, Silver PJ, Ezrin AM, et al: The effects of iodixanol and iopamidol on hemodynamic and cardiac electrophysiologic parameters in vitro and in vivo, *Invest Radiol* 26:715–721, 1991.
17. Feinstein SB, Ten Cate F, Zwehl W, et al: Two-dimensional contrast echocardiography. I. In vitro development and quantitative analysis of echo contrast agents, *J Am Coll Cardiol* 3:14–20, 1984.
18. Ferrucci JT, Stark DD: Iron oxide-enhanced MR imaging of the liver and spleen: review of the first 5 years, *AJR Am J Roentgenol* 155:943–950, 1990.
19. Firschke C, Lindner JR, Wei K, et al: Myocardial perfusion imaging in the setting of coronary artery stenosis and acute myocardial infarction using venous injection of a second generation echocardiographic contrast agent, *Circulation* 96:959–967, 1997.
20. Friedman HZ, DeBoe SF, McGillem MJ, et al: Immediate effects of graded ionic and nonionic contrast injections on coronary blood flow and myocardial function. Implications for digital coronary angiography, *Invest Radiol* 22:722–727, 1987.
21. Gillam LD, Kaul S, Fallon JT, et al: Functional and pathologic effects of multiple echocardiographic contrast injections on the myocardium, brain and kidney, *J Am Coll Cardiol* 6:687–694, 1985.
22. Gong Z, Giraud G, Pantely G, et al: Time course of chamber and myocardial contrast opacification with Echogen: a videodensitometric study in monkeys with microvascular visualization studies in a cat mesentery model, *Circulation* 90:I–556, 1994 (abstract).
23. Gould RG: Perfusion quantitation by ultrafast computed tomography, *Invest Radiol* 27Suppl 2:S18–S21, 1992.
24. Grayburn PA, Erickson JM, Escobar J, et al: Peripheral intravenous myocardial contrast echocardiography using a 2% dodecafluoropen-

tane emulsion: identification of myocardial risk area and infarct size in the canine model of ischemia, *J Am Coll Cardiol* 26:1340–1347, 1995.
25. Haase A, Matthaei D, Bartkowski R, et al: Inversion recovery snapshot FLASH MR imaging, *J Comput Assist Tomogr* 13:1036–1040, 1989.
26. Hellebust H, Christiansen C, Skotland T: Biochemical characterization of air-filled albumin microsphere, *Biotechnol Appl Biochem* 18:227–229, 1993.
27. Higgins CB, Saeed M, Wendland M: Contrast enhancement for the myocardium, *Magn Reson Med* 22:347–353, 1991.
28. Hine AL, Lui D, Dawson R: Contrast media osmolality and plasma volume changes, *Acta Radiol [Diagn] (Stockh)* 26:753–756, 1985.
29. Ismail S, Jayaweera AR, Camarano G, et al: Relation between air-filled albumin microbubble and red blood cell rheology in the human myocardium. Influence of echocardiographic systems and chest wall attenuation, *Circulation* 94:445–541, 1996.
30. Jayaweera AR, Edwards N, Glasheen WP, et al: In vivo myocardial kinetics of air-filled albumin microbubbles during myocardial contrast echocardiography. Comparison with radiolabeled red blood cells, *Circ Res* 74:1157–1165, 1994.
31. Johnston DL, Liu P, Lauffer RB, et al: Use of gadolinium-DTPA as a myocardial perfusion agent: potential applications and limitations for magnetic resonance imaging, *J Nucl Med* 28:871–877, 1987.
32. Karstoft J, Baath L, Jansen I, et al: Calcium antagonistic effects of an angiographic contrast medium in vitro: A comparison of the effects of iohexol with the effects of nifedipine in isolated arteries, *Invest Radiol* 30:21–27, 1995.
33. Keller MW, Glasheen WP, Kaul S: Albunex: a safe and effective commercially produced agent for myocardial contrast echocardiography, *J Am Soc Echocardiogr* 2:48–52, 1989.
34. Keller MW, Glasheen WP, Teja K, et al: Myocardial contrast echocardiography without significant hemodynamic effects or reactive hyperemia: a major advantage in the imaging of regional myocardial perfusion, *J Am Coll Cardiol* 12:1039–1047, 1988.
35. Keller MW, Segal SS, Kaul S, et al: The behavior of sonicated albumin microbubbles within the microcirculation: a basis for their use during myocardial contrast echocardiography, *Circ Res* 65:458–467, 1989.
36. Klopp R, Niemer W, Schippel W, et al: Changes in the microcirculation of the intact rat heart after iodinated and gadolinium-containing contrast media, *Invest Radiol* 30:69–74, 1995.
37. Kraitchman DL, Wilke N, Hexeberg E, et al: Myocardial perfusion and function in dogs with moderate coronary stenosis, *Magn Reson Med* 35:771–780, 1996.
38. Larsson HBW, Stubgaard M, Sondergaard L, et al: In vivo quantification of the unidirectional influx constant for Gd-DTPA diffusion across the myocardial capillaries with MR imaging, *J Magn Reson Imaging* 4:433–440, 1994.
39. Lang RM, Borow KM, Neumann A, et al: Effects of intracoronary injections of sonicated microbubbles on left ventricular contractility, *Am J Cardiol* 60:166–171, 1987.
40. Lindner JR, Firschke C, Wei K, et al: Myocardial perfusion characteristics and hemodynamic profile of MRX-115, a venous echocardiographic contrast agent during acute myocardial infarction, *J Am Soc Echocardiogr* 11:36–46, 1998.
41. Linka A, Ates G, Wei K: Three-dimensional myocardial contrast echocardiography validation of in-vivo risk area and infarct size, *J Am Coll Cardiol* 30:1892–1899, 1997.
42. Liu YH, Shu NH, Ritman EL: A fast computed tomographic imaging method for myocardial perfusion, *Am J Card Imaging* 7:301–308, 1993.
43. Ludman PF, Darby M, Tomlinson N, et al: Cardiac flow measurement by ultrafast CT: validation of continuous and pulsatile flow, *J Comput Assist Tomogr* 16:795–803, 1992.
44. Manning WJ, Atkinson DJ, Grossman W, et al: First-pass nuclear magnetic resonance imaging studies using gadolinium-DTPA in patients with coronary artery disease, *J Am Coll Cardiol* 18:959–965, 1991.
45. Meyers WW, Honig CR: Number and distribution of capillaries as determinants of myocardial oxygen tension, *Am J Physiol* 207:653–660, 1964.

46. Meza M, Greener Y, Hunt R, et al: Myocardial contrast echocardiography: reliable, safe, and efficacious myocardial perfusion assessment after intravenous injections of a new echocardiographic contrast agent, *Am Heart J* 132:871–881, 1996.

47. Miller DD, Holmvang G, Gill JB, et al: MRI detection of myocardial perfusion changes by gadolinium-DTPA infusion during dipyridamole hyperemia, *Magn Reson Med* 10:246–255, 1989.

48. Moore CA, Smucker ML, Kaul S: Myocardial contrast echocardiography in humans: I. Safety—a comparison with routine coronary arteriography, *J Am Coll Cardiol* 8:1066–1072, 1986.

49. Nishimura T, Kobayashi H, Ohara Y, et al: Serial assessment of myocardial infarction by using gated MR imaging and Gd-DTPA, *Am J Roentgenol* 153:715–720, 1989.

50. Pflugfelder PW, Wendland MF, Holt WW, et al: Acute myocardial ischemia: MR imaging with Mn-TP, *Radiology* 167:129–133, 1988.

51. Pomeroy OH, Wendland M, Wagner S, et al: MRI of acute myocardial ischemia using a manganese chelate, Mn-DPDP, *Invest Radiol* 531–536, 1989.

52. Ratner AV, Okada RD, Newell JB, et al: The relationship between proton nuclear magnetic resonance relaxation parameters and myocardial perfusion with acute coronary arterial occlusion and reperfusion, *Circulation* 71:823–828, 1985.

53. Revel D, Chambon C, Havard P, et al: Iodinated polymer as blood-pool contrast agent. Computed tomography evaluation in rabbits, *Invest Radiol* 26 Suppl 1:S57–S59, 1991.

54. Rumberger JA, Bell MR, Feiring AJ, et al: *Measurement of myocardial perfusion using fast computed tomography.* In Marcus M, Schelbert HR, Skorton DJ, et al, eds: *Cardiac Imaging,* Philadelphia, 1991, WB Saunders Company.

55. Rumberger JA, Feiring AJ, Lipton MJ, et al: Use of ultrafast computed tomography to quantitate regional myocardial perfusion: a preliminary report, *J Am Coll Cardiol* 9:59–69, 1987.

56. Saeed M, Wendland MF, Masui T, et al: Myocardial infarction: assessment with an intravascular MR contrast medium. Work in progress, *Radiology* 180:153–160, 1991.

57. Saeed M, Wendland MF, Takehara Y, et al: Reversible and irreversible injury in the reperfused myocardium: differentiation with contrast material-enhanced MR imaging, *Radiology* 175:633–637, 1990.

58. Schaefer S, Malloy CR, Katz J, et al: Gadolinium-DTPA-enhanced nuclear magnetic resonance imaging of reperfused myocardium: identification of the myocardial bed at risk, *J Am Coll Cardiol* 12:1064–1072, 1988.

59. Schmiedl U, Ogan M, Paajanen H, et al: Albumin labeled with Gd-DTPA as an intravascular, blood pool-enhancing agent for MR imaging: biodistribution and imaging studies, *Radiology* 162 (1 Pt 1): 205–210, 1987.

60. Sheu SH, Hwang MH, Piao ZE, et al: Effects of contrast media on coronary hemodynamics and myocardial metabolism, *Invest Radiol* 30:28–32, 1995.

61. Skyba DM, Camarano G, Goodman NC, et al: Hemodynamic characteristics, myocardial kinetics and microvascular rheology of FS-069, a second-generation contrast agent capable of producing myocardial opacification from a venous injection, *J Am Coll Cardiol* 28: 1292–1300, 1996.

62. Skyba DM, Jayaweera AR, Goodman NC, et al: Quantification of myocardial perfusion with myocardial contrast echocardiography during left atrial injection of contrast. Implications for venous injection, *Circulation* 90:1513–1521, 1994.

63. Stehling MK, Turner R, Mansfield P: Echo-planar imaging: magnetic resonance imaging in a fraction of a second, *Science* 154:43–50, 1991.

64. Strich G, Hagan PL, Gerber KH, et al: Tissue distribution and magnetic resonance spin lattice relaxation effects of gadolinium-DTPA, *Radiology* 154:723–726, 1985.

65. Ten Cate FJ, Widimsky P, Cornel JH, et al: Intracoronary albunex. Its effect on left ventricular hemodynamics, function, and coronary sinus flow in humans, *Circulation* 88(5 pt 1):2123–2127, 1993.

66. Unger E, Fritz T, Shen DK, et al: Manganese-based liposomes. Comparative approaches, *Invest Radiol* 28:933–938, 1993.

67. van der Wall EE, Vliegen HW, de Roos A, et al: Magnetic resonance imaging in coronary artery disease, *Circulation* 92:2723–2739, 1995.

68. van Dijkman PRM, Doornbos J, de Roos A, et al: Improved detection of acute myocardial infarction by magnetic resonance imaging using gadolinium-DTPA, *Int J Card Imaging* 5:1–8, 1989.

69. van Dijkman PRM, van der Wall EE, de Roos A, et al: Acute, subacute, and chronic myocardial infarction: quantitative analysis of gadolinium-enhanced MR images, *Radiology* 180:147–151, 1991.

70. van Hecke P, Marchal G, Bosmans H: NMR imaging study of the pharmacodynamics of polylysine-gadolinium-DTPA in the rabbit and the rat, *Magn Reson Imaging* 9:313–321, 1991.

71. van Rugge FP, Boreel JJ, van der Wall EE, et al: Cardiac first-pass and myocardial perfusion in normal subjects assessed by sub-second Gd-DTPA enhanced MR imaging, *J Comput Assist Tomogr* 15:959–965, 1991.

72. Walday P, Tolleshaug H, Gjoen T, et al: Biodistributions of air-filled albumin microspheres in rats and pigs, *Biochem J* 299(Pt 2):437–443, 1994.

73. Wang T, Wu X, Chung N, et al: Myocardial blood flow estimated by synchronous, multislice, high-speed computed tomography, *IEEE Trans Med Imaging* 8:70–77, 1989.

74. Wei K, Jayaweera AR, Firoozan S, et al: Quantification of myocardial blood flow with ultrasound-induced destruction of microbubbles administered as a constant venous infusion, *Circulation* 97:473–483, 1998.

75. Wei K, Skyba DM, Firschke C, et al: Interactions between microbubbles and ultrasound: in vitro and in vivo observations, *J Am Coll Cardiol* 29:1081–1088, 1997.

76. Weinmann HJ, Brasch RC, Press WR, et al: Characteristics of gadolinium-DTPA complex: a potential NMR contrast agent, *AJR Am J Roentgenol* 142:619–624, 1984.

77. Weiss RM, Otoadese EA, Noel MP, et al: Quantitation of absolute regional myocardial perfusion using cine computed tomography, *J Am Coll Cardiol* 23:1186–1193, 1994.

78. Wendland MF, Saeed M, Higgins CB: Strategies for differential enhancement of myocardial ischemia using echoplanar imaging, *Invest Radiol* 26Suppl 1:S236–S238, 1991.

79. Wesbey GE, Higgins CB, McNamara MT, et al: Effect of gadolinium DTPA on the magnetic relaxation times of normal and infarcted myocardium, *Radiology* 153:165–169, 1984.

80. Wilke N, Jerosch-Herold M, Stillman AE, et al: Concepts of myocardial perfusion imaging in magnetic resonance imaging, *Magn Reson Q* 10:249–286, 1994.

81. Wilke N, Kroll K, Merkle H, et al: Regional myocardial blood volume and flow: first-pass MR imaging with polylysine-Gd-DTPA, *J Magn Reson Imaging* 5:227–237, 1995.

82. Wilke N, Simm C, Zhang J, et al: Contrast-enhanced first pass myocardial perfusion imaging: correlation between myocardial blood flow in dogs at rest and during hyperemia, *Magn Reson Med* 29:485–497, 1993.

83. Wolf GL: *Contrast agents for cardiac MRI.* In Marcus ML, Schelbert HR, Skorton DJ, et al, eds: *Cardiac imaging,* Philadelphia, 1991, WB Saunders Company.

84. Wolfkiel CJ, Brundage BH: Transfer-function analysis of UFCT myocardial time-density curves by time-varying recursive least squares analysis, *IEEE Trans Biomed Eng* 41:69–76, 1994.

85. Wolfkiel CJ, Ferguson JL, Chomka EV, et al: Measurement of myocardial blood flow by ultrafast computed tomography, *Circulation* 76:1262–1273, 1987.

86. Wu XS, Ewert DL, Liu YH, et al: In vivo relation of intramyocardial blood volume to myocardial perfusion. Evidence supporting microvascular site for autoregulation, *Circulation* 85:730–737, 1992.

87. Zelis R, Caudill CC, Baggette K, et al: Reflex vasodilation induced by coronary angiography in human subjects, *Circulation* 53:490–493, 1976.

Chapter 24

Assessment of revascularization

Robert C. Hendel

Coronary artery revascularization is a key strategy in the modern management of ischemic heart disease. Coronary artery bypass graft (CABG) surgery was, until recently, the most frequently performed surgical procedure in the United States, with more than 300,000 operations performed annually.[128] The number of CABG procedures has been surpassed by the number of percutaneous transluminal coronary angioplasties (PTCA).[17,128] The remarkable growth of these revascularization techniques since their inception 30 years ago not only has provided the clinician with new treatments for coronary disease but has also introduced new variables into the use of noninvasive techniques, such as myocardial perfusion imaging and radionuclide angiography.

Coronary angiography provides a clinically valuable measure of the severity of ischemic heart disease and is the gold standard to which noninvasive methods are often compared. However, angiography provides anatomic evaluation only and cannot assess the physiologic significance of an individual coronary lesion. The estimation of the potential for a given lesion to cause myocardial ischemia is one of the key applications of myocardial scintigraphy. The two primary techniques used in nuclear cardiology for the evaluation of patients before and after coronary revascularization are myocardial perfusion imaging and radionuclide angiography. Despite the obvious differences in these methods and their specific applications, true distinctions have become somewhat blurred, with the advent of functional assessment (first-pass angiography and gated single-photon emission computed tomography [SPECT]) as part of perfusion imaging.

Nuclear cardiology pioneered the movement toward an outcome-based approach to the assessment and treatment of ischemic heart disease. The field has demonstrated its ability to be a valuable marker of cardiac risk and has extended the applications of nuclear methods beyond the boundaries of detection of coronary artery disease. Perhaps the greatest value of perfusion imaging and radionuclide angiography is their ability to predict future cardiac events and identify high-risk patients who may benefit from additional therapies.[20] This is of critical importance when the diagnosis of coronary artery disease is already established. Thus, in patients being considered for revascularization or those who have had CABG surgery or coronary angioplasty, the value of noninvasive testing is primarily related to the ability of the procedure to provide prognostic information.

In the current climate of accelerating health care costs and the need to strive for cost-effectiveness, it is also crucial that nuclear cardiology methods demonstrate incremental value beyond that obtained with less expensive methods, such as electrocardiographic stress testing. Several studies examining the incremental value of perfusion imaging have shown that it adds significantly to the prediction of cardiac events and is superior to coronary angiography for risk stratification.[75,143] A normal myocardial perfusion imaging study yields a very low risk for a cardiac event (<0.05% per year), thus potentially obviating the need for revascularization in such patients. Alternatively, high-risk patients may then be selected for angioplasty or bypass surgery.

SELECTION FOR REVASCULARIZATION

The overall value of myocardial perfusion imaging and radionuclide angiography for identification of the severity and extent of coronary artery disease is beyond the scope of this chapter. However, these findings, along with the determination of myocardial viability and other factors, are important considerations with regard to the selection of patients for PTCA or CABG surgery (Box 24-1). To maximize the potential benefits of coronary revascularization and to reduce the risk associated with the procedure, selection of the most appropriate patients must be based on the clear evidence of the benefits of revascularization.

Despite the undisputed clinical value of cardiac catheterization, the degree of a given stenosis may vary greatly with regard to the physiologic risk it confers and the potential for the lesion to cause myocardial ischemia. The need to assess the physiologic importance of angiographic stenosis of intermediate severity is a common clinical problem.[176] Andreas Gruentzig, the forefather of coronary angioplasty, and his colleagues emphasized the need to examine more than coronary anatomy and concluded that "imaging post-catheterization permits evaluation of the physiologic significance of an observed lesion."[58] Evaluation of the ischemia-producing potential of individual coronary arteries is thus of vital importance when considering coronary revascularization. Myocardial perfusion imaging is more valuable for determining the importance of a specific stenosis before angioplasty than CABG surgery, in which all potentially significant lesion are bypassed.[150]

The ability to identify the "culprit" lesion with myocardial perfusion imaging was first demonstrated by Hirzel et al,[69] who examined the value of perfusion imaging before and after revascularization with PTCA and CABG surgery. Planar exercise thallium imaging was able to identify the ischemic zone that corresponded to a coronary stenosis in 88% of lesions. Similarly, other studies have confirmed that myocardial perfusion imaging accurately identifies the culprit stenosis in 80% to 93% of patients.[18,69,83,110,156] Identification of the culprit lesion allows the performance of limited angioplasty in patients with multivessel coronary disease. This in turn enables a strategy of incomplete revascularization to be undertaken with the potential for the successful relief of symptoms. Recently, it was shown that the identification of ischemic perfusion defects is

correlated with alterations in coronary blood flow reserve as determined by intravascular Doppler flow measurements (another physiologic marker).[33,34,88,122]

The correlation of the amount of ischemic myocardium subtended by a given stenosis is often difficult to determine by angiographic assessment alone. This is seen in the setting of acute myocardial infarction, in which angiography significantly overestimates the area at risk compared with SPECT.[74] The extent of ischemia may be determined by scintigraphic techniques, such as administration of the perfusion imaging agent during total coronary occlusion in angioplasty balloon inflation.[14,15] However, as previously noted, only a moderate correlation exists between angiographic methods and technetium-99m (^{99m}Tc) sestamibi imaging (Fig. 24-1).[61] The true estimation of ischemic risk has potentially important clinical ramifications; identification of patients with large areas of myocardium at risk enables closer surveillance in such patients and consideration of earlier revascularization.[61]

The ability of myocardial perfusion imaging to demonstrate and objectify the presence of myocardial ischemia is desirable when considering revascularization for the relief of anginal pain because the presence, location, and extent of ischemia may be delineated.[14,18] The clinician may then be able to determine whether coronary revascularization would relieve symptoms.[9] For more than 20 years, preoperative thallium-201 (^{201}Tl) scintigraphy has demonstrated the ability to predict improvement in not only perfusion but also left ventricular function after CABG surgery.[55] Gibson et al[55] showed that the presence of defect reversibility on an exercise redistribution thallium study or a mild or moderate (>50% thallium activity) persistent abnormality was associated with postoperative improvement in perfusion and function.[55]

Myocardial perfusion imaging has also shown substantial prognostic value in its ability to delineate patients at increased risk for cardiac events.[20] Not only does perfusion imaging have independent predictive value with regard to future events but it has incremental value beyond that obtained with clinical and electrocardiographic stress testing data and superior to that obtained with coronary angiography.[75,143] This may be of substantial assistance in the decision-making process for coronary revascularization. The finding of high-risk markers, such as transient ischemic dilation of the left ventricle,[174] several perfusion defects,[103] or increased lung uptake of ^{201}Tl,[56] identifies patients who are likely to benefit the most from revascularization (in terms of mortality) and indicates a more urgent need for these procedures.[20,21,93]

A problematic decision about the need for angiography and revascularization remains after thrombolytic therapy is administered for acute myocardial infarction. In this regard, sequential ^{99m}Tc sestamibi imaging (before and after administration of thrombolytic therapy) may provide information on the occurrence of coronary reperfusion and the status of vessel patency in the infarct-related artery distribution.[158,170] Because vessel patency is associated with improved outcome, perfusion imaging may indicate the presence of additional myocardium at risk

---

Box 24-1.   Value of nuclear cardiology testing before revascularization

Determination of presence of ischemia
Objective documentation of ischemia
Stratification of equivocal lesions
Identification of "culprit" lesion
Definition of the severity and extent of ischemia
Identification of high-risk patients
Detection of myocardial viability
Prediction of functional recovery

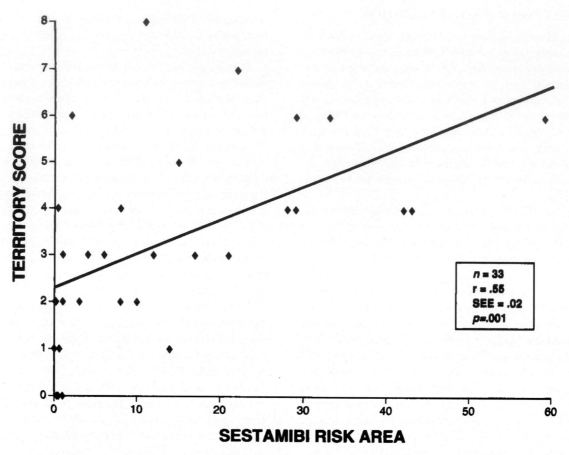

Fig. 24-1. Correlation between risk zones defined by technetium-99m sestamibi and angiography, with wide range of scintigraphic defect scores for a similar angiographic score. (Reproduced with permission from Haronian HL, Remetz MS, Sinusas AJ, et al: Myocardial risk area defined by technetium-99m sestamibi imaging during percutaneous transluminal coronary angioplasty: comparison with coronary angiography, *J Am Coll Cardiol* 22:1033-1043, 1993.)

and the need for coronary angiography and revascularization after myocardial infarction. Another example of the application of myocardial perfusion imaging was provided by Lew et al,[106] who demonstrated that a reversible rest-redistribution thallium defect after acute myocardial infarction identifies patients who may benefit from early angioplasty.

Like myocardial perfusion imaging, exercise radionuclide angiography may be used to identify patients who are at high risk for cardiac events and who may benefit most from surgical revascularization.[87,95,99,109] An abnormal functional response to exercise is associated with patients who have extensive coronary artery disease. Patients with the greatest amount of exercise-induced left ventricular dysfunction are likely to derive the greatest benefit from CABG surgery. The preoperative response to exercise predicts the postoperative improvement in exercise performance,[99] because left ventricular function at peak exercise increases substantially after CABG surgery.[95,109]

It is increasingly apparent that functional improvement after coronary revascularization may be predicted by the delineation of myocardial viability on perfusion imaging,[55,145,163] echocardiography,[4,23] or position emission tomography (PET).[169] Quantiatation of the intensity of the myocardial perfusion de-

fect seems to be important.[55,145,163] In addition, experience with PET has revealed that the improvements in systolic function noted after revascularization are correlated with a reduction in symptoms and improved survival.[36,41] Thus, methods for enhanced detection of myocardial viability are important for the evaluation of patients with left ventricular dysfunction. Numerous methods have been used; these are detailed in the chapter on myocardial viability. The increasing use of techniques to identify myocardial viability has substantial impact on the selection of patients for revascularization, especially CABG surgery.[35,36,41,145,163] The symptomatic improvement of patients with heart failure after CABG surgery is directly related to the extent and magnitude of myocardial ischemia and viability in patients with cardiomyopathy.[35] Patients with severe left ventricular dysfunction receive the most benefit with regard to improvement in function,[38,79,129,145] symptoms,[35] and overall event-free survival.[36,41] In fact, candidates for cardiac transplantation may be reevaluated by scintigraphic methods and subsequently referred for revascularization instead of transplantation on the basis of the finding of viability. Clearly, this has ramifications for resource utilization and overall health care costs.[113]

CORONARY ARTERY BYPASS GRAFT SURGERY

Coronary artery bypass graft surgery is currently the most commonly performed surgical procedure in the United States[17] and is highly effective for the reduction of symptoms and improvement of left ventricular function and survival.[180] In addition to assisting in the selection of patients for surgical revascularization, nuclear cardiology techniques may be used in patients after CABG surgery to 1) document intraoperative cardiac injury, 2) document improvement in perfusion or function after revascularization, 3) demonstrate or predict graft disease and stenosis, and 4) predict subsequent cardiac events. With regard to documentation of intraoperative cardiac injury, nuclear techniques may be particularly valuable as traditional methods (such as electrocardiography and cardiac enzymes) for the detection of perioperative infarction may be problematic in the setting of recent cardiac surgery. Infarct-avid imaging, such as indium-111 antimyosin imaging, may be of particular value, especially early in the postoperative period.[165] This radiolabeled monoclonal antibody reveals uptake only at sites where irreversible injury has occurred and is not confounded by the surgery and the use of cardiopulmonary bypass (as may occur with cardiac enzyme analysis or determinations of ventricular function).

The primary value of myocardial perfusion imaging and radionuclide angiography after CABG surgery lie in the value of these techniques for identification of graft disease or occlusion. Initial studies of graft patency rates revealed that 10% to 31% of grafts were occluded at 1 year after surgery; vein graft stenosis was 10% at 1.5 years.[47,59,126] A recent article reviewing results in more than 1300 patients reported a graft occlusion rate of approximately 2.1% per year; at 5 years, more than 48% of patients had significant graft disease, and at 15 years, 81%.[47] The risk for graft closure is approximately 12% to 20% after the first year and an additional 5% reveals significant stenosis.[48] In additionally, recurrent angina frequently develops in CABG patients,[52] because of incomplete revascularization, native disease progression, or significant graft disease.

Radionuclide angiography

After CABG surgery, radionuclide angiography may show no change from the preoperative resting left ventricular ejection fraction, even though improvement or deterioration may occur. Many reasons account for this variability, including: 1) inability to improve when preoperative function is normal, 2) perioperative infarction, 3) inability to improve function of previously infarcted myocardium, 4) functional improvement after resolution of resting ischemia (hibernation), or 5) lack of improvement of global function despite regional changes. Most often, the resting left ventricular function reveals little postoperative improvement.[53,95,109] A reduction in the resting left ventricular ejection fraction or the presence of a new wall-motion abnormality after surgery is usually indicative of an intraoperative myocardial infarction. Ideally, post-CABG evaluation of left ventricular function should be performed 3 months after surgery, when alterations in fluid status, hematocrit, and neuro-

hormone levels have resolved.[53,99] Hellman et al[66] found that 16 of 19 patients with resting left ventricular ejection fraction of less than 40% had improvement of the resting left ventricular ejection fraction and a more normal functional response to exercise, without deterioration of regional wall motion. The three patients who failed to have functional improvement were subsequently found to have had incomplete revascularization.

Even when improvement of ventricular function is noted, which may be as early as 8 days after revascularization,[5] the recovery of ventricular function after CABG surgery is often delayed.[53] The study by Ghods et al[53] revealed that functional recovery often revealed further improvement with time after revascularization, and almost 50% of patients had improved function 2 months after surgery. Therefore, the timing of the postoperative assessment of left ventricular function is important when dysfunction is present preoperatively, because an early evaluation may underestimate the benefits of coronary revascularization.[53]

After CABG surgery, impairment of the global and regional functional responses to exercise may improve substantially.* The degree of postoperative improvement is usually correlated with the severity of the compromise of preoperative function. Although in most circumstances the resting left ventricular ejection fraction fails to improve after CABG surgery[109] (especially when it is normal before surgery), most patients with an abnormal left ventricular ejection fraction response to exercise had improvement.[5,95,153] The prediction of improvement after revascularization by using radionuclide angiography was initially reported by Rozanski et al.[153] These investigators noted that postoperative recovery of function in asynergic segments was predicted by improvement in wall motion immediately after exercise. In the study by Lim et al,[109] surgical correction of stress-induced ischemia resulted in an increase in the mean peak exercise left ventricular ejection fraction from 53% to 63% (Fig. 24-2).

A common finding that was first described with radionuclide angiography but has also been noted with echocardiography and gated SPECT perfusion imaging is abnormal septal motion after CABG surgery.[151] It has been suggested that the septal abnormality may be caused by the use of cardiopulmonary bypass or myocardial preservation techniques.[2] This idea is based on the finding that abnormal septal motion is present in almost all patients after cardiopulmonary bypass, but rarely occurs outside this setting, even when CABG surgery is performed. The precise cause for this phenomenon is not known. It was initially thought that akinesis or dyskinesis of the septum might be caused by perioperative injury to the septum. However, both radionuclide angiography and gated SPECT show that although septal wall motion is paradoxical, myocardial thickening is still present, suggesting that only the pattern of contraction, not septal viability, is altered. Consistent with this observation are results of studies showing that septal perfusion and viability as

---

*References 5, 66, 95, 99, 109, 172.

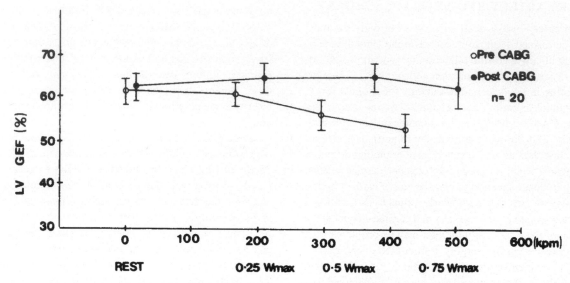

Fig. 24-2. Mean left ventricular ejection fraction during bicycle exercise before and after coronary artery bypass graft *(CABG)* surgery. (Reproduced with permission from Lim YL, Kalff V, Kelly MJ, et al: Radionuclide angiographic assessment of global and segmental left ventricular function at rest and during exercise after coronary artery bypass graft surgery, *Circulation* 66:972-979, 1982.)

assessed by thallium rest-redistribution imaging are normal in most postoperative patients, despite the presence of abnormal septal motion in almost all post-bypass patients.[133] Therefore, it seems that perioperative infarction is not the cause of septal dysfunction. It is also unlikely that myocardial stunning explains this abnormality, because severe ischemia is unlikely to cause wall-motion abnormality that persists for years after the ischemic event. Other theories advanced to explain the abnormal septal motion include increased anterior motion of the heart after CABG surgery or the presence of an open pericardium.[96,133]

Overall, events that occur early after CABG surgery seem to be dependent on left ventricular function and the completeness of revascularization. Residual disease is an important factor after surgery that affects early postoperative cardiac function.[78] Late events are more dependent on disease progression and graft disease or occlusion. After surgical revascularization, the prognostic value of radionuclide angiography is high, and exercise left ventricular ejection fraction seems to be the best predictor of mortality and total events.[76,172] In the study by Wallis, Supino, and Boer,[172] 192 patients underwent exercise radionuclide angiography at least 1 month after CABG surgery. The change in left ventricular ejection fraction with exercise was found to be the most important predictor of cardiac death, major nonsurgical cardiac events, and cardiac event–free or surgery-free survival[172] (Fig. 24-3). In this study, cardiac death rates were increased more than twofold for each 10% decrease in the change of left ventricular ejection fraction with exercise. These results confirm that left ventricular function with exercise, as determined by exercise radionuclide angiography, is an important marker of prognosis after CABG surgery.[86]

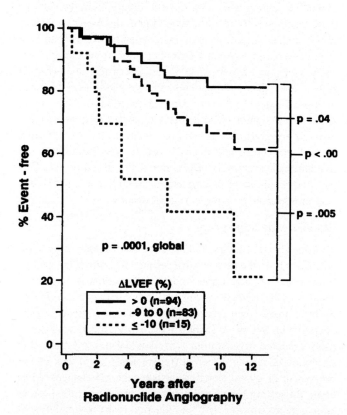

Fig. 24-3. Relation of event-free survival (cardiac death and myocardial infarction) to the change in left ventricular ejection fraction with exercise. (Reproduced with permission from Wallis J, Supino P, Borer J: Prognostic value of left ventricular ejection fraction response to exercise during long-term follow-up after coronary artery bypass graft surgery, *Circulation* 88(52):II99-II109, 1993.)

Because it is difficult to correlate wall motion with specific vascular territories, exercise radionuclide angiography is limited in its ability to predict the patency of bypass grafts. The accurate prediction of the patency of a graft and the presence of significant disease was accomplished in less than one half of 59 grafts analyzed in a study using biplane rest and exercise radionuclide angiography.[67] Thus, it seems that myocardial perfusion imaging may be better suited for the assessment of graft patency because this technique, especially when performed tomographically, can more accurately pinpoint graft disease.

Myocardial perfusion imaging

In the absence of perioperative injury or abrupt graft closure, myocardial perfusion imaging after CABG surgery will probably show improvement of coronary perfusion.[55,149,155,166] In early studies, a high correlation was noted between improvements in perfusion and the performance of successful bypass surgery.[149,155] For example, Verani et al[166] revealed that 19 of 23 post–CABG surgery patients had improved thallium uptake. However, few patients had complete normalization of thallium activity. However, lack of complete scan normalization did not preclude relief of angina and improved exercise tolerance.[166] The more reversible the stress-induced perfusion, the more likely an improvement in postoperative perfusion will occur.[55] Furthermore, if a persistent defect had a less than 50% reduction in thallium activity, improvement was noted in 57% of defects after CABG surgery compared with only 21% of defects if they were severe[55] (Fig. 24-4). Thus, even in 1983, the value of quantitation of tracer activity was demonstrated for detection of viable myocardium and its subsequent recovery of function after revascularization.

An interesting phenomenon that occurs with surprising frequency in post–CABG surgery patients was described by Watarida et al.[173] Reverse redistribution of ^{201}Tl, which has been noted 1 to 3 months after CABG surgery, occurred in 48% of the group studied. Patients with reverse redistribution after surgery had significant improvement in left ventricular function markers of viability. The cause for this may be the reestablishment of adequate coronary blood flow in regions with previous infarction. These regions were predominantly viable myocardium, as evidenced by postoperative recovery of ventricular function; thus, the presence of reverse redistribution may be a marker of potential functional improvement after CABG surgery.

The presence of new scintigraphic perfusion abnormalities often marks the development of CABG stenosis or occlusion.* Hirzel[70] et al found that 81% of patients have improved regional thallium perfusion after bypass surgery in contrast to only a 15% graft patency rate if the result of myocardial perfusion imaging is worse after surgery. Stenosis or occlusion of a bypass graft is therefore usually associated with the persistence or worsening of a preoperative perfusion abnormality. Various additional studies showed that planar ^{201}Tl imaging has been

*References 5, 70, 77, 149, 155, 182.

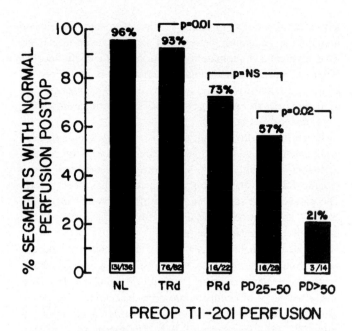

Fig. 24-4. Relation of preoperative and postoperative perfusion to the amount of thallium-201 activity, indicating that the most severe defects are less likely to demonstrate improved perfusion after bypass surgery. NL = normal; PD = persistent defect (25% to 50% or >50%); PRd = partial redistribution; TRd = total redistribution. (Reproduced with permission from Gibson RG, Watson DD, Taylor GJ, et al: Prospective assessment of regional myocardial perfusion before and after coronary revascularization surgery by quantitative thallium-201 scintigraphy, *J Am Coll Cardiol* 1:804-815, 1983.)

successfully used to detect early graft stenosis,[77,146,166,171] with diagnostic sensitivities ranging from 65% to 86%. One important limitation of perfusion imaging was noted by Wainwright et al,[171] who noted a low predictive value for vessel patency when assessing the revascularized artery subtending an infarct zone.

In an important early trial, Pfisterer et al[138] examined patients 1 year after CABG surgery and found that planar thallium imaging provided valuable information about the patency status of the aortocoronary grafts, with a sensitivity, specificity, and accuracy of 80%, 88%, and 86%, respectively. However, localization of the occluded graft was correct in only 61% of patients. This deficiency may be related to the use of planar imaging, and substantial improvement in localization of graft occlusion may be possible with SPECT. To evaluate the value of tomographic imaging, Lakkis et al[104] performed SPECT thallium imaging in 50 patients a mean of 51 months after surgery. All patients developed chest pain, although atypical symptoms were noted in 40% of the patients. The sensitivity (80%), specificity (87%), and accuracy (82%) of SPECT thallium imaging in this trial were similar to those found by Pfisterer et al with planar imaging.[138] However, the sensitivity for individual vascular territories was substantially higher with SPECT imaging—82% for the left anterior descending coronary artery, 92% for the right coronary artery, and 75% for the left circumflex coronary artery.[104] Thus, myocardial perfusion imaging can accurately detect graft stenoses, even in patients with atypical symptomatology, and can effectively localize stenoses, especially if tomographic imaging is performed. In addition, the sensitivity and accuracy of ^{201}Tl scintigraphy for graft stenosis are superior to those of electrocardiographic stress testing[104] (Fig. 24-5).

Regardless of the conduit used for coronary bypass surgery, graft patency has been assessed accurately with myocardial perfusion imaging, and a high correlation between scintigraphic findings and angiographic patency has been shown. The patency of a saphenous vein graft,[182] internal mammary artery,[84] and gastroepiploic artery[101] have all correlated with the results of perfusion imaging.

The development of chest pain or the presence of electrocardiographic abnormalities with stress testing are poor markers for the presence of coronary graft disease. Clinical markers of graft stenosis or occlusion are often inaccurate; new development or recurrence of chest pain provides a sensitivity of only 60% and a specificity of 20%.[57] Likewise, routine stress testing fails to detect a large number of graft stenoses or occlusions (low sensitivity)[7,57,171] despite high specificity (86%).[57] This may be due in part to the reduced functional capacity of the patients or a lack of electrocardiographic changes with exercise.[7] Overall, myocardial perfusion imaging has substantially higher sensitivity than electrocardiographic exercise stress testing or clinical markers for the detection of graft stenosis or occlusion.[57] In addition, perfusion imaging permits localization of the perfusion defect and correlation with the coronary anatomy and the location of grafts.

Other imaging methods have been used to detect coronary bypass graft stenoses. Both computed tomography[125] and magnetic resonance imaging[175] have been used successfully for the detection and prediction of graft disease. Positron emission tomography may also be used to detect graft stenosis. Marwick et al[117] compared dipyridamole stress testing with rubidium-82 and thallium SPECT imaging in 50 consecutive patients late after coronary artery bypass graft (6.5 years). Rubidium PET demonstrated a similar or slightly better detection rate for important graft disease than did SPECT (91% and 73%, respectively).[117]

Perhaps more important than the detection or prediction of bypass graft occlusion is the potential prognostic value of myocardial perfusion imaging for late cardiac events after CABG surgery. To evaluate the value of perfusion imaging in this context, Palmas et al[136] examined a cohort of patients who had undergone CABG surgery a minimum of 5 years earlier.[136] During the 31-month follow-up, 14% of the patients had nonfatal myocardial infarction or cardiac death and an additional 10% underwent additional revascularization at least 60 days after the initial surgery. The only clinical factors that were predictive of cardiac events were shortness of breath and peak heart rate with treadmill exercise. When scintigraphic variables from the exercise thallium study were incorporated into the predictive model, the global chi-square value more than doubled, in-

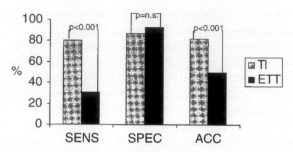

Fig. 24-5. Comparative sensitivity *(SENS)*, specificity *(SPEC)*, and overall accuracy *(ACC)* for exercise testing compared with exercise thallium-201 imaging for the detection of graft stenosis after bypass surgery. (Derived from Lakkis NM, Mahmarian JJ, Verani MS: Exercise thallium-201 single photon emission computed tomography for evaluation of coronary artery bypass graft patency, *Am J Cardiol* 76:107-111, Copyright 1995 by Excerpta Medica Inc.)

dicating the incremental value of ^{201}Tl data. The perfusion scan variables related to cardiac events were increased lung uptake and the summed reversibility score; these variables increased the odds of a cardiac event by 80% and 10%, respectively. The latter measure is a marker that reflects both the extent and severity of viable myocardium at ischemic risk (Fig. 24-6). Thus, myocardial perfusion imaging after CABG surgery has important independent prognostic value and is incrementally valuable above and beyond clinical and electrocardiographic variables, as has been shown in other patient cohorts.[75,143]

Almost all of the studies published to date examining the value of myocardial perfusion imaging in the postsurgical patient have used ^{201}Tl as the imaging agent. Iskandrian et al[80] have recently demonstrated the value of ^{99m}Tc sestamibi imaging in predicting cardiac events following bypass surgery. They report their results in only a small group of patients. Despite this limitation, it is likely that many papers will be available in the future describing the value of imaging with ^{99m}Tc agents in post-CABG patients. The greatest value with these newer agents may be the ability to determine myocardial perfusion and left ventricular function simultaneously.[80] After surgery, a direct correlation between improvement in perfusion and regional and global left ventricular function may be observed as part of the same noninvasive study.[80] As stated earlier, left ventricular function remains a principal determinant of long-term outcome in patients undergoing CABG surgery.[26,86] It is rational that improvements in perfusion are associated with increases in regional and global left ventricular function, with a resultant improvement in patient prognosis. The abnormal septal motion noted with radionuclide angiography is also present with gated SPECT or first-pass acquisitions in myocardial perfusion imaging. Although the septum appears kinetic or even dyskinetic, myocardial thickening and brightening are present on gated SPECT imaging.[96]

The use of nuclear cardiology methods for the evaluation of newer techniques in surgical coronary revascularization is not well documented. Essentially no information is available about

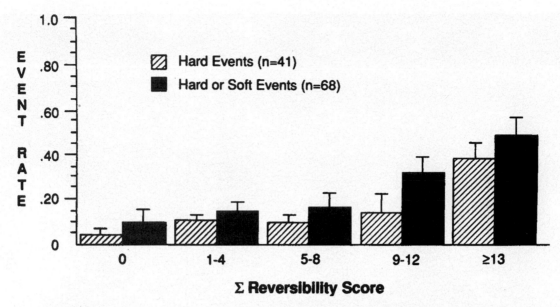

Fig. 24-6. Event rate in relation to the summed reversibility score. Hard = myocardial infarction and cardiac death; soft = hard events and revascularization. (Reproduced from Palmas W, Bingham S, Diamma GA, et al: Incremental prognostic value of exercise thallium-201 myocardial single-photon emission computed tomography late after coronary artery bypass surgery, *J Am Coll Cardiol* 25:403-409, 1995.)

prognostic utility in patients after minimally invasive ("keyhole") surgery. Furthermore, although myocardial perfusion imaging has demonstrated the potential benefits of laser revascularization, these data remain preliminary. Nonetheless, they seem to document the improvement in myocardial perfusion after laser drilling of the left ventricle.[115]

In summary, myocardial perfusion imaging may be valuable in assessing the presence, location, extent, and severity of myocardial ischemia after bypass surgery and may clarify the meaning of a positive result on an electrocardiographic stress test. Perfusion imaging may assist in the determination of whether findings are related to incomplete revascularization, new disease, or graft stenosis.[149,166] Nuclear cardiology techniques should be used only if recurrent symptoms are present; they cannot be advocated as a routine procedure in asymptomatic patients after CABG surgery.[150]

PERCUTANEOUS TRANSLUMINAL CORONARY ANGIOPLASTY (PTCA)

More than 500,000 PTCAs are performed in the United States each year.[162] The rapid rate of technical advances and improved operator expertise have enabled his technique to gain more widespread application. Despite the large number of PTCAs performed yearly, preprocedure documentation of myocardial ischemia is uncommon, occurring in only 29% of patients.[162] Thus, despite the obvious value of nuclear cardiology to detect, localize, and define the extent of ischemia, this procedure appears underutilized before performance of percutaneous revascularization. It is unclear whether this reflects an underutilization of noninvasive methods to objectively justify the performance of PTCA or whether the addi-

tion of such techniques as myocardial perfusion imaging is considered superfluous.

Pre-PTCA myocardial perfusion imaging

Myocardial perfusion imaging provides information on the extent and location of myocardial ischemia that supplements the mere detection of myocardial ischemia. The assessment of jeopardized myocardium may be performed during temporary balloon occlusion of a coronary artery and provides a measure of the relative value of PTCA in terms of the amount of jeopardized myocardium.[14-16,98,139] By intravenous injection of ^{99m}Tc sestamibi during angioplasty balloon inflation, Braat et al[15] were able to visualize the extent of myocardial ischemia supplied by a given coronary artery in 11 of 13 patients. The two patients who did not show a perfusion defect had extensive collaterals noted on angiography, thus demonstrating the potential importance of such vessels. It has also been suggested that collateral circulation protects myocardium and, when present, may cause balloon occlusion perfusion imaging to fail to reveal ischemic defects.[139]

Another use of myocardial perfusion tracer injection during angioplasty is to accurately delineate the area subtended by a specific stenosis and to provide data on the area at risk and the relative benefits of angioplasty.[98] The location of the stenosis may dictate the area at risk; this follows from the finding that the extent and severity of perfusion defects were significantly smaller in patients with proximal compared with distal left anterior descending coronary artery occlusions.[139] Sestamibi and other agents that show no clinically relevant redistribution are ideally suited to such applications, because the tracer distribution will not change between injection and imaging.[14,132] In a

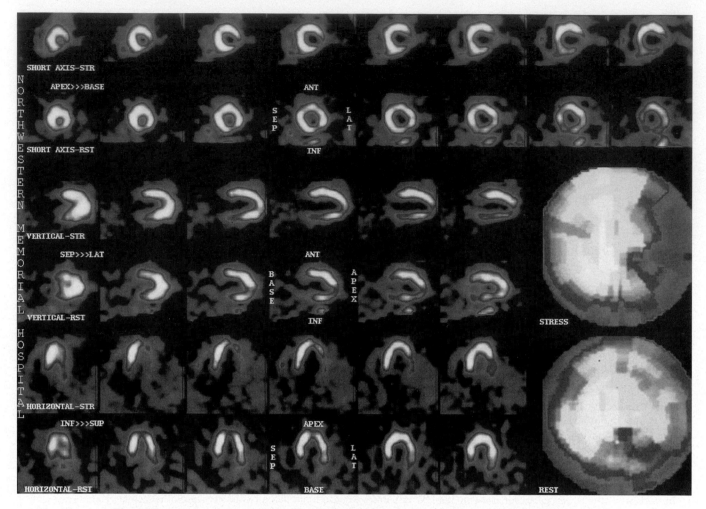

Fig. 24-7. Exercise technetium-99m sestamibi *(top)* and resting thallium-201 images obtained as part of an exercise dual-isotope protocol in a man with recent-onset chest pain, demonstrating a moderate-sized region of severely decreased activity in the lateral wall. The patient was subsequently found to have 95% stenosis of the proximal left circumflex coronary artery. He underwent successful coronary angioplasty of this vessel.

recent study by Borges-Neto et al,[14] the area at risk during balloon inflation was well delineated and correlated well with the extent of dipyridamole-induced ischemia. Heller et al[65] imaged patients by using ^{99m}Tc teboroxime during and after balloon occlusion and demonstrated that the culprit vessel could be accurately identified in 93% of cases. After PTCA, these investigators noted that the perfusion defects seen during balloon occlusion resolved, indicating that imaging provided an assessment of vessel patency.

The aforementioned value of tomographic myocardial perfusion imaging to accurately localize coronary stenoses is of critical importance when considering revascularization, because the culprit lesion may be accurately identified with perfusion imaging.[18,69,83,110,156] The localization and definition of the ischemic burden before PTCA provide objective data on which to base clinical decisions (Fig. 24-7). Coronary intervention may thus be targeted at a specific lesion, even in the setting of multivessel coronary disease. Although this approach may

provide incomplete revascularization, angioplasty of the ischemic lesion may obviate the need (at least temporarily) for a surgical solution. Breisblatt et al[18] examined the value of exercise thallium imaging before angioplasty in 85 patients with multivessel disease. Although only 31% of patients had initial perfusion abnormalities in multiple vascular territories, 38 patients had evidence of ischemia in a second vascular distribution within 1 month after PTCA. However, among the 37 patients with no further ischemia, only 13% required an angioplasty of a second coronary artery. Therefore, myocardial perfusion imaging after angioplasty may reveal new perfusion defects not noted previously because of the limiting nature of the stenosis.[18] With the higher workload achieved after PTCA, these areas become apparent on repeated perfusion imaging.

The objectification of ischemia plays an important role in the decision to proceed with angioplasty of a coronary artery with an intermediate level of narrowing, although few conclusive data are available about this common practice.[98] Additional methods, including intracoronary Doppler flow assessment of flow reserve, may also be used to examine equivocal lesions.[33,34,88,122] Doppler flow wire measurements correlate well with myocardial perfusion imaging using [99mTc] sestamibi[122] or [201Tl] scintigraphy[33,88] and provide an alternative invasive method for the physiologic assessment of an intermediate (40% to 70%) coronary stenosis. In the study by Joye et al,[88] 94% concordance was demonstrated between [201Tl] SPECT imaging and intracoronary Doppler flow measurements.[88] One potential advantage of using a Doppler flow wire is the ability to obtain this physiologic determination of lesion severity while the patient is in the cardiac catheterization laboratory and to use these data immediately in making decisions about interventional therapy.

The delineation of the area at risk is another important factor that may be defined by perfusion imaging before angioplasty, in a manner similar to that used to assess the area at risk in acute myocardial infarction.[54,158] Electrocardiography during acute infarction or balloon inflation has a poor correlation with the area at risk, as defined by perfusion imaging.[159] It seems that ST-segment changes primarily reflect the severity of ischemia rather than its extent. Because long-term prognosis is dependent on the amount of myocardium at risk, myocardial perfusion imaging with sestamibi or other [99mTc] tracers may greatly assist in decision making, both during the acute procedure and in the event of suspected restenosis.[159] Perfusion imaging may also be used to identify patients who may be at high risk for subsequent events after treatment for acute infarction. Data suggest that a reversible rest-redistribution thallium defect may benefit from early PTCA.[106]

Therefore, perfusion imaging after coronary angioplasty can identify the culprit vessel and enable incomplete revascularization to be considered. In addition, the presence and extent of perfusion defects may affect the decision to perform PTCA by allowing consideration of medical or surgical options in the context of the scintigraphic abnormalities found.

Assessment of improvement in perfusion after PTCA

To confirm improvement in coronary perfusion after coronary angioplasty, it may be worthwhile to compare the perfusion images obtained before the procedure with those obtained afterward. The direct comparison of scintigraphic flow patterns provides objective evidence of the beneficial effects of PTCA. After coronary angioplasty, myocardial perfusion imaging usually demonstrates improvement of regional myocardial perfusion; in most cases, this improvement is substantial.* In the classic study of coronary blood flow after PTCA, Hirzel et al[69] examined patients with single-vessel disease who underwent successful PTCA.[69] Significant improvement in perfusion was noted in 28 of the 30 patients within 3 weeks. The only patients with abnormal images 6 months after angioplasty were shown to have restenosis. Similarly, quantitative [201Tl] scintigraphy

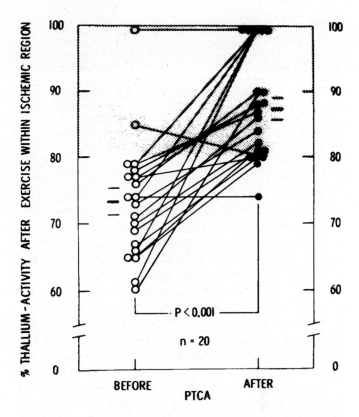

Fig. 24-8. Thallium-201 activity after exercise within the ischemic region, expressed as a percentage of maximal thallium activity before and after successful percutaneous transluminal coronary angioplasty. (Reproduced with permission from Hirzel HO, Nuesch K, Gruentzig AR, et al: Thallium-201 exercise scintigraphy after percutaneous transluminal angioplasty of coronary artery stenoses, *Med Clin North Am* 64:163-176, 1980.)

shows significant increases in thallium activity after successful angioplasty[68,91,167] (Fig. 24-8).

However, despite the potential for substantial improvement of coronary blood flow patterns after angioplasty, many studies show that not all patients have normalization of perfusion. Partially reversible or persistent defects have been noted in many patients shortly after PTCA† (Table 24-1). In fact, reversible defects consistent with ischemia may be found with myocardial perfusion imaging in 18% to 47% of patients.‡ Resolution of these perfusion defects is often noted on subsequent stress tests.[69,114,156] For example, Scholl et al[156] performed exercise thallium testing before and at 1 and 6 months after PTCA in 36 patients. The initial post-PTCA perfusion images were abnormal in 6 patients, 3 of whom were later found to have restenosis. The remaining 3 patients had normal studies at 6 months.[156] It is apparent that the timing of the imaging procedure after angioplasty is a crucial factor in terms of persistence of perfusion abnormalities. However, resolution of ischemic-type perfusion defects occurs in most studies. The use of a submaximal exer-

---

*References 18, 19, 25, 40, 60, 69, 81, 83, 91, 107, 110, 111, 114, 123, 124, 144, 147, 156, 160, 167, 177, 178.

†References 25, 81, 110, 111, 114, 156.
‡References 25, 30, 60, 83, 140, 177.

Table 24-1. Possible causes of abnormal perfusion images after angioplasty

Reversible defect	Persistent defect
Incomplete revascularization	Previous infarction
Disease progression	Procedural infarction
Residual stenosis	Artifact
Dissection or thrombus	Severe ischemia
Restenosis	Stunning
Abnormal coronary flow reserve	

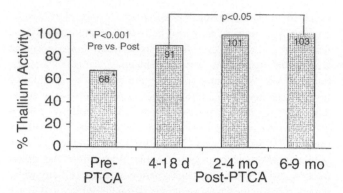

Fig. 24-9. Serial changes in regional thallium activity before and at three times after percutaneous transluminal coronary angioplasty. d = days; mo = months. (Modified with permission from Manyari DE, Knudtson M, Kloiben R, et al: Sequential thallium-201 myocardial perfusion studies after successful percutaneous transluminal coronary angioplasty: delayed resolution of exercise-induced scintigraphic abnormalities, *Circulation* 77:86-95, 1988.)

cise study may prevent the identification of the abnormal coronary flow at peak hyperemia.[69]

Just as reversible perfusion abnormalities may improve or resolve, persistent (fixed) perfusion defects (formerly synonymous with the presence of myocardial scar) may also improve after PTCA.[40,111] Liu et al[111] noted that 85% of the reversible defects present before angioplasty and 75% of the persistent abnormalities became normal when studied 2 weeks after successful coronary angioplasty. In another study involving 141 patients, 112 of whom had not had infarction, Cloninger et al[25] performed exercise thallium imaging before and 1 to 4 days after angioplasty. Partial redistribution was noted in more than three fourths of the studies before angioplasty. Of the patients without previous infarction, 66% of patients had a perfusion defect after PTCA; repeated imaging at 8 to 24 hours showed improvement in most of these patients.[25] It was therefore concluded that incomplete thallium redistribution occurs frequently early after PTCA and does not necessarily imply infarction.

The resolution of persistent myocardial perfusion defects as described above may in part reflect the scintigraphic technique used. It is probable that many fixed defects do not reflect myocardial scar but remain viable and will show recovery of regional or global left ventricular function after revascularization.[11,38,97,111,131] Scintigraphic techniques aimed at the enhanced detection of myocardial viability, such as delayed thallium imaging or thallium reinjection, may be useful. These methods have previously been shown to differentiate patients who truly have myocardial scar from those who are likely to show subsequent improvement in perfusion and function after PTCA.[37,38,97,111,131]

In addition to documenting improvements in myocardial perfusion after PTCA, radiopharmaceuticals and instrumentation can now be used in gated SPECT and first-pass perfusion imaging, allowing the assessment of ventricular function as part of the perfusion study. Although there is limited experience in postrevascularization patients, improved perfusion and function have been reported with these techniques after PTCA.[135]

It is well established that perfusion imaging is valuable in documenting improvements in perfusion after PTCA of native vessels. As the application of PTCA has grown, it is now well accepted that PTCA of grafts is feasible and efficacious.[27] In 55 post-CABG patients who underwent graft angioplasty, Reed et

al[147] demonstrated that thallium imaging after angioplasty revealed reduced lung activity and a reduction of the magnitude and extent of ischemic perfusion abnormalities. Of the 38% of patients with thallium redistribution after angioplasty, all subsequently developed recurrent chest pain; restenosis was the most common cause of the thallium redistribution defect.

Timing of post-PTCA testing

As discussed above, the value of myocardial perfusion imaging shortly after PTCA has been questioned.* Illustrating the potential problems encountered with early myocardial perfusion imaging after PTCA, Manyari et al[114] studied 43 patients after PTCA with serial exercise planar thallium studies, all of whom had single-vessel disease. All patients had a successful procedure and were confirmed to be without restenosis on angiography. The patients underwent testing before angioplasty, within 18 days after PTCA and 2 to 4 months and 6 to 9 months after PTCA. Although perfusion was improved in most patients even days after angioplasty, 12 patients (28%) had ischemia shortly after the procedure. These 12 patients and 5 patients with fixed defects showed improvement on subsequent thallium stress tests (Fig. 24-9). Therefore, thallium scintigraphy reveals a delayed improvement after PTCA, and abnormal early results (within 18 days) do not correlate with restenosis or the presence of a residual lesion. These results were confirmed by Breisblatt et al,[19] who showed that thallium imaging within 2 weeks of PTCA is not predictive of restenosis. Four of 7 patients who had early abnormal studies had normal images at 4 to 6 weeks. However, by 4 weeks, perfusion imaging was predictive of restenosis; 87% of patients were identified, even if they were asymptomatic at the time of imaging.

Although several investigators have expressed concern about the value of perfusion imaging soon after PTCA, others have shown that early perfusion imaging after PTCA is accu-

*References 19, 25, 30, 31, 110, 111, 114, 156.

rate and usually confirms the success of the procedure.* In fact, early testing may identify patients at risk for restenosis or subsequent cardiac events early after angioplasty. The ability to perform early risk stratification after angioplasty (12 to 24 hours) has obvious potential benefits, because high-risk patients may be considered for altered medical treatment or additional efforts at revascularization. Pharmacologic stress may be particularly useful for early postprocedural evaluation of patients[82,107] and is discussed at length in the section on pharmacologic stress perfusion imaging. Alternatively, very early post-PTCA assessment may also be accomplished with myocardial perfusion imaging in conjunction with transesophageal atrial pacing.[60] Both atrial pacing and pharmacologic stress testing may be done safely after arterial puncture or with the sheaths in situ.

*References 40, 60, 81, 83, 123, 160, 178.

Thus, although a perfusion study showing lack of ischemia is useful after PTCA, concern should remain about the implications of an abnormal study within the first 4 to 6 weeks after the procedure (Fig. 24-10). However, early testing is feasible and may provide the maximum clinical value.

Potential mechanisms for abnormal post-PTCA perfusion images

The potential reasons for an abnormal perfusion scan after PTCA are many (Table 24-1). After angioplasty, an abnormal myocardial perfusion imaging study may accurately reflect ischemia resulting from 1) disease progression, 2) incomplete revascularization, 3) residual stenosis, 4) dissection or local trauma, 5) restenosis, or 6) postprocedural ischemia (stunning). A persistent perfusion abnormality is noted when a periprocedural infarction has occurred or when there was previous myocardial infarction. It is also well documented that persistent

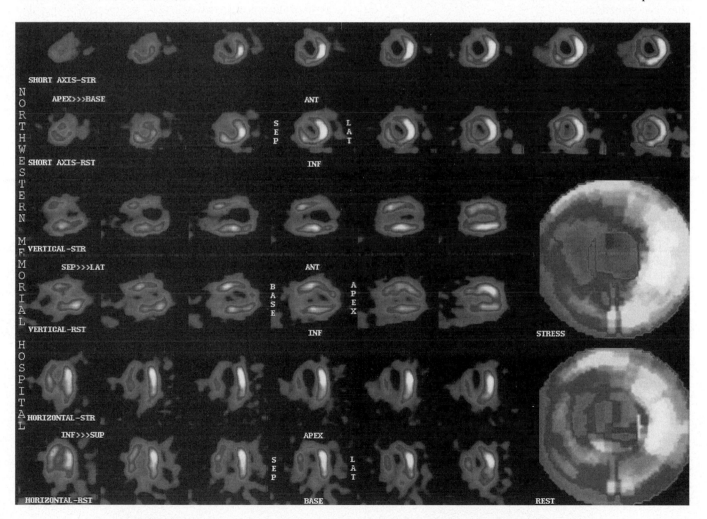

Fig. 24-10. Dual-isotope images of a 47-year-old man who presented 5 days earlier with acute myocardial infarction and underwent successful percutaneous transluminal coronary angioplasty of the left anterior descending and first diagonal arteries. A moderately large defect of moderate severity is noted in the anterior, apical, and septal walls, with substantial (albeit not complete) reversibility. Because of recurrent symptoms 2 weeks later, he underwent repeated angiography, which revealed widely patent vessels. This study reveals the potential for a false-positive examination shortly after angioplasty.

abnormalities may reflect ischemia, and additional methods are often required to fully elucidate the presence of myocardial viability.[37,116]

Perfusion defects may not resolve after angioplasty, especially when imaging is performed within the first several weeks after the procedure. There are several possible explanations for the continued presence of a reversible defect. Firstly, the angioplasty may not have been completely successful, and post-PTCA angiography may be an imperfect assessment of the degree of success. Alternatively, the mechanism of the delayed return of normal perfusion images may be due to a hibernating or stunned state or local trauma to the angioplasty site.[114] Abnormal biochemistry, which may be present in these altered states, may resolve slowly, affecting the uptake of the perfusion agent and producing an abnormality. Other explanations include the possibility that the autoregulation of the arterioles distal to the stenosis may be abnormal, resulting in impedance to flow even after successful dilation.

Substantial evidence shows that the lack of resolution of perfusion abnormalities after PTCA is related to persistent perturbations in coronary flow reserve despite the appearance of angiographic success. Although several investigators using digital angiography have demonstrated that significant improvement of coronary flow reserve occurs immediately after balloon dilation of a coronary stenosis,[71,141] it is not uniformly agreed that this effect is immediate. Despite improvements in flow reserve noted in patients after angioplasty, a subnormal value was common early after the procedure.* Persistent perturbation of coronary blood flow reserve has been hypothesized as the explanation of the failure of immediate postangioplasty imaging to demonstrate angiographic success.[105] This is consistent with the observation of the poor correlation between intracoronary Doppler flow measurement of coronary flow reserve and angiographic patency when assessed early after angioplasty.[85,179,181] An abnormal Doppler-derived coronary flow reserve was found immediately after PTCA by Wilson et al[179] in more than one half of patients (Fig. 24-11).[179] In the four patients in that study who had subnormal flow reserve immediately after PTCA but did not subsequently develop restenosis, the coronary flow reserve returned to normal approximately 7 months later. This finding has been confirmed by other investigators.[164,181]

Despite the lack of correlation between epicardial coronary diameter and coronary flow reserve, a significant association has been documented between flow reserve and myocardial perfusion imaging.[88,122] Doppler-derived measurements agree with results of myocardial perfusion imaging in 89% to 94% of patients.[122] The aforementioned alterations in coronary flow reserve and correlation of myocardial perfusion imaging with this variable explain the lack of immediate improvement on perfusion imaging and the failure to normalize myocardial perfusion soon after PTCA.[19,114,156] The etiology of reduced coronary

*References 8, 71, 85, 127, 164, 181.

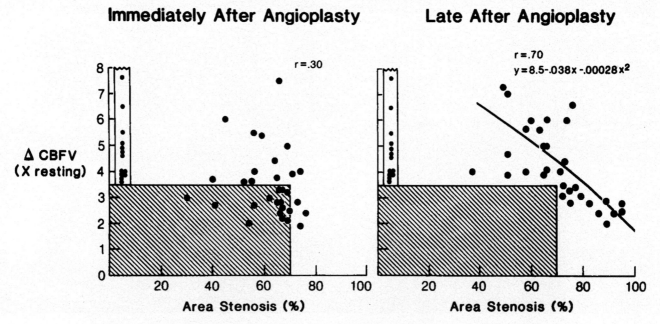

Fig. 24-11. Relation between area stenosis and coronary flow reserve *(ΔCBFV)* in vessels immediately and later after percutaneous transluminal coronary angioplasty (PTCA). The bar in the upper left of each panel displays the ΔCBFV in normal vessels. The left panel shows that immediately after PTCA, ΔCBFV was unrelated to area stenosis. The right panel demonstrates a significant relation and a normal flow reserve if the lesion produced less than a 70% area stenosis. (Reproduced with permission from Wilson RF, Johnson MR, Marcus ML: The effect of coronary angioplasty on coronary flow reserve, *Circulation* 77:873-885, 1988.)

flow reserve early after PTCA is unclear but may involve 1) an absolute increase in resting flow due to hyperemia related to balloon inflation,[127] 2) the presence of a residual stenosis, or 3) changes in the arteriolar dilation as a result of proximal arterial injury.

In conclusion, the importance of the timing of perfusion imaging after angioplasty is unclear with regard to results and the true time course necessary for the resolution of transient post-PTCA perfusion abnormalities. A normal maximal exercise perfusion study seems to be a useful marker for a good outcome and low risk for recurrent symptoms or restenosis, even when performed very early after angioplasty. However, when an abnormal result on myocardial perfusion imaging is noted shortly after angioplasty, the accuracy of these early abnormal results can be questioned. It therefore seems rational to defer imaging for at least 4 to 6 weeks after PTCA. This delay will also permit the safe performance of maximal exercise testing in many patients, providing an assessment of functional ability and the likelihood of provoking symptoms.

Recurrent symptoms and clinical events

The return of anginal symptoms after revascularization usually raises important concerns for the patient and clinician. When typical symptoms are present in the first 3 to 6 months after angioplasty, restenosis at the site of PTCA is usually the problem. The ability of perfusion imaging to identify and predict restenosis is discussed in the section on restenosis. However, when angina returns more than 6 months after the procedure, disease progression is most often the cause.

Exercise ^{201}Tl scintigraphy has been shown to be useful after angioplasty for predicting which patients will develop recurrent symptoms[147,160,177,178] or clinical cardiac events, such as myocardial infarction or cardiac death. Regardless of whether clinically silent or symptomatic, an abnormal result on thallium imaging increased the risk for readmission to the hospital or for myocardial infarction. Several additional studies have shown that the only noninvasive procedure to accurately predict postangioplasty events within several weeks after PTCA was exercise thallium scintigraphy.[123,160] This is similar to the value of myocardial perfusion imaging for prediction of restenosis,* which is highlighted in the following section.

To examine the value of early exercise quantitative thallium imaging for the prediction of recurrent chest pain, Stuckey et al[160] studied 68 asymptomatic patients a mean of 2.2 weeks after PTCA. During follow-up, 34% of patients developed typical chest pain; the only significant independent predictor of this event was the presence of thallium redistribution (Fig. 24-12). However, despite a high specificity of thallium imaging (91%), only 9 of the 23 symptomatic patients had abnormal results on thallium studies, yielding a sensitivity of 39%. Despite the disappointing performance of thallium perfusion imaging, it was still superior to ST-segment changes during treadmill exercise testing. Similar findings were reported by Wijns et al,[177] who

*References 19, 60, 63, 81, 83, 107, 116, 123, 140, 148, 156.

performed symptom-limited exercise thallium testing a mean of 4.7 weeks after PTCA. Thallium testing was shown to be superior for the prediction of restenosis (74%) and recurrent angina (66%) compared with exercise testing (50% on restenosis and 38% on angina recurrence) (Fig. 24-13).

Somewhat conflicting data were presented in a recent study that failed to demonstrate the value of noninvasive testing in patients with recurrence of symptoms more than 1 year after angioplasty. Klein et al[98] concluded that neither clinical nor noninvasive testing variables were predictive of changes in coronary anatomy, and catheterization was advised for all symptomatic patients regardless of the time of symptom recurrence. However, only patients who underwent angiography were included in this study, and the authors admitted that myocardial perfusion imaging may serve as a means of eliminating the need for catheterization in many patients. Furthermore, the authors stated that perfusion imaging may be of substantial value in the evaluation of an equivocal coronary stenosis.

Therefore, an abnormal thallium study is associated with a high incidence of recurrent symptoms and late cardiac events, while a normal study is associated with a good prognosis. Thus, patients with abnormal post-PTCA perfusion studies require close clinical surveillance. It seems advisable that if recurrent symptoms develop in the setting of an abnormal perfusion study, coronary angiography should be undertaken.[160,177] Although it has not yet been examined, myocardial perfusion imaging in postangioplasty patients may play a role in resource allocation (coronary angiography and additional revascularization) and the optimization of cost-effective management.

Restenosis

Successful coronary angioplasty is frequently complicated by the development of a restenosis of the artery at the same site of the previously dilated lesion. Although the actual frequency of restenosis varies by patient, location of the dilated lesion, and devices used, the incidence seems to range from 30% to 40%.[17,58,100,130,157] However, since the advent of intracoronary stenting, this rate has substantially decreased.[46] Most often, restenosis occurs early (within 3 to 6 months) after PTCA and is usually heralded by the return of preangioplasty symptoms. After 6 months or if atypical symptoms occur, restenosis is less likely. The precise cause of restenosis is unknown, but it probably results from local injury with plaque disruption, intimal tearing, endothelial hematoma, thrombus formation, fibrin deposition, and smooth-muscle and intimal proliferation.[49] In addition, arterial remodeling may contribute to restenosis.

Several studies have demonstrated the value of myocardial perfusion imaging or prediction of restenosis after coronary angioplasty.* Both planar† and tomographic‡ imaging techniques

*References 19, 44, 60, 63, 64, 69, 83, 107, 114, 116, 120, 123, 140, 156, 160, 177.
†References 60, 69, 114, 123, 140, 160, 177.
‡References 19, 63, 64, 81, 83, 107, 116, 120.

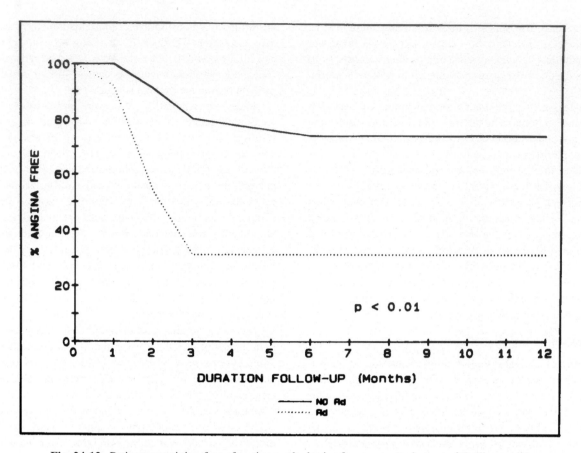

Fig. 24-12. Patients remaining free of angina on the basis of presence or absence of thallium redistribution *(Rd)*. (Reproduced with permission from Stuckey TD, Burwell LR, Nygaard TW, et al: Quantitative exercise thallium-201 scintigraphy for predicting angina recurrence after percutaneous transluminal coronary angioplasty, *Am J Cardiol* 63:517-521, Copyright 1989 by Excerpta Medica Inc.)

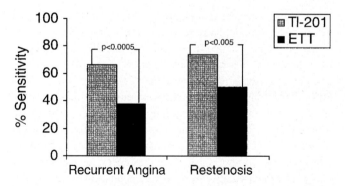

Fig. 24-13. Comparison of the sensitivity for the prediction of restenosis or recurrent angina based on exercise electrocardiographic data or exercise thallium scintigraphy. (Derived from Wijns W, Serruy PW, Reiber JH, et al: Early detection of restenosis after successful percutaneous transluminal coronary angioplasty by exercise-redistribution thallium scintigraphy, *Am J Cardiol* 55:357-361, 1985.)

have been used successfully to this end, and symptomatic and asymptomatic restenosis may be detected by myocardial perfusion imaging[64,116,140] (Fig. 24-14).

In an early study by Breisblatt et al,[19] exercise planar thallium imaging was used to predict coronary restenosis in 121 patients after successful PTCA. Serial thallium studies were performed at 4 to 6 weeks, 3 to 6 months, and 1 year. Reversible perfusion defects were noted in 25% of asymptomatic patients at 4 to 6 weeks; 86% and 96% of these patients developed restenosis at 6 months and 1 year, respectively. Of equal importance is that the 74 patients with a negative perfusion study at 3 to 6 months had a very low probability of developing symptoms of restenosis. This study also showed that of the 19 patients with recurrent chest pain but a negative thallium study, only 1 had angiographic restenosis.[19] Therefore, a normal perfusion study after PTCA provides excellent negative predictive value for the development of restenosis. The potential value of perfusion imaging was further demonstrated in a subsequent study in which approximately 50% of the early reversible defects occurred in patients who developed late restenosis. In that study, thallium redistribution was found to be the most powerful predictor of restenosis.[60]

In one of the largest trials, Pfisterer et al[140] examined 405 patients who underwent exercise planar thallium imaging after angioplasty. Ischemia was noted in 28% of patients and was associated with restenosis in a high number of patients, by a specificity of 97%. Perhaps most important was that restenosis was accurately detected by perfusion imaging in this patient

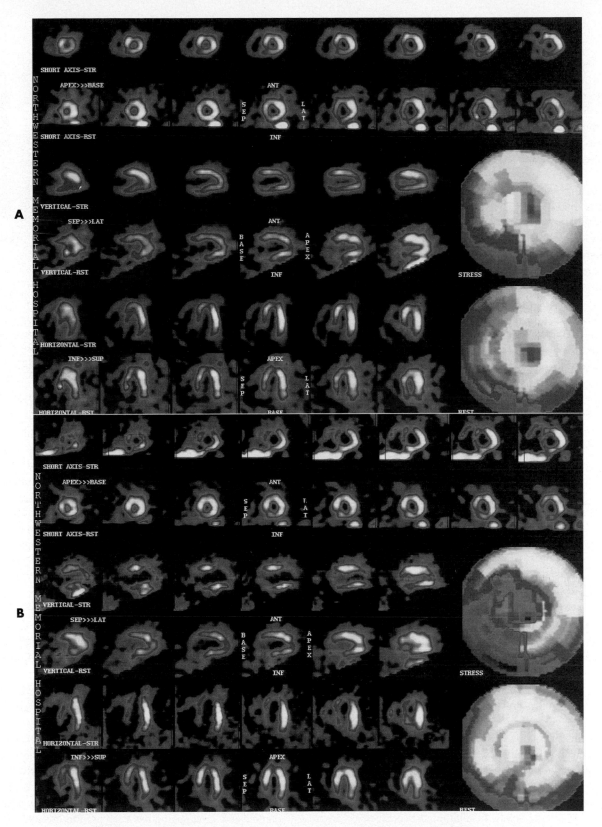

Fig. 24-14. These images are of a 52-year-old man who sustained an anterior wall myocardial infarction, treated urgently with an angioplasty of the left anterior descending *(LAD)* coronary artery. **A,** The first dual-isotope perfusion study *(top)* was obtained approximately 3 weeks later and was thought to be normal except for diaphragmatic attenuation. His chest pain subsequently recurred, and at 3.5 months after the initial event, he underwent a second perfusion study. These images *(middle)* show a large, reversible perfusion defect in the anterior, septal, and apical walls. In addition, the ejection fraction measured by gated single-photon emission computed tomography decreased from 51% on the first study to 40% on the second. Repeated angiography demonstrated restenosis in the proximal LAD, for which angioplasty was performed and a stent was placed. **B,** Repeated perfusion imaging after percutaneous transluminal coronary angioplasty and stent placement demonstrates resolution of ischemia.

group, even though it was clinically silent in 60% of thallium studies that showed redistribution. Furthermore, regardless of whether restenosis was silent or symptomatic, an abnormal result on thallium imaging was associated with an increased risk for hospital readmission or myocardial infarction.[140]

It has been noted that not all persistent perfusion abnormalities after PTCA reflect the presence of myocardial necrosis.[11,38,97,111,131] To maximize detection of a reversible defect, Marie et al[116] studied 62 consecutive post-PTCA patients with bicycle exercise SPECT imaging using stress ^{201}Tl imaging with resting reinjection.[116] Testing was performed within 6 months after PTCA. The discrimination of angiographic findings based on the results of the perfusion images was impressive: A reversible defect was present in 94% of patients with restenosis and was seen in only 16% of patients without angiographic restenosis.[116]

As suggested in two of the aforementioned reports,[19,140] the presence of angina pectoris and the provocation of chest pain with exercise testing are insensitive markers of postangioplasty restenosis. When patients are examined with follow-up angiography, a substantial number (19% to 33%) are found to have clinically silent restenosis.[44,64,118,157] Therefore, the finding that restenosis may occur in the absence of recurrent angina is clinically important and implies a potentially crucial role for myocardial perfusion imaging in the management of patients after angioplasty.

Even the development of chest pain during an exercise stress test is a poor marker for restenosis, with a sensitivity of only 24% to 63%.[10,19,63,116,140] Furthermore, electrocardiographic changes with exercise fail to accurately detect angiographic restenosis, with a sensitivity of 26% to 52%.[10,63,116,140,178] However, one study that included a small number of patients demonstrated excellent predictive value for coronary restenosis with an electrocardiographic stress test.[43] A possible explanation for the discrepancy may be bias in the literature reflecting the fact that not all patients achieved the target heart rate.[10,63] However, in general, it seems that electrocardiographic stress testing lacks optimal diagnostic value for the detection of coronary restenosis.

When comparing the value of exercise testing with and without perfusion imaging, most reports show that myocardial perfusion imaging is superior to exercise testing alone for the detection and prediction of restenosis after PTCA.* In one such study, Hecht et al[63] compared exercise testing with and without perfusion imaging in 116 patients, almost half of whom had multivessel disease (Fig. 24-15). The sensitivities for exercise testing and perfusion imaging for detection of restenosis were 53% and 93%, respectively. In addition, the specificity of myocardial perfusion imaging was found to be higher than that of exercise electrocardiography (77% compared with 64%). These results were similar regardless of whether single-vessel or multivessel coronary disease was noted and were not altered according to whether complete revascularization was performed.

*References 19, 44, 60, 63, 64, 69, 83, 114, 116, 123, 140, 156, 157, 160, 177.

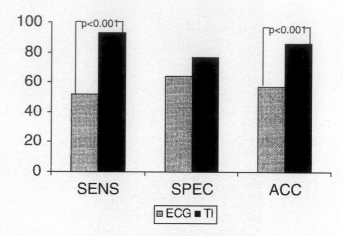

Fig. 24-15. Comparative sensitivity *(SENS),* specificity *(SPEC),* and overall accuracy *(ACC)* for exercise testing and exercise thallium-201 imaging for the detection of restenosis after coronary angioplasty. (Derived from Hecht HS, Shaw RE, Bruce TR, et al: Usefulness of tomographic thallium-201 imaging for detection of restenosis after percutaneous transluminal coronary angioplasty, *Am J Cardiol* 66:1314-1318, Copyright 1990 by Excerpta Medica Inc.)

In a subsequent study by the same group, the ability of exercise SPECT thallium imaging to detect restenosis was evaluated in 41 asymptomatic and 77 symptomatic patients.[64] Restenosis occurred with the same frequency regardless of symptoms, and the sensitivity and specificity for the detection of restenosis did not depend on symptomatology. For detection of angina, exercise testing was not nearly as sensitive as thallium scintigraphy.

Despite the concern raised by several authors about the presence of false positive perfusion defects early after angioplasty,[19,114] data support the diagnostic accuracy of perfusion imaging even when it is performed very early after angioplasty.[40,60,81] Clearly, the sooner a patient who has the potential for restenosis is identified, the earlier treatment may be administered. Thus, performance of perfusion imaging before or shortly after hospital discharge may be valuable. Testing should probably incorporate nonexercise methods of stress testing because of the problems that may be encountered with strenuous exercising in a patient who has recently undergone femoral artery cannulation.

Although most studies have examined the efficacy of exercise myocardial perfusion imaging in predicting coronary restenosis, other stress techniques have been performed in patients early after angioplasty or in those who are unable to perform adequate exercise. Pharmacologic testing with dipyridamole and atrial pacing has been used to this end.[60,83,107] Jain et al[83] demonstrated that the induction of a reversible thallium defect after oral dipyridamole was associated with a 71% restenosis rate, whereas only 11.5% of patients without an ischemic defect had angiographic restenosis. Thallium scintigraphy in conjunction with atrial pacing may predict late restenosis even when it is performed within 24 hours after angioplasty[60,107] (sensitivity, 77%; specificity, 67%). Conversely, the absence of a reversible defect was associated with a low risk for restenosis (14%).[60] This technique may be used almost immediately after PTCA (37 ± 16 minutes) with similar results.[107]

Few data are currently available on the value of myocardial perfusion imaging after intracoronary stent implantation. Two preliminary reports including more than 300 patients indicate that myocardial perfusion imaging after stent implantation provides valuable clinical information on the prediction of restenosis, with positive and negative predictive values ranging from 81% to 95% and 83% to 85%, respectively.[121,137] A recent study in 17 patients with isolated left anterior descending coronary artery disease revealed that whereas PTCA was associated with the presence of thallium redistribution early after revascularization in 8 patients, a few patients treated with stenting had early hypoperfusion that was also less severe.[168] These findings occurred in the absence of restenosis. It is conceivable that these differences in post-PTCA patients and in patients who received stent perfusion were caused by the absence of a residual lesion after stenting.[168]

After PTCA, techniques other than exercise testing and myocardial perfusion imaging may be used to detect coronary restenosis. As discussed later in this chapter, echocardiographic stress testing has been used successfully for this purpose.[62,142] Some authors have advocated the routine use of coronary angiography at designated intervals after angioplasty. The combination of variables has been shown to be a highly accurate method for predicting coronary restenosis on the basis of a logistic model composed of clinical, angiographic, exercise, and scintigraphic variables.[148] This method provided near-optimal diagnostic accuracy for restenosis; with a positive predictive value of 100% for the high-risk group and a negative predictive value of 94% for the low-risk group, it outperformed both exercise test variables or clinical information alone. The superiority of this approach—combining angiographic and scintigraphic data to improve the prediction of late results after PTCA—was recently confirmed.[107] A normal result on myocardial perfusion imaging immediately or early after PTCA in combination with a larger lumen diameter was associated with a better late angiographic result than was angiographic data alone.

In conclusion, myocardial perfusion imaging seems to be the most diagnostically useful noninvasive technique for the detection of coronary restenosis after routine balloon angioplasty. Perfusion imaging is useful not only in native coronary arteries for the detection of restenosis but also in bypass grafts[147] (Fig. 24-16). Despite the value of myocardial perfusion imaging for the detection and prediction of restenosis after PTCA, the precise method for the optimal use of this technique is not clear.

Pharmacologic stress perfusion imaging

Many patients are unable to perform an adequate exercise test before or after revascularization, potentially limiting the diagnostic value of perfusion imaging.[70,82] In addition, early exercise testing after angioplasty is complicated by the fact that

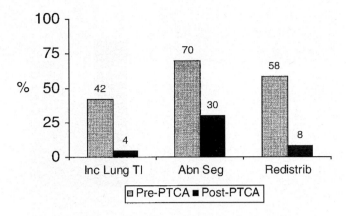

Fig. 24-16. Changes in thallium-201 imaging characteristics in post–coronary artery bypass graft surgery patients with recurrent angina who underwent successful percutaneous transluminal coronary angioplasty (PTCA). All differences between pre-PTCA and post-PTCA values have a *P* value greater than 0.005. Abn Seg = percentage of abnormal scan segments; Inc Lung Tl = increased thallium activity in lung; Redistrib = redistribution present. (Modified from Reed DC, Beller GA, Nygaard TW, et al: The clinical efficacy and scintigraphic evaluation of post-coronary bypass patients undergoing transluminal coronary angioplasty for recurrent angina pectoris, *Am Heart J* 117:60-71, 1989.)

these patients have recently undergone arterial puncture, increasing the risk for bleeding and hematoma formation during vigorous exercise and causing soreness in the groin. Pharmacologic stress testing provides an alternative to exercise myocardial perfusion imaging and may be performed in conjunction with a vasodilator infusion (adenosine or dipyridamole) or with dobutamine.[82] Furthermore, pharmacologic testing is not affected by medications that may frequently be administered after revascularization, such as calcium-channel antagonists or β-blockers, thus providing a more thorough assessment of residual ischemia. Recently, it has been shown that the extent of the defect, as delineated by vasodilator stress ^{99m}Tc sestamibi imaging, is highly correlated with the extent of the defect noted during balloon occlusion of the culprit lesion,[14] thus providing an accurate assessment of the amount of jeopardized myocardium.

Pharmacologic stress testing has been studied early after PTCA, and early assessment has been done of the physiology under conditions of maximal stress.[40,81,83] It has been suggested that the determination of coronary flow reserve after angioplasty as determined by vasodilator SPECT imaging is not altered, as is often seen with exercise testing shortly after PTCA.[81] Eichhorn et al[40] demonstrated that dipyridamole thallium testing within 1 week after PTCA was associated with improvement in 94% of patients with reversible perfusion defects before PTCA; some fixed defects also improved after PTCA. These latter findings support the well-documented finding of underestimation of myocardial viability with stress-redistribution thallium scintigraphy.[11,38,40,97,131] Jain et al[83] studied 53 patients who underwent tomographic thallium imaging after oral dipyridamole administration before and very soon after PTCA

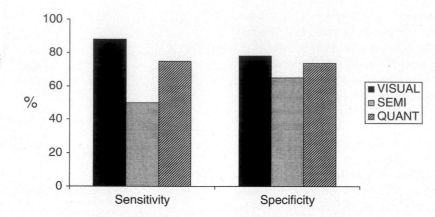

Fig. 24-17. Sensitivity and specificity of bicycle exercise technetium-99m sestamibi imaging for the detection of restenosis after percutaneous transluminal coronary angioplasty using visual, semiquantitative *(SEMI)*, and quantitative (polar map [*QUANT*]) techniques. (Reprinted by permission of the Society of Nuclear Medicine. Modified from Milan E, Zoccarato O, Terzi A, et al: Technetium-99m-sestamibi SPECT to detect restenosis after successful percutaneous coronary angioplasty, *J Nucl Med* 37:1300-1305, 1996.)

(<3 days). They showed that 35% of patients still had ischemic perfusion defects, which were associated with a worse outcome. Of the 14 patients with ischemic thallium defects, 71% developed restenosis, compared with 11.5% of patients without this type of defect. Therefore, these authors suggest that vasodilator-induced perfusion defects early after PTCA identify a group of patients at high risk for restenosis. Likewise, Pirelli et al,[142] using high-dose dipyridamole planar thallium imaging, found an 83% sensitivity and 84% specificity for the detection of restenosis. Iskandrian et al[81] also provided evidence for the value of early adenosine thallium imaging performed less than 1 week after PTCA and a logical explanation was found for the more than 35% of patients with an abnormal post-PTCA study (dissection, myocardial infarction, or residual stenosis). Therefore, vasodilator perfusion imaging seems to have excellent diagnostic accuracy regardless of when the procedure is performed in relation to angioplasty. This finding contrasts with results noted after exercise scintigraphy and supports the differential mechanism of pharmacologic stress and its impact on coronary flow reserve.[81,82]

Technetium-99m agents

To date, few data have been published on ^{99m}Tc agents in the postrevascularization setting.[72,120] Thus far, the results seem to be encouraging and consistent with those found for ^{201}Tl scintigraphy. Technetium-99m sestamibi has been shown to have substantial value in delineating risk zones with myocardial infarction and documenting myocardial salvage after reperfusion.[54,158,170] In addition, post-PTCA improvement in myocardial perfusion has been shown with ^{99m}Tc sestamibi.[22,135] Milan et al[120] examined 37 patients after PTCA with bicycle exercise sestamibi perfusion imaging for the detection of restenosis. All patients underwent angiography 1 month after the initial procedure. Visual, semiquantitative, and quantitative methods were used and revealed substantial diagnostic value

for the presence or absence of restenosis (Fig. 24-17). Visual interpretation of ^{99m}Tc SPECT images was at least as good as quantitative methods. Of clinical importance is that no patient had a previous perfusion imaging study, which resembles the usual clinical situation.

Perhaps the most valuable aspect of postangioplasty perfusion imaging with ^{99m}Tc agents is the ability to evaluate the functional status of the left ventricle both globally and regionally after revascularization.[6,50,80,135] Such agents as ^{99m}Tc sestamibi allow the simultaneous assessment of left and right ventricular function and the presence and extent of perfusion abnormalities. This may be of value in the evaluation of post-CABG patients. Iskandrian et al[80] found good correction between left ventricular ejection fraction and the extent of perfusion defects with the use of simultaneous first-pass and myocardial perfusion imaging, although considerable variation was noted. Gallik et al[50] studied the relation between left ventricular function using first-pass imaging and perfusion imaging during balloon occlusion in 35 patients undergoing PTCA. Although a significant correlation was noted between perfusion imaging and left ventricular function, it was not strong (Fig. 24-18), and substantial individual variation existed for both methods with regard to the specific artery involved. Substantially more patients developed perfusion abnormalities during balloon inflation than had wall-motion abnormalities. These findings suggest that perfusion imaging is more sensitive than the evaluation of regional wall motion for the detection of ischemia.[50]

In addition to first-pass imaging for the determination of left ventricular function, gated SPECT has been used in patients undergoing coronary revascularization. Pace et al[135] demonstrated improvement in fractional shortening and wall thickening after PTCA with the use of planar gated SPECT imaging. Recently, the value of gated SPECT with ^{99m}Tc sestamibi imaging was evaluated before and 3 months after PTCA.[6] Of 21 patients ex-

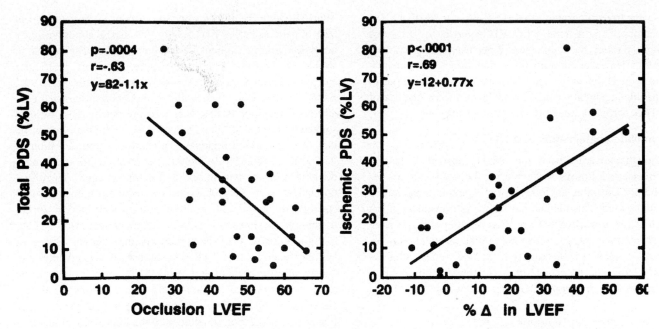

Fig. 24-18. Correlation between left ventricular ejection fraction *(LVEF; left)* and total perfusion defect score *(PDS)* and the change (Δ) in LVEF *(right)* from baseline to coronary occlusion and extent of reversible PDS. (Reproduced with permission from Gallik DM, Obermueller SD, Swama US, et al: Simultaneous assessment of myocardial perfusion and left ventricular function during transient coronary occlusion, *J Am Coll Cardiol* 25:1529-1538, 1995.)

amined, 18 had ischemic perfusion defects and 19 had abnormal ventricular function. All of the patients who subsequently developed restenosis had abnormal function after angioplasty on gated SPECT, and 3 of 4 had abnormal perfusion images. However, the relative or incremental value of gated SPECT was not assessed. A new development in gated SPECT is the ability to provide accurate quantitation of global left ventricular function.[51] This may be of substantial clinical importance and may assist in the evaluation of patients being considered for myocardial revascularization.

Summary of coronary angioplasty and perfusion imaging

The use of preangioplasty myocardial perfusion imaging, although often not critical, is valuable for the confirmation and delineation of ischemia and for the selection of patients for revascularization. After angioplasty, the pre-PTCA study provides a basis for comparison with subsequent tests and is especially useful in asymptomatic patients. Therefore, patients without clear coronary symptoms and those at high risk (such as those in whom a large area is at risk or those who have multivessel disease) should probably undergo routine myocardial perfusion imaging after PTCA. An early scan may also help to unmask a defect in a second vascular territory.

After percutaneous revascularization, myocardial perfusion imaging has an excellent negative predictive value for restenosis and clinical events. Prediction or accurate identification of coronary restenosis after PTCA assists in implementing treatment. Therefore, the earlier that restenosis is identified, the bet-

ter the theoretical outcome. The value of a positive perfusion study early after PTCA is limited. Conversely, normal perfusion scan after angioplasty has substantial clinical value, especially when the preangioplasty study was abnormal, and indicates 1) a successful procedure, 2) a low risk for chest pain and recurrent cardiac events, and 3) a reduced probability of late restenosis. In these patients, such procedures as angiography may be deferred and antianginal therapy may be avoided. By its ability to identify the location and extent of ischemia, myocardial perfusion imaging may permit a relatively conservative approach in patients with only a small region of ischemia. However, this approach is somewhat controversial. This strategy was recently supported by a position paper from the American Heart Association (AHA) and the American College of Cardiology (ACC) stating that "In the absence of symptoms, a modest reversible defect on stress perfusion scintigraphy may not justify repeat angiography."[154] Thus, myocardial perfusion imaging is likely to have substantial cost-effectiveness in the care of the post-PTCA patient, although no data currently support this approach. The routine use of myocardial perfusion imaging in asymptomatic patients after PTCA who were previously symptomatic is probably not justified. Early myocardial perfusion imaging seems to be indicated in the setting of a suboptimal CABG or angioplasty procedure, such as incomplete revascularization or coronary dissection after angioplasty.

The AHA/ACC Task Force on Assessment of Diagnostic and Therapeutic Cardiovascular Procedures stressed the value of myocardial perfusion imaging for 1) detection of restenosis in asymptomatic patients, 2) added specificity compared with exercise electrocardiography, and 3) excellent predictive value for restenosis.[154] In general, when PTCA has been performed for symptom relief, the routine use of perfusion imaging is not justified.[150] However, despite these and other recommendations, as well as the well-established role of myocardial perfusion imaging in patients with ischemic heart disease, the role of post-PTCA perfusion imaging remains controversial.

Radionuclide angiography and PTCA

Although myocardial perfusion imaging currently is the preferred nuclear cardiology technique for the assessment of patients before and after angioplasty, radionuclide angiography may also be used. This method has shown improvement in left ventricular functional response to exercise after PTCA.* Kent et al[94] showed a marked improvement in the mean left ventricular ejection fraction with exercise from 51% to 62% after angioplasty. However, no change in the resting ejection fraction was noted as seen in post–CABG surgery patients (Fig. 24-19).

*References 13, 29, 31, 44, 94, 105, 108, 112, 152.

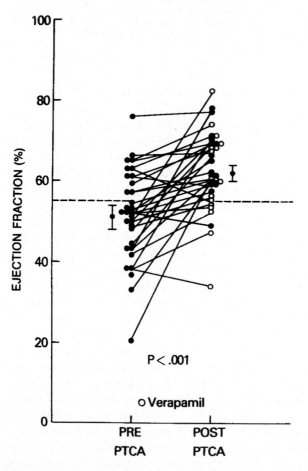

Fig. 24-19. Left ventricular ejection fraction before and after successful angioplasty. (Reproduced with permission from Kent KM, Bonow RO, Rosing DR, et al: Improved myocardial function during exercise after successful percutaneous transluminal coronary angioplasty, *N Engl J Med* 306:441-446, Copyright 1982 Massachusetts Medical Society. All rights reserved.)

Thus, although the ejection fraction response was abnormal in 87% of patients before PTCA, only 19% had an abnormal study afterward. Similar findings have been noted in other studies, in which an abnormal preangioplasty exercise left ventricular ejection fraction response resolved in most patients.[29,108,152,161] Exercise-induced regional wall-motion abnormalities that usually resolved after PTCA were also present in most patients studied by Kent et al[94] and DePuey et al.[29] Explanations for the lack of resolution of regional or global wall-motion responses with exercise after PTCA include previous infarction, left bundle-branch block, female sex, and advanced age.[31] Therefore, normalization of the global ejection fraction response to exercise and the resolution of stress-induced wall-motion abnormalities are reasonably sensitive markers of successful PTCA.

In addition to the aforementioned improvements noted in systolic function after PTCA, radionuclide angiography may document improvement of diastolic function after angioplasty, as shown in the study by Bonow et al[13] in 25 patients with single-vessel coronary disease but without abnormal systolic function at rest. Moreover, in addition to the improvement noted in diastolic function after exercise, an association was also shown between the reduction of exercise-induced ventricular dysfunction after PTCA and improved resting diastolic function.

A sensitive measure of left ventricular dysfunction is the pulmonary blood volume ratio, which is the relative change of pulmonary blood volume from a resting to an exercise state. In a study examining the effects of angioplasty on the pulmonary blood volume ratio, Liu et al[112] revealed that 85% of the 31 patients had an abnormal pulmonary blood volume ratio; this proportion decreased to 38% within 2 weeks after angioplasty.[112] These results were diagnostically superior to the improvement noted in global left ventricular ejection function, suggesting that the pulmonary blood volume ratio, like a diastolic variable,[13] seems to be a sensitive indicator of successful angioplasty.

The value of radionuclide angiography for predicting restenosis was examined by DePuey et al,[32] who performed radionuclide angiography before PTCA 4 days and 4 to 12 months after PTCA in 41 patients with single-vessel coronary disease. All patients underwent recatheterization, regardless of their symptoms. On the basis of early post-PTCA radionuclide angiography, only 18% of patients without restenosis did not have an increase in exercise ejection fraction of at least 5%; among patients with restenosis, 75% had an abnormal exercise response. On late follow-up radionuclide angiography, the exercise ejection fraction response correlated with the presence of restenosis and was a better predictor than symptoms or exercise electrocardiographic changes (Fig. 24-20). Most of the patients without restenosis (73%) had a normal result on exercise radionuclide angiography, whereas 88% of those with restenosis had an abnormal exercise ejection fraction response. The value of exercise radionuclide angiography for the prediction of restenosis after PTCA was confirmed by other investigators.[90,134] O'Keefe et al[134] performed exercise radionuclide angiography in 48 patients within 1 month after PTCA and found a negative predictive value of 100%. Thus, patients may be ef-

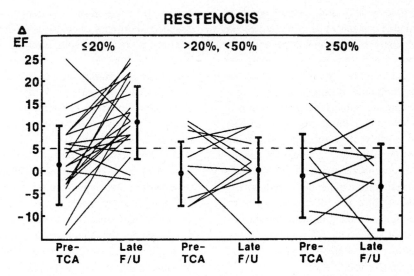

Fig. 24-20. The change in the ejection fraction *(ΔEF)* with exercise before *(pre)* and 4 to 12 months of follow-up *(F/U)* after angioplasty *(PTCA)*. Patients are grouped on the basis of the degree of angiographic stenosis at the time of radionuclide angiography. (Reproduced with permission from DePuey EG, Leatherman LL, Leachman RD, et al: Restenosis after transluminal coronary angioplasty detected with exercise-gated radionuclide ventriculography, *J Am Coll Cardiol* 4:1107, 1984.)

fectively stratified into groups that are at low and high risk for restenosis according to radionuclide angiographic results,[32,90,134] although this technique is best suited for the identification of a group at low risk for restenosis.

Ernst et al[44] evaluated 25 patients with single-vessel disease before PTCA and again at 14 days and 4 to 8 months after angioplasty. They directly compared radionuclide angiography data with data obtained with thallium scintigraphy. Both techniques accurately identified the presence of ischemia before PTCA was performed. Despite the trend noted in changes in left ventricular ejection fraction, thallium imaging demonstrated a diagnostic accuracy for the prediction of restenosis superior to that achieved with radionuclide angiography. The differences noted between radionuclide angiography and myocardial perfusion imaging in this study probably resulted from the inherent differences between these two nuclear cardiology methods, including the superior localization of coronary ischemia with myocardial perfusion imaging.

Thus, after coronary angioplasty, radionuclide ventriculography may show the resolution of ischemia and an improved functional response to exercise. In addition, the improvement in the diastolic properties of the left ventricle may be substantiated, and radionuclide angiography may predict restenosis after PTCA (Box 24-2).

COMPARISON WITH OTHER METHODS
Exercise stress testing

For approximately 25 years, exercise electrocardiographic stress testing has been used for the evaluation of patients undergoing CABG surgery.[39] This method of noninvasive evaluation provides important clinical information about the frequent

---

Box 24-2. Value of nuclear cardiology testing after revascularization

Documentation of therapeutic improvement
Identification of residual ischemia
Detection and prediction of graft stenosis
Detection and prediction of restenosis
Determination of disease progression

---

problems of graft disease and occlusion.[7,57,171] Recently, Lakkis[104] directly compared the diagnostic accuracy of electrocardiographic stress testing with that of exercise myocardial perfusion imaging in 50 patients after CABG. Overall, a significant increase in sensitivity for the detection of graft stenosis was noted with thallium scintigraphy compared with electrocardiographic stress testing (80% and 31%), with a resultant increase in overall accuracy (82% and 50%) (Fig. 24-5). Radionuclide angiography also showed the superiority of exercise testing for the prediction of long-term prognosis after bypass surgery; exercise left ventricular fraction was the most important noninvasive determinant of event-free survival.[76,172]

Exercise testing without imaging was shown to be useful in the prediction of restenosis in a study of 31 patients with a positive study before angioplasty.[43] Of the patients who subsequently developed restenosis, 93% had a positive treadmill test 3 to 6 months after PTCA, but none of the 17 patients without restenosis had an abnormal result on exercise electrocardiography. Thus, the authors concluded that radionuclide angiography or myocardial perfusion imaging was not necessary. However, the study was highly selected—only patients who had positive exercise tests before angioplasty and single-vessel coronary artery disease were included. Laarman et al[102] examined the value of electrocardiographic stress testing in 141 patients after PTCA by using coronary angiography as the standard for restenosis. The positive and negative predictive values for restenosis with electrocardiographic testing were 15% and 87%, respectively. The prognostic value for the prediction of further cardiac events was low (35%); this is consistent with results of other studies.[10] In a study of more than 300 patients who underwent exercise testing after PTCA, Bengston demonstrated that exercise-induced angina, recurrent chest pain, and a positive treadmill exercise test were independent predictors of restenosis.[10] However, 20% of patients with restenosis had recurrent angina or exercise-induced ischemia, thus demonstrating an important limitation of sensitivity for exercise testing. The authors suggested that the exercise treatment test "must be supplemented by a more definitive test."[10]

Although exercise testing has the advantage of widespread availability and relatively low cost, myocardial perfusion imaging has distinct advantages for the treatment of patients before or after coronary revascularization. Perfusion imaging has clear superiority with regard to specificity and predictive value for postrevascularization events.[25,123,160,178] Exercise stress testing does not contribute to the prediction of recurrent chest pain or myocardial infarction beyond data obtained with scintigraphy.[178] Furthermore, many studies have demonstrated improved prediction of restenosis after PTCA with perfusion imaging compared with exercise testing alone.* The sensitivity for restenosis detection with exercise testing ranges from 40% to 74% compared with 67% to 97% for perfusion imaging.† In addition, the positive predictive value of an abnormal stress test is substantially less than comparable values for the presence of thallium redistribution[177] (Fig. 24-13).

Therefore, nuclear cardiology techniques provide important prognostic information about the development of recurrent symptoms or cardiac events and predict restenosis or bypass graft disease. An additional advantage is that nonexercise stress testing may be performed in patients who are unable to exercise or who have a potentially confounding electrocardiogram (see the section on pharmacologic testing). Perhaps most important, the exercise electrocardiogram does not permit the determination of location of the ischemia, nor does it accurately assess the extent of ischemia; these factors are often crucial in the decision-making process in the post–CABG surgery or post-PTCA patient. Although no clear validation for this approach can be found in the literature, management decisions are likely to be more appropriate when they are guided by scintigraphic testing.[154]

Stress echocardiography

Echocardiography, in conjunction with exercise or pharmacologic stress testing, recently demonstrated diagnostic and prognostic value in the assessment of patients with known or suspected coronary artery disease. Both before and after PTCA, exercise echocardiography provides a useful functional assessment and has a high concordance with thallium scintigraphy.[45] The functional significance of a lesion may also be determined with echocardiography.[28,92] With regard to the evaluation of patients after coronary revascularization, echocardiography has demonstrated the success of angioplasty by documenting the resolution of dobutamine-induced wall-motion abnormalities in 31 of 35 patients.[3] Both exercise[89] and dobutamine[42] echocardiography have been shown to detect graft stenosis or disease progression after bypass surgery. In the largest series, Kafka et al[89] demonstrated a sensitivity of 70% and specificity of 82% for post-CABG disease. However, echocardiography has a low sensitivity for the detection of multivessel disease.[42,89]

Furthermore, exercise echocardiography may predict the development of recurrent ischemia after PTCA, with a sensitivity of 83% and specificity of 85%.[119] For noninvasive detection of coronary restenosis, exercise,[62] dipyridamole,[142] and dobutamine[12] echocardiography have shown a diagnostic accuracy similar to that seen with thallium scintigraphy and had an acceptable sensitivity (75% to 87%) and a very high specificity (84% to 95%)[62,142] (Fig. 24-21). In addition, a good correlation was noted with regard to the site, severity, and extent of the abnormalities.[142] Similarly, transesophageal atrial pacing and [99mTc] sestamibi imaging had a comparable efficacy for the detection of restenosis; the sensitivity and specificity of both techniques was 84% to 86%.[72]

Low-dose dobutamine echocardiography has been successfully used to detect myocardial viability based on improved contractile function. Comparative studies abound on myocardial perfusion imaging and dobutamine echocardiography, and essentially all of the studies show the general comparability of the techniques for the detection of viability and the prediction of functional recovery after CABG surgery[4,23,24] and PTCA.[1,92]

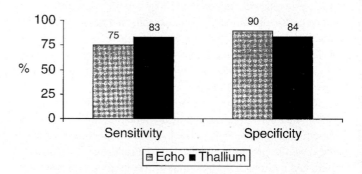

Fig. 24-21. Comparative sensitivity and specificity for the detection of asymptomatic restenosis after coronary angioplasty, based on thallium-201 imaging or stress echocardiography *(Echo).* (Reproduced with permission from Pirelli S, Danzi GB, Massa D, et al: Exercise thallium scintigraphy versus high-dose dipyridamole echocardiography testing for detection of asymptomatic restenosis in patients with positive exercise tests after coronary angioplasty, *Am J Cardiol* 71:1052-1056, Copyright 1993 by Excerpta Medica Inc.)

*References 19, 44, 60, 63, 64, 116, 140, 156.
†References 81, 83, 123, 148, 177, 178.

Therefore, although few comparative studies of nuclear cardiology techniques and stress echocardiography have been performed in patients after revascularization, the results seem similar. However, the usual limitations of echocardiography remain, such as an inadequate acoustic window and the reduced ability to localize abnormalities. The use of transesophageal imaging all but eliminates the problem of poor endocardial visualization. A study recently confirmed that transesophageal echocardiography was superior to transthoracic echocardiography for the detection of ischemia after CABG surgery, with the sensitivity increasing from 78% to 93%.[73] Echocardiography with the administration and visualization of contrast material offers the potential for improved visualization of the endocardial surfaces as a result of acoustic opacification of the left ventricle. No data are currently available on the use of contrast stress echocardiography in patients after revascularization.

SUMMARY AND RECOMMENDATIONS

Coronary revascularization by means of CABG surgery or with PTCA is frequently used in the care of patients with ischemic heart disease. Before revascularization is performed, radionuclide angiography and myocardial perfusion imaging may assist in management decisions by demonstrating the presence of myocardial ischemia and viability and delineating the severity and extent of coronary artery disease. The presence of myocardial ischemia may provide an indication for revascularization, even in asymptomatic persons.[154] The significance of equivocal lesions may be determined and the culprit vessel may be successfully defined by perfusion imaging before angioplasty or CABG.

After revascularization, coronary anatomy and physiology are altered, and many of the markers and findings in patients before revascularization may have different clinical value afterward. Both perfusion scintigraphy and radionuclide angiography usually demonstrate improvement of perfusion or functional response to exercise. Noninvasive testing has been studied far less extensively in post-PTCA and post–CABG surgery patients, but it seems that nuclear cardiology techniques accurately predict events in patients after revascularization. In addition, the determination and prediction of coronary restenosis after angioplasty and graft disease after CABG surgery may be determined by scintigraphic techniques. The finding that restenosis may occur in the absence of recurrent symptoms[44,140] is clinically relevant and implies a potentially crucial role for myocardial perfusion imaging in the management of patients after angioplasty. An examination demonstrating myocardial ischemia early after PTCA may be of limited value because of reduced specificity during the first 4 to 6 weeks after angioplasty, but performance of a nonischemic study makes restenosis much less likely.

Beyond the documentation of improved cardiac perfusion and function and the prediction of restenosis after revascularization, both perfusion imaging and radionuclide angiography have demonstrated prognostic value for the prediction of long-term event-free survival. For perfusion imaging, these findings have been shown regardless of the method selected and include the use of ^{201}Tl or ^{99m}Tc radiopharmaceuticals or after varying modes of stress testing. In addition, nuclear cardiology techniques have obvious superiority for diagnostic accuracy of graft disease or angiographic restenosis compared with clinical assessment alone or in conjunction with electrocardiographic stress testing.

The recent recommendations by the joint AHA/ACC Task Force seem rational and well supported by the previously reviewed literature[150] (Table 24-2). The definition of culprit vessels before PTCA by perfusion imaging is a class I recommendation (appropriate and useful). Likewise, the determination by thallium scintigraphy of myocardial viability in patients being considered for revascularization is also a class I recommendation. After revascularization, perfusion imaging is thought to be useful and appropriate for 1) the determination of restenosis after angioplasty in patients who are symptomatic, 2) evaluation

Table 24-2. Recommendations for the use of radionuclide testing in association with revascularization*

Indication	Test	Class†
Viability assessment before revascularization	Thallium imaging	I
Pre-PTCA detection of ischemia	Exercise or pharmacologic MPI	I
	Exercise radionuclide angiography	IIa
Assessment of restenosis in symptomatic patients after angioplasty	Exercise or pharmacologic MPI	I
	Exercise radionuclide angiography	IIa
Assessment of ischemia in symptomatic patients after CABG surgery	Exercise or pharmacologic MPI	I
	Exercise radionuclide angiography	IIa
Asymptomatic patients after revascularization with abnormal or indeterminant stress test	Exercise and pharmacologic MPI	I
	Exercise radionuclide angiography	IIa
Routine assessment of asymptomatic patients after revascularization	All tests	III

*CABG = coronary artery bypass graft; MPI = myocardial perfusion imaging; PTCA = percutaneous transluminal coronary angioplasty.
†I = usually appropriate and considered useful; IIa = weight of evidence in favor of usefulness; III = generally not appropriate.
Modified from Richie J, et al, AHA/ACC Task Force: Guidelines for clinical use of cardiac radionuclide imaging, *Circulation* 91:1278-1302, 1995.

of ischemia in symptomatic post–CABG surgery patients, and 3) asymptomatic post-revascularization patients who have an abnormal or uninterpretable electrocardiographic response to exercise. For all of these indications, radionuclide angiography is considered a class IIa recommendation, in which the weight of the evidence favors the usefulness of the technique. However, all radionuclide testing was felt not to be appropriate for the routine assessment of asymptomatic patients after revascularization.

REFERENCES

1. Afridi I, Kleiman NS, Raizner AE, et al: Dobutamine echocardiography in myocardial hibernation. Optimal dose and accuracy in predicting recovery of ventricular function after coronary angioplasty, *Circulation* 91:663–670, 1995.
2. Akins CN, Boucher CA, Pohost GM: Preservation of interventricular septal function in patients having coronary artery bypass grafts without cardiopulmonary bypass, *Am Heart J* 107:304–309, 1984.
3. Akosah KO, Porter TR, Simon R, et al: Ischemia-induced regional wall motion abnormality is improved after coronary angioplasty: demonstration by dobutamine stress echocardiography, *J Am Coll Cardiol* 21:584–589, 1993.
4. Arnese M, Cornel JH, Salustri A, et al: Prediction of improvement of regional left ventricular function after surgical revascularization. A comparison of low-dose dobutamine echocardiography with ^{201}Tl single-photon emission computed tomography, *Circulation* 91: 2748–2752, 1995.
5. Austin EH, Oldman HN Jr, Sabiston DC Jr, et al: Early assessment of rest and exercise left ventricular function following coronary artery surgery, *Ann Thorac Surg* 35:159–169, 1983.
6. Avery PG, Hudson NM, Hubner PJ: Assessment of myocardial perfusion and function using gated methoxy-isobutyl-isonitrile scintigraphy to detect restenosis after coronary angioplasty, *Coron Artery Dis* 4:1097–1102, 1993.
7. Bartel AG, Behar VS, Peter RH, et al: Exercise stress testing in evaluation of aortocoronary bypass surgery. Report of 123 patients, *Circulation* 48:141–148, 1973.
8. Bates ER, Aueron FM, Legrand V, et al: Comparative long-term effects of coronary artery bypass graft surgery and percutaneous transluminal coronary angioplasty on regional coronary flow reserve, *Circulation* 72:833–839, 1985.
9. Beller GA, Gibson RS, Watson DD: Radionuclide methods of identifying patients who may require coronary artery bypass surgery, *Circulation* 72(6 Pt 2):V9–V22, 1985.
10. Bengtson JR, Mark DB, Honan MB, et al: Detection of restenosis after elective percutaneous transluminal coronary angioplasty using the exercise treadmill test. *Am J Cardiol* 65:28–34, 1990.
11. Blood DK, McCarthy DM, Sciacca RR, et al: Comparison of single-dose and double-dose thallium-201 myocardial perfusion scintigraphy for the detection of coronary artery disease and prior myocardial infarction, *Circulation* 58:777–788, 1978.
12. Bolognese L, Antoniucci D, Rovai D, et al: Myocardial contrast echocardiography versus dobutamine echocardiography for predicting functional recovery after acute myocardial infarction treated with primary coronary angioplasty, *J Am Coll Cardiol* 28:1677–1683, 1996.
13. Bonow RO, Kent KM, Rosing DR, et al: Improved left ventricular diastolic filling in patients with coronary artery disease after percutaneous transluminal coronary angioplasty, *Circulation* 66:1159–1167, 1982.
14. Borges-Neto S, Watson JE, Miller MJ: Tc-99m sestamibi cardiac SPECT imaging during coronary artery occlusion in humans: comparison with dipyridamole stress studies, *Radiology* 198:751–754, 1996.
15. Braat SH, de Swart H, Rigo P, et al: Value of technetium Mibi to detect short lasting episodes of severe myocardial ischaemia and to estimate the area at risk during coronary angioplasty, *Eur Heart J* 12:30–33, 1991.
16. Braat SH, de Swart H, Janssen JH, et al: Use of technetium-99m sestamibi to determine the size of the myocardial area perfused by a coronary artery, *Am J Cardiol* 66:85E–90E, 1990.
17. Braunwald EE: *Heart disease: a textbook of cardiovascular medicine*, ed 5, Philadelphia, 1997, WB Saunders Co.
18. Breisblatt WM, Barnes JV, Weiland F, et al: Incomplete revascularization in multivessel percutaneous transluminal coronary angioplasty: the role for stress thallium-201 imaging, *J Am Coll Cardiol* 11:1183–1190, 1988.
19. Breisblatt WM, Weiland FL, Spaccavento LJ: Stress thallium-201 imaging after coronary angioplasty predicts restenosis and recurrent symptoms, *J Am Coll Cardiol* 12:1199–1204, 1988.
20. Brown KA: Prognostic value of thallium-201 myocardial perfusion imaging. A diagnostic tool comes of age, *Circulation* 83:363–381, 1991.
21. Brown KA, Boucher CA, Okada RD, et al: Prognostic value of exercise thallium-201 imaging in patients presenting for evaluation of chest pain, *J Am Coll Cardiol* 1:994–1001, 1983.
22. Carvalho PA, Vekshtein VI, Tumeh SS, et al: Tc-99m MIBI SPECT in the assessment of myocardial perfusion after percutaneous transluminal coronary angioplasty, *Clin Nucl Med* 16:819–825, 1991.
23. Charney R, Schwinger ME, Chun J, et al: Dobutamine echocardiography and resting-redistribution thallium-201 scintigraphy predicts recovery of hibernating myocardium after coronary revascularization, *Am Heart J* 128:864–869, 1994.
24. Cigarroa CG, deFilippi CR, Brinker ME, et al: Dobutamine stress echocardiography identifies hibernating myocardium and predicts functional recovery of left ventricular function after coronary revascularization. *Circulation* 88:430–436, 1993.
25. Cloninger KG, DePuey EG, Garcia EV, et al: Incomplete redistribution in delayed thallium-201 single photon emission computed tomographic (SPECT) images: an overestimation of myocardial scarring, *J Am Coll Cardiol* 12:955–963, 1988.
26. McCormick JR, Schick EC Jr, McCabe CH, et al: Determinants of operative mortality and long term survival in patients with unstable angina. The CASS experience, *J Thorac Cardiovasc Surg* 89: 683–688, 1985.
27. Cote G, Myler RK, Stertzer SH, et al: Percutaneous transluminal angioplasty of stenotic coronary artery bypass grafts: 5 years experience, *J Am Coll Cardiol* 9:8–17, 1987.
28. Davila-Roman VG, Wong AK, Li D, et al: Usefulness of dobutamine stress echocardiography for the prospective identification of the physiologic significance of coronary narrowings of moderate severity in patients undergoing evaluation for percutaneous transluminal coronary angioplasty, *Am J Cardiol* 76:245–249, 1995.
29. DePuey EG, Boskovic D, Krajcer Z, et al: Exercise radionuclide ventriculography in evaluating successful transluminal coronary angioplasty, *Cathet Cardiovasc Diagn* 9:153–166, 1983.
30. DePuey EG, Roubin G, Cloninger K, et al: Correlates of PTCA parameters and quantitative thallium-201 tomography, *J Invest Cardiol* 1:40–49, 1988.
31. DePuey EG: Radionuclide methods to evaluate percutaneous transluminal coronary angioplasty, *Semin Nucl Med* 21:102–115, 1991.
32. DePuey EG, Leatherman LL, Leachman RD, et al: Restenosis after transluminal coronary angioplasty detected with exercise-gated radionuclide ventriculography, *J Am Coll Cardiol* 4:1103–1113, 1984.
33. Deychak YA, Segal J, Reiner JS, et al: Doppler guide wire flow-velocity indexes measured distal to coronary stenoses associated with reversible thallium perfusion defects, *Am Heart J* 129:219–227, 1995.
34. Deychak YA, Segal J, Reiner J, et al: Doppler guide wire-derived coronary flow reserve distal to intermediate stenoses used in clinical

decision making regarding interventional therapy, *Am Heart J* 128:178–181, 1994.

35. Di Carli MF, Asgarzadie F, Schelbert, HR, et al: Quantitative relation between myocardial viability and improvement in heart failure symptoms after revascularization in patients with ischemic cardiomyopathy, *Circulation* 92:3436–3444, 1995.

36. Di Carli MF, Davidson M, Little R, et al: Value of metabolic imaging with positron emission tomography for evaluating prognosis in patients with coronary artery disease and left ventricular dysfunction, *Am J Cardiol* 73:527–533, 1994.

37. Dilsizian V, Bonow RO: Current diagnostic techniques of assessing myocardial viability in patients with hibernating and stunned myocardium, *Circulation* 87:1–20, 1993.

38. Dilsizian V, Rocco TP, Freedman NM, et al: Enhanced detection of ischemic but viable myocardium by the reinjection of thallium after stress-redistribution imaging, *N Engl J Med* 323:141–146, 1990.

39. Dodek A, Kassebaum DG, Griswold HE: Stress electrocardiography in the evaluation of aortocoronary bypass surgery, *Am Heart J* 86:292–307, 1973.

40. Eichhorn EJ, Konstam MA, Salem DN, et al: Dipyridamole thallium-201 imaging pre- and post-coronary angioplasty for assessment of regional myocardial ischemia in humans, *Am Heart J* 117:1203–1209, 1989.

41. Eitzman D, al-Aouar Z, Kanter HL, et al: Clinical outcome of patients with advanced coronary artery disease after viability studies with positron emission tomography, *J Am Coll Cardiol* 20:559–565, 1992.

42. Elhendly A, Geleijnse ML, Roelandt JR, et al: Assessment of patients after coronary artery bypass grafting by dobutamine stress echocardiography, *Am J Cardiol* 77:1234–1236, 1996.

43. el-Tamimi H, Davies GJ, Hackett D, et al: Very early prediction of restenosis after successful coronary angioplasty: anatomic and functional assessment, *J Am Coll Cardiol* 15:259–264, 1990.

44. Ernst SM, Hillebrand FA, Klein B, et al: The value of exercise tests in the follow-up of patients who underwent transluminal coronary angioplasty, *Int J Cardiol* 7:267–279, 1985.

45. Fioretti PM, Pozzi MM, Ilmer B, et al: Exercise echocardiography versus thallium-201 SPECT for assessing patients before and after PTCA, *Eur Heart J* 13:213–219, 1992.

46. Fischman DL, Leon MB, Baim DS, et al: A randomized comparison of coronary-stent placement and balloon angioplasty in the treatment of coronary artery disease. Stent Restenosis Study Investigators, *N Engl J Med* 331:496–501, 1994.

47. Fitzgibbon GM, Kafka HP, Leach AJ, et al: Coronary bypass graft fate and patient outcome: angiographic follow-up of 5,065 grafts related to survival and reoperation in 1,388 patients during 25 years, *J Am Coll Cardiol* 26:616–626, 1996.

48. Fitzgibbon GM, Leach AJ, Kafka HP, et al: Coronary bypass graft fate: long term angiographic study, *J Am Coll Cardiol* 17:1075–1080, 1991.

49. Fuster V, Badimon L, Badimon JJ, et al: The pathogenesis of coronary artery disease and the acute coronary syndrome (1), *N Engl J Med* 326:242–259, 1992.

50. Gallik DM, Obermueller SD, Swarna US, et al: Simultaneous assessment of myocardial perfusion and left ventricular function during transient coronary occlusion, *J Am Coll Cardiol* 25:1529–1538, 1995.

51. Germano G, Kiat H, Kavanaugh PB, et al: Automatic quantitation of ejection fraction from gated myocardial perfusion SPECT, *J Nucl Med* 36:2138–2147, 1995.

52. Gershlick AH, Lyons JP, Wright JE, et al: Long term clinical outcome of coronary surgery and assessment of the benefit obtained with postoperative aspirin and dipyridamole, *Br Heart J* 60:111–116, 1988.

53. Ghods M, Pancholy SP, Cave V, et al: Serial changes in left ventricular function after coronary artery bypass: implications in viability assessment, *Am Heart J* 129:20–23, 1995.

54. Gibbons RJ, Verani MS, Behrenbeck T, et al: Feasibility of tomographic 99mTc-hexakis-2-methoxy-2-methylpropyl-isonitrile imaging for the assessment of myocardial area at risk and the effect of treatment in acute myocardial infarction, *Circulation* 80:1277–1286, 1989.

55. Gibson RS, Watson DD, Taylor GJ, et al: Prospective assessment of regional myocardial perfusion before and after coronary revascularization surgery by quantitative thallium-201 scintigraphy, *J Am Coll Cardiol* 1:804–815, 1983.

56. Gill JB, Ruddy TD, Newell JB, et al: Prognostic importance of thallium uptake by the lungs during exercise in coronary artery disease, *N Engl J Med* 317:1486–1489, 1987.

57. Greenberg BH, Hart R, Botvinick EH, et al: Thallium-201 myocardial perfusion scintigraphy to evaluate patients after coronary bypass surgery, *Am J Cardiol* 42:167–176, 1978.

58. Gruentzig AR, King SB 3d, Schlumpf M, et al: Long-term follow-up after percutaneous transluminal coronary angioplasty. The early Zurich experience, *N Engl J Med* 316:1127–1132, 1987.

59. Hamby RI, Aintablian A, Handler M, et al: Aortocoronary saphaneous vein bypass grafts. Long-term patency, morphology and blood flow in patients with patent grafts early after surgery, *Circulation* 60: 901–909, 1979.

60. Hardoff R, Shefer A, Gips S, et al: Predicting late restenosis after coronary angioplasty by very early (12 to 24 h) thallium-201 scintigraphy: implications with regard to mechanisms of late coronary restenosis, *J Am Coll Cardiol* 15:1486–1492, 1990.

61. Haronian HL, Remetz MS, Sinusas AJ, et al: Myocardial risk area defined by technetium-99m sestamibi imaging during percutaneous transluminal coronary angioplasty: comparison with coronary angiography, *J Am Coll Cardiol* 22:1033–1043, 1993.

62. Hecht HS, DeBord L, Shaw R, et al: Usefulness of supine bicycle stress echocardiography for detection of restenosis after percutaneous transluminal coronary angioplasty, *Am J Cardiol* 71:293–296, 1993.

63. Hecht HS, Shaw RE, Bruce TR, et al: Usefulness of tomographic thallium-201 imaging for detection of restenosis after percutaneous transluminal coronary angioplasty, *Am J Cardiol* 66:1314–1318, 1990.

64. Hecht HS, Shaw RE, Chin HL, et al: Silent ischemia after coronary angioplasty: evaluation of restenosis and extent of ischemia in asymptomatic patients by tomographic thallium-201 exercise imaging and comparison with symptomatic patients, *J Am Coll Cardiol* 17: 670–677, 1991.

65. Heller LI, Villegas BJ, Weiner BH, et al: Sequential teboroxime imaging during and after balloon occlusion of a coronary artery, *J Am Coll Cardiol* 21:1319–1327, 1993.

66. Hellman C, Schmidt DH, Kamath ML, et al: Bypass graft surgery in severe left ventricular dysfunction, *Circulation* 62 (2 Pt 2):103–110, 1980.

67. Higginbotham MB, Belkin RN, Morris KG, et al: Value and limitation of biplane rest and exercise radionuclide angiography for assessing individual bypass grafts: a prospective study, *J Am Coll Cardiol* 7:1004–1014, 1986.

68. Hirzel HO, Nuesch K, Gruentzig AR, et al: Thallium-201 exercise scintigraphy after percutaneous transluminal angioplasty of coronary artery stenoses, *Med Clin North Am* 64:163–176, 1980.

69. Hirzel HO, Nuesch K, Gruentzig AR, et al: Short- and long-term changes in myocardial perfusion after percutaneous transluminal coronary angioplasty assessed by thallium-201 exercise scintigraphy, *Circulation* 63:1001–1007, 1981.

70. Hirzel HO, Nuesch K, Sialer G, et al: Thallium-201 exercise myocardial imaging to evaluate myocardial perfusion after coronary artery bypass surgery, *Br Heart J* 43:426–435, 1980.

71. Hodgson JM, Riley RS, Most AS, et al: Assessment of coronary flow reserve using digital angiography before and after successful percutaneous transluminal coronary angioplasty, *Am J Cardiol* 60:61–65, 1987.

72. Hoffmann R, Kleinhans H, Lambertz H, et al: Transesophageal pacing echocardiography for detection of restenosis after percutaneous transluminal coronary angioplasty, *Eur Heart J* 15:823–831, 1994.

73. Hoffmann R, Lethen H, Falter F, et al: Dobutamine stress echocardiography after coronary artery bypass grafting. Transthoracic vs biplane transesophageal imaging, *Eur Heart J* 17:222–229, 1996.

74. Huber KC, Bresnahan JF, Bresnahan DR, et al: Measurement of myocardium at risk by technetium-99m sestamibi: correlation with coronary angiography, *J Am Coll Cardiol* 13:67–73, 1992.

75. Iskandrian AS, Chae SC, Heo J, et al: Independent and incremental prognostic value of exercise single-photon emission computed tomographic (SPECT) thallium imaging in coronary artery disease, *J Am Coll Cardiol* 22:665–670, 1993.

76. Iskandrian AS, Friedman T, Hakki A, et al: Evaluation of left ventricular function during exercise after coronary artery bypass surgery, *Cardiovasc Rev Rep* 138, 1984.

77. Iskandrian AS, Haaz W, Segal B, et al: Exercise thallium 201 scintigraphy in evaluating aortocoronary bypass surgery, *Chest* 80:11–15, 1981.

78. Iskandrian AS, Hakki AH, Nestico PF, et al: Effects of residual coronary artery disease on results of coronary artery bypass grafting, *Int J Cardiol* 6:537–545, 1984.

79. Iskandrian AS, Hakki AH, Kane SA, et al: Rest and redistribution thallium-201 myocardial scintigraphy to predict improvement in left ventricular function after coronary arterial bypass grafting, *Am J Cardiol* 51:1312–1316, 1983.

80. Iskandrian AE, Kegel JG, Tecce MA, et al: Simultaneous assessment of left ventricular perfusion and function with technetium-99m sestamibi after coronary artery bypass grafting, *Am Heart J* 126: 1199–1203, 1993.

81. Iskandrian AS, Lemlek J, Ogilby JD, et al: Early thallium imaging after percutaneous transluminal coronary angioplasty: tomographic evaluation during adenosine-induced coronary hyperemia, *J Nucl Med* 33:2086–2089, 1993.

82. Iskandrian AS, Verani MS, Heo J: Pharmacologic stress testing: mechanism of action, hemodynamic responses, and results in detection of coronary artery disease, *J Nucl Cardiol* 1:94–111, 1994.

83. Jain A, Mahmarian JJ, Borges-Neto S, et al: Clinical significance of perfusion defects by thallium-201 single photon emission tomography following oral dipyridamole early after coronary angioplasty, *J Am Coll Cardiol* 11:970–976, 1988.

84. Johnson AM, Kron IL, Watson DD, et al: Evaluation of postoperative flow reserve in internal mammary artery bypass grafts, *J Thorac Cardiovasc Surg* 92:822–826, 1986.

85. Johnson M, Wilson R, Skorton D, et al: Coronary lumen area immediately after angioplasty does not correlate with coronary vasodilator reserve: a videodensitometric study, *Circulation* 74 (suppl):II-193, 1986.

86. Johnson WD, Brenowitz JB, Kayser KL: Factors influencing long-term (10-year to 15-year) survival after a successful coronary artery bypass operation, *Ann Thorac Surg* 48:19–24, 1989.

87. Jones EL, Craver JM, Hurst JW, et al: Influence of left ventricular aneurysm on survival following the coronary bypass operation. *Ann Surg* 193:733–742, 1981.

88. Joye JD, Schulman DS, Lasorda D, et al: Intracoronary Doppler guide wire versus stress single-photon emission computed tomographic thallium-201 imaging in assessment of intermediate coronary stenoses, *J Am Coll Cardiol* 24:940–947, 1994.

89. Kafka H, Leach AJ, Fitzgibbon GM: Exercise echocardiography after coronary artery bypass surgery: correlation with coronary angiography, *J Am Coll Cardiol* 25:1019–1023, 1995.

90. Kanemoto N, Hor G, Kober G, et al: Noninvasive assessment of left ventricular performance following transluminal coronary angioplasty, *Int J Cardiol* 3:281–294, 1983.

91. Kanemoto N, Hor G, Kober G, et al: Quantitative evaluation of exercise Tl-201 myocardial scintigraphy before and after transluminal coronary angioplasty. A preliminary report, *Jpn Heart J* 24:891–907, 1983.

92. Kao HL, Wu CC, Ho YL, et al: Dobutamine stress echocardiography predicts early wall motion improvement after elective percutaneous transluminal coronary angioplasty, *Am J Cardiol* 76:652–665, 1995.

93. Kaul S, Lilly DR, Gascho JA, et al: Prognostic utility of the exercise thallium-201 test in ambulatory patients with chest pain: comparison with cardiac catheterization, *Circulation* 77:745–758, 1988.

94. Kent KM, Bonow RO, Rosing DR, et al: Improved myocardial function during exercise after successful percutaneous transluminal coronary angioplasty, *N Engl J Med* 306:441–446, 1982.

95. Kent KM, Borer JS, Green MV, et al: Effects of coronary-artery bypass on global and regional left ventricular function during exercise, *N Engl J Med* 298:1434–1439, 1978.

96. Kerber RE, Litchfield R: Postoperative abnormalities of interventricular septal motion: two dimensional and M-mode echocardiographic correlations, *Am Heart J* 104(2 Pt 1):263–268, 1982.

97. Kiat H, Berman DS, Maddahi J, et al: Late reversibility of tomographic myocardial thallium-201 defects: an accurate marker of myocardial viability, *J Am Coll Cardiol* 12:1456–1463, 1988.

98. Klein LW, Avula SB, Uretz E, et al: Utility of various clinical, noninvasive, and invasive procedures for determining the causes of recurrence of myocardial ischemia or infarction ≥1 year after percutaneous transluminal coronary angioplasty, *Am J Cardiol* 75:1003–1006, 1995.

99. Kronenberg MW, Pederson RW, Harston WE, et al: Left ventricular performance after coronary artery bypass surgery. Prediction of functional benefit, *Ann Intern Med* 99:305–313, 1983.

100. Kuntz RE, Baim DS: Defining coronary restenosis. Newer clinical and angiographic paradigms, *Circulation* 88:1310–1323, 1993.

101. Kusukawa J, Hirota Y, Kawamura K, et al: Efficacy of coronary artery bypass surgery with gastroepiploic artery. Assessment with thallium 201 myocardial scintigraphy, *Circulation* 80(3 Pt 1):I135–I140, 1989.

102. Laarman G, Luijten HE, Van Zeyl LG, et al: Assessment of "silent" restenosis and long term follow-up after successful angioplasty in single vessel coronary artery disease: the value of quantitative exercise electrocardiography and quantitative coronary angiography, *J Am Coll Cardiol* 16:578–585, 1990.

103. Ladenheim ML, Pollock BH, Rozanski A, et al: Extent and severity of myocardial hypoperfusion as predictors of prognosis in patients with suspected coronary artery disease, *J Am Coll Cardiol* 7:464–471, 1986.

104. Lakkis NM, Mahmarian JJ, Verani MS: Exercise thallium-201 single photon emission computed tomography for evaluation of coronary artery bypass graft patency, *Am J Cardiol* 76:107–111, 1995.

105. Legrand V, Aueron FM, Bates ER, et al: Value of exercise radionuclide ventriculography and thallium-201 scintigraphy in evaluating successful coronary angioplasty: comparison with coronary flow reserve, translesion gradient and percent diameter stenosis, *Eur Heart J* 8:329–339, 1987.

106. Lew AS, Maddahi J, Shah K, et al: Critically ischemic myocardium in clinically stable patients following thrombolytic therapy for acute myocardial infarction: potential implications for early coronary angioplasty in selected patients, *Am Heart J* 120:1015–1025, 1990.

107. Lewis BS, Hardoff R, Merdler A, et al: Importance of immediate and very early postprocedural angiographic and thallium-201 single photon emission computed tomographic perfusion measurements in predicting late results after coronary intervention, *Am Heart J* 130(3 Pt 1):425–432, 1995.

108. Lewis JF, Verani MS, Poliner LR, et al: Effects of transluminal coronary angioplasty on left ventricular systolic and diastolic function at rest and during exercise, *Am Heart J* 109:792–798, 1985.

109. Lim YL, Kalff V, Kelly MJ, et al: Radionuclide angiographic assessment of global and segmental left ventricular function at rest and during exercise after coronary artery bypass graft surgery, *Circulation* 66:972–979, 1982.

110. Lim YL, Okada RD, Chesler DA, et al: A new approach to quantitation of exercise thallium-201 scintigraphy before and after an intervention: application to define the impact of coronary angioplasty on

regional myocardial perfusion, *Am Heart J* 108(4 Pt 1):917–925, 1984.

111. Liu P, Kiess MC, Okada RD, et al: The persistent defect on exercise thallium imaging and its fate after myocardial revascularization: does it represent scar or ischemia? *Am Heart J* 110:996–1001, 1985.

112. Liu P, Kiess MC, Strauss HW, et al: Comparison of ejection fraction and pulmonary blood volume ratio as markers of left ventricular function after coronary angioplasty, *J Am Coll Cardiol* 8:511–516, 1986.

113. Maddahi J, Blitz A, Phelps M, et al: The use of positron emission tomography imaging in the management of patients with ischemic cardiomyopathy, *Adv Card Surg* 7:163–188, 1996.

114. Manyari DE, Knudtson M, Kloiber R, et al: Sequential thallium-201 myocardial perfusion studies after successful percutaneous transluminal coronary angioplasty: delayed resolution of exercise-induced scintigraphic abnormalities, *Circulation* 77:86–95, 1988.

115. March R, Ali A, Bouzoukis M, et al: Effects of transmyocardial laser revascularization on myocardial perfusion, *J Am Coll Cardiol* 29:121A, 1997 (abstract).

116. Marie PY, Danchin N, Karcher G, et al: Usefulness of exercise SPECT-thallium to detect asymptomatic restenosis in patients who had angina before coronary angioplasty, *Am Heart J* 126(3 Pt 1): 571–577, 1993.

117. Marwick TH, Lafont A, Go RT, et al: Identification of recurrent ischemia after coronary artery bypass surgery: a comparison of positron emission tomography and single photon emission computed tomography, *Int J Cardiol* 35:33–41, 1992.

118. Mata LA, Bosch X, David PR, et al: Clinical and angiographic assessment 6 months after double vessel percutaneous coronary angioplasty, *J Am Coll Cardiol* 6:1239–1244, 1985.

119. Mertes H, Erbel R, Nixdorff U, et al: Exercise echocardiography for the evaluation of patients after nonsurgical coronary artery revascularization, *J Am Coll Cardiol* 21:1087–1093, 1993.

120. Milan E, Zoccarato O, Terzi A, et al: Technetium-99m-sestamibi SPECT to detect restenosis after successful percutaneous coronary angioplasty, *J Nucl Med* 37:1300–1305, 1996.

121. Milavertz J, TD M, Hodge D, et al: SPECT myocardial perfusion imaging in patients who have undergone coronary artery stenting, *J Am Coll Cardiol* 29:228A, 1997 (abstract).

122. Miller DD, Donohue TJ, Younis LT, et al: Correlation of pharmacological ^{99m}Tc-sestamibi myocardial perfusion imaging with post-stenotic coronary flow reserve in patients with angiographically intermediate coronary stenoses, *Circulation* 89:2150–2160, 1994.

123. Miller DD, Liu P, Strauss HW, et al: Prognostic value of computer-quantitated exercise thallium imaging early after percutaneous transluminal coronary angioplasty, *J Am Coll Cardiol* 10:275–283, 1987.

124. Miller DD, Verani MS: Current status of myocardial perfusion imaging after percutaneous transluminal coronary angioplasty, *J Am Coll Cardiol* 24:260–266, 1994.

125. Muhlberger V, Knapp E, zur Nedden D: Predictive value of computed tomographic determination of the patency rate of aortocoronary venous bypassess in relation to angiographic results, *Eur Heart J* 11:380–388, 1990.

126. Murphy ML, Hultgren HN, Detre K, et al: Treatment of chronic stable angina. A preliminary report of survival data in the randomized Veterans Administration cooperative study, *N Engl J Med* 297: 621–627, 1977.

127. Nanto S, Kodama K, Hori M, et al: Temporal increase in resting coronary blood flow causes an impairment of coronary flow reserve after coronary angioplasty, *Am Heart J* 123:28–36, 1992.

128. National Heart, Lung, and Blood Institute Alert. 21:1995.

129. Nienaber CA, Brunken RC, Sherman CT, et al: Metabolic and function recovery of ischemic human myocardium after coronary angioplasty, *J Am Coll Cardiol* 18:966–978, 1981.

130. Nobuyoshi M, Kimura T, Nosaka H: Restenosis after successful percutaneous transluminal coronary angioplasty: serial angiographic follow-up of 229 patients, *J Am Coll Cardiol* 12:616–623, 1988.

131. Ohtani H, Tamaki N, Yonekura Y, et al: Value of thallium-201 reinjection after delayed SPECT imaging for predicting reversible ischemia after coronary artery bypass grafting, *Am J Cardiol* 66:394–399, 1990.

132. Okada RD, Glover D, Gaffney T, et al: Myocardial kinetics of technetium-99m-hexakis-2-methoxy-2-methyl-propyl-isonitrile, *Circulation* 77:491–498, 1988.

133. Okada RD, Murphy JH, Boucher CA, et al: Relationship between septal perfusion, viability, and motion before and after coronary artery bypass surgery, *Am Heart J* 124:1190–1195, 1992.

134. O'Keefe JH Jr, Lapeyre AC 3d, Holmes DJ Jr, Gibbons RJ: Usefulness of early radionuclide angiography for identifying low-risk patients for late restenosis after percutaneous transluminal coronary angioplasty, *Am J Cardiol* 61:51–54, 1988.

135. Pace L, Betocchi S, Piscione F, et al: Evaluation of myocardial perfusion and function by technetium-99m methoxy isobutyl isonitrile before and after percutaneous transluminal coronary angioplasty. Preliminary results, *Clin Nucl Med* 18:286–290, 1993.

136. Palmas W, Bingham S, Diamond GA, et al: Incremental prognostic value of exercise thallium-201 myocardial single-photon emission computed tomography late after coronary artery bypass surgery, *J Am Coll Cardiol* 25:403–409, 1995.

137. Petrakian A, Ahmad A, Badruddin S, et al: Value of myocardial perfusion tomography in the assessment of post-stent coronary restenosis, *J Am Coll Cardiol* 29:228A, 1997 (abstract).

138. Pfisterer M, Emmenegger H, Schmitt HE, et al: Accuracy of serial myocardial perfusion scintigraphy with thallium-201 for prediction of graft patency early and late after coronary artery bypass surgery. A controlled prospective study, *Circulation* 66:1017–1024, 1982.

139. Pfisterer M, Muller-Brand J, Spring P, et al: Assessment of the extent of jeopardized myocardium during acute coronary artery occlusion followed by reperfusion in man using technetium-99m isonitrile imaging, *Am Heart J* 122(1 Pt 1):7–12, 1991.

140. Pfisterer M, Rickenbacher P, Kiowski W, et al: Silent ischemia after percutaneous transluminal coronary angioplasty: incidence and prognostic significance, *J Am Coll Cardiol* 22:1446–1454, 1993.

141. Pijls NH, Aengevaeren WR, Uijen GJ, et al: Concept of maximal flow ratio for immediate evaluation of percutaneous transluminal coronary angioplasty result by videodensitometry, *Circulation* 83:854–865, 1991.

142. Pirelli S, Danzi GB, Massa D, et al: Exercise thallium scintigraphy versus high-dose dipyridamole echocardiography testing for detection of asymptomatic restenosis in patients with positive exercise tests after coronary angioplasty, *Am J Cardiol* 71: 1052–1056, 1993.

143. Pollock SG, Abbott RD, Boucher CA, et al: Independent and incremental prognostic value of tests performed in hierarchical order to evaluate patients with suspected coronary artery disease. Validation of models based in those tests, *Circulation* 85:237–248, 1992.

144. Powelson S, et al: Discordance of coronary angiography and 201-thallium tomography early after transluminal coronary angioplasty, *J Nucl Med* 27:900, 1986.

145. Ragosta M, Beller GA, Watson DD, et al: Quantitative planar rest-redistribution ^{201}Tl imaging in detection of myocardial viability and prediction of improvement in left ventricular function after coronary artery bypass surgery in patients with severely depressed left ventricular function, *Circulation* 87:1630–1641, 1993.

146. Rasmussen SL, Nielsen SL, Amtorp O, et al: 201-Thallium imaging as an indicator of graft patency after coronary artery bypass surgery, *Eur Heart J* 5:494–499, 1984.

147. Reed DC, Beller GA, Nygaard TW, et al: The clinical efficacy and scintigraphic evaluation of post-coronary bypass patients undergoing transluminal coronary angioplasty for recurrent angina pectoris, *Am Heart J* 117:60–71, 1989.

148. Renkin J, Melin J, Robert A, et al: Detection of restenosis after successful coronary angioplasty: improved clinical decision making with

use of a logistic model combining procedural and follow-up variables, *J Am Coll Cardiol* 16:1333–1340, 1990.

149. Ritchie JL, Narahara KA, Trobaugh GB, et al: Thallium-201 myocardial imaging before and after coronary revascularization: assessment of regional myocardial blood flow and graft patency, *Circulation* 56:830–836, 1977.

150. Richie JL, Bateman TM, Bonow RO, et al: Guidelines for clinical use of cardiac radionuclide imaging. A report of the American Heart Association/American College of Cardiology Task Force on Assessment of Diagnostic and Therapeutic Cardiovascular Procedures, Committee in Radionuclide Imaging, developed in collaboration with the American Society of Nuclear Cardiology, *Circulation* 91:1278–1303, 1995.

151. Righetti A, Crawford MH, O'Rourke RA, et al: Interventricular septal motion and left ventricular function after coronary artery bypass surgery: evaluation with echocardiography and radionuclide angiography, *Am J Cardiol* 39:372–377, 1977.

152. Rosing DR, Cannon RO 3d, Watson RM, et al: Three year anatomic, functional and clinical follow-up after successful percutaneous transluminal coronary angioplasty, *J Am Coll Cardiol* 9:1–7, 1987.

153. Rozanski A, Berman D, Gray A, et al: Preoperative prediction of reversible myocardial asynergy by postexercise radionuclide ventriculography, *N Engl J Med* 307:212–216, 1982.

154. Guidelines for percutaneous transluminal coronary angioplasty. A report of the American College of Cardiology/American Heart Association Task Force on Assessment of Diagnostic and Therapeutic Cardiovascular Procedures (Committee on Percutaneous Transluminal Coronary Angioplasty), *J Am Coll Cardiol* 22:2033–2054, 1993.

155. Sbarbaro JA, Karunaratne H, Cantez S, et al: Thallium-201 imaging in assessment of aortocoronary artery bypass graft patency, *Br Heart J* 42:553–556, 1979.

156. Scholl JM, Chaitman BR, David PR, et al: Exercise electrocardiography and myocardial scintigraphy in the serial evaluation of the results of percutaneous transluminal coronary angioplasty, *Circulation* 66:380–389, 1982.

157. Serruys PW, Luijten HE, Beatt KJ, et al: Incidence of restenosis after successful coronary angioplasty: a time-related phenomenon. A quantitative angiographic study in 342 consecutive patients at 1, 2, 3, and 4 months, *Circulation* 77:361–371, 1988.

158. Gibson WS, Christian TF, Pellikka PA, et al: Serial tomographic imaging with technetium-99m-sestamibi for the assessment of infarct-related arterial patency following reperfusion therapy, *J Nucl Med* 33:2080–2085, 1992.

159. Steg PG, Faraggi M, Himbert D, et al: Comparison using dynamic vectorcardiography and MIBI SPECT of ST-segment changes and myocardial MIBI uptake during percutaneous transluminal coronary angioplasty of the left anterior descending coronary artery, *Am J Cardiol* 75:998–1002, 1995.

160. Stuckey TD, Burwell LR, Nygaard TW, et al: Quantitative exercise thallium-201 scintigraphy for predicting angina recurrence after percutaneous transluminal coronary angioplasty, *Am J Cardiol* 63:517–521, 1989.

161. Swigart U, Grbic M, Essinger A, et al: Improvement of left ventricular function after percutaneous transluminal coronary angioplasty, *Am J Cardiol* 49:651–657, 1982.

162. Topol EJ, Ellis SG, Cosgrove DM, et al: Analysis of coronary angioplasty practice in the United States with an insurance-claims data base, *Circulation* 87:1489–1497, 1993.

163. Udelson JE, Coleman PS, Metherall J, et al: Predicting recovery of severe regional ventricular dysfunction. Comparison of resting scintigraphy with ^{201}Tl and ^{99m}Tc sestamibi, *Circulation* 89:2552–2561, 1994.

164. Uren NG, Crake T, Lefroy DC, et al: Delayed recovery of coronary resistive vessel function after coronary angioplasty, *J Am Coll Cardiol* 21:612–621, 1993.

165. van Vlies B, van Royen EA, Visser CA, et al: Frequency of myocardial indium-111 antimyosin uptake after uncomplicated coronary artery bypass grafting, *Am J Cardiol* 66:1191–1195, 1990.

166. Verani MS, Marcus ML, Spoto G, et al: Thallium-201 myocardial perfusion scintigrams in the evaluation of aorto-coronary saphenous bypass surgery, *J Nucl Med* 19:765–772, 1978.

167. Verani MS, Tadros S, Raizner AE, et al: Quantitative analysis of thallium-201 uptake and washout before and after transluminal coronary angioplasty, *Int J Cardiol* 13:109–124, 1986.

168. Versaci F, Tomai F, Nudi F, et al: Differences of regional coronary flow reserve assessed by adenosine thallium-201 scintigraphy early and six months after successful percutaneous transluminal coronary angioplasty or stent implantation, *Am J Cardiol* 78:1097–1102, 1996.

169. von Dahl J, Altehoefer C, Sheehan FH, et al: Recovery of regional left ventricular dysfunction after coronary revascularization. Impact of myocardial viability assessed by nuclear imaging and vessel patency at follow-up angiography, *J Am Coll Cardiol* 28:948–958, 1996.

170. Wackers FJ, Gibbons RJ, Verani MS, et al: Serial quantitative planar technetium-99m isonitrile imaging in acute myocardial infarction: efficacy for noninvasive assessment of thrombolytic therapy, *J Am Coll Cardiol* 14:861–873, 1989.

171. Wainwright RJ, Brennand-Roper DA, Maisey MN, et al: Exercise thallium-201 myocardial scintigraphy in the follow-up of aortocoronary bypass graft surgery, *Br Heart J* 43:56–66, 1980.

172. Wallis JB, Supino PG, Borer JS: Prognostic value of left ventricular ejection fraction response to exercise during long-term follow-up after coronary artery bypass graft surgery, *Circulation* 88(5 Pt 2):II99–II109, 1993.

173. Watarida S, Onoe M, Sugita T, et al: Clinical significance of reverse redistribution phenomenon after coronary artery bypass grafting, *Ann Thorac Surg* 59:1528–1532, 1995.

174. Weiss AT, Berman DS, Lew AS, et al: Transient ischemic dilation of the left ventricle on stress thallium-201 scintigraphy: a marker of severe and extensive coronary artery disease, *J Am Coll Cardiol* 9:752–759, 1987.

175. White R, Capito G, Mark A, et al: Evaluation of coronary artery bypass graft patency by magnetic resonance imaging, *Radiology* 164:681–686, 1987.

176. White CW, Wright CB, Doty DB, et al: Does visual interpretation of the coronary arteriogram predict the physiologic importance of a coronary stenosis? *N Engl J Med* 310:819–824, 1984.

177. Wijns W, Serruys PW, Reiber JH, et al: Early detection of restenosis after successful percutaneous transluminal coronary angioplasty by exercise-redistribution thallium scintigraphy, *Am J Cardiol* 55:357–361, 1985.

178. Wijns W, Serruys PW, Simoons ML, et al: Predictive value of early maximal exercise test and thallium scintigraphy after successful percutaneous transluminal coronary angioplasty, *Br Heart J* 53:194–200, 1985.

179. Wilson RF, Johnson MR, Marcus ML: The effect of coronary angioplasty on coronary flow reserve, *Circulation* 77:873–885, 1988.

180. Yusef S, Zucker D, Peduzzi P, et al: Effect of coronary artery bypass graft surgery on survival: overview of 10-year results from randomised trials by the Coronary Artery Bypass Graft Surgery Trialists Collaboration, *Lancet* 344:563–570, 1994.

181. Zijlstra F, den Boer A, Reiber JS, et al: Assessment of immediate and long-term functional results of percutaneous transluminal coronary angioplasty, *Circulation* 78:15–24, 1988.

182. Zimmermann R, Tillmanns H, Knapp WH, et al: Noninvasive assessment of coronary artery bypass patency: determination of myocardial thallium-201 washout rates, *Eur Heart J* 9:319–327, 1988.

PERFUSION IMAGING IN ACUTE ISCHEMIC SYNDROMES

Chapter 25

Myocardium at risk and the effect of reperfusion therapy in acute myocardial infarction: new insights from technetium-99m sestamibi

Timothy F. Christian and **Raymond J. Gibbons**

The care of acute myocardial infarction has undergone a revolution during the past decade. The use of early reperfusion therapy with intravenous thrombolytic agents, as well as direct and ancillary coronary angioplasty, is now commonplace. Multiple randomized trials have demonstrated that early mortality in myocardial infarction is reduced by acute therapy with several different intravenous thrombolytic agents.* This improvement in mortality is maintained for at least 12 months after the acute event.[2,42,113] The reduction in mortality is thought to be related in part to a reduction in infarct size, because reperfusion is presumed to salvage some myocardium that would become infarcted in the absence of reperfusion therapy. Various end points have been used to detect this reduction in infarct size, including the electrocardiogram,[22,31,45,46] resting ejection fraction after infarction,† myocardial perfusion defect size measured by

*References 1, 3, 41, 53, 54, 96.
†References 44, 58, 59, 61, 75, 83, 84, 96.

thallium-201 (^{201}Tl) scintigraphy after infarction,[26,27,84,85] change in resting ejection fraction measured during and after infarction,[44,75,96] and regional wall motion assessed during and after infarction.[93,94,105] Although some studies have demonstrated a consistent significant benefit in both the total study group and major patient subgroups,[53,96] other studies have not been able to detect a treatment effect in any subgroup of patients.[58,59,83,84] Although several studies have found that treatment benefit is restricted to patients with anterior infarction,[58,96] the Global Utilization of Streptokinase and Tissue Plasminogen Activator for Occluded Coronary Arteries (GUSTO) angiographic substudy found a consistent relation among mortality, infarct-related artery patency, and left ventricular function in all groups.[103] The discrepancy between the well-demonstrated reduction in patient mortality and the inconsistent results with other end points that reflect infarct size has generated considerable debate. Possible explanations for this discrepancy include 1) the absence of infarct size measurements on patients who die acutely,[107] 2) other beneficial effects from the restoration of arterial patency,[34,50,88] the so-called "open artery" hypothesis,[8] or 3) potential limitations of the techniques used to measure infarct size. This chapter will review the utility of perfusion imaging with technetium-99m (^{99m}Tc) sestamibi in acute myocardial infarction as it applies to clinical management and clinical trials.

MYOCARDIUM AT RISK

Animal studies

The limitations of the end points used to detect a reduction in infarct size in clinical trials are readily evident from a careful review of the literature. Multiple animal studies have demonstrated that infarct size varies greatly[60,63,81,82] and that this variability is closely related to the anatomic area at risk.[63,81] Most studies have measured the anatomic area at risk by using postmortem injections to define the myocardial region supplied by the occluded coronary artery. The Animal Models for Protecting Ischemic Myocardium program,[81] sponsored by the National Heart, Lung, and Blood Institute, was undertaken in three well-recognized laboratories to achieve a better understanding of the major factors that determine infarct size. In an unconscious dog model,[81] coronary reperfusion was performed after 3 hours of left circumflex occlusion. Histologic infarct size varied widely, with a mean of 26% and a standard deviation of 14% of the left ventricle. The variation in the anatomic area at risk accounted for 77% of the variation in infarct size (Fig. 25-1). In a conscious dog model of permanent left circumflex occlusion performed as part of the same program,[60] infarct size again varied greatly, with a mean of 22% and a standard deviation of 14% of the left ventricle. The variation in the anatomic area at risk accounted for 66% of the variation in infarct size in this model. Both models demonstrated that the anatomic area at risk from left circumflex occlusion is highly variable. Compelling evidence from animal models shows that the amount of myocardium at risk from a given coronary occlusion varies greatly and is a major determinant of final infarct size.

Although it has long been recognized clinically that there is a wide range of infarct sizes, clinical measurements of myocardium at risk were performed for the first time only recently. The first such measurements were performed by Feiring et al,[32] who used intracoronary injections of macroaggregated albumin in patients with acute myocardial infarction who had not yet received reperfusion therapy. They subsequently performed gated planar imaging and quantitated the acute perfusion defect. They demonstrated that patients with acute myocardial infarction vary greatly in the amount of myocardium at risk, even when coronary occlusion occurs in a similar location, thus confirming the earlier results in animal models (Fig. 25-2). This variability in myocardium at risk in the clinical setting presumably reflects both the variability in the actual territory supplied by the native coronary arteries and the effect of collaterals in chronic coronary artery disease. Feiring et al[32] also demonstrated a close relation between myocardium at risk and the ejection fraction at 4 days, which they used as an estimate of infarct size. In patients who were not successfully reperfused, the correlation between myocardium at risk and the 4-day ejection fraction was very close ($r = 0.91$), presumably because almost all of the myocardium at risk underwent infarction. In the group of patients who were successfully reperfused, the correlation between myocardium at risk and the 4-day ejection fraction was not quite as close ($r = 0.77$), presumably because some of the myocardium at risk had been salvaged.

Properties of technetium-99m sestamibi

The technique used by Feiring et al[32] is clearly not practical for more widespread use, because it requires acute catheterization and a delay in reperfusion therapy. Technetium-99m ses-

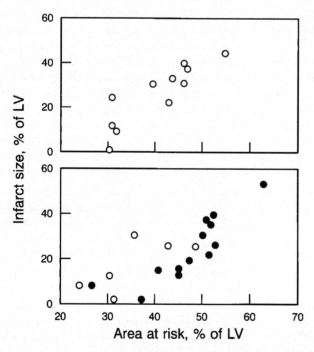

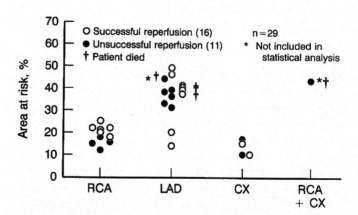

Fig. 25-1. Relation between infarct size and area at risk assessed by postmortem angiography in an unconscious model. Reperfusion was performed after 3 hours of occlusion. The linear correlation coefficient was 0.88. (Reproduced with permission from Reimer KA, Jennings RB, Cobb FR, et al: Animal models for protecting ischemic myocardium: results of the NHLBI Cooperative Study. Comparison of unconscious and conscious dog models, *Circ Res* 56:651-665, 1985.)

Fig. 25-2. Area of myocardium at risk compared with the site of coronary occlusion. Myocardium at risk, which was assessed by intracoronary injections of technetium-99m macroaggregated albumin, was highly variable. CX = left circumflex coronary artery; LAD = left anterior descending coronary artery; RCA = right coronary artery. (Reproduced with permission from Feiring AJ, Johnson MR, Kioschos JM, et al: The importance of the determination of the myocardial area at risk in the evaluation of the outcome of acute myocardial infarction in patients, *Circulation* 75:980-987, 1987.)

tamibi has properties that permit a more practical approach to the measurement of myocardium at risk. This radiopharmaceutical can be injected intravenously and is rapidly cleared from the blood with an effective half-time of 2.2 minutes.[110] It is taken up by the myocardium in direct proportion to myocardial blood flow,[62,73] although its extraction fraction is somewhat lower than that of ^{201}Tl[64] or ^{99m}Tc teboroxime.[66] The radiopharmaceutical is concentrated within the mitochondria of myocardial cells.[4,80] The activity within the myocardium peaks early after intravenous injection, although the ratio of heart activity to liver activity and heart activity to lung activity continues to increase over the next several hours.[110]

The most important property of the radiopharmaceutical for measurement of myocardium at risk is the presence of very slow washout from the myocardium, which is independent of myocardial blood flow.[27,73] As a result, in contrast to ^{201}Tl or ^{99m}Tc teboroxime, this agent undergoes minimal redistribution over time. De Coster et al[27] confirmed minimal redistribution in an animal model of reperfusion. They injected ^{99m}Tc sestamibi during a 90- to 120-minute occlusion and compared the activity in myocardial biopsy samples obtained during occlusion and after 2 to 3 hours of reperfusion. The ^{99m}Tc sestamibi activity in the sample obtained after reperfusion was similar to the activity present during occlusion (Fig. 25-3). Tomographic images of the heart obtained during occlusion and after reperfusion had almost identical count profiles. Eighty-eight percent of the tomographic myocardial segments had less than 10% variation in activity between the images obtained during occlusion and after reperfusion. As a result of this property, when ^{99m}Tc sestamibi is injected during coronary occlusion, imaging can be delayed for several hours and still provide accurate information

about the distribution of myocardial perfusion at the time of the initial injection.

Several clinical studies have reported a small amount of redistribution of ^{99m}Tc sestamibi when this agent is used in conjunction with stress imaging.[28,101] Although redistribution 1 and 3 hours after injection was quantifiable, it was not visually apparent.[101] In contrast to stress imaging, assessment of ischemia due to coronary occlusion often produces fivefold differences between normal and ischemic territories. Consequently, the small amount of redistribution seen in stress imaging will have minimal impact on the quantification of risk area during acute myocardial infarction.

The 140 keV emission and the administered dose of 20 to 30 mCi of this agent provide high-count density images that can be easily quantitated. In an animal model of permanent occlusion, Li et al[62] demonstrated that the circumferential count profile on tomographic ^{99m}Tc sestamibi images correlated closely with the distribution of microspheres. Actual sestamibi activity consistently exceeded microspheres to a small degree in regions of very low flow. The counts recorded in tomographic images of the same regions were even higher because of the effects of scatter, attenuation, and filtered back-projection. The overestimation of flow at severely reduced levels probably reflects enhanced tissue extraction. Other investigators have consistently reproduced this phenomenon.[19,27,62]

Several approaches to quantify defect size have been described.[47,70] O'Connor, Hammell, and Gibbons[70] reported a relatively simple method for the quantitation of the area of absent perfusion on tomographic ^{99m}Tc sestamibi images. In a detailed series of static cardiac phantom experiments, they measured the region of absent perfusion from selected short-axis slices by us-

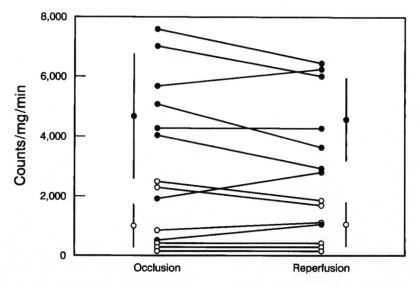

Fig. 25-3. Technetium-99m sestamibi activity in biopsy samples obtained from normal *(closed circles)* and ischemic *(open circles)* regions during occlusion and reperfusion. There was little change in activity after reperfusion. (Reproduced with permission from De Coster DM, Wijns W, Cauwe F, et al: Area-at-risk determination by technetium-99m-hexakis-2-methoxyisobutyl isonitrile in experimental reperfused myocardial infarction, *Circulation* 82:2152-2162, 1990.)

ing different threshold values of normalized counts, as first described by Tamaki et al.[102] O'Connor, Hammell, and Gibbons found a very close correlation between true defect size and the measured region of absent perfusion over a range of threshold values from 50% to 70% of peak counts. A threshold of 60% gave a correlation coefficient of 0.99 and a regression equation that closely approximated the line of identity [measured defect = 1.01 × (true defect) − 1.135].[70] The use of ^{201}Tl in similar phantom studies was associated with a loss of image contrast, making it far more difficult to define the boundaries of the perfusion defect.[69] However, with scatter correction techniques, accurate estimates of infarct size with a 60% threshold have been quantified from tomographic ^{201}Tl images through enhanced contrast.[69]

Multiple animal studies have validated the use of ^{99m}Tc sestamibi for the measurement of myocardium at risk and final infarct size. In an animal model of permanent occlusion, Verani et al[108] found a close correlation between the perfusion defect measured ex vivo on tomographic ^{99m}Tc sestamibi images and the subsequent measurement of histologic infarction by using triphenyl tetrazolium chloride staining. In an animal model of reperfusion, Sinusas et al[97] found that the perfusion defect measured by autoradiography when ^{99m}Tc sestamibi was injected during occlusion correlated closely with the area at risk measured by postmortem angiography (Fig. 25-4). The uptake of ^{99m}Tc sestamibi also correlated closely with microsphere mea-

surements of flow when it was injected during occlusion. When the radiopharmaceutical was injected after reperfusion, its uptake no longer correlated with flow, but the perfusion defect measured by autoradiography correlated closely with histologic infarct size (Fig. 25-5). Thus, when the radiopharmaceutical was injected after reperfusion, its uptake primarily reflected viability rather than flow and measured final infarct size. These same investigators have subsequently reported measurements using tomographic scanning and a threshold technique similar to that already described.[47,97] The correlation between sestamibi uptake and myocardium at risk ($r = 0.92$) remains close.[97] The available animal data therefore suggest that this radiopharmaceutical can accurately measure both myocardium at risk and final infarct size.

Clinical studies using technetium-99m sestamibi

The feasibility of using this technique in clinical studies of acute myocardial infarction was supported by an early case report[57] and subsequent series using tomographic[38] and planar[111] imaging. Twenty to 30 mCi of ^{99m}Tc sestamibi was administered intravenously in the emergency department to patients who presented with ischemic chest pain of at least 30 minutes' duration, had a ST elevation of at least 0.1 mV in two electrocardiographic leads, and had no historical or electrocardiographic evidence of previous myocardial infarction. One to 8 hours later, tomographic imaging was performed when the pa-

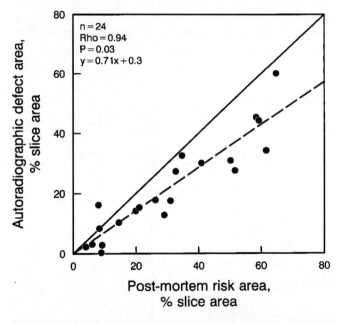

Fig. 25-4. Relation between autoradiographic defect size measured by technetium-99m sestamibi and angiographic area at risk assessed by postmortem angiography in an animal model of reperfusion. Technetium-99m sestamibi was injected during the occlusion phase. (Reproduced with permission from Sinusas AJ, Trautman KA, Bergin JD, et al: Quantification of "area at risk" during coronary occlusion and degree of myocardial salvage after reperfusion using cardiac imaging technetium-99m-methoxy isobutyl isonitrile, *Circulation* 82:1424-1437, 1990.)

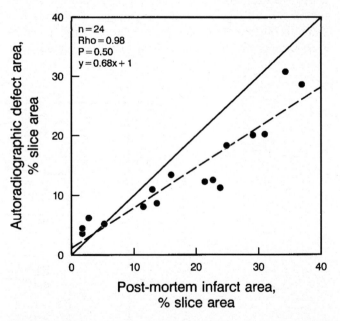

Fig. 25-5. Relation between autoradiographic defect size measured by technetium-99m sestamibi and pathologic infarct size in an animal model of reperfusion. Technetium-99m sestamibi was injected after reperfusion. (Reproduced with permission from Sinusas AJ, Trautman KA, Bergin JD, et al: Quantification of "area at risk" during coronary occlusion and degree of myocardial salvage after reperfusion using cardiac imaging technetium-99m-methoxy isobutyl isonitrile, *Circulation* 82:1424-1437, 1982.)

tient was clinically stable (Fig. 25-6). The percentage of the left ventricle that was at risk for infarction because it had absent perfusion was quantitated by using the five-slice method described elsewhere.[70]

Preliminary clinical studies measuring myocardium at risk in acute infarction are shown in Fig. 25-7. These data demonstrated the feasibility of tomographic imaging after acute injection of ^{99m}Tc sestamibi for the quantitative assessment of myo-

cardium at risk in acute myocardial infarction. They confirmed the previous results of the animal studies and of the clinical studies by Feiring et al:[32] that is, that myocardium at risk varies widely even for a coronary occlusion in a similar location. This finding has been replicated with controlled coronary occlusions during elective coronary angioplasty with ^{99m}Tc sestamibi injected during balloon inflation. Braat et al[6] and Haronian et al[47] demonstrated that the correlation between the occluded vessel

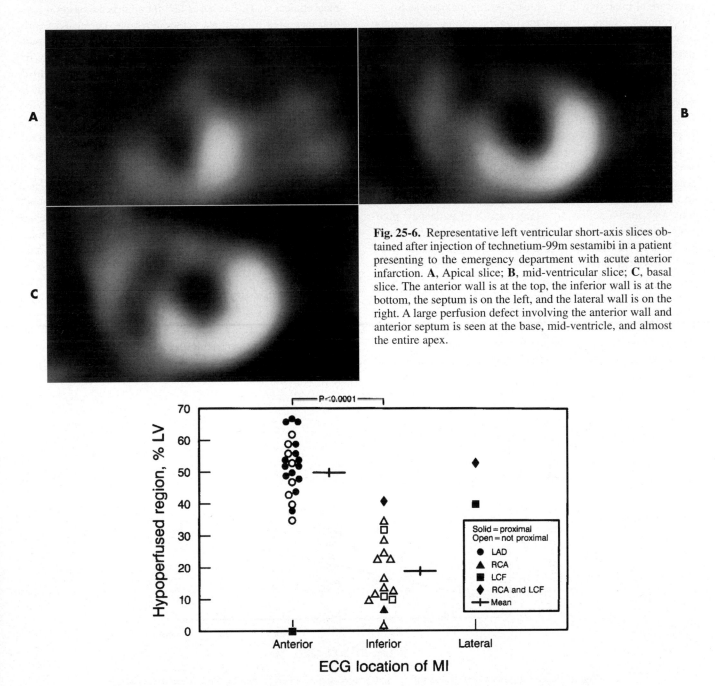

Fig. 25-6. Representative left ventricular short-axis slices obtained after injection of technetium-99m sestamibi in a patient presenting to the emergency department with acute anterior infarction. **A**, Apical slice; **B**, mid-ventricular slice; **C**, basal slice. The anterior wall is at the top, the inferior wall is at the bottom, the septum is on the left, and the lateral wall is on the right. A large perfusion defect involving the anterior wall and anterior septum is seen at the base, mid-ventricle, and almost the entire apex.

Fig. 25-7. Initial hypoperfused region (myocardium at risk) for each of 40 patients injected with technetium-99m sestamibi during acute myocardial infarction. The results are displayed according to the location of infarction; patients with anterior infarction had more myocardium at risk. (Reproduced with permission from Gibbons RJ: Technetium 99m sestamibi in the assessment of acute myocardial infarction, *Semin Nucl Med* 21:213-222, 1991.)

and location of the sestamibi perfusion defect was excellent. However, as in studies of acute infarction, the region at risk varied greatly for each of the three major arteries during coronary angioplasty.

Other techniques

Alternative techniques that may be used to estimate the amount of myocardium at risk during the early stages of acute myocardial infarction in the clinical setting include electrocardiography,[24] global ejection fraction,[32] regional wall-motion assessment,[87] and coronary angiography.[51] Clements et al[22] examined the association between multiple different electrocardiographic variables and myocardium at risk measured by ^{99m}Tc sestamibi. Only two electrocardiographic variables correlated with myocardium at risk in patients with anterior infarction: the sum of ST displacement and the sum of ST displacement normalized to the sum of the R waves. However, the correlation between these two variables and myocardium at risk was quite weak ($r = 0.58$), and the standard error of the estimate was very large, suggesting that these variables had little value in the prediction of myocardium at risk in individual patients with anterior infarction. In a larger series of patients,[29] myocardium at risk was significantly greater in patients with inferior infarction who had anterior ST depression than in those with inferior infarction without ST elevation. This difference was due to extension of the risk zone up the lateral wall of the left ventricle. The opposite scenario of inferior ST depression in anterior infarction was not associated with a greater extent of the risk area but more lateral extension of the anterior perfusion defect.[33] Christian et al[15] found that the magnitude of ST elevation on acute 12-lead electrocardiography correlated modestly with the severity of the perfusion defect but only very weakly with the extent.[15] Consequently, electrocardiography has only limited ability to predict myocardium at risk.

The potential value of global ejection fraction has been assessed in both animal and clinical studies. In an animal model of anterior myocardial infarction, Jang et al[55] found that the ejection fraction measured by contrast ventriculography was not significantly associated with subsequent infarct size. In their clinical study, Feiring et al[32] found that the ejection fraction measured by contrast ventriculography correlated poorly with myocardium at risk. The failure of acute global ventricular function to represent myocardium at risk presumably reflects the effects of many other influences, including preload, afterload, duration of myocardial ischemia, and hyperkinesia in normal segments, which all contribute to its extreme variability during the first 24 hours of infarction.[112] The minimal improvement seen in patients with successful reperfusion therapy in global left ventricular ejection fraction at 1 week is probably due to persistent stunning.[7]

Regional wall motion has been most carefully investigated using two-dimensional echocardiography in animal models.[37,68,77,105] The quantitative methods have varied considerably among studies. The correlation between two-dimensional echocardiographic measurements and final infarct size in animal models of permanent occlusion (which presumably reflects the risk area) has been good, ranging from 0.60 to 0.92. However, several potential limitations of this technique have been identified. Echocardiographic measurements tend to overestimate risk area[68] (Fig. 25-8). Small infarcts are often not detected using either systolic wall thickening or endocardial wall motion.[77] The extent of regional dysfunction changes signifi-

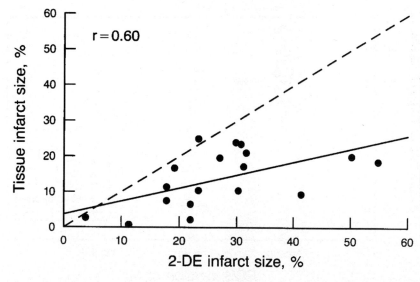

Fig. 25-8. Relation between tissue infarct size (expressed as a percentage of the left ventricle) and infarct size assessed by two-dimensional echocardiography *(2-DE)* in an animal model of permanent occlusion. Echocardiography overestimated infarct size. (Reproduced with permission from Nieminen M, Parisi AF, O'Boyle JE, et al: Serial evaluation of myocardial thickening and thinning in acute experimental infarction: identification and quantification using two-dimensional echocardiography, *Circulation* 66:174-180, 1982.)

cantly over time in animal models of permanent occlusion, increasing from the time of acute measurements to 48 hours later and subsequently decreasing steadily over the following 3 to 6 weeks[37] (Fig. 25-9). Clinical studies have used sequential two-dimensional echocardiography to assess the results of thrombolysis,[105] and early studies reported on the ability of acute echocardiography to measure myocardium at risk in the clinical setting.[71] The use of contrast agents to define the risk area has demonstrated modest correlations with pathologic risk area,[109] but the addition of dobutamine infusion may improve the correlation.[100] However, such an approach is not likely to be practical in the acute setting of infarction.

Regional wall motion can also be assessed by using contrast ventriculography. In an animal model of permanent occlusion, Jang et al[55] found only a weak relation between the extent of regional dysfunction and subsequent histologic infarction. The GUSTO investigators found a significant difference between the extent of regional wall-motion abnormalities at 90 minutes that was maintained at 5 to 7 days.[103] The pattern showing less regional abnormality in the tissue plasminogen activator group paralleled the mortality results, suggesting a relation between this measure and final infarct size.[103] However, the TIMI (Thrombolysis in Myocardial Infarction) investigators noted that changes in global and regional function are small during the postinfarction hospitalization phase in patients treated with thrombolytic therapy, possibly because of persistence of myocardial stunning. They found that infarct artery patency and, to a greater extent, resolution of acute wall-motion abnormalities were the best predictors of functional recovery in infarct size; but neither provided clinically reliable predictions. Although regional wall-motion assessment by contrast ventriculography has been measured in clinical trials,[72,93,94,96] it has not yet been

compared with radioisotope measurements of myocardium at risk in clinical studies.

As indicated previously, postmortem angiography is routinely used in animal models to assess the anatomic area at risk. A small study[51] suggested that there is excellent overall correlation between angiographic assessment and myocardium at risk measured by ^{99m}Tc sestamibi, although most of the correlation reflects the effects of infarct location. In subgroups of patients with anterior and inferior infarcts, the correlation between angiographic assessment and myocardium at risk is modest ($r = 0.60$) and the ability to predict myocardium at risk in individual patients is limited.[51]

FINAL INFARCT SIZE AND MYOCARDIAL SALVAGE

Measurement by technetium-99m sestamibi

Repeated tomographic images after reinjection of ^{99m}Tc sestamibi can be performed at the time of hospital discharge to determine final infarct size. As discussed above, animal models of permanent occlusion and reperfusion suggest that the perfusion defect measured after late injection of this radiopharmaceutical correlates closely with histologic infarct size.[27,97,108] In clinical studies, the close relation between the final defect size measured at discharge by this technique and both regional and global function confirms the validity of the discharge defect as a measurement of infarct size.[38] In the initial patient study, defect size at discharge correlated closely ($r = -0.82$) with ejection fraction at discharge (Fig. 25-10), as well as with discharge regional wall-motion score in the infarct segment ($r = -0.97$ for inferior infarction; $r = -0.74$ for anterior infarction).[38] In a subsequent larger series of patients, Christian et al[11] showed that this close correlation between global ejection fraction and regional wall-motion persisted 6 weeks later (Fig. 25-11). In longer-term follow-up, end-diastolic volume, end-systolic volume, and ejection fraction at 1 year all correlated closely with the defect size at discharge[13] as measured by electron-beam computed tomography.[10] Of note, infarct size measured by ^{99m}Tc sestamibi at hospital discharge after acute myocardial infarction was significantly associated with left ventricular remodeling in the year after the index infarction (Fig. 25-12).[10] Consequently, there is ample evidence that infarct size measured by ^{99m}Tc sestamibi accurately reflects mechanical indices of left ventricular function (Table 25-1).

Ample data are also available regarding this measure as a true reflection of actual pathologic infarction. Several well-designed animal studies have shown an excellent correlation between tomographic defect size and the extent of pathologic infarction at autopsy.[97,108] In an important clinical study, Medrano et al[65] injected ^{99m}Tc sestamibi in patients undergoing cardiac transplantation just before explantation of the native heart.[65] There was an excellent correlation between both tomographic and explanted short-axis slice defects and pathologic infarction by histology (Fig. 25-13). Udelson et al[106] found that a definition of infarction as 60% of maximal counts on tomographic imaging provided an accurate separation of myocardial

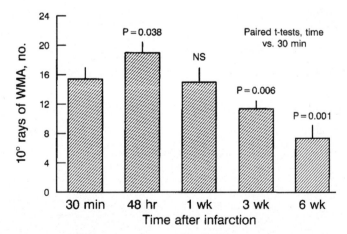

Fig. 25-9. Two-dimensional echocardiographic infarct size expressed as the number of 10° rays with wall-motion abnormalities (*WMA*) and time after infarction in an animal model of permanent occlusion. Significant changes were seen in the echocardiographic infarct size measured at different times. (Reproduced with permission from Gibbons EF, Hogan RD, Franklin TA, et al: The natural history of regional dysfunction in a canine preparation of chronic infarction, *Circulation* 71:394-402, 1985.)

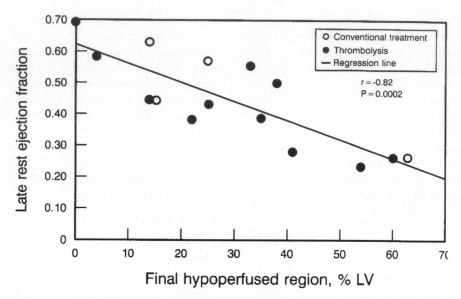

Fig. 25-10. Relation of final hypoperfused region (infarct size) with late (discharge) resting ejection fraction, demonstrating a close correlation. (Reproduced with permission from Gibbons RJ, Verani MS, Behrenbeck T, et al: Feasibility of tomographic technetium-99m-hexakis-2-methoxy-2-methyl-propyl-isonitrile imaging for the assessment of myocardial area at risk and the effect of acute treatment in myocardial infarction, *Circulation* 80:1277-1286, 1989.)

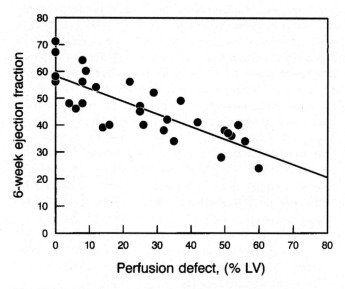

Fig. 25-11. Relation of technetium-99m sestamibi perfusion defect at discharge expressed as a percentage of the left ventricle *(LV)* and the ejection fraction measured 6 weeks later, demonstrating a close correlation. (Reproduced with permission from Christian TF, Behrenbeck T, Pellikka PA, et al: Mismatch of left ventricular function and perfusion with Tc-99m-isonitrile following reperfusion therapy for acute myocardial infarctions: identification of myocardial stunning and hyperkinesia, *J Am Coll Cardiol* 16:1632-1638, 1990, and the American College of Cardiology.)

Table 25-1. Clinical validation of infarct size measurement by technetium-99m sestamibi single-photon emission computed tomography

Measurement	Correlation coefficient	*P* Value
Left ventricular ejection fraction		
At discharge	0.80	<0.0001
At 6 weeks	−0.81	<0.0001
At 1 year	−0.76	<0.0001
End-systolic volume at 1 year*	0.80	<0.0001
Regional wall motion†		
At discharge	−0.75	<0.0001
At 6 weeks	−0.81	<0.0001
Peak creatine kinase levels	0.78	0.002
Thallium infarct size	0.87	<0.0001

*Measured by electron-beam computed tomography.
†Measured by guided radionuclide ventriculography.

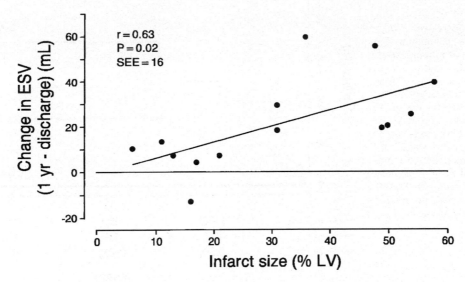

Fig. 25-12. The change in end-systolic volume by electron-beam computed tomography in the year following the index infarction as a function of infarct size at hospital discharge. There is a significant association between these variables, with larger infarcts showing a strong propensity for remodeling. (Reprinted from Chareonthaitawee P, Christian TF, Hirose K, et al: Relation of initial infarct size to extent of left ventricular remodeling in the year after acute myocardial infarction, *J Am Coll Cardiol* 25:567-573, 1995. With permission from the American College of Cardiology.)

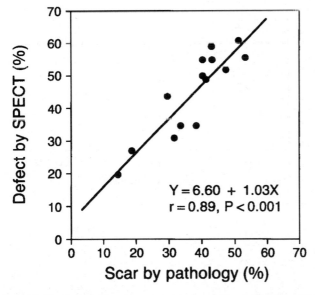

Fig. 25-13. Correlation between tomographic technetium-99m sestamibi defect size and actual extent of pathologic scarring by histology in explanted hearts of patients undergoing cardiac transplantation. Technetium-99m sestamibi injection was performed just before explantation. (From Medrano R, Lowry RW, Young UB, et al: Assessment of myocardial viability with Tc99m sestamibi in patients undergoing cardiac transplantation, *Circulation* 94:1013-1017, 1996. Reproduced with permission from the American Heart Association.)

segments with improvement in contractility after revascularization from those segments with no improvement.

Final infarct size (measured on or after day 5) has been shown to be a powerful predictor of survival (Fig. 25-14). In a series of 274 patients, Miller et al[67] found that survival was significantly better in patients with a small (<12% of the left ventricle) versus large (≥12% of the left ventricle) infarct size at discharge in patients treated with reperfusion therapy for acute myocardial infarction. Consistent with previous observations,[16] infarct size was greater for patients with anterior compared with inferior infarction.[67] This phenomenon is due to the greater amount of myocardium at risk in patients with anterior infarction (approximately 50% of the left ventricle) compared with those with inferior infarction (approximately 20% of the left ventricle) (Fig. 25-15). The absolute benefit of reperfusion therapy is therefore greater for patients with anterior infarction, although the proportion of the area at risk salvaged is not different. Thus, considerable evidence from animal and clinical data show that perfusion defect size assessed by tomographic imaging with ^{99m}Tc sestamibi is a valid measure of actual infarct size.

Because the size of the perfusion defect on acute tomographic imaging with ^{99m}Tc sestamibi is a measure of myocardium at risk and the size of the defect on discharge imaging is a measure of infarct size, the change in the defect size between acute and discharge imaging would seem to provide a measure of treatment effect or myocardial salvage. Gibbons et al[38] reported the first data from sequential tomographic imaging,[38] and Wackers et al[111] used planar imaging to assess this

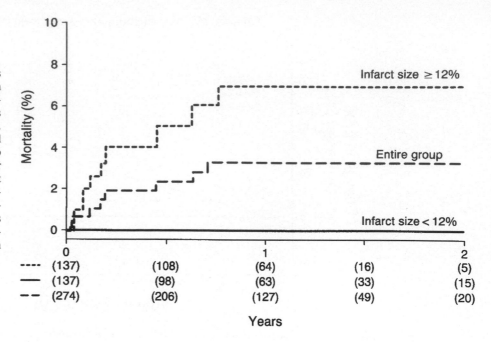

Fig. 25-14. Survival curves over 2 years for 274 patients with technetium-99m sestamibi measurement of infarct size after acute myocardial infarction. Images were acquired before hospital discharge. The patient population was dichotomized by the median infarct size for the group (12% of the left ventricle). (From Miller TD, Christian TF, Hopfenspirger MR, et al: Infarct size after acute myocardial infarction measured by quantitative tomographic 99mTc sestamibi imaging predicts subsequent mortality, *Circulation* 92:334-341, 1995. Reproduced with permission from the American Heart Association.)

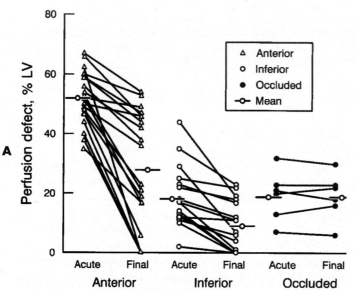

A

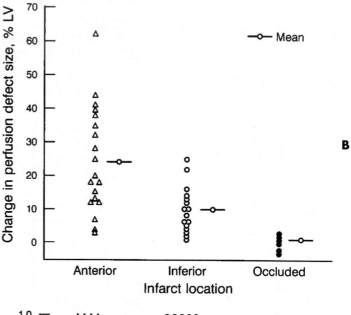

B

Fig. 25-15. A, The acute and final perfusion defect size as a percentage of the left ventricle *(LV)* according to infarct location and arterial patency. Perfusion defect size significantly decreased after reperfusion in both anterior and inferior myocardial infarction. There was no significant change in those patients with persistent occlusion of the infarct-related artery. **B,** The change in perfusion defect size between acute and discharge images expressed as a percentage of the left ventricle *(LV)* according to infarct location and arterial patency. This estimate of myocardial salvage was significantly greater in patients with anterior infarction than in patients with inferior infarction (*p*<0.01). This estimate was also significantly greater for patients with inferior infarction than for those patients with a persistent arterial occlusion (*p* = 0.001). **C,** Salvage index (the ratio of the change in the perfusion defect to the acute perfusion defect) according to infarct location and arterial patency. Anterior and inferior infarcts did not differ from the salvage index. Salvage index was significantly greater in both groups than in patients with persistent arterial occlusion. (Reproduced from Christian TF, Gibbons RJ, Gersh BJ, et al: Effect of infarct location on myocardial salvage assessed by technetium-99m isonitrile, *J Am Coll Cardiol* 17:1303-1308, 1991. With permission from the American College of Cardiology.)

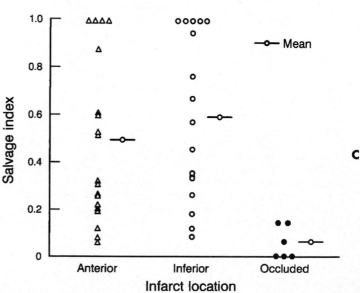

C

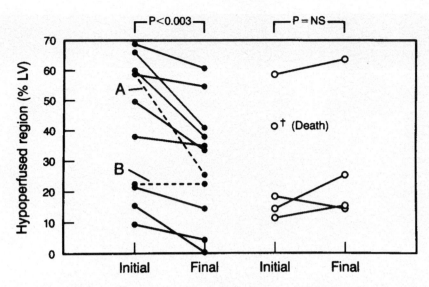

Fig. 25-16. Initial hypoperfused region (myocardium at risk) and final hypoperfused region (infarct size) for patients treated with thrombolysis and those treated with conventional therapy and no thrombolysis. A significant change in perfusion defect size was seen in patients treated with thrombolysis. (Reproduced with permission from Gibbons RJ, Verani MS, Behrenbeck T, et al: Feasibility of tomographic technetium-99m-hexakis-2-methoxy-2-methylpropyl-isonitrile imaging for the assessment of myocardial area at risk and the effect of acute treatment in myocardial infarction, *Circulation* 80:1277-1286, 1989.)

potential measurement tool. A highly significant decrease in defect size was seen for patients treated with thrombolytic therapy; no significant change in defect size was seen for the conventional treatment group (Fig. 25-16). The added power to detect beneficial responses to any given therapy for acute infarction is evident from the patients highlighted in this figure. Examples of acute and discharge images for two patients are shown in Figs. 25-17 and 25-18.

These promising initial results were confirmed in a second tomographic study by Santoro et al[90] using a different quantitative technique. These investigators found that the final defect size correlated closely with enzymatic infarct size and that the percentage decrease in perfusion defect size between acute and late imaging was closely associated with the decrease in asynergy assessed by two-dimensional echocardiography. Wackers et al[111] also demonstrated good agreement between the findings obtained on redistribution ^{201}Tl scintigraphy and those obtained on a resting predischarge ^{99m}Tc sestamibi.

A correlate of the ability to assess myocardial salvage was to use this measure as an end point in comparative trials. Gibbons et al[40] used the change in ^{99m}Tc sestamibi defect size as the primary end point in a randomized prospective trial comparing the use of thrombolytic therapy with direct coronary angioplasty for acute myocardial infarction. Both therapies were effective for salvaging jeopardized myocardium. There was no significant difference in this end point between the two strategies even though the study had adequate power to detect such a difference (Fig. 25-19). Gibson et al[89] demonstrated that the

serial change in the extent and severity of a ^{99m}Tc sestamibi perfusion defect was highly predictive of coronary artery patency in patients treated with thrombolytic therapy, thus providing a noninvasive method to assess this important factor.

COMPARISON WITH OTHER END POINTS

Many other end points have been used in various studies to assess the efficacy of acute reperfusion therapy in myocardial infarction. The late electrocardiogram, late resting ejection fraction, and late thallium perfusion defect are all end points that measure only final infarct size. They therefore cannot possibly adjust for the broad variability in myocardium at risk. As a result, they are very limited in their ability to assess efficacy in individual patients, because the myocardium at risk in an individual patient may have been greater than, equal to, or even less than the final infarct size. In groups of patients, the variability in myocardium at risk will tend to obscure any treatment benefit measured by these end points, unless very large sample sizes are employed to ensure that the distribution of myocardium at risk is similar in each treatment group.

The late electrocardiogram and late resting ejection fraction have potential limitations in the quantitation of final infarct size. In the pre-thrombolytic era, various measurements from the resting electrocardiogram were used to estimate infarct size and validated by correlation with left ventricular ejection fraction, regional wall motion, and cardiac enzyme levels.[49,76] However, in a consecutive series of 43 patients with acute infarction who received reperfusion therapy, Christian et al[12]

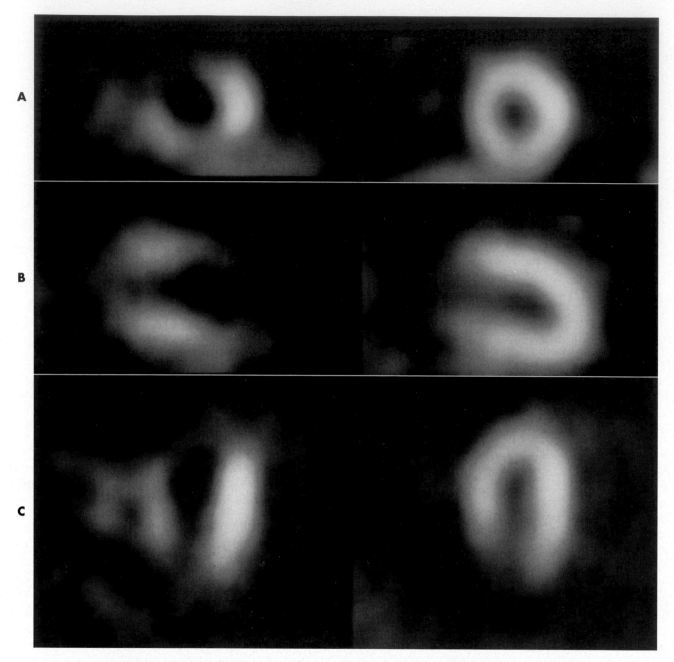

Fig. 25-17. A, Representative midventricular short-axis slices, **B,** vertical long-axis slices, and **C,** horizontal long-axis slices from a patient with acute anterior infarction. The image on the left in each panel was acquired after injection of technetium-99m sestamibi in the emergency department. The image on the right in each panel was acquired at the time of discharge. A large acute anterior, septal, and apical perfusion defect occurred that resolved completely by the time of discharge. (Reproduced with permission from Gibbons RJ: Technetium 99m sestamibi in the assessment of acute myocardial infarction, *Semin Nucl Med* 21:213-222, 1991.)

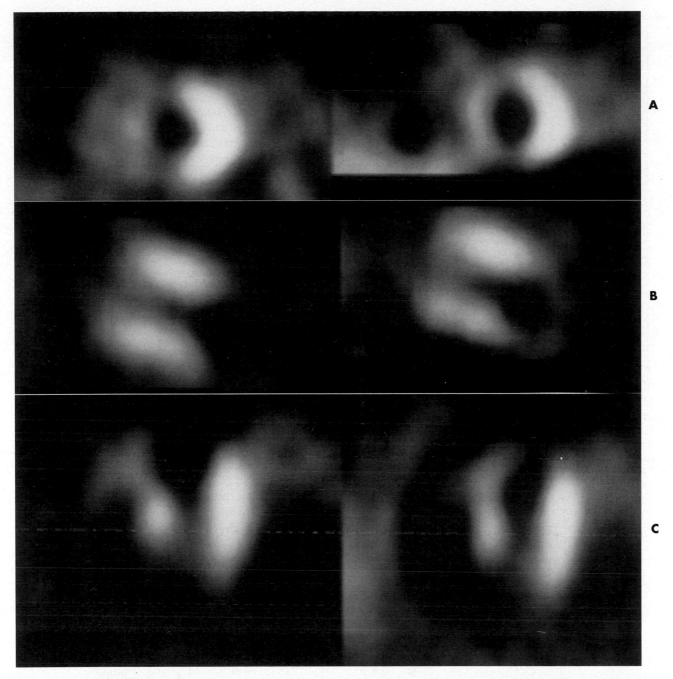

Fig. 25-18. Representative midventricular short-axis slices (**A**), vertical long-axis slices (**B**), and horizontal long-axis slices (**C**) from a patient with acute anterior infarction. The image on the left in each panel was acquired after injection of technetium-99m sestamibi in the emergency department. A large anterior, septal, and apical perfusion defect occurred that improved minimally 1 week later.

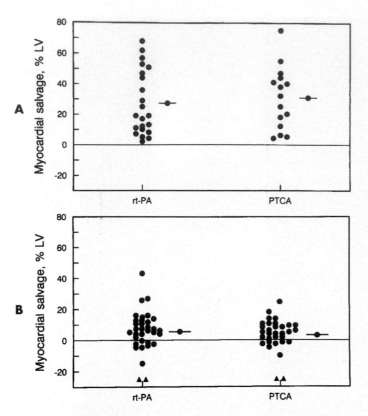

Fig. 25-19. Myocardial salvage by infarct location in patients treated with thrombolytic therapy or direct coronary angioplasty for acute myocardial infarction. **A**, anterior infarcts; **B**, inferior infarcts. The groups did not differ significantly despite adequate statistical power. (From Gibbons RJ, Holmes DR, Reeder GS, et al: Immediate angioplasty compared with the administration of a thrombolytic agent followed by conservative treatment for myocardial infarction, *N Engl J Med* 328:685-691, 1993. Copyright 1993. Reproduced by permission of Massachusetts Medical Society. All rights reserved.)

found little correlation between the Selvester QRS score and radionuclide measurements of left ventricular function and perfusion, either at discharge or after 6 weeks (Fig. 25-20). Although this study suggested that electrocardiography does not provide a reliable estimate of infarct size after reperfusion therapy, conflicting results were reported by Haasche et al,[45] who found a reasonable correlation between ^{201}Tl resting defect size after infarction by using a more extensive version of the Selvester scoring system for infarct size.

Global ejection fraction also has substantial limitations as a measure of infarct size. The standard deviation on repeated measurements of resting ejection fraction is approximately 0.04[79] and presumably reflects the variable effects of loading conditions, drug therapy, and sympathetic activation. The presence of coexistent valvular heart disease and myopathic processes may reduce the accuracy of ejection fraction as a measurement of infarct size. Measurements of ejection fraction at discharge may also be affected by stunning or compensatory hyperkinesia. In a series of 32 patients studied with ^{99m}Tc sestamibi at discharge, Christian et al[11] found that five patients had a significant (>0.08) increase in ejection fraction from discharge to 6 weeks later; at discharge, these patients had ejection fractions that were significantly lower than expected on the basis of perfusion defect size, suggesting that they had stunning at the time of discharge. In the same study, Christian et al[11] identified six patients who had a significant decrease in ejection fraction 6 weeks later; these patients had ejection fractions at discharge that were higher than expected on the basis of their perfusion defect size, suggesting the presence of compensatory hyperkinesia. Thus, this small study suggested that approximately one third of patients will have either stunning or compensatory hyperkinesia at discharge; this condition will reduce the accuracy of ejection fraction as a measure of infarct size at that time. These findings have subsequently been verified by a

Fig. 25-20. Correlation coefficients for the associations between different radionuclide estimates of infarct size and ejection fraction *(EF)* at discharge, ejection fraction 6 weeks later, QRS score at discharge, and QRS score after discharge. There was generally little association between QRS score and the infarct size measured by radionuclide techniques. * = $p<0.001$; † = $p<0.005$; ‡ = $p<0.05$. (Reproduced with permission from Christian TF, Clements IP, Behrenbeck T, et al: Limitations of the electrocardiogram in estimating infarction size after acute reperfusion therapy for myocardial infarction, *Ann Intern Med* 114:264-270, 1991.)

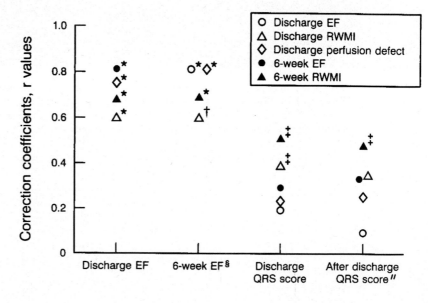

larger series of patients who underwent perfusion imaging post infarction and serial assessment of LV function.[43] Sinusas et al[99] confirmed in an animal model of reperfusion that the cellular uptake and kinetics of ^{99m}Tc sestamibi are unaffected by myocardial stunning. These results have important implications regarding the assessment of infarct size early after myocardial infarction, particularly when perfusion imaging is compared with mechanical estimates.

In the measurement of global or regional left ventricular function during infarction and later, some attempt is made to adjust for myocardium at risk and therefore permit the assessment of benefit in individual patients. However, as discussed above, neither ejection fraction nor regional wall motion is an accurate measure of myocardium at risk. In addition, global and regional function are subject to other influences—preload, afterload, catecholamines, and cardiomyopathy—that do not influence the measurement of infarct size. These influences produce considerable variability in these characteristics in patients with little or no infarction. A detailed discussion of clinical trial design is beyond the scope of this chapter, and a detailed analysis of the sample size required for trials using sestamibi perfusion imaging as an end point has been published.[39] The required sample size using ventricular function end points is approximately 2.5-fold greater than that required using perfusion imaging.

Death and recurrent myocardial infarction are definitive end points that have been used in large clinical trials to establish the efficacy of thrombolytic therapy. However, such end points are of limited value in the assessment of individual patients, because they can never detect any differential benefit in survivors who do not have recurrent myocardial infarction and are very costly to perform. Given the power of myocardial perfusion imaging (myocardial salvage or infarct size), this approach can

be useful to study new therapies on a pilot basis before proceeding with large mortality trials.

The limitations of all other available end points for the assessment of treatment benefit in acute myocardial infarction are evident. It would therefore seem that early and late imaging with ^{99m}Tc sestamibi is the best measurement tool currently available for the assessment of the efficacy of acute therapy.

Clinical studies

Acute and serial perfusion imaging using ^{99m}Tc sestamibi has been used in several clinical studies.[5,78,89] Pellikka et al[78] assessed the time course of recovery of perfusion after reperfusion therapy in 25 patients who underwent tomographic imaging acutely, at 18 to 48 hours, and at discharge. At 5 days, perfusion defect size was significantly reduced in successfully reperfused patients, but only half of such patients showed improvement on the early scan done at 18 to 24 hours. Myocardial salvage was not apparent until at least 5 days later in these patients. Gibson et al[89] found a high degree of correlation between infarct vessel patency and the reduction in perfusion defect size at 5 days, but this finding was not consistent at 18 to 48 hours.[89]

Most patients with acute myocardial infarction do not present with ST elevation and therefore do not qualify for intravenous thrombolytic therapy according to the current criteria.[56] One population-based study suggested that only 22% of patients with acute myocardial infarction would be eligible for thrombolytic therapy if ST elevation was required.[86] Christian et al[14] performed a pilot study in 14 patients with myocardial infarction and no ST elevation to assess the potential value of ^{99m}Tc sestamibi in this setting (Fig. 25-21). Thirteen of the 14 patients had acute perfusion defects that ranged from 2% to 53% of the left ventricle. The mean for the entire group was

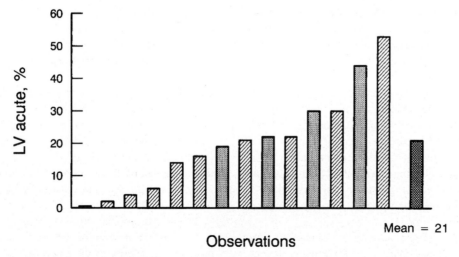

Fig. 25-21. Acute perfusion defect expressed as a percentage of the left ventricle *(LV)* for 14 patients with acute myocardial infarction and without electrocardiographic ST elevation. Shaded bars represent patients with previous myocardial infarction. Acute perfusion defect ranged from 0% to 53% of the left ventricle (mean, 21%). (Reproduced with permission from Christian TF, Gibbons RJ, Gush BJ, et al: Effect of infarct location on myocardial salvage assessed by technetium-99m isonitrile, *J Am Coll Cardiol* 17:1303-1308, 1991, and the American College of Cardiology.)

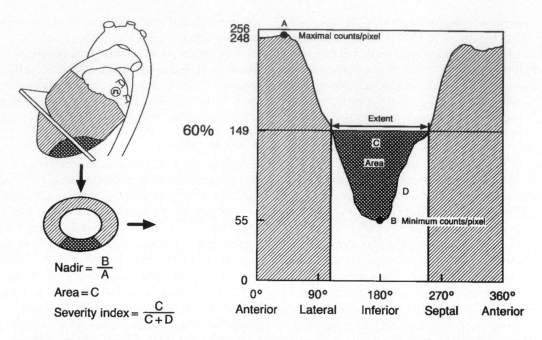

Fig. 25-22. Schematic representation of a count profile curve from a short-axis slice in a patient with acute inferior infarction. The arrows define the extent of the defect. Severity of the defect was measured by using the three methods shown. Note that the severity index and area methods constitute a measure of both severity and extent. Severity is hypothesized to be inversely proportional to the degree of collateral flow within the jeopardized zone. (Reproduced from Christian TF, Gibbons RJ, Clements IP, et al: Estimates of myocardiomate risk and collateral flow in acute myocardial infarction using electrocardiographic indexes with comparison to radionuclide and angiographic measures, *J Am Coll Cardiol* 26:388-393, 1995. With permission from the American College of Cardiology.)

21% of the left ventricle, a value that is similar to the size of the acute perfusion defect measured in patients with inferior myocardial infarction and ST elevation. More important, on subsequent coronary angiography, 11 of the 13 patients in whom the infarct-related artery could be determined had arterial occlusion. These data suggest that many patients with acute myocardial infarction who present without ST elevation have coronary artery occlusion and may therefore potentially benefit from thrombolytic therapy.

The acute use of ^{99m}Tc sestamibi has been successfully used as a form of triage in the hospital and particularly in the emergency department in several studies. In one small study, the positive predictive value of an abnormal scan during chest pain was 90% and the negative predictive value of a normal scan was 100%.[48] Several institutions now incorporate acute perfusion imaging in the triage of patients with chest pain. This strategy is likely to be cost effective, given the large percentage of patients admitted with chest pain who are ultimately proven not to have cardiac disease.

Serial imaging with ^{99m}Tc sestamibi has provided a way to assess the validity of clinical markers of reperfusion therapy. Christian et al[13] found a significant association between the magnitude of relief of chest pain and the amount of myocardial salvage in patients receiving reperfusion therapy.[17] However, there was no correlation between the severity of pain and the extent of the area of risk. Of interest, in patients in whom pain

had resolved but ST elevation was still present, the amount of salvage was substantial (11% ± 11% of the left ventricle) when reperfusion therapy was given.

Extensions of the methodology

The ability to accurately quantify infarct size and estimate myocardial salvage are important features of perfusion imaging with ^{99m}Tc sestamibi in acute myocardial infarction. Although the extent of myocardium at risk is the strongest predictor of infarct size, the duration of coronary occlusion and any residual blood flow to the risk zone to sustain viability during occlusion are also important contributors. The estimation of the duration of coronary occlusion in patients is readily available but is imprecise. However, the estimation of residual flow has been problematic to obtain. Residual flow may come from antegrade flow or collateral flow, or both. Flow can be estimated somewhat successfully by acute coronary angiography (before reperfusion therapy), but this approach is not practical in all patients.

In patients with no residual antegrade flow (TIMI grade 0 or 1), collateral flow to the risk zone could be estimated on the basis of the severity of the count profile curve (Fig. 25-22) of an acute perfusion defect.[21] This approach postulates that the greater the residual flow to the risk zone, the less severe the perfusion defect. Christian, Schwartz, and Gibbons[21] assessed three ways to measure defect severity (Fig. 25-22). They found a consistent relation between defect severity and angiographic

Table 25-2. Invasive and noninvasive models predictive of infarct size

Invasive model*		Noninvasive model	
Variable	P Value	Variable	P Value
Myocardium at risk	<0.0001	Myocardium at risk	0.0007
Collateral grade†	<0.0005	Collateral flow‡	<0.0001
Collateral grade and infarct location†	0.003	Collateral flow and infarct location‡	0.008
Time to reperfusion	0.04	Time to reperfusion	0.01

*$R^2 = 0.70$.
†Measured by acute coronary angiography.
‡Measured by the severity of acute technetium-99m sestamibi perfusion image.

Table 25-3. Comparison of perfusion-based with mortality-based trials of new therapies in acute myocardial infarction*

Variable	Sestamibi trial	GUSTO trial
Area at risk	Yes	No
Collateral flow	Yes	No
Time	Yes	Yes
Infarct size	Yes	No
Patients per treatment arm, n	140	10,000
Estimated direct trial cost, $	2 million	35 million

*GUSTO = Global Utilization of Streptokinase and Tissue Plasminogen Activator for Occluded Coronary Arteries

collateral grade, as well as subsequent final infarct size, by using any of these methods. Furthermore, defect severity was an independent predictor of infarct size when used as a measure of collateral flow in addition to myocardium at risk, infarct location, and the time to reperfusion therapy (Table 25-2).[21] Clements et al[23] extended this relation by incorporating the degree of antegrade flow into the model and including patients with higher grades of antegrade flow.[23] The ability to estimate residual flow from the severity of the acute perfusion defect has been confirmed in a multicenter acute imaging trial.[9] In addition, two separate animal studies have validated this approach.[18,95] Therefore, a noninvasive method to prospectively evaluate residual blood flow in patients may be possible. Such information will be most useful for patients who present relatively late in the course of infarction or who have relative contraindications to reperfusion therapy.

Clinical trials

Although knowledge of the extent of the risk zone can be clinically beneficial in patients with clear evidence of acute myocardial infarction with ST elevation, its delineation is not essential for institution of reperfusion therapy. However, it provides a powerful method for assessment of new treatment strategies in acute myocardial infarction. Myocardium at risk accounts for 70% of the variability in infarct size in animal models of reperfusion.[81] Consequently, a large portion of the determinants of infarct size in patients can be accounted for when comparing new treatments. Myocardium at risk was the strongest predictor of infarct size in 89 patients treated with thrombolytic therapy or direct coronary angioplasty (Table 25-2).[21] Incorporation of a measure of collateral flow (either invasively by acute coronary angiography or noninvasively from the severity of the acute sestamibi perfusion defect) and the elapsed time to reperfusion accounted for approximately 70% of the variability in infarct size; this value approaches those seen in the controlled setting of the animal laboratory.[21,81]

Because of the ability to control for important variables that determine infarct size and patient outcome, comparative trials of treatment strategies in myocardial infarction can be per-

formed with relatively few patients. Gibbons et al[39] demonstrated that a new therapy that was 30% more effective than a comparable therapy would result in an increase in late left ventricular ejection fraction of only 1.0 ejection fraction point in patients with inferior infarction and 3.8 ejection fraction points in patients with anterior infarction. Clearly, more sensitive techniques are needed to detect differences in outcome. In a comparative study of direct coronary angioplasty and intravenous thrombolytic therapy by Gibbons et al,[38] no difference in myocardial salvage with ^{99m}Tc sestamibi was reported. Fifty patients per treatment arm were included, which provided 80% power to detect a true difference.[38] This method has been extended to other comparative trials in acute infarction.[74,92]

Because it is possible to account for multiple variables that determine infarct size and, to a large extent, patient outcome, comparative trials can be conducted with fewer patients using perfusion imaging with ^{99m}Tc sestamibi and at lower cost. Table 25-3 compares two approaches to clinical trials in acute myocardial infarction: a perfusion imaging–based trial and a well-known mortality trial. There is no question that an adequately powered mortality trial, such as the GUSTO study,[104] is the optimal scientific approach for comparing therapies. However, the cost of conducting such a study is prohibitive and is clearly beyond what independent institutions can fund. Technetium-99m sestamibi imaging provides a way to conduct adequately powered studies at a substantially lower cost. Larger mortality trials can be reserved for therapies that are shown by these smaller, low-cost studies to have significant benefit. It is likely to be in this area that risk assessment in acute infarction in patients who otherwise meet criteria for reperfusion therapy will remain important. However, it is clear that the detection of jeopardized myocardium in patients with nondiagnostic electrocardiograms will continue to be an important clinical triage procedure.

Limitations

Several practical difficulties must be acknowledged in the acute use of ^{99m}Tc sestamibi in patients with acute myocardial infarction and as a means to triage patients with chest pain. The current kit, which requires 30 minutes for preparation according to the instructions in the package insert, has an official shelf-life of 6 hours. Ready availability of the isotope can be problematic. Although a rapid preparation and quality control protocol can be performed in 5 minutes,[35,52] the presence of someone trained for this procedure is necessary and can be a source of delay. Two alternatives include preparing a dose every 6 to 8 hours, with substantial waste of the isotope, or to have it delivered on demand by a commercial vendor. All three approaches have associated problems.

Perfusion imaging usually requires transportation of potentially critically ill patients from the coronary care unit or emergency department to the nuclear cardiology laboratory. In patients in whom the indications for acute reperfusion therapy are clear, the available time window of 1 to 8 hours for acute imaging generally permits stabilization of the patient before imaging. However, in patients without ST elevation, in whom the results of imaging may influence early therapy, imaging must be performed as soon as possible and at a time when ventricular arrhythmias are common. Most laboratories will have to adjust their procedures and personnel to accommodate such patients.

Noncardiac uptake of the radiopharmaceutical in the lungs, gallbladder, and bowel can present technical difficulties. These difficulties can usually be overcome by waiting a sufficient amount of time after injection for imaging, properly positioning the patient, and processing images carefully to exclude noncardiac uptake. Despite these steps, in the occasional patient, a very high loop of bowel in the splenic flexure may preclude adequate separation of the inferior wall and bowel for quantitative measurements. In such patients, it may be necessary to repeat the images several hours later when more bowel clearance has occurred. Unfortunately, the use of narcotics in many patients with acute myocardial infarction tends to slow bowel transit.

Currently, there is no consistently reliable method to distinguish new myocardium at risk from previous myocardial infarction. This is particularly important when the method is used to detect myocardium at risk in patients with chest pain who are known to have had infarction and have nondiagnostic electrocardiograms.[14] Clearly, spatially distinct defects can be individually quantified; however, contiguous defects are problematic. All imaging methods currently share this limitation.

The detection of hibernating myocardium is also problematic using this method. It has been reported that significantly delayed reductions in perfusion defect size can occur 2 to 5 days after acute assessment of myocardium at risk.[78] Despite accurate assessment of infarct size in most patients who undergo ^{99m}Tc sestamibi tomographic imaging at hospital discharge (Table 25-1), further reductions in infarct size have been noted in the months after infarction, presumably because of resolution of hibernating myocardium.[36] Because uptake of ^{99m}Tc sestamibi is proportional to flow but has minimal redistribution characteristics,[4,73] it is conceivable that in viable myocardium served by a vessel with a critical obstruction to flow, a perfusion defect may overestimate infarct size from low blood flow because there is no mechanism of delayed redistribution.[91] This

Table 25-4. Insights into myocardial infarction provided by technetium-99m sestamibi

Limited ability of acute electrocardiography (except for infarct location) to predict myocardium at risk in individual patients
Limited ability of coronary angiography to predict myocardium at risk in individual patients
Potential value of direct angiography in patients who are not candidates for thrombolysis
Presence of acute coronary occlusion and significant myocardium at risk in patients without ST elevation
Large differences in myocardium at risk and final infarct size in patients with anterior and inferior myocardial infarction
Frequent presence of stunning and compensatory hyperkinesia at discharge, reducing the value of discharge ventricular function as a measure of infarct size
Lack of value of discharge electrocardiography as a measure of infarct size

scenario is most likely present in patients with severe residual stenosis after thrombolysis.

The extent to which severe wall-motion abnormalities can affect assessment of the area at risk remains unclear. Sinusas et al[98] demonstrated that perfusion defects can be created on the basis of significant contractile abnormalities without any reduction in blood flow.[98] Other investigators have reported similar findings, suggesting that partial volume effects may lead to overestimation of the area at risk.[30] However, gating of the images, which corrects to an extent for partial volume effects, demonstrated no difference in the assessment of the area at risk compared with conventional tomographic imaging in patients who underwent imaging after reperfusion therapy.[20,25] The significance of partial volume effects in the clinical setting remains to be established.

CONCLUSIONS

The available evidence from both basic laboratory and clinical studies suggests that ^{99m}Tc sestamibi is a new, superior measurement tool for assessment of myocardium at risk, final infarct size, and myocardial salvage in acute myocardial infarction. It has definite advantages over the other methods that have been used to assess the efficacy of acute therapy. It has already provided numerous important insights into myocardial infarction (Table 25-4). Further studies with this unique method should add to our understanding of the variability in the response to acute reperfusion therapy and the role of collaterals and reperfusion injury. This technique should permit the performance of future clinical trials comparing different therapies with smaller and more practical sample sizes. It should therefore speed the search for the most effective therapy for myocardial infarction and facilitate the optimal treatment of as many patients as possible, thereby reducing the morbidity and mortality associated with one of leading public health problems in the United States.

REFERENCES

1. Effect of intravenous APSAC on mortality after acute myocardial infarction: preliminary report of a placebo-controlled clinical trial AIMS Trial Study Group, *Lancet* 1:545–549, 1988.

2. Long-term effects of intravenous anistreplase in acute myocardial infarction: final report of the AIMS study AIMS Trial Study Group, *Lancet* 335:427–431, 1990.

3. Wilcox RG, von derLippe G, Olsson CG, et al: Trial of tissue plasminogen activator for mortality reduction in acute myocardial infarction. Anglo-Scandinavian Study of Early Thrombolysis (ASSET), *Lancet* 2:525–530, 1988.

4. Beanlands RSB, Dawood F, Wen WH, et al: Are the kinetics of technetium-99m methoxyisobutyl isonitrile affected by cell metabolism and viability? *Circulation* 82:1802–1814, 1990.

5. Behrenbeck T, Pellikka PA, Huber KC, et al: Primary angioplasty in myocardial infarction: assessment of improved myocardial perfusion with technetium-99m isonitrile, *J Am Coll Cardiol* 17:365–372, 1991.

6. Braat SH, de Swart H, Janssen JH, et al: Use of technetium-99m sestamibi to determine the size of the myocardial area perfused by a coronary artery, *Am J Cardiol* 66:85E–90E, 1990.

7. Califf RM, Harrelson-Woodlief L, Topol EJ: Left ventricular ejection fraction may not be useful as an end point of thrombolytic therapy comparative trials. *Circulation* 82:1847–1853, 1990.

8. Califf RM, Topol EJ, Gersh BJ: From myocardial salvage to patient salvage in acute myocardial infarction: The role of reperfusion therapy, *J Am Coll Cardiol* 14:1382–1388, 1989.

9. Chareonthaitawee P, Christian TF, O'Connor MK, et al: Noninvasive prediction of residual blood flow within the risk area during acute myocardial infarction: a multicenter validation study of patients undergoing direct coronary angioplasty, *Am Heart J* 134:639–646, 1997.

10. Chareonthaitawee P, Christian TF, Hirose K, et al: Relation of initial infarct size to extent of left ventricular remodeling in the year after myocardial infarction, *J Am Coll Cardiol* 25:567–573, 1995.

11. Christian TF, Behrenbeck T, Pellikka PA, et al: Mismatch of left ventricular function and infarct size demonstrated by technetium-99m-isonitrile imaging after reperfusion therapy for acute myocardial infarction: identification of myocardial stunning and hyperkinesia, *J Am Coll Cardiol* 16:1632–1638, 1990.

12. Christian TF, Clements IP, Behrenbeck T, et al: Limitations of the electrocardiogram in estimating infarction size after acute reperfusion therapy for myocardial infarction, *Ann Intern Med* 114:264–270, 1991.

13. Christian TF, Behrenbeck T, Gersh BJ, et al: Relation of left ventricular volume and function over one year after acute myocardial infarction to infarct size determined by technetium-99m sestamibi, *Am J Cardiol* 68:21–26, 1991.

14. Christian TF, Clements IP, Gibbons RJ: Noninvasive identification of myocardium at risk in patients with acute myocardial infarction and nondiagnostic electrocardiograms using technetium-99m-sestamibi, *Circulation* 83:1615–1620, 1991.

15. Christian TF, Gibbons RJ, Clements IP, et al: Estimates of myocardium at risk and collateral flow in acute myocardial infarction using electrocardiographic indexes with comparison to radionuclide and angiographic measures, *J Am Coll Cardiol* 26:388–393, 1995.

16. Christian TF, Gibbons RJ, Gersh BJ: Effect of infarct location on myocardial salvage assessed by technetium-99m isonitrile, *J Am Coll Cardiol* 17:1303–1308, 1991.

17. Christian TF, Gibbons RJ, Hopfenspirger MR, et al: Severity and response of chest pain during thrombolytic therapy for acute myocardial infarction: a useful indicator of myocardial salvage and infarct size, *J Am Coll Cardiol* 22:1311–1316, 1993.

18. Christian TF, O'Connor MK, Schwartz RS, et al: Technetium-99m MIBI to assess coronary collateral flow during acute myocardial infarction in two closed-chest animal models, *J Nucl Med* 38:1840–1846, 1997.

19. Christian TF, O'Connor MK, Gibbons RJ, et al: The effect of high and low collateral flow states and tissue viability on the distribution of Tc99m sestamibi, *Circulation* 92:I-449, 1995 (abstract).

20. Christian TF, O'Connor MK, Glynn RB, et al: The influence of gating on measurements of myocardium at risk and infarct size during acute myocardial infarction by tomographic technetium-99m labeled sestamibi imaging, *J Nucl Cardiol* 2:207–216, 1995.

21. Christian TF, Schwartz RS, Gibbons RJ: Determinants of infarct size in reperfusion therapy for acute myocardial infarction, *Circulation* 86:81–90, 1992.

22. Clements IP, Kaufmann UP, Bailey KR, et al: Electrocardiographic prediction of myocardial area at risk, *Mayo Clin Proc* 66:985–990, 1991.

23. Clements IP, Christian TF, Higano ST, et al: Residual flow to the infarct zone as a determinant of infarct size after direct angioplasty, *Circulation* 88(4 Part 1):1527–1533, 1993.

24. Clemmensen P, Grande P, Saunamaki K, et al: Effect of intravenous streptokinase on the relation between initial ST-predicted size and final QRS-estimated size of acute myocardial infarcts, *J Am Coll Cardiol* 16:1252–1257, 1990.

25. Das A, Christian TF, O'Connor MK, et al: Are partial volume effects important for the quantification of Tc99m sestamibi defect extent in the assessment of myocardium at risk during coronary occlusion? *Circulation* 92:I-448, 1995 (abstract).

26. De Coster PM, Melin JA, Detry JM, et al: Coronary artery reperfusion in acute myocardial infarction: assessment by pre- and postintervention thallium-201 myocardial perfusion imaging, *Am J Cardiol* 55:889–895, 1985.

27. De Coster PM, Wijns W, Cauwe F, et al: Area-at-risk determination by technetium-99m-hexakis-2-methoxyisobutyl isonitrile in experimental reperfused myocardial infarction, *Circulation* 82:2152–2162, 1990.

28. Dilsizian V, Arrighi JA, Diodati JG, et al: Myocardial viability in patients with chronic coronary artery disease. Comparison of 99mTc-sestamibi with thallium reinjection and [18 F] fluorodeoxyglucose, *Circulation* 89:578–587, 1994.

29. Edmunds JJ, Gibbons RJ, Bresnahan JF, et al: Significance of anterior ST depression in inferior wall acute myocardial infarction, *Am J Cardiol* 73:143–148, 1994.

30. Eisner RL, Schmarkey LS, Martin SE, et al: Detects on SPECT "perfusion" images can occur due to abnormal segmental contraction, *J Nucl Med* 35:638–643, 1994.

31. Ellis SG, Debowey D, Bates ER, et al: Treatment of recurrent ischemia after thrombolysis and successful reperfusion for acute myocardial infarction: effect on in-hospital mortality and left ventricular function, *J Am Coll Cardiol* 17:752–757, 1991.

32. Feiring AJ, Johnson MR, Kioschos JM, et al: The importance of the determination of the myocardial area at risk in the evaluation of the outcome of acute myocardial infarction in patients, *Circulation* 75:980–987, 1987.

33. Fletcher WO, Gibbons RJ, Clements IP: The relationship of inferior ST depression, lateral ST elevation, and left precordial ST elevation to myocardium at risk in acute anterior myocardial infarction, *Am Heart J* 126:526–535, 1993.

34. Force T, Kemper A, Leanitt M, et al: Acute reduction in functional infarct expansion with late coronary reperfusion: assessment with quantitative two-dimensional echocardiography, *J Am Coll Cardiol* 11:192–200, 1988.

35. Gagnon A, Taillefer R, Bavaria G, et al: Fast labeling of technetium-99m-sestamibi with microwave oven heating, *J Nucl Med Technol* 19:90–93, 1991.

36. Galli M, Maressa C, Bolli R, et al: Spontaneous delayed recovery of perfusion and contraction after the first 5 weeks after anterior infarction. Evidence for the presence of hibernating myocardium in the infarcted area, *Circulation* 90:1386–1397, 1994.

37. Gibbons EF, Hogan RD, Franklin TD, et al: The natural history of regional dysfunction in a canine preparation of chronic infarction, *Circulation* 71:394–402, 1985.

38. Gibbons RJ, Verani MS, Behrenbeck T, et al: Feasibility of tomographic ^{99m}Tc-hexakis-2-methoxy-2-methylpropyl-isonitrile imaging for the assessment of myocardial area at risk and the effect of treatment in acute myocardial infarction, *Circulation* 80:1277–1286, 1989.

39. Gibbons RJ, Christian TF, Hopfenspirger M, et al: Myocardium at risk and infarct size after thrombolytic therapy for acute myocardial infarction: implications for the design of randomized trials of acute intervention, *J Am Coll Cardiol* 24:616–623, 1994.

40. Gibbons RJ, Holmes DR, Reeder GS, et al: Immediate angioplasty compared with the administration of a thrombolytic agent followed by conservative treatment for myocardial infarction. The Mayo Coronary Care Unit and Catheterization Laboratory Groups, *N Engl J Med* 328:685–691, 1993.

41. Effectiveness of intravenous thrombolytic treatment in acute myocardial infarction. Gruppa Italiano per lo Studio della Streptokinasi nell'Infarto Miocardico (GISSI), *Lancet* 1:397–402, 1986.

42. Long-term effects of intravenous thrombolysis in acute myocardial infarction: final report of the GISSI study. Gruppo Italiano per lo Studio della Streptokinasi nell'Infarto Miocardico (GISSI), *Lancet* 2:871–874, 1987.

43. Gitter MJ, Christian TF, Gibbons RJ: Technetium-99m sestamibi distinguishes stunned from infarcted myocardium and predicts 6 week left ventricular ejection fraction after acute myocardial infarction, *J Am Coll Cardiol* 476A, 1994 (abstract).

44. Guerci AD, Gerstenblith G, Brimker JA, et al: A randomized trial of intravenous tissue plasminogen activator for acute myocardial infarction with subsequent randomization to elective coronary angioplasty, *N Engl J Med* 17:1613–1618, 1987.

45. Hasche ET, Fernandes C, Freedman SB, et al: Relation between ischemia time, infarct size, and left ventricular function in humans, *Circulation* 92:710–719, 1995.

46. Hackworthy RA, Vogel MB, Harris PJ: Influence of infarct artery patency on the relation between initial ST segment elevation and final infarct size, *Br Heart J* 156:222–225, 1986.

47. Haronian HL, Remetz MS, Sinusas AJ, et al: Myocardial risk area defined by technetium-99m sestamibi imaging during percutaneous transluminal coronary angioplasty: comparison with coronary angiography, *J Am Coll Cardiol* 22:1033–1043, 1993.

48. Hilton TC, Thompson RC, Williams HJ, et al: Technetium-99m sestamibi myocardial perfusion imaging in the emergency room evaluation of chest pain, *J Am Coll Cardiol* 23:1016–1022, 1994.

49. Hindman N, Grande P, Harrele FE Jr, et al: Relation between electrocardiographic and enzymatic methods of estimating acute myocardial infarct size, *Am J Cardiol* 58:31–35, 1986.

50. Hochman JS, Choo H: Limitation of myocardial infarction expansion by reperfusion independent of myocardial salvage, *Circulation* 75:299–306, 1987.

51. Huber KC, Bresnahan JF, Bresnahan DR, et al: Measurement of myocardium at risk by technetium-99m sestamibi: correlation with coronary angiography, *J Am Coll Cardiol* 19:67–73, 1992.

52. Hung JC, Wibon ME, Bronn ML, et al: Rapid preparation and quality control method for technetium-99m 2-methoxy isobutyl isonitrile technetium-99m (sestamibi), *J Nucl Med* 32:2162–2168, 1991.

53. A prospective trial of intravenous streptokinase in acute myocardial infarction (I.S.A.M.). Mortality, morbidity, and infarct size at 21 days. The I.S.A.M. Study Group, *N Engl J Med* 314:1465–1471, 1986.

54. Randomised trial of intravenous streptokinase, oral aspirin, both, or neither among 17,187 cases of suspected acute myocardial infarction: ISIS-2. ISIS-2 (Second International Study of Infarct Survival) Collaborative Group, *Lancet* 2:349–360, 1988.

55. Jang IK, van de Werf F, Vanhaecke J, et al: Comparison of angiographic methods for the assessment of the extent of experimental anterior myocardial infarction in dog hearts, *Int J Cardiol* 82:179–190, 1990.

56. Karlson BW, Herlitz J, Edvardsson N, et al: Eligibility for intravenous thrombolysis in suspected acute myocardial infarction, *Circulation* 82:1140–1146, 1990.

57. Kayden DS, Mattera JA, Zaret BL, et al: Demonstration of reperfusion after thrombolysis with technetium-99m isonitrile myocardial imaging, *J Nucl Med* 29:1865–1867, 1988.

58. Kennedy JW, Martin GV, Davis KB, et al: The Western Washington Intravenous Streptokinase in Acute Myocardial Infarction Randomized Trial, *Circulation* 77:345–352, 1988.

59. Khaja F, Walton JA Jr, Brymer JF, et al: Intracoronary fibrinolytic therapy in acute myocardial infarction. Report of a prospective randomized trial, *N Engl J Med* 308:1305–1311, 1983.

60. Klonar RA, Braunwald E: Observation on experimental myocardial ischaemia, *Cardiovasc Res* 14:371–395, 1980.

61. Leiboff RH, Katz RJ, Wesserman AG, et al: A randomized, angiographically controlled trial of intracoronary streptokinase in acute myocardial infarction, *Am J Cardiol* 53:404–407, 1984.

62. Li QS, Franc TL, Franceschi D, et al: Technetium-99m methoxyisobutyl isonitrile (RP30) for quantification of myocardial ischemia and reperfusion in dogs, *J Nucl Med* 29:1539–1548, 1988.

63. Lowe JE, Reimer KA, Jennings RB: Experimental infarct size as a function of the amount of myocardium at risk, *Am J Pathol* 90:363–379, 1978.

64. Marshall RC, Leidholdt EM Jr, Zhang DY, et al: Technetium-99m hexakis 2-methoxy-2-isobutyl isonitrile and thallium-201 extraction, washout, and retention at varying coronary flow rates in rabbit heart, *Circulation* 82:998–1007, 1990.

65. Medrano R, Lowry RW, Young JB, et al: Assessment of myocardial viability with ^{99m}Tc sestamibi in patients undergoing cardiac transplantation. A scintigraphic/pathological study, *Circulation* 94:1010–1017, 1996.

66. Leppo JA, Meerdink DJ: Comparative myocardial extraction of two technetium-labeled BATO derivatives (SQ30217, SQ30214) and thallium, *J Nucl Med* 31:67–74, 1990.

67. Miller TD, Christian TF, Hopfenspirger MR, et al: Infarct size after acute myocardial infarction measured by quantitative tomographic ^{99m}Tc-sestamibi imaging predicts subsequent mortality, *Circulation* 92:334–341, 1995.

68. Nieminen M, Parisi AF, O'Boyle JE, et al: Serial evaluation of myocardial thickening and thinning in acute experimental infarction: identification and quantification using two-dimensional echocardiography, *Circulation* 66:174–180, 1982.

69. O'Connor MK, Caiati C, Christian TF, et al: Effects of scatter correction on the measurement of infarct size from SPECT cardiac phantom studies, *J Nucl Med* 36:2080–2086, 1995.

70. O'Connor MK, Hammell TC, Gibbons RJ: In vitro validation of a simple tomographic technique for estimation of percentage myocardium at risk using methoxyisobutyl isonitrile technetium 99m (sestamibi), *Eur J Nucl Med* 17:69–76, 1990.

71. Oh JK, Gibbons RJ, Christian TF, et al: Correlation of regional wall motion abnormalities detected by two-dimensional echocardiography with perfusion defect determined by technetium 99m sestamibi imaging in patients treated with reperfusion therapy during acute myocardial infarction, *Am Heart J* 131:32–37, 1996.

72. Ohman EM, Califf RM, Topol EJ, et al: Consequences of reocclusion after successful reperfusion therapy in acute myocardial infarction. TAMI Study Group, *Circulation* 82:781–791, 1990.

73. Okada RD, Glover D, Gaffrey T, et al: Myocardial kinetics of technetium-99m-hexakis-2-methoxy-2-methylpropyl-isonitrile, *Circulation* 77:491–498, 1988.

74. O'Keefe JH, Grines CL, DeWood MA, et al: Poloxamer-188 as an adjunct to primary percutaneous transluminal coronary angioplasty for acute myocardial infarction, *Am J Cardiol* 78:747–750, 1996.

75. O'Rourke M, Baron D, Keogh A, et al: Limitation of myocardial in-

farction by early infusion of recombinant tissue-type plasminogen activator, *Circulation* 77:1311–1315, 1988.

76. Palmeri ST, Harrison DG, Gobb FR, et al: A QRS scoring system for assessing left ventricular function after myocardial infarction, *N Engl J Med* 306:4–9, 1982.

77. Pandian NG, Skorton DJ, Collins SM, et al: Myocardial infarct size threshold for two-dimensional echocardiographic detection: sensitivity of systolic wall thickening and endocardial motion abnormalities in small versus large infarcts, *Am J Cardiol* 55:551–555, 1985.

78. Pellikka PA, Behrenbecke T, Verani MS, et al: Serial changes in myocardial perfusion using tomographic technetium-99m-hexakis-2-methoxy-2-methylpropyl-isonitrile imaging following reperfusion therapy of myocardial infarction, *J Nucl Med* 31:1269–1275, 1990.

79. Pfisterer ME, Battler A, Swanson SM, et al: Reproducibility of ejection-fraction determinations by equilibrium radionuclide angiography in response to supine bicycle exercise: concise communication, *J Nucl Med* 20:491–495, 1979.

80. Piwnica-Worms D, Kronauge JF, Chi ML: Uptake and retention of hexakis (2-methoxyisobutyl isonitrile) technetium(I) in cultured chick myocardial cells. Mitochondrial and plasma membrane potential dependence, *Circulation* 82:1826–1838, 1990.

81. Reimer KA, Jennings RB, Cobb FR, et al: Animal models for protecting ischemic myocardium: results of the NHLBI Cooperative Study. Comparison of unconscious and conscious dog models, *Circ Res* 56:651–665, 1985.

82. Reimer KA, Ideker RE, Jennings RB: Effect of coronary occlusion site on ischaemic bed size and collateral blood flow in dogs, *Cardiovasc Res* 15:668–674, 1981.

83. Rentrop KP, Feit F, Blanke H, et al: Effects of intracoronary streptokinase and intracoronary nitroglycerin infusion on coronary angiographic patterns and mortality in patients with acute myocardial infarction, *N Engl J Med* 311:1457–1463, 1984.

84. Ritchie JL, Davis KB, Williams DL, et al: Global and regional left ventricular function and tomographic radionuclide perfusion: the Western Washington Intracoronary Streptokinase in Myocardial Infarction Trial, *Circulation* 70:867–875, 1984.

85. Ritchie JL, Cerqueira MN, Maynard C, et al: Ventricular function and infarct size: the Western Washington Intravenous Streptokinase in Myocardial Infarction Trial, *J Am Coll Cardiol* 11:689–697, 1988.

86. Rouan GW, Lee TH, Cook EF, et al: Clinical characteristics and outcome of acute myocardial infarction in patients with initially normal or nonspecific electrocardiograms (a report from the Multicenter Chest Pain Study), *Am J Cardiol* 64:1087–1092, 1989.

87. Sabia P, Afrookteh A, Touchstone DA, et al: Value of regional wall motion abnormality in the emergency room diagnosis of acute myocardial infarction. A prospective study using two-dimensional echocardiography, *Circulation* 84:I85–I92, 1991.

88. Sager PT, Perlmutter RA, Rosenfeld LE, et al: Electrophysiologic effects of thrombolytic therapy in patients with a transmural anterior myocardial infarction complicated by left ventricular aneurysm formation, *J Am Coll Cardiol* 12:19–24, 1988.

89. Gibson WS, Christian TF, Pellikka PA, et al: Serial tomographic imaging with technetium-99m-sestamibi for the assessment of infarct-related arterial patency following reperfusion therapy, *J Nucl Med* 33:2080–2085, 1992.

90. Santoro GM, Bisi G, Sciagra R, et al: Single photon emission computed tomography with technetium-99m hexakis 2-methoxyisobutyl isonitrile in acute myocardial infarction before and after thrombolytic treatment: assessment of salvaged myocardium and prediction of late functional recovery, *J Am Coll Cardiol* 15:301–314, 1990.

91. Sawada SG, Allman KC, Muzik O, et al: Positron emission tomography detects evidence of viability in rest technetium-99m defects, *J Am Coll Cardiol* 23:92–98, 1994.

92. Schaer GL, Spaccavento LJ, Browne KF, et al: Beneficial effects of RheothRx injection in patients receiving thrombolytic therapy for acute myocardial infarction. Results of a randomized, double-blind, placebo-controlled trial, *Circulation* 94:298–307, 1996.

93. Sheehan FH, Mathey DG, Schofer J, et al: Effect of interventions in salvaging left ventricular function in acute myocardial infarction: a study of intracoronary streptokinase, *Am J Cardiol* 52:431–438, 1983.

94. Sheehan FH, Braunwald E, Canner P, et al: The effect of intravenous thrombolytic therapy on left ventricular function: a report on tissue-type plasminogen activator and streptokinase from the Thrombolysis in Myocardial Infarction (TIMI Phase I) Trial, *Circulation* 75:817–829, 1987.

95. Lin YH, Sinusas AJ, Shi CQX, et al: Quantification of technetium 99m-labeled sestamibi single-photon emission computed tomography based on mean counts improved accuracy for assessment of relative regional blood flow: experimental validation in a canine model, *J Nucl Cardiol* 3:312–320, 1996.

96. Simoons ML, Serruys PW, van den Brand M, et al: Early thrombolysis in acute myocardial infarction: limitation of infarct size and improved survival, *J Am Coll Cardiol* 7:717–728, 1986.

97. Sinusas AJ, Trautman KA, Bergin JD, et al: Quantification of area at risk during coronary occlusion and degree of myocardial salvage after reperfusion using cardiac imaging with technetium-99m-methoxyisobutyl isonitrile, *Circulation* 82:1424–1437, 1990.

98. Sinusas AJ, Shi Q, Vitols PJ, et al: Impact of regional ventricular function, geometry, and dobutamine stress on quantitative ^{99m}Tc-sestamibi defect size, *Circulation* 88(5 Pt 1):2224–2234, 1993.

99. Sinusas AJ, Watson DD, Cannon JM Jr, et al: Effect of ischemia and postischemic dysfunction on myocardial uptake of technetium-99m labeled methoxyisobutyl isonitrile and thallium-201, *J Am Coll Cardiol* 14:1785–1793, 1989.

100. Sklenar J, Ismail S, Villanueva FS, et al: Dobutamine echocardiography for determining the extent of myocardial infarction after reperfusion. An experimental evaluation, *Circulation* 90:1502–1512, 1994.

101. Taillefer R, Primeau M, Costi P, et al: Technetium-99m-sestamibi myocardial perfusion imaging in detection of coronary artery disease: comparison between initial (1-hour) and delayed (3-hour) postexercise images, *J Nucl Med* 32:1961–1965, 1991.

102. Tamaki S, Nakajima H, Murakami T, et al: Estimation of infarct size by myocardial emission computed tomography with thallium-201 and its relation to creatine kinase-MB release after myocardial infarction in man, *Circulation* 66:994–1001, 1982.

103. The effects of tissue plasminogen activator, streptokinase, or both on coronary-artery patency, ventricular function, and survival after acute myocardial infarction. The GUSTO Angiographic Investigators, *N Engl J Med* 329:1615–1622, 1993.

104. An international randomized trial comparing four thrombolytic strategies for acute myocardial infarction. The GUSTO Investigators, *N Engl J Med* 329:673–682, 1993.

105. Touchstone DA, Beller GA, Nygaard TW, et al: Effects of successful intravenous reperfusion therapy on regional myocardial function and geometry in humans: a tomographic assessment using two-dimensional echocardiography, *J Am Coll Cardiol* 13:1506–1513, 1989.

106. Udelson JE, Coleman PS, Metherall J, et al: Predicting recovery of severe regional dysfunction. Comparison of resting scintigraphy with ^{201}Tl and ^{99m}Tc-sestamibi, *Circulation* 89:2552–2561, 1994.

107. Van de Werf F: Discrepancies between the effects of coronary reperfusion on survival and left ventricular function, *Lancet* 1:1367–1369, 1989.

108. Verani MS, Jeroudi MO, Mahmarian JJ, et al: Quantification of myocardial infarction during coronary occlusion and myocardial salvage after reperfusion using cardiac imaging with technetium-99m hexakis 2-methoxyisobutyl isonitrile, *J Am Coll Cardiol* 12:1573–1581, 1988.

109. Villanueva FS, Glasheen WP, Sklenar J, et al: Assessment of risk area during coronary occlusion and infarct size after reperfusion with myocardial contrast echocardiography using left and right atrial injections of contrast, *Circulation* 88:596–604, 1993.

110. Wackers FJTh, Berman DS, Maddahi J, et al: Technetium-99m hexakis 2-methoxyisobutyl isonitrile: human biodistribution, dosimetry, safety, and preliminary comparison to thallium-201 myocardial imaging, *J Nucl Med* 30:301–311, 1989.

111. Wackers FJ, Gibbons RJ, Verani MS, et al: Serial quantitative planar technetium-99m isonitrile imaging in acute myocardial infarction: efficacy for noninvasive assessment of thrombolytic therapy, *J Am Coll Cardiol* 14:861–873, 1989.

112. Wackers FJ, Berjen HJ, Weinberg MA, et al: Spontaneous changes in left ventricular function over the first 24 hours of acute myocardial infarction: implications for evaluating early therapeutic interventions, *Circulation* 66:748–754, 1982.

113. Wilcox RG, von der Lippe G, Olsson CG, et al: Effects of alteplase in acute myocardial infarction: 6-month results from the ASSET study. Anglo-Scandinavian Study of Early Thrombolysis, *Lancet* 335: 1175–1178, 1990.

Chapter 26

Risk stratification after acute myocardial infarction by using noninvasive radionuclide imaging

George A. Beller

Radionuclide techniques can be clinically useful in the evaluation of patients who have had infarction with respect to determining infarct size, assessing the degree of myocardial salvage after reperfusion, and determining myocardial viability in infarct zones of resting asynergy. These techniques can also be used in conjunction with exercise or pharmacologic stress for risk stratification.[5] Myocardial perfusion imaging can be done with thallium-201 (^{201}Tl) or one of the new technetium-99m (^{99m}Tc) imaging agents to identify residual ischemia within or remote from the infarct zone. Submaximal exercise testing can be done as early as 4 to 5 days after admission or pharmacologic stress imaging can be performed 48 to 72 hours after onset of symptoms.[23] The latter approach permits earlier hospital discharge in patients deemed to be at low risk for subsequent cardiac events on the basis of scintigraphic findings. The goal of early risk stratification is to better select patients who will truly benefit from an invasive strategy comprising early angiography and, when indicated, coronary revascularization. In this chapter, data from the literature will be reviewed on the value of risk assessment with radionuclide techniques in patients with uncomplicated myocardial infarction.

PROGNOSIS AFTER ACUTE INFARCTION
Assessment of resting left ventricular function

Prognosis in survivors of acute myocardial infarction is related to the degree of left ventricular dysfunction, the extent and severity of coronary artery disease, and the presence of residual myocardial ischemia. One of the best prognostic measurements that can be derived by radionuclide angiography in patients with acute infarction is the left ventricular ejection fraction. In the Multicenter Postinfarction Research Group (MPRG) study, which included 799 patients with acute infarction who underwent predischarge radionuclide angiography, the 1-year cardiac mortality rate increased exponentially as the resting left ventricular ejection fraction decreased to less than 40% (Fig. 26-1).[47] The importance of left ventricular ejection fraction as a prognostic variable in postinfarction patients has been sustained in patients who received thrombolytic therapy or primary angioplasty to attain reperfusion.[7,13,17,31,59] Postinfarction patients treated with thrombolysis, however, may have an improved survival rate at any value of left ventricular ejection fraction compared with the mortality rate relative to left ventricular ejection fraction in patients treated in the prethrombolytic era (Fig. 26-2).[7,73] Simoons et al[59] showed that the 5-year mortality rate exceeded 50% in patients who were receiving thrombolytic therapy at the time of hospital admission but were discharged with left ventricular ejection fraction of less than 30%. In that study, patients with left ventricular ejection fraction at rest that exceeded 40% had an annual mortality rate of approximately 2%.

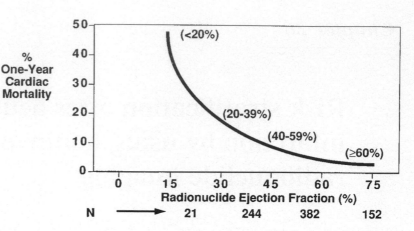

% One-Year Cardiac Mortality

Fig. 26-1. One-year cardiac mortality rate related to the predischarge radionuclide ejection fraction in patients who survived acute myocardial infarction. (Reprinted by permission of *The New England Journal of Medicine*. Risk stratification and survival after myocardial infarction, *N Engl J Med* 309:331-336, 1983. Copyright 1983 by the Massachusetts Medical Society.)

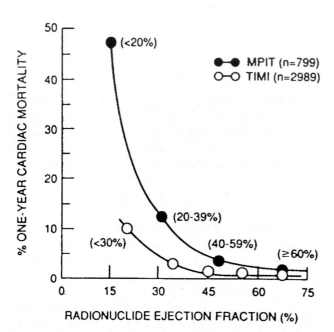

Fig. 26-2. One-year cardiac mortality rate and radionuclide ejection fraction in the Thrombolysis in Myocardial Infarction (TIMI) study *(dark solid circles)* and the Multicenter Postinfarction Research Group trial *(MPIT)* *(lightly shaded circles)*. The mortality rate is lower for any given resting ejection fraction in the TIMI study, in which all patients received thrombolytic therapy at the time of hospital admission. (Reproduced from Bonow RO: Prognostic assessment in coronary artery disease: role of radionuclide angiography, *J Nucl Cardiol* 11:280-291, 1994. With permission. Copyright 1994 American Society of Nuclear Cardiology.)

Rogers et al[52] investigated variables that were predictive of a good outcome after thrombolytic therapy in the Thrombolysis in Myocardial Infarction (TIMI)-II pilot study. In the group of patients randomized to the 18- to 48-hour early angioplasty group, variables independently predictive of survival were a resting left ventricular ejection fraction of more than 50%, few leads with ST-segment elevation on admission, younger age, rapid normalization of ST segments with dramatic relief of chest pain during thrombolysis, absence of arrhythmias within the first 24 hours of treatment initiation, absence of previous in-

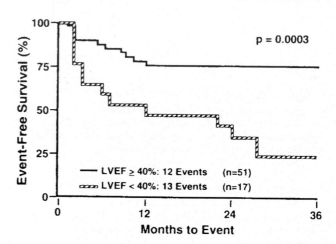

Fig. 26-3. Kaplan–Meier curve showing event-free survival as a function of left ventricular ejection fraction *(LVEF)* in patients who received thrombolytic therapy during acute myocardial infarction. (From Dakik HA, Mahmarian JJ, Kimball KT, et al: Prognostic value of exercise ^{201}Tl tomography in patients treated with thrombolytic therapy during acute myocardial infarction, *Circulation* 94:2735-2742, 1996. Reproduced with permission from *Circulation*. Copyright 1996 by the American Heart Association.)

farction, and being a nonsmoker at entry. Dakik et al[17] found that the estimated risk for a cardiac event doubled for every 10% decrease in the left ventricular ejection in postinfarction patients who received thrombolytic therapy. Figure 26-3 shows the event-free survival in patients with left ventricular ejection fraction of 40% or more compared with those with left ventricular ejection fraction of less than 40%.

The Canadian Assessment of Myocardial Infarction (CAMI) study sought to evaluate in-hospital and postdischarge mortality among patients with acute myocardial infarction in the 1990s.[55] When factors influencing 1-year postdischarge mortality were considered together by multivariate statistical analysis, only advancing age, a history of hypertension, diabetes, previous myocardial infarction, preinfarction coronary artery bypass graft (CABG) surgery, and Killip class were correlated with mortality, and in-hospital CABG surgery

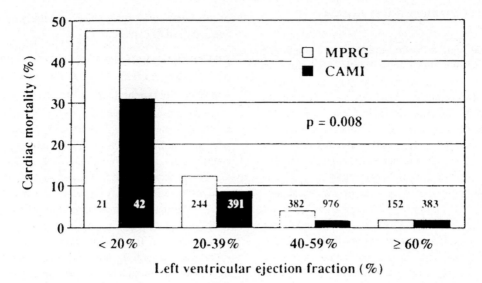

Fig. 26-4. Cardiac mortality related to left ventricular ejection fraction in patients enrolled in The Canadian Assessment of Myocardial Infarction *(CAMI)* study compared with mortality rate and ejection fraction in the Multicenter Postinfarction Research Group *(MPRG)* trial, which was performed in the prethrombolytic era. The major difference in mortality rate between the two groups was seen in patients in whom left ventricular ejection fraction was less than 20%. (From Rouleau JL, Talajik M, Sussex B, et al: Myocardial infarction patients in the 1990s—their risk factors, stratification and survival in Canada: The Canadian Assessment of Myocardial Infarction [CAMI] study, *J Am Coll Cardiol* 27:1119-1127, 1996. Reprinted with permission from the American College of Cardiology.)

or percutaneous transluminal coronary angioplasty (PTCA) in thrombolysis use was inversely correlated with mortality. As seen in the MPRG study,[47] the 1-year postdischarge cardiac mortality rate in the CAMI study increased progressively with decreasing left ventricular ejection fraction (Fig. 26-4).[55] As seen with the TIMI data (Fig. 26-2), the CAMI study showed that for a given ejection fraction less than 60%, the cardiac mortality rate was lower than that observed in the MPRG study,[47] which was performed in the prethrombolytic era. Thus, the studies cited above indicate that left ventricular ejection fraction at the time of discharge remains a potent predictor of subsequent mortality.

Patients treated with thrombolytic therapy in whom TIMI grade 3 flow is achieved in the infarct vessel have a higher left ventricular ejection fraction compared with patients in whom reflow in the infarct-related artery is not established.[28] In the Global Utilization of Streptokinase and Tissue Plasminogen Activator for Occluded Arteries (GUSTO) trial,[28] the average left ventricular ejection fraction was 61% in patients who had TIMI grade 3 flow in the infarct vessel and 54% in patients with TIMI grade 1 flow. In that trial, the mortality rate at 30 days was 4% among patients with a 90-minute left ventricular ejection fraction more than 45%, but was 15% among those with left ventricular ejection fraction of 45% or less. In 542 patients reported by Harrison et al,[30] patients with TIMI grade 0 flow were less likely than patients with patent infarct-related arteries to have improved regional function. Of interest, the correlation between time to reperfusion and improvement in function was not great.

The use of left ventricular ejection fraction measurement as a predictor of outcome in the very early acute phase of myocardial infarction has some limitations. Some patients may demonstrate substantial hyperkinesis of the normally perfused zone, which influences global performance to some degree. This may falsely elevate the left ventricular ejection fraction. With resolution of remote hyperkinesis in the weeks after the acute event, the true effect of infarct size on global cardiac performance becomes evident. The measurement of ejection fraction at 10 to 14 days after infarction in patients receiving thrombolytic therapy will more truly reflect global performance in the long term and will therefore be a more sensitive predictor for ultimate prognosis. This is because of resolution of myocardial stunning resulting from reperfusion. Resting ^{201}Tl scintigraphy can provide important information for distinguishing asynergy in the infarct zone due to myocardial stunning from myocardial necrosis. The greater the uptake of ^{201}Tl in the infarct zone, the greater the probability of improved left ventricular ejection fraction at 3 weeks after infarction.[38]

Routine revascularization of patent but stenotic arteries does not seem to improve resting global left ventricular function in patients with acute myocardial infarction. In the TIMI study, the left ventricular ejection fraction at 6 weeks after infarction was similar in patients randomly allocated to receive a conservative strategy and those randomized to an "invasive" strategy.[63] In the Should We Intervene Following Myocardial Infarction trial (SWIFT),[60] no difference was seen left ventricular ejection fraction in patients randomized to an invasive strategy compared with a conservative strategy after thrombolysis.

Influence of extent of coronary artery disease on prognosis

The extent of underlying coronary artery disease is a major risk variable in patients who have had infarction. Schulman et al[57] followed a group of 143 postinfarction patients of whom 50% had triple-vessel coronary artery disease. Multivariate analysis showed that the combination of left anterior descending and right coronary artery disease, left ventricular ejection fraction, and the number of risk segments in the distribution of stenotic vessels were significant predictors of outcome. The angiographic variables provided significant prognostic information that supplemented clinical variables for prediction of subsequent cardiac events. De Feyter et al[18] described a significant interaction between left ventricular ejection fraction and extent of angiographic coronary artery disease for predicting outcome after discharge in patients with an uncomplicated infarction. The mortality rate was 22% in infarct survivors with left ventricular ejection fraction less than 30% or triple-vessel coronary artery disease and 1% in patients with a left ventricular ejection fraction of 30% or more and single- or double-vessel disease.

The number of coronary artery stenoses remains a major risk variable in myocardial infarction patients who have received thrombolytic therapy. In the TIMI-II trial,[2] triple-vessel disease was a significant risk variable for death and recurrent nonfatal infarction in patients who underwent coronary angioplasty. The mortality rate increased threefold during follow-up after angioplasty in patients with triple-vessel disease compared with patients with single-vessel disease. Similar findings were reported from the Thrombolysis and Angioplasty in Myocardial Infarction (TAMI) database.[46] Significantly increased mortality was seen among patients with multivessel coronary artery disease compared with those with single-vessel disease (11.4% and 4.2%; $P < 0.001$). Data from the GUSTO trial[28] also showed that patients with triple-vessel disease had a significant increase in mortality rate compared with those who had stenoses of a lesser extent.

Clearly, the role of noninvasive stress testing with or without cardiac imaging is to identify patients with multivessel disease and patients with depressed left ventricular function, regardless of the extent of coronary artery disease, who are at risk for premature cardiac death with medical therapy. Patients with depressed function due to a large infarct should show low exercise tolerance and extensive nonreversible defects compared with patients who have had significant myocardial salvage with reperfusion therapy. Patients with small infarcts will show better exercise tolerance and have smaller defects. Patients with multivessel coronary artery disease and a first infarction may have inducible ischemia with myocardial defects identified remote from the zone of infarction. These defects should be reversible in the absence of previous infarction. Residual ischemia in a zone of infarction should be readily detected by demonstration of a mild to moderate initial postexercise defect with subsequent reversibility on the resting study. Nonimaging variables derived from treadmill testing, such as abnormal heart rate and blood pressure changes, should also reflect the degree of left ventricular dysfunction and the extent of angiographic coronary artery disease.

PREDISCHARGE EXERCISE IMAGING FOR RISK STRATIFICATION AFTER INFARCTION
Exercise electrocardiographic stress testing

In the prethrombolytic era, exercise testing was shown to be useful in separating high-risk and low-risk subsets of patients with myocardial infarction on the basis of functional and stress electrocardiographic end points.[21] Box 26-1 summarizes the exercise electrocardiographic stress test variables associated with an increased risk for a future cardiac event after acute infarction. Perhaps the most important of these variables relates to failure to achieve a workload of more than 4 metabolic equivalents (METs). Patients who have a flat blood pressure response or an exercise-induced decrease in blood pressure are at increased risk for an adverse outcome after discharge. Ischemic ST-segment depression of more than 1.0 mm, especially if observed at a low exercise heart rate or workload, is associated with an increased mortality rate during follow-up. In the prethrombolytic era, approximately 30% of patients with uncomplicated myocardial infarction exhibited exercise-induced ST-segment depression on predischarge submaximal exercise testing.[26] The cardiac mortality rate was approximately 15% in patients who had ischemic ST-segment depression on testing compared with 5% in patients who did not manifest an ischemic ST-segment response.

The incidence of exercise-induced ST-segment depression on predischarge stress testing is lower among patients who receive thrombolytic therapy. In the TIMI-IIB multicenter trial, the prevalence of exercise-induced ST-segment depression at discharge was 17.7% in patients randomly allocated to receive the conservative strategy.[63] By 6 weeks after discharge, the incidence of ST-segment depression was 19.4%. This value is lower than the approximately 30% prevalence of inducible ST-segment depression cited previously for patients studied in the prethrombolytic era.[21] The specificity of the ST-segment depression response for inducible ischemia in postinfarction patients is problematic. Froelicher et al[22] performed a meta-analysis of various studies that investigated exercise test responses after myocardial infarction and found that exercise-induced ST-segment depression was only predictive of increased risk in pa-

---

Box 26-1. High-risk exercise electrocardiographic stress test variables after acute myocardial infarction

Failure to achieve a workload of ≥4 metabolic equivalents
Exercise-induced limiting angina
A horizontal or downsloping ST-segment depression of ≥1mm in leads without Q waves
Exercise-induced decrease in blood pressure
Ventricular tachycardia

tients with inferior or posterior Q-wave infarction and not in those with anterior Q-wave infarction. This is because ST-segment depression in the presence of anterior precordial Q waves is not predictive of an increased ischemic event rate. Dakik et al[17] found that none of the variables derived from exercise stress testing contributed to predicting risk in a cohort of patients who underwent thrombolysis and achieved a mean treadmill exercise time of 7.3 ± 2.5 minutes when testing was performed a median of 13 days after the index infarction. Patients with ST-segment depression are more likely to have multivessel disease than single-vessel disease, and the greater the magnitude of ST-segment depression, the greater the likelihood of extensive coronary artery disease.

Of interest, the highest mortality rate is seen in patients who are deemed ineligible for predischarge exercise testing.[14,68] In the Gruppo Italiano per lo Studio della Sopravvivenza nell'Infarto Miocardico (GISSI)-II trial,[68] in which the rate of revascularization after infarction treated with thrombolytic therapy was low, the mortality rate at 6 months was 1.17 among patients with a negative result on exercise stress test, compared with 1.7% among patients with a positive test result. The mortality rate was 9.87 among patients deemed ineligible for testing.

Some observers have found that symptom-limited exercise testing is preferable to submaximal testing for identifying patients with residual myocardial ischemia after uncomplicated infarction. Juneau et al[33] performed low-level and symptom-limited exercise tests in patients with uncomplicated infarction of whom slightly more than 50% received thrombolytic therapy. The symptom-limited test was associated with a greater exercise duration (554 compared with 389 seconds), a higher peak workload (5.7 compared with 4.2 METs), and a higher peak exercise heart rate (121 compared with 108 beats/min), as compared with the low-level stress test. The number of patients who developed ischemic ST-segment depression increased from 56 to 89 when the symptom-limited test was compared with the low-level test. The number of patients who had at least 2.0 mm of ST-segment depression increased 86%.

Exercise myocardial perfusion imaging

Variables derived from low-level exercise perfusion imaging after acute myocardial infarction provide additional prognostic information over clinical and electrocardiographic stress test variables for separating high-risk and low-risk subsets.[34] Several reasons explain the enhanced predictive value of perfusion imaging over electrocardiographic stress testing alone for prognostication. First, perfusion imaging is more sensitive than exercise electrocardiographic stress testing alone for detection of ischemia at low exercise heart rates. Second, perfusion imaging is superior to exercise electrocardiography in localizing the regions of stress-induced ischemia, which permits better assessment of area at risk and identification of patients with multivessel disease. This is important because stress-induced reversible defects remote from the zone of infarction are associated with a substantially higher risk for a subsequent cardiac

event compared with the demonstration of defects solely in the zone perfused by the infarct-related artery.[24] The location of ST-segment depression in the limb leads or the precordial leads does not have high localizing value for distinguishing various coronary supply zones.

Certain variables derived from perfusion imaging have been associated with an increased risk for an adverse outcome (Box 26-2). A large defect in the zone of the infarct-related artery showing no residual viability would reflect a large infarct with an increased propensity for left ventricular remodeling, progressive cardiac dilatation with consequent congestive heart failure, and an increased rate of cardiac death. A second prognostic variable on stress perfusion imaging is a large zone of inducible ischemia (>10% of the left ventricular area). A third variable is demonstration of defects both within and remote from the infarct zone. This finding indicates underlying multivessel disease. A fourth variable related to the use of ^{201}Tl scintigraphy is abnormally increased lung uptake of ^{201}Tl. A high lung-to-heart ^{201}Tl ratio on the anterior view planar image is indicative of exercise-induced pulmonary edema, which predominantly results from combination of depressed resting left ventricular function and superimposed inducible ischemia with a further acute decrease in systolic performance. These pathophysiologic alterations result in a rise in left ventricular filling pressure as the heart dilates to maintain stroke volume during exercise. Transient left ventricular cavity dilation from the exercise to the resting images is a fifth imaging variable associated with an adverse outcome. This is most likely caused by stress-induced diffuse subendocardial ischemia with subsequent filling of the underperfused region in the resting state, leading to a visual finding of a decrease in the size of the left ventricular cavity.

In the prethrombolytic era, approximately 50% of patients with an uncomplicated infarction who were younger than 65 years of age and who had a multivessel disease scan pattern, a reversible perfusion defect within or outside the infarct zone, or abnormal lung uptake of ^{201}Tl on predischarge submaximal imaging subsequently experienced cardiac death, nonfatal infarction, or rehospitalization for class III or IV angina.[24] In this study by Gibson et al, the cardiac event rate was only 6% for postinfarction patients who had a normal scan or nonreversible

---

Box 26-2. High-risk myocardial perfusion imaging variables after acute myocardial infarction

Defect size >20% of left ventricular area
Large zone of reversible ischemia
Reversible defects remote from the zone of infarction (multivessel disease scan pattern)
Increased lung uptake of thallium-201
Transient ischemic left ventricular cavity dilation
Multiple areas of decreased wall thickening on gated single-photon emission computed tomography

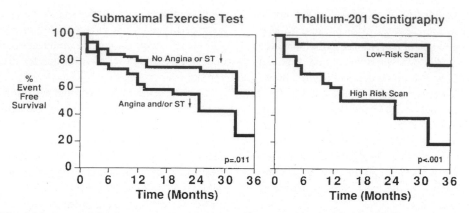

Fig. 26-5. Event-free survival after uncomplicated myocardial infarction in the prethrombolytic era related to exercise electrocardiographic stress tests *(left)* and thallium-201 scintigraphy *(right)* in 140 patients followed for an average of 15 months after infarction. High- and low-risk subsets were better separated by thallium-201 scintigraphic variables than by submaximal exercise stress test variables. ST ↓ = ST-segment depression. (From Gibson RS, Watson DD: Value of ^{201}Tl imaging in risk stratification of patients recovering from acute myocardial infarction, *Circulation* 84(Suppl I):I148-I162, 1991. Reproduced with permission by *Circulation.* Copyright 1991 by the American Heart Association.)

defects confined to the infarct zone. Figure 26-5 shows the rate of event-free survival after uncomplicated myocardial infarction related to exercise electrocardiographic stress test and ^{201}Tl scintigraphic data in 140 patients who were studied for an average of 15 months. High-risk and low-risk subsets were better identified by ^{201}Tl scintigraphic variables than by variables derived from submaximal exercise testing. Twenty-six percent of patients with a low-risk exercise electrocardiographic stress test experienced a cardiac event during follow-up. Figure 26-6 is an example of a high-risk single-photon emission computed tomographic (SPECT) imaging study in a patient with inferior myocardial infarction who had a nonreversible inferior defect and a reversible defect in the supply zone of the left anterior descending coronary artery. These findings are indicative of a multivessel disease scan pattern.

Brown and coworkers[10] examined the prognostic implications of ischemia within the territory of a previous acute myocardial infarction versus ischemia at a distance that developed late after infarction. In a group of 61 consecutive patients who underwent both exercise ^{201}Tl planar imaging and cardiac catheterization after discharge from the hospital after acute infarction, 29 had ^{201}Tl redistribution confined to the infarct zone and 16 had redistribution outside of the infarct zone. Stepwise multivariate logistic regression analysis revealed that the presence of both ^{201}Tl redistribution defect and multivessel angiographic coronary disease were significant predictors of total events during 10 months of follow-up. However, when coronary revascularization was excluded as an end point, ^{201}Tl redistribution limited to the infarct zone was the only significant predictor of cardiac events. As expected, reversible perfusion defects and inducible ST-segment depression were observed more frequently after non–Q-wave infarction than after Q-wave infarction.

Exercise perfusion imaging in the thrombolytic era

Controversy exists about the value of exercise electrocardiographic testing and exercise myocardial perfusion imaging for risk stratification in the thrombolytic era.[3] The controversy primarily focuses on the perception of a lower predictive value of high-risk stress imaging variables in postthrombolytic patients who undergo predischarge exercise imaging and are followed up. It should be pointed out that in patients who have undergone thrombolytic therapy, reversible defects on ^{201}Tl exercise scintigraphy are still more prevalent than ST-segment depression on treadmill testing. Tilkemeier et al[61] reported a 42% prevalence of ^{201}Tl redistribution compared with 15% for ischemic ST-segment depression in postinfarction patients who received thrombolytic therapy. Haber et al[29] reported that ^{201}Tl redistribution was seen in 48% of postinfarction patients who had undergone thrombolytic therapy compared with a 14% prevalence of inducible ST-segment depression. More recently, Dakik et al[17] found a 15% prevalence of exercise-induced ST-segment depression in postthrombolysis patients, whereas 38% of these patients had scintigraphic evidence of ischemia. Although exercise perfusion imaging remains more sensitive than exercise electrocardiographic stress testing alone after thrombolytic therapy, the prevalence of redistribution defects is lower than that seen in the prethrombolytic era.[29] When a prethrombolytic cohort was compared with a thrombolytic cohort in the same institution, the prevalence of ^{201}Tl redistribution decreased from 59% to 48%.[26] Several explanations account for the apparent reduction in ischemic responses on stress imaging in postinfarction patients receiving thrombolytic therapy. One important explanation may be a significantly lower prevalence of triple-vessel disease (10% to 13%) in patients who are enrolled in thrombolytic trials from which information about prevalence of ischemic responses is derived.

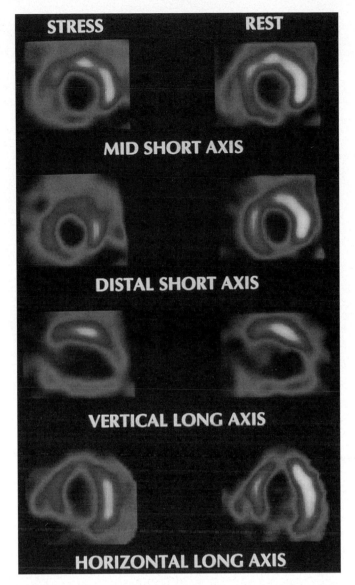

Fig. 26-6. Stress *(left row)* and rest *(right row)* technetium-99m sestamibi SPECT images obtained in a patient who underwent submaximal exercise testing 1 week after an uncomplicated acute myocardial infarction. Note the nonreversible inferior defect consistent with the patient's inferior myocardial infarction. A defect in the anterior wall and intraventricular septum can be seen that demonstrates reversibility on the resting tomograms. This is consistent with remote ischemia in the supply region of the left anterior descending coronary artery.

Multivessel disease detection

Multivessel coronary artery disease is one of the most important prognostic variables for identifying high-risk patients who survive an acute infarction. One of the primary goals of risk assessment is to identify patients with multivessel disease and residual myocardial ischemia who might benefit from triage for early coronary angiography and revascularization if coronary anatomy is suitable. Haber et al[29] reported that 35% of patients treated with thrombolytic therapy had underlying multivessel disease by angiography, and only 13% had triple-

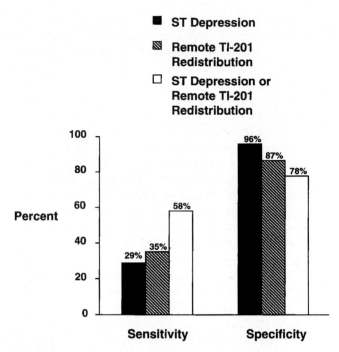

Fig. 26-7. Detection of multivessel coronary artery disease with exercise myocardial perfusion imaging after uncomplicated acute myocardial infarction. Both the sensitivity of exercise-induced ST-segment depression (29%) and that of a redistribution technetium-99m defect remote from the zone of infarction *(cross-hatched bar)* are lower than the sensitivity reported for multivessel disease detection by these variables in the prethrombolytic era. The presence of 1.0 mm or more of ST-segment depression or defects remote from the infarct zone had a sensitivity of 58% and a specificity of 78% for detecting multivessel disease in these thrombolytic patients.

vessel disease. A ^{201}Tl defect identified remote from the infarct zone was observed in only 35% of patients with multivessel disease (Fig. 26-7). Fifty-eight percent of patients with angiographic multivessel disease had either a remote ^{201}Tl defect or ST-segment depression, whereas only 22% of patients with single-vessel disease manifested one or both of these conditions.

In the prethrombolytic era, the sensitivity of ^{201}Tl scintigraphy for detecting multivessel disease was approximately 70% and approximately 59% of patients with multivessel disease had exercise-induced ischemic ST-segment depression.[4] Thus, the detection rate of multivessel disease by using exercise stress scintigraphy in postinfarction patients who received thrombolytic therapy on admission seems to be less than the detection rate for multivessel disease reported in prethrombolytic patient cohorts.

Potential explanations for the diminished sensitivity of exercise scintigraphy for identifying multivessel disease in patients receiving thrombolytic therapy are as follows:

1. Prethrombolytic populations of acute infarction patients had a 55% to 60% prevalence of underlying multivessel disease compared with a 35% prevalence of multivessel disease in a series of patients reported from thrombolytic trials.[66] In these trials, the prevalence of triple-

vessel disease ranges from only 10% to 15%. In the TIMI-II trial, the prevalence of triple-vessel disease was 5% in the routine catheterization subset and 11% in the selective catheterization subset.[53] In the GUSTO angiographic trial, only 14% of patients had triple-vessel disease (Fig. 26-8).[28] Because a defect remote from the infarct zone is more likely to be induced by submaximal exercise perfusion imaging in the setting of triple-vessel disease than in the setting of double-vessel disease, it is not surprising that the sensitivity of remote defects for multivessel disease identification is lower in thrombolytic patient populations. Postinfarction patients with triple-vessel disease would be expected to have more extensive perfusion defects remote from the infarct zone than patients with single-vessel or double-vessel disease.

2. Another explanation relates to the fact that the prevalence of previous infarction is lower in patients enrolled in trials that include thrombolytic therapy than in patients enrolled in series in the prethrombolytic era.[24] A previous infarction remote from the infarct zone of new myocardial damage would be associated with a greater probability of a multivessel disease scan pattern.

3. A final reason for the lower sensitivity for multivessel disease detection in the thrombolytic patients relates to the observation that patients with non–Q-wave infarct accounted for a substantial percentage of patient series reported in the prethrombolytic era.[25] Patients without ST-segment elevation on admission electrocardiography make up a smaller percentage of patients reported in series of thrombolytic therapy. Patients with non–Q-wave infarction have an extent of angiographic coronary disease similar to that in patients with Q-wave infarction

but have a higher prevalence of stress-induced ischemia.[25] In addition, because of less myocardial necrosis in the infarct zone, patients with non–Q-wave infarction may exercise to higher peak workloads. This should yield a greater probability of inducing ischemia remote from the infarct zone in the supply region of a second stenotic vessel.

Thus, the diminished sensitivity of myocardial perfusion imaging for identification of multivessel disease in the thrombolytic era may be attributed to a change in the patient population undergoing testing and being reported. Patients enrolled in thrombolytic series turn out to be a lower-risk population with more single-vessel disease and less triple-vessel disease than patients reported in series in the prethrombolytic era.

Separation of high-risk and low-risk subsets

Some observers have stated that exercise myocardial perfusion imaging is of little value for risk stratification in patients with acute myocardial infarction in the thrombolytic era.[35,43,45] Krone et al[35] reported that exercise testing with or without ^{201}Tl perfusion imaging added little to the overall prediction of primary cardiac events in 936 patients who recovered from acute infarction or unstable angina. As shown in Table 26-1, 31% of the patients in this study underwent thrombolytic therapy, 67% underwent coronary angiography before noninvasive testing, and 39% had coronary angioplasty before testing. Patients were enrolled an average of 2.7 months after the index event, and those excluded from enrollment had undergone coronary bypass surgery after the index event, were takings digitalis or other drugs that were thought to probably induce false-positive or nondiagnostic ST-segment changes on exercise electrocardiographic recordings, or had resting ST-T–wave changes on

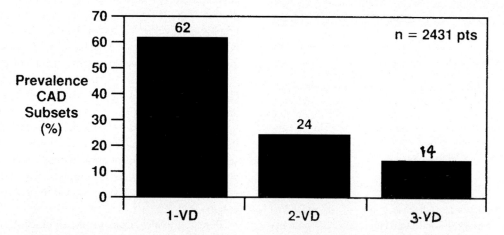

Fig. 26-8. Presence of single-vessel disease *(1-VD)*, double-vessel disease *(2-VD)*, and triple-vessel disease *(3-VD)* in 2431 patients enrolled in the Global Utilization of Streptokinase and Tissue Plasminogen Activator for Occluded Arteries *(GUSTO)* angiographic trial. Only 14% of patients with acute myocardial infarction who received thrombolytic therapy had triple-vessel disease on acute coronary angiography. (Reprinted with permission of the publisher, from Gibson RS, Beller GA: *Value of predischarge myocardial perfusion scintigraphy.* In Fuster V, Ross R, Topol EJ, eds: *Atherosclerosis and coronary artery disease,* vol 2, Philadelphia, 1996, Lippincott–Raven. Copyright 1996 by Lippincott–Raven.)

the baseline electrocardiogram. As would be expected in a patient population in which most high-risk patients were either not enrolled in the first place or underwent coronary angiography or angioplasty before enrollment, the cardiac mortality rate at 1 year was only 1.2%. It should also be pointed out that 21% of the patients underwent early postexercise test revascularization, most likely on the basis of high-risk stress test findings. Thus, no matter how sensitive and specific a noninvasive test may be for detecting high-risk and low-risk subgroups of postinfarction patients, it cannot accurately identify the few patients in the subgroup with a subsequent mortality rate of only 1.2%.

Miller et al[43] also sought to determine the prognostic value of ^{201}Tl exercise treadmill testing performed early after myocardial infarction in patients treated with thrombolysis. Their study cohort comprised 131 patients treated with thrombolytic therapy alone and 79 patients who underwent thrombolytic therapy and coronary angioplasty. At 2 years, survival free of any cardiac event did not differ for patients with a high-risk or low-risk ^{201}Tl scan who were treated with thrombolysis alone or with both thrombolysis and coronary angioplasty. No single exercise or ^{201}Tl variable was predictive of outcome. However, 73% of these patients underwent coronary angiography before exercise ^{201}Tl stress testing and 38% underwent pretest coronary angioplasty (Table 26-1). Another 26% underwent early posttest revascularization, presumably on the basis of high-risk noninvasive test findings. The annual mortality rate in this cohort was 1.5%. As seen in the study by Krone et al,[35] no noninvasive test is capable of identifying a subgroup of postinfarction patients with such a low mortality rate. As the authors themselves stated, "For a population with a very low event rate, it is unlikely that any test will be accurate enough to identify the few cases in which future events occur."

In contrast, some investigators have reported the prognostic utility of exercise myocardial perfusion imaging in the thrombolytic era. Candell-Riera et al[12] performed exercise ^{201}Tl scintigraphy, resting radionuclide angiography, and resting echocardiography in 115 consecutive patients with a first myocardial infarction younger than 65 years of age. The combina-

tion of the exercise electrocardiographic stress test and ^{201}Tl scintigraphy with resting two-dimensional echocardiography provided the greatest probability of predicting severe complications during follow-up. Major variables found to identify high-risk patients were a resting ejection fraction of less than 45%, maximal systolic blood pressure less than 150 mm Hg with exercise, and presence of pulmonary uptake of [201]Tl. Thallium-201 variables were superior to variables derived from cardiac catheterization for predicting severe complications (88% vs. 66%). Subsequently, these authors reported the 5-year follow-up for these 115 patients to further evaluate the prognostic role of predischarge cardiac noninvasive studies.[48] The combination of exercise ^{201}Tl scintigraphy and resting radionuclide ventriculography yielded an 87% positive predictive value and 91% negative predictive value for severe complications (cardiac death, reinfarction, development of severe angina, development of severe heart failure, or late coronary revascularization). The addition of cardiac catheterization did not improve the predictive power of these noninvasive studies. Dakik et al[17] found that the absolute extent of left ventricular ischemia defined risk when it was dichotomized at 10%. Fifty percent of postinfarction patients who received thrombolytic therapy and had an ischemic defect larger than 10% had a subsequent cardiac event compared with 26% of patients with a defect 10% or smaller. The risk for a cardiac event was 1.36 times higher for every 10% increase in the size of the SPECT perfusion defect. Figure 26-9 shows the event-free survival in patients with a defect smaller than 20% compared with a 20% or larger defect in this study.

Travin and coworkers[67] found that exercise ^{99m}Tc sestamibi SPECT imaging after myocardial infarction often reveals resid-

Table 26-1. Studies concluding that postmyocardial infarction exercise thallium-201 stress imaging has "limited usefulness" or "limited prognostic value"*

Variable	Miller et al[43] (n = 210)	Krone et al[35] (n = 936)
	%	
Thrombolysis	100	31
Pretest angiography	73	67
Pretest PTCA	38	39
Early posttest revascularization	17	21
Late revascularization	9	–
Annual mortality rate	1.5	1.2

*PTCA = percutaneous transluminal coronary angioplasty.

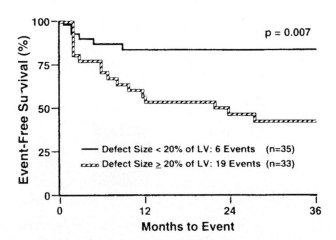

Fig. 26-9. Kaplan–Meier curve showing event-free survival as a function of perfusion defect size in patients who received thrombolytic therapy during myocardial infarction. LV = left ventricle. (From Dakik HA, Mahmarian JJ, Kimball KT, et al: Prognostic value of exercise ^{201}Tl tomography in patients treated with thrombolytic therapy during acute myocardial infarction, *Circulation* 94:2735-2742, 1996. Reproduced with permission by *Circulation.* Copyright 1996 by the American Heart Association.)

ual ischemia and is superior to clinical information and exercise electrocardiographic stress data alone in identifying patients with a high probability of a subsequent cardiac event. By Cox regression analysis of all variables, the number of ischemic defects on SPECT ^{99m}Tc sestamibi imaging was the only significant correlate of future cardiac events. Patients with 3 or more reversible ^{99m}Tc sestamibi defects had an event rate of 38% (Fig. 26-10). As previously mentioned, ischemia was detected more often with ^{99m}Tc sestamibi imaging than with exercise ST-segment depression. In conclusion, these data suggest that exercise perfusion imaging is still useful for risk stratification after uncomplicated acute myocardial infarction.

Reduction in late heart failure after infarction

Predischarge exercise myocardial perfusion imaging is also useful for predicting which patients are prone to develop early or late congestive heart failure after an uncomplicated acute anterior wall myocardial infarction. Lystash et al[39] studied patients who developed early-onset congestive heart failure after

anterior infarction and found that such patients were likely to have had a large area of myocardial damage reflected by a larger number of persistent ^{201}Tl defects (3.4 ± 1.2) compared with patients with late-onset (2.1 ± 1.2) or no (1.8 ± 1.1) heart failure (Fig. 26-11). Patients with late-onset congestive heart failure after discharge had significantly greater myocardial ischemia on predischarge submaximal exercise testing as assessed by the number of segments demonstrating redistribution (Fig. 26-11). A total of 1.4 ± 1.1 segments in patients with late-onset heart failure showed redistribution compared with 0.4 ± 1.1 segments in patients with early-onset congestive heart failure. During follow-up (mean, 49 months), 50% of patients developed late-onset heart failure after a recurrent myocardial infarction. Of interest, none of the 26 patients with anterior infarction who underwent CABG surgery for management of postinfarction myocardial ischemia developed late-onset heart failure. This observation supports the concept that an increased amount of myocardium at jeopardy is an important variable contributing to late heart failure. The decreased incidence of

Fig. 26-10. Cardiac event rate related to the number of reversible defects on exercise technetium-99m sestamibi myocardial perfusion imaging after uncomplicated acute myocardial infarction. Patients with 3 or more reversible technetium-99m sestamibi defects had a significantly higher event rate than patients with normal scans or patients with only one or two reversible defects.

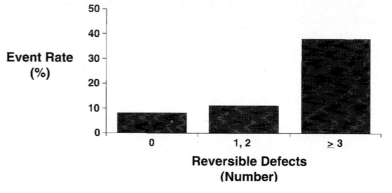

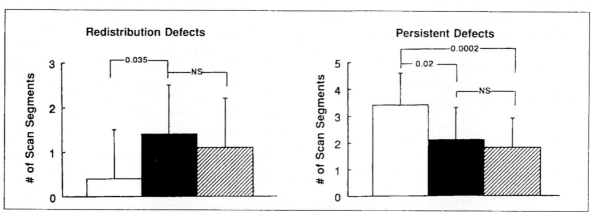

Fig. 26-11. Number of scan segments showing thallium-201 redistribution defects *(left)* and persistent defects *(right)* on predischarge submaximal exercise scintigraphy in patients who developed early *(open bars)*, late *(solid bars)*, and no *(slashed bars)* congestive heart failure after acute myocardial infarction. Patients who developed early heart failure following hospital discharge after acute myocardial infarction had significantly more persistent defects and fewer redistribution defects than did patients who developed late heart failure after discharge. Fifty percent of patients who developed late heart failure had an antecedent recurrent myocardial infarction. NS = not significant. (Reprinted by permission of the publisher, from Lystash JC, Gibson RS, Watson DD, et al: Early versus late congestive heart failure after initially uncomplicated anterior wall acute myocardial infarction, *Am J Cardiol* 75:653–658, 1995. Copyright 1995 by Excerpta Medica, Inc.)

late heart failure in the surgical cohort may be secondary to amelioration of ischemia, thereby reducing extent of myocardium at jeopardy and lowering the subsequent reinfarction rate that contributes to development of heart failure.

PREDISCHARGE VASODILATOR STRESS IMAGING FOR RISK STRATIFICATION AFTER INFARCTION

Dipyridamole thallium-201 scintigraphy

Vasodilator stress perfusion imaging has proven to be an excellent alternative to exercise stress imaging for prognostication after acute myocardial infarction. In the prethrombolytic era, Leppo et al[37] were the first to show that dipyridamole ^{201}Tl scintigraphy could be performed safely 1 to 2 weeks after admission in patients who had had uncomplicated infarction. In that study, 11 of 12 patients who died or sustained a recurrent nonfatal myocardial infarction during follow-up demonstrated dipyridamole-induced reversible defects on predischarge testing. Among all clinical and perfusion variables evaluated, the presence of ^{201}Tl redistribution was the only significant predictor of subsequent cardiac events and was more sensitive than exercise ST-segment depression in predicting outcome. Brown et al[11] showed that dipyridamole ^{201}Tl scintigraphy was safe even when performed very soon after admission for acute infarction. These investigators performed dipyridamole scintigraphy an average of 62 ± 21 hours after hospitalization. By stepwise multivariate logistic regression analysis, the best and only statistically significant predictor of in-hospital ischemic cardiac events was the presence of dipyridamole-induced ^{201}Tl redistribution within the infarct zone. Bosch et al[9] performed dipyridamole ^{201}Tl scintigraphy on the morning of the third day after myocardial infarction in 114 consecutive patients. Logistic regression analysis showed that of all clinical, scintigraphic, and angiographic variables, the presence of ^{201}Tl redistribution on the dipyridamole perfusion scan was the only independent predictor of cardiac events, showing a six fold increase in risk.

Pirelli et al[50] also performed early dipyridamole ^{201}Tl imaging in 35 patients with uncomplicated myocardial infarction. Seven of 11 patients who had redistribution defects developed angina, and 5 required bypass surgery for severe angina that was refractory to medical therapy. Six of the 7 patients who developed angina had multivessel coronary artery disease. A more recent report by this group extends these earlier observations on the prognostic value of dipyridamole ^{201}Tl very early after infarction.[51] In this later study, dipyridamole imaging was performed 4 days after admission in patients who were initially treated with thrombolytic therapy and followed for an average of 14 months after discharge. As observed with previous studies, no major complications occurred when using vasodilator stress testing this early after infarction. The authors found that an ischemic response in these early images was predictive of both in-hospital and late postdischarge cardiac events.

Adenosine stress myocardial perfusion imaging

Adenosine can be substituted for dipyridamole as a vasodilator for stress perfusion imaging and has a comparable safety profile.[40,41] Mahmarian et al[40] determined the prognostic value of adenosine SPECT perfusion imaging for identifying high-risk postinfarction patients soon after hospitalization. Adenosine perfusion defects were significantly larger in patients who had in-hospital cardiac events (45% ± 18%) compared with those who had no events (22% ± 15%). The overall sensitivity for detecting individual coronary stenoses with adenosine SPECT imaging was 87%. Sixty-three percent of patients with double-vessel disease and 91% of patients with triple-vessel disease had a multivessel disease scan pattern. In a subsequent long-term follow-up study from the same group of investigators,[41] univariate predictors of cardiac events over 15.7 months of follow-up included quantified perfusion defect size, absolute extent of left ventricular ischemia, and ejection fraction. Of interest, adenosine ^{201}Tl imaging variables were equally predictive of events in patients who underwent early reperfusion therapy and in those who did not (Fig. 26-12).

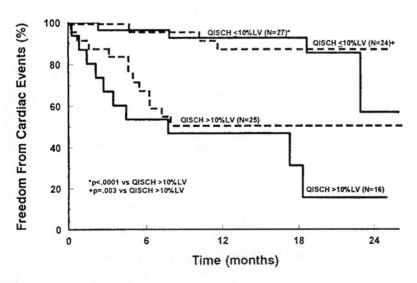

Fig. 26-12. Quantified extent of ischemia *(QISCH)* and freedom from cardiac events in patients who received early reperfusion therapy *(solid lines)* or no reperfusion therapy *(dashed lines)* during acute myocardial infarction. Extent of ischemia was quantitated by adenosine thallium-201 SPECT imaging. LV = left ventricle. (From Mahmarian JJ, Mahmarian AC, Marks JF, et al: Role of adenosine thallium-201 tomography for defining long-term risk in patients after acute myocardial infarction, *J Am Coll Cardiol* 25:1333-1340, 1995.)

Adenosine ^{99m}Tc sestamibi SPECT imaging has also proven clinically useful for the early assessment of jeopardized myocardium after acute myocardial infarction.[15] In 53 consecutive patients with acute myocardial infarction, of whom 42 received thrombolytic therapy, adenosine ^{99m}Tc SPECT had positive predictive value of 88% for identifying jeopardized myocardium, defined as a residual viable myocardium supplied by a vessel with a significant stenosis. The technique also had negative predictive value of 88% for identifying the absence of residual viable myo-cardium.

In summary, stress perfusion imaging with dipyridamole or adenosine is an adequate alternative to exercise stress imaging for separating high-risk and low-risk subsets of patients after uncomplicated infarction. Patients with residual jeopardized myocardium can be detected by demonstration of reversible defects within or remote from the infarct zone. It seems that vasodilator stress imaging is useful for assessing prognosis in patients who undergo reperfusion therapy at the time of admission. Few data are available on the use of dobutamine stress imaging for predischarge risk assessment in patients with uncomplicated myocardial infarction. Nevertheless, for patients who are not eligible for vasodilator stress imaging (such as those receiving theophylline), dobutamine stress can be used with careful patient monitoring.

EXERCISE RADIONUCLIDE ANGIOGRAPHY FOR RISK STRATIFICATION AFTER ACUTE MYOCARDIAL INFARCTION

Determination of the peak ejection fraction during exercise as well as the change in ejection fraction from rest to exercise can be used for risk stratification in patients after uncomplicated myocardial infarction.* Morris et al[44] found that left ventricular ejection fraction was inversely correlated with subsequent mortality in 106 consecutive survivors of acute myocardial infarction evaluated in the prethrombolytic era. Using the Cox regression model, they showed that as the ejection fraction fell below 45%, mortality increased substantially. Corbett et al[16] observed that the change in ejection fraction from rest to

*References 1, 8, 16, 19, 32, 42, 44, 69, 70.

exercise in postinfarction patients was the most important prognostic variable in predicting the combined events of death, recurrent infarction, refractory angina, and heart failure. Abraham et al[1] reported that when the exercise ejection fraction was less than 50%, the 2-year survival rate free of medical complications was 42% compared with 83% for patients whose exercise in whom the ejection fraction exceeded 50%.

Exercise radionuclide angiography for prognostication has been undertaken in postinfarction patients initially treated with thrombolytic agents. In the TIMI-II trial, patients randomly assigned to the invasive strategy group more frequently had normal exercise ejection fraction responses (29.7%) than did patients randomized to the conservative strategy (25.8%; $P = 0.01$).[72] Peak exercise ejection fraction and peak infarct zone regional ejection fraction were also greater in patients who received the invasive strategy. Nevertheless, at 6 weeks of follow-up, the differences between the conservative and invasive strategy groups were no longer evident. In a subsequent report from the TIMI investigators,[73] exercise radionuclide angiography was not found to be as predictive for identifying high-risk patients among those receiving thrombolytic therapy. In this report by Zaret et al,[73] peak exercise ejection fraction did not provide appreciable prognostic information beyond that obtained with measurement of the resting ejection fraction alone. It should be pointed out, however, that among the 2143 patients for whom both rest and exercise data were available, the 1-year mortality rate was only 1.7%. Thus, the cohort seemed to be a low-risk group. The mortality rate was substantially higher (5.8%) in the 1045 patients in whom no exercise study was performed within 14 days (Fig. 26-13). It is possible that if these patients deemed not eligible for exercise stress had undergone vasodilator stress myocardial perfusion imaging, high-risk and low-risk subsets would have been well separated on the basis of such variables as defect size and extent of defect reversibility. Patients who are judged unable to exercise early after myocardial infarction should be considered for pharmacologic stress perfusion imaging for risk stratification.

Postinfarction transient left ventricular dysfunction can be detected by using a radionuclide left ventricular function monitor, which permits continuous measurement of left ventricular

Fig. 26-13. Mortality rate versus peak exercise left ventricular ejection fraction as determined by radionuclide angiography in postinfarction patients who received thrombolytic therapy. The highest mortality rate (5.8%) was seen among patients who did not undergo an exercise radionuclide angiographic study within 14 days. (From Zaret BL, Wackers FJ, Terrin ML, et al: Value of radionuclide rest and exercise left ventricular ejection fraction in assessing survival of patients after thrombolytic therapy for acute myocardial infarction: results of Thrombolysis in Myocardial Infarction (TIMI) phase II study. TIMI Study Group, *J Am Coll Cardiol* 26:73-79, 1995. Reprinted with permission from the American College of Cardiology.)

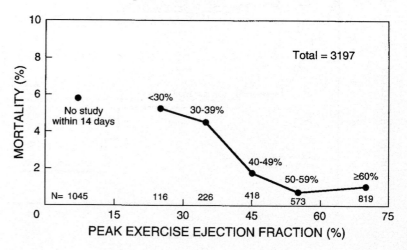

ejection fraction during normal activity. Kayden et al[34] prospectively investigated the occurrence and significance of transient left ventricular dysfunction in 33 ambulatory patients who underwent thrombolytic therapy after myocardial infarction. At an average of 19 months of follow-up, cardiac events had occurred in 8 of 12 patients with transient left ventricular dysfunction but in only 3 of 21 patients without this condition ($P < 0.01$). During submaximal supine bicycle exercise, only 2 patients showed a decrease in ejection fraction of more than 5% at peak exercise, and neither patient had a subsequent cardiac event. These authors concluded that silent myocardial ischemia is common in patients treated with thrombolysis after myocardial infarction and is associated with poor outcome. Furthermore, they concluded that continuous left ventricular function monitoring during normal activity may provide prognostic data not available from submaximal exercise radionuclide angiography.

ROUTINE CORONARY ANGIOGRAPHY FOR RISK STRATIFICATION AFTER UNCOMPLICATED MYOCARDIAL INFARCTION

The principal objective of predischarge risk stratification in patients who have survived an uncomplicated myocardial infarction is to identify high-risk patients who will derive survival benefit from coronary revascularization and to identify patients at low risk who can be treated medically, regardless of the status of the infarct-related vessel or the extent of coronary anatomic disease. Controversy exists about the most cost-effective approach to risk stratification in the thrombolytic era. Many patients who undergo reperfusion early and who have uncomplicated courses are candidates for early hospital discharge. Some observers have asserted that early routine coronary angiography is the most cost effective approach to risk stratification because it permits identification of lack of patency of the infarct-related artery and detection of multivessel disease.

Results of randomized trials have indicated that immediate or delayed elective angioplasty of the infarct-related vessel after thrombolytic therapy in asymptomatic postinfarction patients who have no spontaneous or inducible ischemia did not improve outcome or enhance left ventricular function.* Immediate PTCA after thrombolysis did not improve the extent of left ventricular global or segmental functional recovery. Immediate balloon dilatation of residual infarct-related stenoses was associated with an increased risk for procedural complications without a reduction in subsequent reocclusion or reinfarction. In fact, a trend was seen toward an increase in hospital mortality.[65]

Deferred angioplasty after thrombolytic therapy has not been shown to be superior to a "watchful waiting" noninvasive strategy, as was indicated in several other clinical trials. In the TIMI-IIB study,[63] the cumulative 6-week mortality rate was 5.2% in the group that received invasive therapy compared with 4.7% in the group randomly assigned to receive conservative treatment. At discharge, reinfarction was observed in

*References 20, 58, 60, 62, 63, 65.

5.9% of the invasive therapy group and 5.4% of patients in the conservatively treated group. When follow-up was extended to 3 years after discharge, the mortality and reinfarction rates were similar in the invasive therapy and the conservative treatment groups. Similar findings were observed in the SWIFT study.[60] In this trial, the cumulative 1-year mortality rate was 5.8% in the intervention group compared with 5.0% in the conservative therapy group, with reinfarction rates of 5.1% and 12.9%, respectively. Finally, the Treatment of Post-Thrombolytic Stenoses trial showed no functional or clinical benefit of routine late PTCA after myocardial infarction treated with thrombolytic agents in patients with a negative result on a functional stress test before randomization.[20] The actuarial 12-month infarction-free survival rate was 97.8% in the no-PTCA group and 90.5% in the PTCA group. Similarly, in the TIMI-IIIB study,[64] patients with non–Q-wave infarction or unstable angina who were randomly assigned to receive an invasive strategy showed no enhanced survival or lower reinfarction rate compared with patients who underwent a noninvasive strategy. Recent data from the VANQWISH trial, in which 920 patients with non–Q-wave infarction were randomly assigned to receive an initial invasive strategy or an initial conservative strategy (in which angiography was only performed for spontaneous ischemia or ischemia on stress ^{201}Tl imaging), showed that at 1 year after discharge, the two groups did not differ for cardiac death or recurrent infarction.[16]

Outcome studies reported in the literature have shown no relation between use of invasive cardiac procedures and the subsequent mortality rate in patients with uncomplicated acute myocardial infarction. Rouleau et al[54] reported that although coronary angiography was more commonly performed in the United States than in Canada (68% and 35%), as were revascularization procedures after infarction (31% and 12%), no difference in mortality (22% in Canada and 23% in the United States) or rate of reinfarction (14% in Canada and 13% in the United States) was observed during a mean follow-up of 42 months. However, angina was more prevalent in Canada than in the United States (33% and 27%). Guadagnoli et al[27] found significant regional variation in the use of cardiac procedures after acute myocardial infarction without a difference in measures of outcome. Coronary angiography was performed after acute myocardial infarction more often in Texas than in New York (45% and 30%), but the adjusted likelihood of death was lower in New York than in Texas. These authors concluded that on average, performing the procedures at the higher rate used in Texas had no advantage with respect to mortality and health-related quality of life.

New data from the OASIS registry showed no difference in outcome for postinfarction patients admitted to hospitals with on-site cardiac catheterization facilities (rate of catheterization, 66%) compared with those admitted to hospitals with no on-site catheterization facilities (rate of catheterization, 34%).[71]

Kuntz et al[36] evaluated the cost-effectiveness of routine coronary angiography after acute myocardial infarction by using a decision-analytic model for acute myocardial infarction in

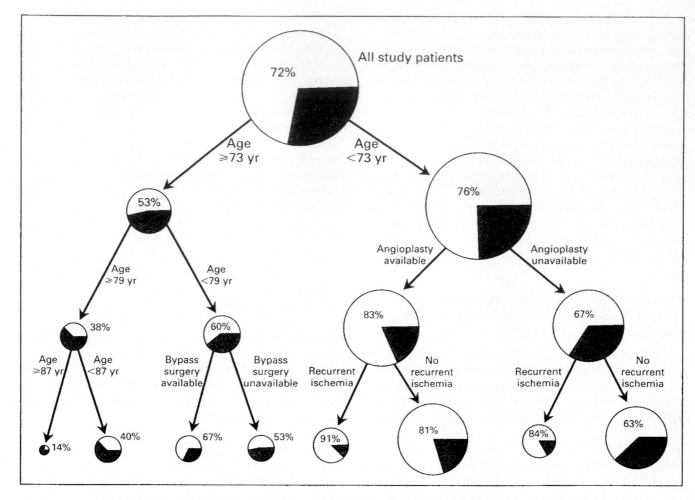

Fig. 26-14. Classification and regression tree *(CART)* model showing the variables used to discriminate between subgroups of postinfarction patients in the Global Utilization of Streptokinase and Tissue Plasminogen Activator for Occluded Arteries (GUSTO) trial according to the likelihood that the patient would undergo coronary angiography after thrombolysis. The white area of each pie chart represents the percentage of patients in that subgroup in whom angiography was performed, and the overall area of the pie chart indicates the size of the subgroup relative to the total population. Among the 21,772 U.S. patients in the trial, 71% underwent coronary angiography before discharge. Age was the variable most predictive of angiography. In hospitals in which angioplasty was available, 81% of the patients with no recurrent ischemia still underwent coronary angiography. (Reprinted by permission of *The New England Journal of Medicine.* Pilote L, Miller DP, Califf RM, et al: Determinants of the use of coronary angiography and revascularization after thrombolysis for acute myocardial infarction, *N Engl J Med* 335:1198-1205, 1996. Copyright 1996 by the Massachusetts Medical Society.)

representative patient subgroups. They identified two clinical factors that were particularly influential in determining favorable cost-effectiveness ratios for coronary angiography in patients of all ages after acute myocardial infarction: acute inducible myocardial ischemia (defined as severe postinfarction angina or a strongly positive exercise treadmill test) and history of infarction before the current infarction. In general, the incremental cost-effectiveness ratio for coronary angiography and treatment guided by its results compared with no angiography for patients in whom both of these factors were present was $17,000 to $44,000 per quality-adjusted year of life gained. In contrast, for most patient subgroups with a negative exercise

test, the incremental cost-effectiveness ratios for coronary angiography were more than $50,000 per quality-adjusted year of life gained.

Although clinical trials and epidemiologic studies indicate that routine angiography offers no clinical benefit over selective angiography on the basis of high-risk clinical variables or evidence of residual postinfarction ischemia, a large number of patients still undergo angiography after uncomplicated myocardial infarction in the United States. Among the 21,772 U.S. patients in the GUSTO trial, 71% underwent coronary angiography before hospital discharge.[49] Of these patients, 58% underwent revascularization, of whom three quarters received angioplasty. All of these patients had received thrombolytic therapy. Younger age and the availability of procedures seemed to be the major determinants of angiography use (Fig. 26-14), whereas coronary anatomy largely determined the use and type of revascularization. The authors concluded that the use of invasive cardiac procedures after thrombolysis for acute myocardial infarction in the GUSTO trial was more prevalent than would be expected from current guidelines. Instead of the presence of high-risk clinical variables or recurrent myocardial ischemia, which have been associated with greater benefit from revascularization, younger age seemed to be the primary predictor of the use of coronary angiography, which was performed in many low-risk patients. Aside from age as the major determinant, the mere availability of facilities for invasive procedures predominantly determined the use of angiography.

COST-EFFECTIVE DECISION-MAKING ALGORITHM

On the basis of the data reviewed in this chapter and from other reports in the literature, a decision-making algorithm, such as that described below, may be useful for prognostic evaluation of postinfarction patients. Patients who are clinically at high risk with cardiogenic shock, congestive heart failure, postinfarction angina, or previous myocardial infarction would be candidates for direct referral for coronary angiography. A substantial number of patients without congestive heart failure but with left ventricular ejection fraction less than 40% after infarction could benefit from myocardial perfusion imaging for the determination of both viability and inducible ischemia. For example, rest ^{201}Tl imaging could identify asynergic segments that have a high probability of showing improved function after revascularization. Zones of asynergy that showed markedly reduced tracer activity would be unlikely to show improved systolic function after angioplasty or bypass surgery.

Patients at intermediate risk by clinical criteria would be candidates for noninvasive risk assessment strategy, regardless of whether they had undergone thrombolytic therapy. These patients would benefit from submaximal exercise stress perfusion imaging performed 4 to 5 days after onset of symptoms or from vasodilator perfusion imaging as early as 3 days after admission. High-risk patients with residual ischemia in the infarct zone or a multivessel disease scan pattern would be eligible for referral for invasive strategies, whereas patients with low-risk noninvasive findings (lack of inducible ischemia at completion of a submaximal exercise test or lack of reversible defects with vasodilator stress) would be candidates for medical therapy. In such patients, symptom-limited exercise electrocardiographic stress testing at 6 weeks after infarction might provide more information on additional myocardium at jeopardy.

Patients who are classified as low risk by clinical criteria might be best assessed by submaximal exercise electrocardiographic stress testing alone as the first step. These patients most often undergo reperfusion therapy within several hours after onset of symptoms and have preserved left ventricular function, no spontaneous angina, and no postinfarction heart failure. Pa-

tients with previous myocardial infarction and those older than 70 years of age who are deemed unable to adequately exercise would be excluded from this low-risk group. If patients judged to be at low risk by clinical criteria who underwent exercise electrocardiographic stress testing alone achieved more than 4 METs with no inducible chest pain or ST-segment depression, no further testing would be required, and they could be followed medically with, perhaps, repeated maximal testing at 6 weeks. The mortality rate among these clinically low-risk patients is 2% mortality rate during follow-up.

In the United States, only 30% to 40% of patients with acute myocardial infarction undergo reperfusion therapy. Many patients are not eligible to receive thrombolytic agents and do not undergo early catheterization with direct angioplasty. These patients have been successfully risk stratified in the thrombolytic era by using noninvasive strategies. Many of these patients have underlying multivessel disease. This proposed algorithm is consistent with the most recent American College of Cardiology/American Heart Association Guidelines for Management of Patients with Acute Myocardial Infarction.[56]

ACKNOWLEDGMENT

I am very grateful to Mr. Jerry Curtis for his editorial assistance in writing this chapter.

REFERENCES

1. Abraham RD, Harris PJ, Roubin GS, et al: Usefulness of ejection fraction response to exercise one month after acute myocardial infarction in predicting coronary anatomy and prognosis, *Am J Cardiol* 60:225–230, 1987.
2. Baim DS, Diver DJ, Feit F, et al: Coronary angioplasty performed within the Thrombolysis in Myocardial Infarction II study, *Circulation* 85:93–105, 1992.
3. Beller GA: Noninvasive assessment of prognosis after acute myocardial infarction in the thrombolytic era and age of interventional cardiology, *J Nucl Cardiol* 2:159–162, 1995 (editorial).
4. Beller GA: *Radionuclide imaging in acute myocardial infarction.* In Beller GA: *Clinical nuclear cardiology,* Philadelphia, 1995, W.B. Saunders.
5. Beller GA: *Radionuclide imaging in acute myocardial infarction.* In Gersh BJ, Rahimtoola SH, eds: *Acute myocardial infarction,* ed 2. New York, (in press), Chapman & Hall.
6. Boden WE, O'Rourke RA, Dai H, et al: Improved clinical outcomes in non-Q-wave infarction patients randomized to a conservative "ischemia-guided" strategy compared to an invasive/interventional strategy: results of the multicenter VA Non-Q-wave Infarction Strategies In-Hospital (VANQWISH) trial, *Circulation* 96 (Suppl I):I207, 1997 (abstract).
7. Bonow RO: Prognostic assessment in coronary artery disease: role of radionuclide angiography, *J Nucl Cardiol* 1:280–291, 1994.
8. Borer JS, Miller D, Schreiber T, et al: Radionuclide cineangiography in acute myocardial infarction: role in prognostication, *Semin Nucl Med* 17:89–94, 1987.
9. Bosch X, Magrina J, March R, et al: Prediction of in-hospital cardiac events using dipyridamole-thallium scintigraphy performed very early after acute myocardial infarction, *Clin Cardiol* 19:189–196, 1996.
10. Brown KA, Weiss RM, Clements JP, et al: Usefulness of residual ischemic myocardium within prior infarct zone for identifying patients at high risk late after acute myocardial infarction, *Am J Cardiol* 60:15–19, 1987.

11. Brown KA, O'Meara J, Chambers CE, et al: Ability of dipyridamole-thallium-201 imaging one to four days after acute myocardial infarction to predict in-hospital and late recurrent myocardial ischemic events. Am J Cardiol 65:160–167, 1990.

12. Candell-Riera J, Permanyer-Miralda G, Castele J, et al: Uncomplicated first myocardial infarction: strategy for comprehensive prognostic studies, J Am Coll Cardiol 18:1207–1219, 1991.

13. Cerqueira MD, Maynard C, Ritchie JL, et al: Long-term survival in 618 patients from the Western Washington Streptokinase in Myocardial Infarction trials, J Am Coll Cardiol 20:1452–1459, 1992.

14. Chaitman BR, McMahon RP, Terrin M, et al: Impact of treatment strategy on predischarge exercise test in the Thrombolysis in Myocardial Infarction (TIMI) II trial, Am J Cardiol 71:131–138, 1993.

15. Claeys MJ, Vrints CJ, Khy B, et al: Adenosine technetium-99m sestamibi (SPECT) for the early assessment of jeopardized myocardium after acute myocardial infarction, Eur Heart J 16:1186–1194, 1995.

16. Corbett JR, Dehmer GJ, Lewis SE, et al: The prognostic value of submaximal exercise testing with radionuclide ventriculography before hospital discharge in patients with recent myocardial infarction, Circulation 64:535–544, 1981.

17. Dakik HA, Mahmarian JJ, Kimball KT, et al: Prognostic value of exercise ^{201}Tl tomography in patients treated with thrombolytic therapy during acute myocardial infarction, Circulation 94:2735–2742, 1996.

18. De Feyter PJ, van Eenige MJ, Dighton DH, et al: Prognostic value of exercise testing, coronary angiography and left ventriculography 6–8 weeks after myocardial infarction, Circulation 66:527–536, 1982.

19. Dewhurst NG, Muir AL: Comparative prognostic value of radionuclide ventriculography at rest and during exercise in 100 patients after first myocardial infarction, Br Heart J 49:111–121, 1983.

20. Ellis SG, Mooney MR, George BS, et al: Randomized trial of late elective angioplasty versus conservative management for patients with residual stenoses after thrombolytic treatment of myocardial infarction. Treatment of Post-Thrombolytic Stenoses (TOPS) Study Group, Circulation 86:1400–1406, 1992.

21. Froelicher VF, Perdue ST, Atwood JE, et al: Exercise testing of patients recovering from myocardial infarction, Curr Probl Cardiol 11:369–444, 1986.

22. Froelicher VF, Perdue S, Perven W, et al: Application of meta-analysis using an electronic spread sheet to exercise testing in patients after myocardial infarction, Am J Med 83:1045–1054, 1987.

23. Gibson RS, Beller GA: Value of predischarge myocardial perfusion scintigraphy. In Fuster V, Ross R, Topol EJ, eds: Atherosclerosis and coronary artery disease, vol 2, Philadelphia, 1996, Lippincott–Raven.

24. Gibson RS, Watson DD, Craddode GB, et al: Prediction of cardiac events after uncomplicated myocardial infarction: a prospective study comparing predischarge exercise thallium-201 scintigraphy and coronary angiography, Circulation 68:321–336, 1983.

25. Gibson RS, Beller GA, Gheoghiade M, et al: The prevalence and clinical significance of residual myocardial ischemia 2 weeks after uncomplicated non-Q wave infarction: a prospective natural history study, Circulation 73:1186–1198, 1986.

26. Gimple LW, Beller GA: Assessing prognosis after acute myocardial infarction in the thrombolytic era. J Nucl Cardiol (2 Pt 1):198–209, 1994.

27. Guadagnoli E, Hauptman PJ, Ayanian JZ, et al: Variation in the use of cardiac procedures after acute myocardial infarction, N Engl J Med 333:573–578, 1995.

28. The effects of tissue plasminogen activator, streptokinase, or both on coronary-artery patency, ventricular function, and survival after acute myocardial infarction. The GUSTO Angiographic Investigators, N Engl J Med 329:1615–1622, 1993.

29. Haber HL, Beller GA, Watson DD, et al: Exercise thallium-201 scintigraphy after thrombolytic therapy with or without angioplasty for acute myocardial infarction. Am J Cardiol 71:1257–1261, 1993.

30. Harrison JK, Califf RM, Woodlief LH, et al: Systolic left ventricular function after reperfusion therapy for acute myocardial infarction.

Analysis of determinants of improvement. The TAMI Study Group, Circulation 87:1531–1541, 1993.

31. Holmes DR Jr, Califf RM, Topol EJ: Lessons we have learned from the GUSTO trial. Global Utilization of Streptokinase and Tissue Plasminogen Activator for Occluded Arteries, J Am Coll Cardiol 25(Suppl):10S–17S, 1995.

32. Hung J, Goris ML, Nash E, et al: Comparative value of maximal treadmill testing, exercise thallium myocardial perfusion scintigraphy and exercise radionuclide ventriculography for distinguishing high- and low-risk patients soon after acute myocardial infarction, Am J Cardiol 53:1221–1227, 1984.

33. Juneau M, Colles P, Theroux P, et al: Symptom-limited versus low level exercise testing before hospital discharge after myocardial infarction, J Am Coll Cardiol 20:927–933, 1992.

34. Kayden DS, Wackers FJTh, Zaret BL: Silent left ventricular dysfunction during routine activity after thrombolytic therapy for acute myocardial infarction, J Am Coll Cardiol 15:1500–1507, 1990.

35. Krone RJ, Gregory JJ, Freedland KE, et al: Limited usefulness of exercise testing and thallium scintigraphy in evaluation of ambulatory patients several months after recovery from an acute coronary event: implications for management of stable coronary heart disease. Multicenter Myocardial Ischemia Research Group, J Am Coll Cardiol 24:1274–1281, 1994.

36. Kuntz KM, Tsevat J, Goldman L, et al: Cost-effectiveness of routine coronary angiography after acute myocardial infarction. Circulation 94:957–965, 1996.

37. Leppo JA, O'Brien J, Rothendler JA, et al: Dipyridamole-thallium-201 scintigraphy in the prediction of future cardiac events after acute myocardial infarction. N Engl J Med 310:1014–1018, 1984.

38. Lomboy CT, Schulman DS, Grill HP, et al: Rest-redistribution thallium-201 scintigraphy to determine myocardial viability early after myocardial infarction, J Am Coll Cardiol 25:210–217, 1995.

39. Lystash JC, Gibson RS, Watson DD, et al: Early versus late congestive heart failure after initially uncomplicated anterior wall acute myocardial infarction, Am J Cardiol 75:653–658, 1995.

40. Mahmarian JJ, Pratt CM, Nishimura S, et al: Quantitative adenosine ^{201}Tl single-photon emission computed tomography for the early assessment of patients surviving acute myocardial infarction, Circulation 87:1197–1210, 1993.

41. Mahmarian JJ, Mahmarian AC, Marks JF, et al: Role of adenosine thallium-201 tomography for defining long-term risk in patients after acute myocardial infarction, J Am Coll Cardiol 25:1333–1340, 1995.

42. Mazzotta G, Camerini A, Scopinaro G, et al: Predicting severe ischemic events after uncomplicated myocardial infarction by exercise testing and rest and exercise radionuclide ventriculography, J Nucl Cardiol 1:246–253, 1994.

43. Miller TD, Gersh BJ, Christian TF, et al: Limited prognostic value of thallium-201 exercise treadmill testing early after myocardial infarction in patients treated with thrombolysis, Am Heart J 130:259–266, 1995.

44. Morris KG, Palmeri ST, Califf RM, et al: Value of radionuclide angiography for predicting specific cardiac events after acute myocardial infarction, Am J Cardiol 55:318–324, 1985.

45. Moss AJ, Goldstein RE, Hall WJ, et al: Detection and significance of myocardial ischemia in stable patients after recovery from an acute coronary event. Multicenter Myocardial Ischemia Research Group, JAMA 269:2379–2385, 1993.

46. Muller DW, Topol EJ, Ellis SG, et al: Multivessel coronary artery disease: a key predictor of short-term prognosis after reperfusion therapy for acute myocardial infarction. Thrombolysis and Angioplasty in Myocardial Infarction (TAMI) Study Group, Am Heart J 121(4 pt 1):1042–1049, 1991.

47. Risk stratification and survival after myocardial infarction. N Engl J Med 309:331–336, 1983.

48. Olona M, Candell-Riera J, Permanger-Miralda G, et al: Strategies for

prognostic assessment of uncomplicated first myocardial infarction: 5-year follow-up study, *J Am Coll Cardiol* 25:815–822, 1995.

49. Pilote L, Miller DP, Califf RM, et al: Determinants of the use of coronary angiography and revascularization after thrombolysis for acute myocardial infarction, *N Engl J Med* 335:1198–1205, 1996.

50. Pirelli S, Zuglese E, Suppa M, et al: Dipyridamole-thallium 201 scintigraphy in the early post-infarction period. (Safety and accuracy in predicting the extent of coronary disease and future recurrence of angina in patients suffering from their first myocardial infarction), *Eur Heart J* 9:1324–1331, 1988.

51. Pirelli S, Mores A, Piccolo G, et al: Dipyridamole thallium-201 imaging very early after uncomplicated acute myocardial infarction in patients treated with thrombolytic therapy, *Eur Heart J* 18:927–930, 1997.

52. Rogers WJ, Bourge RC, Pappapietro SE, et al: Variables predictive of good functional outcome following thrombolytic therapy in the Thrombolysis in Myocardial Infarction phase II (TIMI II) pilot study, *Am J Cardiol* 63:503–512, 1989.

53. Rogers WJ, Babb JD, Baim DS, et al: Selective versus routine predischarge coronary arteriography after therapy with recombinant tissue-type plasminogen activator, heparin and aspirin for acute myocardial infarction. TIMI II Investigators, *J Am Coll Cardiol* 17:1007–1016, 1991.

54. Rouleau JL, Moye LA, Pfeffer MA, et al: A comparison of management patterns after acute myocardial infarction in Canada and the United States. The SAVE Investigators, *N Engl J Med* 328:779–784, 1993.

55. Rouleau JL, Talajik M, Sussex B, et al: Myocardial infarction patients in the 1990s—their risk factors, stratification and survival in Canada: The Canadian Assessment of Myocardial Infarction (CAMI) Study, *J Am Coll Cardiol* 27:1119–1127, 1996.

56. Ryan TJ, Anderson JL, Antman EM, et al: ACC/AHA guidelines for the management of patients with acute myocardial infarction: executive summary. A report of the American College of Cardiology/American Heart Association Task Force on Practice Guidelines (Committee on Management of Acute Myocardial Infarction), *Circulation* 94:2341–2350, 1996.

57. Schulman SP, Achuff JC, Griffith LS, et al: Prognostic cardiac catheterization variables in survivors of acute myocardial infarction: a five year prospective study, *J Am Coll Cardiol* 11:1164–1172, 1988.

58. Simoons ML, Arnold AE, Betrin A, et al: Thrombolysis with tissue plasminogen activator in acute myocardial infarction: no additional benefit from immediate percutaneous coronary angioplasty, *Lancet* 1:197–203, 1988.

59. Simoons ML, Vos J, Tijssen JG, et al: Long-term benefit of early thrombolytic therapy in patients with acute myocardial infarction: 5 year follow-up of a trial conducted by the Interuniversity Cardiology Institute of the Netherlands, *J Am Coll Cardiol* 14:1609–1615, 1989.

60. SWIFT trial of delayed elective intervention vs conservative treatment after thrombolysis with anistreplase in acute myocardial infarction. SWIFT (Should We Intervene Following Thrombolysis?) Trial Study Group, *BMJ* 302:555–560, 1991.

61. Tilkemeier PL, Gutney TE, LaRaia PJ, et al: Prognostic value of predischarge low-level exercise thallium testing after thrombolytic treatment of acute myocardial infarction, *Am J Cardiol* 66:1203–1207, 1990.

62. Immediate vs delayed catheterization and angioplasty following thrombolytic therapy for acute myocardial infarction. TIMI II A results. The TIMI Research Group, *JAMA* 260:2849–2858, 1988.

63. Comparison of invasive and conservative strategies after treatment with intravenous tissue plasminogen activator in acute myocardial infarction. Results of the Thrombolysis in Myocardial Infarction (TIMI) phase II trial. The TIMI Study Group, *N Engl J Med* 320:618–627, 1989.

64. Effects of tissue plasminogen activator and a comparison of early invasive and conservative strategies in unstable angina and non-Q-wave myocardial infarction. Results of the TIMI IIIB trial. Thrombolysis in Myocardial Ischemia, *Circulation* 89:1545–1556, 1994.

65. Topol EJ, Califf RM, George BS, et al: A randomized trial of immediate versus delayed elective angioplasty after intravenous tissue plasminogen activator in acute myocardial infarction, *N Engl J Med* 317:581–588, 1987.

66. Topol EJ, Holmes DR, Rogers WJ: Coronary angiography after thrombolytic therapy for acute myocardial infarction, *Ann Intern Med* 114:877–885, 1991.

67. Travin MI, Dessouki A, Cameron T, et al: Use of exercise technetium-99m sestamibi SPECT imaging to detect residual ischemia and for risk stratification after acute myocardial infarction, *Am J Cardiol* 75:665–669, 1995.

68. Volpi A, De Vita C, Franzosi MG, et al: Determinants of 6-month mortality in survivors of myocardial infarction after thrombolysis. Results of the GISSI-2 data base. The Ad Hoc Working Group of the Gruppo Italiano per lo Studio della Sopravvivenza nell'Infarto Miocardico (GISSI)-2 Data Base, *Circulation* 88:416–429, 1993.

69. Wallis JB, Holmes JR, Borer JS: Prognosis in patients with coronary artery disease and low ejection fraction at rest: impact of the exercise ejection fraction, *Am J Card Imaging* 4:1, 1990.

70. Wasserman AG, Katz RJ, Cleary P, et al: Noninvasive detection of multivessel disease after myocardial infarction by exercise radionuclide ventriculography, *Am J Cardiol* 50:1242–1247, 1982.

71. Yusuf S, Flather MD, Pogue JM, et al: Factors affecting the use of invasive facilities in patients with unstable angina or suspected non Q wave infarction, *Circulation* 96 (Suppl I):I535–I536, 1997 (abstract).

72. Zaret BL, Wackers FJ, Terrin ML, et al: Assessment of global and regional left ventricular performance at rest and during exercise after thrombolytic therapy for acute myocardial infarction: results of the Thrombolysis in Myocardial Infarction (TIMI) II Study, *Am J Cardiol* 69:1–9, 1992.

73. Zaret BL, Wackers FJ, Terrin ML, et al: Value of radionuclide rest and exercise left ventricular ejection fraction in assessing survival of patients after thrombolytic therapy for acute myocardial infarction: results of Thrombolysis in Myocardial Infarction (TIMI) phase II study. The TIMI Study Group, *J Am Coll Cardiol* 26:73–79, 1995.

Chapter 27

Emergency department triage and imaging of patients with acute chest pain

James L. Tatum and **Robert L. Jesse**

Difficulties with the evaluation of the acute chest pain patient have been evident for more than a decade. One result is an unacceptable number of patients who are discharged from emergency departments and are later found to have had myocardial infarction. The rate of myocardial infarction reported in the recent literature ranges from 2% to 10%, with 4% to 5% quoted most often.* The Acute Myocardial Infarction Study, published in 1996 by the Physician Insurers Association of America, noted that 2045 claims and suits involving myocardial infarction have been filed since 1985. Almost 38% of claims result in an indemnity payment to the claimant, and claims that have been closed since January 1994 have averaged $222,000. Frequently litigated errors include no treatment, delay in admission to the hospital, and failure to use or delay in administering thrombolytics.

*References 58, 71, 85, 86, 94, 110.

Concern over litigation is one factor promoting the practice of admitting large numbers of patients to expensive critical care units in order to rule out myocardial infarction. In a 1992 survey, the National Institute of Health estimated that 5.5 million patients were evaluated for chest pain in emergency departments that year, representing approximately 6% of all emergency department visits, but 10% of all hospital admissions through the emergency department. Most of these admissions do not lead to a diagnosis of myocardial infarction.[23] Instead, more than half of the patients admitted for suspected ischemic chest pain are discharged without a diagnosis of myocardial infarction or unstable angina.[57] A report published by the Agency for Health Care Policy and Research (AHCPR) estimated that the cost of U.S. hospital care for ischemic heart disease in 1987 was approximately $8.8 billion.[3] This figure includes the emergency department evaluation and subsequent admission of patients presenting with chest pain or other symptoms suggestive of ischemia but does not include the costs of myocardial infarction. When myocardial infarction was included, the total exceeded $13 billion.

These costs are expected to increase as the population ages and as public awareness of the need for rapid evaluation and treatment of chest pain grows. This will amplify the intensity of the current conflict in health care policy: that is, the requirement that high-risk patients be identified and treated earlier while fewer resources are used to screen the population at risk.

PATHOPHYSIOLOGY OF ACUTE CORONARY SYNDROMES

Acute coronary syndromes, which include unstable angina and non–Q-wave and Q-wave myocardial infarction, are precipitated by rupture of an atherosclerotic plaque and propagation of an associated thrombus, resulting in an abrupt reduction of blood flow. Plaque vulnerability may be related to intrinsic properties of the plaque constituents, such as the types of cells, lipid composition, extent of inflammation, and amount of connective tissue and fibrosis present. Small, soft plaques with a thin cap overlying a lipid pool seem to be more prone to rupture than larger, relatively more stable, fibrotic plaques.[54] Activated monocytes and macrophages within the plaque seem to secrete enzymes that can degrade the fibrous cap[131] and may also contribute to the activation of thrombosis through release of free radicals and lipid peroxides, as well as through elaboration of tissue factor–like compounds.[101] When the structural integrity of the cap, which seems to be especially vulnerable at the junction of the fibrous cap and normal arterial wall,[91] has been compromised, other elements such as increased sympathetic tone may then contribute to rupture. Acute coronary syndromes are associated with rapid progression of arteriographically mild coronary lesions.[2] In approximately two thirds of myocardial infarctions, the culprit lesion is a stenosis of less than 50% on angiography performed within the preceding 6 months.[61,62]

Plaque rupture may be much more common than was previously realized. It seems likely that many ruptured plaques reseal, incorporating the thrombus without generating overt clinical symptoms. The presence of layered thrombi overlying plaques in patients who had unstable angina followed by myocardial infarction or sudden death,[16] as well as the presence of fibrin and platelet-derived products within plaques, are both suggestive of recurrent rather than single thrombotic events. The process of rupture, thrombus formation, and healing is one possible mechanism of plaque growth.

This repetitive sequence also suggests that plaque rupture may often be silent. It is only when impaired blood flow causes symptomatic myocardial ischemia, even transiently, that the clinical syndrome is unstable angina. If the ischemic episode lasts long enough to compromise myocardial viability and cause necrosis, the syndrome progresses to myocardial infarction. The balance of the factors discussed above determines whether the event is silent or is manifested clinically as unstable angina, non–Q-wave myocardial infarction, or Q-wave myocardial infarction. From a clinical perspective, it is important to understand that the acute coronary syndrome, whether manifested as unstable angina or myocardial infarction, results from a single dynamic pathophysiologic process.

Clinical evidence of this process is provided by outcome data in patients with unstable angina. Karlson et al[48] reported that of 715 patients admitted with unstable angina, 27% (192) developed myocardial infarction during the first 3 days and 38% (255) experienced this event during the first year. Several studies of cardiac mortality have demonstrated that patients with unstable angina who present with suspected myocardial infarction or transient ST-segment changes are at a risk for cardiac death similar to patients who rule in for myocardial infarction.[36,56,64,100] Therefore, when designing strategies for triage, diagnosis, and treatment of the acute chest pain patient, the focus should be on the entirety of the acute coronary syndrome, with a diagnostic hierarchy that first rules in myocardial infarction, then rules in unstable angina. The strategy should identify not only patients with acute myocardial infarction but also patients with unstable angina who are at increased risk and, according to recent studies, may benefit from aggressive medical management.[112,117]

EVALUATION OF THE ACUTE CHEST PAIN SYNDROME

Differentiating between cardiac and noncardiac chest pain is often difficult. Only one third of misdiagnosed myocardial infarctions can be explained by misinterpretation of the electrocardiogram.[58,71,82,97] Misdiagnosis has also been associated with patients who are younger or have atypical presentations[58,82,97] and with physician inexperience.[97] Physicians with more experience generally have a lower threshold for admission, which increases the sensitivity for admitting patients with myocardial infarction but does not increase the specificity or diagnostic accuracy.[113] Physicians tend to overestimate the probability of infarction in high-risk patients and underestimate it in lower-risk patients, especially those thought to be at the lowest risk. In one study, the group of patients predicted to have an infarct rate of less than 5% had an actual rate of 11% to 12%.[27,28]

Patients often are asymptomatic or do not attribute their symptoms to cardiac causes. Various studies estimate that more than 30% of myocardial infarctions go unrecognized at the time they occur and are discovered incidentally later.[47,67,72] Only about half of these patients are retrospectively able to recall symptoms that were consistent with myocardial infarction.[47] In addition, most of these studies have relied on the development of new Q waves on yearly electrocardiography as the indicator of myocardial infarction, which probably underestimates the actual incidence of unrecognized infarction.[102,133]

Clinical presentation and early risk stratification

In 1994, the AHCPR published guidelines for the management of unstable angina, in which angina was categorized as high risk, intermediate risk, and low risk.[8] These guidelines discuss diagnostic and therapeutic strategies for the different risk levels, including the relative merits of invasive and conservative approaches. The AHCPR makes it clear that risk stratification and the ability to affect outcomes should be the focus of patient management. Rapid treatment of patients with acute myocardial infarction has been well documented to affect patient outcomes[26,32,128] and therefore drives the evaluation of all patients to identify those who are candidates for thrombolysis or primary angioplasty. Thus, the immediate goal for the evaluation of the patient presenting with acute chest pain is risk stratification, because clinical imperatives are dictated by risk and the ability to intervene effectively.

Presenting chest pain

Chest pain characteristics, such as location, quality, intensity, and presence of associated signs and symptoms, may be useful in some cases for identifying patients who have a higher probability of cardiac ischemia. Some characteristics are more frequently associated with noncardiac causes, including very short or very long duration of symptoms, localization of discomfort to a very small area, and onset of worsening of symptoms with respiration or other movement of the thorax. Ischemic pain is often described as viselike, heavy, tight, crushing, pressing, burning, or aching. Unfortunately, the quality of the pain is not sensitive enough to differentiate between ischemic and nonischemic causes. Hofgren et al[40] were unable to distinguish between patients with and without myocardial infarction among those who described their pain as pressing, aching, burning, or cramping. Associated symptoms that are more common in patients with myocardial infarction include nausea or vomiting[30,42,45]; diaphoresis[28,45,95,111]; and radiation of pain to the arm,[29,95] neck, or shoulder,[27,29] although radiation of pain is not uncommon in patients without myocardial infarction.[29,99] Although some investigators have demonstrated a correlation between the acute coronary syndrome and certain symptoms, including the character of chest pain,[57] a diagnostic challenge persists because the number of patients with noncardiac chest pain who have typical anginal symptoms is greater than the total number of patients with myocardial infarction or unstable angina.

Risk factors

The clinical variables associated with a higher risk for cardiovascular disease include increased age, male sex, hypercholesterolemia, diabetes mellitus, tobacco use, hypertension, and family history of premature coronary disease.[96] The value of these cardiovascular risk factors in the acute evaluation of chest pain is overestimated by most physicians; in fact, only age, sex, and documented presence of coronary artery disease are consistently found to be significant. Even when electrocardiographic findings are excluded from the predictive algorithm, risk factors do not have high predictive value. The multicenter ACI-TIPI (Acute Cardiac Ischemia Time Sensitive Predictive Instrument) study found that family history and diabetes were significant in men, but no risk factors were significant in women.[43] In a subgroup of patients from the multicenter Chest Pain database[95] who did not have diagnostic changes on electrocardiography, the univariate predictors of myocardial infarction included age older than 60 years, male sex, diaphoresis, previous myocardial infarction or angina, and pain described as pressure or radiating to the neck, arm, shoulder, or jaw. In these instances, the relative risks were low, with none greater than 2.0. Unfortunately, although cardiovascular risk factors can be used to predict the development of coronary disease in populations over time, they have limited ability to discriminate an ischemic event in an individual patient presenting to the emergency department with chest pain.

Presenting electrocardiography

Serial electrocardiography performed over 2 to 3 days is highly sensitive and specific for the detection of acute myocardial infarction. This is not true, however, for the single electrocardiogram at the initial presentation, because only 50% to 60% of patients with acute myocardial infarction have diagnostic changes on electrocardiography.[137] Young et al[134] found that 44% of patients with acute myocardial infarction had no change from a previous electrocardiogram, including patients with normal initial electrocardiograms. However, the initial electrocardiogram seems to have short-term prognostic value. Patients in whom myocardial infarction is subsequently diagnosed who have normal or nonspecific presenting electrocardiograms have a lower rate of serious in-hospital complications and in-hospital mortality than those with ischemia on electrocardiography; however, when these patients are inadvertently discharged from the emergency department, they have a mortality rate approximately twice that of admitted patients.[95]

The initial electrocardiogram also provides long-term prognostic information. Patients with myocardial infarction but without ST-segment elevation were found to have a 6-month event-free survival rate of 86% compared with 73% in those who had ST-segment elevation on admission.[55]

The presenting electrocardiogram may also offer risk stratification in patients at the other extreme of the acute coronary syndrome. Although 38% of patients with unstable angina have been shown to have normal or nondiagnostic ECGs,[57] Cohen et al[12] found that for patients with unstable angina or non–Q-wave myocardial infarction, the presence of ST-segment changes more than 1 mm/lead in two or more leads was a reliable predictor of major clinical events over the following 3 months. Other studies have also found that the initial electrocardiogram can define high-risk and low-risk patient populations.*

Myocardial markers

Symptoms, physical examination, and electrocardiographic changes are important in the initial evaluation of patients with chest pain, but they are not sufficient, either alone or in combination, to confirm the diagnosis. Biochemical assessment has therefore become the gold standard for the diagnosis of myocardial infarction. The first biochemical markers used for detecting myocardial necrosis were enzymes that appear in the serum after myocardial cell death. The diagnosis provided by these early tests was retrospective and led to the concept of ruling out myocardial infarction if the results of serial tests were negative. Because retrospective diagnoses are often no longer adequate, these confirmatory tests are being replaced with assays that provide real-time information that helps guide patient management. The diagnosis of acute myocardial infarction by biochemical markers is predicated on the assumptions that the appearance of these specific compounds in the circulation reflects cardiac myocyte death and that ischemia alone will not cause leakage of these compounds. New markers that are currently under investigation may be able to detect other components of the acute coronary syndrome that do not require myocardial necrosis for release, including intracoronary thrombus formation, plaque rupture, or activation of inflammatory processes within the plaque.†

---

*References 17, 74, 79, 103, 135, 136.
†References 5, 31, 46, 63, 77, 84, 87, 88, 90, 115.

The diagnostic accuracy of any marker depends on its kinetics and the time after onset of the infarct that the sample is drawn. Some of the timing issues can be circumvented by using combinations of markers, thereby capitalizing on the differences in kinetics. However, acute coronary occlusion is a dynamic process that easily lends itself to errors due to sampling mistakes. The negative predictive value of the initial sample for all currently available markers is not adequate to exclude acute myocardial infarction, much less rule out an unstable coronary syndrome. Bakker et al[6] reported that among 153 patients presenting within 10 hours of acute myocardial infarction, sensitivity was 60% for creatine kinase-MB by mass assay, 35% for creatine kinase-MB activity, 40% for myoglobin, and 64% for troponin T. To rule out myocardial infarction, serial sampling of markers is required. Traditional protocols do this over 18 to 24 hours, but rapid serial sampling is now being evaluated. Gibler et al[24] reported a sensitivity of 80% for serial studies obtained at admission and hourly for 3 hours among patients with nondiagnostic electrocardiograms. In a similar study of 313 patients who sustained 71 acute myocardial infarctions, the baseline sample had a sensitivity of only 76% and a specificity of 72%; serial sampling increased the sensitivity to 92% and the specificity to 96%. The sensitivity and specificity of two samples two hours apart were 94% and 91%, respectively.[68]

Creatine kinase isoenzyme is recognized as highly sensitive (95%) and specific (98%) for the diagnosis of myocardial infarction when serial sampling is performed and is the current gold standard. However, the sensitivity and specificity of a single sample, especially one obtained at presentation, is far less reliable. Even when the creatine kinase-MB fraction is considered with the results of initial electrocardiography, the combination may miss more than 20% of acute myocardial infarctions.[134] Newer, more sensitive creatine kinase-MB assays allow identification of lower concentrations of creatine kinase-MB. Elevations that are only slightly above the normal range, even with normal total creatine kinase concentration, have been associated with increased risk for cardiac events in some[15] but not all studies.[83,90]

Myoglobin is released rapidly from necrotic myocytes. It can usually be detected in serum 1 to 2 hours after onset of infarction and often peaks within 3 to 5 hours. It is eliminated through renal filtration, so it has a limited biological half-life and therefore may be nondiagnostic in patients who present late. No difference in cardiac and skeletal muscle myoglobin can be detected, resulting in a lower specificity for this marker. Specificity can be even lower in patients with renal insufficiency, which falsely elevates serum levels because of impaired clearance. Despite this drawback, the need to rapidly exclude myocardial infarction has rekindled interest in using myoglobin for early diagnosis of this event.[22,51]

Troponins are structural and regulatory proteins, including the binding protein troponin and the inhibitory protein troponin I, which form the tropomyosin complex. The cardiac troponin and troponin isoenzymes are immunologically distinct from those found in skeletal muscle and are almost undetectable under normal circumstances. Cardiac levels of troponin T and troponin I seem to be highly sensitive and specific,[1] to increase quickly, and to remain elevated for prolonged periods, all of which may substantially improve the ability to detect myocardial necrosis. Katus et al.[49] reported a sensitivity of 100% for troponin T in the diagnosis of acute myocardial infarction but an unexpectedly low specificity of 78% (compared with 92% for creatine kinase). However, when patients with the clinical diagnosis of unstable angina were excluded, the specificity improved to 97% because 40% to 50% of these patients were positive for troponin T.

Small elevations of troponin T seem to predict an increased short-term risk for myocardial infarction and death in patients in whom unstable angina is clinically diagnosed; larger elevations predict higher levels of risk. Lindahl, Venge, and Wallentin[60] reported that risk increased relative to the maximal level of troponin T found during the first 24 hours, ranging from 4.3% in the lowest quartile (<0.06 ng/ml) to 16% in the highest quartile (>0.18 ng/ml). Its prognostic value was independent of whether the event was classified clinically as myocardial infarction or unstable angina. Wu and Lane[132] performed a meta-analysis to confirm the predictive value of troponin T in ischemic heart disease. In seven studies with follow-up ranging from hospital discharge to 6 months, the cumulative odds ratio for myocardial infarction or death with elevated troponin T levels was 4.3 (95% CI, 2.8 to 6.8). Similar findings have been shown with troponin I. Although these findings seemed promising, they still required serial sampling and had limited value in a single presentation sample for risk stratification.

Point-of-care testing and rapid assays for the detection of myocardial necrosis are also subjects of increasing interest. Mach et al[66] evaluated a semiquantitative rapid bedside assay for troponin T (Boehringer Mannheim) and showed that results were available almost immediately, with a sensitivity and specificity of 100% and 86%, respectively. Antman, Goudzien, and Sacko[4] reported a similar sensitivity and specificity for the rapid bedside troponin T assay and showed that the relative risk for death or nonfatal myocardial infarction was 6.8 in patients with a positive result. The clinical value of rapid assays will be determined by the ability to use the information quickly and effectively. The added expense of these assays can only be justified if it can be demonstrated that rapid confirmation of myocardial necrosis drives early intervention that improves patient outcomes. Limited early reports suggest that this may be the case, but further large-scale evaluations are needed.

IMAGING IN THE ACUTE SETTING

Presenting symptoms, history, physical examination, and electrocardiography, even when considered together, have limitations and cannot accurately identify all patients with cardiac ischemia among the many patients who present with chest pain. Increased sensitivity and specificity for early diagnosis could provide substantial advantages for patients with nondiagnostic electrocardiograms, including early initiation of appropriate therapy in those with myocardial infarction or unstable angina (Fig. 27-1), reduction in the inadvertent discharge of patients with ongoing ischemia, and reduction in the length of stay and the number of unnecessary admissions for patients with noncardiac chest pain. In the absence of the laboratory tests to provide the needed information, myocardial perfusion and function imaging are under intense investigation.

Echocardiography

Several studies have documented high sensitivity of echocardiography in the detection of myocardial infarction. Gibson et al,[25] who studied 75 patients with acute myocardial infarction who underwent echocardiography within 8 hours of admission, found a sensitivity of 100%. Horowitz et al[41] studied 80 patients within 12 hours of admission and found that only 2 of the 33 patients (6%) in whom myocardial infarction was diagnosed had normal wall motion. Both of these patients had nontransmural infarctions. Other investigators have determined that infarctions involving less than 20% of the ventricular wall thickness[59,80] or small transmural infarctions involving less than 5% of the left ventricular mass may be below the threshold required to produce detectable wall-motion abnormalities.[80,129] Wall-motion abnormalities are observed on echocardiography in 89% to 100% of patients with transmural infarction and in approximately 79% to 86% of patients with nontransmural or subendocardial infarction.[69]

Sabia et al[98] performed acute echocardiography in 180 chest pain patients within 4 hours of presentation to the emergency department. Six percent of the studies (11 patients) were not technically adequate. Sixty patients had no regional wall-motion abnormalities, including 2 (4%) who had uncomplicated myocardial infarction. Global left ventricular systolic dysfunction without regional wall-motion abnormalities was detected in 22 patients (none of whom had had acute myocardial infarction), and regional wall-motion abnormalities were noted in 87 patients, including 27 (31%) who subsequently received a diagnosis of myocardial infarction. One of the patients with myocardial infarction had an uninterpretable study. Sensitivity for detecting myocardial infarction was high (93%), but specificity was limited, in part because of the 31 patients with previous myocardial infarction.

The utility of echocardiography in identifying patients with unstable angina has been studied less thoroughly. Nixon, Brown, and Smitherman[78] evaluated 19 chest pain patients without previous myocardial infarction by performing echocardiography at admission and before discharge. The authors found that a lack of improvement in wall-motion score between the admission and discharge study was associated with a more complicated postdischarge course. Peels et al[81] compared echocardiography and angiography in 43 patients with no history of myocardial infarction or coronary disease who were admitted to the hospital after presenting to the emergency department with chest pain and found that the presence of regional wall-motion abnormalities was associated with a sensitivity of 88% and a specificity of 78% for the diagnosis of significant coronary disease. Three patients with normal echocardiograms had significant coronary disease, but all had single-vessel disease with stenoses only in branch vessels. Kontos et al[53] performed echocardiography in the emergency department in 140 patients with possible cardiac ischemia. Among the patients with normal wall motion, 1 had myocardial infarction and 5 had significant stenosis on angiography or abnormal stress perfusion imaging. The sensitivity for predicting infarction or significant cardiac disease was 84%. Stein et al[105] found that admission echocardiography had a sensitivity of 92% and specificity of 69% for predicting major in-hospital complications in 63 patients admitted for unstable angina. In contrast, Gibler et al[23] found that echocardiography used as part of a diagnostic pathway had excellent specificity and negative predictive value but had limited sensitivity, which may have been compromised because studies were performed late (at the end of a 9-hour rule-out protocol).

Echocardiographic studies also provide data on the time course of wall-motion abnormalities in unstable angina. Persistence of wall-motion abnormalities may be related to the duration or severity of the ischemic insult or to the size of the risk zone. In patients with prolonged ischemia, myocardial stunning or hibernation may result in persistent regional wall-motion abnormalities, whereas patients with shorter episodes of ischemia, such as those induced during stress testing, are likely to experience resolution more quickly. Jeroudi et al[44] performed serial echocardiography in six patients who were admitted with chest pain in whom myocardial infarction was excluded. In the two patients in whom pain lasted less than 10 minutes, wall-motion abnormalities normalized on repeated echocardiography 2 hours after relief of pain, whereas in three patients in whom pain listed more than 20 minutes, the abnormalities remained 24 hours after relief of pain. Although radionuclide studies have demonstrated a rapid return to normal function after the recurrence of exercise-induced wall-motion abnormality, these echocardiographic data suggest that this rapid recovery may not occur in acute coronary syndromes, including severe unstable angina; rather, wall-motion abnormalities may persist for much longer periods.

The acute use of echocardiography for evaluating chest pain has limitations. These include poor echocardiographic windows in some patients, which may limit the ability to obtain adequate images, and the lack of wall-motion abnormalities seen in patients with small, especially nontransmural, infarctions. Also, abnormal septal motion in patients with right ventricular volume overload, left bundle-branch block, or the Wolff–Parkinson–White syndrome, as well as focal wall-motion abnormalities occasionally present in patients with myocarditis,[73] may lead to false-positive results.

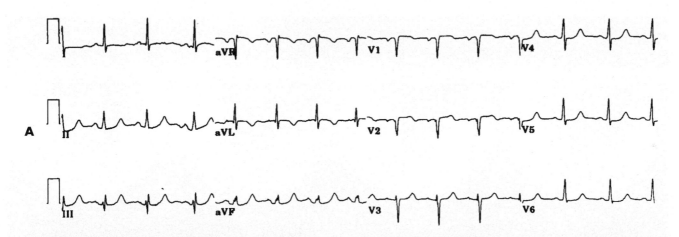

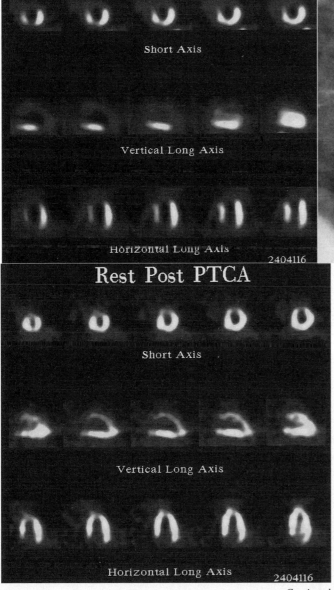

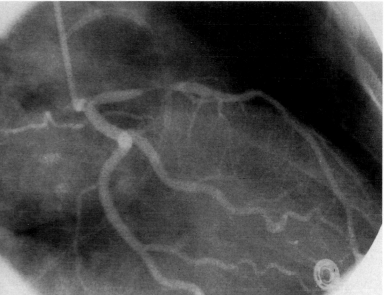

Fig. 27-1. A 32-year-old woman who experienced intermittent chest pain for 3 days. The presenting electrocardiogram (**A**) showed only T-wave changes that were considered suspicious but nonspecific. The patient was assigned to Acute Cardiac Team level 4. Acute technetium-99m sestamibi single-photon emission computed tomography (SPECT) (**B**) showed an extensive high-grade anteroseptal defect, and cardiac catheterization (**C**) demonstrated a high-grade proximal left anterior descending defect that led to immediate percutaneous transluminal coronary angioplasty (PTCA). Repeated resting sestamibi SPECT MIBI before hospital discharge (day 5) (**D**) demonstrates significant salvage of myocardium compared with the acute risk area.

Continued

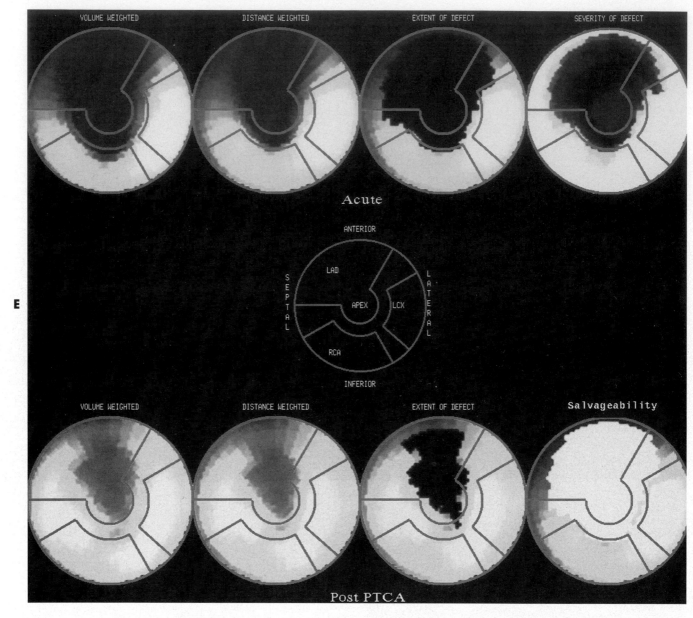

Fig. 27-1, cont'd. This is also seen when comparing the acute and post-PTCA polar maps with salvageability displayed in lower right corner (**E**).

MYOCARDIAL PERFUSION IMAGING IN THE ACUTE CORONARY SYNDROME

Thallium-201 planar imaging

More than 20 years ago, several investigators reported the visualization of myocardial infarctions by using various isotopes.[9,10,93] Among these early reports was one of the first applications of perfusion imaging to the acute coronary syndrome: the noninvasive identification of acute myocardial infarction with thallium-201 (^{201}Tl).[126] The following year, Wackers et al[122] reported a 96% sensitivity (92 of 96 patients) for the detection of acute myocardial infarction by using planar ^{201}Tl imaging within the first 24 hours. Sensitivity was 82% (165 of 200 patients) overall, but this value decreased over time; sensitivity was 100% (44 of 44 patients) within the first 6 hours, which decreased to 79% when imaging was performed later than 48 hours. The authors suggested that early sensitivity was in part related to early periinfarct ischemia, because 28 patients had significant reductions in infarct size on repeated imaging done 24 hours later. Subsequently, Smitherman, Osborn, and Narahara demonstrated that serial imaging after a single injection of ^{201}Tl could be used to separate the ischemic component from infarction. In patients with definite acute myocardial infarction, defects on delayed images (4 to 8 hours) corresponded to infarct size on technetium-99m (^{99m}Tc) pyrophosphate imaging, whereas images obtained immediately tended to overestimate the extent of infarction.

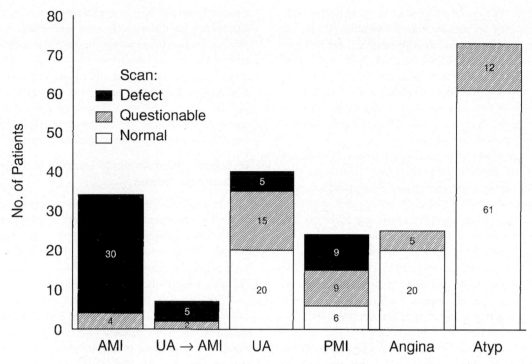

Fig. 27-2. Final diagnosis compared with results of thallium-201 rest planar perfusion imaging in 203 patients referred to the coronary care unit. AMI = acute myocardial infarction; Atyp, atypical complaints; PMI = previous myocardial infarction; UA = unstable angina; UA → AMI = unstable angina progressing to acute myocardial infarction. (Adapted from Wackers FJ, Lie KI, Liem KL, et al: Potential value of thallium-201 scintigraphy as a means of selecting patients for the coronary care unit, *Br Heart J* 41:111-117, 1979.)

However, Wackers et al[124] concluded that this seeming lack of specificity for acute myocardial infarction did not reduce the clinical usefulness of acute imaging; rather, it identified a high-risk group of patients, including those with acute myocardial infarction and unstable angina. Among 98 patients with unstable angina who were injected with ^{201}Tl during a pain-free period within 18 hours of symptom resolution planar imaging demonstrated a sensitivity of 76% for identifying patients with a complicated hospital course. When imaging results were combined with electrocardiographic findings, the investigators were able to assign patients to the high-risk group with a sensitivity of 94%. As had been previously demonstrated with acute myocardial infarction, the incidence of abnormal perfusion studies decreased as the time after resolution of pain increased; 84% of the studies were abnormal at 0 to 6 hours, but only 19% were abnormal at 12 to 18 hours.[124]

In 1979, Wackers et al[125] evaluated the risk stratification capability of ^{201}Tl planar imaging in patients with no evidence of previous myocardial infarction and normal or nondiagnostic electrocardiograms who were admitted to rule out myocardial infarction. Although in some cases, imaging was delayed for as long as 10 hours after the last pain episode, all 34 patients presenting with acute myocardial infarction had abnormal perfusion studies, whereas none of the 98 patients with atypical chest pain or stable angina had abnormal studies. Of the 47 patients

who were subsequently discharged with a diagnosis of unstable angina, 27 had an abnormality noted on perfusion imaging; however, in the subset of patients presenting with unstable angina that progressed to myocardial infarction, the sensitivity was 100% (Fig. 27-2).

Van der Wieken et al[116] also evaluated acute ^{201}Tl planar imaging as a decision tool. Patients were injected as soon as possible, and no patient was injected longer than 12 hours after resolution of pain. Among 149 patients with no history of myocardial infarction and normal or equivocal electrocardiograms, only 1 of the 79 patients with a normal imaging study developed myocardial infarction. When equivocal and abnormal studies were grouped together, the authors reported a sensitivity of 97%, a specificity of 71%, a negative predictive value of 99%, and a positive predictive value of 54% for the detection of acute myocardial infarction. For the detection of coronary artery disease, the sensitivity was 96%, the specificity was 79%, the negative predictive value was 97%, and the positive predictive value was 71%.

Freeman et al[19] examined the relation between the results of acute ^{201}Tl planar imaging and the severity of coronary artery disease in 66 patients admitted to the hospital with unstable angina who were injected 5.6 ± 5.1 hours after rest pain. Perfusion abnormalities were seen in 83% of patients with stenoses 50% or more but in only half of patients with less severe disease. The authors also correlated perfusion abnormality with coronary morphology and demonstrated a significantly higher incidence of defects in association with complex stenoses ($p<$ 0.002). Of note, 61% of patients (11 of 18) with in-hospital events had perfusion abnormalities, whereas only 32% of those without events had abnormal studies. Hakki et al[33] also demonstrated a correlation between the degree of stenosis and the presence of perfusion defects on rest ^{201}Tl imaging when patients were injected while free of pain.

Two studies reported varying results of mobile ^{201}Tl planar imaging in the emergency department. Mace[65] concluded that ^{201}Tl perfusion imaging in the emergency department was useful in the differential diagnosis of acute myocardial infarction in high-risk patients when other variables are inconclusive. Among the 20 patients examined, none of the 13 with normal perfusion imaging were ruled in for myocardial infarction, and all 7 patients with abnormal studies demonstrated some cardiac abnormality, although only 3 had acute myocardial infarction. In contrast, Henneman et al[35] reported a 75% sensitivity and 42% specificity, yielding a negative predictive value of 95% and a positive predictive value of only 11%.

These initial studies with ^{201}Tl planar imaging in the acute setting demonstrated a high sensitivity for the detection of acute myocardial infarction and a remarkable but less favorable sensitivity for the detection of unstable angina, especially in the face of frequent long delays between pain and injection.

Planar imaging compared with single-photon emission computed tomography

All of the early acute perfusion imaging studies used ^{201}Tl planar imaging; but compelling data now suggest that planar imaging may not be optimal in this setting. Planar imaging has been demonstrated to have a lower sensitivity than single-photon emission computed tomography (SPECT) imaging for the detection of small infarction,[92,107] including non–Q-wave myocardial infarction.[127] Planar imaging also has a relatively poor sensitivity in the posterior (circumflex) distribution.[13,18] The importance of this weakness is amplified when patients with nondiagnostic or normal electrocardiograms undergo acute imaging, because the posterior distribution is most likely to be electrically silent on the presenting electrocardiogram. In our experience, 58% of the patients with acute myocardial infarction who had normal or nondiagnostic electrocardiograms and underwent acute myocardial perfusion imaging had defects in the posterior distribution.

For various reasons, neither planar nor SPECT ^{201}Tl imaging gained widespread clinical use in the acute setting. The most plausible explanation is that the standard of care for the treatment of suspected myocardial infarction did not justify additional risk stratification. In the late 1970s, early intervention was not routinely performed and thrombolytic agents were not available. Therefore, in an environment in which rapid diagnosis provided no great treatment advantage and there was no pressure to reduce admissions or length of stay, additional triage aids were unnecessary. In the ensuing years, a different

standard evolved, one in which rapid identification and early intervention are known to improve outcomes. However, the recent acceptance of an economic policy that strongly discourages inappropriate admissions has further increased the complexity of rapid evaluation and triage. These conflicting goals of economic policy and health care standards create an environment in which effective diagnostic tools that assist in rapid risk stratification may have substantial incremental value with respect to improved outcomes and cost.

Technetium-99m sestamibi imaging in acute coronary syndromes

While radical changes in the treatment of acute myocardial infarction were occurring, significant developments in myocardial perfusion imaging were taking place. Among these was the introduction of technetium-based myocardial perfusion imaging agents, of which ^{99m}Tc sestamibi (Cardiolite [DuPont Pharma]) has had the widest clinical use.

[99m]Tc sestamibi has been extensively studied in models of coronary occlusion and reperfusion, both in animals[34,119] and in human thrombolytic trials.[21,50,120,123] These studies reveal that when ^{99m}Tc sestamibi is injected during occlusion, the perfusion image accurately defines the risk area without changing significantly for several hours after the initial injection, even when reperfusion occurs. This characteristic forms the physiologic basis for the use of sestamibi imaging in the evaluation of conditions in the acute coronary syndrome, from unstable angina to acute myocardial infarction.[11] However, one of the greatest advantages of technetium-based perfusion imaging agents may be the ability to assess perfusion and function simultaneously. Recently, DePuey and Rozanski[14] documented enhanced specificity of perfusion imaging when functional evaluation was performed simultaneously. In a recent report by Nicholson et al[76] of 102 studies performed in the acute setting, the addition of simultaneous functional evaluation by gating the resting sestamibi SPECT study provided a substantial improvement in specificity (69% to 97%) and positive predictive value (38% to 97%).

One of the most important studies of the use of perfusion imaging in patients with unstable angina was published by Bilodeau et al,[7] who focused on the diagnostic capability of resting sestamibi SPECT perfusion imaging to detect significant coronary artery disease. The results of sestamibi SPECT with injection during active chest pain and pain-free periods were compared with coronary anatomy in 45 patients. In patients injected during a pain episode, SPECT perfusion imaging had a 96% sensitivity and a 79% specificity for detection of significant coronary artery disease. This was significantly higher than the 65% sensitivity of electrocardiography done during a pain episode (Fig. 27-3). Although this study demonstrates a high diagnostic potential, it must be interpreted in the setting of a selected group of patients, all of whom were hospitalized with unstable angina and were awaiting angiography.

Varetto et al[118] were among the first to address the use of acute radionuclide imaging in the population of interest: emer-

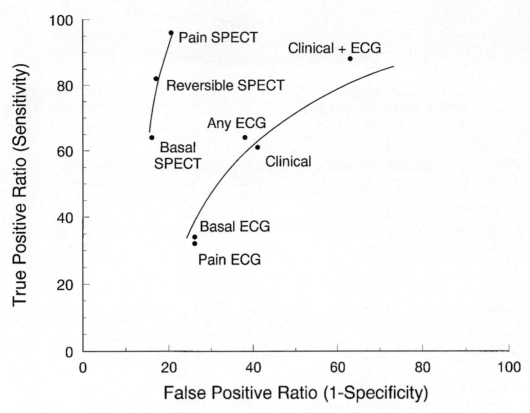

Fig. 27-3. Technetium-99m (^{99m}Tc) sestamibi single-photon emission computed tomographic (SPECT) studies obtained during the pain-free state *(Basal)* had a higher sensitivity than electrocardiography *(ECG)* done during *(Pain)* or between *(Basal)* episodes of pain and a sensitivity similar to that of any electrocardiographic changes *(Any ECG)* and that of the presence of typical symptoms of angina *(Clinical)*. Injection of ^{99m}Tc sestamibi during chest pain shows a higher sensitivity than any other combination. The presence of a reversible ^{99m}Tc sestamibi defect *(Reversible)* also has a high sensitivity. The specificity of the ^{99m}Tc sestamibi SPECT studies is higher than that of any of the clinical and electrocardiographic criteria. (Adapted from Bilodeau L, Theroux P, Grejoine J, et al: Technetium-99m sestamibi tomography in patients with spontaneous chest pain: correlations with clinical, electrocardiographic and angiographic findings, *J Am Coll Cardiol* 18:1684-1691, 1991.)

gency department patients at low to moderate risk who had normal or nondiagnostic electrocardiograms. This study assessed diagnostic and prognostic accuracy in a small population ($n = 64$) and demonstrated remarkable results. None of the 34 patients with normal sestamibi SPECT studies were subsequently diagnosed with significant coronary artery disease or sustained a significant cardiac event over the subsequent 18 months. On the other hand, among the 30 patients with significant perfusion defects, 13 received a diagnosis of myocardial infarction and 14 received a diagnosis of unstable angina without infarction (Fig. 27-4). In addition, six cardiac events occurred during follow-up in the group with abnormal studies. The negative predictive value for both long-term and short-term events was 100%. Among the 14 patients without acute myocardial infarction, 12 had complete normalization on follow-up imaging 24 hours after the acute event, providing additional evidence that acute myocardial perfusion imaging is a useful tool for the identification of the acute coronary syndrome without infarction in this population.

This study also reported that most of the patients with unstable angina (11 of 14) were injected after remission of chest pain (mean, 4.7 hours; range, 2 to 8 hours), suggesting the existence of a window of opportunity after an ischemic event during which diagnostic accuracy is not compromised. It is clear that the extent, duration, severity, and reperfusion status of the ischemic insult affect the degree of perfusion abnormality that persists after an ischemic event. Therefore, reliable detection of coronary artery disease that has produced a transient ischemic event will require injection during an episode of pain.[106] However, the observation of significant perfusion abnormalities several hours after remission of chest pain suggests a far more significant ischemic insult with serious prognostic implications.[33,70]

Hilton et al[38] specifically evaluated the risk stratification and prognostic potential of acute myocardial perfusion imaging in 102 patients presenting to the emergency department with active typical anginal chest pain and nondiagnostic or normal electrocardiograms. Imaging results were graded as normal,

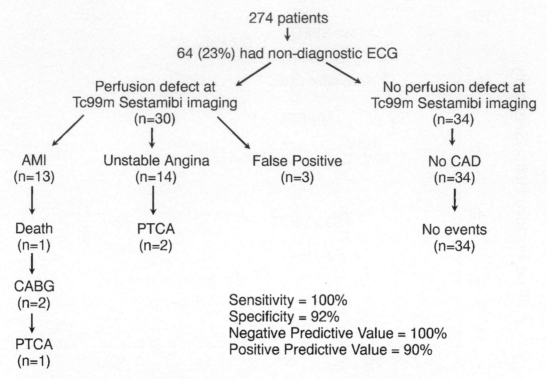

Fig. 27-4. Flow chart showing the breakdown of final diagnoses and the occurrence of cardiac events at follow-up compared with results of technetium-99m (*Tc99m*) sestamibi perfusion imaging. AMI = acute myocardial infarction; CABG = coronary artery bypass graft surgery; CAD = coronary artery disease; ECG = electrocardiography; PTCA = percutaneous transluminal coronary angioplasty. (Adapted from Varetto T, Cantalupi D, Altieri A, et al: Emergency room technetium-99m sestamibi imaging to rule out acute myocardial ischemic events in patients with nondiagnostic electrocardiograms, *J Am Coll Cardiol* 22:1804-1808, 1993.)

equivocal, or clearly abnormal. Among the 70 patients with normal perfusion studies, only 1 (1.5%) had a significant cardiac event (coronary revascularization), whereas patients with clearly abnormal studies had an event rate of 71% (12 of 17 patients). The risk level was intermediate in those with equivocal studies; as two of the 15 patients (13%) sustained events (Fig. 27-5). Hilton et al[37] and Varetto et al[118] demonstrated that an unequivocally normal result on resting sestamibi SPECT in patients injected during a pain episode indicated a good short-term prognosis, with no events observed within 90 days of follow-up.

Kjoller et al[52] studied 134 patients injected with ^{99m}Tc sestamibi within 2 hours of resolution of chest pain. The authors concluded that acute perfusion imaging was not useful in the diagnosis of acute myocardial infarction and therefore could not be used to direct therapy. However, this study differs greatly from those discussed above in three key ways:

1. Portable planar imaging rather than SPECT was performed in the coronary unit.
2. The study population was very high risk, with a high percentage of patients having had a previous (40%) or acute (54%) myocardial infarction.
3. Acute myocardial infarction was the only end point. As would be expected in this population, the sensitivity

was high (96%) but the specificity was poor (8%); 57 of 62 (92%) patients without acute myocardial infarction had perfusion defects. The low specificity clearly relates to the choice of acute myocardial infarction as the only end point. As the authors themselves point out, many perfusion defects seemed to be related to ischemia in the absence of infarction.

Appropriate selection of patients in whom acute myocardial perfusion imaging will be useful is extremely important. Acute perfusion imaging has little incremental value in patients who have diagnostic electrocardiograms or have a presentation that otherwise dictates invasive evaluation. The greatest impact on patient care occurs when acute perfusion imaging is used in populations at low to moderate risk, allowing appropriate management of the small but significant percentage of patients with high-risk perfusion patterns while directing patients at lower risk to less expensive therapies. The data in the few studies to date that used acute rest sestamibi SPECT demonstrate substantial risk stratification potential, with a high sensitivity for detection of acute myocardial infarction and an excellent negative predictive value in patients with normal studies (Table 27-1).

The risk stratification potential of acute perfusion imaging

Table 27-1. Accuracy of technetium-99m single-photon emission computed tomography in the acute evaluation of chest pain

Study*	Patients	Follow-up	Sensitivity		Negative Predictive Value	
			Acute myocardial infarction†	Cardiac events‡	Acute myocardial infarction†	Cardiac events‡
	n	*mo*		*n/n (%)*		
Varetto et al[118]	64	18	13/13 (100)	15/15 (100%)	34/34 (100)	34/34 (100)
Hilton et al[38]	102	3	12/12 (100)	15/16 (93.8%)	70/70 (100)	69/70 (98.5)
Tatum et al[108]	438	12	7/7 (100)	42/52 (80.8%)	338/338 (100)	328/338 (97)
Total	604	–	32/32 (100)	72/83 (86.7%)	442/442 (100)	431/442 (97.5)

*Patients in all three studies presented to the emergency department with a chief complaint of chest pain and a normal or nondiagnostic electrocardiogram. All patients were injected with technetium-99m sestamibi in the emergency department. Patients in the studies by Varetto et al and Tatum et al did not require the presence of active chest pain at the time of injection.
†Associated with index evaluation.
‡Cardiac death, nonfatal myocardial infarction, or revascularization during follow-up.

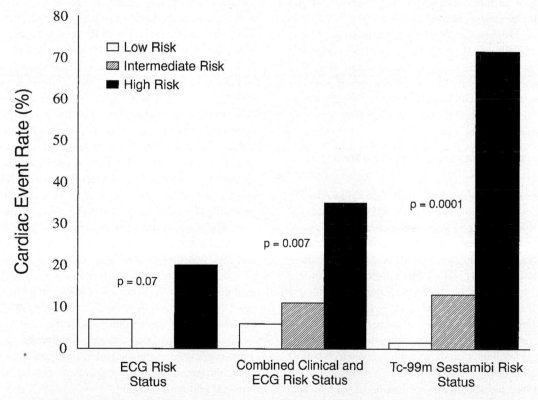

Fig. 27-5. Risk status determined from results of electrocardiography *(ECG)* (normal or abnormal but nondiagnostic), a combination of clinical and electrocardiographic variables, and the results of the technetium *(Tc)*–99m sestamibi scan (normal [low risk, *open bars*], equivocal [intermediate risk, *hatched bars*], and abnormal [high risk, *solid bars*]). Technetium-99m sestamibi imaging identifies both a lower (<2%) and a higher (>70%) risk groups than electrocardiography alone or in combination with clinical variables. (Adapted from Hilton TC, Thompson RC, Williams HJ, et al: Technetium-99m sestamibi myocardial perfusion imaging in the emergency room evaluation of chest pain. *J Am Coll Cardiol* 23:1016-1022, 1994.)

has also been demonstrated in a multicenter study that used ^{99m}Tc tetrofosmin.[121] In this blinded acute perfusion imaging study, although the incidence of acute myocardial infarction with negative perfusion imaging was higher than that reported in nonblinded studies, a negative study indicated a small infarction and was associated with a good prognosis. Of note, the negative predictive value of a normal study for exclusion of acute myocardial infarction remained high (98%).

Clinical considerations

Any diagnostic or prognostic tool is used most effectively through a systematic and comprehensive approach. Each test must be evaluated for the incremental value that it adds to patient care, with specific attention to its ability to guide therapy and affect outcomes, as well as to its cost effectiveness. It is important to identify the specific situations in which each test will have maximal value and to avoid those in which it has little to no value. Appropriate use of testing should drive therapy or management, because this is the key to cost effectiveness.

An excellent example of effective use of diagnostic testing within a systematic strategy for chest pain is the 9-hour rule-out protocol reported by Gibler et al.[23] Patients thought to be at low risk on the basis of the initial history, physical examination, and electrocardiography were evaluated over 9 hours by using serial markers and continuous ST-segment monitoring. At the completion of the 9-hour rule-out protocol, patients underwent echocardiography and exercise stress testing. More than 80% of the 1010 patients studied were safely discharged from the chest pain evaluation unit. Studies using this and similar protocols have demonstrated substantial cost savings compared with routine admissions for chest pain.[39,114]

The Acute Cardiac Team strategy for evaluation and triage

The guidelines for unstable angina published by the AHCPR in March of 1994 state that patients without known coronary artery disease who are judged in the initial evaluation to be at low risk for adverse outcomes can often be evaluated as outpatients. The subsequent evaluation should focus on determining the cause of the symptoms and evaluating the risk for future cardiac events. It is clear from these guidelines that effective identification of the low-risk patient can provide options other than routine admission of all patients with chest pain.

In recognition of these guidelines, a multispecialty Acute Cardiac Team at Virginia Commonwealth University/Medical College of Virginia developed a risk-based, systematic strategy for the rapid triage and subsequent evaluation of patients presenting to the emergency department with chest pain (Fig. 27-6). The goal of the strategy is to risk stratify patients according to their probability of acute myocardial infarction or the acute coronary syndrome. Risk assessment is based on the initial presentation, consisting of a brief history, description of chest pain, and the presenting electrocardiogram. Risk level is assigned within 30 minutes of the initial encounter in the emergency department. Each of the five risk levels is defined by a critical pathway that directs subsequent evaluation and intervention (if appropriate). Each patient progresses along a diagnostic hierarchy designed to first rule in myocardial infarction, then rule in the acute coronary syndrome, then rule out significant coronary artery disease. Level 1 (high probability of myocardial infarction) patients are clearly identified by an initial electrocardiogram showing classic ST-segment elevation or new left bundle-branch block and are slated for immediate revascularization (thrombolysis or percutaneous transluminal coronary angioplasty). At the other extreme, level 5 (noncardiac chest pain) patients have a clear noncoronary cause of their chest pain and are given an appropriate outpatient referral. Patients in levels 2 through 4, however, require the use of other diagnostic schemes within the evaluation to meet the goals of the diagnostic hierarchy. In level 2 patients, ischemic changes on the presenting electrocardiogram define a population at high risk for the acute coronary syndrome and moderate risk for acute myocardial infarction. Because the risk in this level is considered high enough to make invasive procedures likely and revascularization probable, the diagnostic tools consist primarily of myocardial markers and serial electrocardiography.

Patients assigned to level 3 are thought to be at lower risk for acute myocardial infarction and at moderate risk for the acute coronary syndrome. The presenting electrocardiogram in these patients is usually normal or nondiagnostic, but other characteristics suggest a higher probability of significant underlying coronary artery disease. Traditionally, these patients would be admitted directly to the coronary care unit, as the level 2 patients would be. In the risk-based strategy, however, this group is admitted into a fast-track rule-out protocol in which the entire sequence of goals as defined above is completed within 23 hours. At this level, as well as at the lower risk level 4, acute myocardial perfusion imaging at rest is used for further risk stratification. An integral part of the level 3 pathway is the injection of a tracer dose of ^{99m}Tc sestamibi in the emergency department as soon as possible after, if not during, chest pain. The result of the gated perfusion imaging study becomes a pivotal decision-making element in the subsequent critical pathway. A definitive abnormal study with a significant perfusion defect and associated wall-motion abnormality is considered consistent with acute myocardial infarction and leads to rapid revascularization in most cases (Fig. 27-7). Normal or equivocal studies are combined with the results of serial electrocardiography and markers obtained over the next 8 hours. If markers are normal and the electrocardiograms are negative for ischemia, patients undergo a standard exercise treadmill stress test with perfusion imaging.

Patients considered to be at extremely low risk for acute myocardial infarction but a moderate probability for the acute coronary syndrome are assigned to level 4. Patients assigned to level 4 are most likely to present with atypical chest pain and normal or nondiagnostic electrocardiogram. The diagnostic goals at this level are to find the unsuspected patient at high risk because of evolving silent myocardial infarction or unstable

ACT Strategy for Chest Pain Evaluation and Triage
Risk Based and Goal-Driven

Level Assignment Based on CP Character, History, and Initial ECG

Level	Risk	Goal	Disposition	Diagnostic Strategy
1	Very High	Intervention	Treat and Admit CICU	Presenting ECG
2	High	Intervention	Admit CICU	Serial ECGs and Markers
3	Moderate	R/in ACS	"Fast Track"	Serial ECGs Acute Perfusion Imaging
4	Low	Risk Stratification	ED Workup	Acute Perfusion Imaging
5	Very Low	Alternate Diagnosis	Home	Appropriate Referral

(RISK axis, increasing upward, shown at left)

Acute Cardiac Team (ACT) Medical College of Virginia Hospitals / VCU / Richmond, Va.

Fig. 27-6. The Acute Cardiac Team triage strategy is risk-based and goal-driven. Patients are assigned to one of five levels on the basis of initial risk determination. The diagnostic strategy and disposition are then directed by critical pathways.

acute coronary syndrome and to exclude significant underlying coronary artery disease. Acute myocardial perfusion imaging is the primary diagnostic tool. Previous studies have established the risk stratification ability of acute perfusion imaging, as well as its potential for high diagnostic accuracy for excluding coronary artery disease when patients are injected during an episode of pain. Therefore, patients are injected with sestamibi at rest in the emergency department as soon as triage assignment is made. Imaging with gating is performed approximately 90 minutes later to provide combined information on perfusion and function. Patients with equivocal or markedly abnormal studies are admitted to the hospital and are assigned to level 2 or 3, as appropriate (Fig. 27-8). Patients with normal studies (normal perfusion and function) are discharged and are scheduled to return within the next 72 hours for a follow-up stress test with perfusion imaging. The results of the subsequent stress study are combined with those of the normal resting study to form one perfusion imaging study. Therefore, in the time from initial encounter to the completion of the stress test, all three goals are satisfied.

Since March 1994, acute myocardial perfusion imaging using gated sestamibi SPECT has been routinely performed as an element of this triage protocol at the Medical College of Virginia/Virginia Commonwealth University.[75,109] More than 5000 emergency department patients have been evaluated by using this strategy, including more than 3000 patients assigned to low or moderate risk levels in whom acute myocardial perfusion imaging was performed. We recently reported results from a consecutive population triaged between 1 June 1994 and 6 October 1994.[108] During this time, 1187 patients with chest pain were evaluated in the emergency department. On the basis of their initial evaluation, 438 patients were triaged into the moderate-risk or low-risk groups (levels 3 or 4) and underwent acute myocardial perfusion imaging with injection of sestamibi in the emergency department. Patients were followed for 1 year to determine the incidence of significant cardiac events. Among the 338 patients with normal studies, no acute myocardial infarction or deaths occurred and only 10 revascularizations (3%) were performed over the next year. On the other hand, among the 100 patients with abnormal or equivocal perfusion studies,

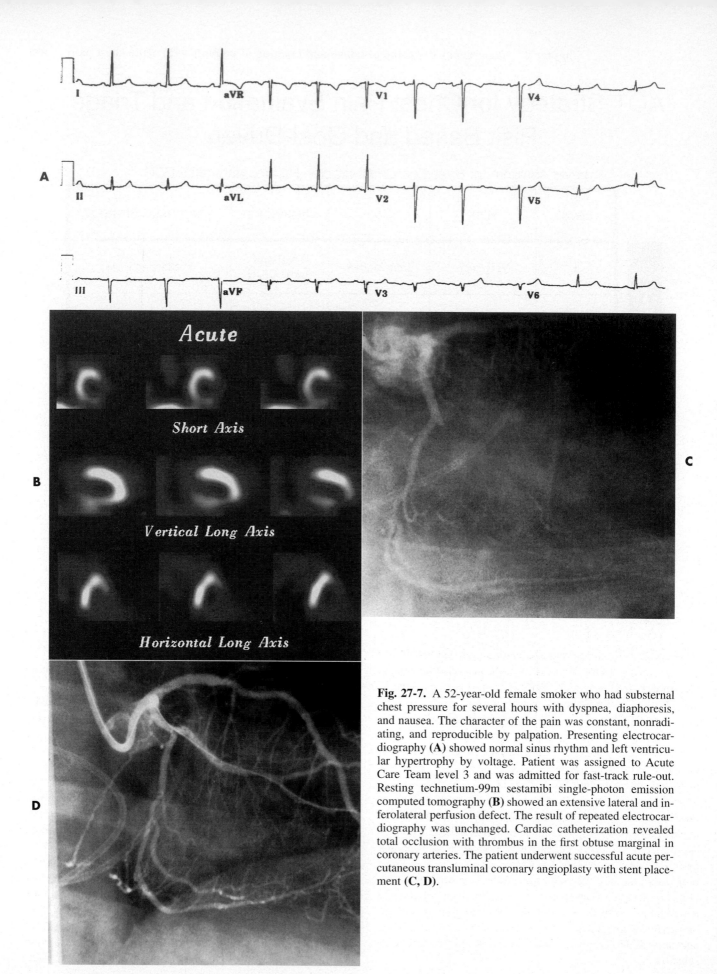

Fig. 27-7. A 52-year-old female smoker who had substernal chest pressure for several hours with dyspnea, diaphoresis, and nausea. The character of the pain was constant, nonradiating, and reproducible by palpation. Presenting electrocardiography (**A**) showed normal sinus rhythm and left ventricular hypertrophy by voltage. Patient was assigned to Acute Care Team level 3 and was admitted for fast-track rule-out. Resting technetium-99m sestamibi single-photon emission computed tomography (**B**) showed an extensive lateral and inferolateral perfusion defect. The result of repeated electrocardiography was unchanged. Cardiac catheterization revealed total occlusion with thrombus in the first obtuse marginal in coronary arteries. The patient underwent successful acute percutaneous transluminal coronary angioplasty with stent placement (**C, D**).

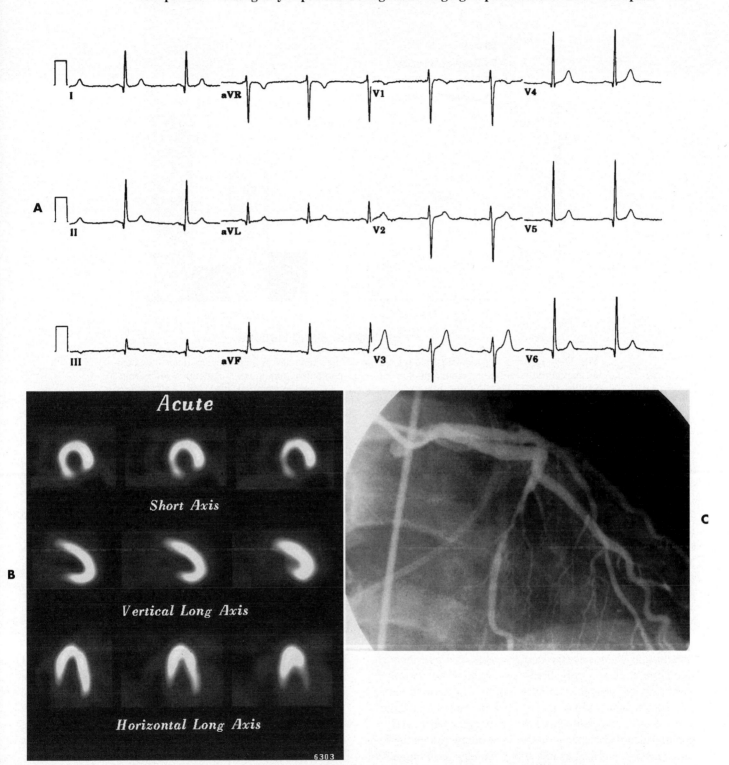

Fig. 27-8. A 54-year-old man with known hypertension had had intermittent chest pain for 2 days. The burning character of the pain was attributed to eating spicy foods. Presenting electrocardiography (**A**) demonstrated normal sinus rhythm with left ventricular hypertrophy by voltage. The patient was assigned to Acute Cardiac Team level 4. Resting technetium-99m sestamibi single-photon emission computed tomography (**B**) showed an extensive high-grade inferior perfusion defect. The patient was admitted to the coronary intensive care unit. Two hours later, he developed ST elevation and received tissue plasminogen activator. Cardiac catheterization performed 24 hours later (**C**) revealed a long high-grade circumflex lesion. The patient underwent successful percutaneous transluminal coronary angioplasty and had an uneventful postintervention course.

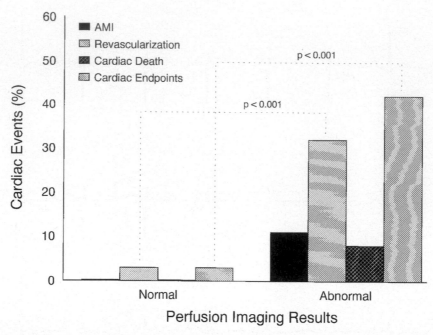

Fig. 27-9. Lower-risk patients triaged into Acute Cardiac Team levels 3 or 4 underwent acute gated technetium-99m sestamibi single-photon emission computed tomography. Patients with normal studies (*n* = 383) had a significantly lower event rate (no acute myocardial infarction *[AMI]* or cardiac death) than did those with abnormal studies (*n* = 100).

there were 11 myocardial infarctions, 32 revascularizations, and 9 cardiac deaths, for a combined cardiac event rate of 42% (Fig. 27-9). A comparison between the patients with abnormal sestamibi SPECT results and those assigned to level 2 revealed no significant difference in event rate: that is, patients at low risk on initial presentation who had an abnormal sestamibi SPECT result were at a risk similar to that in patients who presented with ischemic ST-segment changes (Fig. 27-10). Most patients (224 of 253) in the low-risk group (level 4) were discharged home from the emergency department and were scheduled for follow-up stress testing within 72 hours. In the group of patients discharged home after a normal acute resting perfusion imaging study, no acute cardiac events occurred, although significant coronary artery disease leading to revascularization was found in 7 patients. However, 5 of the 7 underwent revascularization more than 1 month after the initial evaluation. These data seem to substantiate the safety of outpatient evaluation in patients who are considered to be at low risk on the basis of history, physical examination, and electrocardiography and have a normal acute myocardial perfusion imaging study in association with chest pain.

In addition to short-term risk assessment, acute resting myocardial perfusion imaging with chest pain seems to provide substantial prognostic information on the basis of a 1-year evaluation of the event rate in our study. For this analysis, patients who underwent revascularization less than 1 month after the index evaluation were excluded to prevent diagnostic testing influence on soft events (that is, revascularization). If this correc-

tion for test bias is applied to the follow-up studies, a normal result on sestamibi SPECT was associated with an annual event rate of less than 1% (3 revascularizations), whereas an abnormal study carried an event rate of 21% (9 deaths, 4 myocardial infarctions, and 2 late revascularizations). As might have been anticipated, cardiac deaths were strongly associated with extensive perfusion defects and depressed left ventricular systolic function on acute rest sestamibi SPECT.

Cost effectiveness

To date, only two studies have addressed the cost effectiveness of using acute myocardial perfusion imaging in the emergency department.[89,130] The first study evaluated the impact of acute imaging on the disposition of patients. Cost savings were calculated by comparing the cost of the original disposition to that of the perfusion imaging study plus the altered disposition that resulted. The authors calculated a potential cost savings of $785.92 per patient due to more appropriate triage of patients after imaging. Similar results were reported in a larger study by Radensky et al[89] for Medicare source data and institutional source data. These authors compared the actual costs of two triage strategies; one included acute perfusion imaging (scan) and one did not (no scan). This study included a sensitivity analysis that concluded that for patients presenting to the emergency department with chest pain and nondiagnostic electrocardiograms the no-scan strategy would be less costly only if the subsequent cardiac event rate in these patients exceeded 60%.

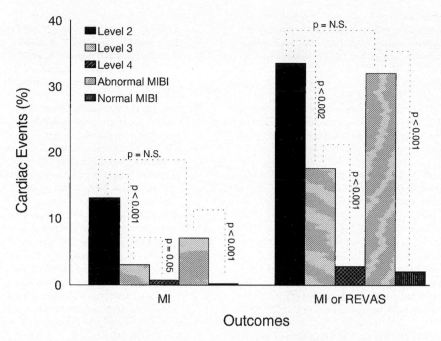

Fig. 27-10. Comparison of outcomes by Acute Cardiac Team triage levels (2 to 4) and results of acute myocardial perfusion. There was significant difference in all levels ($P < 0.05$), except between levels 3 and 4 for myocardial infarction *(MI)* ($P = 0.05$). Normal and abnormal results on technetium-99m sestamibi single-photon emission computed tomography *(MIBI)* also differed significantly ($P < 0.001$) for both MI and MI or revascularization *(REVAS)*. However, an abnormal MIBI result did not differ significantly from level 2 for MI and MI or REVAS.

Although the results of larger and more comprehensive cost effectiveness studies are anticipated in the near future, numerous previous studies have shown that strategies that allocate resources in accordance with risk stratification enable more cost-effective management of patients presenting with chest pain.[20,39] The greatest savings have been demonstrated when patients can be discharged from the emergency department to home with subsequent outpatient evaluation.[20]

REFERENCES

1. Adams JE 3d, Bodor G3, Davila-Roman VG, et al: Cardiac troponin I. A marker with high specificity for cardiac injury, *Circulation* 88:101–106, 1993.

2. Ambrose JA, Tannenbaum MA, Alexopoulos D, et al: Angiographic progression of coronary artery disease and the development of myocardial infarction, *J Am Coll Cardiol* 12:56–62, 1988.

3. Andrews RM, Fox S, Elixhauser A, et al: *The national bill for diseases treated in U.S. hospitals: 1987,* Agency for Health Care Policy and Research Pub No 94-0002, Rockville, MD, 1994, Public Health Service.

4. Antman EM, Grudzien C, Sacks DB: Evaluation of a rapid bedside assay for detection of serum cardiac troponin T, *JAMA* 273: 1279–1282, 1995.

5. Ardissino D, Merlini PA, Gamba G, et al: Thrombin activity and early outcome in unstable angina pectoris, *Circulation* 93:1634–1639, 1996.

6. Bakker AJ, Koelemay MJ, Gorgels JP, et al: Failure of new biochemical markers to exclude acute myocardial infarction at admission, *Lancet* 342:1220–1222, 1993.

7. Bilodeau L, Theroux P, Gregoire J, et al: Technetium-99m sestamibi tomography in patients with spontaneous chest pain: correlations with clinical, electrocardiographic and angiographic findings, *J Am Coll Cardiol* 18:1684–1691, 1991.

8. Braunwald E, Mark DB, Jones RH: *Unstable angina: diagnosis and management.* In *Clinical practice guideline number 10* (amended), AHCPR Pub No 94-0602, Rockville, MD, 1994, Agency for Health Care Policy and Research and the National Heart, Lung, and Blood Institute, Public Health Service, U.S. Department of Health and Human Services.

9. Carr EAJ, Beierwalters WH, Wegst AV, et al: Myocardial scanning with rubidium-86, *J Nucl Med* 3:76–82, 1962.

10. Carr EAJ, Gleason G, Shaw J, et al: The direct diagnosis of myocardial infarction by photoscanning after administration of cesium-131, *Am Heart J* 68:627–636, 1964.

11. Christian TF, Clements IP, Gibbons RJ: Noninvasive identification of myocardium at risk in patients with acute myocardial infarction and nondiagnostic electrocardiograms with technetium-99m-sestamibi, *Circulation* 83:1615–1620, 1991.

12. Cohen M, Hawkins L, Greenberg S, et al: Usefulness of ST-segment changes in ≥2 leads on the emergency room electrocardiogram in either unstable angina pectoris or non-Q-wave myocardial infarction in predicting outcome, *Am J Cardiol* 67:1368–1373, 1991.

13. DePasquale EE, Nody AC, DePuey EG, et al: Quantitative rotational thallium-201 tomography for identifying and localizing coronary artery disease, *Circulation* 77:316–327, 1988.

14. DePuey EG, Rozanski A: Using gated technetium-99m-sestamibi SPECT to characterize fixed myocardial defects as infarct or artifact, *J Nucl Med* 36:952–955, 1995.

15. de Winter RJ, Koster RW, Schotveld JH, et al: Prognostic value of troponin T, myoglobin, and CK-MB mass in patients presenting with chest pain without acute myocardial infarction, *Heart* 75:235–239, 1996.

16. Falk E: Unstable angina with fatal outcome: dynamic coronary thrombosis leading to infarction and/or sudden death. Autopsy evidence of recurrent thrombosis with peripheral embolization culminating in total vascular occlusion, *Circulation* 71:699–708, 1985.

17. Fesmire FM, Percy RF, Wears RL, et al: Risk stratification according to the initial electrocardiogram in patients with suspected acute myocardial infarction, *Arch Intern Med* 149:1294–1297, 1989.

18. Fintel DJ, Links JM, Brinker JA, et al: Improved diagnostic performance of exercise thallium-201 single photon emission computed tomography over planar imaging in the diagnosis of coronary artery disease: a receiver operating characteristic analysis, *J Am Coll Cardiol* 13:600–612, 1989.

19. Freeman MR, Williams AE, Chisholm RJ, et al: Role of resting thallium[201] perfusion in predicting coronary anatomy, left ventricular wall motion, and hospital outcome in unstable angina pectoris, *Am Heart J* 117:306–314, 1989.

20. Gaspoz JM, Lee TH, Weinstein MC, et al: Cost-effectiveness of a new short-stay unit to "rule out" acute myocardial infarction in low risk patients, *J Am Coll Cardiol* 24:1249–1259, 1994.

21. Gibbons RJ, Verani MS, Behrenbeck T, et al: Feasibility of tomographic ^{99m}Tc-hexakis-2-methoxy-2-methylpropyl-isonitrile imaging for the assessment of myocardial area at risk and the effect of treatment in acute myocardial infarction, *Circulation* 80:1277–1286, 1989.

22. Gibler WB, Gibler CD, Weinshenker E, et al: Myoglobin as an early indicator of acute myocardial infarction, *Ann Emerg Med* 16:851–856, 1987.

23. Gibler WB, Runyon JP, Levy RC, et al: A rapid diagnostic and treatment center for patients with chest pain in the emergency department, *Ann Emerg Med* 25:1–8, 1995.

24. Gibler WB, Young GP, Hedges JR, et al: Acute myocardial infarction in chest pain patients with nondiagnostic ECGs: serial CK-MB sampling in the emergency department. The Emergency Cardiac Medicine Research Group, *Ann Emerg Med* 21:504–512, 1992.

25. Gibson RS, Bishop HL, Stamm RB, et al: Value of early two dimensional echocardiography in patients with acute myocardial infarction, *Am J Cardiol* 49:1110–1119, 1982.

26. Effectiveness of intravenous thrombolytic treatment in acute myocardial infarction. Gruppo Italiano per lo Studio della Streptochinosi nell'Infarto Miocardico (GISSI), *Lancet* 1:397–401, 1986.

27. Goldman L, Cook EF, Brand DA, et al: A computer protocol to predict myocardial infarction in emergency department patients with chest pain, *N Engl J Med* 318:797–803, 1988.

28. Goldman L, Weinberg M, Weisberg M, et al: A computer-derived protocol to aid in the diagnosis of emergency room patients with acute chest pain, *N Engl J Med* 307:588–596, 1982.

29. Grijseels EWM, Deckers JW, Hoes AW, et al: Pre-hospital triage of patients with suspected myocardial infarction. Evaluation of previously developed algorithms and new proposals, *Eur Heart J* 16:325–332, 1995.

30. Grijseels EWM, Deckers JW, Hoes AW, et al: Implementation of a pre-hospital decision rule in general practice. Triage of patients with suspected myocardial infarction, *Eur Heart J* 17:89–95, 1996.

31. Gurfinkel E, Bozovich G, Cerda M, et al: Time significance of acute thrombotic reactant markers in patients with and without silent myocardial ischemia and overt unstable angina pectoris, *Am J Cardiol* 76:121–124, 1995.

32. An international randomized trial comparing four thrombolytic strategies for acute myocardial infarction. The GUSTO Investigators, *N Engl J Med* 329:673–682, 1993.

33. Hakki A-H, Iskandrian AS, Kane SA, et al: Thallium-201 myocardial scintigraphy and left ventricular function at rest in patients with rest angina pectoris, *Am Heart J* 108:326–332, 1984.

34. Haronian HL, Remetz MS, Sinusas AJ, et al: Myocardial risk area defined by technetium-99m sestamibi imaging during percutaneous transluminal coronary angioplasty: comparison with coronary angiography, *J Am Coll Cardiol* 22:1033–1043, 1993.

35. Henneman PL, Mena IG, Rothstein RJ, et al: Evaluation of patients with chest pain and nondiagnostic ECG using thallium-201 myocardial planar imaging and technetium-99m first-pass radionuclide angiography in the emergency department, *Ann Emerg Med* 21:545–550, 1992.

36. Herlitz J, Hjalmarson A, Karlson BW, et al: Long-term morbidity in patients where the initial suspicion of myocardial infarction was not confirmed, *Clin Cardiol* 11:209–214, 1988.

37. Hilton TC, Fulmer H, Abuan T, et al: Ninety-day follow-up of patients in the emergency department with chest pain who undergo initial single-photon emission computed tomographic perfusion scintigraphy with technetium 99m-labeled sestamibi, *J Nucl Cardiol* 3:308–311, 1996.

38. Hilton TC, Thompson RC, Williams HJ, et al: Technetium-99m sestamibi myocardial perfusion imaging in the emergency room evaluation of chest pain, *J Am Coll Cardiol* 23:1016–1022, 1994.

39. Hoekstra JW, Gibler WB, Levy RC, et al: Emergency-department diagnosis of acute myocardial infarction and ischemia: a cost analysis of two diagnostic protocols, *Acad Emerg Med* 1:103–110, 1994.

40. Hofgren C, Karlson BW, Gaston-Johansson F, et al: Word descriptors in suspected acute myocardial infarction: a comparison between patients with and without confirmed myocardial infarction, *Heart Lung* 23:397–403, 1994.

41. Horowitz RS, Morganroth J, Parrotto C, et al: Immediate diagnosis of acute myocardial infarction by two-dimensional echocardiography, *Circulation* 65:323–329, 1982.

42. Ingram DA, Fulton RA, Portal RW, et al: Vomiting as a diagnostic aid in acute ischaemic cardiac pain, *Br Med J* 281:636–637, 1980.

43. Jayes RL Jr, Beshansky JR, D'Agostino RB, et al: Do patients' coronary risk factor reports predict acute cardiac ischemia in the emergency department? A multicenter study, *J Clin Epidemiol* 45:621–626, 1992.

44. Jeroudi MO, Cherif J, Habib GB, et al: Prolonged wall motion abnormalities after chest pain at rest in patients with unstable angina: a possible manifestation of myocardial stunning, *Am Heart J* 127:1241–1250, 1994.

45. Jonsbu J, Rollag A, Aase O, et al: Rapid and correct diagnosis of myocardial infarction: standardized case history and clinical examination provide important information for correct referral to monitored beds, *J Intern Med* 229:143–149, 1991.

46. Kanda T, Hirao Y, Oshima S, et al: Interleukin-8 as a sensitive marker of unstable coronary artery disease, *Am J Cardiol* 77:304–307, 1996.

47. Kannel WB, Abbott RD: Incidence and prognosis of unrecognized myocardial infarction. An update on the Framingham Study, *N Engl J Med* 311:1144–1147, 1984.

48. Karlson BW, Herlitz J, Pettersson P, et al: One-year prognosis in patients hospitalized with a history of unstable angina pectoris, *Clin Cardiol* 16:397–402, 1993.

49. Katus HA, Remppis A, Neumann FJ, et al: Diagnostic efficiency of troponin T measurements in acute myocardial infarction, *Circulation* 83:902–912, 1991.

50. Kayden DS, Mattera JA, Zaret BL, et al: Demonstration of reperfusion after thrombolysis with technetium-99m isonitrile myocardial imaging, *J Nucl Med* 29:1865–1867, 1988.

51. Kilpatrick WS, Wosornu D, McGuinness JB, et al: Early diagnosis of acute myocardial infarction: CK-MB and myoglobin compared, *Ann Clin Biochem* 30(Pt 5):435–438, 1993.

52. Kjoller E, Nielsen SL, Carlsen J, et al: Impact of immediate and delayed myocardial scintigraphy on therapeutic decisions in suspected acute myocardial infarction, *Eur Heart J* 16:909–913, 1995.

53. Kontos MC, Arrowood JA, Paulsen WH, et al: Early echocardiography can predict cardiac events in emergency department patients with chest pain, *Ann Emerg Med* 31:550–557, 1998.

54. Kragel AH, Gertz SD, Roberts WC: Morphologic comparison of frequency and types of acute lesions in the major epicardial coronary arteries in unstable angina pectoris, sudden coronary death and acute myocardial infarction, *J Am Coll Cardiol* 18:801–808, 1991.

55. Laji K, Wilkinson P, Ranjadayalan K, et al: Prognosis in acute myocardial infarction: comparison of patients with diagnostic and nondiagnostic electrocardiograms, *Am Heart J* 130:705–710, 1995.

56. Launbjerg J, Fruergaard P, Madsen JK, et al: Three-year mortality in patients suspected of acute myocardial infarction with and without confirmed diagnosis. The Danish Study Group on Verapamil in Myocardial Infarction, *Am Heart J* 122:1270–1273, 1991.

57. Lee TH, Cook EF, Weisberg M, et al: Acute chest pain in the emergency room. Identification and examination of low-risk patients, *Arch Intern Med* 145:65–69, 1985.

58. Lee TH, Rouan GW, Weisberg MC, et al: Clinical characteristics and natural history of patients with acute myocardial infarction sent home from the emergency room, *Am J Cardiol* 60:219–224, 1987.

59. Lieberman AN, Weiss JL, Jugdutt BI, et al: Two-dimensional echocardiography and infarct size: relationship of regional wall motion and thickening to the extent of myocardial infarction in the dog, *Circulation* 63:739–746, 1981.

60. Lindahl B, Venge P, Wallentin L: Relation between troponin T and the risk of subsequent cardiac events in unstable coronary artery disease. The FRISC Study Group, *Circulation* 93:1651–1657, 1996.

61. Little WC: Angiographic assessment of the culprit coronary artery lesion before acute myocardial infarction, *Am J Cardiol* 66:44G–47G, 1990.

62. Little WC, Constantinescu M, Applegate RJ, et al: Can coronary angiography predict the site of a subsequent myocardial infarction in patients with mild-to-moderate coronary artery disease? *Circulation* 78(5 Pt 1):1157–1166, 1988.

63. Liuzzo G, Biasucci LM, Gallimore JR, et al: The prognostic value of C-reactive protein and serum amyloid a protein in severe unstable angina, *N Engl J Med* 331:417–424, 1994.

64. Lopes MG, Spivack AP, Harrison DC, et al: Prognosis in coronary care unit noninfarction cases, *JAMA* 228:1558–1562, 1974.

65. Mace SE: Thallium myocardial scanning in the emergency department evaluation of chest pain, *Am J Emerg Med* 7:321–328, 1989.

66. Mach F, Lovis C, Chevrolet J-C, et al: Rapid bedside whole blood cardiospecific troponin T immunoassay for the diagnosis of acute myocardial infarction, *Am J Cardiol* 75:842–845, 1995.

67. Margolis JR, Kannel WB, Feinleib M, et al: Clinical features of unrecognized myocardial infarction—silent and symptomatic. Eighteen year follow-up: the Framingham Study, *Am J Cardiol* 32:1–7, 1973.

68. Marin MM, Teichman SL: Use of rapid serial sampling of creatine kinase MB for very early detection of myocardial infarction in patients with acute chest pain, *Am Heart J* 123:354–361, 1992.

69. Marshall SA, Picard MH, Ray PA, et al: Ventricular morphology and function in acute non Q-wave myocardial infarction, *Circulation* 82:III–73, 1993.

70. Marwick TH, Nemec JJ, Pashkow FJ, Accuracy and limitations of exercise echocardiography in a routine clinical setting, *J Am Coll Cardiol* 19:74–81, 1992.

71. McCarthy BD, Beshansky JR, D'Agostino RB, et al: Missed diagnoses of acute myocardial infarction in the emergency department: results from a multicenter study, *Ann Emerg Med* 22:579–582, 1993.

72. Medalie JH, Goldbourt U: Unrecognized myocardial infarction: five-year incidence, mortality, and risk factors, *Ann Intern Med* 84:526–531, 1976.

73. Medina R, Panidis IP, Morganroth J, et al: The value of echocardiographic regional wall motion abnormalities in detecting coronary artery disease in patients with or without a dilated left ventricle, *Am Heart J* 109:799–803, 1985.

74. Metcalfe MJ, Rawles JM, Shirreffs C, et al: Six year follow up of a consecutive series of patients presenting to the coronary care unit with acute chest pain: prognostic importance of the electrocardiogram, *Br Heart J* 63:267–272, 1990.

75. Nicholson CS, Roberts CS, Tatum JL, et al: A systematic approach to the evaluation of chest pain in the emergency department: a prospective risk assessment and treatment protocol based on patient presentation, ECG and rest technetium-99m sestamibi, *J Am Coll Cardiol* 25:211A, 1995.

76. Nicholson CS, Tatum JL, Jesse RL, et al: The value of gated tomographic Tc-99m sestamibi perfusion imaging in acute ischemic syndromes, *J Nucl Cardiol* 2:S57, 1995.

77. Nieuwenhuizen W: Soluble fibrin as a molecular marker for a pre-thrombotic state: a mini-review, *Blood Coagul Fibrinolysis* 4:93–96, 1993.

78. Nixon JV, Brown CN, Smitherman TC: Identification of transient and persistent segmental wall motion abnormalities in patients with unstable angina by two-dimensional echocardiography, *Circulation* 65:1497–1503, 1982.

79. Nyman I, Areskog M, Areskog N-H, et al: Very early risk stratification by electrocardiogram at rest in men with suspected unstable coronary heart disease. The RISC Study Group, *J Intern Med* 234:293–301, 1993.

80. Pandian NG, Skorton DJ, Collins SM, et al: Myocardial infarct size threshold for two-dimensional echocardiographic detection: sensitivity of systolic wall thickening and endocardial motion abnormalities in small versus large infarcts, *Am J Cardiol* 55:551–555, 1985.

81. Peels CH, Visser CA, Kupper AJ, et al: Usefulness of two-dimensional echocardiography for immediate detection of myocardial ischemia in the emergency room, *Am J Cardiol* 65:687–691, 1990.

82. Pelberg AL: Missed myocardial infarction in the emergency room, *Qual Assur Util Rev* 4:39–42, 1989.

83. Pettersson T, Ohlsson O, Tryding N: Increased CKMB (mass concentration) in patients without traditional evidence of acute myocardial infarction. A risk indicator of coronary death, *Eur Heart J* 13:1387–1392, 1992.

84. Phadke KV, Phillips RA, Clarke DT, et al: Anticardiolipin antibodies in ischaemic heart disease: marker or myth? *Br Heart J* 69:391–394, 1993.

85. Pozen MW, D'Agostino RB, Selker HP, et al: A predictive instrument to improve coronary-care-unit admission practices in acute ischemic heart disease. A prospective multicenter trial, *N Engl J Med* 310:1273–1278, 1984.

86. Puleo PR, Meyer D, Wathen C, et al: Use of a rapid assay of subforms of creatine kinase-MB to diagnose or rule out acute myocardial infarction, *N Engl J Med* 331:561–566, 1994.

87. Qiu S, Theroux P, Marcil M, et al: Plasma endothelin-1 levels in stable and unstable angina, *Cardiology* 82:12–19, 1993.

88. Rabitzsch G, Mair J, Lechleitner P, et al: Isoenzyme BB of glycogen phosphorylase b and myocardial infarction, *Lancet* 341:1032–1033, 1993.

89. Radensky PW, Hilton TC, Fulmer H, et al: Potential cost effectiveness of initial myocardial perfusion imaging for assessment of emergency department patients with chest pain, *Am J Cardiol* 79:595–599, 1997.

90. Ravkilde J, Nissen H, Horder M, et al: Independent prognostic value of serum creatine kinase isoenzyme MB mass, cardiac troponin T and myosin light chain levels in suspected acute myocardial infarction. Analysis of 28 months of follow-up in 196 patients; *J Am Coll Cardiol* 25:574–581, 1995.

91. Richardson PD, Davies MJ, Born GV: Influence of plaque configuration and stress distribution on fissuring of coronary atherosclerotic plaques, *Lancet* 2:941–944, 1989.

92. Ritchie JL, Williams DL, Harp G, et al: Transaxial tomography with thallium-201 for detecting remote myocardial infarction. Comparison with planar imaging; *Am J Cardiol* 50:1236–1241, 1982.

93. Romhilt DW, Adolph RJ, Sodd VJ, et al: Cesium-129 myocardial scintigraphy to detect myocardial infarction, *Circulation* 48:1242–1251, 1973.

94. Rouan GW, Hedges JR, Toltzis R, et al: A chest pain clinic to improve the follow-up of patients released from an urban university teaching hospital emergency department, *Ann Emerg Med* 16:1145–1150, 1987.

95. Rouan GW, Lee TH, Cook EF, et al: Clinical characteristics and outcome of acute myocardial infarction in patients with initially normal or nonspecific electrocardiograms (a report from the Multicenter Chest Pain Study), *Am J Cardiol* 64:1087–1092, 1989.

96. Rouleau JL, Talajic M, Sussex B, et al: Myocardial infarction patients in the 1990s—their risk factors, stratification and survival in Canada: the Canadian Assessment of Myocardial Infarction (CAMI) Study, *J Am Coll Cardiol* 27:1119–1127, 1996.

97. Rusnak RA, Stair TO, Hansen KN, et al: Litigation against the emergency physician: common features in cases of missed myocardial infarction, *Ann Emerg Med* 18:1029–1034, 1989.

98. Sabia PJ, Afrookteh A, Touchstone DA, et al: Value of regional wall motion abnormality in the emergency room diagnosis of acute myocardial infarction. A prospective study using two-dimensional echocardiography, *Circulation* 84(3 Suppl):I85–I92, 1991.

99. Sawe U: Pain in acute myocardial infarction. A study of 137 patients in a coronary care unit, *Acta Med Scand* 190:79–81, 1971.

100. Schroeder JS, Lamb IH, Hu M: Do patients in whom myocardial infarction has been ruled out have a better prognosis after hospitalization than those surviving infarction? *N Engl J Med* 303:1–5, 1980.

101. Serneri GGN, Abbate R, Gori AM, et al: Transient intermittent lymphocyte activation is responsible for the instability of angina, *Circulation* 86:790–797, 1992.

102. Sigurdsson E, Thorgeirsson G, Sigvaldason H, et al: Unrecognized myocardial infarction: epidemiology, clinical characteristics, and the prognostic role of angina pectoris. The Reykjavik Study, *Ann Intern Med* 122:96–102, 1995.

103. Sirois JG, Pimentel L: Prognostic value of the emergency department for in-hospital complications of acute myocardial infarction, *Ann Emerg Med* 22:1568–1572, 1993.

104. Smitherman TC, Osborn RC Jr, Narahara KA: Serial myocardial scintigraphy after a single dose of thallium-201 in men after acute myocardial infarction, *Am J Cardiol* 42:177–182, 1978.

105. Stein JH, Neumann A, Preston LM, et al: Admission echocardiography predicts in-hospital cardiac events in patients with unstable angina, *J Am Coll Cardiol* 27:377A, 1996.

106. Stowers SA, Abuan TH, Syzmanski TJ, et al: Technetium-99m sestamibi SPECT and technetium-99m tetrofosmin SPECT in prediction of cardiac events in patients injected during chest pain and following resolution of pain, *J Nucl Med* 36:88P–89P, 1995 (abstract).

107. Tamaki S, Kambara H, Kadota K, et al: Improved detection of myocardial infarction by emission computed tomography with thallium-201. Relation to infarct size, *Br Heart J* 52:621–627, 1984.

108. Tatum JL, Jesse RL, Kontos MC, et al: A comprehensive strategy for the evaluation and triage of the chest pain patient, *Ann Emerg Med* 29:116–125, 1997.

109. Tatum JL, Ornato JP, Jesse RL, et al: A diagnostic strategy using Tc-99m sestamibi for evaluation of patients with chest pain in the emergency room, *Circulation* 90:I367, 1994.

110. Tierney WM, Fitzgerald J, McHenry R, et al: Physicians' estimates of the probability of myocardial infarction in emergency room patients with chest pain, *Med Decis Making* 6:12–17, 1986.

111. Tierney WM, Roth BJ, Psaty B, et al: Predictors of myocardial infarction in emergency room patients, *Crit Care Med* 13:526–531, 1985.

112. Effects of tissue plasminogen activator and a comparison of early invasive and conservative strategies in unstable angina and non-Q-wave myocardial infarction. Results of the TIMI III B trial. Thrombolysis in Myocardial Ischemia, *Circulation* 89:1545–1556, 1994.

113. Ting HH, Lee TH, Soukup JR, et al: Impact of physician experience on triage of emergency room patients with acute chest pain at three teaching hospitals, *Am J Med* 91:401–407, 1991.

114. Tosteson AN, Goldman L, Udvarhelyi IS, et al: Cost-effectiveness of a coronary care unit versus an intermediate care unit for emergency department patients with chest pain, *Circulation* 94:143–150, 1996.

115. Tsuji R, Tanaka T, Sohmiya K, et al: Human heart-type cytoplasmic fatty acid-binding protein in serum and urine during hyperacute myocardial infarction, *Int J Cardiol* 41:209–217, 1993.

116. van der Wieken LR, Kan G, Belfer AJ, et al: Thallium-201 scanning to decide CCU admission in patients with non-diagnostic electrocardiograms, *Int J Cardiol* 4:285–295, 1983.

117. van Miltenburg-van Zijl AJ, Simoons ML, Veerhoek RJ, et al: Incidence and follow-up of Braunwald subgroups in unstable angina pectoris, *J Am Coll Cardiol* 25:1286–1292, 1995.

118. Varetto T, Cantalupi D, Altieri A, et al: Emergency room technetium-99m sestamibi imaging to rule out acute myocardial ischemic events in patients with nondiagnostic electrocardiograms, *J Am Coll Cardiol* 22:1804–1808, 1993.

119. Verani MS, Jeroudi MO, Mahmarian JJ, et al: Quantification of myocardial infarction during coronary occlusion and myocardial salvage after reperfusion using cardiac imaging with technetium-99m hexakis 2-methoxyisobutyl isonitrile, *J Am Coll Cardiol* 12:1573–1581, 1988.

120. Wackers FJ: Thrombolytic therapy for myocardial infarction: assessment of efficacy by myocardial perfusion imaging with technetium-99m sestamibi, *Am J Cardiol* 66:36E–41E, 1992.

121. Wackers FJ: The role of emergency radionuclide imaging in the evaluation of patients with acute chest pain syndromes, *Q J Nucl Med* 41:39–43.

122. Wackers FJ, Sokole EB, Samson G, et al: Value and limitations of thallium-201 scintigraphy in the acute phase of myocardial infarction, *N Engl J Med* 295:1–5, 1976.

123. Wackers FJ, Gibbons RJ, Verani MS, et al: Serial quantitative planar technetium-99m isonitrile imaging in acute myocardial infarction: efficacy for noninvasive assessment of thrombolytic therapy, *J Am Coll Cardiol* 14:861–873, 1989.

124. Wackers FJ, Lie KI, Liem KL, et al: Thallium-201 scintigraphy in unstable angina pectoris, *Circulation* 57:738–742, 1978.

125. Wackers FJ, Lie KI, Liem KL, et al: Potential value of thallium-201 scintigraphy as a means of selecting patients for the coronary care unit, *Br Heart J* 41:111–117, 1979.

126. Wackers FJ, Schoot JB, Sokole EB, et al: Noninvasive visualization of acute myocardial infarction in man with thallium-201, *Br Heart J* 37:741–744, 1975.

127. Whal JM, Hakki A-H, Iskandrian AS, et al: Scintigraphic characterization of Q wave and non-Q-wave acute myocardial infarction, *Am Heart J* 109:769–775, 1985.

128. Weaver WD, Cerqueira M, Hallstrom AP, et al: Prehospital-initiated vs hospital-initiated thrombolytic therapy. The Myocardial Infarction Triage and Intervention Trial, *JAMA* 270:1211–1216, 1993.

129. Weiss JL, Bulkley BH, Hutchins GM, Mason SJ: Two-dimensional echocardiographic recognition of myocardial injury in man: comparison with postmortem studies, *Circulation* 63:401–408, 1981.

130. Weissman IA, Dickinson CZ, Dworkin HJ, et al: Cost-effectiveness of myocardial perfusion imaging with SPECT in the emergency department evaluation of patients with unexplained chest pain, *Radiology* 199:353–357, 1996.

131. Woolf N, Davies MJ: *Interrelationship between atherosclerosis and thrombosis.* In Fuster V, Verstraete M, eds: *Thrombosis in cardiovascular disorders.* Philadelphia, 1992, W.B. Saunders Company.

132. Wu AH, Lane PL: Metaanalysis in clinical chemistry: validation of cardiac troponin T as a marker for ischemic heart diseases, *Clin Chem* 41:1228–1233, 1995.

133. Yano K, MacLean CJ: The incidence and prognosis of unrecognized myocardial infarction in the Honolulu, Hawaii, Heart Program, *Arch Intern Med* 149:1528–1532, 1989.

134. Young GP, Green TR: The role of single ECG, creatine kinase, and CKMB in diagnosing patients with acute chest pain, *Am J Emerg Med* 11:444–449, 1993.

135. Zalenski RJ, Sloan EP, Chen EH, et al: The emergency department ECG and immediately life-threatening complications in initially uncomplicated suspected myocardial ischemia, *Ann Emerg Med* 17:221–226, 1988.

136. Zareba W, Moss AJ, Raubertas RF: Risk of subsequent cardiac events in stable convalescing patients after first non-Q-wave and Q-wave myocardial infarction: the limited role of non-invasive testing. The Multicenter Myocardial Ischemia Research Group, 5:1009–1018, 1994.

137. Zarling EJ, Sexton H, Milnor PJ: Failure to diagnose acute myocardial infarction. The clinicopathologic experience at the large community hospital, *JAMA* 250:1177–1181, 1983.

Chapter 28

Risk stratification in unstable angina pectoris

D. Douglas Miller

Current understanding of the pathophysiology and natural history of unstable angina suggests that the therapeutic window of opportunity is narrow and that reducing delays from admission to the institution where aggressive therapy is given greatly influences mortality and morbidity. Whereas stable angina is characterized by myocardial ischemia secondary to obstructive coronary artery disease, acute ischemic syndromes (including unstable angina) result from an abrupt reduction in coronary flow, frequently after atherosclerotic plaque disruption and with or without associated thrombosis or vasospasm.[15] This rapidly evolving pathophysiology contributes to the labile clinical course of unstable angina, which accelerates clinical decisions often made on the basis of acute studies designed to document myocardial ischemia. Subsequent management generally results in the medical stabilization of patients before performance of diagnostic testing.

Nuclear cardiology studies and, in particular, myocardial perfusion imaging are well established as powerful noninvasive tools for detecting and assessing the severity of stable coronary artery disease and for defining its consequences within the spectrum of chronic or acute ischemic syndromes, including unstable angina pectoris. Many of the principles derived from the application of myocardial perfusion imaging in the setting of acute myocardial infarction have also been successfully applied in the evaluation of unstable angina patients.

Previous myocardial imaging studies of unstable angina have focused on two important areas: 1) the objective demonstration of myocardial ischemia in patients with the clinical syndrome of acute coronary insufficiency in whom ischemic electrocardiographic changes are absent or are obscured by baseline electrocardiographic abnormalities, and 2) the predischarge evaluation of patients with stabilized unstable angina to detect those at the greatest risk for short-term and long-term cardiac events. Of interest, not all patients within the broadly defined clinical syndrome of unstable angina are found to be at increased risk for future cardiac events. Thus, not all patients tested in the context of this diverse clinical entity require special testing. However, among appropriately selected patients in the settings of acute triage and in-hospital risk stratification, the information derived from a nuclear cardiology study can answer unresolved clinical questions and aid in subsequent patient management. Specifically, the presence, location, and extent of ischemically jeopardized myocardium detected during spontaneously occurring acute chest pain or controlled stress testing is an important determinant of 1) the need for admission to an intensive care monitoring unit, 2) the need for and urgency of coronary angiography, and 3) the appropriate use of percutaneous or surgical coronary revascularization procedures.

Although published nuclear cardiology studies are frequently subject to patient selection bias because they often enroll nonconsecutive series of patients with medically stabilized unstable angina from which the most acutely ischemic patients have already been culled, their results have been remarkably consistent. Regardless of the imaging technique or type of stress (exercise or pharmacologic) used, the presence of a reversible myocardial perfusion defect reproducibly identifies a population at more than 20% risk for a subsequent ischemic cardiac event (Table 28-1). Patients without this risk marker have a 1% to 2% risk for a serious adverse outcome. Thus, on the basis of results of acute or predischarge myocardial imaging studies, a clinically useful greater than 10-fold risk differential can be assigned in unstable angina patients with a low to intermediate pretest risk for cardiac events.

Clinical practice guidelines[45] and critical pathways[10] have been developed by national expert panels and health care delivery networks to guide physicians in the appropriate use of expensive medical resources among the large population of pa-

Table 28-1. Unstable angina cardiac event rates—comparison with exercise thallium-201 studies*

Study	Patients	Isotope (imaging technique)	Cardiac event rate	
			Normal scan	Reversible defect
	n			n/n (%)
Madsen et al[30]	158	Thallium (planar)	2/97 (2)	6/29 (21)†
Brown[7]	52	Thallium (planar)	0/15 (0)	6/23 (26)†
Stratmann et al[42]	127	Single-photon emission computed tomography (SPECT)	1/52 (2)	9/41 (22)†

*SPECT = single-photon emission computed tomography
†p < 0.05 vs normal scan

tients presenting with unstable angina pectoris. Although data bearing directly on this issue are limited, these guidelines recommend stress myocardial perfusion imaging for risk assessment of patients with unstable angina patients.

EVOLVING CONCEPTS

Although the degree of risk separation afforded by existing myocardial perfusion imaging studies has traditionally been considered a sufficient criterion for the widespread adoption of any prognostic method, the current health care market places additional demands on potential testing strategies. The standard of care "bar" is constantly being raised by market and medicolegal forces. Prospective studies evaluating the impact of noninvasive testing on patient outcomes within predefined cohorts, treated according to preset and carefully controlled clinical management matrices, would help to validate the existing retrospectively acquired data. In this highly competitive milieu, future studies must critically evaluate the role of nuclear testing strategies for their incremental value compared to the clinical information that is readily available[33] and their cost-effectiveness compared with alternative invasive and noninvasive diagnostic approaches within a proposed management algorithm.

To be maximally cost-effective, a test or treatment should be delivered to patients only when it can be expected to improve on patient outcomes (that is, "when it counts"). In this context, few clinicians doubt the clinical value of early coronary angiography and prophylactic coronary revascularization in patients with truly unstable ("hot") angina who are clearly at high risk for early coronary events. However, compared with more conservative strategies, coronary revascularization in subsets of lower-risk patients with unstable angina may not improve outcomes, even in patients with predischarge evidence of myocardial ischemia,[28] and may dilute the benefits of revascularization by exposing patients to greater procedural risk.[25]

Noninvasive myocardial imaging studies may prove to be of greatest value in the accurate selection of patients for aggressive treatment from the population of patients with clinically undeclared or medically stabilized unstable angina. Future investigations of the cost-effectiveness of test-driven medical or interventional management strategies designed to improve the outcomes of patients with unstable angina must be a priority.

Finally, when considering the cost-effectiveness of a prognostic tool such as myocardial perfusion imaging, particularly when applied in a capitated managed health care system, test performance characteristics assume preeminence. Alternative testing methods, such as echocardiography, should be compared head-to-head with nuclear perfusion imaging for test performance characteristics, including 24-hour-per-day access to testing, technical support requirements, and data quality and reproducibility. Nowhere are these test performance factors more crucial than in the evaluation of patients with acute chest pain syndromes, a clinical population that, by definition, is at high risk for early adverse cardiac events if myocardial ischemia goes undetected and untreated.

CLINICAL DEFINITION AND PATHOPHYSIOLOGY

Unstable angina represents a heterogeneous spectrum of clinical entities between chronic stable angina and acute myocardial infarction.[40] Clinical classifications for unstable angina have been proposed to aid in management and risk stratification. Subsets include acceleration of exertional angina without electrocardiographic changes (class IA), acceleration of exertional angina with electrocardiographic changes (class IB), new-onset exertional angina (class II), new-onset rest angina (class III), and protracted rest angina with electrocardiographic changes (class IV). Previous studies have demonstrated a significant trend toward increasing cardiac events from class I to class IV.[40] Class IV patients have the highest risk for in-hospital adverse events (43%).

Within this heterogeneous clinical population, the degree of underlying coronary artery disease varies considerably.[1] A relatively small percentage of patients with unstable angina remain refractory to in-hospital medical therapy; these patients should undergo urgent coronary angiography and appropriate revascularization. However, most patients stabilize with medical therapy and should therefore only undergo coronary angiography when clinical risk markers or noninvasive testing results suggest significant underlying myocardial ischemic jeopardy.

The pathophysiology of unstable angina has been extensively studied in recent years, providing clues on how to optimize the early diagnosis and risk stratification of patients with this syndrome.[15] In vivo studies have shown the importance of platelet deposition by using indium-111–labeled platelets to image sites of plaque rupture.[32] The underlying plaque is now recognized to be a lipid-laden, macrophage-rich lesion that ruptures secondary to excessive local stresses on the tensile strength of the lesion.[29] Although the angiographic findings in unstable angina have been characterized,[3] the occurrence of plaque rupture cannot be predicted by coronary angiography. However, the consequences of plaque rupture, thrombus formation, and flow deterioration may be detected with scintigraphic techniques.

Plaque rupture is associated with several biochemical and cellular reactions, including the release of troponin T,[26] liberation of inflammatory C-reactive protein and amyloid A,[27] and associated impairment of endothelial vasodilator function, as reflected by circulating endothelin-1 levels.[52] Increased serum levels of these byproducts of plaque rupture have been associated with an increased risk for future cardiac events, including acute myocardial infarction and refractory angina with electrocardiographic changes requiring revascularization. Increased levels of troponin T may be measured within 24 hours of unstable angina and are independently predictive of adverse events compared with clinical risk markers in a multivariate analysis.[26] Low levels of inflammatory proteins are associated with a decreased risk for in-hospital ischemic events and urgent revascularization.[27] These rapidly available and relatively inexpensive biochemical markers have not been compared with noninvasive imaging studies for their predictive value.

CLINICAL RISK ASSESSMENT

Although the incremental value of nuclear imaging compared with clinical risk markers has been amply demonstrated in patients with stable angina, similar data are not yet available for cohorts with unstable angina. Previous studies of Holter electrocardiographic monitoring in patients with acute ischemic syndromes indicate that an increased short-term risk is associated with objective Holter electrocardiographic evidence of myocardial ischemia (ST depression) compared with clinical risk assessment alone.[9] These data suggest that more sensitive and specific myocardial perfusion imaging studies would also provide incremental value for prognostication over a clinical risk assessment alone. However, the relative or incremental predictive value of scintigraphic data compared with clinical, electrocardiographic, and angiographic risk markers has not yet been evaluated in unstable angina patients.

Holter electrocardiography shows that the severity of angina pectoris predicts in-hospital coronary events more accurately than clinical markers do; electrocardiographic ischemia lasting 60 minutes or more per 24 hours was more predictive of coronary events and high-risk coronary anatomy than was recurrent chest pain after admission.[9] A prehospital study of clinical triage compared with resting electrocardiographic analysis in a community hospital demonstrated that electrocardiographic findings were more predictive of acute coronary pathology than was a clinical assessment by general practitioners.[18] Emergency department assessment of clinical[40] and resting electrocardiographic[37] findings has been associated with future severe cardiac events. Specifically, patients with a normal electrocardiogram have 1-year risk for ST elevation of 8%, an 18% risk for ST depression, and a 26% risk for ST elevation and depression.[37] The site of ST changes does not significantly discriminate the future risk for cardiac events (anterior compared with inferior electrocardiographic leads).

The clinical correlates of patients with unstable angina without critical arterial narrowing have been described[12] and include female sex, nonwhite race, and the absence of ST segment deviation on the presenting electrocardiogram. The prognosis of patients with unstable angina without critical coronary obstruction (no stenosis >70% in luminal diameter) is excellent; only 2% of patients die or have myocardial infarction compared with 18% of patients who have at least one critical obstruction. According to the Braunwald classification of unstable angina,[47] among 417 consecutive patients with suspected unstable angina, multivariable analysis demonstrated that advanced age, male sex, hypertension, postinfarction chest pain, and maximal intravenous medical therapy were independent predictors of subsequent cardiac death. Acute angina at rest and electrocardiographic ST changes during chest pain and maximal therapy were associated with reduced infarct-free survival in patients who did not receive early and appropriate interventional treatment. Additional clinical prognostic indices in unstable angina pectoris include recurrent resting pain, previous angina, diabetes, and transient or evolutionary T-wave changes on the admission electrocardiogram.[21]

These studies indicate that unstable angina clinical classifications are highly predictive of in-hospital adverse cardiac events and may have potential value for acute triage decisions about hospital admission and the intensity of early therapy.[40] Risk stratification, when performed according to these strict clinical criteria, is a useful tool for patient selection in clinical trials and for the evaluation of treatment strategies.[47] Although it is not definitive, the early clinical stratification of patients with unstable angina assists clinicians in the early management and treatment of this difficult condition.[21] Noninvasive testing, including Holter electrocardiography and acute myocardial perfusion imaging,[4,19] refines the risk stratification of unstable angina patients compared with clinical assessment and resting electrocardiographic analysis alone.

EMERGENCY IMAGING STUDIES

An aggressive new mindset has developed in the emergency management of patients with acute chest pain. Early coronary artery disease diagnosis and the accelerated risk stratification of patients with chest pain is increasingly viewed as cost-effective. Early and accurate identification of patients with the greatest plaque instability or multivessel coronary disease theoretically facilitates more appropriate acute triage and the prompt institution of aggressive therapy. Coronary angiography can provide much of this information but may not always be practical because of the associated time delays, procedural risks, and costs. The sole reliance on "low-technology" clinical and electrocardiographic assessments reduces the detection of serious ischemia and infarction,[24,31] leading to the inappropriate use of intensive care facilities by patients whose condition evolves to a nonischemic chest pain syndrome.[8,51]

Initial studies of thallium-201 myocardial imaging during

acute chest pain and unstable angina[14,50] showed diagnostic and prognostic promise but were limited by the suboptimal planar imaging characteristics of this radiotracer at rest. Data now support the utility of technetium-99m (^{99m}Tc) perfusion imaging during chest pain as a more accurate technique for detecting acute myocardial ischemia in the emergency department[19] or the coronary care unit.[4] Acute imaging studies during chest pain in patients with unstable angina have been correlated with predischarge angiographic findings. The initial scan results reflect the presence, number, and location of coronary arterial narrowings, accounting for the close relation observed between acute scintigraphic findings and rates of short-term cardiac events.[19,48] This approach seems to be of particular value in acute chest pain patients with nondiagnostic electrocardiographic findings or an uninterpretable electrocardiogram.

Whereas the long-term prognosis and potential benefits of coronary revascularization are closely related to the number and location of coronary stenoses, short-term risk is related to plaque instability, a variable that is not measurable with current noninvasive imaging techniques. Although the above approach has been widely tested for evaluation of patients with chest pain in the emergency department, it may also be used to assess patients with unstable angina admitted to the coronary care unit.[17] In this setting, ^{99m}Tc sestamibi perfusion imaging is three times more sensitive for detection of myocardial ischemia than 12-lead electrocardiography performed during chest pain (Fig. 28-1).

Recent developments underscore the clinical value of imaging studies in the emergency department. Tatum et al[43] demonstrated the safety and efficacy of a triage strategy that included immediate injection of ^{99m}Tc sestamibi on presentation to the emergency department in 1187 consecutive patients who had chest pain. At this urban tertiary referral hospital, each patient was assigned to one of five levels of clinical risk (level 1 = myocardial infarction; level 5 = non-cardiac chest pain) within 60 minutes of presentation. The early imaging study improved the sensitive detection of myocardial infarction and accomplished the sensitive (100%) and specific (78%) detection of myocardial infarction. Patients with an abnormal imaging study had a significantly higher relative risk for subsequent myocardial infarction or revascularization than did those with a normal imaging finding. During 1 year of follow-up, patients with a normal imaging study ($n = 338$) had a 3% rate of revascularization and no myocardial infarction or death. The negative predictive value of a normal imaging study in the emergency department was 97%. Rates of myocardial infarction and cardiac death in patients with an abnormal study were 11% and 8%, respectively.

Jesse and Kontos[20] developed a systematic approach to the use of cardiac imaging in addition to clinical evaluation and en-

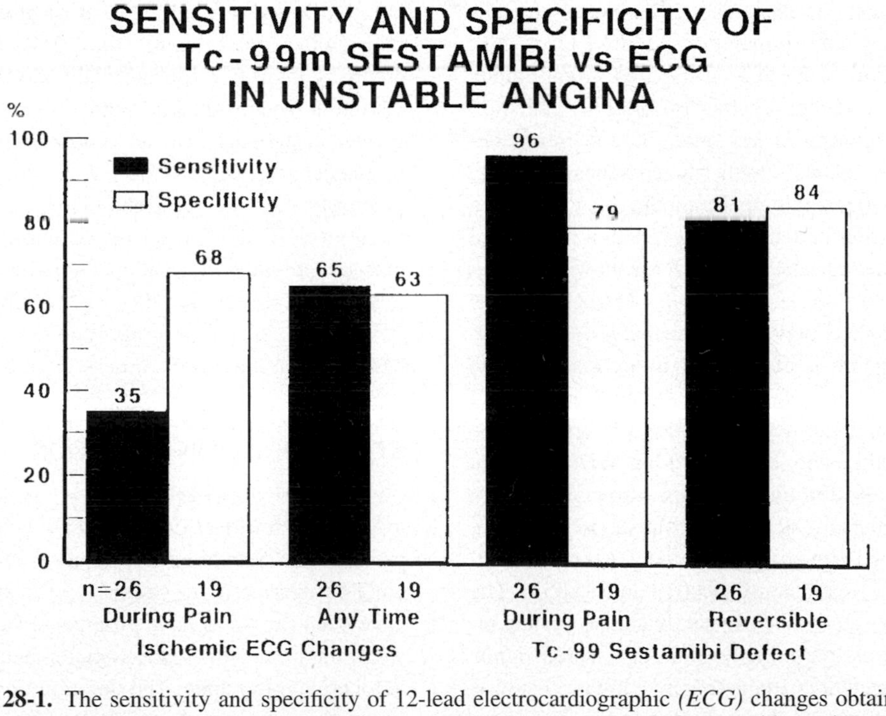

Fig. 28-1. The sensitivity and specificity of 12-lead electrocardiographic *(ECG)* changes obtained during chest pain or anytime during admission to the coronary care unit for unstable angina compared with similar measurements obtained with technetium-99m sestamibi myocardial tomography in the same patients. The sensitivity of a technetium-99m sestamibi perfusion defect or significant coronary artery disease was approximately three-fold greater than that of ischemic ST-segment depression on ECG during pain (96% compared with 35%). (From Varetto T, Cantalupi D, Altieri A, et al: Emergency room technetium-99m sestamibi imaging to rule out acute myocardial ischemic events in patients with nondiagnostic electrocardiograms, *J Am Coll Cardiol* 22:1804-1808, 1993. Reprinted with permission from the American College of Cardiology.)

zymatic studies in the population with acute chest pain. In their comprehensive chest pain evaluation program, patients at high risk are recommended for rapid therapy with thrombolytic agents or primary angioplasty; patients with unstable angina receive aspirin with heparin. Moderate-risk patients require further evaluation to rule out coronary disease and to manage co-morbid conditions before discharge. Low-risk patients can be discharged for further outpatient evaluation once the likelihood of an acute unstable coronary syndrome has been eliminated. The poor predictive accuracy of the history, physical examination, and electrocardiography for classifying subsequent risk in patients with chest pain and suspected acute coronary syndromes was reemphasized, as was the success rate of emergency department imaging studies with ^{99m}Tc radionuclide agents or echocardiography. As recommended by the Agency for Health Care Policy and Research guidelines, exercise or pharmacologic stress imaging should be included in the evaluation of intermediate-risk patients before discharge. On the basis of their literature review, the authors concluded that a careful systematic approach to the evaluation of chest pain can achieve cost-effectiveness and improve patient care.

Radensky et al[39] also addressed the potential cost-effectiveness of emergency room myocardial perfusion imaging in chest pain patients. Their study reemphasized the excellent short-term prognosis of patients with chest pain who had a normal imaging study, which can be a prelude to subsequent outpatient management and evaluation. Their cost-effectiveness models evaluated two strategies in this population. Model 1 used ^{99m}Tc sestamibi single-photon emission computed tomography (SPECT) as a decision point for whether to admit the patient to the hospital or discharge him or her from the emergency department. In the model, patients with normal scans were discharged and others were admitted. In model 2, no imaging study was performed, and patients were evaluated by clinical and electrocardiographic variables alone. Patients with at least three cardiac risk factors or an abnormal electrocardiogram were admitted, and other patients were discharged. When adverse events (death, nonfatal myocardial infarction, or acute coronary intervention) were evaluated for their frequency in terms of cost, it was apparent that the mean costs were greatest among hospital patients who experience an adverse event ($21,375 ± $2,733) compared with patients who could be discharged directly from the emergency department ($715 ± $71). The costs of the model 1 (imaging) and model 2 (no imaging) strategies did not differ significantly ($5,019 and $6,051). The authors concluded that a study that can safely and accurately indicate the need for admission to the hospital can accrue significant cost savings and that a trend towards lower cost was achieved with a strategy that includes ^{99m}Tc myocardial perfusion imaging in the emergency department.

Tosteson et al[44] also evaluated the cost-effectiveness of an intermediate care unit for the evaluation of patients presenting to the emergency department with chest pain compared with traditional care in a coronary care unit. When resource utiliza-tion was estimated on the basis of cost data from an elderly population of 901 of 12,139 patients, the incremental cost-effectiveness achieved by triage to a coronary care unit was shown to be cost-effective because of the higher earlier complication rate in this age group. The authors recommended that admission to the coronary care unit for patients with acute chest pain should be reserved for those with a moderate (>21%) probability of acute myocardial infarction in the absence of other clinical indications for admission to the intensive care unit. Intermediate care units were shown to be most appropriate for patients in whom the risk for myocardial infarction was less than 21%. The authors did not systematically discuss the role of cardiac imaging in the decision to use intermediate care units.

The recent U.S. Food and Drug Administration approval of ^{99m}Tc tetrofosmin for myocardial imaging has prompted its use in the evaluation of patients with chest pain in the emergency department. A multicenter study by Wackers et al[49] examined the clinical relevance of a missed diagnosis of myocardial infarction based on electrocardiographic and chest pain assessment alone in 357 patients undergoing ^{99m}Tc tetrofosmin imaging in the emergency department. These patients were subsequently followed for 30 days for in-hospital events. The result of tetrofosmin imaging was normal in 295 patients (83%) with a nondiagnostic or normal electrocardiogram obtained during chest pain. All patients were admitted for further studies to rule out myocardial infarction. Treating physicians were blinded of the results of the imaging study. The rate of cardiac death and recurring infarction (primary end point) and coronary revascularization (secondary end point) was found to be significantly greater in patients with an abnormal result on emergency department tetrofosmin SPECT than in those with normal or non-diagnostic electrocardiogram (21% and 2% for myo-cardial infarction; 23% and 7% for revascularization; $P < 0.02$ for both events compared with patients who had normal scans). No patient died in this study. Thus, the widely demonstrated value of ^{99m}Tc sestamibi seems to apply to the use of other technetium-based myocardial perfusion agents in this setting.

ALTERNATIVE NONINVASIVE RISK STRATIFICATION METHODS

Various noninvasive testing alternatives have been applied to the risk stratification of patients with unstable angina. The presence and duration (≥60 minutes) of silent myocardial ischemia as measured by Holter electrocardiographic monitoring have been shown to have prognostic value in patients with unstable angina.[22] This value is incremental over that provided by coronary angiography. The duration of the ST shift and the angiographic severity of coronary artery disease are independent predictors of myocardial infarction or death.[22] In the presence of these two variables, left ventricular function does not have independent prognostic value. In this and previous small series of patients with unstable angina, 60 minutes or more of ST shift in 24 hours has been shown to be more predictive of cardiac events and high-risk coronary anatomy than is abnormal left ventricular function[22] or the severity of angina.[9]

Among men undergoing predischarge symptom-limited exercise testing, the presence of stress-induced ST depression provided additional prognostic information about the long-term risk for recurrent angina and coronary events compared with ST shifts on predischarge Holter examination.[23] Ischemia is detected less frequently in women than men undergoing 24-hour Holter electrocardiographic monitoring[35] after an acute coronary event (myocardial infarction or unstable angina). Subsequent cardiac event rates are similar in the sexes.

Exercise echocardiography also provides long-term prognostic information in patients with unstable angina. In a small series (33 patients), a visually scored wall-motion index showed that new or worsening wall-motion abnormalities after exercise were associated with subsequent risk for myocardial infarction and death during 8 years of follow-up (2 deaths, 8 myocardial infarctions). Patients with a normal or near-normal wall-motion score were unlikely to experience a cardiac event.[13] When compared to exercise thallium imaging, stress echocardiography provides complementary prognostic information.[2] When exercise thallium imaging and echocardiography were performed 3 days after admission for unstable angina, fatal and nonfatal cardiac events were predicted by ST depression during exercise, wall-motion score abnormalities during exercise, and the presence and number of myocardial thallium redistribution defects. Patients with wall-motion abnormalities due to previous myocardial infarction, coronary revascularization, left bundle-branch block, or dilated cardiomyopathy, conditions that may compromise the accuracy of echocardiography, were excluded. Thallium redistribution was the only independent risk marker when all exercise echocardiographic and scintigraphic predictors were combined in a multivariate analysis.

Although additional imaging data generally add to the prognostic information in unstable angina patients, a large study of 355 men with unstable angina or non–Q-wave myocardial infarction showed that the number of leads with ST depression during exercise, a low maximal workload, increasing age, and ST elevation all exerted independent and significant prognostic value for future myocardial infarction or death during 8 years of follow-up. The mortality rate among patients with a low-risk exercise response was 0%.[38] Of note, 30% of patients with any of these risk indicators during exercise had incapacitating symptoms that necessitated coronary angiography compared with only 5% of the group without these findings. Thus, medical resource utilization and referral for angiography may be determined by the stress test data alone.

When comparing unstable angina patients with and without previous myocardial infarction, no significant differences were found in the frequency of cardiovascular events despite the fact that rates of hospitalization and coronary revascularization were greater in patients with previous infarction.[11] This study contained only patients with left ventricular ejection fraction of more than 40%. This study suggests that the prognosis of patients with and without previous infarction does not differ when left ventricular function is maintained or slightly decreased, although medical resource utilization is increased in the previous infarction subset.

Other studies examining readmission rates in patients with unstable angina have determined that the predictors of rehospitalization during 2 years after discharge include age older than 70 years, nondiagnostic exercise stress testing, angiographically diffuse coronary artery disease, and noninterventional (medical) management.[16] This finding is consistent with previous studies demonstrating that unstable angina patients who are refractory to intensive medical therapy are at high risk for developing thrombotic complications, including recurrent ischemia and myocardial ischemia due to coronary occlusion during coronary angioplasty.[46]

Prognostic information, in addition to information based on ventricular function, can be derived in patients who are triaged to coronary angiography. Patients with TIMI (Thrombolysis in Myocardial Ischemia) grade flow of 2 or less, without ulceration or thrombus, impaired angiographic filling (microvascular dysfunction), and coronary occlusion, have a worse short-term prognosis than patients with unstable angina who do not have these coronary findings (18% and 2% rate of death or myocardial infarction).[12,46] As in patient subsets with stable coronary disease, the presence of left main or triple vessel coronary disease is a marker of high risk, especially in patients with left ventricular dysfunction.[6] Preliminary data also suggest that abnormal coronary flow reserve detected by Doppler flow techniques may be a marker of increased cardiac events in patients with unstable angina.

NUCLEAR CARDIOLOGY RISK ASSESSMENT

Myocardial perfusion imaging has been useful for risk stratification of patients with previous myocardial infarction and for prediction of outcomes in patients with stable chest pain symptoms. Studies in the unstable angina population have been limited and have focused on a medically stabilized subset of patients at low to intermediate risk. This fact and the inclusion of patients with atypical chest pain who do not have coronary disease may have diluted the study populations and reduced the predictive value of stress imaging studies. There has also been growing clinical pressure to define coronary anatomy early after admission for unstable angina so that the culprit lesion can be treated with interventional therapy (angioplasty). However, few data support the survival benefit of an aggressive interventional approach in medically stabilized patients with unstable angina. In this setting, cardiac imaging has been used as a proxy for coronary angiography for identification of patients with a greater short-term and long-term risk for cardiac events due to multivessel coronary disease.

Dipyridamole[54] and exercise[36] thallium myocardial imaging have been used to risk stratify patients after admission for unstable angina. In patients who were able to perform exercise stress, the Multicenter Myocardial Ischemia Research Group study[36] demonstrated that noninvasive testing with ambulatory electrocardiography, exercise stress testing, and thallium scintigraphy provided important diagnostic data in 936 patients who had been medically stabilized. The only predictor of a primary cardiac event (cardiac death, nonfatal infarction, or unstable angina) was ST depression on the resting electrocardiogram. Other noninvasive findings suggestive of myocardial ischemia were not predictive. However, the presence of a reversible thallium defect and lung uptake of thallium were associated with a significant hazard ratio of 2.8.

Other studies support the value of stress thallium perfusion in post–unstable angina patients.[2,5] In these studies, the presence of reversible or fixed myocardial perfusion defects was associated with early cardiac events. Of 896 patients followed for 1 to 6 months after an acute coronary event (30% of whom had unstable angina), cardiac death and nonfatal infarction were increased in patients with the largest areas of reversible defect.[5] The presence of a fixed defect was associated with a prognosis similar to that of a normal exercise thallium scan in this study.

In patients who are unable to exercise, dipyridamole vasodilator stress imaging is a valuable alternative when combined with thallium imaging.[53,54] In 77 patients with acute ischemic syndromes, dipyridamole thallium stress imaging demonstrated that a reversible defect was predictive of subsequent cardiac events. This and other studies (Table 28-2) led to the recommendation of dipyridamole stress imaging in patients requiring risk stratification who are unable to exercise after admission for unstable angina.[6] To quote the 1994 Unstable Angina Clinical Practice Guidelines, "Patients with widespread ST depression, ECG changes secondary to digoxin, left ventricular hypertrophy, left bundle branch block or significant intraventricular conduction defects should usually be tested using an imaging modality (strength of evidence = B)." The Unstable Angina Clinical Practice Guidelines also recommended that low-risk unstable angina patients undergo outpatient stress imaging or be admitted to an unmonitored bed.

Studies by Madsen et al[30] and Brown[7] demonstrated that the presence of a reversible thallium defect on planar imaging studies is associated with a 21% and 26% likelihood of future serious cardiac events, whereas patients with a normal scan had a 2% and 0% likelihood of a future serious cardiac event (Table 28-1).

The prognostic value of predischarge dipyridamole[41] or exercise[42] ^{99m}Tc sestamibi tomography was recently reported in patients with unstable angina (Table 28-2). As recommended by the Unstable Angina Clinical Practice Guidelines, medically treated intermediate-risk patients with unstable angina who could not exercise underwent predischarge intravenous dipyridamole ^{99m}Tc sestamibi perfusion studies.[41] Cardiac events occurred in 53% of the patients studied during 16 months of follow-up, including unstable angina, nonfatal myocardial infarction, and cardiac death. The cardiac event rate was 10% in patients with a normal sestamibi scan compared with 69% in those with an abnormal perfusion imaging study (Fig. 28-2). Additional clinical variables associated with an increased risk of cardiac events included congestive heart failure, previous myocardial infarction, and diabetes. The relative risk ratio was 1.8 for a reversible ^{99m}Tc sestamibi defect and 2.9 for a fixed perfusion defect.

Exercise ^{99m}Tc sestamibi imaging provided prognostic data comparable to that obtained with dipyridamole stress imaging in a similar population that was hospitalized for unstable angina and medically stabilized.[42] In this study of 126 consecutive men, 12% of patients with a normal sestamibi scan and 39% with an abnormal sestamibi scan had cardiac events during follow-up. Of note, 60% of the patients with a reversible perfusion defect experienced a cardiac event, but only 2% of patients with a normal scan sustained a future nonfatal myocardial infarction or cardiac death. Cardiac event-free survival was significantly decreased in patients with a reversible perfusion defect (Fig. 28-3). From the results of these and other[34] studies, we concluded that like thallium imaging, dipyridamole or exercise ^{99m}Tc sestamibi tomography provides valuable prognostic information in medically stabilized patients with unstable angina. The presence of a reversible or a fixed perfusion defect adds incremental prognostic information over that obtained from the electrocardiographic stress test or clinical variables alone in this population.

Table 28-2. Nuclear risk assessment in acute ischemic syndromes; the St. Louis experience

Study	Patients, *n*	Stress	Tracer	Diagnosis	Risk
Younis et al[53]	77	Dipyridamole	Thallium-201*	Unstable angina, myocardial infarction	Reversible defect
Miller et al[34]	137	Dipyridamole	Technetium-99m sestamibi	Unstable angina, myocardial infarction	Reversible or fixed defect
Stratmann et al[42]	126	Exercise	Technetium-99m sestamibi	Unstable angina	Reversible defect
Stratmann et al[41]	128	Dipyridamole	Technetium-99m sestamibi	Unstable angina†	Reversible or fixed defect

*Planar imaging.
†Intermediate risk.

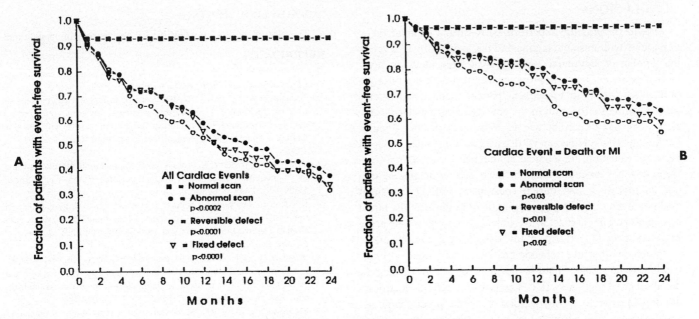

Fig. 28-2. A, Two-year survival curves for occurrence of any cardiac event in patients with normal and abnormal scans. Event-free survival was significantly lower in patients with abnormal scans (p< 0.0002). **B,** Two-year survival curves for occurrence of nonfatal myocardial infarction or cardiac death with patients with normal and abnormal scan results. Event-free survival was significantly less in patients with abnormal scan results (p< 0.03). MI, Myocardial infarction.

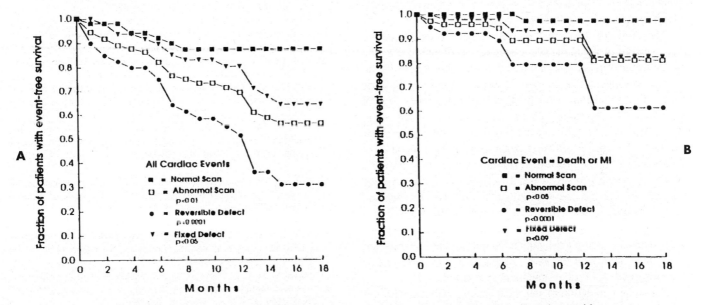

Fig. 28-3. A, Eighteen-month survival curves for occurrence of any cardiac event in patients with normal and abnormal scans. Compared with patients with normal scans, event-free survival was significantly lower in patients with any type of abnormal scan (p< 0.01) and in those with the specific presence of a reversible (p< 0.0001) or fixed (p< 0.05) perfusion defect. **B,** Eighteen-month survival curves for occurrence of a nonfatal myocardial infarction (MI) or cardiac death in patients with normal and abnormal scans. Compared with patients with normal scans, event-free survival was significantly lower in patients with any type of abnormal scan (p< 0.05) and with the specific presence of a reversible defect (p< 0.0001).

CONCLUSIONS

Despite the pressure to perform early cardiac catheterization in patients with unstable angina and the availability of a growing number of alternative noninvasive testing methods, myocardial perfusion imaging provides useful prognostic information which assists in subsequent patient management. Acute imaging during chest pain in the emergency room clarifies the in-hospital risk of cardiac events. Many patients suspected of having unstable angina can be discharged home after an initial clinical evaluation; the clinical confidence for discharge from the emergency department can be increased by the finding of a normal perfusion scan during chest pain. Further outpatient evaluation may be scheduled for up to 72 hours after the initial presentation for patients with clinical symptoms of unstable angina who are judged to be at low risk for early complications.

Patients with acute ischemic heart disease who are at intermediate or high risk should be hospitalized and monitored. In the absence of high-risk clinical events or recurrent electrocardiographic evidence of myocardial ischemia, predischarge assessment of risk by noninvasive testing often leads to selection of appropriate therapy. Predischarge stress myocardial perfusion imaging with exercise or drug stress is a useful proxy for coronary angiography, providing information on cardiac risk and associated high-risk coronary anatomy. Coronary angiography is appropriate for patients who are judged to be at high clinical risk or for patients with evidence of extensive myocardial ischemia on stress imaging studies.

The choice of stress imaging study relates to local expertise and availability and to the cost-effectiveness of alternative noninvasive stress imaging techniques in this setting. Extensive information suggests that stress nuclear perfusion imaging is the best validated technique for predischarge risk stratification of patients with unstable angina who have been medically stabilized. Although definitive data on medical resource utilization are lacking, early information suggests that the avoidance of unncessary coronary revascularization by requiring previous objective evidence of myocardial ischemia is a cost-effective strategy. As was the case with postinfarction risk stratification, early evidence shows that accelerating predischarge stress imaging protocols to within 72 hours of admission permits early detection of high-risk patients requiring angiography and revascularization and the early discharge of low-risk patients who may undergo further outpatient evaluation.

The large population of intermediate-risk patients with unstable angina should be targeted for aggressive medical therapy aimed at medical stabilization. A focus on baseline clinical markers and the subsequent use of noninvasive testing methods assists in the risk stratification and management of these patients. Clinical and noninvasive risk indices help to stratify the heterogeneous unstable angina population, thereby optimizing the use of medical resources in these difficult-to-manage patients. Future studies aimed at the noninvasive identification of plaque instability in this population may further refine the current medical management of this acute coronary syndrome.

ACKNOWLEDGMENTS

The author thanks Lori Gallini for her secretarial assistance.

REFERENCES

1. Amanullah AM: Noninvasive testing in the diagnosis and management of unstable angina, *Int J Cardiol* 47:95–103, 1994.
2. Amanullah AM, Lindvall K, Bevegard S: Prognostic significance of exercise thallium-201 myocardial perfusion imaging compared to stress echocardiography and clinical variables in patients with unstable angina who respond to medical treatment, *Int J Cardiol* 39:71–78, 1993.
3. Ambrose JA, Winters SL, Stern A, et al: Angiographic morphology and the pathogenesis of unstable angina pectoris, *J Am Coll Cardiol* 5:609–616, 1985.
4. Bilodeau L, Theroux P, Gregoire J, et al: Technetium-99m sestamibi tomography in patients with spontaneous chest pain: correlations with clinical electrocardiographic and angiographic findings, *J Am Coll Cardiol* 18:1684–1691, 1991.
5. Bodenheimer MM, Wackers FJ, Schwartz RG, et al: Prognostic significance of a fixed thallium defect one to six months after onset of acute myocardial infarction or unstable angina. Multicenter Myocardial Ischemia Research Group, *Am J Cardiol* 74:1196–1200, 1994.
6. Braunwald E, Jones RH, Mark DB, et al: Diagnosing and managing unstable angina. Agency for Health Care Policy and Research, *Circulation* 90:613–622, 1994.
7. Brown KA: Prognostic value of thallium-201 myocardial perfusion imaging in patients with unstable angina who respond to medical treatment, *J Am Coll Cardiol* 17:1053–1057, 1991.
8. Brush JE Jr, Brand DA, Acampora D, et al: Use of the initial electrocardiogram to predict in-hospital complications of acute myocardial infarction, *N Engl J Med* 312:1137–1141, 1985.
9. Bugiardini R, Borghi A, Pozzati A, et al: Relation of severity of symptoms to transient myocardial ischemia and prognosis in unstable angina, *J Am Coll Cardiol* 25:597–604, 1995.
10. Catherwood E, O'Rourke DJ: Critical pathway management of unstable angina, *Prog Cardiovasc Dis* 37:121–148, 1994.
11. Dini FL, Volterrani C, Giaconi A, et al: Prior myocardial infarction and prognostic outcome in patients with unstable angina in a postdischarge follow-up, *Angiology* 47:321–327, 1996.
12. Diver DJ, Bier JD, Ferreira PE, et al: Clinical and arteriographic characterization of patients with unstable angina without critical coronary arterial narrowing (from the TIMI IIIA Trial), *Am J Cardiol* 74:531–537, 1994.
13. Eriksson SV, Erhardt L, Lindvall K, et al: Long-term prognostic importance of exercise echocardiography after an episode of unstable angina, *Cardiology* 86:426–431, 1995.
14. Freeman MR, Williams AE, Chisholm RJ, et al: Role of resting thallium 201 perfusion in predicting coronary anatomy, left ventricular wall motion, and hospital outcome in unstable angina pectoris, *Am Heart J* 117:306–314, 1989.
15. Fuster V, Stein B, Ambrose JA, et al: Atherosclerotic plaque rupture and thrombosis. Evolving concepts, *Circulation* 82(3 Suppl):1147–1159, 1990.
16. Gonzalez-Fernandez RA, Baez J, Fernandez-Martinez J, et al: Readmission in unstable angina, *P R Health Sci J* 14:7–10, 1995.
17. Gregoire J, Theroux P: Detection and assessment of unstable angina using myocardial perfusion imaging: comparison between technetium-99m sestamibi SPECT and 12-lead electrocardiogram, *Am J Cardiol* 66:42E–46E, 1990.
18. Grijseels EW, Deckers JW, Hoes AW, et al: Pre-hospital triage of patients with suspected myocardial infarction. Evaluation of previously developed algorithms and new proposals, *Eur Heart J* 16:325–332, 1995.
19. Hilton TC, Thompson RC, Williams HJ, et al: Technetium-99m sestamibi myocardial perfusion imaging in the emergency room evaluation of chest pain, *J Am Coll Cardiol* 23:1016–1022, 1994.

20. Jesse RL, Kontos MC: Evaluation of chest pain in the emergency department, *Curr Probl Cardiol* 22:149–236, 1997.

21. Kelly DT, Wilcox I: Determinants of prognosis in unstable angina, *Postgrad Med J* 70 suppl I:S46–S49, 1994.

22. Langer A, Singh N, Freeman MR, et al: Detection of silent ischemia adds to the prognostic value of coronary anatomy and left ventricular function in predicting outcome in unstable angina patients, *Can J Cardiol* 11:117–122, 1995.

23. Larsson H, Areskog M, Areskog NH, et al: The diagnostic and prognostic importance of ambulatory ST recording compared to a predischarge exercise test after an episode of unstable angina or non-Q wave myocardial infarction, *Eur Heart J* 16:888–893, 1995.

24. Lee TH, Rouan GW, Weisberg MC, et al: Clinical characteristics and natural history of patients with acute myocardial infarction sent home from the emergency room, *Am J Cardiol* 60:219–224, 1987.

25. Leeman DE, McCabe CH, Faxon DP, et al: Use of percutaneous transluminal coronary angioplasty and bypass surgery despite improved medical therapy for unstable angina pectoris, *Am J Cardiol* 61:38G–44G, 1988.

26. Lindahl B, Venge P, Wallentin L: Relation between troponin T and the risk of subsequent cardiac events in unstable coronary artery disease. The FRISC study group, *Circulation* 93:1651–1657, 1996.

27. Liuzzo G, Biasucci LM, Gallimore JR, et al: The prognostic value of C-reactive protein and serum amyloid a protein in severe unstable angina, *N Engl J Med* 331:417–424, 1994.

28. Luchi RJ, Scott SM, Deupree RH, et al: Comparison of medical and surgical treatment for unstable angina pectoris. Results of a Veterans Administration Cooperative Study, *N Engl J Med* 316:977–984, 1987.

29. MacIsaac AI, Thomas JD, Topol EJ: Toward the quiescent coronary plaque, *J Am Coll Cardiol* 22:1228–1241, 1993.

30. Madsen JK, Stubgaard M, Utne HE, et al: Prognosis and thallium-201 scintigraphy in patients admitted with chest pain without confirmed acute myocardial infarction, *Br Heart J* 59:184–189, 1988.

31. McCarthy BD, Beshansky JR, D'Agostino RB, et al: Missed diagnoses of acute myocardial infarction in the emergency department: results from a multicenter study, *Ann Emerg Med* 22:579–582, 1993.

32. Miller DD: *Radionuclide labeled monoclonal antibody imaging of atherosclerosis and vascular injury.* In Fuster V, ed: *Syndromes of atherosclerosis: correlations of clinical imaging,* 1996, Futura Publishing Company.

33. Miller DD, Shaw LJ: Incremental prognostic value of stress myocardial perfusion imaging in coronary artery disease: potential for improving patient outcomes, *ACC Educational Highlights* 11:1–5, 1995.

34. Miller DD, Stratmann HG, Shaw L, et al: Dipyridamole technetium 99m sestamibi myocardial tomography as an independent predictor of cardiac event-free survival after acute ischemic events, *J Nucl Cardiol* 1:72–82, 1994.

35. Moriel M, Benhorin J, Brown MW, et al: Detection and significance of myocardial ischemia in women versus men within six months of acute myocardial infarction or unstable angina. The Multicenter Myocardial Ischemia Research Group, *Am J Cardiol* 77:798–804, 1996.

36. Moss AJ, Goldstein RE, Hall WJ, et al: Detection and significance of myocardial ischemia in stable patients after recovery from an acute coronary event. Multicenter Myocardial Ischemia Research Group, *JAMA* 269:2379–2385, 1993.

37. Nyman I, Areskog M, Areskog NH, et al: Very early risk stratification by electrocardiogram at rest in men with suspected unstable coronary heart disease, *J Intern Med* 234:293–301, 1993.

38. Nyman I, Wallentin L, Areskog M, et al: Risk stratification by early exercise testing after an episode of unstable coronary artery disease. The Rise Study Group, *Int J Cardiol* 39:131–142, 1993.

39. Radensky PW, Hilton TC, Fulmer H, et al: Potential cost effectiveness of initial myocardial perfusion imaging for assessment of emergency department patients with chest pain, *Am J Cardiol* 79:595–599, 1997.

40. Rizik DG, Healy S, Margulis A, et al: A new clinical classification for hospital prognosis of unstable angina pectoris, *Am J Cardiol* 75:993–997, 1995.

41. Stratmann HG, Tamesis BR, Younis LT, et al: Prognostic value of predischarge dipyridamole technetium 99m sestamibi myocardial tomography in medically treated patients with unstable angina, *Am Heart J* 130:734–740, 1995.

42. Stratmann HG, Younis LT, Wittry MD, et al: Exercise technetium-99m myocardial tomography for the risk stratification of men with medically treated unstable angina pectoris, *Am J Cardiol* 76:236–240, 1995.

43. Tatum JL, Jesse RL, Kontos MC, et al: Comprehensive strategy for the evaluation and triage of the chest pain patient, *Ann Emerg Med* 29:116–125, 1997.

44. Tosteson AN, Goldman L, Udvarhelyi IS, et al: Cost-effectiveness of a coronary care unit versus an intermediate care unit for emergency department patients with chest pain, *Circulation* 94:143–150, 1996.

45. Unstable angina: diagnosis and management. Clinical practice guideline no. 10, AHCPR publication no. 94-0602, 1994, Department of Health and Human Services, Public Health Service, Agency for Healthcare Policy and Research, National Heart, Lung and Blood Institute.

46. van den Brand MJ, van Miltenburg A, de Boer MJ, et al: Correlation between clinical course and quantitative analysis of the ischemia related artery in patients with unstable angina pectoris, refractory to medical treatment. The European Cooperative Study Group, *Int J Card Imaging* 10:177–185, 1994.

47. van Milenburg-van Zijl AJ, Simoons ML, Veerhoek RJ, et al: Incidence and follow-up of Braunwald subgroups in unstable angina pectoris, *J Am Coll Cardiol* 25:1286–1292, 1995.

48. Varetto T, Cantalupi D, Altieri A, et al: Emergency room technetium-99m sestamibi imaging to rule out acute myocardial ischemic events in patients with nondiagnostic electrocardiograms, *J Am Coll Cardiol* 22:1804–1808, 1993.

49. Wackers FJ, Heller GV, Stowers S, et al: Normal rest tetrofosmin SPECT imaging in patients with chest pain and normal or nondiagnostic ECG in the emergency department is associated with lower need for subsequent cardiac catheterization and revascularization, *J Am Coll Cardiol* 29:196A, 1997.

50. Wackers FJ, Lie KI, Liem KL, et al: Thallium-201 scintigraphy in unstable angina pectoris, *Circulation* 57:738–742, 1978.

51. Weingarten SR, Riedinger MS, Conner L, et al: Practice guidelines and reminders to reduce duration of hospital stay for patients with chest pain. An interventional trial, *Ann Intern Med* 120:257–263, 1994.

52. Wieczorek I, Haynes WG, Webb DJ, et al: Raised plasma endothelin in unstable angina and non-Q wave myocardial infarction: relation to cardiovascular outcome, *Br Heart J* 72:436–441, 1994.

53. Younis LT, Byers S, Shaw L, et al: Prognostic value of intravenous dipyridamole thallium scintigraphy after an acute myocardial ischemic event, *Am J Cardiol* 64:161–166, 1989.

54. Zhu YY, Chung WS, Botvinick EH, et al: Dipyridamole perfusion scintigraphy: the experience with its application in one hundred seventy patients with known or suspected unstable angina, *Am Heart J* 121:33–43, 1991.

VIABILITY/METABOLIC IMAGING

Chapter 29

Assessment of myocardial viability with thallium-201

Robert O. Bonow

In the current era of revascularization surgery and interventional cardiology, the assessment of myocardial viability has become an integral component of the diagnostic evaluation of patients with coronary artery disease and depressed left ventricular function. During the past 15 years, numerous studies have demonstrated that left ventricular dysfunction does not always represent an irreversible process related to previous infarction, as was once widely believed. Instead, regional and global ventricular function may improve substantially and even normalize after reperfusion therapy for acute myocardial infarction[9,14,68,72,78] and after myocardial revascularization procedures in patients with chronic coronary artery disease.[12,25,31,64]

The distinction between viable and nonviable myocardium in patients with left ventricular dysfunction is clinically important in patients who are possible candidates for myocardial revascularization because these procedures are often accompanied by high operative morbidity and mortality in this subset of patients. However, patients with impaired ventricular function also face substantial short-term and long-term risks during medical therapy and have the most to gain in terms of survival from successful revascularization.

The number of patients with left ventricular dysfunction who manifest a substantial improvement in ventricular function after myocardial revascularization is not inconsequential. It has been estimated that 25% to 40% of patients with chronic coronary artery disease and left ventricular dysfunction have the potential for significant improvement in ventricular function after revascularization[12,16,25,31,66] (Fig. 29-1).

Currently, several clinically reliable physiologic markers can be used for the assessment of myocardial viability. Indexes of regional coronary blood flow, regional wall motion, and regional systolic wall thickening are accurate markers of viability if they are normal or near normal, but these indexes have major limitations in identifying viable myocardium when they are reduced or absent. By definition, regional perfusion and systolic function (regional wall motion and wall thickening) are severely reduced or absent in patients with hibernating myocardium,[15,25,61,62,64] despite maintenance of tissue viability. Other patients have preserved blood flow at rest but recurrent ischemic episodes during stress, leading to persistent contractile dysfunction from repetitive stunning.* In these latter patients, indexes of wall motion and wall thickening will also be imprecise markers of viability.

Techniques to assess intact cellular metabolic processes or cell membrane integrity have intrinsic advantages over indexes of resting function and blood flow. During the past decade, numerous studies have demonstrated that nuclear cardiology techniques involving single photon methods, as well as positron emission tomography (PET), can be used to investigate perfusion, cell membrane integrity, and metabolic activity and thus provide critically important information on viability in patients with left ventricular dysfunction. This chapter will focus on the assessment of myocardial viability by using thallium-201 (^{201}Tl) imaging.

The requirements for cellular viability include intact sarcolemmal function to maintain electrochemical gradients across the cell membrane, as well as preserved metabolic activity to generate high-energy phosphates. These processes also require adequate myocardial blood flow to deliver substrates and wash out the metabolites of the metabolic processes. Because the retention of ^{201}Tl is an active process that is a function of cell viability, cell membrane activity, and blood flow, ^{201}Tl should in theory be taken up and retained by viable myo-

*References 9, 20, 32, 40, 67, 80.

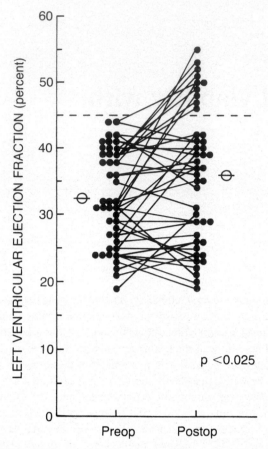

Fig. 29-1. Left ventricular ejection fraction at rest by radionuclide ventriculography before *(Preop)* and 6 months after *(Postop)* coronary artery bypass graft surgery in 43 patients with preoperative left ventricular dysfunction. The dashed line at 45% indicates the lower limit of normal resting ejection fraction. Although surgery resulted in only a small increase in mean ejection fraction, substantial increases in ejection fraction were observed in 15 patients (35%) and postoperative ejection fraction was normal in 10 patients (23%). (Reproduced with permission of W.B. Saunders Co. From Bonow RO, Dilsizian V: Thallium-201 for assessing myocardial viability, *Semin Nucl Med* 21:230-241, 1991.)

cardium regardless of whether systolic function is preserved. Thus, regional thallium activity, even in asynergic regions, should be an accurate marker of viability and should predict improvement of regional contraction after revascularization.*

STRESS-REDISTRIBUTION IMAGING

As noted previously, several recent studies indicate that many patients with chronic coronary artery disease have normal or near normal blood flow under basal conditions in myocardial regions with severe systolic dysfunction, and that systolic function in these regions improves after myocardial revascularization.[9,20,32,67,80] This evidence of perfusion–contraction mismatch suggests that the segmental dysfunction arises from repeated episodes of myocardial ischemia leading

to repetitive stunning rather than true myocardial hibernation, which by definition requires reduced blood flow under basal conditions. Although the relative prevalence of stunning compared with hibernation as a causative mechanism of reversible contractile dysfunction in patients with chronic coronary artery disease is uncertain, it seems that both processes exist, but that most patients have a form of repetitive stunning. In these patients, demonstration of reversible ischemia may be the key to determining the viability of dysfunctional segments, and this may be readily accomplished using stress thallium imaging. Thus, thallium redistribution in an asynergic region with a defect on stress imaging predicts improvement of regional contraction after revascularization[33,64] (Fig. 29-2). However, many regions of severely ischemic or hibernating myocardium have irreversible thallium defects on standard exercise redistribution imaging. It has been demonstrated that up to 50% of regions with "irreversible" thallium defects will improve in function after revascularization.* Thus, standard stress redistribution thallium imaging has an excellent positive predictive value but a suboptimal negative predictive value. It is now generally accepted that stress 4-hour redistribution imaging does not provide satisfactory precision in differentiating left ventricular dysfunction arising from infarcted versus hibernating myocardium because this technique frequently underestimates both the presence of viable myocardium and potential for recovery after revascularization.

This concept is supported by studies directly comparing PET imaging with exercise-redistribution thallium scintigraphy. In 4 studies, 38% to 47% of apparently "irreversible" thallium defects (that would have been identified as scar by stress redistribution thallium imaging) were identified as viable on the basis of regional uptake of ^{18}F-fluorodeoxyglucose (FDG).[17,18,73,74] Although these data suggest that metabolic imaging using PET is superior to thallium imaging in the detection of viable myocardium, two limitations of these particular studies must be emphasized. First, the severity of the reduction in thallium activity within the "irreversible" thallium defects was not assessed. The importance of quantitative analysis of regional thallium activity will be discussed below. Second, the previous comparative studies of thallium scintigraphy and PET performed postexercise thallium imaging followed by a single redistribution study 3 to 4 hours later; as noted above, the limitations of 4-hour redistribution imaging are now well established.

LATE THALLIUM REDISTRIBUTION IMAGING

Several investigators have shown that late imaging at 8 to 72 hours will demonstrate substantial thallium redistribution in many defects that seem to be irreversible at 3 to 4 hours[23,36,45,82] and that this late thallium redistribution is consistent with the presence of viable myocardium.[45,82] Kiat et al,[45] in a study of 21 patients undergoing myocardial revascularization procedures, found that 61% of nonreversible defects at 4

---

*References 7, 8, 11, 38, 40, 42, 65.

*References 33, 36, 45, 47, 50, 53.

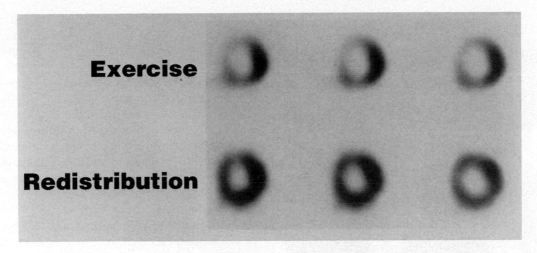

Fig. 29-2. Stress and redistribution (3-hour delay) thallium-201 tomographic images obtained after maximal treadmill exercise, demonstrating a reversible perfusion abnormality in the septal, anterior, and apical regions in a patient with a high-grade stenosis of the left anterior descending coronary artery. The demonstration of reversibly ischemic myocardium is an accurate indicator of viable myocardium.

hours reversed at the time of late (18 to 72 hour) redistribution imaging. The revascularization results in this study, as assessed by post-intervention repeat thallium imaging, provided additional important insights. Among all regions that were nonreversible at 4 hours, 72% showed improvement after revascularization. This result confirms the findings of earlier studies, in which standard 3 to 4 hour thallium redistribution imaging overestimated the prevalence and severity of irreversible myocardial damage. However, among the regions with nonreversible defects at 4 hours, 95% of regions manifesting late redistribution improved after revascularization compared with only 37% of regions that remained nonreversible on late imaging.[45] These findings indicate that myocardial segments with late thallium redistribution represent viable myocardium and that late imaging may considerably improve the identification of viable myocardium in thallium defects that are nonreversible at 3 to 4 hours.

The implications of late thallium redistribution in regard to myocardial viability are similar to those of 3 to 4 hour redistribution. Although many persistent defects at 3 to 4 hours manifest late redistribution, and although the positive predictive value of late redistribution is excellent, the negative predictive value remains poor. As noted above, 37% of persistent defects at 24 hours improved after revascularization in the study by Kiat et al.[45] Moreover, almost 50% of such defects have been shown to be metabolically active with PET imaging.[19] Finally, in a quantitative analysis of regional thallium activity, Kayden et al[44] showed that almost 40% of late persistent defects manifest enhanced thallium uptake when thallium reinjection is performed immediately after the 24-hour redistribution study. This suggests that some ischemic regions may never redistribute, even with late imaging, unless serum thallium levels are augmented.

THALLIUM REINJECTION TECHNIQUES

The reinjection of thallium at rest immediately after standard 4-hour redistribution imaging may overcome several of these limitations and may be used to assess myocardial viability in apparently irreversible thallium defects on standard early or late redistribution images[26,63,75] (Fig. 29-3). Up to 49% of "irreversible" defects on 3- to 4-hour redistribution images demonstrate improved or normal uptake after thallium reinjection.[26] Thus, thallium reinjection at rest after 3- to 4-hour redistribution imaging may be used instead of 24-hour imaging in most patients in whom a persistent thallium defect is observed on conventional redistribution images. Additional redistribution imaging hours after reinjection of thallium seems to provide no further information beyond that obtained by imaging done immediately after reinjection,[27] because less than 5% of myocardial regions with persistent defects on 3- to 4-hour redistribution plus reinjection imaging show evidence of late redistribution. On the other hand, redistribution imaging is important when reinjection is performed. A simple exercise-reinjection protocol without redistribution imaging may miss unique and important information on viability. Thus, if reinjection protocols are used, it is essential to also perform routine 3- to 4-hour redistribution imaging before reinjection or to perform late redistribution imaging in patients with persistent defects on stress reinjection imaging.[28]

The idea that the uptake of thallium after reinjection represents viable myocardium is substantiated in three subgroups of patients. First, in 295 patients with left ventricular dysfunction reported in 9 studies* who were reexamined 3 to 6 months after revascularization, improved wall motion occurred in 69% of segments identified as viable by thallium reinjection before

*References 2, 4, 5, 26, 37, 52, 53, 69, 81.

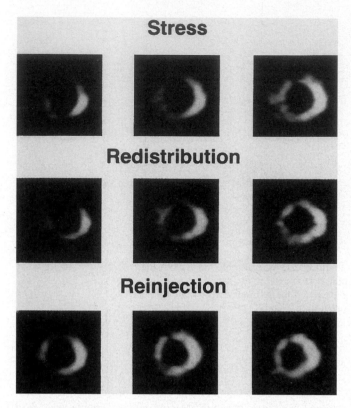

Fig. 29-3. Thallium reinjection imaging. Short-axis thallium single-photon emission computed tomography images obtained after exercise show extensive abnormalities in anterior and septal perfusion that persist on 4-hour redistribution images but improve substantially after reinjection. (Reproduced with permission of the New England Journal of Medicine. From Dilsizian V, Rocco TP, Freedman NM, et al: Enhanced detection of ischemic but viable myocardium by the reinjection of thallium after stress-redistribution imaging, *N Engl J Med* 323:141-146, 1990.)

revascularization. Such improvement occurred in only 11% of segments identified as nonviable by redistribution plus reinjection imaging (Fig. 29-4). Second, in comparative studies with thallium reinjection and PET imaging with FDG, most myocardial segments identified as viable by reinjection showed metabolic evidence of myocardial viability.[10,56,76] The concordance between the thallium reinjection and FDG uptake data was excellent; 51% of regions with severe "irreversible" thallium defects on 4-hour redistribution studies were identified as viable by both thallium reinjection and PET.[10] Third, in patients studied with gated magnetic resonance imaging to assess regional systolic function, an excellent correlation was observed between regional thallium activity and FDG activity in myocardial regions with severely reduced or no wall thickening.[56]

These latter PET data are in keeping with previous studies indicating that up to 50% of regions with "irreversible" thallium defects show evidence of viability according to PET.[17,18,73,74] These data also indicate that thallium reinjection is a convenient, clinically accurate, and relatively inexpensive method with which to identify viable myocardium in patients with chronic coronary artery disease and left ventricular dysfunction.

REST-REDISTRIBUTION THALLIUM IMAGING

The demonstration of exercise-induced ischemia in a patient with left ventricular dysfunction has important prognostic implications that under most conditions identify that patient as a candidate for revascularization therapy. Thus, exercise-redistribution–reinjection thallium protocols are attractive, because they provide important information regarding both jeopardized myocardium and viable myocardium. However, in many patients, the sole clinical issue to be addressed is the viability of one or more regions of dysfunctional left ventricular myocardium, not whether there is also inducible ischemia. In such patients, rest-redistribution thallium imaging is a practical ap-

Fig. 29-4. Likelihood of improved regional left ventricular function after revascularization based on thallium-201 single-photon emission computed tomography. Data are summarized from nine studies using stress-redistribution–reinjection imaging[2,4,5,26,36,51,52,68,80] and four studies using rest-redistribution imaging.[21,56,57,78] The range of values reported from the individual studies is indicated by the horizontal bars connected by vertical lines. The shaded bars represent the positive predictive value, and the open bars represent the inverse of the negative predictive value.

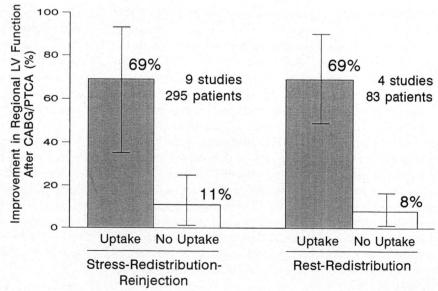

proach that can yield accurate viability data (Fig. 29-5). It is essential to obtain not only initial images (indicating regional perfusion) but also subsequent redistribution images. Although early thallium studies yielded mixed results regarding the predictive accuracy of rest-redistribution imaging,[8,42] recent studies indicate that quantitative analysis of regional thallium activity in rest-redistribution studies predicts recovery of regional left ventricular function with an accuracy virtually identical to that achieved with thallium exercise-reinjection imaging (Fig. 29-4).* These results are comparable to those of PET imaging with FDG; although PET achieves a higher positive predictive value, thallium SPECT imaging achieves a higher negative predictive value.[13]

QUANTITATIVE ANALYSIS OF THALLIUM DATA

In 12 of the 13 SPECT studies summarized in Fig. 29-4, regional thallium activities were analyzed quantitatively rather than by using a visual scoring system, and it is uncertain whether subjective interpretation of images can replicate these results. However, in most cases, the criteria for viability or nonviability in these quantitative studies were based on a threshold level of thallium activity, so that thallium levels greater than 50% or 60% of the activity in normal myocardial segments were considered viable. Although this black-and-white approach to the thallium data—classifying myocardial territories simply as viable or nonviable—achieves reasonable results, it does not take advantage of one of the greatest strengths of perfusion imaging: the ability to view regional tracer activity as a continuum rather than as a simple binary function. Several studies have shown an almost linear relation between regional thallium activity and the likelihood of recovery of regional function after revascularization.[57-59] For example, although all

myocardial segments with thallium activity greater than 50% of normal activity were considered viable in the study by Perrone-Filardi et al,[57] only 56% of segments with thallium activity in the range of 50% to 60% improved after revascularization, whereas 88% of segments with thallium activity greater than 80% showed functional improvement after revascularization (Fig. 29-6). This is one important factor that may explain the wide range of positive predictive values of thallium imaging reported thus far in the individual studies summarized in Fig. 29-4; relative thallium activities in regions considered viable among these studies may have differed considerably. A corollary to this argument is that relative regional thallium activity provides a high degree of certainty at either end of the thallium activity spectrum (Fig. 29-4), but important uncertainty exists when intermediate thallium levels are encountered. Recent data suggest that late redistribution imaging (using a rest-redistribution protocol) may provide greater confidence regarding the potential for recovery of function in a myocardial region with intermediate thallium activity at 3 to 4 hours, as 21% of such regions show increased relative thallium activity at 24 hours.[58]

Regional thallium activity also predicts the response of dysfunctional myocardium to dobutamine stimulation. Dobutamine echocardiography to assess inotropic reserve in viable myocardium has shown considerable promise in assessing myocardial viability, in keeping with the presence of residual inotropic reserve in stunned or hibernating myocardium that may be elicited through catecholamine stimulation.* The available data suggest that thallium imaging is more sensitive but less specific for identifying which myocardial regions and which patients will manifest improved function after revascularization.[13] Regional discordance has also been noted; greater evidence of viability in the anterior and septal regions has been

*References 6, 21, 29, 57, 58, 60, 79.

*References 1-3, 21, 22, 46, 49, 57-59, 70, 71.

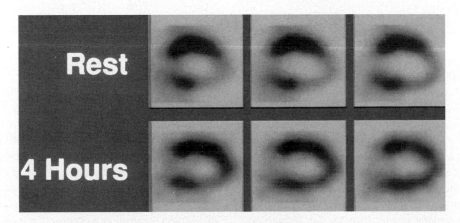

Fig. 29-5. Rest-redistribution thallium imaging in a patient with severe heart failure and severe left ventricular dysfunction (ejection fraction, 29%). Substantial redistribution of thallium is evident in the left ventricular apex. After successful coronary bypass surgery, the symptoms of heart failure resolved and the ejection fraction increased to 40%. (From Hendel RC: Single-photon perfusion imaging for the assessment of myocardial viability, *J Nucl Med* 35(4 Suppl):23S-31S, 1994. Reprinted by permission of the Society of Nuclear Medicine.)

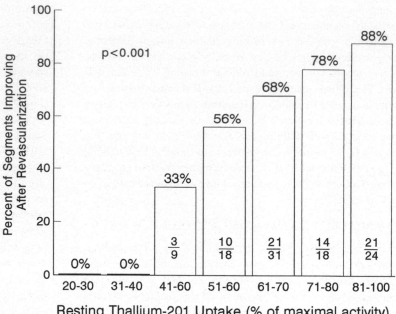

Fig. 29-6. Demonstration of the linear relation between the percentage of peak thallium activity on rest-redistribution imaging and the likelihood of segmental improvement after revascularization. Although various cutoff values have been proposed as thresholds for viability, this figure indicates the continuous nature of this relation. (Reprinted with permission of the American Heart Association. From Perrone-Filardi P, Pace L, Prastaro M, et al: Dobutamine echocardiography predicts improvement of hypoperfused dysfunctional myocardium after revascularization in patients with coronary artery disease, *Circulation* 91:2556-2565, 1995.)

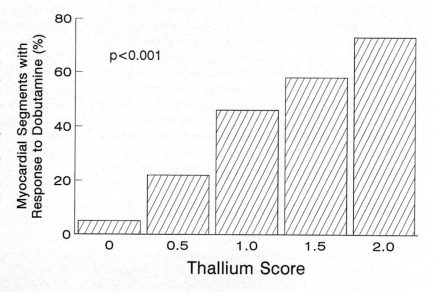

Fig. 29-7. Relation between regional thallium activity (graded on a 5-point visual scale) and the likelihood of inotropic reserve during dobutamine echocardiography. Inotropic reserve is significantly related to regional thallium activity. (Reproduced with permission of the American Heart Association. From Panza JA, Dilsizian V, Laurienzo JM, et al: Relation between thallium uptake and contractile response to dobutamine. Implications regarding myocardial viability in patients with chronic coronary artery disease and left ventricular dysfunction, *Circulation* 91:990–998, 1995.)

demonstrated with thallium scintigraphy than with dobutamine echocardiography.[39] Relative regional thallium activity can be used to determine the likelihood that an asynergic myocardial segment will manifest contractile reserve with dobutamine[55,58] (Fig. 29-7).

Several studies have shown another advantage of quantitative analysis. Regional thallium activity on delayed redistribution imaging seems to be a more important determinant of functional recovery after revascularization and a stronger determinant of dobutamine responsiveness than is the change in regional activity between the initial resting images and the redistribution study.[58,60] Thus, the severity of a thallium defect on redistribution imaging is more predictive of functional outcome than is reversibility of the defect.

One final aspect of quantitative analysis of the thallium data relates to the extent of viable myocardium rather than to the severity of reduction in thallium activity. A meaningful increase in left ventricular ejection fraction after revascularization, rather than merely an improvement in regional ventricular function, is dependent on the mass of myocardium with potentially reversible asynergy. In the study of Ragosta et al,[60] revascularization of seven or more viable but dysfunctional myocardial segments was required for a postoperative increase in left ventricular ejection fraction. This observation is consistent with previous data obtained using preoperative PET imaging with FDG.[51,77] Thus, the extent of viable myocardium in a patient with left ventricular dysfunction may predict the magnitude of recovery in global left ventricular function after revascularization.

VIABILITY ASSESSMENT AND PATIENT OUTCOME

The recovery of left ventricular function after revascularization in patients with evidence of myocardial viability may also translate into an improvement in prognosis. It has been demonstrated with PET imaging that patients with an FDG-to-blood flow mismatch have significantly higher survival rates with myocardial revascularization than with medical therapy. In two separate studies[24,30] involving a total of 87 patients with left ventricular dysfunction (mean ejection fraction, 31%) the 1-year mortality rate in patients who received medical treatment was 33% in one study and 41% in the other. In contrast, the mortality rate was reduced to only 4% in the first study and 12% in the second in patients treated with coronary artery bypass graft surgery or angioplasty. Although the prognostic implications of viability assessment using ^{201}Tl imaging are less well advanced, the available results provide information that parallel the published PET data. Gioia et al[35] demonstrated a borderline (p = 0.06) cardiac event reduction in patients with myocardial viability on thallium imaging who underwent myocardial revascularization compared to those treated medically. Similar results were observed in a multicenter Italian study. Among 161 patients with left ventricular dysfunction (mean ejection fraction, 35%) and thallium evidence of myocardial viability, survival and survival without myocardial infarction were significantly enhanced in patients treated with revascularization as opposed to those treated medically.[34]

These studies have limitations that should be addressed. They represent retrospective, nonrandomized studies involving relatively small numbers of patients. The factors used to refer some patients for revascularization and others for medical therapy are unspecified, and it is unclear whether other predictors of outcome, such as severity of angina or inducible myocardial isch-emia, were used to guide the selection toward revascularization. However, the overall concordance of the results supports the concept that patients with left ventricular dysfunction and evidence of myocardial viability represent a high-risk group with a high rate of cardiac events and that this poor prognosis may be reduced considerably by revascularization of the viable but underperfused myocardium.

Conversely, thallium imaging may also identify patients with left ventricular dysfunction who should not undergo myocardial revascularization. Patients with impaired left ventricular function who have no evidence of residual myocardial viability in dysfunction regions or who have only a small number of viable regions seem to have a significantly greater short-term and long-term postoperative risk of death than do patients who undergo revascularization with evidence of extensive viable myocardium in the dysfunctional segments.[54] These data indicate that assessment of myocardial viability with ^{201}Tl imaging may provide critically important information for risk stratification and revascularization decision making in patients with coronary artery disease and left ventricular dysfunction.

CLINICAL IMPLICATIONS

The assessment of myocardial viability has become an area of intense interest for several reasons. Among these is the rather unique potential of nuclear cardiology techniques to identify viable regions on the basis of perfusion, cell membrane integrity, and metabolic activity, thereby providing greater precision than can be achieved by assessment of regional anatomy or function. However, it must be emphasized that there are unresolved issues regarding the clinical applications of such techniques. First, larger-scale studies comparing PET and ^{201}Tl, using reinjection techniques or resting injection, are required in patients undergoing revascularization to determine the relative efficacy of these two methods in identifying viable myocardium. There may be a subgroup of patients in whom PET provides more accurate and complete data than can be accomplished using thallium imaging, but the characteristics of this subgroup have not yet been defined. Second, further studies are required to assess the relative efficacies of technetium-based perfusion agents, which do not redistribute appreciably, compared with the efficacy of thallium imaging. Although this area of investigation has been controversial and has had mixed results thus far, the most recent studies using quantitative analysis of regional ^{99m}Tc-sestamibi activity have shown considerable promise.[43,48,78] Third, additional studies are needed to assess the accuracy of dobutamine echocardiography to unmask contractile reserve in regions with resting dysfunction compared with the efficacy of thallium imaging. Although dobutamine echocardiography works well in asynergic regions with preserved blood flow (which apparently have repetitive stunning), it may perform less well in regions with reduced blood flow, which may be hibernating.[41,67] Finally, recovery of regional left ventricular function after revascularization, which has long been the gold standard against which noninvasive imaging techniques are compared, may not be the only, or even the most important, benefit of revascularization of viable but dysfunctional myocardium. Even in the absence of improved left ventricular systolic function, revascularization of viable myocardium downstream from a critical coronary artery stenosis may provide clinical benefit by attenuation of left ventricular dilatation and remodeling, reduction in ventricular arrhythmias, and reduction of the risk for subsequent fatal ischemic events.

Whether a clinically relevant change in ventricular performance occurs after myocardial revascularization and whether this event translates into improved lifestyle and prognosis depends on numerous factors, many of which are only poorly defined. The amount of dysfunctional but viable myocardium is certainly one such factor, but the identification of viable myocardium is currently not in and of itself an indication for revascularization. As in any other patient with coronary artery disease, this decision should be based on clinical presentation, coronary anatomy, left ventricular function, and evidence of inducible ischemia. The knowledge that a large region of left ventricular myocardium is viable rather than irreversibly damaged will aid in this decision-making process, but it should not be the primary indication for revascularization.

REFERENCES

1. Afridi I, Kleiman NS, Raizner AE, et al: Dobutamine echocardiography in myocardial hibernation. Optimal dose and accuracy in predicting recovery of ventricular function after coronary revascularization, *Circulation* 91:663–670, 1995.

2. Arnese M, Cornel JH, Salustri A, et al: Prediction of improvement of regional left ventricular function after surgical revascularization. A comparison of low-dose dobutamine echocardiography with ^{201}Tl single-photon emission computed tomography, *Circulation* 91: 2748–2752, 1995.

3. Barilla F, Gheorghiade M, Alam M, et al: Low-dose dobutamine in patients with acute myocardial infarction identifies viable but not contractile myocardium and predicts the magnitude of improvement in wall motion abnormalities in response to coronary revascularization, *Am Heart J* 122:1522–1531, 1991.

4. Bartenstein P: Tl-201 reinjection and improvement of left ventricular function following revascularization, *J Nucl Med* 34:45P, 1993 (abstract).

5. Bax JJ, Cornel JH, Visser FC, et al: Prediction of recovery of regional ventricular dysfunction following revascularization. Comparison of Fluorine-18 fluorodeoxyglucose/thallium-201 SPECT, thallium-201 stress-reinjection SPECT and dobutamine echocardiography, *J Am Coll Cardiol* 28:558–564, 1996.

6. Bax JJ, Cornel JH, Visser FC, et al: Comparison of thallium-201 rest-redistribution SPECT and FDG SPECT in predicting functional recovery after revascularization, *J Am Coll Cardiol* 27:300A, 1996 (abstract).

7. Beller GA: Comparison of 201Tl scintigraphy and low-dose dobutamine echocardiography for the noninvasive assessment of myocardial viability. *Circulation* 94:2681–2684, 1996.

8. Berger BC, Watson DD, Burwell LR, et al: Redistribution of thallium at rest in patients with stable and unstable angina and the effect of coronary artery bypass surgery, *Circulation* 60:1114–1125, 1979.

9. Bolli R: Myocardial 'stunning' in man, *Circulation* 86:1671–1691, 1992.

10. Bonow RO, Dilsizian V, Cuocolo A, et al: Identification of viable myocardium in patients with chronic coronary artery disease and left ventricular dysfunction. Comparison of thallium scintigraphy with reinjection and PET imaging with ^{18}F-fluorodeoxyglucose, *Circulation* 83:26–37, 1991.

11. Bonow RO, Dilsizian V: Thallium-201 for assessing myocardial viability, *Semin Nucl Med* 21:230–241, 1991.

12. Bonow RO: The hibernating myocardium: implications for management of congestive heart failure, *Am J Cardiol* 75:17A–25A, 1995.

13. Bonow RO: Identification of viable myocardium, *Circulation* 94:2674–2680, 1996.

14. Braunwald E, Kloner RA: The stunned myocardium: prolonged, postischemic ventricular dysfunction, *Circulation* 66:1146–1149, 1982.

15. Braunwald E, Rutherford JD: Reversible ischemic left ventricular dysfunction: evidence for "hibernating myocardium," *J Am Coll Cardiol* 8:1467–1470, 1986.

16. Brundage BH, Massie BM, Botvinick EH: Improved regional ventricular function after successful surgical revascularization, *J Am Coll Cardiol* 3:902–908, 1984.

17. Brunken R, Schwaiger M, Grover-McKay M, et al: Positron emission tomography detects tissue metabolic activity in myocardial segments with persistent thallium perfusion defects, *J Am Coll Cardiol* 10:557–567, 1987.

18. Brunken RC, Kottou S, Nienaber CA, et al: PET detection of viable tissue in myocardial segments with persistent defects at Tl-201 SPECT, *Radiology* 65:65–73, 1989.

19. Brunken RC, Mody FV, Hawkins RA, et al: Positron emission tomog-

raphy detects metabolic activity in myocardium with persistent 24-hour single-photon emission computed tomography 201Tl defects, *Circulation* 86:1357–1369, 1992.

20. Buxton DB: Dysfunction in collateral-dependent myocardium. Hibernation or repetitive stunning? *Circulation* 87:1756–1758, 1993.

21. Charney R, Schwinger ME, Chun J, et al: Dobutamine echocardiography and resting-redistribution thallium-201 scintigraphy predicts recovery of hibernating myocardium after coronary revascularization, *Am Heart J* 128:864–869, 1994.

22. Cigarroa CG, deFilippi CR, Brickner ME, et al: Dobutamine stress echocardiography identifies hibernating myocardium and predicts recovery of left ventricular function after coronary revascularization, *Circulation* 88:430–436, 1993.

23. Cloninger KG, et al: Incomplete redistribution in delayed thallium-201 single photon emission computed tomographic (SPECT) images: an overestimation of myocardial scarring, *J Am Coll Cardiol* 12:955–963, 1988.

24. Di Carli MF, Davidson M, Little R, et al: Value of metabolic imaging with positron emission tomography for evaluating prognosis in patients with coronary artery disease and left ventricular dysfunction, *Am J Cardiol* 73:527–533, 1994.

25. Dilsizian V, Bonow RO, Cannon RO 3d, et al: The effect of coronary artery bypass grafting on left ventricular systolic function at rest: evidence for preoperative sublinical myocardial ischemia, *Am J Cardiol* 61:1248–1254, 1988.

26. Dilsizian V, Rocco TP, Freedman NM, et al: Enhanced detection of ischemic but viable myocardium by the reinjection of thallium after stress-redistribution imaging, *N Engl J Med* 323:141–146, 1990.

27. Dilsizian V, Smeltzer WR, Freedman NM, et al: Thallium reinjection after stress-redistribution imaging. Does 24-hour delayed imaging after reinjection enhance detection of viable myocardium? *Circulation* 83:1247–1255, 1991.

28. Dilsizian V, Bonow RO: Differential uptake and apparent 201Tl washout after thallium reinjection. Options regarding early redistribution imaging before reinjection or late redistribution imaging after reinjection, *Circulation* 85:1032–1038, 1992.

29. Dilsizian V, Perrone-Filardi P, Arrijhi JA, et al: Concordance and discordance between stress-redistribution-reinjection and rest-redistribution thallium imaging for assessing viable myocardium. Comparison with metabolic activity by positron emission tomography, *Circulation* 88:941–952, 1993.

30. Eitzman D, al-Aonar Z, Kanter HL, et al: Clinical outcome of patients with advanced coronary artery disease after viability studies with positron emission tomography, *J Am Coll Cardiol* 20:559–565, 1992.

31. Elefteriades JA, Tolis G Jr, Levi E, et al: Coronary artery bypass grafting in severe left ventricular dysfunction: excellent survival with improved ejection fraction and functional state, *J Am Coll Cardiol* 22:1411–1417, 1993.

32. Gerber BL, Vanoverschelde JO, Bol A, et al: Myocardial blood flow, glucose uptake, and recruitment of inotropic reserve in chronic left ventricular ischemic dysfunction. Implications for the pathophysiology of chronic myocardial hibernation, *Circulation* 94:651–659, 1996.

33. Gibson RS, Watson DD, Taylor GJ, et al: Prospective assessment of regional myocardial perfusion before and after coronary revascularization surgery by quantitative thallium-201 scintigraphy, *J Am Coll Cardiol* 1:804–815, 1983.

34. Gimelli A, Marzullo P, Landi P, et al: Value of thallium-201 viability imaging for evaluating prognosis in patients with ischemic left ventricular dysfunction, *J Am Coll Cardiol* 27:90A, 1996 (abstract).

35. Gioia G, Powers J, Heo J, Iskandrian AS: Prognostic value of rest redistribution tomographic thallium-201 imaging in ischemic cardiomyopathy, *Am J Cardiol* 75:759–762, 1995.

36. Gutman J, Berman DS, Freeman M, et al: Time to completed redistribution of thallium-201 in exercise myocardial scintigraphy: relationship to the degree of coronary artery stenosis, *Am Heart J* 106(5 Pt 1):989–995, 1983.

37. Haque T, Furukawa T, Takahashi M, et al: Identification of hibernating myocardium by dobutamine stress echocardiography: comparison with thallium-201 reinjection imaging, *Am Heart J* 130(3 Pt 1):553–563, 1995.

38. Hendel RC: Single-photon perfusion imaging for the assessment of myocardial viability, *J Nucl Med* 35(4 Suppl):23S–31S, 1994.

39. Hendel RC, Chaudhry FA, Parker MA, et al: Regional discordance in myocardial viability assessment with thallium-201 rest-redistribution imaging and low-dose dobutamine echocardiography, *Circulation* 92: I-550, 1995 (abstract).

40. Hendel RC, Chaudhry FA, Bonow RO: Myocardial viability, *Curr Probl Cardiol* 21:145–221, 1996.

41. Hepner AM, Bach DJ, Bolling SF, et al: A positive dobutamine stress echocardiogram predicts viable myocardium in ischemic cardiomyopathy: a comparison with PET, *Circulation* 90:I-117, 1994 (abstract).

42. Iskandrian AS, Haldei AH, Kane SA, et al: Rest and redistribution thallium-201 myocardial scintigraphy to predict improvement in left ventricular function after coronary arterial bypass grafting, *Am J Cardiol* 51:1312–1316, 1983.

43. Kauffman GJ, Boyne TS, Watson DA, et al: Comparison of rest thallium-201 imaging and rest technetium-99m sestamibi imaging for assessment of myocardial viability in patients with coronary artery disease and severe left ventricular dysfunction, *J Am Coll Cardiol* 27:1592–1597, 1996.

44. Kayden DS, Sigal S, Soufer R, et al: Thallium-201 for assessment of myocardial viability: quantitative comparison of 24-hour redistribution imaging with imaging after reinjection at rest, *J Am Coll Cardiol* 18:1480–1486, 1991.

45. Kiat H, Berman DS, Maddahi J, et al: Late reversibility of tomographic myocardial thallium-201 defects: an accurate marker of myocardial viability, *J Am Coll Cardiol* 12:1456–1463, 1988.

46. La Canna G, Alfieri O, Giubbini R, et al: Echocardiography during infusion of dobutamine for identification of reversible dysfunction in patients with chronic coronary artery disease, *J Am Coll Cardiol* 23:617–626, 1994.

47. Liu P, Kiess MC, Okada RD, et al: The persistent defect on exercise thallium imaging and its fate after myocardial revascularization: does it represent scar or ischemia? *Am Heart J* 110:996–1001, 1985.

48. Maes AF, Borgers M, Flameng W, et al: Assessment of myocardial viability in chronic coronary artery disease using technetium-99m sestamibi SPECT. Correlation with histologic and positron emission tomographic studies and functional follow-up, *J Am Coll Cardiol* 29:62–68, 1997.

49. Marzullo P, Parodi O, Reisenhofer B, et al: Value of rest thallium-201/technetium-99m sestamibi scans and dobutamine echocardiography for detecting myocardial viability, *Am J Cardiol* 71:166–172, 1993.

50. Manyari DE, Knudtson M, Kloiber R, et al: Sequential thallium-201 myocardial perfusion studies after successful percutaneous transluminal coronary artery angioplasty: delayed resolution of exercise-induced scintigraphic abnormalities, *Circulation* 77:86–95, 1988.

51. Nienaber CA, Brunken RC, Sherman CT, et al: Metabolic and functional recovery of ischemic human myocardium after coronary angioplasty, *J Am Coll Cardiol* 18:966–978, 1991.

52. Nienaber CA, de la Roche J, Camarius H, et al: Impact of ^{201}thallium reinjection imaging to identify myocardial viability after vasodilation-redistribution SPECT, *J Am Coll Cardiol* 21:283A, 1993 (abstract).

53. Ohtani H, Tamaki N, Yonekura Y, et al: Value of thallium-201 reinjection after delayed SPECT imaging for predicting reversible ischemia after coronary artery bypass grafting, *Am J Cardiol* 66:394–399, 1990.

54. Pagley PR, Beller GA, Watson DD, et al: Improved outcome after coronary artery bypass surgery in patients with ischemic cardiomyopathy and residual myocardial viability, *Circulation* 96:793–800, 1997.

55. Panza JA, Dilsizian V, Laurienzo JM, et al: Relation between thallium uptake and contractile response to dobutamine. Implications regarding myocardial viability in patients with chronic coronary artery disease and left ventricular dysfunction, *Circulation* 91:990–998, 1995.

56. Perrone-Filardi P, Bacharach SL, Dilsizian V, et al: Regional left ventricular wall thickening. Relation to regional uptake of ^{18}F-fluorodeoxyglucose and ^{201}Tl in patients with chronic coronary artery disease and left ventricular dysfunction, *Circulation* 86:1125–1137, 1992.

57. Perrone-Filardi P, Pace L, Prastaro M, et al: Dobutamine echocardiography predicts improvement of hypoperfused dysfunctional myocardium after revascularization in patients with coronary artery disease, *Circulation* 91:2556–2565, 1995.

58. Perrone-Filardi P, Pace L, Prastaro M, et al: Assessment of myocardial viability in patients with chronic coronary artery disease. Rest-4-hour-24-hour ^{201}Tl tomography versus dobutamine echocardiography, *Circulation* 94:2712–2719, 1996.

59. Pierard LA, De Landsheere CM, Berthe C, et al: Identification of viable myocardium by echocardiography during dobutamine infusion in patients with myocardial infarction after thrombolytic therapy: comparison with positron emission tomography, *J Am Coll Cardiol* 15:1021–1031, 1990.

60. Ragosta M, Beller GA, Watson DD, et al: Quantitative planar rest-redistribution ^{201}Tl imaging in detection of myocardial viability and prediction of improvement in left ventricular function after coronary bypass surgery in patients with severely depressed left ventricular function, *Circulation* 87:1630–1641, 1993.

61. Rahimtoola SH: A perspective on the three large multicenter randomized clinical trials of coronary bypass surgery for chronic stable angina, *Circulation* 72(6 pt 2): V123–V135, 1985.

62. Rahimtoola SH: The hibernating myocardium, *Am Heart J* 117:211–221, 1989.

63. Rocco TP, Dilsizian V, McKusick RA, et al: Comparison of thallium redistribution with rest "reinjection" imaging for the detection of viable myocardium, *Am J Cardiol* 66:158–163, 1990.

64. Ross J Jr: Myocardial perfusion-contraction matching. Implications for coronary artery disease and hibernation, *Circulation* 83:1076–1083, 1991.

65. Rozanski A, Berman DS, Gray R, et al: Use of thallium-201 redistribution scintigraphy in the preoperative differentiation of reversible and nonreversible myocardial asynergy, *Circulation* 64:936–944, 1981.

66. Rozanski A, Berman D, Gray R, et al: Preoperative prediction of reversible myocardial asynergy by postexercise radionuclide ventriculography, *N Engl J Med* 307:212–216, 1982.

67. Sawada S, Elsner G, Segar DS, et al: Evaluation of patterns of perfusion and metabolism in dobutamine-responsive myocardium, *J Am Coll Cardiol* 29:55–61, 1997.

68. Sheehan FH, Doerr R, Schmidt WG, et al: Early recovery of left ventricular function after thrombolytic therapy for acute myocardial infarction: an important determinant of survival, *J Am Coll Cardiol* 12:289–300, 1988.

69. Skopicki HA, Weissman NJ, Rose GA, et al: Thallium imaging, dobutamine echocardiography, and positron emission tomography for the assessment of myocardial viability, *J Am Coll Cardiol* 27:162A, 1996 (abstract).

70. Smart SC, Sawada S, Ryan T, et al: Low-dose dobutamine echocardiography detects reversible dysfunction after thrombolytic therapy of acute myocardial infarction, *Circulation* 88:405–415, 1993.

71. Smart SC: The clinical utility of echocardiography in the assessment of myocardial viability. *J Nucl Med* 35(4 Suppl):49S–58S, 1994.

72. Stack RS, Phillips HR 3d, Grierson DS, et al: Functional improvement of jeopardized myocardium following intracoronary streptokinase infusion in acute myocardial infarction, *J Clin Invest* 72:84–95, 1983.

73. Tamaki N, Yonekura Y, Yamashita K, et al: Relation of left ventricular perfusion and wall motion with metabolic activity in persistent defects on thallium-201 tomography in healed myocardial infarction, *Am J Cardiol* 62:202–208, 1988.

74. Tamaki N, Yonekura Y, Yamashita K, et al: SPECT thallium-201 tomography and positron tomography using N-13 ammonia and F-18

fluorodeoxyglucose in coronary artery disease, *Am J Card Imaging* 3:3–9, 1989.

75. Tamaki N, Ohtani H, Yonekura Y, et al: Significance of fill-in after thallium-201 reinjection following delayed imaging: comparison with regional wall motion and angiographic findings, *J Nucl Med* 31: 1617–1623, 1990.

76. Tamaki N, Ohtani H, Yamashita K, et al: Metabolic activity in the areas of new fill-in after thallium-201 reinjection: comparison with positron emission tomography using fluorine-18-deoxyglucose, *J Nucl Med* 32:673–678, 1991.

77. Tillisch J, Brunken R, Marshall R, et al: Reversibility of cardiac wall-motion abnormalities predicted by positron tomography, *N Engl J Med* 314:884–888, 1986.

78. Topol EJ, Weiss JL, Brinker JA, et al: Regional wall motion improvement after coronary thrombolysis with recombinant tissue plasminogen activator: importance of coronary angioplasty, *J Am Coll Cardiol* 6:426–433, 1985.

79. Udelson JE, Coleman PS, Metherall J, et al: Predicting recovery of severe regional ventricular dysfunction. Comparison of resting scintigraphy with ^{201}Tl and ^{99m}Tc sestamibi. *Circulation* 89:2552–2561, 1994.

80. Vanoverschelde JLJ, Wijns W, Depre C, et al: Mechanisms of chronic regional postischemic dysfunction in humans. New insights from the study of noninfarcted collateral-dependent myocardium. *Circulation* 87:1513–1523, 1993.

81. Vanoverschelde JLJ, D'Hondt AM, Marwick T, et al: Head-to-head comparison of exercise-redistribution-reinjection thallium single-photon emission computed tomography and low dose dobutamine echocardiography for prediction of reversibility of chronic left ventricular ischemic dysfunction, *J Am Coll Cardiol* 28:432–442, 1996.

82. Yang LD, Berman DS, Kiat H, et al: The frequency of late reversibility in SPECT thallium-201 stress-redistribution studies, *J Am Coll Cardiol* 15:334–340, 1990.

Chapter 30

Assessment of myocardial viability with technetium-99m–labeled agents

James E. Udelson

A large body of literature has emerged in recent years supporting the use of perfusion and metabolic imaging with positron emission tomography (PET), as well as single-photon emission computed tomography (SPECT) imaging using thallium-201 (^{201}Tl), for the assessment of myocardial viability. Information resulting from such noninvasive assessment often has important implications for the functional and clinical benefits of revascularization in patients with coronary artery disease and regional or global left ventricular dysfunction.

The use of technetium-99m (^{99m}Tc)–labeled agents for tracing myocardial perfusion in SPECT imaging is inherently at-tractive because of the superior imaging characteristics of ^{99m}Tc as a radiolabel for gamma-camera imaging.[77] These attri-butes include the more optimal photon peak of ^{99m}Tc gamma-camera imaging and its shorter half-life and more optimal radiation dosimetry, which allows higher doses to be used compared with ^{201}Tl. Moreover, slightly reduced tissue attenuation accompanies the use of ^{99m}Tc-labeled agents. These factors result in higher count flux and generally more optimal images reflecting myocardial perfusion and tracer uptake.

Although the information provided by ^{99m}Tc-labeled agents for the standard clinical applications of myocardial perfusion imaging has been generally similar to that of ^{201}Tl in the detection of coronary artery disease[51,59,108] and has been superior to that of ^{201}Tl in certain populations,[101] and although the early data on prognostic information inherent in the images seem to parallel data from ^{201}Tl imaging,[44,72] controversy has evolved about the use of the nonredistributing ^{99m}Tc-labeled agents for assessment of myocardial viability. The roots of this controversy lie in several assumptions about the nonredistributing ^{99m}Tc-labeled agents and about the pathophysiology of chronic but reversible left ventricular dysfunction in the setting of severe coronary artery disease. For instance, it is often assumed that the uptake of myocardial perfusion agents accurately reflects myocardial blood flow across wide ranges of flow. Because it is also commonly assumed that chronic left ventricular dysfunction that is reversible with revascularization represents hibernating myocardium and because hibernation is widely believed to be a state of chronic hypoperfusion with matched downregulation of function,[84] it seems logical to conclude that an agent that merely traces myocardial blood flow will show an important uptake defect in an area of hibernating myocardium. In this setting, it is assumed that the redistribution properties of an agent such as ^{201}Tl will more optimally identify an area of viable myocardium with chronic dysfunction on the basis of low-flow ischemia.

Many or all of these assumptions can be challenged by data in the experimental and clinical literature, and a growing body of data suggests that quantitative analysis of regional tracer distribution with nonredistributing ^{99m}Tc-labeled agents, such as sestamibi or tetrofosmin, may provide information on myocardial viability similar to that derived from ^{201}Tl images by using principles of quantitative analysis derived from early studies of ^{201}Tl and myocardial viability.

EXPERIMENTAL BASIS FOR THE USE OF TECHNETIUM-99M–LABELED AGENTS TO ASSESS MYOCARDIAL CELL MEMBRANE INTEGRITY

An important prerequisite for any radiolabeled tracer used to assess myocardial viability is not only delivery through myocardial blood flow to an area of regional dysfunction but also intact myocardial cell membrane integrity to ensure extraction and retention and, thus, to allow clinical imaging. Several studies in cultured myocardial cells and isolated heart preparations support the concept that ^{99m}Tc-labeled agents, such as sestamibi, reflect myocardial cell membrane integrity.

For sestamibi, studies indicate that the major mechanism of myocellular uptake is dependent on passive distribution across sarcolemmal and mitochondrial membranes, driven by transmembrane eletrochemical gradients.[16,22,81] Uptake is significantly diminished in the setting of severe, irreversible injury to the myocardial cell membrane,[3] suggesting that an intact cell membrane is an important component of uptake and retention. Thallium-201 and ^{99m}Tc sestamibi differ in this regard. A significant proportion of the myocellular uptake of ^{201}Tl is dependent on sufficient membrane adenosine triphosphate (ATP) stores and the Na[+], K[+]-ATPase system.[69,82] Inhibition of energy generation by various agents results in distinct changes in uptake and extraction characteristics between ^{201}Tl and ^{99m}Tc sestamibi. Piwnica-Worms et al[80] studied extraction of ^{201}Tl and ^{99m}Tc sestamibi in cultured chick embryo cardiac myocytes after various degrees of cell membrane injury and metabolic inhibition. Mild-to-moderate ATP depletion resulted in diminished cellular extraction of ^{201}Tl but enhanced extraction of ^{99m}Tc sestamibi. These investigators postulated a model in which mild-to-moderate cell membrane injury as a consequence of ischemia would result in differences in uptake of ^{201}Tl and ^{99m}Tc sestamibi uptake (Fig. 30-1). This would correspond to changes that may be present in the setting of chronic hypoperfusion and reversibly ischemic myocardium, and this concept suggests that any advantage of redistribution of ^{201}Tl in low-flow ischemic areas may be offset by a potential increase in extraction of ^{99m}Tc sestamibi. Similar findings regarding diminished ^{201}Tl uptake relative to sestamibi in the setting of metabolic inhibition have also been reported by other investigators.[65]

EXPERIMENTAL STUDIES IN INTACT HEART MODELS OF REPERFUSION AND LOW-FLOW ISCHEMIA

The relation of ^{99m}Tc sestamibi uptake to blood flow has been assessed using intact perfused heart models. Canby et al[15] reported that the uptake of ^{99m}Tc sestamibi was higher than ex-

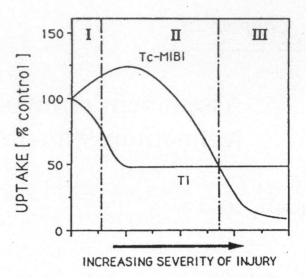

Fig. 30-1. Schematic representation of the effect of increasing degrees of cell membrane ischemic injury on the initial uptake rates of sestamibi *(Tc-MIBI) (x axis)* and thallium-201 *(Tl) (y axis)*. At mild-to-moderate levels of postulated ischemic cell membrane injury, *(zones I to II)* uptake of sestamibi would be enhanced, possibly because of membrane hyperpolarization, and the uptake of thallium-201 becomes depressed owing to depletion of cell membrane adenosine triphosphate levels. (From Piwnica-Worms D, Chiu ML, Kronauge JF: Divergent kinetics of ^{201}Tl and ^{99m}Tc-SESTAMIBI in cultured chick ventricular myocytes during ATP depletion, *Circulation* 85:1531-1541, 1992. Reprinted with permission.)

pected based on radiolabeled microspheres when flow was reduced to 10% to 40% of nonischemic zones (Fig. 30-2). This finding is similar to those reported earlier by Li and coworkers.[56] An analogous overestimation of flow in zones of moderate-to-severe ischemia was also seen using [201]Tl.[15]

Uptake and retention of ^{99m}Tc sestamibi does not seem to be affected importantly by states of coronary blood flow that would correspond to the clinical settings relevant to the study of myocardial viability (reperfusion after coronary occlusion or a more sustained state of low-flow ischemia). When ^{201}Tl and ^{99m}Tc sestamibi were injected during coronary occlusion or during reperfusion after occlusion in an experimental setting, the regional activities of both isotopes were similar soon after injection and were linearly related to flow determined by radiolabeled microspheres.[98] This and other studies[5,33,56] suggest that uptake and retention of ^{99m}Tc sestamibi are maintained even when this agent is administered in the setting of stunned myo-cardium and profound systolic dysfunction.

An important potential limitation of the use of ^{201}Tl imaging early after reperfusion following coronary occlusion is that the apparent uptake of ^{201}Tl, of necessity imaged soon after injection following reperfusion, overestimates the degree of myocardial salvage (viability) and is more closely related to the often-seen hyperemic flow conditions.[32,42,71] In a dog model of occlusion–reperfusion, Sinusas et al[97] found that ^{99m}Tc sestamibi activity after injection during reperfusion was signifi-

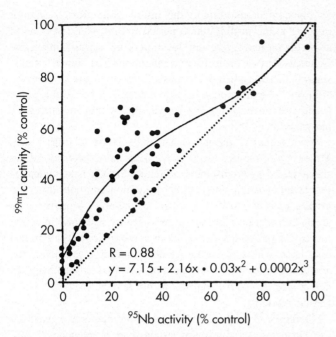

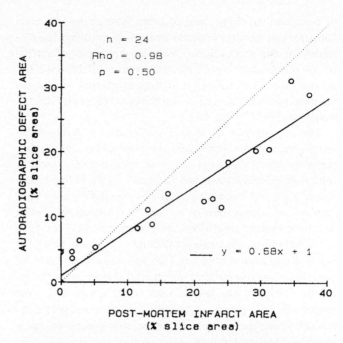

Fig. 30-2. Overestimation of myocardial blood flow in low flow territories by technetium-99m sestamibi. In a plot of the relation between sestamibi (^{99m}Tc-MIBI, y axis) and microsphere-determined myocardial blood flow (percent control, x axis), the relation of sestamibi uptake to blood flow is nonlinear at lower flow ranges. In these low-flow ranges, blood flow is consistently overestimated. (From Canby RC, Silber S, Pohost GM: Relations of myocardial imaging agents ^{99m}Tc-MIBI and ^{201}Tl to myocardial blood flow in a canine model of myocardial ischemic insult, *Circulation* 81:289-296, 1990. Reprinted with permission.)

Fig. 30-3. The relation between uptake of technetium-99m sestamibi following injection during postocclusion hyperemic flow and histologic infarct zone viability in a dog model. Uptake of isotope is significantly reflective of regional infarct zone viability, even during a high-flow state. (From Sinusas AF, Trautman KA, Bergin JD, et al: Quantification of area at risk during coronary occlusion and degree of myocardial salvage after reperfusion and technetium-99m methoxyisobutyl isonitrile, *Circulation* 82:1424-1437, 1990. Reprinted with permission.)

cantly less than reperfusion flow as assessed by radiolabeled microspheres and that the defect area on postmortem studies defined by the sestamibi uptake on autoradiographs of the postmortem ventricular slices correlated very highly with the histopathologically determined postmortem infarct area (Fig. 30-3). These investigators concluded that the degree of myocardial salvage following reperfusion can be assessed by sestamibi imaging, a potential tool for assessing the extent of myocardial viability in the infarct zone after myocardial infarction.

In an animal model of short-term low-flow ischemia accompanied by regional dysfunction without infarction, simulating the clinical situation of chronic but reversible left ventricular dysfunction in severe coronary disease, Sinusas et al[94] injected thallium and sestamibi at rest and performed regional counting of activities 3 hours after injection. Contrary to the expectation of higher thallium activity at this time point on basis of the property of ^{201}Tl redistribution, the activities of ^{201}Tl and sestamibi were equivalent at 3 hours after injection across all levels of reduced flow (as determined by radioactive microspheres). The activities of both agents at 3 hours after injection similarly overestimated regional flow and were more consistent with the activities of agents marking cell membrane integrity. These data suggest that overextraction at low flows[15] or a significant component of redistribution of sestamibi must have

been operative. Such studies suggest that by quantifying regional activity, these agents should similarly report the status of regional myocardial viability.

EXPERIMENTAL AND CLINICAL STUDIES OF ASSESSING INFARCT ZONE SALVAGE AND VIABILITY AFTER REPERFUSION THERAPY IN MYOCARDIAL INFARCTION

The relative lack of redistribution of sestamibi after initial uptake allows imaging to be performed hours after injection, with the result that imaging will represent blood flow at the time of injection. Thus, serial imaging following separate rest injections administered before and after thrombolytic therapy may provide important information on the extent of myocardial salvage. When sestamibi is injected before thrombolysis, the resulting defect, imaged up to several hours after successful thrombolysis and restoration of flow, represents the risk area of the occluded artery.[39,97,106] Even if thrombolysis is successful, imaging may be performed hours later, and on the basis of the relative lack of redistribution, the imaging pattern will remain stable despite restoration of flow. The accuracy of such imaging for delineating the area at risk during coronary occlusion has been confirmed by numerous investigators.[39,97,106] Subsequently, a second injection of sestamibi at rest with imaging can be done, and the change in defect size between the two scans will represent the magnitude of salvaged myocardium. The feasibility of this approach for detecting the results of thrombolytic therapy, not only for the patency status of the vessel but for true myocardial salvage (and, thus, myocardial viability in the infarct zone), has been shown for both planar and SPECT techniques[39,106,109] (Fig. 30-4).

The concept that the change in defect size during serial imaging represents true myocardial salvage and viability is supported by the correlation of defect size to predischarge and late follow-up ejection fraction and volume.[17,18] This finding is consistent with the experimental studies correlating autoradiographic[97] or scintigraphic defect size[106] to histopathologically determined infarct area. Moreover, patients who have a significant decrease in defect size between the acute study (injection before reperfusion therapy) and the follow-up study were far more likely to have a patent infarct-related artery after thrombolytic therapy.[39] The improvement in infarct zone regional function in these patients further supports the concept that the amount of salvage as shown by this scintigraphic technique is related to the extent of regional myocardial viability.

Thus, serial sestamibi imaging in the course of reperfusion therapy (thrombolytic therapy or primary angioplasty) for myocardial infarction may provide clinically relevant information on myocardial viability in the infarct zone. Rest sestamibi imaging in the postinfarction period will provide information about the presence, size, and location of myocardial infarction. Concepts derived from basic preparations and animal models suggest that the altered kinetics of sestamibi uptake and the "roll-off" of extraction at high flow rates may be advantageous in the assessment of myocardial viability within and surrounding the infarct zone.

With regard to prognosis and the relation to infarct size, Miller et al[73] showed a significant association between infarct size assessed by predischarge sestamibi SPECT using quantitative techniques after myocardial infarction and both total and cardiac mortality over long-term follow-up.[73] Moreover, the area of myocardium at risk (as assessed by sestamibi injection just before thrombolytic therapy or acute angioplasty) was also associated with subsequent cardiac mortality. However, the amount of myocardium salvaged (as assessed by the change in defect size on serial images) was not associated with total or cardiac mortality.[73]

Scintigraphic techniques for assessing infarct size generally use cut-points or thresholds established in phantom,[76] animal,[97,106] or human models to differentiate predominantly viable from nonviable myocardium in order to determine the extent of an infarct zone. However, histologic studies of myocar-

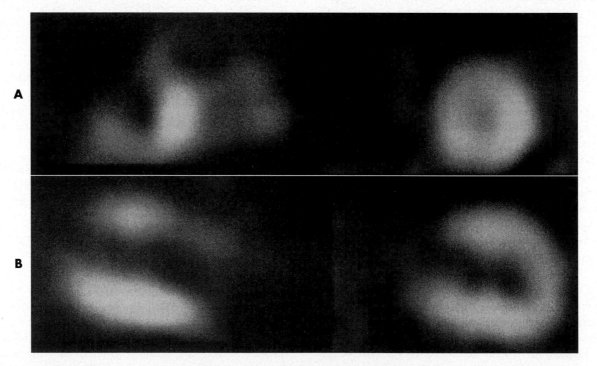

Fig. 30-4. Serial technetium-99m sestamibi single-photon emission computed tomographic images with injection performed just before thrombolytic therapy (*left,* **A** and **B**) and several days later (*right*). In the first image, the large defect in the short-axis (*top*) and long-axis (*bottom*) images represents the area at risk for infarction. In the right panels, the defect has almost completely resolved. The major change in defect size between images represents myocardial salvage resulting from reperfusion therapy. (From Gibbons RJ, Verani MS, Behrenbeck T, et al: Feasibility of tomographic ^{99m}Tc-hexakis-2-methoxy-2-methylpropylisonitrile imaging for the assessment of myocardial area at risk and the effect of treatment in acute myocardial infarction, *Circulation* 80:1277-1286. Reprinted with permission.)

dial tissue after infarction suggest that a continuum of tissue viability exists within an identifiable infarct zone. In a preliminary report, Vannan et al[105] demonstrated that within an infarct zone defined by standard thresholds using sestamibi SPECT in patients early after a first anterior infarction, the presence of moderately preserved viability (as determined by quantitative analysis of sestamibi activity) was associated with an attenuation of susequent remodeling in the course of 1 year (increasing left ventricular volumes and decreasing ejection fraction) compared with patients who had severe reduction of infarct zone viability. Thus, viability within an infarct zone should not necessarily be conceptualized as an all-or-nothing phenomenon; rather, a continuum exists in which physiologically relevant effects of preserved myocardial tissue may be seen.

STUDIES IN CHRONIC CORONARY ARTERY DISEASE AND LEFT VENTRICULAR DYSFUNCTION

Correlation with regional tissue viability

Much of the focus in the use of myocardial perfusion and cell membrane integrity tracers, such as ^{201}Tl or ^{99m}Tc sestamibi, is on the prediction of functional recovery after revascularization, since these tracers are imaged after uptake by individual viable myocardial cells. Therefore, the various thresholds or cut-points that are used to formulate predictive values for functional recovery are merely markers for a mass of viable myocardial tissue sufficient to support regional function after restoration of blood flow. In that regard, an important point of validation of these tracers for the assessment of myocardial viability is the correlation with the magnitude of viable myocardial cells within a dysfunctional territory. Several reports have investigated quantitative measures of regional uptake of these agents for their association with the magnitude of preserved tissue viability within dysfunctional territories.

Zimmerman et al[112] performed myocardial biopsies of dysfunctional anterior wall zones during bypass surgery in patients who had undergone planar thallium scintigraphy with thallium reinjection before surgery. Excellent correlation was seen between the quantitated thallium regional activity within the anterior wall from the planar images after reinjection and the percentage of fibrosis within the biopsy specimens of those walls (Fig. 30-5, *A*), suggesting that the quantitative analysis of thallium uptake on the planar scintigrams reflected the degree of regional tissue viability.

Two studies have examined this issue by using ^{99m}Tc sestamibi. Medrano et al[70] injected sestamibi at rest in patients with severe ischemic cardiomyopathy just before heart transplantation. After explantation of the recipient's severely dysfunctional heart, these investigators found that the magnitude of sestamibi defect severity (on imaging of the sliced pathologic specimens of the explanted heart) was closely correlated with the percentage of scarring within those same segments on pathologic examination (Fig. 30-5, *B*). In addition, well counting of myocardial specimens for sestamibi activity correlated well with the presence of viable myocardium by microscopy.

These data suggest that even in the setting of severe ischemic cardiomyopathy (average ejection fraction in this study, 24% ± 6%) and dysfunctional territories supplied by severely stenosed coronary arteries, quantitative sestamibi activity correlates well with the magnitude of preserved regional tissue viability within the dysfunctional territories. The data on sestamibi defect severity were, however, gathered from imaging specimens of the already explanted heart, leaving open the question of whether these elegant data can be generalized to in vivo clinical planar imaging or SPECT.

In a subsequent study, Maes et al[60] demonstrated that similar data could indeed be derived from SPECT imaging. Thirty patients with severe left anterior descending coronary artery stenosis and significant anterior wall dysfunction underwent resting sestamibi SPECT, and the resulting data were analyzed by using quantitative polar maps. All patients subsequently underwent bypass surgery, and intraoperative biopsies were performed. Excellent correlation was seen between the quantitated sestamibi activity within the anterior wall from the preoperative SPECT images and the percentage of fibrosis seen in the biopsy specimen (Fig. 30-5, *C*). These investigators concluded that the amount of sestamibi uptake is inversely related to the amount of interstitial fibrosis (and, thus, directly to the magnitude of preserved tissue viability) and that ^{99m}Tc sestamibi activity reflects not only flow but also regional tissue viability. These data have been independently confirmed by Dakik et al,[21] who also used an intraoperative biopsy technique for direct analysis of regional tissue viability compared with preoperative sestamibi SPECT.

When considered together, the results of the studies of Medrano et al,[70] Maes et al,[60] and Dakik et al[21] show correlations between measures of sestamibi uptake and measures of regional tissue viability similar to that demonstrated in the earlier study by Zimmerman et al[112] using ^{201}Tl reinjection (Fig. 30-5), suggesting that these agents comparably report the degree of preserved myocardial tissue viability in severe coronary disease and regional ventricular dysfunction. The data from all of these studies emphasize the idea that regional isotope activity in dysfunctional myocardium should be viewed as a continuum of values related to the degree of tissue viability and intact myocardial cell membranes. Whether functional recovery occurs after revascularization is, in turn, related to the mass of preserved myocardial tissue, and threshold or cut-points of regional isotope activity merely reflects that sufficient mass of tissue.[4,39,53]

Comparisons with thallium-201

Several studies directly compared uptake of ^{99m}Tc sestamibi with uptake of ^{201}Tl using various ^{201}Tl protocols in patients with left ventricular dysfunction. Using visual analysis of planar ^{201}Tl images after reinjection and stress and rest sestamibi images, in 20 patients with an average ejection fraction of 30% ± 8%, Cuocolo et al[20] found more reversible defects with ^{201}Tl reinjection than with stress and rest sestamibi studies and concluded that thallium reinjection may be more optimal for

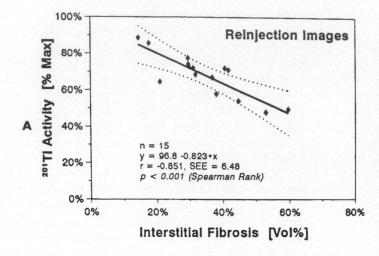

A

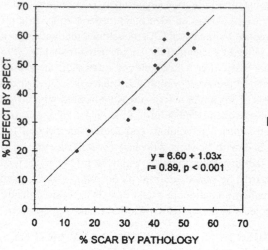

B

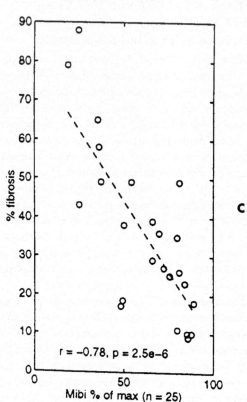

C

Fig. 30-5. A, Plot of the relation between thallium-201 activity, assessed by quantitative analysis of planar images following reinjection after stress-redistribution imaging *(y axis),* and the percentage of interstitial fibrosis, quantitated by histopathology after biopsy of anterior wall segments during coronary bypass surgery *(x axis).* Very good correlation is demonstrated. (From Zimmermann R, Mall G, Rauch B, et al: Residual ^{201}Tl activity in irreversible defects as a marker of myocardial viability. Clinicopathological study, *Circulation* 91:1016–1021, 1995. Reprinted with permission.) **B,** Relation between percentage of defect size by single-photon emission computed tomography of explanted heart slices *(y axis)* following sestamibi administration before heart transplantation, and the percentage of scar by pathology of the explanted heart *(x axis).* Good correlation was found between the defect size, as determined by ex vivo sestamibi SPECT, and the percentage of scar, measured by histopathology. (From Medrano R, Lowry R, Young J, et al: Assessment of myocardial viability with ^{99m}Tc sestamibi in patients undergoing cardiac transplantation. A scintigraphic/pathologic study, *Circulation* 94:1010–1017, 1996. Reprinted with permission.) **C,** Relation between sestamibi activity on preoperative quantitative analysis of SPECT images *(MIBI % of max, x axis)* and the percentage of fibrosis on anterior wall biopsy specimens in patients undergoing bypass surgery *(y axis).* Good correlation was seen from in vivo clinical SPECT and an indirect measure of measure of myocardial viability. (From Maes AF, Borgers M, Flameng W, et al: Assessment of myocardial viability in chronic coronary artery disease using technetium-99m sestamibi SPECT. Correlation with histologic and positron emission tomographic studies and functional follow-up, *J Am Coll Cardiol* 29:62-68, 1997. Reprinted with permission from the American College of Cardiology.)

detection of viability. The results of this study must be viewed in light of the absence of quantitative analysis, as well as the absence of any gold standard to determine which isotope was supplying the more accurate information. Other studies that found a slightly greater extent of stress defect reversibility with various thallium protocols compared with resting sestamibi uptake similarly lacked quantitative analysis or a reference standard.[86] Using quantitative analysis to compare regional activity of ^{201}Tl during redistribution after rest injection with sestamibi activity after rest injection, Maurea et al[66] reported that regional activity was slightly but significantly higher than with sestamibi in akinetic or dyskinetic segments (73% ± 12% and 67% ± 14% of the peak value; $p < 0.001$) and concluded that

^{201}Tl more accurately identifies viable myocardium on the basis of this difference in activity. However, such conclusions must be constrained in the absence of a reference standard, such as recovery of wall motion after revascularization. Functional recovery may not occur in up to 30% of dyssynergic myocardial segments with normal ^{201}Tl uptake.[83]

The importance of a reference standard when directly comparing two isotopes is also emphasized by the preliminary report of DePuey et al.[23] These investigators found apparent ^{201}Tl uptake or "fill-in" in the territory of a sestamibi defect in a phantom model, a finding that would usually be interpreted in a clinical study as showing the superiority of ^{201}Tl for identification of myocardial viability. However, these investigators

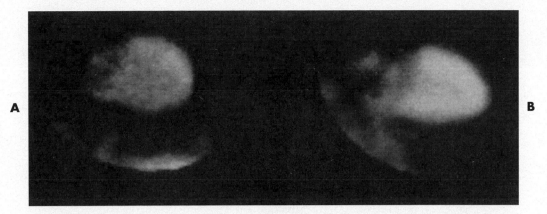

Fig. 30-6. Anterior planar views of a patient before (**A**) and after (**B**) coronary bypass surgery following a resting injection of technetium-99m sestamibi. **A,** An inferior defect is seen that is mild by visual or quantitative analysis, suggesting a significant mass of preserved viability and uptake of sestamibi. After bypass surgery, inferior wall perfusion in normal. (From Rocco TP, Dilsizian V, Strauss HW, et al: Technetium-99m isonitrile myocardial uptake at rest. II. Relation to clinical markers of potential viability, *J Am Coll Cardiol* 14:1678-1684, 1989. Reprinted with permission from the American College of Cardiology.)

demonstrated that this pattern may in part be related to differing resolution effects of the two agents. In this SPECT study of a phantom with an anterior defect, sestamibi more correctly identified the true defect inherent in the phantom, and apparent ^{201}Tl uptake was due to the poorer contrast resolution with that agent. When these data were applied to human studies, only about 10% of severe sestamibi defects demonstrated an extent of thallium uptake beyond that expected from the phantom study. This result is within the range of expected discordance when two tracers are compared for any purpose. Thus, the demonstration of a moderate degree of thallium uptake cannot, per se, be taken as evidence of functionally significant regional viability. These data reinforce the importance of independent gold standards.

The importance of quantitation of regional isotope activity was shown in an earlier investigation comparing sestamibi uptake with clinically available markers of myocardial viability. Rocco et al[85] reported that visual analysis of sestamibi uptake often demonstrated apparent defects in segments with preserved wall motion or in reversibly dysfunctional territories; when regional activity was subjected to quantitative analysis, however, the correlation improved significantly (Fig. 30-6). The figure supports an important concept in the analysis of scintigraphic images for the purpose of assessing viability: If this preoperative image is read as merely demonstrating an inferior defect (Fig. 30-6, left), the improvement in perfusion seen in *B* after revascularization would imply that the preoperative image underestimated the extent of viability within the inferior wall. If, however, the image in *A* was interpreted as showing a defect of only mild-to-moderate severity, thus consistent with significant retention of regional myocardial viability and associated with a high probability of postrevascularization recovery of perfusion or function or preserved metabolism (a concept derived from numerous studies of ^{201}Tl imag-

ing[11,26,83]) a more correct prediction of the perfusion pattern in *B* would be achieved.

A subsequent analysis used quantitation of ^{201}Tl and ^{99m}Tc sestamibi activity for comparison and PET as a gold standard for myocardial viability. In this study, Dilsizian et al[26] studied 54 patients with moderate left ventricular dysfunction and severe coronary disease with stress-redistribution–reinjection ^{201}Tl SPECT and separate-day stress–rest sestamibi SPECT. By visual analysis, 70% of segments with stress-induced defects were concordant with regard to reversibility of those defects by either the redistribution or reinjection technique ^{201}Tl or rest sestamibi SPECT. Among the discordant segments, most were found to be reversible by ^{201}Tl imaging but irreversible by sestamibi imaging, suggesting that the latter agent underestimated the extent of myocardial ischemia and viability. However, when the magnitude of defect severity was assessed quantitatively for both the ^{201}Tl and the sestamibi images in patients who also underwent PET, a 93% concordance was reported between the thallium and the sestamibi data (Table 30-1). The correctness of the separation of the mild-to-moderate ^{201}Tl or sestamibi defects as viable compared with the more severe defects as predominantly nonviable was supported by the PET data on flow and glucose metabolism. These data were the first to suggest that quantitative analysis of regional isotope activity was important to optimize the information on detection of myocardial viability by ^{99m}Tc-labeled agents using PET as an independent gold standard. The data were also consistent with the findings of Rocco et al[85] with regard to the use of quantitative analysis. Other studies using quantitative analysis to compare the magnitude of defect severity assessed by ^{201}Tl in various protocols with that of ^{99m}Tc sestamibi are listed in Table 30-1. They generally show high concordance when defect severity is classified by using discrete thresholds.

Data from studies describing the relation between isotope

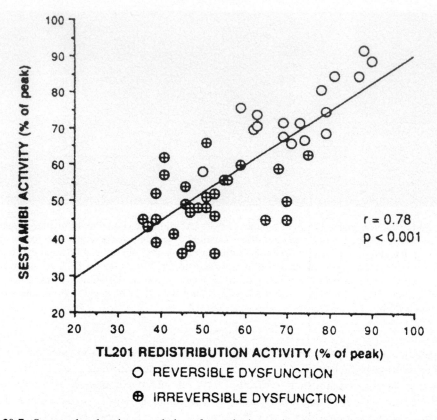

O REVERSIBLE DYSFUNCTION

⊕ IRREVERSIBLE DYSFUNCTION

Fig. 30-7. Scatter plot showing correlation of quantitative regional activities of thallium-201 at redistribution imaging after rest injection *(x axis)* and regional activities of technetium-99m sestamibi after rest injection *(y axis)* among segments with significant regional dysfunction in 18 patients undergoing revascularization. The open symbols represent segments with improved regional dysfunction (reversible dysfunction) after revascularization; the closed symbols represent segments with irreversible ventricular dysfunction. (From Udelson JE, Coleman PS, Metherall J: Predicting recovery of severe regional ventricular dysfunction. Comparison of resting scintigraphy with ^{201}Tl and ^{99m}Tc-sestamibi, *Circulation* 89:2552-2561, 1994. Reprinted with permission.)

Table 30-1. Concordance between abnormal thallium-201 and technetium-99m-sestamibi regions in studies using quantitative analysis

Author	Threshold	Concordance	Protocol
	%		
Dilsizian et al[26]	50	93	Stress-redistribution–reinjection compared with stress–rest
Rossetti et al[86]	50	91	Rest-redistribution compared with rest
	60	78	
Udelson et al[104]	50	92	Rest-redistribution compared with rest
	65	79	
Kauffman et al[52]	50	88	Rest-redistribution compared with rest

uptake using ^{201}Tl or ^{99m}Tc sestamibi and measures of regional tissue viability on histopathology[60,70,112] suggest that isotope content can also be viewed as a continuous variable rather than as separated into discrete categories. When viewed in this manner, a good correlation has been reported between quantitated regional activities in dysfunctional myocardial segments on [201]Tl (at redistribution after rest injection) and ^{99m}Tc sestamibi (1 hour after rest injection) imaging in patients with severe coronary artery disease (Fig. 30-7).[104] These

data suggest that the activities of ^{201}Tl and ^{99m}Tc sestamibi should be generally similar in reversibly or irreversibly dysfunctional myocardium.

In that regard, Marzullo et al[62] studied 14 patients before and after revascularization. Changes in wall motion were analyzed with echocardiography. Before surgery, all patients underwent rest and redistribution ^{201}Tl imaging and rest sestamibi imaging. The quantitative regional activities seen on planar images were similar for ^{201}Tl and ^{99m}Tc sestamibi in reversibly

Table 30-2. Regional activities of thallium-201 and technetium-99m sestamibi after rest injection in dysfunctional myocardium*

	Reversible dysfunction		Irreversible dysfunction	
	Thallium-201†	Technetium-99m sestamibi	Thallium 201†	Technetium-99m sestamibi
Study (imaging method)	% of peak value			
Marzullo et al[62] (planar)	67 ± 9	67 ± 13	46 ± 6	48 ± 10
Udelson et al[104] (SPECT)	72 ± 11	75 ± 9	51 ± 11	50 ± 8

*Values are given as the mean ± SD. SPECT = single-photon emission computed tomography.
†^{201}Tl activity based on the redistribution study after rest injection.

Table 30-3. Technetium-99m sestamibi activity in reversible rest thallium-201 defects*

		Thallium-201			Technetium-99m	
		Rest	Redistribution	P value†	sestamibi	P value‡
Author	Segments	% of peak value			% of peak value	
Udelson et al[104]	Rest thallium defect	64 ± 10	80 ± 10	<0.001	78 ± 10	NS
Kauffman et al[52]	Mildly decreased viability§	62 ± 5	67 ± 9	<0.05	68 ± 12	NS
	Severely decreased viability§	37 ± 8	43 ± 9	<0.05	44 ± 11	NS

*Values are given as the mean ± SD. NS = not significant.
†Rest compared with redistribution.
‡Sestamibi compared with redistribution.
§By thallium-201 criteria.

and irreversibly dysfunctional segments (Table 30-2). Udelson et al[104] reported similar results using SPECT rather than planar imaging: Among segments demonstrating significant reversibility of regional dysfunction after revascularization, mean ^{201}Tl activity at redistribution was 72% ± 11% of the peak value and sestamibi activity was 75% ± 9% of the peak value (P value not significant) (Table 30-2). Among segments with irreversible dysfunction, the redistribution activity of ^{201}Tl was 51% ± 11% of the peak value and that of sestamibi was 50% ± 8% (p value not significant).

Tc-99m sestamibi activity in reversible resting ^{201}Tl defects. The redistribution kinetics of ^{201}Tl theoretically give this agent an advantage in viable territories with resting hypoperfusion in that tracer accumulation over time and delayed imaging should allow better identification of ultimate tracer uptake, manifested scintigraphically as a reversible resting ^{201}Tl defect.[6,36,49] Two studies directly compared resting ^{99m}Tc sestamibi quantitative regional activity (approximately 1 hour after resting injection) with ^{201}Tl redistribution activity in segments in which significant redistribution into an initially resting ^{201}Tl defect occurred.[52,104] Contrary to expectation, in both studies, sestamibi activity in these segments was found to be similar to ^{201}Tl redistribution activity rather than to ^{201}Tl resting activity (Table 30-3). Although somewhat unexpected, these consistent data from two laboratories using similar study designs and analytic protocols are concordant with data from previous investigations in animal models of low-flow ischemia that demonstrated higher-than-expected ^{99m}Tc sestamibi activity compared with radiolabeled microsphere–based flow measurements and activity similar to that of ^{201}Tl redistribution activity.[94] The results in animal models and human studies suggest that the initial uptake or subsequent handling of sestamibi cannot be explained by the kinetics of a pure flow tracer with no redistribution.

The similarity of ^{99m}Tc sestamibi activity to ^{201}Tl redistribution activity in these studies[52,94,104] may be explained by any one or a combination of mechanisms: increased extraction in low-flow territories (possibly based on longer diffusibility times[94]), higher individual cell extraction compared with ^{201}Tl based on mildly ischemic injury to cell membranes,[80] or a greater-than-expected degree of redistribution of sestamibi after initial injection and uptake.[57,88,94]

Comparisons with positron emission tomography

In a group of 20 patients with previous myocardial infarction, Sawada et al[89] compared sestamibi activity after resting injection and SPECT imaging with PET information provided by nitrogen-13 ammonia (NH$_3$) and fluorine-18 fluorodeoxyglucose (FDG) imaging. Using a threshold of 60%, concordant activities between sestamibi and FDG were seen in 68% of all segments analyzed, suggesting a significant amount of discordance. Among the segments with severe sestamibi defects,

50% had preserved FDG activity (greater than or equal to 60% of peak), suggesting an underestimation of viability. However, among the segments with severe FDG defects (less than 60% of peak uptake), 46% had preserved sestamibi activity (greater than 60%). Thus, the significant discordance between the two agents was associated with only a slight excess of preservation of FDG uptake within discordant segments. An important potential underlying factor in the discrepancy among these tracers and techniques for identifying regional uptake consistent with viability may be that of the 20 patients in this study, 16 had a history of an inferior myocardial infarction; thus, the inferior wall was a territory of interest. Differences in attenuation between single-photon agents and positron emission techniques are likely to lead to differences in the ability to identify the magnitude of tracer uptake in the inferior wall. This suggests that distinct criteria for viability might be required in evaluating inferior wall segments when using single-photon techniques. This concept has not been adequately investigated in published studies.

The concept that the inferior wall territory may be problematic when directly comparing SPECT and PET agents was further emphasized by Soufer et al.[100] These investigators directly compared PET NH_3 and FDG data with resting sestamibi uptake in a group of 37 patients with a wide range of left ventricular ejection fractions (16% to 67%). A concordance of 71% was found between the sestamibi and PET data on segmental viability; thus, the amount of discordance was 29%. Among the discordant segments, most (72%) were considered nonviable by sestamibi criteria but viable by PET criteria. Most of these segments were found in the inferior wall. It is conceivable (but unproven) that application of various attenuation correction techniques to SPECT sestamibi data may improve the correlation with PET in such patients.

The importance of examining the full spectrum of tracer activities quantitatively rather than merely examining ^{201}Tl uptake or metabolic activity in sestamibi defects was shown by Altehoefer et al[2] in a series of 111 patients with coronary artery disease and resting wall-motion abnormalities who underwent resting sestamibi SPECT and FDG PET. A strong general correlation was seen between the quantitated values of sestamibi uptake 1 to 2 hours after resting injection and the percentage of segments within each category that were viable or nonviable by FDG PET criteria (Fig. 30-8). An important feature of this study was the recognition that PET imaging may distinguish viable from nonviable territories on the basis of the magnitude of FDG uptake, but an "intermediate zone" exists in which FDG uptake is 50% to 70% of normal. In such segments, the prevalence of functionally significant viability is itself intermediate.

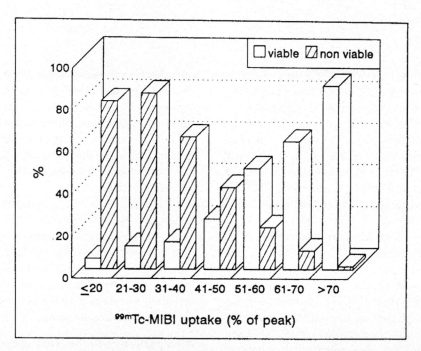

Fig. 30-8. Segments classified by quantitative regional activity of sestamibi after rest injection (^{99m}Tc-*MIBI uptake, x axis*) and the percentage of segments within each category that were viable or nonviable by fluorine-18 fluorodeoxyglucose (FDG) positron emission tomographic criteria. A general correlation was seen between the quantitative activity of sestamibi and the probability of viability by FDG criteria. Segments were classified as viable if the FDG peak activity was greater than 70% and as nonviable if the FDG activity was less than 50%. Segments with an FDG uptake of 50% to 70% were classified as intermediate (not shown in the figure). (From Altehoefer C, von Dahl J, Biedermann M, et al: Significance of defect severity in technetium-99m-MIBI SPECT at rest to assess myocardial viability: comparison with fluorine-18-FDG PET, *J Nucl Med* 35:569-574, 1994. Reprinted with permission.)

As shown in Table 30-4, among segments with "intermediate" regional sestamibi activity (41% to 60%), most also had "intermediate" viability by FDG criteria. Among the very severe sestamibi defects, the prevalence of PET viability by FDG criteria was low and was similar to the degree of PET nonviability among segments with clearly preserved sestamibi uptake. These data can be interpreted as suggesting that sestamibi and PET data are generally concordant regarding myocardial viability.

All studies show some discordance between uptake of any tracer and various measures of regional myocardial viability, which range from up to 23% segmental recovery of function in PET match segments[103] to 27% recovery of regional dysfunctional in segments with severe rest-redistribution ^{201}Tl defects.[83] Data from several studies comparing sestamibi uptake with PET evaluation of regional myocardial viability show similar correlations,[2,89,99] except for a higher degree of discordance when analyzing inferior wall segments, in which the attenuation correction capabilities of PET are advantageous.

Prediction of functional recovery after revascularization in regional or global left ventricular dysfunction

Several published studies have examined the ability of sestamibi uptake in dysfunctional myocardial regions to predict improvement in regional or global left ventricular function in patients with coronary artery disease undergoing revascularization. The results of published studies in which such data could be ascertained and in which quantitative or semiquantitative analysis was used to assess sestamibi uptake are listed in Table 30-5. The range of positive and negative predictive values for functional recovery (or lack thereof) are generally similar to that reported in a recent review of thallium SPECT studies and other techniques.[10] The studies listed in Table 30-5 involved relatively modest numbers of patients; used different acquisition and analytic techniques; and, of note, used different criteria for classifying segments or patients preoperatively as predominantly viable or nonviable.

Two studies directly compared resting ^{99m}Tc sestamibi data and rest-redistribution ^{201}Tl data by quantitative analytical criteria for predicting functional recovery in the same group of patients. Using planar techniques in 14 patients, Marzullo et al[62] showed a slighter higher sensitivity and specificity for the redistribution ^{201}Tl data compared with rest ^{99m}Tc sestamibi data in the assessment of functional recovery. However, the confidence limits around the point estimates for sensitivity and specificity overlapped widely, suggesting that no statistical difference existed between the two agents. This limitation is inherent to many studies that involve only modest numbers of patients. Subsequently, using SPECT techniques and quantitative analysis, Udelson and et al[104] demonstrated no difference in positive (75% and 80%) or negative predictive value (92% and 96%) between redistribution ^{201}Tl data after rest injection and resting ^{99m}Tc sestamibi data in predicting regional functional

Table 30-4. Relation of fluorine-18 fluorodeoxyglucose uptake and severity of technetium-99m sestamibi defect*

Imaging method and status	Percentage of peak technetium-99m sestamibi uptake			
	≤20 (n = 20)	% 21–40 (n = 108)	% 41–60 (n = 362)	% ≥61 (n = 953)
PET viable (FDG uptake >70%), %	5	12	37	82
PET nonviable (FDG uptake <50%), %	80	70	29	4
PET intermediate (FDG uptake 50% to 70%), %	15	18	34	14

*FDG = fluorine-18 fluorodeoxyglucose; PET = positron emission tomography.

Table 30-5. Predictive values for functional recovery after revascularization using technetium-99m sestamibi

Study	Patients n	Criteria threshold (% of peak)	Unit of recovery	Positive predictive value	Negative predictive value
				%	
Marzullo et al[62]	14	55%	Improvement in segmental function	79	76
Udelson et al[104]	18	60%	Improvement in segmental function	80	96
Maublant et al[64]	25	Semiquantitative severe defect	Improvement in segmental function	91	100
Bisi et al[9]	48	70%	Improvement in segmental uptake	62	78
vom Dahl et al[107]	72	50%	Vascular territory	45	59
Maes et al[60]	30	50%	Anterior-wall regional ejection fraction	75	86
Dakik et al[21]	21	55%	Improvement in segmental function	79	100
Sciagra et al[92]*	35	65%	Improvement in segmental function	79	74

*With nitrates.

recovery in a group of 18 patients with left ventricular dysfunction undergoing revascularization.

In the study by Udelson et al,[104] the predictive value of both isotopes across a wide range of uptake activity levels was examined in relation to functionally important myocardial viability. The probability of functionally significant viability was high among segments with clearly preserved uptake of ^{201}Tl or ^{99m}Tc sestamibi (Fig. 30-9) and was low among segments with very severe defects. In the intermediate range of uptake (40% to 60%), the probability of functionally important viability was intermediate, as described in previous studies that of rest-redistribution ^{201}Tl imaging when analyzed in a similar manner.[83] As suggested by the PET data obtained by Tamaki et al[102] and vom Dahl et al[107] it is conceivable that in segments within the intermediate ranges of uptake, further stratification into segments more or less likely to improve function might be made possible by PET FDG data or demonstration of reversible hypoperfusion or inducible ischemia. How often an entire decision about revascularization for an individual patient will revolve entirely around one such segment or group of segments is unclear from the literature.

In a study of one of the largest patient groups reported to date, vom Dahl et al[107] examined 72 patients by using resting ^{99m}Tc sestamibi SPECT and PET. Functional recovery was assessed by serial left ventricular contrast angiography, and quantitative analysis of changes in regional wall motion was done by using the centerline method.[93] Modest positive and negative predictive values of 45% and 59%, respectively, were reported in this study; these are similar to the least optimal values reported for ^{201}Tl SPECT.[10] This interesting study was one of the only investigations to analyze entire vascular territories as the

unit of functional recovery, and this aspect of the study design highlights the important issue of defining the relevant end-point in studies of myocardial viability. Like the previous study by Tamaki et al,[102] the PET FDG data in this study were most helpful in differentiating the probability of functional recovery among segments in the intermediate range of ^{99m}Tc sestamibi uptake.

Thus, the data in the literature regarding the predictive value of ^{99m}Tc sestamibi imaging for functional recovery after revascularization suggest that when quantitative analysis is used, predictive values across a range similar to those reported for ^{201}Tl imaging are possible. As in reports of other agents and techniques, most studies examined the outcome of individual segments rather than of large territories or patients (with some exceptions[60,107]). It would be expected that as patients are selected for revascularization on the basis of the scintigraphic data, specificity and predictive values will decrease because of posttest referral bias.[87] Moreover, how well the published data on the prediction of recovery of function using SPECT or PET, predominantly reported from studies of patients with moderate left ventricular dysfunction, extrapolate to patients with more severe left ventricular dysfunction is unclear.

Alternative protocols: technetium-99m sestamibi redistribution and infusion

Data from numerous animal models have clearly demonstrated that sestamibi does not behave like a "chemical microsphere": that is, as a pure flow tracer across all ranges of flows with 100% retention after initial uptake. In animal models in which resting hypoperfusion was induced with subsequent regional dysfunction in the absence of necrosis, a

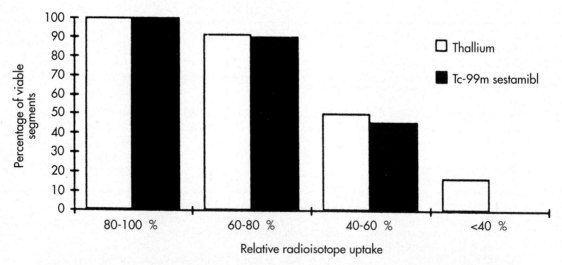

Fig. 30-9. Bar graphs showing the percentage of segments falling into quantitative quintiles of regional activity that represent viable myocardium (defined by preserved wall motion or improved wall motion after revascularization) for thallium-201 or technetium-99m sestamibi in 216 segments from 18 patients studied before and after revascularization. The probability of a scintigraphic segment representing viable myocardium is related to the magnitude of regional activity. (From Udelson JE, Coleman PS, Metherall J, et al: Predicting recovery of severe regional ventricular dysfunction. Comparison of resting scintigraphy with ^{201}Tl and ^{99m}Tc-sestamibi, *Circulation* 89:2552-2561, 1994. Reprinted with permission.)

change over time is seen in the ischemic-to-normal zone count-activity ratio, or "redistribution."[56,88,94] The magnitude of the change in activity is smaller than that seen with ^{201}Tl but is demonstrable in these models. Sinusas et al[94] demonstrated that regional activity of sestamibi quantitated 3 hours after injection in the setting of low-flow ischemia was similar to that of [201]Tl 3 hours after injection (that is, at redistribution). They also showed that the regional activities of both tracers were higher than the values for regional myocardial blood flow as measured by radiolabeled microspheres. Likewise, Sansoy et al[88] demonstrated that regional activity of sestamibi was higher than early ^{201}Tl activity after rest injection and was more similar to redistribution ^{201}Tl activity after 2 to 3 hours. Thus, not only are the cellular uptake and retention of sestamibi maintained in states of low-flow ischemia that mimic the classically defined clinical situation of hibernation, but the reported data also suggest that in low-flow territories, this agent acts more as a marker of cell membrane integrity than of myocardial blood flow. Whether the phenomenon of apparent redistribution of sestamibi is predominantly due to continuing arterial input into an initially severely hypoperfused zone or to differential washout between normal and hypoperfused zones is not entirely clear from animal models.

Studies in humans with left ventricular dysfunction have also demonstrated this phenomenon in a subset of patients with severe coronary artery disease after rest sestamibi injection[26,68] and seem to support the potential of clinically relevant sestamibi redistribution suggested by animal models. In a group of 18 patients reported by Dilsizian et al,[26] 16 myocardial segments among 55 stress-induced defects were found to be irreversible by stress and rest sestamibi imaging but viable by ^{201}Tl reinjection criteria. Of these 16 segments, 6 had visually apparent redistribution of sestamibi when resting imaging was repeated several hours after the first acquisition (Fig. 30-10), thus improving the concordance with ^{201}Tl reinjection data for assessment of myocardial viability. At least one segment showing sestamibi redistribution was seen in 4 of the 18 patients (22%). Similar data were reported by Maurea et al[68]: among 31 patients with coronary artery disease and left ventricular dysfunction who underwent rest and subsequent delayed sestamibi SPECT imaging several hours later, 28% of moderate sestamibi defects and 24% of initially severe sestamibi defects (by quantitative analysis) demonstrated an apparent increase in activity on delayed images. The segments with such "redistribution" were found to often improve in function following revascularization, thus confirming their viability. At least one segment demonstrating this phenomenon was seen in most of the patients studied.

Thus, the available data suggest that in patients in whom there are questions about myocardial viability, redistribution or delayed imaging after rest injection of sestamibi may provide important information. Larger studies are needed to examine the incremental importance of this finding compared with rest imaging alone in these patients, in whom clinical decisions revolve around the magnitude of isotope uptake and detection of regional viability.

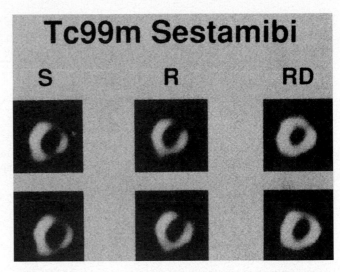

Fig. 30-10. Short-axis single-photon emission tomographic images at stress *(S)* and rest *(R)* as well as redistribution *(RD)* after sestamibi injection at stress and rest. An apparent fixed defect of the anterolateral wall after stress–rest imaging demonstrates a degree of reversibility on the redistribution images, which also show more complete reversibility of the partially reversible inferolateral defect. (From Dilsizian V, Arrighi JA, Diodati JG, et al: Myocardial viability in patients with chronic coronary artery disease. Comparison of ^{99m}Tc-sestamibi with thallium reinjection and [^{18}F] fluorodeoxyglucose, *Circulation* 89:678-687, 1994. Reprinted with permission.)

Tc-99m sestamibi infusion. The magnitude of ^{201}Tl redistribution into a severely hypoperfused region seems to be at least in part related to the blood level of ^{201}Tl during the time period of redistribution.[13,75] In reports of small numbers of cases, it appears that by maintaining a relatively high ^{201}Tl blood level during the time period of redistribution by the process of a several hour infusion of ^{201}Tl, the identification of hypoperfused but viable segments may be improved.[14] A similar concept has been applied by a prolonged infusion of sestamibi in an attempt to enhance the arterial input function of this tracer into a presumably hypoperfused zone. In a patient with severe coronary artery disease and left ventricular dysfunction, Worsley et al[110] demonstrated superior defect reversibility in an apparent fixed defect by using a prolonged sestamibi infusion; this is analogous to findings with ^{201}Tl infusion. The defect reversibility correctly identified the viable segments, as demonstrated by postrevascularization studies of stress and rest sestamibi perfusion. Further investigation in a series of patients with coronary artery disease and left ventricular dysfunction may be warranted to fully evaluate this potentially interesting technique.

USE OF NITRATES TO ENHANCE DETECTION OF MYOCARDIAL VIABILITY BY TECHNETIUM-99M TRACERS

Because it is commonly thought that areas of hibernating myocardium are associated with reduced resting myocardial blood flow,[84] treatment with nitrates before tracer injection is being extensively investigated for the possibility of enhanced

Table 30-6. Use of nitrates with technetium-99m–labeled agents in the assessment of myocardial viability*

Author	Agent	End-point	Result
Galli et al[35]	Sestamibi	Size and severity of the perfusion defect	Decreased size of perfusion defect in 56% of patients
Maurea et al[67]	Sestamibi	Sestamibi uptake, rest-redistribution thallium-201	Increased uptake in 27% of severe sestamibi defects
Sciagra et al[91]	Sestamibi	Functional recovery	Increased ROC curve area with nitrates and sestamibi
Li et al[58]	Sestamibi	Sestamibi uptake, functional recovery	Increased uptake in 47% of segments
Bisi et al[8]	Teboroxime	Defect reversibility compared with thallium-201	Change from fixed defect to reversible defect in 4 of 11 segments

*ROC = receiver-operating characteristic.

ability to assess myocardial viability. It has been well documented that nitrates can improve regional myocardial blood flow in ischemic areas through a combination of vasodilation of the epicardial coronary arteries and recruitment of collateral flow into the ischemic zone.[12,31]

Several investigators have examined the use of nitrates in conjunction with sestamibi or teboroxime injection to assess stress defect reversibility or myocardial viability. The results of these studies are summarized in Table 30-6.[8,35,58,67,91] These studies involved heterogeneous patient populations and analytical techniques, as well as differing end-points. A potentially important analytical issue is the timing of nitrate administration relative to imaging and the duration of the effects of nitrate. Because wall motion affects the apparent severity of a perfusion defect in SPECT or planar imaging[48] (as originally demonstrated with ^{201}Tl[37] and, more recently, with sestamibi,[28,96] it is possible that the improvement in perfusion or apparent activity seen in conjunction with nitrate administration is to some degree a function of improved wall motion in a previously akinetic segment (which, of course, would assist in the identification of segmental viability) or may merely be a consequence of having a smaller ventricle.[37] The latter possibility would be most important in studies where defect extent rather than severity is an end-point.[7] This concept emphasizes the importance of comparing isotope activity during nitrates administration to an independent gold standard rather than merely demonstrating an increase in apparent tracer activity.

In an analysis that used receiver-operating characteristic (ROC) curves to assess the discriminative ability of the resting sestamibi data alone compared with the nitrate sestamibi data for the prediction of functional recovery in dysfunctional segments, Sciagra et al[91] demonstrated a statistically significant improvement in the area under the ROC curve for the combination of baseline and nitrate-enhanced sestamibi data compared with rest sestamibi data alone (Fig. 30-11). This suggests that the combination of nitrate-enhanced and rest sestamibi data is associated with an increased ability to discriminate reversible from irreversible regional dysfunction. This type of analysis (that is, one that incorporates an independent standard of viability) is important in assessing the actual value of nitrate-induced changes in uptake, because the magnitude of the ob-

served changes of tracer uptake in several of these studies has been relatively small. Moreover, whether nitrate-enhanced data alone or in combination with rest tracer uptake data provide important incremental information beyond that obtained with resting tracer uptake data alone for the prediction of functional recovery has not been fully explored. For instance, in the study by Maurea et al,[67] segments that showed improvement in quantitated sestamibi uptake after nitrate administration had significantly higher resting sestamibi uptake at baseline compared with segments that showed no improvement after nitrate administration. However, the increase in the area under the ROC curve found by Sciagra et al[91] (Fig. 30-11) suggests that the use of nitrates may be an important strategy for optimal detection of viability. Larger studies of nitrate-induced changes in the uptake of nonredistributing ^{99m}Tc-labeled agents in patients with significant degrees of left ventricular dysfunction are warranted.

OTHER TECHNETIUM-99M–LABELED AGENTS
Technetium-99m teboroxime

Technetium-99m–labeled teboroxime has been used as a perfusion agent for myocardial imaging because of its very high extraction compared with ^{201}Tl and ^{99m}Tc sestamibi.[74] Studies in animal models have demonstrated a more rapid clearance of this tracer from reperfused infarcted zones than from noninfarcted zones[78] and a significantly reduced uptake compared with reperfusion blood flow after coronary occlusion.[1] These characteristics suggest that intact cell membrane integrity may be necessary for teboroxime uptake and retention and for clinical imaging. Other preliminary studies, however, have suggested that the relation between retained infarct zone viability and teboroxime regional activity after reperfusion may be less precise than that seen with ^{201}Tl or sestamibi.[32,45]

Few studies have directly examined the relation of teboroxime uptake to standard markers of regional myocardial viability in appropriate patients with left ventricular dysfunction. However, several investigations have suggested that teboroxime may be somewhat useful for this purpose.

In animal models with a fixed coronary stenosis, washout or redistribution of teboroxime after a stress injection has been documented,[43] although the extent of these effects is less than

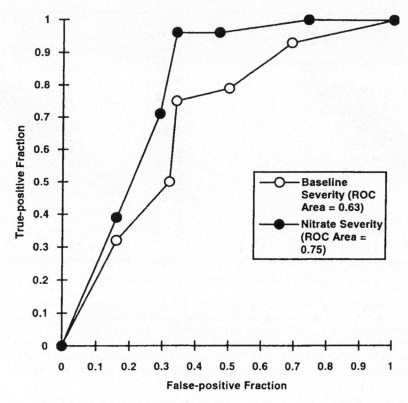

Fig. 30-11. Receiver-operating characteristic *(ROC)* curves for baseline single-photon emission computed tomography (SPECT) sestamibi imaging *(open circles)* and nitrate-enhanced SPECT sestamibi imaging *(closed circles),* indicating the diagnostic accuracy for the quantitative analysis of defect severity in discriminating reversible from irreversible regional dysfunction. (From Sciagra R, Bisi G, Santoro GM, et al: Influence of the assessment of defect severity and intravenous nitrate administration during tracer injection on the detection of viable hibernating myocardium with database quantitative technetium 99m-labeled sestamibi single-photon emission computed tomography, *J Nucl Cardiol* 3:221-230, 1996. Reprinted with permission.)

that seen with [201]Tl. This suggests that redistribution or washout imaging may be of some value as a substitute for subsequent rest injection in detecting ischemic but viable myocardium. In an attempt to demonstrate this finding in human subjects, Henzlova and Machac[47] examined 56 patients referred for standard myocardial perfusion imaging for clinical purposes. They found that teboroxime washout imaging acquired immediately after adenosine stress SPECT acquisition demonstrated a reversibility of stress-induced perfusion abnormalities similar to that of subsequent rest teboroxime imaging. However, other studies that directly compared stress–rest teboroxime scans with stress-redistribution–reinjection ^{201}Tl imaging have shown a smaller degree of stress defect reversibility with serial teboroxime imaging compared with ^{201}Tl reinjection.[46]

Clearly, the data on teboroxime for examination of myocardial viability are limited, and little if any information exists in the patients in whom such assessment is most appropriate: that is, those with significant left ventricular dysfunction. The development of multi-headed cameras and the potential for more rapid SPECT image acquisition suggests that further research into this issue, taking advantage of the kinetics of teboroxime, may be of value.

Technetium-99m tetrofosmin

Recently approved by the U.S. Food and Drug Administration, ^{99m}Tc tetrofosmin is, like sestamibi, a lipophilic cationic complex. Several studies have shown that this imaging agent is extracted by viable myocardial tissue in proportion to blood flow[95] and requires cellular viability for uptake and retention.[41] In a large multicenter trial, tetrofosmin was found to have an accuracy comparable to that of ^{201}Tl for the detection of angiographically significant coronary artery disease.[111]

Unlike ^{201}Tl, but like ^{99m}Tc sestamibi, tetrofosmin seems to have limited redistribution after initial uptake into the myocardium. This aspect of the kinetics of this agent raises questions about its ability to trace myocardial viability in low-flow ischemia. In an animal model of sustained low-flow ischemia, Koplan et al[55] compared the relative uptake of radiolabeled microspheres, ^{201}Tl, and ^{99m}Tc tetrofosmin. A previous study of sestamibi used an analogous design.[94] The results showed slightly but significantly less tetrofosmin activity in low-flow territories compared with ^{201}Tl redistribution activity at 2 hours. However, when quantitative analysis was used, the relative activity of tetrofosmin was higher than would be expected on the basis of the radiolabeled microsphere flow values alone,

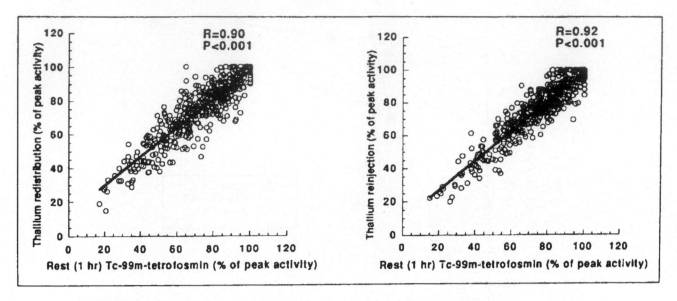

Fig. 30-12. Scatter plots demonstrating the correlation between regional tracer activities by quantitative analysis between 1-hour post–rest injection technetium-99m tetrofosmin imaging *(x axes)* and redistribution thallium-201 activity after rest injection *(left, y axis)* or reinjection thallium-201 imaging after stress and redistribution imaging (right, *y axis*). Good correlation is seen in both settings. (From Matsunari I, Fujino S, Taki J, et al: Myocardial viability assessment with technetium-99m tetrofosmin and thallium-201 reinjection in coronary artery disease, *J Nucl Med* 36:1961-1967, 1995.)

suggesting that quantitative analysis of regional uptake of this agent may provide information on myocardial viability[55] similar to that seen with sestamibi.

In a study of 25 patients with left ventricular dysfunction, Matsunari et al[63] compared both visual and quantitative analysis of exercise–rest tetrofosmin studies with stress-redistribution–reinjection ^{201}Tl imaging. On visual analysis, a greater prevalence of reversible stress-induced defects was seen with the ^{201}Tl reinjection protocol than with the exercise–rest tetrofosmin protocol. However, as in previous studies comparing ^{201}Tl with sestamibi,[26,52,104] when defect severity was taken into account by quantitative analytical methods, the concordance between the ^{201}Tl and tetrofosmin data regarding myocardial viability (magnitude of defect severity) increased significantly to 90%. This value is similar to the 93% concordance between ^{201}Tl and sestamibi reported by Dilsizian et al.[26] Moreover, excellent correlation was seen between the quantitative regional activity of tetrofosmin on 1-hour post–rest injection studies and ^{201}Tl redistribution or reinjection quantitative activities in individual segments (Fig. 30-12). This correlation is similar to that between redistribution ^{201}Tl activity after rest injection and sestamibi activity reported by Udelson et al.[104] Other preliminary data on tetrofosmin support these findings.[34]

Thus, it seems that despite the lack of redistribution compared with ^{201}Tl, tetrofosmin may be capable of providing significant information on myocardial viability when clinical studies are assessed quantitatively for the relative magnitude of defect severity. This concept, originally derived from studies of

[201]Tl stress and redistribution imaging,[40] seems to be an important analytical requisite that influences the ability of nonredistributing agents to assess regional myocardial viability.

Technetium-99m NOET

Technetium-99m NOET [bis(N-ethoxy, N-ethyldithiocarbamato) nitrido] is a neutral lipophilic myocardial imaging agent that carries the favorable imaging characteristics associated with the ^{99m}Tc radiolabel but seems in preliminary studies to have redistribution characteristics after injection similar to those of [201]Tl. In a canine model of partial coronary ligature in which dipyridamole infusion was used to induce hyperemia, an excellent linear correlation was seen between myocardial ^{99m}Tc NOET activity and radiolabeled microsphere flow determination across a wide range of coronary blood flow values early after injection.[38] However, after discontinuation of partial arterial occlusion, a poor linear relation with initial coronary blood flow was seen, which had been apparent at the time of injection, and it seemed that significant and almost complete redistribution of ^{99m}Tc NOET activity had ensued.[38]

In a group of 25 patients in whom coronary angiography was used as a gold standard, ^{99m}Tc NOET activity was compared at multiple time points after stress injection with ^{201}Tl in a stress-redistribution–reinjection protocol.[30] Both agents showed similar sensitivity and specificity for the detection of coronary artery disease in these patients, and good correlation was seen for the classification of stress defect reversibility between the thallium stress-redistribution–reinjection protocol

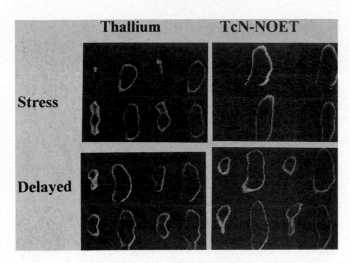

Fig. 30-13. Stress and 4-hour redistribution images ("*Delayed*") using thallium-201 *(left).* A large apical and septal defect with redistribution in the septum can be seen. Stress and 4-hour redistribution ("*Delayed*") technetium-99m NOET images *(right)* also demonstrate a severe apical and a more severe septal defect; the septal defect shows evidence of redistribution at 4-hour delayed imaging similar to that seen with thallium-201. (From Fagret D, Marie PY, Brunotte F, et al: Myocardial perfusion imaging with technetium-99m-Tc NOET: comparison with thallium-201 and coronary angiography, *J Nucl Med* 36:936-943, 1995. Reprinted with permission.)

and the stress-redistribution NOET images (Fig. 30-13). In a subset of patients in this study who underwent ^{99m}Tc NOET injection at rest, apparent redistribution was noted several hours later within resting defects.[30] Of interest and somewhat contrary to expectations, image quality was reported to be slightly less optimal with ^{99m}Tc-labeled NOET than with ^{201}Tl after stress injection.

These data suggest that this new agent may combine the favorable characteristics of the ^{99m}Tc label with the redistribution characteristics of ^{201}Tl and may be of interest for the assessment of myocardial viability in left ventricular dysfunction. It is important to note that of the 25 patients in this study,[30] only 9 had a history of myocardial infarction, and the presence or absence of left ventricular dysfunction was not reported. Thus, with regard to the assessment of myocardial viability, larger studies are needed in more relevant patient populations for this purpose. Data must be compared with various end-points for myocardial viability, including results of positron emission tomography, functional recovery after revascularization, and patient-related outcomes. It is not certain that the presence of redistribution is associated with enhanced viability information from this agent; much of the work on adapting ^{201}Tl protocols and analysis to optimize the assessment of viability* has been driven by the limitations of the redistribution process for this purpose.

*References 4, 10, 27, 40, 54, 66.

ANALYTICAL ISSUES IN STUDIES OF MYOCARDIAL VIABILITY
Interpretive differences in studies

It is of interest that in the literature on PET, thallium, and sestamibi for assessment of regional myocardial viability, similar data have been interpreted differently. Marzullo et al[62] reported that 25% of segments with severe wall-motion abnormalities and severe reduction in sestamibi activity had improved wall motion after revascularization. From these data, the authors concluded that sestamibi underestimates viability according to wall-motion criteria. However, similar data have been reported for rest-redistribution thallium imaging and for PET imaging, two methods widely thought to provide accurate information about viability (and often used as gold standards). In the study by Ragosta et al,[83] 27% of severely dyssynergic segments with severe reduction in ^{201}Tl activity had improved function after revascularization. Because this study demonstrated a general correlation between thallium uptake in dyssynergic segments and the probability of improvement in function after revascularization, it is widely (and appropriately) cited as supporting the use of rest-redistribution thallium imaging for this purpose. Tamaki et al[103] reported that 23% of dyssynergic segments with concordant reduction in perfusion and FDG activity (usually considered PET evidence of scar) demonstrated improved wall motion after revascularization. Despite this finding, a general correlation was seen between FDG activity and the potential for improved regional function after revascularization. This study is among those cited to support the use of PET to assess myocardial viability.[90] Indeed, in four of seven FDG PET studies reviewed by Schelbert,[90] 20% or more of segments with absent FDG uptake showed improved wall motion after revascularization.

Thus, similar data obtained with different techniques have been interpreted from distinct perspectives, and these differing conclusions have entered the conventional wisdom. When examining the results of individual studies, a perspective on the wide range of predictive values reported for all techniques[10] is important for context. All techniques both overestimate and underestimate functionally significant viability to some degree. Some of this variability may be ascribed to limitations in tracers or acquisition methods, but another component is the "noise" introduced into such studies by the potential misregistration of segments when comparing SPECT or PET techniques with echocardiographic or radionuclide ventriculographic wall-motion studies.

Is gated imaging helpful?

It is axiomatic that detection of wall thickening is synonymous with myocardial viability; a thickening wall must by definition be viable. Thus, the use of gated planar imaging or SPECT to detect the presence of wall motion or thickening can aid in the detection of myocardial viability and may, in some cases, be a substitute for rest imaging. In theory, if a gated acquisition is performed after stress injection, the presence of visually or quantitatively apparent wall motion or thickening within the territory of a stress perfusion defect should mean that the defect is an ischemic but viable territory that would be reversible on rest imaging. Several studies support this concept.[19,50,61,99] However, these studies also showed that the absence of apparent wall thickening by gated sestamibi SPECT does not always correspond to the absence of defect reversibility on rest imaging.[19,99] These territories may represent dysfunctional but viable (stunned or hibernating) regions.

Detection of regional wall motion with gated perfusion imaging can also be helpful in differentiating irreversible defects that represent true infarcts from artifacts, such as breast attenuation of the anterior or anterolateral wall or diaphragmatic attenuation of the inferior wall.[24,101] The presence of apparent wall motion or thickening on a gated study in the area of an irreversible defect (usually of only mild-to-moderate severity) signals that the area is unlikely to be an infarct; rather, the area is viable myocardium, and the irreversible defect probably represents an attenuation artifact.

There is another, untested mechanism by which gated SPECT using ^{99m}Tc-labeled agents may examine myocardial viability. Apparent regional tracer activity during clinical imaging is related not only to the actual regional tracer concentration but also to wall thickness.[28,37,48,96] Thus, in a patient with regional left ventricular dysfunction, analysis of tracer activity in a summed image will reveal more activity in a region that is thickening than in an akinetic region, even if the tracer concentration is the same in the two regions. It is therefore conceivable that if the effect of wall thickening on apparent regional activity can be removed, a more true representation of regional tracer concentration would be obtained, improving the ability to assess the extent of preserved viable myocardial tissue. This could be accomplished in a gated SPECT acquisition by quantitative assessment of the end-diastolic frame alone, in which the effects of wall thickening would be obviated because the regional wall thickness of akinetic but viable territories and normal territories would be at their most evenly matched point.

What are appropriate end-points for viability studies?

In the early assessment of a new agent for its ability to act as a probe of myocardial viability, cross-correlation is usually examined by comparing the new agent with ^{201}Tl in various protocols or with PET.* Because each tracer is associated with an error rate of approximately 20% or more for the prediction of functional recovery,[4,10,90] discordances between tracers should not necessarily be assumed to represent an advantage of one tracer over another in the absence of an independent standard of viability.

Given that the usual purpose of assessing the presence and extent of myocardial viability in a patient with coronary artery disease and left ventricular dysfunction is to select patients who will most benefit from revascularization, it would be appropriate to examine patient outcomes after viability assessment. Two studies of patients undergoing PET concordantly demonstrated

*References 20, 46, 52, 63, 89, 100.

that revascularization in the setting of PET evidence of viability is associated with more favorable event-free survival than is medical therapy in similar patients.[25,29] Data also suggest that rest-redistribution ^{201}Tl imaging has the same implications.[79] To date, ^{99m}Tc-labeled agents have not been examined in this regard.

Whether regional or global functional recovery after revascularization represent the most important or relevant clinical end-point for viability studies is not entirely certain. Whereas significant improvement in left ventricular ejection fraction is likely to be associated with favorable clinical and prognostic outcomes, revascularization may be associated with many favorable clinical effects such as relief of ischemic symptoms, improved exercise tolerance related to diminished inducible ischemia, and stabilization of remodeling and the electrophysiologic milieu, even in the absence of ventricular functional improvement. Large studies examining the relation between left ventricular functional change and outcomes will be of great interest in this area.

SUMMARY

Although the total number of patients studied with ^{99m}Tc-labeled agents for myocardial viability using quantitative analytic techniques and independent standards of viability is relatively small at this time and predominantly involves ^{99m}Tc sestamibi, the data at hand suggest performance characteristics within the ranges reported for other techniques and agents.[10] To the extent that myocardial hibernation is associated with a resting decrease in myocardial blood flow, the theoretical disadvantage of the lack of redistribution of most ^{99m}Tc agents seems to be at least in part overcome by the apparent overextraction at low flows and, possibly, by some degree of redistribution. Future studies will examine the generalizability of the smaller initial reports to larger populations and to patients with more severe degrees of left ventricular dysfunction, as well as the prognostic significance of viability defined by ^{99m}Tc agents in that setting.

REFERENCES

1. Abraham SA, Mirecki FN, Levine D, et al: Myocardial technetium-99m-teboroxime activity in acute coronary artery occlusion and reperfusion: relation to myocardial blood flow and viability, *J Nucl Med* 36:1062–1068, 1995.
2. Altehoefer C, vom Dahl J, Biedermann M, et al: Significance of defect severity in technetium-99m-MIBI SPECT at rest to assess the myocardial viability: comparison with fluorine-18-FDG PET, *J Nucl Med* 35:569–574, 1994.
3. Beanlands RS, Dawood F, Wen WH, et al: Are the kinetics of technetium-99m methoxyisobutyl isonitrile affected by cell metabolism and viability? *Circulation* 82:1802–1814, 1990.
4. Beller GA: Comparison of ^{201}Tl scintigraphy and low-dose dobutamine echocardiography for the noninvasive assessment of myocardial viability, *Circulation* 94:2681–2684, 1996.
5. Beller GA, Glover DK, Edwards NC, et al: ^{99m}Tc-sestamibi uptake and retention during myocardial ischemia and reperfusion, *Circulation* 87:2033–2042, 1993.
6. Berger BC, Watson DD, Burwell LR, et al: Redistribution of thallium at rest in patients with stable and unstable angina and the effect of coronary artery bypass surgery, *Circulation* 60:1114–1125, 1979.

7. Bisi G, Sciagra R, Santoro GM, et al: Rest technetium-99m sestamibi tomography in combination with short-term administration of nitrates: feasibility and reliability for prediction of postrevascularization outcome of asynergic territories, *J Am Coll Cardiol* 24: 1282–1289, 1994.

8. Bisi G, Sciagra R, Santoro GM, et al: Sublingual isosorbide dinitrate to improve technetium-99m-teboroxime perfusion defect reversibility, *J Nucl Med* 35:1274–1278, 1994.

9. Bisi G, Sciagra R, Santoro GM, et al: Technetium-99m-sestamibi imaging with nitrate infusion to detect viable hibernating myocardium and predict postrevascularization recovery, *J Nucl Med* 36:1994–2000, 1995.

10. Bonow RO: Identification of viable myocardium, *Circulation* 94: 2674–2680, 1996.

11. Bonow RO, Dilsizian V, Cuocolo A, et al: Identification of viable myocardium in patients with chronic coronary artery disease and left ventricular dysfunction. Comparison of thallium scintigraphy with reinjection and PET imaging with ^{18}F-fluorodeoxyglucose, *Circulation* 83:26–37, 1991.

12. Brown BG, Bolson E, Petersen RB, et al: The mechanisms of nitroglycerin action: stenosis vasodilatation as a major component of the drug response, *Circulation* 64:1089–1097, 1981.

13. Budinger TF, Pohost GM: Thallium "redistribution"—an explanation, *J Nucl Med* 27:996, 1986 (abstract).

14. Burns RJ, Wright LM, Lumsden CH, et al: Hibernating myocardium: detection by rest ^{201}Tl infusion SPECT, *Circulation* 88:I-534, 1993 (abstract).

15. Canby RC, Silber S, Pohost GM: Relations of the myocardial imaging agents ^{99m}Tc-MIBI and ^{201}Tl to myocardial blood flow in a canine model of myocardial ischemic insult, *Circulation* 81:289–296, 1990.

16. Chiu ML, Kronauge JF, Piwnica-Worms D: Effect of mitochondrial and plasma membrane potentials on accumulation of hexakis (2-methoxyisobutylisonitrile) technetium (I) in cultured mouse fibroblasts, *J Nucl Med* 31:1646–1653, 1990.

17. Christian TF, Behrenbeck T, Gersh BJ, et al: Relation of left ventricular volume and function over one year after acute myocardial infarction to infarct size determined by technetium-99m-sestamibi, *Am J Cardiol* 68:21–26, 1991.

18. Christian TF, Behrenbeck T, Pellikka PA, et al: Mismatch of left ventricular function and infarct size demonstrated by technetium-99m isonitrile imaging after reperfusion therapy for acute myocardial infarction: identification of myocardial stunning and hyperkinesia, *J Am Coll Cardiol* 16:1632–1638, 1990.

19. Chua T, Kiat H, Germano G, et al: Gated technetium-99m sestamibi for simultaneous assessment of stress myocardial perfusion, postexercise regional ventricular function and myocardial viability. Correlation with echocardiography and rest thallium-201 scintigraphy, *J Am Coll Cardiol* 23:1107–1114, 1994.

20. Cuocolo A, Pace L, Ricciardelli B, et al: Identification of viable myocardium in patients with chronic coronary artery disease: comparison of thallium-201 scintigraphy with reinjection and technetium-99m-methoxyisobutyl isonitrile, *J Nucl Med* 33:505–511, 1992.

21. Dakik HA, Howell JF, Lawrie GM, et al: Assessment of myocardial viability with ^{99m}Tc-sestamibi tomography before coronary bypass graft surgery: correlation with histopathology and postoperative improvement in cardiac function, *Circulation* 96:2892–2898, 1997.

22. Delmon-Moingeon LI, Piwnica-Worms D, Van den Abbeele AD, et al: Uptake of the cation hexakis(2-methoxyisobutylisonitrile)-technetium-99m by human carcinoma cell lines in vitro, *Cancer Res* 50:2198–2202, 1990.

23. DePuey EG, Nichols K, Rozanski A, et al: Defect reversibility with dual isotope SPECT: viability or just poorer contrast resolution with Tl201? *J Nucl Med* 35:103P, 1994 (abstract).

24. DePuey EG, Rozanski A: Using gated technetium-99m-sestamibi SPECT to characterize fixed defects as infarct or artifact, *J Nucl Med* 36:952–955, 1995.

25. Di Carli MF, Davidson M, Little R, et al: Value of metabolic imaging with positron emission tomography for evaluating prognosis in patients with coronary artery disease and left ventricular dysfunction, *Am J Cardiol* 73:527–533, 1994.

26. Dilsizian V, Arrighi JA, Diodati JG, et al: Myocardial viability in patients with chronic coronary artery disease. Comparison of ^{99m}Tc-sestamibi with thallium reinjection and [^{18}F] fluorodeoxyglucose, *Circulation* 89:578–587, 1994.

27. Dilsizian V, Rocco TP, Freedman NM, et al: Enhanced detection of ischemic but viable myocardium by the reinjection of thallium after stress-redistribution imaging, *N Engl J Med* 323:141–146, 1990.

28. Eisner RL, Schmarkey LS, Martin SE, et al: Defects on SPECT "perfusion" images can occur due to abnormal segmental contraction, *J Nucl Med* 35:638–643, 1994.

29. Eitzman D, al-Aouar Z, Kanter HL, et al: Clinical outcome of patients with advanced coronary artery disease after viability studies with positron emission tomography, *J Am Coll Cardiol* 20:559–565, 1992.

30. Fagret D, Marie PY, Brunotte F, et al: Myocardial perfusion imaging with technetium-99m-Tc NOET: comparison with thallium-201 and coronary angiography, *J Nucl Med* 36:936–943, 1995.

31. Fallen EL, Nahmias C, Scheffel A: Redistribution of myocardial blood flow with topical nitroglycerin in patients with coronary artery disease, *Circulation* 91:1381–1388, 1995.

32. Forman R, Kirk ES: Thallium-201 accumulation during reperfusion of ischemic myocardium: dependence on regional blood flow rather than viability, *Am J Cardiol* 54:659–663, 1984.

33. Freeman I, Grunwald A, Hoory S, et al: Effect of coronary occlusion and myocardial viability on myocardial activity of technetium-99m-sestamibi, *J Nucl Med* 32:292–298, 1991.

34. Galassi AR, Centomore G, Liberti F, et al: Quantitative SPECT Tc99m-tetrafosmin for the assessment of myocardial viability in patients with severe left ventricular dysfunction, *J Nucl Cardiol* 2:S23, 1995 (abstract).

35. Galli M, Marcassa C, Imparato A, et al: Effects of nitroglycerin by technetium-99m sestamibi tomoscintigraphy on resting regional myocardial hypoperfusion in stable patients with healed myocardial infarction, *Am J Cardiol* 74:843–848, 1994.

36. Gewirtz H, Beller GA, Strauss HW, et al: Transient defects of resting thallium scans in patients with coronary artery disease, *Circulation* 59:707–713, 1979.

37. Gewirtz H, Grotte GJ, Strauss HW, et al: The influence of left ventricular volume and wall motion in myocardial images, *Circulation* 59:1172–1177, 1979.

38. Ghezzi C, Fagret D, Arvieux CC, et al: Myocardial kinetics of TcN-NOET: a neutral lipophilic complex tracer of regional myocardial blood flow, *J Nucl Med* 36:1069–1077, 1995.

39. Gibbons RJ, Verani MS, Behrenbeck T, et al: Feasibility of tomographic ^{99m}Tc-hexakis-2-methoxy-2-methylpropyl-isonitrile imaging for the assessment of myocardial area at risk and the effect of treatment in acute myocardial infarction, *Circulation* 80:1277–1286, 1989.

40. Gibson RS, Watson DD, Taylor GJ, et al: Prospective assessment of regional myocardial perfusion before and after coronary revascularization surgery by quantitative thallium-201 scintigraphy, *J Am Coll Cardiol* 1:804–815, 1983.

41. Glover DK, Ruiz M, Allen TR, et al: Assessment of myocardial viability by Tc-99m tetrofosmin in a canine model of coronary occlusion and reperfusion, *J Am Coll Cardiol* 23:475A, 1994 (abstract).

42. Granato JE, Watson DD, Flanagan TL, et al: Myocardial thallium-201 kinetics during coronary occlusion and reperfusion: influence of method of reflow and timing of thallium-201 administration, *Circulation* 73:150–160, 1986.

43. Gray WA, Gewirtz H: Comparison of ^{99m}Tc-teboxime with thallium for myocardial imaging in the presence of a coronary artery stenosis, *Circulation* 84:1796–1807, 1991.

44. Heller GV, Herman SD, Travin MI, et al: Independent prognostic

value of intravenous dipyridamole with technetium-99m sestamibi tomographic imaging in predicting cardiac events and cardiac-related hospital admissions, *J Am Coll Cardiol* 26:1202–1208, 1995.

45. Heller LI, Villegas BJ, Weiner BH, et al: Use of sequential teboroxime imaging for the detection of coronary artery occlusion and reperfusion in ischemic and infarcted myocardium, *Am Heart J* 127:779–785, 1994.

46. Hendel RC, Dahlberg ST, Weinstein H, et al: Comparison of teboroxime and thallium for the reversibility of exercise-induced myocardial perfusion defects, *Am Heart J* 126:856–862, 1993.

47. Henzlova MJ, Machac J: Clinical utility of technetium-99m-teboroxime myocardial washout imaging, *J Nucl Med* 35:575–579, 1994.

48. Hoffman EJ, Huang SC, Phelps ME: Quantitation in positron emission computed tomography: 1. Effect of object size, *J Comput Assist Tomogr* 3:299–308, 1979.

49. Iskandrian AS, Hakki AH, Kane SA, et al: Rest and redistribution thallium 201 myocardial scintigraphy to predict improvement in left ventricular function after coronary arterial bypass grafting, *Am J Cardiol* 51:1312–1316, 1983.

50. Kahn JK, Henderson EB, Akers MS, et al: Prediction of reversibility of perfusion defects with a single post-exercise technetium-99m RP-30A gated tomographic image: the role of residual systolic thickening, *J Am Coll Cardiol* 11:31A, 1988.

51. Kahn JK, McGhie I, Akers MS, et al: Quantitative rotational tomography with ^{201}Tl and ^{99m}Tc 2-methoxy-isobutyl-isonitrile. A direct comparison in normal individuals and patients with coronary artery disease, *Circulation* 79:1282–1293, 1989.

52. Kauffman GJ, Boyne TS, Watson DD, et al: Comparison of rest thallium-201 imaging and rest technetium-99m sestamibi imaging for assessment of myocardial viability in patients with coronary artery disease and severe left ventricular dysfunction, *J Am Coll Cardiol* 27:1592–1597, 1996.

53. Kaul S: Response of dysfunctional myocardium to dobutamine. "The eyes see what the mind knows!" *J Am Coll Cardiol* 27:1608–1611, 1996.

54. Kiat H, Berman DS, Maddahi J, et al: Late reversibility of tomographic myocardial thallium-201 defects: an accurate marker of myocardial viability, *J Am Coll Cardiol* 12:1456–1463, 1988.

55. Koplan BA, Beller GA, Ruiz M, et al: Comparison between thallium-201 and technetium-99m-tetrofosmin uptake with sustained low flow and profound systolic dysfunction, *J Nucl Med* 37:1398–1402, 1996.

56. Li QS, Frank TL, Franceschi D, et al: Technetium-99m methoxyisobutyl isonitrile (RP30) for quantification of myocardial ischemia and reperfusion in dogs, *J Nucl Med* 29:1539–1548, 1988.

57. Li QS, Solot G, Frank TL, et al: Myocardial redistribution of technetium-99m-methoxyisobutyl isonitrile (SESTAMIBI), *J Nucl Med* 31:1069–1076, 1990.

58. Li ST, Liu XJ, Lu ZL, et al: Quantitative analysis of technetium 99m 2-methoxyisobutyl isonitrile single-photon emission computed tomography and isosorbide dinitrate infusion in assessment of myocardial viability before and after revascularization, *J Nucl Cardiol* 3:457–463, 1996.

59. Maddahi J, Kiat H, Van Train KF, et al: Myocardial perfusion imaging with technetium-99m sestamibi SPECT in the evaluation of coronary artery disease, *Am J Cardiol* 66:55E–62E, 1990.

60. Maes AF, Borgers M, Flameng W, et al: Assessment of myocardial viability in chronic coronary artery disease using technetium-99m sestamibi SPECT. Correlation with histologic and positron emission tomographic studies and functional follow-up, *J Am Coll Cardiol* 29:62–68, 1997.

61. Marzullo P, Marcassa C, Sambuceti G, et al: The clinical usefulness of electrocardiogram-gated Tc-99m methoxy-isobutyl-isonitrile images in the detection of basal wall motion abnormalities and reversibility of stress induced perfusion defects, *Int J Card Imaging* 8:131–141, 1992.

62. Marzullo P, Parodi O, Reisenhofer B, et al: Value of rest thallium-201/technetium-99m sestamibi scans and dobutamine echocardiography for detecting myocardial viability, *Am J Cardiol* 71:166–172, 1993.

63. Matsunari I, Fujino S, Taki J, et al: Myocardial viability assessment with technetium-99m-tetrofosmin and thallium-201 reinjection in coronary artery disease, *J Nucl Med* 36:1961–1967, 1995.

64. Maublant JC, Citron B, Lipiecki J, et al: Rest technetium 99m-sestamibi tomoscintigraphy in hibernating myocardium, *Am Heart J* 129:306–314, 1995.

65. Maublant JC, Gachon P, Moins N: Hexakis (2-methoxy isobutylisonitrile) technetium-99m and thallium-201 chloride: uptake and release in cultured myocardial cells, *J Nucl Med* 29:48–54, 1988.

66. Maurea S, Cuocolo A, Pace L, et al: Left ventricular dysfunction in coronary artery disease: comparison between rest-redistribution thallium 201 and resting technetium 99m methoxyisobutyl isonitrile cardiac imaging, *J Nucl Cardiol* 1:65–71, 1994.

67. Maurea S, Cuocolo A, Soricelli A, et al: Enhanced detection of viable myocardium by technetium-99m-MIBI imaging after nitrate administration in chronic coronary artery disease, *J Nucl Med* 36:1945–1952, 1995.

68. Maurea S, Cuocolo A, Soricelli A, et al: Myocardial viability index in chronic coronary artery disease: technetium-99m-methoxy isobutyl isonitrile redistribution, *J Nucl Med* 36:1953–1960, 1995.

69. McCall D, Zimmer LJ, Katz AM: Kinetics of thallium exchange in cultured rat myocardial cells, *Circ Res* 56:370–376, 1985.

70. Medrano R, Lowry RW, Young JB, et al: Assessment of myocardial viability with ^{99m}Tc sestamibi in patients undergoing cardiac transplantation. A scintigraphic/pathologic study, *Circulation* 94:1010–1017, 1996.

71. Melin JA, Becker LC, Bulkley BH: Differences in thallium-201 uptake in reperfused and nonreperfused myocardial infarction, *Circ Res* 53:414–419, 1983.

72. Miller DD, Stratmann HG, Shaw L, et al: Dipyridamole technetium 99m sestamibi myocardial tomography as an independent predictor of cardiac event-free survival after acute ischemic events, *J Nucl Cardiol* 1:72–82, 1994.

73. Miller TD, Christian TF, Hopfenspirger MR, et al: Infarct size after acute myocardial infarction measured by quantitative tomographic ^{99m}Tc sestamibi imaging predicts subsequent mortality, *Circulation* 92:334–341, 1995.

74. Narra RK, Nunn AD, Kuczynski BL, et al: A neutral technetium-99m complex for myocardial imaging, *J Nucl Med* 30:1830–1837, 1989.

75. Nelson CW, Wilson RA, Angello DA, et al: Effect of thallium-201 blood levels on reversible myocardial defects, *J Nucl Med* 30:1172–1175, 1989.

76. O'Connor MK, Hammell T, Gibbons RJ: In vitro validation of a simple tomographic technique for estimation of percentage myocardium at risk using methoxyisobutyl isonitrile technetium 99m (sestamibi), *Eur J Nucl Med* 17:69–76, 1990.

77. Okada RD, Glover D, Gaffney T, et al: Myocardial kinetics of technetium-99m-hexakis-2-methoxy-2-methylpropyl-isonitrile, *Circulation* 77:491–498, 1988.

78. Okada RD, Glover DK, Moffett JD, et al: Kinetics of technetium-99m-teboroxime in reperfused nonviable myocardium, *J Nucl Med* 38:274–279, 1997.

79. Pagley PR, Beller GA, Watson DD, et al: Improved outcome after coronary bypass surgery in patients with ischemic cardiomyopathy and residual myocardial viability, *Circulation* 96:793–800, 1997.

80. Piwnica-Worms D, Chiu ML, Kronauge JF: Divergent kinetics of ^{201}Tl and ^{99m}Tc-sestamibi in cultured chick ventricular myocytes during ATP depletion, *Circulation* 85:1531–1541, 1992.

81. Piwnica-Worms D, Kronauge JF, Chiu ML: Uptake and retention of hexakis (2-methoxyisobutyl isonitrile) technetium (I) in cultured chick myocardial cells. Mitochondrial and plasma membrane potential dependence, *Circulation* 82:1826–1838, 1990.

82. Piwnica-Worms D, Kronauge JF, Delmon L, et al: Effect of metabolic

inhibition on technetium-99m-MIBI kinetics in cultured chick myocardial cells, *J Nucl Med* 31:464–472, 1990.

83. Ragosta M, Beller GA, Watson DD, et al: Quantitative planar rest-redistribution ^{201}Tl imaging in detection of myocardial viability and prediction of improvement in left ventricular function after coronary bypass surgery in patients with severely depressed left ventricular function, *Circulation* 87:1630–1641, 1993.

84. Rahimtoola SH: A perspective on the three large multicenter randomized clinical trials of coronary bypass surgery for chronic stable angina, *Circulation* 72:V123–V135, 1985.

85. Rocco TP, Dilsizian V, Strauss HW, et al: Technetium-99m isonitrile myocardial uptake at rest. II. Relation to clinical markers of potential viability, *J Am Coll Cardiol* 14:1678–1684, 1989.

86. Rossetti C, Landoni C, Lucignani G, et al: Assessment of myocardial perfusion and viability with technetium-99m methoxyisobutylisonitrile and thallium-201 rest redistribution in chronic coronary artery disease, *Eur J Nucl Med* 22:1306–1312, 1995.

87. Rozanski A, Diamond GA, Berman D, et al: The declining specificity of exercise radionuclide ventriculography, *N Engl J Med* 309:518–522, 1983.

88. Sansoy V, Glover DK, Watson DD, et al: Comparison of thallium-201 resting redistribution with technetium-99m-sestamibi uptake and functional response to dobutamine for assessment of myocardial viability. *Circulation* 92:994–1004, 1995.

89. Sawada SG, Allman KC, Muzik O, et al: Positron emission tomography detects evidence of viability in rest technetium-99m sestamibi defects, *J Am Coll Cardiol* 23:92–98, 1994.

90. Schelbert HR: Metabolic imaging to assess myocardial viability, *J Nucl Med* 35(4 Suppl):8S–14S, 1994.

91. Sciagra R, Bisi G, Santoro GM, et al: Influence of the assessment of defect severity and intravenous nitrate administration during tracer injection on the detection of viable hibernating myocardium with data-based quantitative technetium 99m-labeled sestamibi single-photon emission computed tomography, *J Nucl Cardiol* 3:221–230, 1996.

92. Sciagra R, Bisi G, Santoro GM, et al: Comparison of baseline-nitrate technetium-99m sestamibi with rest-redistribution thallium-201 tomography in detecting viable hibernating myocardium and predicting postrevascularization recovery, *J Am Coll Cardiol* 30:384–391, 1997.

93. Sheehan FH, Bolson EL, Dodge HT, et al: Advantages and applications of the centerline method for characterizing regional ventricular function, *Circulation* 74:293–305, 1986.

94. Sinusas AJ, Bergin JD, Edwards NC, et al: Redistribution of ^{99m}Tc-sestamibi and ^{201}Tl in the presence of a severe coronary artery stenosis, *Circulation* 89:2332–2341, 1994.

95. Sinusas AJ, Shi Q, Saltzberg MT, et al: Technetium-99m-tetrofosmin to assess myocardial blood flow: experimental validation in an intact canine model of ischemia, *J Nucl Med* 35:664–671, 1994.

96. Sinusas AJ, Shi Q, Vitols PJ, et al: Impact of regional ventricular function, geometry, and dobutamine stress on quantitative ^{99m}Tc-sestamibi defect size, *Circulation* 88:2224–2234, 1993.

97. Sinusas AJ, Trautman KA, Bergin JD, et al: Quantification of area at risk during coronary occlusion and degree of myocardial salvage after reperfusion with technetium-99m methoxyisobutyl isonitrile, *Circulation* 82:1424–1437, 1990.

98. Sinusas AJ, Watson DD, Cannon JM Jr, et al: Effect of ischemia and postischemic dysfunction on myocardial uptake of technetium-99m-

labeled methoxyisobutyl isonitrile and thallium-201, *J Am Coll Cardiol* 14:1785–1793, 1989.

99. Snapper HJ, Shea NL, Konstam MA, et al: Combined analysis of resting regional wall thickening and stress perfusion with electrocardiographic-gated technetium-99m-labeled sestamibi single-photon emission computed tomography: prediction of stress defect reversibility, *J Nucl Cardiol* 4:3–10, 1997.

100. Soufer R, Dey HM, Ng CK, et al: Comparison of sestamibi single-photon emission computed tomography with positron emission tomography for estimating left ventricular myocardial viability, *Am J Cardiol* 75:1214–1219, 1995.

101. Taillefer R, DePuey EG, Udelson JE, et al: Comparative diagnostic accuracy of Tl-201 and Tc-99m sestamibi SPECT imaging (perfusion and ECG-gated SPECT) in detecting coronary artery disease in women, *J Am Coll Cardiol* 29:69–77, 1997.

102. Tamaki N, Kawamoto M, Tadamura E, et al: Prediction of reversible ischemia after revascularization. Perfusion and metabolic studies with positron emission tomography, *Circulation* 91:1697–1705, 1995.

103. Tamaki N, Yonekura Y, Yamashita K, et al: Positron emission tomography using fluorine-18 deoxyglucose in evaluation of coronary artery bypass grafting, *Am J Cardiol* 64:860–865, 1989.

104. Udelson JE, Coleman PS, Metherall J, et al: Predicting recovery of severe regional ventricular dysfunction. Comparison of resting scintigraphy with ^{201}Tl and ^{99m}Tc-sestamibi, *Circulation* 89:2552–2561, 1994.

105. Vannan M, Kettle A, Coakley A, et al: Influence of infarct zone viability on left ventricular remodeling in the year following anterior myocardial infarction, *Circulation* 92:I-286, 1995.

106. Verani MS, Jeroudi MO, Mahmarian JJ, et al: Quantification of myocardial infarction during coronary occlusion and myocardial salvage after reperfusion using cardiac imaging with technetium-99m hexakis 2-methoxyisobutyl isonitrile, *J Am Coll Cardiol* 12:1573–1581, 1988.

107. vom Dahl J, Altehoefer C, Sheehan FH, et al: Recovery of regional left ventricular dysfunction after coronary revascularization. Impact of myocardial viability assessed by nuclear imaging and vessel patency at follow-up angiography, *J Am Coll Cardiol* 28:948–958, 1996.

108. Wackers FJTh, Berman DS, Maddahi J, et al: Technetium-99m hexakis 2-methoxyisobutyl isonitrile: human biodistribution, dosimetry, safety, and preliminary comparison to thallium-201 for myocardial perfusion imaging, *J Nucl Med* 30:301–311, 1989.

109. Wackers FJ, Gibbons RJ, Verani MS, et al: Serial quantitative planar technetium-99m isonitrile imaging in acute myocardial infarction: efficacy for noninvasive assessment of thrombolytic therapy, *J Am Coll Cardiol* 14:861–873, 1989.

110. Worsley DF, Fung AY, Jue J, et al: Identification of viable myocardium with technetium-99m-MIBI infusion, *J Nucl Med* 36:1037–1039, 1995.

111. Zaret BL, Rigo P, Wackers FJ, et al: Myocardial perfusion imaging with 99mTc tetrofosmin. Comparison to ^{201}Tl imaging and coronary angiography in a phase III multicenter trial. Tetrofosmin International Trial Study Group, *Circulation* 91:313–319, 1995.

112. Zimmermann R, Mall G, Rauch B: Residual ^{201}Tl activity in irreversible defects as a marker of myocardial viability. Clinicopathological study, *Circulation* 91:1016–1021, 1995.

Chapter 31

Metabolic assessment of myocardial viability: a physiologic perspective

Christophe Depre and **Heinrich Taegtmeyer**

PRINCIPLES OF ENERGY TRANSFER IN HEART MUSCLE

The development of methods for the regional assessment of myocardial blood flow and metabolism provides an unprecedented opportunity to image substrate metabolism in the intact, beating heart in vivo. Positron emission tomography (PET) of labeled substrates offers a glimpse at the intricate and complex system of energy conversion in myocardial cells. To understand the mechanisms underlying the metabolic assessment of reversible cell damage, or "viability," it is necessary to review the principles of energy transfer under normal and ischemic conditions. Such knowledge provides a background for the salient features of reversible ischemic injury and an understanding of the usefulness and the limitations of noninvasive methods for the assessment of myocardial viability.

The myocardium requires a continuous supply of chemical energy for the synthesis of adenosine triphosphate (ATP) to support its contractile activity. The main energy-providing substrates are fatty acids, carbohydrates, and ketone bodies. Although the heart is an "omnivore," competition exists among these different substrates, which is regulated by their plasma concentrations, the workload to be performed, and the hormonal and dietary status of the organism.[113,168,171] In the fed (postprandial) state, blood glucose and insulin concentrations are increased, fatty acid concentrations are low, and the contribution of glucose to the energy needs of the heart is dominant.[112] In the fasting state, glycolysis is inhibited and the oxidation of fatty acids and ketone bodies prevails.[134] During exercise, lactate may provide all of the energy needed to support the high workload of the heart.[73]

The amount of ATP used and produced by the human heart has been estimated to be about 35 kg each day.[170] Most of the ATP is produced from substrate oxidation through the tricarboxylic acid cycle and the electron transport chain. In most physiologic conditions, the heart preferably oxidizes fuels other than glucose when they are available. However, a major metabolic adaptation occurs when the heart is subjected to conditions restricting oxidative metabolism, as in myocardial ischemia. Under such conditions, glycolysis is dramatically increased and becomes the main pathway for anaerobic production of ATP.[141,190]

In this chapter, we describe the biochemical basis for the use of metabolic tracers. To accomplish this goal, we first describe the metabolic characteristics of the different substrates for the heart and their interactions in the regulation of cardiac function and metabolism.

ENERGY-PROVIDING SUBSTRATES FOR THE HEART

The different substrates used for energy provision in the heart are shown in Fig. 31-1. The main circulating fuels are fatty acids, glucose, lactate, and ketone bodies. We make a distinction between glucose and lactate, which yield pyruvate, and fatty acids and ketone bodies, which yield acetyl coenzyme A (CoA). The importance of this distinction is underlined in the discussion of the pivotal role of pyruvate. Another important feature seen in Fig. 31-1 is the fact that lactate, fatty acids, and

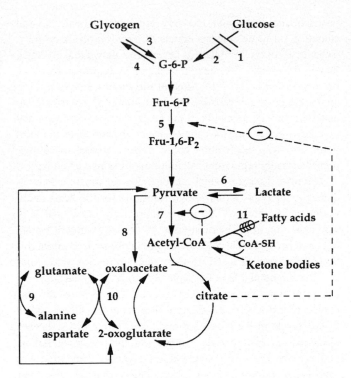

Fig. 31-1. Metabolic pathways and fuel interactions in the heart. 1, Glucose transporter; 2, hexokinase; 3, glycogen phosphorylase; 4, glycogen synthase; 5, phosphofructokinase; 6, lactate dehydrogenase; 7, pyruvate dehydrogenase; 8, pyruvate carboxylase; 9, glutamate–pyruvate transaminase; 10, glutamate–oxaloacetate trans-aminase; 11, β-oxidation. Dotted lines represent feedback inhibitions.

ketone bodies all inhibit glycolysis. Glucose is in equilibrium with glycogen, which can be considered as an intracellular store of glucose moieties and, hence, a special form of energy reserve.

Carbohydrates

The main carbohydrates used by the heart are glucose, arising from exogenous and endogenous sources, and lactate, produced mainly by skeletal muscle when rates of glycolysis in this tissue exceed rates of glucose oxidation.

Glucose. The concentration of glucose in the blood remains constant under most physiologic conditions, except diabetic ketoacidosis.[167] Glucose uptake by the cardiomyocyte occurs along a steep gradient between its extracellular (high) and intracellular (low) concentrations. It is mediated by the combined action of the glucose transport system and hexokinase, resulting in the formation of glucose 6-phosphate. As in other organs, glucose 6-phosphate is found at a metabolic branch point that leads to glycolysis, glycogen synthesis, or the pentose phosphate pathway. The latter pathway is not shown in Fig. 31-1. Although it is important for the synthesis of ribose, the pentose phosphate pathway is of minor importance for energy transfer. Glycolysis usually represents the major fate of glucose in the heart. Major regulatory sites of glycolysis are the reactions catalyzed by phosphofructokinase, glyceraldehyde

3-phosphate dehydrogenase, and the pyruvate dehydrogenase complex.

Glucose transport. Under most physiologic conditions, the rate of glucose transport is slower than the rate of glucose phosphorylation,[102] thus maintaining a gradient in favor of glucose entry.[94] Glucose transport determines the rate of glycolysis. Only when glucose transport is stimulated (for example, after insulin administration), hexokinase becomes rate limiting, and free glucose accumulates inside the cell.[74,130] Glucose transport is regulated by specific transporter proteins. Research done in the last decade has elucidated many salient features of these transporters. The specific glucose transporters (GLUT) in the heart belong to a family of carriers that are encoded by different genes.[59,107,128,161] The glucose transporter that is predominantly expressed at the surface of the adult cardiomyocyte is the GLUT 4 isotype, which is the insulin-sensitive transporter also expressed in adipose tissue and skeletal muscle.[59,107] The GLUT 1 transporter, which predominates in the fetal cardiomyocyte,[161] is also present in adult cardiomyocytes, although it is about 5-10 times less abundant than GLUT 4.[82,128]

The number of transporters at the surface of the cardiomyocytes results from an equilibrium among endocytosis, recycling, and de novo synthesis. In short-term regulation, the number increases by recruitment of the transporters from intracellular stores, whereas in long-term regulation, the rates of synthesis and degradation of the transporters are modified.* The number of transporters at the surface of the cell is increased by insulin, catecholamines, and thyroid hormones,[49,154,183] by workload,[111,137,197] and by ischemia.[165,186] Glucose transporter activity is generally decreased by competing fuels,† but it is not known whether this decrease is related to a change in the density of transporters at the surface of the cell (that is, a decrease in the Vmax for glucose) or covalent modification of the transporter protein.

Hexokinase. The heart contains two isoenzymes of hexokinase: hexokinase I and II.[62] Both have a K_m for glucose of about 0.1 mM and are inhibited by their reaction product, glucose 6-phosphate. Although it is thought that hexokinase is allosterically regulated, the actual mechanism of its inhibition remains unclear; increased rates of glucose phosphorylation are observed despite an accumulation of glucose 6-phosphate when the extracellular concentration of glucose is increased, when insulin is administered, or when oxygen tension is lowered.[34] Similarly, in hearts perfused with lactate (see below), glucose uptake is not completely abolished despite an increased concentration of glucose 6-phosphate.[37] This lack of inhibition of glucose phosphorylation by glucose 6-phosphate in heart cells may be the result of a translocation of hexokinase II from the cytosol to the mitochondria.[11] Hexokinase translocation does occur in isolated heart preparations when glucose uptake is

*References 9, 10, 42, 79, 157, 158, 163.
†References 37, 48, 63, 115, 170, 187, 191.

stimulated by insulin,[143] but the mechanism that induces this translocation is also still not known.

Phosphofructokinase. A major regulatory site of glycolysis resides in phosphofructokinase, the enzyme that catalyzes the phosphorylation of fructose 6-phosphate into fructose 1,6-bisphosphate (Fig. 31-1), because this enzyme is under complex allosteric control by various effectors. One of its substrates, ATP, behaves as a negative allosteric effector.[95,96] The inhibition by ATP can be relieved by an excess of fructose 6-phosphate acting as a positive effector. Citrate and protons are negative effectors,[54,175] whereas fructose 2,6-bisphosphate and adenosine monophosphate (AMP) are the most important positive effectors.[68,108,127,176] Fructose 2,6-bisphosphate represents a major activator of the enzyme under normoxic conditions, whereas AMP seems to be the main activator of phosphofructokinase during ischemia.[34] As discussed below, the citrate-mediated allosteric inhibition of phosphofructokinase (Fig. 31-1) provides a mechanism for the inhibition of glycolysis by competing substrates.

Glycogen metabolism. Glucose 6-phosphate is also the substrate for glycogen synthesis. Although glycogen occupies up to 2% of the cell volume of the cardiomyocyte, the importance and regulation of myocardial glycogen metabolism is still not completely understood. The glycogen content of the heart is greater in the fasted than in the fed state.[47,117,150] Glycogen synthesis is increased by insulin, as in the postprandial state.[29] Glycogen synthesis is also stimulated during exercise because lactate uptake by the heart is increased.[86] Glycogen is broken down by adrenaline[113] and glucagon[57] or during ischemia.[26,47] Glycogenolysis is mainly regulated by glycogen phosphorylase.[104,105] The stimulation of glycogenolysis by ischemia results from the accumulation of AMP, an allosteric stimulator, and inorganic phosphate (Pi), the substrate of glycogen phosphorylase.[39,105] In the isolated glucose-perfused heart, only a small part of extracellular glucose taken up by the cell is first incorporated into glycogen before entering the glycolytic pathway.[57] This incorporation rate seems to be higher in vivo[191] when competing substrate and hormones are present.

Several recent investigations dealt with the role of glycogen as an energy-providing fuel in the heart under normoxic and ischemic conditions. The role of glycogen as a metabolic substrate in the normoxic heart has been studied in the isolated working rat heart.[56] In contrast to extracellular glucose, glucosyl moieties coming from glycogen breakdown are preferentially oxidized rather than converted to lactate.[56] Those observations support the hypothesis that glucose metabolism is compartmentalized in the heart,[185] and that the fate of glucose is shared between glucosyl units coming from extracellular glucose, which are metabolized to lactate and which probably regulates the ionic pumps of the plasma membrane, and glucosyl units coming from glycogen, which are preferably oxidized and sustain the production of ATP necessary for contraction. Such a hypothesis could explain the tight correlation found between glycogen content and ATP concentration in perfused hearts.

The role of glycogen in the ischemic heart and its effect on postischemic functional recovery are controversial. Several studies point to deleterious effects of glycogenolysis on postischemic recovery,[3,110] whereas others have shown that glycogen lessens the effects of ischemia, as shown by improved recovery on reperfusion.[27,58,85,97,149] Most of the studies, however, conclude that glycogen remains the most important contributor to anaerobic energetic supply of the heart. Because glycogen and glycogen-related enzymes are located on the endoplasmic reticulum,[46,129] this localization could also contribute to cellular homeostasis by regulating calcium fluxes during ischemia.[193]

Lactate. Lactate, which accumulates in the bloodstream during exercise, is a physiologic substrate for the heart under normoxic conditions.[43,73] Lactate inhibits glycolysis and fatty acid oxidation in the heart in vivo.[44,56,73,177] Addition of lactate to hearts perfused with glucose induces dose-dependent inhibition of glycolysis (Fig. 31-1). Despite the inhibition of glycolysis, glucose uptake is not completely inhibited by lactate,[37,171] except at supraphysiologic concentrations.[63] As a result, glucose is redirected from oxidation to glycogen synthesis when lactate levels in the blood are high. This effect of lactate has also been observed in vivo.[86] In addition, fatty acids and ketone bodies have been shown to inhibit glycolysis and to favor glycogen synthesis.[115,159] At physiologic concentrations, fatty acids decrease myocardial glucose uptake to a higher extent than does lactate.[55,191] Like glucose, lactate is an essential substrate for the heart because after transformation into pyruvate, it produces both acetyl-CoA and oxaloacetate, the two molecules needed to form citrate and to sustain the cycling of tricarboxylic acids (Fig. 31-1). In contrast, fatty acids and ketone bodies produce acetyl-CoA only and therefore are not sufficient to maintain the full activity of the tricarboxylic acid cycle (Fig. 31-1).

Fatty acids

Fatty acids are the predominant fuel for myocardial respiration. Fatty acids are mobilized with fasting from the pool of triglycerides, stored mainly in the adipose tissue. After crossing the plasma membrane, fatty acids bind to fatty acid–binding proteins and are activated in their CoA derivatives by acyl-CoA synthetase (Fig. 31-2). At this point, activated fatty acids can either remain in the cytosol, where they are incorporated in the myocardial triglyceride pool, or cross the mitochondrial membrane to be oxidized through β-oxidation and in the tricarboxylic acid cycle. The transfer of acyl moiety into mitochondria is catalyzed by carnitine palmitoyltransferases (CPT 1 and CPT 2). Once in the mitochondrial matrix, fatty acids undergo β-oxidation (Fig. 31-2). The rate of fatty acid oxidation is controlled by the rate of transfer into the mitochondria. Carnitine palmitoyl[8,89,98] transferase-1 is inhibited by malonyl-CoA, which is formed from acetyl-CoA by acetyl-CoA carboxylase. Recent studies have shown that the proportion of the carboxylase in the active, dephosphorylated form controls fatty acid oxidation in the heart.[89,146] This production of malonyl-CoA that arises from an excess of acetyl-CoA explains the relative inhibition of β-oxidation in the presence of glucose[171] or lactate.[177] No de novo fatty acid synthesis occurs in heart muscle.

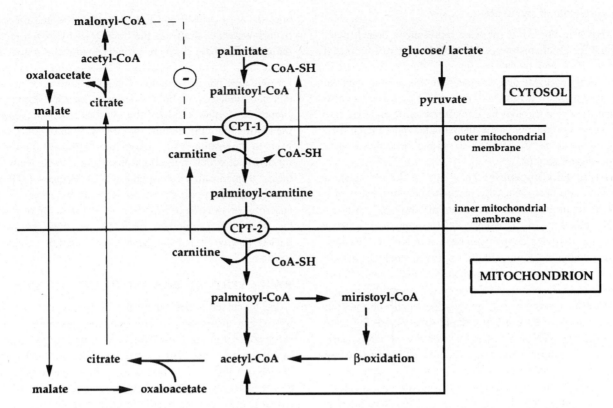

Fig. 31-2. Metabolism of fatty acids. Oxidation of fatty acids is regulated by malonyl-coenzyme A (CoA), produced by acetyl-CoA carboxylase.

During myocardial ischemia, lack of oxygen blocks β-oxidation. Therefore, long-chain acyl-CoA accumulates in the mitochondria, where it exerts a toxic effect on the energetic metabolism by inhibiting the mitochondrial ATP translocase.[160] This deleterious effect can be lessened by administration of L-carnitine, which binds to the activated acyl moieties. Moreover, by liberating CoA-SH from acyl-CoA, L-carnitine decreases the ratio of acetyl-CoA to CoA-SH and, therefore, relieves the feedback inhibition of pyruvate dehydrogenase by acetyl-CoA (Fig. 31-1), resulting in increased oxidation of glucose.[16]

The inhibitory effect of fatty acids on glucose oxidation is far better known than the inhibitory effect of glucose or lactate on fatty acid oxidation.[171] Fatty acids inhibit glucose metabolism at several different sites. First, they inactivate pyruvate dehydrogenase through the production of acetyl-CoA (Fig. 31-1). Second, they induce an accumulation of citrate, which inhibits phosphofructokinase.[54] This inhibition is reinforced by an inhibition of the production of fructose 2,6-bisphosphate, a potent stimulator of phosphofructokinase.[69] Finally, fatty acids also decrease glucose transport in the heart.[1,2,103,135] These three inhibitory effects combine in a concerted action to result in a glucose-sparing and rerouting effect, leading to net glycogen accumulation during fasting. In the presence of physiologic concentrations of fatty acids during fasting, glucose transport is inhibited by about 30% and phosphofructokinase by 60%, whereas pyruvate dehydrogenase is almost completely inactivated.[53,109,126,135]

Ketone bodies

Ketone bodies, represented by acetoacetate and β-hydroxybutyrate, are produced by the catabolism of fatty acids in the liver when acetyl-CoA production exceeds the capacity of the Krebs cycle, mainly during starvation and in diabetic ketoacidosis. Therefore, ketone bodies do not have the same physiologic importance as carbohydrates or fatty acids. However, in contrast to the latter two substrates, when ketone bodies are present in high concentrations, they gain immediate access to the mitochondrial matrix and their metabolism is less regulated. Under extreme conditions, ketone bodies may become the predominant fuel for respiration.

As for fatty acids, the metabolism of ketone bodies inhibits glycolysis by feedback inhibition of phosphofructokinase and pyruvate dehydrogenase mediated by citrate and acetyl-CoA, respectively (Fig. 31-1). Besides this inhibition of glucose metabolism, physiologic concentrations of ketone bodies inhibit fatty acid oxidation both in vitro and in vivo,[23,181] probably because the CoA-SH moieties needed for β-oxidation are consumed by 3-oxoacyl-CoA transferase.

The metabolism of ketone bodies induces a sequestration of CoA-SH in the form of acetyl-CoA, which cannot further be used as a substrate for 2-oxoglutarate dehydrogenase, the enzyme of the tricarboxylic acid cycle that transforms 2-oxoglutarate into succinyl-CoA. This inhibition of the cycle explains why the heart cannot sustain its contractile activity in vitro when ketone bodies are the only substrate available.[144,171]

The pivotal role of pyruvate

As shown in Fig. 31-1, pyruvate represents a branch point for several metabolic pathways. Most of the pyruvate produced from glycolysis and lactate oxidation is further oxidized in acetyl-CoA by pyruvate dehydrogenase and is used to feed the Krebs cycle. However, Fig. 31-1 shows that pyruvate can also replenish the cycle through its transformation to oxaloacetate by pyruvate carboxylation, a mechanism known as anaplerosis. Finally, pyruvate is also related to amino acid metabolism through transaminations.

Pyruvate dehydrogenase. The oxidative decarboxylation of pyruvate into acetyl-CoA by pyruvate dehydrogenase is a point of no return in glucose and lactate metabolism.[133] Understandably, much research has been done on the elucidation of this enzyme. Pyruvate dehydrogenase is a mitochondrial multienzyme complex composed of pyruvate dehydrogenase proper, acetylhydrolipoyl acetyltransferase, and dihydrolipoyl dehydrogenase. The activity of the enzyme is submitted to tight control by effectors and by phosphorylation–dephosphorylation regulation, the active form being dephosphorylated. Pyruvate dehydrogenase kinase is stimulated by acetyl-CoA and NADH, because it occurs during fatty acid oxidation, and is inhibited by pyruvate (or its analogue dichloroacetate), as after feeding.[31,76,90,100,136] In contrast, pyruvate dehydrogenase phosphatase is stimulated by Mg^{2+} and Ca^{2+}.[30,172] The concentration of the latter increases when the heart is subjected to an increased workload, which explains the activation of pyruvate dehydrogenase observed under this condition.[81,137,188]

Pyruvate carboxylation. In normoxic conditions, glucose and lactate provide substrates to the tricarboxylic acid cycle not only through the production of acetyl-CoA but also by the transformation of pyruvate to oxaloacetate (Fig. 31-1), either directly by pyruvate carboxylase or indirectly by malic enzyme. This mechanism, known as anaplerosis, has been characterized in the isolated perfused heart.[144,145,170] It allows both a "refeeding" of several Krebs cycle intermediates and a recycling of carbon dioxide. This is particularly important during prolonged oxidation of fatty acids and ketone bodies, which can "unspan" the Krebs cycle by the sequestration of CoA-SH, as described above.[133,166] This may explain why glucose uptake in vivo is never completely inhibited in hearts perfused with fatty acids or ketone bodies. The inhibition at the level of α-ketoglutarate dehydrogenase also explains the retention of labeled acetate by glutamate, giving rise to a biexponential clearance rate of [^{11}C] acetate from the myocardium (see below).

Transaminations. The two aminotransferases are present in the heart. One of their roles is to feed the tricarboxylic acid cycle through the reactions shown in Fig. 31-1. Perhaps more important is the role of amino acids in the transfer of the reducing equivalents from the cytosol to the mitochondria through the malate–aspartate shuttle. The malate–aspartate shuttle acts through two carriers: the dicarboxylate carrier, which exchanges malate and 2-oxoglutarate, and the aspartate–glutamate shuttle, which exchanges these two amino acids. The anion exchange by these carriers preserves the ionic balance between cytosol and mitochondria. The net effect of the malate–aspartate shuttle is the transfer of hydrogen ions from the cytosol, where they are produced, into the mitochondria, where they sustain the activity of the electron transport chain for oxidative phosphorylation. Finally, amino acids are important intermediary metabolites during ischemia. When pyruvate cannot be further oxidized by pyruvate dehydrogenase, its transformation into alanine by transamination of glutamate leads to the synthesis of 2-oxoglutarate (Fig. 31-1), the transformation of which in the tricarboxylic acid cycle leads to synthesis of guanosine triphosphate (GTP). Because GTP can be readily transphosphorylated to ATP, transaminations allow anaerobic production of ATP. Enhanced utilization of glutamate has been demonstrated in reversibly ischemic human heart muscle in vivo[106] and has been used to identify viable myocardium.[198]

REGULATION OF NORMAL HEART METABOLISM

As explained above, heart metabolism is mainly regulated by oxygen availability, energy demand, hormones, and substrate concentration. The interactions among various substrates have been described. There is growing recognition that the regulation of substrate flux through metabolic pathways is shared by the pathway enzymes ("distributive control")[74] and that efficient energy transfer occurs through a series of moiety-conserved cycles.[170] The critical role of oxygen in heart metabolism is described below.

Increasing the workload imposed on the heart stimulates glycolysis[67,111] from both extracellular glucose and glycogen.[34,56] This increased glycolytic flux implies the stimulation of glucose transport and glycogenolysis,[74] phosphofructokinase,[34,87] and pyruvate dehydrogenase.[81] The increased energy demand to sustain cardiac work during exercise is matched by increased energy production from the oxidation of lactate, which is produced by skeletal muscle.[73,86]

The hormonal regulation of heart metabolism is mainly exerted by catecholamines, insulin, and thyroid hormones, all of which stimulate glucose metabolism in the heart. Adrenaline stimulates glycogenolysis and glucose transport so that glycolysis is fed from glycogen and exogenous glucose.[120] Adrenaline action is mediated by cyclic AMP, which activates the glycogenolytic cascade through a specific protein kinase.[40,139] It has also been proposed that adrenaline may activate phosphofructokinase by phosphorylation[24,25] but this remains a subject of debate. In the heart, the effect of adrenaline corresponds to a stress situation that, if maintained, leads to deleterious effects on heart metabolism and function because the vasoconstrictive properties of adrenaline induce ischemia.[120]

Insulin stimulates both glycolysis and glycogen synthesis in the heart. This metabolic shift from fatty acids to glucose by insulin and the inhibition of glucose oxidation by fatty acids represent the key elements of the glucose–fatty acids cycle.[134] The stimulation of glycolysis by insulin results from concerted regulation at different levels.[29] It implies stimulation of glucose transport and phosphorylation,[102,130,183] as well as stimulation of phosphofructokinase.[44,87] As explained above, pyruvate dehydrogenase activity in the heart does not seem to be directly modified by insulin but rather by the changes in concentration of enzyme activators (such as NAD, pyruvate, and CoA-SH) and inhibitors (such as acetyl-CoA and NADH) consecutive to the metabolic shift induced by the glucose–fatty acids cycle.

Thyroid hormones stimulate glycolysis.[153,154] In hypothyroid rats, a four-fold decrease in phosphofructokinase activity has been reported.[61] Congenital hypothyroidism impairs the transition from the fetal to the adult forms of glucose transporters.[22]

The effects of adenosine on heart metabolism are being widely studied but are still not fully understood. In isolated perfused heart preparations, a stimulation of glucose uptake has been found,[4,91,192] but this could be due to the vasodilatory effect of adenosine in such preparations, because adenosine has no clear-cut effect on glucose transport in isolated cardiomyocytes.[28] In contrast, adenosine definitely seems involved in the adaptation of the heart to ischemia, a phenomenon known as ischemic preconditioning.

METABOLISM OF THE ISCHEMIC HEART

A hallmark of metabolism in the ischemic myocardium is the transformation of cyclic pathways to linear pathways.[170] The lack of oxygen greatly stimulates glycolysis, which is then the only metabolic pathway able to produce ATP.[64,122] The rate of ATP production by anaerobic glycolysis cannot meet the energy required by the beating heart; thus the work performed rapidly decreases under these conditions.[84,124] However, the stimulation of glycolytic flux during severe ischemia delays the onset of irreversible injury,* probably because residual ATP production from glycolysis allows for some ionic homeostasis. Similarly, the stimulation of glycolytic flux at reperfusion decreases myocardial stunning (defined as reversible contractile dysfunction with normal coronary flow) and improves functional recovery.†

The stimulation of glycolysis under anaerobic conditions, known as the reversal of the Pasteur effect,[83] has been observed in many tissues and involves a stimulation of glycogenolysis, glucose transport, and phosphofructokinase activity.‡ The decrease in ATP concentration in the ischemic heart, together with the large increase in AMP concentration, may be responsible for the stimulation of phosphofructokinase.[116] However, the stimulation of glucose uptake rapidly reaches maximal rates, whereas the change in ATP concentration is progressive and relatively linear[35,121,178,179] because, during early ischemia, the concentration of ATP remains constant at the expense of the phosphocreatine pool.[114] Other mechanisms should thus be invoked to explain the burst in glycolytic activity. For instance, changes in cyclic nucleotides (cyclic AMP and cyclic guanosine monophosphate [GMP]) have been reported in ischemic

hearts.[33] The change in cyclic GMP concentration, which results from an ischemia-induced activation of cardiac nitric oxide synthase, may take part in the metabolic adaptation of the heart to ischemia.[35]

Whereas fatty acids play a major role in the metabolism of the normoxic heart, glucose becomes the major substrate for the myocardium under ischemic conditions.

Translocation of the insulin-responsive glucose transporter GLUT4 from an intracellular storage pool to the sarcolemma occurs during acute low-flow ischemia in vivo (50% reduction in distal coronary artery perfusion pressure). GLUT1 is also translocated. Thus, translocation of glucose transporters is an important regulatory site for ischemia-induced myocardial glucose uptake in vivo. With ischemia, the glycolytic flux is initially maximally stimulated, probably in an effort to maintain production of ATP. Such stimulation does not prevent the functional decline of the heart, because glycolysis offers a relatively limited quantity of high-energy equivalents compared with the tricarboxylic acid cycle; however, glycolysis delays as long as possible the onset of ischemic contracture. Irreversible ischemic damage arises only when glycogen stores are exhausted and glucose uptake decreases (Fig. 31-3). This suggests that even if glucose cannot fully meet the energy demand of the ischemic heart, it can delay or prevent irreversible damage. It is likely that the smaller quantity of ATP synthesized by glycolysis allows sustained activity of ionic pumps and, therefore, limits intracellular accumulation of calcium.[123] When glycolytic activity stops, ischemic contracture develops rapidly because of an irreversible alteration of the intracellular ion homeostasis. Taken together, these data suggest that glucose uptake and glycolytic flux in ischemia can be regarded as markers of cell survival, as long as such end-products as lactate and protons can be extruded from the cell.[27] For this reason, glucose tracers are

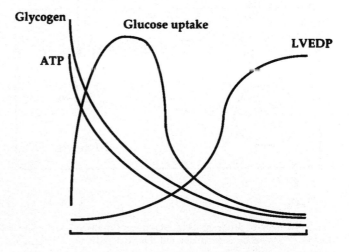

Duration of low-flow ischemia

Fig. 31-3. Evolution during low-flow ischemia of glycogen content, glucose uptake, and rise of left ventricular end-diastolic pressure (*LVEDP*).

---

*References 5, 15, 45, 77, 78, 142, 178, 179.
†References 45, 71, 72, 77, 93, 178, 179.
‡References 26, 47, 84, 132, 141, 190.

used in clinical practice as markers of myocardial viability to assess the reversibility of ischemic injury in patients with left ventricular ischemic dysfunction who are being considered for revascularization.

USE OF METABOLIC TRACERS TO ASSESS MYOCARDIAL VIABILITY

Positron emission tomography allows the tracing of several of the metabolic pathways described above with labeled substrates or their analogues in all regions of the heart. The tracers, usually produced by a cyclotron, are either taken up, metabolized, and cleared from the myocardium or are taken up, metabolized, and retained by the heart. The metabolic tracers currently used with PET imaging assess the metabolism of fatty acids, glucose uptake, or the activity of the tricarboxylic acid cycle (Fig. 31-4). The ability of PET to quantitate regional blood flow with different tracers permits the independent assessment of regional myocardial blood flow and metabolism and forms the basis for the concept of flow–metabolism mismatch in myocardial areas with maintained metabolic activity despite decreased blood flow.

The metabolism of fatty acids is investigated by using ^{11}C palmitate. Clearance of the tracer follows biexponential kinetics. The first part is a rapid decrease due to immediate oxidation and the elimination of carbon dioxide. The second part is a slow and progressive decrease of the tracer, reflecting its incorporation into triglycerides, its release, and its subsequent oxidation.[148,189] In ischemia, the elimination kinetics of ^{11}C palmitate are decreased owing to the slower oxidation of fatty

acids.[152] In contrast, with increased cardiac work, overall elimination of the tracer is accelerated because the oxidative metabolism of the heart is stimulated. The main disadvantages of this kind of tracer are the very fast degradation of fatty acids by β-oxidation, allowing only a very short time of analysis, and the fact that palmitate can leave the cell before complete oxidation occurs. Therefore, iodinated or phenylated derivatives have been synthesized.[50] These analogues are taken up and retained by the myocardium. Their rate of uptake is proportional the rate of uptake of the substance being traced (long-chain fatty acids).

With only two carbons, acetate is the shortest of the fatty acids. Acetate gains immediate access to the mitochondrial matrix, where it is activated to acetyl-CoA for oxidation in the citric acid cycle (Fig. 31-4). Carbon-11 acetate has therefore been used as a tracer of cardiac oxidative metabolism. With regard to ^{11}C palmitate, the kinetics of ^{11}C acetate are degressive because this substance is used as a substrate for the citric acid cycle[88] and is eliminated from the cell as ^{11}CO$_2$ (Fig. 31-4). The elimination kinetics is thus directly proportional to the oxidative activity of the myocardium. Lack of oxygen, one of the major consequences of ischemia, strongly affects the clearance of acetate. Conversely, the clearance of ^{11}C acetate may be used as an index of oxygen consumption by the myocardium,[18] as validated by the measurement of ^{11}CO$_2$ production with any oxidizable substrate.[7,17-20] This correlation may be assumed as long as the coupling between oxygen consumption and ATP production is preserved. The turnover of the tricarboxylic acid cycle is thus assessed very accurately in most conditions, even when cardiac metabolism is enhanced (such as by the administration of dobutamine).[65] [^{11}C] acetate has also been used as a marker of viability; dysfunctional myocardium with sustained oxidative capacity presents a better functional recovery after revascularization than myocardium with poor oxidative activity.[60] It has not been determined whether ^{11}C acetate is as accurate as ^{18}F-fluorodeoxyglucose (FDG) for the detection of myocardial viability in clinical practice.

The glucose tracer analog FDG is the best known of all metabolic tracers and is used to assess glucose uptake. Like 2-deoxyglucose, FDG is phosphorylated by hexokinase to FDG 6-phosphate and is trapped in the cell because it is not dephosphorylated. Fluorodeoxyglucose 6-phosphate does not permeate the cell membrane and is not a substrate for the next enzyme in the glycolytic pathway, hexose 6-phosphate isomerase. At a constant input function, FDG retention by the isolated working rat heart is linear over time (Fig. 31-5). Note the importance of the input function of FDG (perfusate) for the slope of FDG retention by the heart (Fig. 31-6). Patlak graphical analysis corrects for changes in the input function (Fig. 31-6, *inset*). The addition of insulin, however, changes the ratio of tracer to the substance being traced (Fig. 31-7). Such changes also occur during reperfusion in the isolated perfused heart.

As described above, glucose uptake is stimulated in the postprandial state, when insulin is secreted and fatty acid levels are low. This phenomenon is also observed in vivo[101] and with

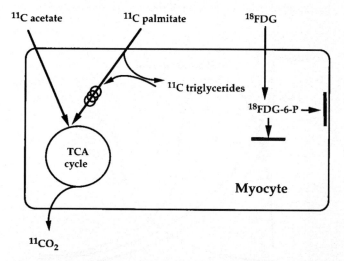

Fig. 31-4. Fate of different metabolic tracers in the myocyte. Carbon-11 (^{11}C) acetate is oxidized and released as ^{11}CO$_2$. ^{11}C palmitate can be oxidized by the same way but is also in equilibrium with the triglyceride pool. Fluorine-18 fluorodeoxyglucose (FDG) is phosphorylated by hexokinase in FDG-6-P and is trapped as such in the cell; it cannot go further in any metabolic pathway of glucose, it cannot leave the cell because it is phosphorylated, and it is only slowly dephosphorylated.

the use of the hyperinsulinemic euglycemic clamp, which improves the quality of PET imaging with FDG[80] but may underestimate the rate of glucose uptake.[63] Moreover, the use of FDG has corroborated in vivo the glucose–fatty acids cycle,[119] first described in vitro in the perfused heart (see above).

FLUORODEOXYGLUCOSE AND THE PATHOPHYSIOLOGY OF HIBERNATING MYOCARDIUM

In addition to these physiologic conditions, an increase in FDG uptake is usually observed in acute and chronic ischemic reversible contractile dysfunction.[21,147,151,194] As described earlier, glycolytic activity during severe ischemia does not sustain normal contractile activity but represents a signal of metabolic activity in tissue with the potential to resume normal contraction with reperfusion. This signal is observed in acute and chronic ischemic dysfunction. In acute ischemic dysfunction, such as that observed after myocardial

infarction, hypoperfused segments with preserved FDG uptake have a better functional recovery than hypoperfused segments without FDG uptake.[151] In chronic ischemic dysfunction, increased FDG uptake is considered the gold standard of viability. Chronic left ventricular ischemic dysfunction does not always result from irreversible injury and can be reversed by revascularization. This reversible ischemic dysfunction led to the principle of myocardial hibernation, a term introduced by Rahimtoola.[131] Neither the degree of dysfunction nor the amount of blood flow reduction can accurately differentiate myocardial necrosis from hibernation. The distinction between irreversibly injured tissue and hibernating myocardium constitutes the main purpose of investigations of myocardial viability and is clinically relevant. The surgical revascularization of hibernating tissue leads to a decreased mortality rate compared with medical treatment, whereas revascularization of irreversibly injured tissue does not prevent further decline in function.[38]

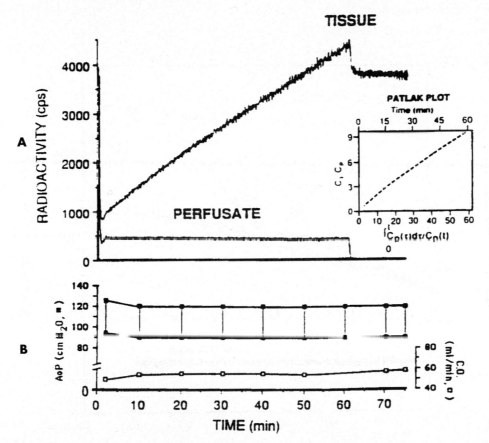

Fig. 31-5. Time–activity curves obtained for a heart perfused at intermediate workload (afterload = 100 cm H_2O; preload = 15 cm H_2O) with Krebs–Henseleit saline containing glucose (10 mM) and 2-[^{18}F]fluoro-2-deoxy-D-glucose (2-FDG) (350 μCi/200 mL perfusate) for first 60 min (A). **A,** *Top tracing,* myocardial retention of 2-FDG; *bottom tracing,* 2-FDG activity in recirculating perfusate. A Patlak plot obtained from graphical analysis of decay-corrected tissue and perfusate curves is shown in *inset.* **B,** Physiologic performance of heart in terms of aortic pressure (*AoP,* expressed in cm H_2O) and cardiac output (*CO,* expressed in ml/min). Note that at 60 minutes, radioactive perfusate was changed to a nonradioactive medium containing only glucose (10 mM). (Reproduced from Nguyen VTB, Mossberg KA, Tewson TJ, et al: Temporal analysis of myocardial glucose metabolism by 2-[^{18}F]-fluoro-2-deoxy-D-glucose, *Am J Physiol* 259:H1022-H1031, 1990; with permission.)

Fig. 31-6. Time–activity curves of a heart perfused at intermediate workload with glucose (10 mM) and stepwise increase in 2-[^{18}F]-fluoro-2-deoxy-D-glucose (2-FDG) activity, followed by a 40-minute washout phase with a nonradioactive medium containing glucose (10 mM). The tracer 2-FDG was added to recirculating perfusion system at 0, 15, and 30 minutes at 376 µCi, 344 µCi, and 334 µCi, respectively. Slope of tissue curve increased with each increment of 2-FDG added (0.166, 0.323, and 0.402 µCi Σ ml–1 Σ min^{-1}). A Patlak plot *(inset)* showed a near-linear and stable increase in the fractional rate of 2-FDG phosphorylation. The performance of the heart was stable for duration of experiment (data not shown). (Reproduced from Nguyen VTB, Mossberg KA, Tewson TJ, et al: Temporal analysis of myocardial glucose metabolism by 2-[^{18}F]-fluoro-2-deoxy-D-glucose, *Am J Physiol* 259:H1022-H1031, 1990; with permission.)

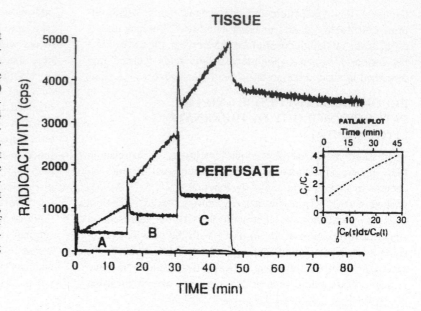

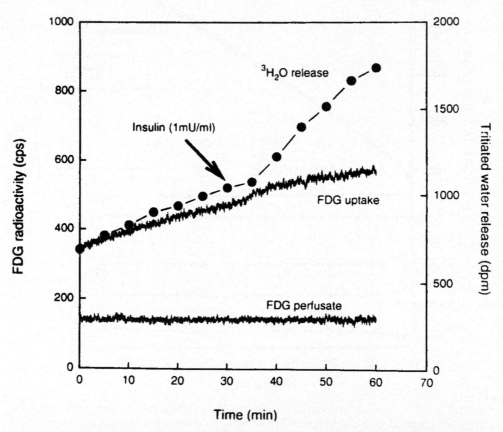

Fig. 31-7 Differential effect of insulin (1 mU/ml) on the uptake of glucose and [^{18}F]2-glucose-2-fluoro-D-glucose (FDG). Time–activity curves of myocardial uptake of FDG are simultaneously compared with time–activity curves of tritiated water released from [2-^{3}H]glucose. Release of ^{3}H$_2$O from [2-^{3}H]glucose measures glucose transport and phosphorylation. The activity of FDG in the perfusate (input function) remains constant throughout the experiment. The uptake of [2-^{3}H]glucose increased after a delay of about 5 minutes when insulin was added at 30 minutes of perfusion. No significant change was observed in the uptake of FDG. (Reproduced from Hariharan R, Bray M, Ganim R, et al: Fundamental limitations of [^{18}F]2-deoxy-2-fluoro-D-glucose for assessing myocardial glucose uptake, *Circulation* 91:2435-2444, 1995; with permission.)

The concept of myocardial hibernation, born from clinical observations, is defined as a reduction of contractile function in response to a reduction of flow. This hypocontractility, which is supposed to decrease energy requirements and delay the onset of irreversible injury, can be reversed by restoration of blood flow, i.e., by revascularization.[14] Most of these postulates have been confirmed in animal experiments. The decrease of coronary perfusion pressure in isolated heart preparations induces a concomitant reduction of contractility and oxygen consumption without the onset of specific signs of ischemia, such as a decrease in ATP content or an accumulation of lactate.[12,75] The downregulation of energy requirement in hibernating tissue has been demonstrated both in humans and in animal models; mild prolonged ischemia does not prevent the ability of the heart to produce phosphocreatine and to preserve the ratio of ATP to adenosine diphosphate,[6,52,124] thereby demonstrating that the mitochondrial oxidative capacity is maintained in this condition. This scenario differs from acute severe ischemia, in which the pool of purine nucleotides is rapidly and irreversibly degraded.[70]

The exact pathophysiologic mechanism leading to myocardial hibernation remains unknown. The original concept of a constant reduction of blood flow with concomitant reduction of contractility has been challenged. More recent observations suggest that hibernating myocardium is submitted to repetitive episodes of ischemic stunning, leading to delayed functional recovery during each reperfusion period despite normalization of blood flow. This mechanism has been seen both in human studies[182] and in animal models.[118,156]

A strong correlation has been found between FDG uptake and myocardial viability. Therefore, FDG has been used to predict myocardial viability before revascularization in patients with chronic ventricular ischemic dysfunction,[174,195] but the significance of the FDG signal in the ischemic heart is still a matter of research. In acute ischemia, the increase in FDG uptake is mainly explained by the stimulation of glucose uptake in hypoxic myocardium consecutive to the reversal of the Pasteur effect, as described above. In myocardial hibernation, the significance of the FDG signal has not been fully explained. Such myocardium presents profound morphologic alterations,[13,51] mainly characterized by a loss of contractile filaments and an accumulation of glycogen in the cytosol (Fig. 31-8). These alterations are also found in fetal heart,[155,162,173] suggesting that hibernation may be a dedifferentiation process accompanied by a glucose dependency of the heart similar to that observed in fetal heart. Indeed, the absolute regional FDG uptake in patients with hibernating myocardium has been shown to be directly related to the intensity of cellular alterations and glycogen accumulation in corresponding areas (Fig. 31-9).[36]

The FDG signal observed in hibernating myocardium could, in theory, correspond to several physiologic processes, such as increased glucose uptake, a shift in glucose transporters expression, translocation of hexokinase, or a change in glycogen metabolism. These hypotheses have been tested in vivo and in vitro. As described above, the induction of myocardial ischemia

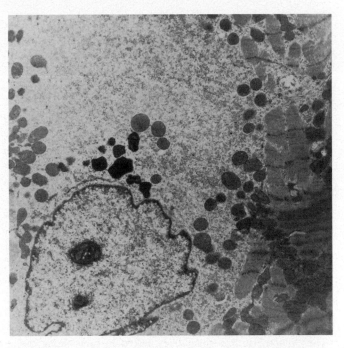

Fig. 31-8. Cellular alterations observed in hibernating myocardium. This cardiomyocyte, observed by electron microscopy (×3600) from a biopsy of human myocardium, displays the major adaptations of hibernating tissue, namely a loss of contractile material and an accumulation of glycogen in the cytosol. The nucleus, seen in the lower left corner, is still active and the plasma membrane (not shown) is normal. This cell is therefore still living.

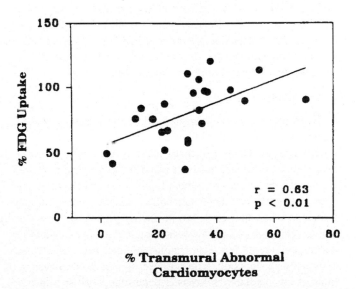

Fig. 31-9. A scatter plot showing the relation between the relative fluorine-18-fluorodeoxyglucose uptake and the area of abnormal cardiac myocytes showing excess glycogen obtained by biopsy in the same region. (Reproduced from Depre C, Vanoverschelde JL, Melin JA, et al: Structural and metabolic correlates to the reversibility of chronic left ventricular ischemic dysfunction in humans, *Am J Physiol* 268:H1265-H1275, 1995; with permission.)

is accompanied by increased glucose uptake, which may explain the FDG signal observed in hibernating areas. However, regional blood flow and oxygen consumption are close to normal in myocardium with chronic ischemic dysfunction.[181] Therefore, no evidence exists of a reversed Pasteur effect leading to a permanent stimulation of glucose uptake in such a condition. Moreover, a study of isolated heart preparation showed that glucose uptake remains unchanged in reversible low-flow ischemia but glucose extraction is increased.[12] It has also been proposed that the increased FDG signal could be due to a shift in the messenger RNA expression of glucose transporters from GLUT4 to GLUT1 but this has not been confirmed. During hyperinsulinemic clamp, hibernating myocardium displays an increase of FDG uptake similar to that of normal remote myocardium,[92] suggesting that the insulin-regulatable GLUT-4 transporter remains the predominant glucose transporter in such tissue. Another possibility to explain the FDG signal is that a translocation of hexokinase from the cytosol to the mitochondria could occur in hibernating myocardium; this phenomenon has been demonstrated in stress conditions in vitro (see above). This hypothesis has never been tested in hibernating tissue, probably because of the difficulty of obtaining a reliable animal model of hibernation. Finally, the role of glycogen metabolism in hibernating myocardium also needs further investigation. As described above, a striking glycogen accumulation is observed in chronically ischemic myocardium; this correlates with increased FDG uptake in these areas. Therefore, the FDG signal in hibernating myocardium may be related to a stimulation of glycogen synthesis. This hypothesis is reinforced by the recent observation that glycogen synthase, the rate-limiting enzyme of glycogen synthesis, is activated in vivo in hearts submitted to low-flow ischemia.[99] Regardless of the underlying metabolic activities, the uptake and retention of FDG define myocardium that is viable and capable of returning to normal oxidative energy production once blood flow is restored.

CONCLUSIONS

Heart metabolism is characterized by the transformation of various substrates into ATP, which, in turn, sustains the contractile activity. Control of metabolism is exerted by substrate availability, workload, hormones, and oxygen tension. We reviewed the major sites of cellular regulation of myocardial glucose metabolism. A major metabolic adaptation occurs during ischemia, when the restriction of energy production consecutive to decreased blood flow does not allow the maintenance of normal contractile function, leading to either acute or chronic contractile dysfunction. The purpose of metabolic investigations of myocardial viability is to determine whether ischemic myocardium can improve functionally after revascularization or reperfusion. Therefore, several metabolic tracers are now available to study the metabolic fate of substrates and the oxidative capacity of the heart in vivo. Among these tracers, FDG is currently the most popular for determining the potential functional recovery after revascularization of myocardium presenting with acute or chronic ischemic dysfunction. However, it may not be possible to quantitate regional blood glucose uptake with FDG under non–steady state conditions; indeed, an increased FDG signal is observed in ischemic myocardium with preserved metabolic activity. In acute ischemia, this signal corresponds to a stimulation of extracellular glucose uptake caused by stimulation of glucose metabolism by oxygen deprivation. In chronic ventricular ischemic dysfunction, increased FDG uptake correlates with dysfunctional but viable myocardium, also termed hibernating myocardium. Myocardial hibernation represents a state of morphologic and energetic adaptation of the heart to ischemia that must be treated by revascularization to avoid a natural trend towards irreversible ischemic damage. In this situation, the actual significance of increased FDG signal, which may correspond to various metabolic steps of glucose metabolism, remains to be determined with accuracy.

ACKNOWLEDGMENT

Work from the authors' laboratory was supported in part by U.S. Public Health Service grant R01-HL 43133.

REFERENCES

1. Abdel-aleem S, Badr M, Perez-Tamayo, RA, et al: Stimulation of myocyte insulin-responsive glucose transporters by the inhibition of fatty acid oxidation, *Diabetes Res* 22:11–19, 1993.
2. Abdel-aleem S, Li X, Anstadt MP, et al: Regulation of glucose utilization during the inhibition of fatty acid oxidation in rat myocytes, *Horm Metab Res* 26:88–91, 1994.
3. Allard MF, Emanuel PG, Russell JA, et al: Preischemic glycogen reduction or glycolytic inhibition improves postischemic recovery of hypertrophied rat hearts, *Am J Physiol* 267:H66–H74, 1994.
4. Angello DA, Berne RM, Coddington NM: Adenosine and insulin mediate glucose uptake in normoxic rat hearts by different mechanisms, *Am J Physiol* 265:H880–H885, 1993.
5. Apstein CS, Gravino FN, Haudenschild CC: Determinants of a protective effect of glucose and insulin on the ischemic myocardium. Effects on contractile function, diastolic compliance, metabolism, and ultrastructure during ischemia and reperfusion, *Circ Res* 52:515–526, 1983.
6. Arai AE, Pantely GA, Anselone CG, et al: Active downregulation of myocardial energy requirements during prolonged moderate ischemia in swine, *Circ Res* 69:1458–1469, 1991.
7. Armbrecht JJ, Buxton DB, Schelbert HR: Validation of [$^{1-11}$C] acetate as a tracer for noninvasive assessment of oxidative metabolism with positron emission tomography in normal, ischemic, post-ischemic, and hyperemic canine myocardium, *Circulation* 81: 1594–1605, 1990.
8. Awan MM, Saggerson ED: Malonyl-CoA metabolism in cardiac myocytes and its relevance to the control of fatty acid oxidation, *Biochem J* 295:61–66, 1993.
9. Bashan N, Burdett E, Guma A, et al: Mechanisms of adaptation of glucose transporters to changes in the oxidative chain of muscle and fat cells, *Am J Physiol* 264:C430–C440, 1993.
10. Bashan N, Burdett E, Hundal HS: Regulation of glucose transport and GLUT1 glucose transporter expression by O_2 in muscle cells in culture, *Am J Physiol* 262:C682–C690, 1992.
11. Bessman SP: A molecular basis for the mechanism of insulin action, *Am J Med* 40:740–749, 1966.
12. Bolukoglu H, Goodwin GW, Guthrie PH, et al: Metabolic fate of glucose in reversible low-flow ischemia of the isolated working rat heart, *Am J Physiol* 270:H817–H826, 1996.
13. Borgers M, Thoné F, Wouters L, et al: Structural correlates of regional myocardial dysfunction in patients with critical coronary artery stenosis: chronic hibernation? *Cardiovasc Pathol* 2:237–245, 1993.

14. Braunwald E, Rutherford JD: Reversible ischemic left ventricular dysfunction: evidence for the "hibernating myocardium," *J Am Coll Cardiol* 8:1467–1470, 1986.

15. Bricknell OL, Daries PS, Opie LH: A relationship between adenosine triphosphate, glycolysis and ischemic contracture in the isolated rat heart, *J Mol Cell Cardiol* 13:941–945, 1981.

16. Broderick TL, Quinney HA, Lopaschuk GD: Carnitine stimulation of glucose oxidation in the fatty acid perfused isolated working rat heart, *J Biol Chem* 267:3758–3763, 1992.

17. Brown M, Marshall DE, Sobel BE: Delineation of myocardial oxygen utilization with carbon-11-labeled acetate, *Circulation* 76:687–696, 1987.

18. Brown MA, Myears DW, Bergmann SR: Validity of estimates of myocardial oxidative metabolism with carbon-11 acetate and positron emission tomography despite altered patterns of substrate utilization, *J Nucl Med* 30:187–193, 1989.

19. Buxton DB, Schwaiger M, Nguyen A, et al: Radiolabeled acetate as a tracer of myocardial tricarboxylic acid cycle flux, *Circ Res* 63: 628–634, 1988.

20. Buxton D, Schwaiger M, Vaghaiwalla Mody F, et al: Regional abnormality of oxygen consumption in reperfused myocardium assessed with ($^{1-11}$C) acetate and positron emission tomography, *Am J Card Imaging* 3:276–287, 1989.

21. Camici P, Ferrannini E, Opie LH: Myocardial metabolism in ischemic heart disease: basic principles and application to imaging by positron emission tomography, *Prog Cardiovasc Dis* 32:217–238, 1989.

22. Castello A, Rodriguez-Manzaneque JC, Camps M, et al: Perinatal hypothyroidism impairs the normal transition of GLUT4 and GLUT1 glucose transporters from fetal to neonatal levels in heart and brown adipose tissue. Evidence for tissue-specific regulation of GLUT4 expression by thyroid hormone, *J Biol Chem* 269: 5905–5912, 1994.

23. Chen V, Wagner G, Spitzer JJ: Regulation of substrate oxidation in isolated myocardial cells by β-hydroxybutyrate, *Horm Metab Res* 16:243–247, 1984.

24. Clark MG, Patten GS: Epinephrine activation of phosphofructokinase in perfused rat heart independent of changes in effector concentrations, *J Biol Chem* 256:27–30, 1981.

25. Clark MG, Patten GS: Adrenergic control of phosphofructokinase and glycolysis in rat heart, *Curr Top Cell Regul* 23:127–176, 1984.

26. Cornblath M, Randle PJ, Parmeggiani A, et al: Regulation of glycogenolysis in muscle. Effects of glucagon and anoxia on lactate production, glycogen content, and phosphorylase activity in the perfused isolated rat heart, *J Biol Chem* 238:1592–1597, 1963.

27. Cross HR, Opie LH, Radda GK, et al: Is a high glycogen content beneficial or detrimental to the ischemic rat heart? A controversy resolved, *Circ Res* 78:482–491, 1996.

28. Dale WE, Hale CC, Kim HD, et al: Myocardial glucose utilization. Failure of adenosine to alter it and inhibition by the adenosine analogue N⁶-(L-2-phenylisopropyl)adenosine, *Circ Res* 69:791–799, 1991.

29. Denton RM: Early events in insulin actions, *Adv Cyclic Nucleotide Protein Phosphorylation Res* 20:293–341, 1986.

30. Denton RM, McCormack JG: Ca²⁺ transport by mammalian mitochondria and its role in hormone action, *Am J Physiol* 249: E543–E554, 1985.

31. Denton RM, Randle PJ, Bridges BJ, et al: Regulation of mammalian pyruvate dehydrogenase, *Mol Cell Biochem* 9:27–53, 1975.

32. Depre C, Fierain L, Hue L: Activation of nitric oxide synthase by ischemia in the perfused heart, *Cardiovasc Res* 33:82–87, 1997.

33. Depre C, Hue L: Cyclic GMP in the perfused rat heart. Effect of ischemia, anoxia and nitric oxide synthase inhibitor, *FEBS Lett* 345:241–245, 1994.

34. Depre C, Rider MH, Veitch K, et al: Role of fructose 2,6-bisphosphate in the control of heart glycolysis, *J Biol Chem* 268: 13274–13279, 1993.

35. Depre C, Vanoverschelde JL, Goudemant JF, et al: Protection against ischemic injury by nonvasoactive concentrations of nitric oxide synthase inhibitors in the perfused rabbit heart, *Circulation* 92: 1911–1918, 1995.

36. Depre C, Vanoverschelde JL, Melin JA, et al: Structural and metabolic correlates of the reversibility of chronic left ventricular ischemic dysfunction in humans, *Am J Physiol* 268:H1265–H1275, 1995.

37. Depre C, Veitch K, Hue L: Role of fructose 2,6-bisphosphate in the control of glycolysis. Stimulation of glycogen synthesis by lactate in the isolated working rat heart, *Acta Cardiol* 48:147–164, 1993.

38. Di Carli MF, Davidson M, Little R, et al: Value of metabolic imaging with positron emission tomography for evaluating prognosis in patients with coronary artery disease and left ventricular dysfunction, *Am J Cardiol* 73:527–533, 1994.

39. Dobson JG Jr, Mayer SE: Mechanisms of activation of cardiac glycogen phosphorylase in ischemia and anoxia, *Circ Res* 33:412–420, 1973.

40. Dobson JG Jr, Ross J Jr, Mayer SE: The role of cyclic adenosine 3',5'-monophosphate and calcium in the regulation of contractility and glycogen phosphorylase activity in guinea pig papillary muscle, *Circ Res* 39:388–395, 1976.

41. Doenst T, Taegtmeyer H: Profound underestimation of glucose uptake by [¹⁸F]2-deoxy-2-fluoroglucose in reperfused rat heart muscle, *Circulation* 97:2454–2462, 1998.

42. Doria-Medina CL, Lund DD, Pasley A, et al: Immunolocalization of GLUT-1 glucose transporter in rat skeletal muscle and in normal and hypoxic cardiac tissue, *Am J Physiol* 265:E454–E464, 1993.

43. Drake AJ, Haines JR, Noble MIM: Preferential uptake of lactate by the normal myocardium in dogs, *Cardiovasc Res* 14:65–72, 1980.

44. Dunaway GA, Kasten TP, Naqui D: Insulin-mediated regulation of heart atrial and ventricular 6-phosphofructo-1-kinase, *J Biol Chem* 261:7831–7833, 1986.

45. Eberli FR, Weinberg EO, Grice WN, et al: Protective effect of increased glycolytic substrate against systolic and diastolic dysfunction and increased coronary resistance from prolonged global underperfusion and reperfusion in isolated rabbit hearts perfused with erythrocyte suspensions, *Circ Res* 68:466–481, 1991.

46. Entam ML, Kanike K, Goldstein MA, et al: Association of glycogenolysis with cardiac sarcoplasmic reticulum, *J Biol Chem* 251:3140–3146, 1976.

47. Evans G: The glycogen content of the rat heart, *J Physiol* 82: 468–480, 1934.

48. Fischer Y, Rose H, Kammermeier H: Possible involvement of alanine and pyruvate in the regulation of glucose transport in heart muscle cells, *FEBS Lett* 274:127–130, 1990.

49. Fischer Y, Thomas J, Holman GD, et al: Contraction-independent effects of catecholamines on glucose transport in isolated rat cardiomyocytes, *Am J Physiol* 39:C1204–C1210, 1996.

50. Fischman A, et al: Myocardial fatty acid imaging: rationale, comparison of 11-C and 123-I labeled fatty acids and potential clinical utility, *Am J Card Imaging* 3:288–296, 1989.

51. Flameng W, Vanhaecke J, Van Belle H, et al: Relation between coronary artery stenosis and myocardial purine metabolism, histology and regional function in humans, *J Am Coll Cardiol* 9:1235–1242, 1987.

52. Flameng W, Wouters L, Sergeant P, et al: Multivariate analysis of angiographic, histologic, and electrocardiographic data in patients with coronary heart disease, *Circulation* 70:7–17, 1984.

53. Garland PB, Randle PJ: Regulation of glucose uptake by muscles. 10. Effects of alloxan-diabetes, starvation, hypophysectomy and adrenelectomy, and of fatty acids, ketone bodies and pyruvate, on the glycerol output and concentrations of free fatty acids, long-chain fatty acyl-coenzyme A, glycerol phosphate and citrate-cycle intermediates in rat heart and diaphragm muscles, *Biochem J* 93:678–687, 1964.

54. Garland PB, Randle PJ, Newsholme EA: Citrate as an intermediary in the inhibition of phosphofructokinase in rat heart muscle by fatty

acids, ketone bodies, pyruvate, diabetes and starvation, *Nature* 200:169–170, 1963.

55. Gertz EW, Wisneski JA, Stanley WC, et al: Myocardial substrate utilization during exercise in humans. Dual carbon-labeled carbohydrate isotope experiments, *J Clin Invest* 82:2017–2025, 1988.

56. Goodwin GW, Ahmad F, Taegtmeyer H: Preferential oxidation of glycogen in isolated working rat heart, *J Clin Invest* 97:1409–1416, 1996.

57. Goodwin GW, Arteaga JR, Taegtmeyer H: Glycogen turnover in the isolated working rat heart, *J Biol Chem* 270:9234–9240, 1995.

58. Goodwin GW, Taegtmeyer H: Metabolic recovery of isolated working rat heart after brief global ischemia, *Am J Physiol* 267:H462–H470, 1994.

59. Gould GW, Holman GD: The glucose transporter family: structure, function and tissue-specific expression, *Biochem J* 295:329–341, 1993.

60. Gropler RJ, Geltman EM, Sampathkumaran K, et al: Functional recovery after coronary revascularization for chronic coronary artery disease is dependent on maintenance of oxidative metabolism, *J Am Coll Cardiol* 20:569–577, 1992.

61. Gualberto A, Molinero P, Sobrino F: The effect of experimental hypothyroidism on phosphofructokinase activity and fructose 2,6-bisphosphate concentrations in rat heart, *Biochem J* 244:137–142, 1987.

62. Hansen R, Pilkis SJ, Krahl ME: Properties of adaptive hexokinase isozymes of the rat, *Endocrinology* 81:1397–1404, 1967.

63. Hariharan R, Bray M, Ganim R, et al: Fundamental limitations of [^{18}F]2-deoxy-2-fluoro-D-glucose for assessing myocardial glucose uptake, *Circulation* 91:2435–2444, 1995.

64. Hearse DJ, Chain EB: The role of glucose in the survival and 'recovery' of the anoxic isolated perfused rat heart, *Biochem J* 128:1125–1133, 1972.

65. Henes CG, Bergmann SR, Walsh MN, et al: Assessment of myocardial oxidative metabolic reserve with positron emission tomography and carbon-11 acetate, *J Nucl Med* 30:1489–1499, 1989.

66. Henning SL, Wambolt RB, Schonekess BO, et al: Contribution of glycogen to aerobic myocardial glucose utilization, *Circulation* 93:1549–1555, 1996.

67. Hornby L, Hamilton N, Marshall D, et al: Role of cardiac work in regulating myocardial biochemical characteristics, *Am J Physiol* 258:H1482–H1490, 1990.

68. Hue L, Rider MH: Role of fructose 2,6-bisphosphate in the control of glycolysis in mammalian tissues, *Biochem J* 245:313–324, 1987.

69. Hue L, Maisin L, Rider MH: Palmitate inhibits liver glycolysis. Involvement of fructose 2,6-bisphosphate in the glucose/fatty acid cycle, *Biochem J* 251:541–545, 1988.

70. Jennings RB, Reimer KA, Hill ML, et al: Total ischemia in dog hearts, in vitro. 1. Comparison of high energy phosphate production, utilization and depletion, and of adenine nucleotide catabolism in total ischemia *in vitro* vs. severe ischemia *in vivo*, *Circ Res* 49:892–900, 1981.

71. Jeremy RW, Ambrosio G, Pike MM, et al: The functional recovery of post-ischemic myocardium requires glycolysis during early reperfusion, *J Mol Cell Cardiol* 25:261–276, 1993.

72. Jeremy RW, Koretsune Y, Marban E, et al: Relation between glycolysis and calcium homeostasis in postischemic myocardium, *Circ Res* 70:1180–1190, 1992.

73. Kaijser L, Berglund B: Myocardial lactate extraction and release at rest and during heavy exercise in healthy men, *Acta Physiol Scand* 144:39–45, 1992.

74. Kashiwaya Y, Sato K, Tsuchiya N, et al: Control of glucose utilization in working perfused rat heart, *J Biol Chem* 269:25502–25514, 1994.

75. Keller AM, Cannon PJ: Effects of graded reductions of coronary pressure and flow on myocardial metabolism and performance: a model of "hibernating" myocardium, *J Am Coll Cardiol* 17:1661–1670, 1991.

76. Kerbey AL, Randle PJ, Cooper RH, et al: Regulation of pyruvate dehydrogenase in rat heart. Mechanism of regulation of proportions of dephosphorylated and phosphorylated enzyme by oxidation of fatty acids and ketone bodies and of effects of diabetes: role of coenzyme A, acetyl-coenzyme A, and nicotinamide-adenine dinucleotide, *Biochem J* 154:327–348, 1976.

77. King LM, Boucher F, Opie LH: Coronary flow and glucose delivery as determinants of contracture in the ischemic myocardium, *J Mol Cell Cardiol* 27:701–720, 1995.

78. Kingsley PB, Sako EY, Yang MQ, et al: Ischemic contracture begins when anaerobic glycolysis stops: a ^{31}P-NMR study of isolated rat hearts, *Am J Physiol* 261:H469–H478, 1991.

79. Klip A, Tsakiridis T, Marette A, et al: Regulation of expression of glucose transporters by glucose: a review of studies in vivo and in cell cultures, *FASEB J* 8:43–53, 1994.

80. Knuuti MJ, Nuutila P, Ruotsalainen U, et al: Euglycemic hyperinsulinemic clamp and oral glucose load in stimulating myocardial glucose utilization during positron emission tomography, *J Nucl Med* 33:1255–1262, 1992.

81. Kobayashi K, Neely JR: Mechanism of pyruvate dehydrogenase activation by increased cardiac work, *J Mol Cell Cardiol* 15:369–382, 1983.

82. Kraegen EW, Sowden JA, Halstead MB, et al: Glucose transporters and in vivo glucose uptake in skeletal and cardiac muscle: fasting, insulin stimulation and immunoisolation studies of GLUT1 and GLUT4, *Biochem J* 295:287–293, 1993.

83. Krebs HA: The Pasteur effect and the relation between respiration and fermentation, *Essays Biochem* 8:1–34, 1972.

84. Kübler W, Spieckermann PG: Regulation of glycolysis in the ischemic and the anoxic myocardium, *J Mol Cell Cardiol* 1:351–377, 1970.

85. Lagerstrom CF, Walker WE, Taegtmeyer H: Failure of glycogen depletion to improve left ventricular function of the rabbit heart after hypothermic ischemic arrest, *Circ Res* 63:81–86, 1988.

86. Laughlin MR, Taylor J, Chesnick AS, et al: Nonglucose substrates increase glycogen synthesis in vivo in dog heart, *Am J Physiol* 267:H219–H223, 1994.

87. Lawson JWR, Uyeda K: Effects of insulin and work on fructose 2,6-bisphosphate content and phosphofructokinase activity in perfused rat hearts, *J Biol Chem* 262:3165–3173, 1987.

88. Lear JL, Ackermann RF: Quantification of patterns of regional cardiac metabolism, *Radiology* 176:659–664, 1990.

89. Lopaschuk GD, Gamble J: The 1993 Merck Frosst Award. Acetyl-CoA carboxylase: an important regulator of fatty acid oxidation in the heart, *Can J Physiol Pharmacol* 72:1101–1109, 1994.

90. Lyn D, Coore HG: Pyruvate inhibition of pyruvate dehydrogenase is a physiological variable, *Biochem Biophys Res Commun* 126:992–998, 1985.

91. Mainwaring R, Lasley R, Rubio R, et al: Adenosine stimulates glucose uptake in the isolated rat heart, *Surgery* 103:445–449, 1988.

92. Mäki M, Luotolahti M, Nuutila P, et al: Glucose uptake in the chronically dysfunctional but viable myocardium, *Circulation* 93:1658–1666, 1996.

93. Mallet RT, Hartman DA, Bünger R: Glucose requirement for postischemic recovery of perfused working heart, *Eur J Biochem* 188:481–493, 1990.

94. Manchester J, Kong X, Nerbonne J: Glucose transport and phosphorylation in single cardiac myocytes: rate-limiting steps in glucose metabolism, *Am J Physiol* 266:E326–E333, 1994.

95. Mansour TE: Studies on heart phosphofructokinase: purification, inhibition and activation, *J Biol Chem* 238:2285–2292, 1963.

96. Mansour TE, Ahlfors CE: Studies on heart phosphofructokinase. Some kinetic and physical properties of the crystalline enzyme, *J Biol Chem* 243:2523–2533, 1968.

97. McElroy DD, Walker WE, Taegtmeyer H: Glycogen loading improves left ventricular function of the rabbit heart after hypothermic ischemic arrest, *J Appl Cardiol* 4:455–465, 1989.

98. McMillin JB, Hudson EK, Van Winkle WB: Evidence for malonyl-CoA-sensitive carnitine acyl-CoA transferase activity in sarcoplasmic reticulum of canine heart, *J Mol Cell Cardiol* 24:259–268, 1992.

99. McNulty PH, Luba MC: Transient ischemia induces regional myocardial glycogen synthase activation and glycogen synthesis in vivo, *Am J Physiol* 268:H364–H370, 1995.

100. McVeigh JJ, Lopaschuk GD: Dichloroacetate stimulation of glucose oxidation improves recovery of ischemic rat hearts, *Am J Physiol* 259:H1079–H1085, 1990.

101. Merhige ME, Mossberg K, Taegtmeyer H, et al: Catecholamine stimulation, substrate competition, and myocardial glucose uptake in conscious dogs assessed with positron emission tomography, *Circ Res* 61(5 Pt 2):II124–II129, 1987.

102. Morgan HE, Cadenas E, Regen DE, et al: Regulation of glucose uptake in muscle. II. Rate-limiting steps and effects of insulin and anoxia in heart muscle from diabetic rats, *J Biol Chem* 236:262–268, 1961.

103. Morgan HE, Neely JR, Kira Y: Factors determining the utilization of glucose in isolated rat hearts, *Basic Res Cardiol* 79:292–299, 1984.

104. Morgan HE, Parmeggiani A: Regulation of glycogenolysis in muscle. II. Control of glycogen phosphorylase reaction in isolated perfused heart, *J Biol Chem* 239:2435–2439, 1964.

105. Morgan HE, Parmeggiani A: Regulation of glycogenolysis in muscle. III. Control of muscle glycogen phosphorylase activity, *J Biol Chem* 239:2440–2445, 1964.

106. Mudge GH, Mills RM, Taegtmeyer H, et al: Alterations of myocardial amino acid metabolism in chronic ischemic heart disease, *J Clin Invest* 58:1185–1192, 1976.

107. Mueckler M: Facilitative glucose transporters, *Eur J Biochem* 219:713–725, 1994.

108. Narabayashi H, Lawson JWR, Uyeda K: Regulation of phosphofructokinase in perfused rat heart. Requirement for fructose 2, 6-bisphosphate and a covalent modification, *J Biol Chem* 260:9750–9758, 1985.

109. Neely JR, Denton RM, England PJ, et al: The effects of increased heart work on the tricarboxylate cycle and its interactions with glycolysis in the perfused rat heart, *Biochem J* 128:147–159, 1972.

110. Neely JR, Grotyohann LW: Role of glycolytic products in damage to ischemic myocardium. Dissociation of adenosine triphosphate levels and recovery of function of reperfused ischemic hearts, *Circ Res* 55:816–824, 1984.

111. Neely JR, Liebermeister H, Morgan HE: Effect of pressure development on membrane transport of glucose in isolated rat heart, *Am J Physiol* 212:815–822, 1967.

112. Neely JR, Morgan HE: Relationship between carbohydrate and lipid metabolism and the energy balance of heart muscle, *Annu Rev Physiol* 36:413–459, 1974.

113. Neely JR, Rovetto MJ, Oram JF: Myocardial utilization of carbohydrate and lipids, *Prog Cardiovasc Dis* 15:289–329, 1972.

114. Neely JR, Rovetto MJ, Whitmer JT, et al: Effects of ischemia on function and metabolism of the isolated working rat heart, *Am J Physiol* 225:651–658, 1973.

115. Neely JR, Whitfield CF, Morgan HE: Regulation of glycogenolysis in hearts: effects of pressure development, glucose, and FFA, *Am J Physiol* 219:1083–1088, 1970.

116. Newsholme EA: The regulation of phosphofructokinase in muscle, *Cardiology* 56:22–34, 1971.

117. Nguyen VTB, Mossberg KA, Tewson TJ, et al: Temporal analysis of myocardial glucose metabolism by 2-[^{18}F] fluoro-2-deoxy-D-glucose, *Am J Physiol* 259:H1022–H1031, 1990.

118. Nicklas JM, Becker LC, Bulkley BH: Effects of repeated brief coronary occlusion on regional left ventricular function and dimension in dogs, *Am J Cardiol* 56:473–478, 1985.

119. Nuutila P, Koivisto VA, Knuuti J, et al: Glucose-free fatty acid cycle operates in human heart and skeletal muscle in vivo, *J Clin Invest* 89:1767–1774, 1992.

120. Opie LH: Metabolism of the heart in health and disease. I, *Am Heart J* 76:685–698, 1968.

121. Opie LH: Effects of regional ischemia on metabolism of glucose and fatty acids. Relative rates of aerobic and anaerobic energy production during myocardial infarction and comparison with effects of anoxia, *Circ Res* 38:I52–I74, 1976.

122. Opie LH: Hypothesis: glycolytic rates control cell viability in ischemia, *J Appl Cardiol* 3:407–414, 1988.

123. Opie LH: Cardiac metabolism—emergence, decline, and resurgence. Part I, *Cardiovasc Res* 26:721–733, 1992.

124. Owen P, Dennis S, Opie LH: Glucose flux rate regulates onset of ischemic contracture in globally underperfused rat hearts, *Circ Res* 66:344–354, 1990.

125. Pantely GA, Malone SA, Rhen WS, et al: Regeneration of myocardial phosphocreatine in pigs despite continued moderate ischemia, *Circ Res* 67:1481–1493, 1990.

126. Parmeggiani A, Bowman RH: Regulation of phosphofructokinase activity by citrate in normal and diabetic muscle, *Biochem Biophys Res Commun* 12:268–272, 1963.

127. Passoneau JV, Lowry OH: Phosphofructokinase and the Pasteur effect, *Biochem Biophys Res Commun* 7:10–15, 1962.

128. Pessin JE, Bell GI: Mammalian facilitative glucose transporter family: structure and molecular regulation, *Annu Rev Physiol* 54:911–930, 1992.

129. Pierce GN, Philipson KD: Binding of glycolytic enzymes to cardiac sarcolemmal and sarcoplasmic reticular membranes, *J Biol Chem* 260:6862–6870, 1985.

130. Post RL, Morgan HE, Park CR: Regulation of glucose uptake in muscle. III. The interaction of membrane transport and phosphorylation in the control of glucose uptake, *J Biol Chem* 236:269–272, 1961.

131. Rahimtoola SH: A perspective on the three large multicenter randomized clinical trials of coronary bypass surgery for chronic stable angina, *Circulation* 72:V123–V135, 1985.

132. Ramaiah A: Pasteur effect and phosphofructokinase, *Curr Top Cell Regul* 8:297–345, 1974.

133. Randle PJ: Regulation of glycolysis and pyruvate oxidation in cardiac muscle, *Circ Res* 38(5 Suppl 1):I8–I15, 1976.

134. Randle PJ, Garland PB, Hales CN, et al: The glucose fatty-acid cycle, *Lancet* 1:785–789, 1963.

135. Randle PJ, Newsholme EA, Garland PB: Regulation of glucose uptake by muscle. 8. Effects of fatty acids, ketone bodies and pyruvate, and of alloxan-diabetes and starvation, on the uptake and metabolic fate of glucose in rat heart and diaphragm muscles, *Biochem J* 93:652–665, 1964.

136. Randle PJ, Sugden PH, Kerbey AL, et al: Regulation of pyruvate oxidation and the conservation of glucose, *Biochem Soc Symp* 43:47–67, 1978.

137. Rattigan S, Appleby GJ, Clark MG: Insulin-like action of catecholamines and Ca^{2+} to stimulate glucose transport and GLUT4 translocation in perfused rat heart, *Biochim Biophys Acta* 1094:217–223, 1991.

138. Reinauer H, Muller-Ruchholtz ER: Regulation of the pyruvate dehydrogenase activity in the isolated perfused heart of guinea-pigs, *Biochim Biophys Acta* 444:33–42, 1976.

139. Robison GA, Butcher RW, Sutherland EW: Cyclic AMP, *Annu Rev Biochem* 37:149–174, 1968.

140. Rogers WJ, Stanley AW Jr, Breinig JB, et al: Reduction of hospital mortality rate of acute myocardial infarction with glucose-insulin-potassium infusion, *Am Heart J* 92:441–454, 1976.

141. Rovetto MJ, Whitmer JT, Neely JR: Comparison of the effects of anoxia and whole heart ischemia on carbohydrate utilization in isolated working rat hearts, *Circ Res* 32:699–711, 1973.

142. Runnman EM, Lamp ST, Weiss JN: Enhanced utilization of exogenous glucose improves cardiac function in hypoxic rabbit ventricle without increasing total glycolytic flux, *J Clin Invest* 86:1222–1233, 1990.

143. Russell RR 3d, Mrus JM, Mommessin JI, et al: Compartmentation of hexokinase in rat heart. A critical factor for tracer kinetic analysis of myocardial glucose metabolism, *J Clin Invest* 90:1972–1977, 1992.

144. Russell RR 3d, Taegtmeyer H: Changes in citric acid cycle flux and anaplerosis antedate the functional decline in isolated rat hearts utilizing acetoacetate, *J Clin Invest* 87:384–390, 1991.

145. Russell RR 3d, Taegtmeyer H: Pyruvate carboxylation prevents the decline in contractile function of rat hearts oxidizing acetoacetate, *Am J Physiol* 261:H1756–H1762, 1991.

146. Saddik M, Gamble J, Witters LA, et al: Acetyl-CoA carboxylase regulation of fatty acid oxidation in the heart, *J Biol Chem* 268:25836–25845, 1993.

147. Schelbert HR, Buxton D: Insights into coronary artery disease gained from metabolic imaging, *Circulation* 78:496–505, 1988.

148. Schelbert HR, Henze E, Sochor H: Effects of substrate availability on myocardial C-11 palmitate kinetics by positron emission tomography in normal subjects and patients with ventricular dysfunction, *Am Heart J* 111:1055–1064, 1986.

149. Scheuer J, Stezoski SW: Protective role of increased myocardial glycogen stores in cardiac anoxia in the rat, *Circ Res* 27:835–849, 1970.

150. Schneider CA, Nguyen VTB, Taegtmeyer H: Feeding and fasting determine postischemic glucose utilization in isolated working rat hearts, *Am J Physiol* 260:H542–H548, 1991.

151. Schwaiger M, Brunken R, Grover-McKay M, et al: Regional myocardial metabolism in patients with acute myocardial infarction assessed by positron emission tomography, *J Am Coll Cardiol* 8:800–808, 1986.

152. Schwaiger M, Fishbein MC, Block M, et al: Metabolic and ultrastructural abnormalities during ischemia in canine myocardium: noninvasive assessment by positron emission tomography, *J Mol Cell Cardiol* 19:259–269, 1987.

153. Segal J: Acute effect of thyroid hormone on the heart: an extranuclear increase in sugar uptake, *J Mol Cell Cardiol* 21:323–334, 1989.

154. Seymour AM, Eldar H, Radda GK: Hyperthyroidism results in increased glycolytic capacity in the rat heart. A ^{31}P-NMR study, *Biochim Biophys Acta* 1055:107–116, 1990.

155. Sharp WW, Terracio L, Borg TK, et al: Contractile activity modulates actin synthesis and turnover in cultured neonatal rat heart cells, *Circ Res* 73:172–183, 1993.

156. Shen YT, Vatner SF: Mechanism of impaired myocardial function during progressive coronary stenosis in conscious pigs. Hibernation versus stunning? *Circ Res* 76:479–488, 1995.

157. Shetty M, Ismail-Beigi N, Loeb JN, et al: Induction of GLUT1 mRNA in response to inhibition of oxidative phosphorylation, *Am J Physiol* 265:C1224–C1229, 1993.

158. Shetty M, Loeb JN, Ismail-Beigi F: Enhancement of glucose transport in response to inhibition of oxidative metabolism: pre- and posttranslational mechanisms, *Am J Physiol* 262:C527–C532, 1992.

159. Shipp JC, Opie LH, Challoner D: Fatty acid and glucose metabolism in the perfused heart, *Nature* 189:1018–1019, 1961.

160. Shrago E, Shug AL, Sul H, et al: Control of energy production in myocardial ischemia, *Circ Res* 38:175–179, 1976.

161. Silverman M: Structure and function of hexose transporters, *Annu Rev Biochem* 60:757–794, 1991.

162. Simpson P, Savion S: Differentiation of rat myocytes in single cell cultures with and without proliferating nonmyocardial cells, *Circ Res* 50:101–116, 1982.

163. Sivitz WI, Lund DD, Yorek B, et al: Pretranslational regulation of two cardiac glucose transporters in rats exposed to hypobaric hypoxia, *Am J Physiol* 263:E562–E569, 1992.

164. Sodi-Pallares D, Testelli MR, Fishleder BL, et al: Effects of intravenous infusion of a potassium-glucose-insulin solution on the electrocardiographic signs of myocardial infarction, *Am J Cardiol* 9:166–181, 1962.

165. Sun D, Nguyen N, DeGrado TR, et al: Ischemia induces translocation of the insulin-responsive glucose transporter GLUT4 to the plasma membrane of cardiac myocytes, *Circulation* 89:793–798, 1994.

166. Taegtmeyer H: On the inability of ketone bodies to serve as the only energy providing substrate for rat heart at physiological work load, *Basic Res Cardiol* 78:435–450, 1983.

167. Taegtmeyer H: Six blind men explore an elephant: aspects of fuel metabolism and the control of tricarboxylic acid cycle activity in heart muscle, *Basic Res Cardiol* 79:322–336, 1984.

168. Taegtmeyer H: Carbohydrate interconversions and energy production, *Circulation* 72(5 Pt 2):IV1–IV8, 1985.

169. Taegtmeyer H: The use of hypertonic glucose, insulin and potassium (GIK) in myocardial preservation, *J Appl Cardiol* 6:255–259, 1991.

170. Taegtmeyer H: Energy metabolism of the heart: from basic concepts to clinical applications, *Curr Probl Cardiol* 19:59–113, 1994.

171. Taegtmeyer H, Hems R, Krebs HA: Utilization of energy-providing substrates in the isolated working rat heart, *Biochem J* 186:701–711, 1980.

172. Thomas AP, Diggle TA, Denton RM: Sensitivity of pyruvate dehydrogenase phosphate phosphatase to magnesium ions. Similar effects of spermine and insulin, *Biochem J* 238:83–91, 1986.

173. Thompson EW, Marino TA, Uboh CE, et al: Atrophy reversal and cardiocyte redifferentiation in reloaded cat myocardium, *Circ Res* 54:367–377, 1984.

174. Tillisch J, Brunken R, Marshall R, et al: Reversibility of cardiac wall motion abnormalities predicted by positron tomography, *N Engl J Med* 314:884–888, 1986.

175. Uyeda K: Phosphofructokinase, *Adv Enzymol Relat Areas Mol Biol* 48:193–244, 1979.

176. Van Schaftingen E, Jett MF, Hue L, et al: Control of liver 6-phosphofructokinase by fructose 2,6-bisphosphate and other effectors, *Proc Natl Acad Sci USA* 78:3483–3486, 1981.

177. van der Vusse GJ, Glatz JFC, Stam HCG, et al: Fatty acid homeostasis in the normoxic and ischemic heart, *Physiol Rev* 72:881–940, 1992.

178. Vanoverschelde JL, Janier MF, et al: The relative importance of myocardial energy metabolism compared with ischemic contracture in the determination of ischemic injury in isolated perfused rabbit hearts, *Circ Res* 74:817–828, 1994.

179. Vanoverschelde JL, Janier MF, Bakke JE, et al: Rate of glycolysis during ischemia determines extent of ischemic injury and functional recovery after reperfusion, *Am J Physiol* 267:H1785–H1794, 1994.

180. Vanoverschelde JL, Wijns W, Kolanowski J, et al: Competition between palmitate and ketone bodies as fuels for the heart: study with positron emission tomography, *Am J Physiol* 264:H701–H707, 1993.

181. Vanoverschelde JL, Wijns W, Depré C, et al: Mechanisms of chronic regional postischemic dysfunction in humans. New insights from the study of noninfarcted collateral-dependent myocardium, *Circulation* 87:1513–1523, 1993.

182. Vanoverschelde JL, Wijns W, Borgers M, et al: Chronic myocardial hibernation: From bedside to bench, *Circulation* 95:1961–1971, 1997.

183. Watanabe T, Smith MM, Robinson FW, et al: Insulin action on glucose transport in cardiac muscle, *J Biol Chem* 259:13117–13122, 1984.

184. Weinstein SP, Haber RS: Differential regulation of glucose transporter isoforms by thyroid hormone in rat heart, *Biochim Biophys Acta* 1136:302–308, 1992.

185. Weiss J, Hiltbrand B: Functional compartmentation of glycolytic versus oxidative metabolism in isolated rabbit heart, *J Clin Invest* 75:436–447, 1985.

186. Wheeler TJ: Translocation of glucose transporters in response to anoxia in heart, *J Biol Chem* 263:19447–19454, 1988.

187. Wheeler TJ, Fell RD, Hauck MA: Translocation of two glucose transporters in heart: effects of rotenone, uncouplers, workload, palmitate, insulin and anoxia, *Biochim Biophys Acta* 1196:191–200, 1994.

188. Wieland OH: The mammalian pyruvate dehydrogenase complex: structure and regulation, *Rev Physiol Biochem Pharmacol* 96: 123–170, 1983.

189. Wyns W, Schwaiger M, Huang SC, et al: Effects of inhibition of fatty acids oxidation on myocardial kinetics of ^{11}C-labeled palmitate, *Circ Res* 65:1787–1797, 1989.

190. Williamson JR: Glycolytic control mechanisms. II. Kinetics of intermediate changes during the aerobic-anoxic transition in perfused rat heart, *J Biol Chem* 241:5026–5036, 1966.

191. Wisneski JA, Gertz EW, Neese RA, et al: Metabolic fate of extracted glucose in normal human myocardium, *J Clin Invest* 76:1819–1827, 1985.

192. Wyatt DA, Edmunds MC, Rubio R, et al: Adenosine stimulates glycolytic flux in isolated perfused rat hearts by A1-adenosine receptors, *Am J Physiol* 257:H1952–H1957, 1989.

193. Xu KY, Zweier JL, Becker LC: Functional coupling between glycolysis and sarcoplasmic reticulum Ca^{2+} transport, *Circ Res* 77:88–97, 1995.

194. Yonekura Y, Tamaki N, Kambara H, et al: Detection of metabolic alterations in ischemic myocardium by F-18-fluorodeoxyglucose uptake with positron emission tomography, *Am J Card Imaging* 2:122–132, 1988.

195. Yoshida K, Gould KL: Quantitative relation of myocardial infarct size and myocardial viability by positron emission tomography to left ventricular ejection fraction and 3-year mortality with and without revascularization, *J Am Coll Cardiol* 22:984–997, 1993.

196. Young LH, Renfu Y, Russell R, et al: Low-flow ischemia leads to translocation of canine heart GLUT-4 and GLUT-1 glucose transporters to the sarcolemma in vivo, *Circulation* 95:415–422, 1997.

197. Zaninetti D, Greco-Perotto R, Jeanrenaud B: Heart glucose transport and transporters in rat heart: regulation by insulin, workload and glucose, *Diabetologia* 31:108–113, 1988.

198. Zimmerman R, Tillman SH, Knopp WH: Regional myocardial ^{13}N-glutamate uptake in patients with coronary artery disease, *J Am Coll Cardiol* 11:549–556, 1988.

Chapter 32

Assessment of viability with fluorine-18 fluorodeoxyglucose positron emission tomography

Andreas J. Morguet and **Heinrich R. Schelbert**

Metabolic imaging using 2-[^{18}F]fluoro-2-deoxy-D-glucose ([18]FDG) is widely considered to be a gold standard for assessing myocardial viability. This is primarily because of the central role of glucose for myocardial energy metabolism and the unique properties of [18]FDG in conjunction with positron emission tomography (PET). Myocardial uptake of [18]FDG has been investigated extensively in various experimental and clinical situations. The comprehensive data that have been accumulated so far should allow a valid evaluation of myocardial [18]FDG imaging. From a clinical standpoint, this is an issue of major relevance for two reasons. First, the aggressive modern treatment of acute myocardial infarction with thrombolytic and interventional reperfusion results in a substantial number of patients with incomplete myocardial infarction. In the subacute phase of the disease, the therapeutic strategy will then crucially depend on the detection of jeopardized residual viable myocardium within the area at risk. In addition, several alternative imaging methods competing with [18]FDG PET have emerged and confront the clinician with the problem of selecting the optimal procedure for evaluation of patients after infarction.

This chapter will first briefly outline the synthesis and production of [18]FDG. Next, the pharmacokinetics of the tracer will be discussed and the in-vivo quantitation of myocardial [18]FDG uptake will be addressed. Finally, the clinical value of [18]FDG PET will be discussed and compared with the value of other imaging approaches currently available for the assessment of myocardial viability.

PRODUCTION OF [18]FDG

The positron emitter ^{18}F is generated in a cyclotron, preferably near the PET scanner because the radioisotope has a short physical half-life (109.7 minutes). Usually, oxygen-15 (^{15}O)–enriched water is bombarded with protons, inducing the nuclear reaction [15]O(p,n)[18]F, with a neutron as an ejectile.[75] The radiopharmaceutical itself is commonly synthesized in a closed automatic unit according to the modified Jülich procedure.[35] The starting compound tetraacetylated trifluormethansulfonyl-mannose is subjected to nucleophilic substitution with tetrabutylammonium-hydrogen carbonate as a phase transfer catalyst, resulting in [18]FDG (Fig. 32-1). A radiochemical yield of approximately 50% to 60% with a purity close to 98.5% can be achieved. The specific activity of the tracer reaches more than 370 GBq/μmol (10 Ci/μmol). The physical half-life of ^{18}F, about 2 hours, permits delivery of the tracer through regional commercial distribution centers.

KINETICS OF [18]FDG
[18]FDG in normal myocardium

Cardiomyocytes are capable of metabolizing various substrates, in particular free fatty acids, glucose, and lactate. In the fasting state under resting conditions, free fatty acids are the predominant source of energy, and glucose follows in second place. The metabolizing ratio between the various myocardial substrates varies markedly with the actual substrate levels in the blood pool. If, for instance, serum glucose levels increase after a carbohydrate-rich meal, glucose becomes the major fuel for the cardiac muscle.[59]

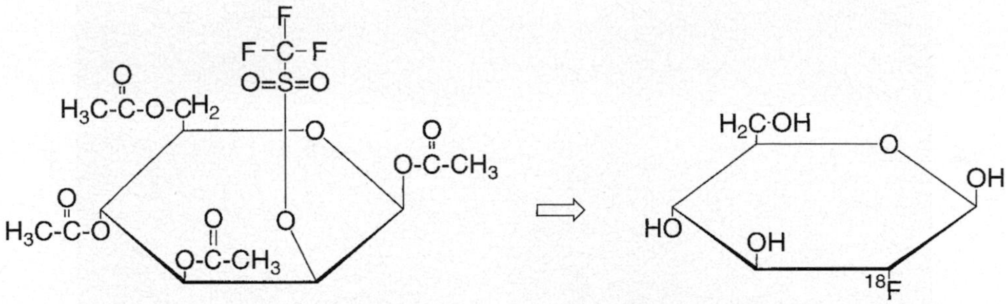

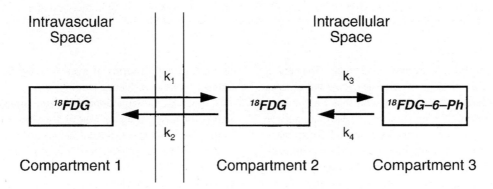

Fig. 32-1. Production of 2-[^{18}F]fluoro-2-deoxy-D-glucose (^{18}FDG). Nucleophilic substitution of 1,3,4,6-tetra-O-acetyl-2-O-trifluoromethansulfonyl-β-mannopyranose (**A**) with tetrabutylammonium-hydrogen carbonate as a phase transfer catalyst provides ^{18}FDG (**B**).

Intravascular Space   Intracellular Space

k_1 k_3

^{18}FDG ^{18}FDG ^{18}FDG–6–Ph

k_2 k_4

Compartment 1   Compartment 2   Compartment 3

Fig. 32-2. Chart of a three-compartment model for ^{18}FDG. The tracer in the intravascular space *(compartment 1)* passes the sarcoplasmic membrane into the cytoplasm *(compartment 2)* and is phosphorylated to 2-[^{18}F]fluoro-2-deoxy-D-glucose (^{18}FDG)-6-phosphate *(^{18}FDG-6-Ph, compartment 3)* by hexokinase. Exchange of ^{18}FDG between the compartments is characterized by the rate constants k_1, k_2, k_3, and k_4.

As a glucose analogue, ^{18}FDG also passes the myocellular membrane through facilitated diffusion. In the intact sarcolemma, this passive transport is mediated predominantly by the insulin-sensitive carrier protein GLUT-4.[82,96] The tracer is subsequently subjected to the first step of glycolysis and is phosphorylated by hexokinase. However, ^{18}FDG is not accepted as substrate by the more specific phosphohexose isomerase. In contrast to ordinary D-glucose, the compound is metabolically trapped within the cytosol.[38,42,65] Moreover, deoxyglucose cannot be incorporated into glycogen. On account of these tracer kinetics, ^{18}FDG is selected intentionally because its biological behavior can be approximated by a three-compartment model (Fig. 32-2).

To enhance ^{18}FDG utilization and, consequently, visualization of the myocardium, most centers stimulate glucose uptake into the myocardium before imaging. This can be done by administering an oral glucose load or performing an euglycemic-hyperinsulinemic clamp technique. Fifty to 75 g of glucose are usually administered for an oral glucose load. Next, ^{18}FDG is injected 1 to 2 hours later, as soon as the stimulation of pancreatic insulin secretion has led to stable plasma glucose and has decreased free fatty acid levels (Fig. 32-3).[34] To avoid uptake

competition between abnormally high glucose levels after an oral glucose load and ^{18}FDG injection in patients with impaired glucose tolerance, the general application of 50 g of glucose combined with 22 g of protein, which also stimulates insulin secretion, has been recommended[34] but has obviously not been evaluated systematically. An alternate approach to increasing myocardial ^{18}FDG uptake is simultaneous intravenous administration of insulin and glucose by using euglycemic-hyperinsulinemic clamping.[17,39] This technique does not diminish the marked interindividual variation in myocardial glucose utilization but does double regional myocardial glucose utilization and enhances image quality compared with oral glucose loading.[39] However, because of the logistic demands of the method, which add to those of ^{18}FDG PET itself, euglycemic-hyperinsulinemic clamping has not replaced oral glucose loading in most laboratories for routine clinical ^{18}FDG PET studies in nondiabetic patients.

^{18}FDG in diabetic patients

Markedly reduced myocardial glucose uptake has been observed in the diabetic rat.[1] In a retrospective analysis, 28% of patients with diabetes mellitus (64% had type I diabetes and

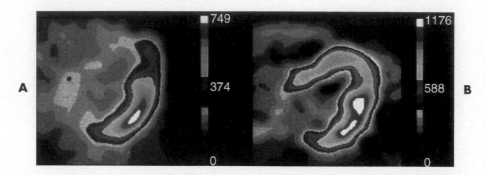

Fig. 32-3. Transversal myocardial positron emission tomographic sections showing distribution of 2-[^{18}F]fluoro-2-deoxy-D-glucose in a normal volunteer under fasting conditions (**A**) and after oral glucose loading (**B**). The markedly diminished tracer accumulation in the septum under fasting conditions improves after glucose loading. (Reprinted by permission of the author and the Society of Nuclear Medicine from: Gropler RJ, Siegel BA, Lee KJ, et al. Nonuniformity in myocardial accumulation of fluorine-18-FDG in normal fasted humans. *J Nucl Med* 31:1749-1756, 1990.)

36% had type II diabetes) exhibited inadequate myocardial ^{18}FDG uptake, possibly because of altered myocardial glucose utilization with a target-to-background ratio that was too low for valid image analysis.[92] Unfortunately, these patients are particularly prone to coronary heart disease and constitute a significant portion of persons who may eventually benefit from the assessment of myocardial viability, because diabetic microangiopathy often involves the coronary circulation. However, it has been shown in young patients with insulin-dependent diabetes mellitus that imaging with the euglycemic-hyperinsulinemic clamp technique yields an accumulation of ^{18}FDG similar to that seen in healthy persons.[92] Recently, predictive values for regional functional improvement after revascularization comparable with those in normal persons have been found in persons with type II diabetes when glucose levels were lowered by 20% with intravenous short-acting insulin, thereby avoiding euglycemic-hyperinsulinemic clamping.[77] Thus, it seems that some degree of metabolic standardization helps to circumvent the problems of ^{18}FDG PET intrinsic to diabetic patients.

^{18}FDG in ischemic and postischemic myocardium

The metabolizing ratio among the various myocardial fuel substrates not only depends on substrate availability but is also markedly influenced by the regional metabolic state of the cardiac muscle. During myocardial ischemia, myocardial fatty acid uptake and oxidation decrease,[58,60] whereas glucose utilization increases above normal levels.[44,60] This phenomenon, which is also observed in eukaryotic cells other than myocytes and is commonly referred to as the Pasteur effect, forms the basis for the assessment of myocardial viability using ^{18}FDG PET. From a teleological point of view, switching from fatty acid oxidation to glycolysis makes it easier for the cell to continue generation of adenosine triphosphate despite oxygen depletion because the phosphorylation:oxidation ratio is higher for glucose (3.17) than for fatty acids (for example 2.83 for palmitate).[59] Glycolysis can also proceed anaerobically—albeit

less effectively in terms of energy—with production of pyruvate and release of lactate (Fig. 32-4).

Chronically dysfunctional but viable myocardium may contain truly hibernating or repeatedly stunned myocardium, or both. Therefore, tracer uptake in two different types of cardiac tissue must be discussed in order to elucidate the role of ^{18}FDG PET in the assessment of viable myocardium. We first consider hibernating myocardium. The concept of myocardial hibernation postulates downregulation of myocardial metabolism and function to match chronically reduced blood flow.[70,71] Such adaptational processes would explain the clinical observation that some chronically dysfunctional ventricular wall segments demonstrate functional recovery after restoration of blood flow. According to the alterations of glucose metabolism in ischemic cardiac tissue discussed above, ^{18}FDG PET imaging should be able to identify these ischemic but viable regions by showing enhanced ^{18}FDG uptake relative to blood flow. However, it is not certain whether these metabolic alterations seen in acute ischemia can be extrapolated to the state of chronic hypoperfusion associated with hibernation. Genuine myocardial hibernation has not yet been demonstrated unequivocally in humans, and animal models of chronic hibernation are difficult to create, even though considerable progress has been made in this regard.[16,24] Porcine preparations with prolonged ischemia for 3 to 24 hours showed metabolic adaptation over time with respect to lactate production.[16,25,28] Because generation of lactate is closely related to glycolysis, these findings may imply a certain degree of resetting in glucose metabolism during long-term ischemia. However, preliminary results in a porcine model of hibernation over 3 months indicated increased ^{18}FDG uptake in chronic ischemia as well.[24]

The second issue that must be discussed in view of myocardial viability is tracer uptake in stunned myocardium. In contrast to hibernation, which is triggered by chronic hypoperfusion, the notion of myocardial stunning implies restored blood flow. A recent study in 26 patients with chronic occlusion of a major coronary artery showed similar almost-normal resting

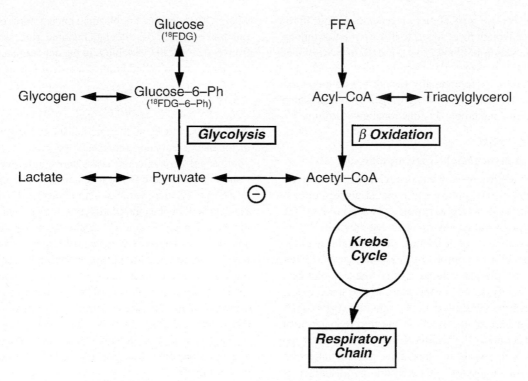

Fig. 32-4. Biochemical pathways of glucose and free fatty acids *(FFA)*, the two most important substrates for myocardial energy metabolism. Glycolysis through glucose-6-phosphate *(Glucose-6-Ph)* progresses to the production of pyruvate, which is decarboxylated by pyruvate dehydrogenase to acetyl-coenzyme A *(CoA)*, fueling the Krebs cycle. Under anaerobic conditions, glucose uptake into the sarcoplasm increases. However, pyruvate dehydrogenase is inhibited by elevated $NADH_2$ levels, leading to increased lactate formation. 2-[^{18}F]fluoro-2-deoxy-D-glucose (^{18}FDG) is converted to ^{18}FDG-6-phosphate (^{18}FDG-6-Ph), which does not undergo subsequent glycolytic pathways and is essentially trapped in the cytosol.

blood flow assessed with nitrogen-13 (^{13}N) ammonia in collateral-dependent left ventricular wall segments with and without regional wall-motion abnormalities.[90] Dysfunctional regions, however, revealed a reduced flow reserve after administration of intravenous dipyridamole. This suggests that chronic wall-motion abnormalities in these cases may not necessarily result from hibernation but from repetitive stunning due to transient ischemic episodes.[90] This concept may serve as an additional or an alternate explanation for reversible chronic wall-motion abnormalities.[91] In addition, ^{18}FDG PET should be able to disclose stunned myocardium as viable. In a canine model of 3-hour coronary occlusion and long-term reperfusion, postischemic glucose utilization in stunned myocardium as measured with ^{18}FDG was elevated after 24 hours of reperfusion, then decreased gradually along with functional improvement.[79] Because this enhanced postischemic ^{18}FDG uptake is paralleled by release of lactate from cardiomyocytes, it has been attributed to a genuine increase in (anaerobic) glycolysis rather than to replenishment of sarcoplasmic glycogen stores.[14,80] Increased postischemic glucose utilization was also documented in humans within the region of stress-induced perfusion defects when ^{18}FDG was injected during the recovery period 20 to 30 minutes after exercise, when the perfusion defects had already

resolved.[13] Thus, ^{18}FDG PET should reveal viable myocardium in chronic dysfunctional wall segments regardless of whether hibernation or stunning is responsible for the wall-motion abnormalities.

The intracellular signal transduction that induces enhanced ^{18}FDG uptake is not known, but some new experimental clues have been found with regard to the underlying mechanisms of the phenomenon itself on a cellular level. Experimental evidence indicates that a translocation of the insulin-sensitive glucose carrier GLUT-4 from a nonaccessible intracellular compartment to the myocellular membrane occurs in ischemia, which could partially explain the increase in glucose metabolism.[85,95] It has also been shown that the insulin-insensitive fetal GLUT-1 carrier is reexpressed in the rat heart in hypobaric hypoxia[82] and that GLUT-1 is translocated to the sarcolemma in ischemic canine cardiomyocytes,[95] which may provide further glucose transport capacities and, therefore, account for the increased glucose uptake in ischemic myocardium as well. To date, it has been impossible to define a clear morphologic basis for the increased uptake of ^{18}FDG in chronically dysfunctional but viable myocardium. This is mainly because of great variations and inconsistencies in the histochemical and ultrastructural findings in myocardium obtained from dysfunctional regions with respect to myocellular degeneration and fibrosis.[12,26,81,84] Even though there seems to be a correlation among the degree of reduction in blood flow, presence of myocellular fibrosis, and [18]FDG uptake,[12,26,84] there has been no clear evidence that the tracer is preferentially bound, as one might expect, in degenerated myocytes with glycogen granules, which have been identified in chronic dysfunctional myocardium.[18,47]

IMAGING OF [18]FDG

Quantitation of myocardial [18]FDG uptake

Because PET allows assessment of regional tissue activity in absolute terms, [18]FDG uptake and regional glucose utilization can be quantitated as long as certain assumptions about the kinetics of the tracer and its environment can be made. To describe the biokinetics of deoxyglucose in the brain, a three-compartment model was proposed by Sokoloff et al,[83] with deoxyglucose in the plasma volume as the first compartment (plasma pool), deoxyglucose in the intracellular space as the second compartment (precursor pool), and deoxyglucose-6-phosphate in the intracellular space as the third compartment (metabolic product pool).[83] This model assumes that the tissue is homogenous with respect to blood flow, rates of intercompartmental substrate transport, and concentrations of intracompartmental substrate concentrations; that the concentrations of deoxyglucose and deoxyglucose-6-phosphate are small compared with their physiologic counterparts; that carbohydrate metabolism in tissue is in a steady state; and that the tissue extraction fraction for glucose and deoxyglucose is small. Another prerequisite of this model is that material exchanges among the three compartments follow first-order kinetics. This implies that the coefficients k_1, k_2, k_3, and k_4 governing forward and reverse transport among compartments remain constant throughout the measurements (Fig. 32-2). In addition, deoxyglucose needs to be completely trapped in the tissue; that is, the rate of dephosphorylation of deoxyglucose-6-phosphate is negligible and the rate constant k_4 can be assumed to equal zero. When these requirements are met, the total tissue concentration of deoxyglucose, C_i, at any given time $t = \tau$ is related to the time course of the tracer plasma concentration $C_p(t)$ as

$$C_i(\tau) = k_1 e^{-(k_2+k_3)\tau} \int_0^\tau C_p(t) e^{(k_2+k_3)t} dt + k_1 k_3 \int_0^T \left(e^{-(k_2+k_3)T} \int_0^T C_p(t) e^{(k_2+k_3)t} dt \right) dT \quad (1)$$

As soon as the time course of the deoxyglucose plasma concentration $C_p(t)$ from time $t = 0$ to $t = \tau$ and the tissue concentration C_i at time $t = \tau$ are known, equation 1 allows us to determine the rate constants k_1, k_2, and k_3 by using a non-linear fitting routine.[83] Net regional glucose utilization, R_i, in the tissue is then given by

$$R_i(\tau) = \frac{C_i(\tau) - k_1 e^{-(k_2+k_3)\tau} \int_0^\tau C_p(t) e^{(k_2+k_3)t} dt}{L \left(\int \frac{C_p(t)}{C'_p(t)} dt - e^{-(k_2+k_3)\tau} \int_0^\tau \frac{C_p(t)}{C'_P(t)} e^{(k_2+k_3)t} dt \right)} \quad (2)$$

where $C'_p(t)$ denotes the plasma concentration of glucose as a function of time.[83] To calculate regional glucose utilization, R_i, from equation 2 the variable L in the denominator has to be determined. The so-called lumped constant L is defined as

$$L = \frac{k_1/(k_2 + k_3)}{k'_1/(k'_2 + k'_3\Phi)} \frac{V_m K'_m}{V'_m K_m} \Phi^{-1} \quad (3)$$

With k'_1, k'_2, and k'_3 as the rate constants for glucose, the first factor of this equation represents the ratio of the distribution volumes for deoxyglucose and glucose in tissue.[37,83] The constant Φ reflects the fraction of glucose further metabolized after phosphorylation, which is set to unity in this model because the degree of dephosphorylation is assumed to be negligible. In the second factor, V_m and V'_m denote the maximum velocity, K_m and K'_m the apparent Michaelis–Menten constants for deoxyglucose and glucose phosphorylation, respectively (that is, for the transition from compartment 2 to compartment 3). Equation 3 provides the basis for a general physiologic interpretation of the lumped constant L, an operational definition that is only valid, however, when the plasma concentration of deoxyglucose C_p has been maintained at a constant (in addition to the plasma concentration of glucose C'_p) over a sufficient period of time:[83]

$$L = \frac{C_A - C_V}{C'_A - C'_V} \frac{C_p'}{C_p} \quad (4)$$

In addition to the (constant) plasma concentrations of deoxyglucose and glucose, this equation for the lumped constant L requires only the arteriovenous differences $C_A - C_V$ and $C'_A - C'_V$ for deoxyglucose and glucose, respectively. The lumped constant for deoxyglucose in rat brain was found to be 0.483 ± 0.022.[83] Values in the same order of magnitude were determined with [18]FDG for the human brain.[29,37,65,73] The lumped constant for myocardium tended to be somewhat higher in rabbits[42] and was found to be 0.67 ± 0.10 in dogs.[72] This value was found to be stable over a wide range of glucose metabolic rates and in excellent agreement with the metabolic rate of glucose determined by the Fick method.[72] It is accepted by most PET centers and may be used to calculate the regional glucose utilization R_i of the myocardium with equation 2. The discussed tracer kinetic model has been extended to the situation in which dephosphorylation for deoxyglucose is accounted for and the rate constant $k_4 \neq 0$.[37]

Another approach that is independent from the number of compartments selected and does not require a constant plasma concentration of tracer was developed by Patlak et al.[61,62] Their graphical analysis applies primarily to a unidirectional system with complete trapping of the tracer in a final irreversible compartment.[62] Even though this model has also been adapted to the situation when all compartments are reversible, such as when dephosphorylation of deoxyglucose is not neglected,[61] we focus on the unidirectional solution. If C_p is the tracer plasma concentration, V_p is the effective plasma volume in the tissue sampled, V_e is the steady-state volume in the reversible compartments, f is the fraction of tracer back-diffusing from the reversible compartments at steady state, and K is the global tracer influx constant, the total amount of tracer in tissue A_m as a function of time t can be expressed as

$$A_m(t) = K \int_0^t C_p(\tau)d\tau + (V_p + fV_e)C_p(t) \qquad (5)$$

However, this relation holds only when the measurements are not taken before the reversible compartments have reached an effective steady state with the plasma space.[62] Rearrangement of the terms to

$$\frac{A_m(t)}{C_p(t)} = K \frac{\int_0^t C_p(\tau)d\tau}{C_p(t)} + (V_p + fV_e) \qquad (6)$$

yields a straight line equation when A_m/C_p is plotted against $\int_0^t C_p d\tau/C_p$. Strict linearity suggests a truly unidirectional system; otherwise, concave deviation occurs.[62] From the graph obtained with equation 6, the slope K and the intercept $(V_p + fV_e)$ can be determined. In the case of a three-compartment system, the slope K relates to the rate constants k_1, k_2, and k_3 as follows:[61]

$$K = \frac{k_1 k_3}{k_2 + k_3} \qquad (7)$$

When the steady-state plasma glucose concentration C_p' and the lumped constant L of the tissue is known, net regional glucose utilization R_i can finally be calculated using the formula

$$R_i = \frac{k_1 k_3}{k_2 + k_3} \frac{C_p'}{L} \qquad (8)$$

This equation was derived from a unidirectional three-compartment model in a steady state.[37] The described graphical analysis has been widely accepted for the quantification of ^{18}FDG PET imaging data. The method has also been adapted to measure myocardial ^{18}FDG uptake using a region of interest over the left ventricle to obtain the required tracer input function $C_p(t)$.[28]

However, although quantification of glucose utilization by using ^{18}FDG PET proved to be a powerful research tool, its clinical value has not been verified. In a study of 70 nondiabetic patients with previous myocardial infarction, the interindividual variation of regional myocardial glucose utilization in normal remote myocardium (SD = 31%) was found to exceed the intraindividual variation (SD = 11%).[40] The authors suggested that static imaging and semiquantitative analysis with intraindividual normalization would be sufficient for the clinical assessment of myocardial viability with ^{18}FDG.[40] This conclusion seems to be in keeping with the everyday practice of most PET laboratories.

Combination of ^{18}FDG with a perfusion tracer

For the assessment of myocardial viability in a patient presenting without precise information about regional myocardial abnormalities, metabolic PET imaging with ^{18}FDG alone is not sufficient and should be supplemented by a perfusion study. Myocardial blood flow is usually examined by means of ^{13}N ammonia, ^{15}O water, rubidium-82 (^{82}Rb), or a single-pho-

ton–emitting radioisotope. There are several reasons for this dual metabolism–perfusion approach.

1. Perfusion images are essential to define normally perfused remote myocardium that serves as a reference region for the normalization of ^{18}FDG uptake.[7]
2. Without perfusion data, ventricular wall segments consisting of an admixture of scar tissue and a clinically significant mass of hibernating but viable myocardium may be missed. In such a segment, regional ^{18}FDG uptake might be mildly reduced over the whole segment compared with normal zones. However, the concomitant decrease in perfusion will usually exceed metabolic reduction suggestive of an overall viable segment.
3. Finally, ^{18}FDG uptake has been shown to be inhomogeneous throughout the normal ventricular wall,[32] also suggesting the implementation of a second, independent functional factor, such as regional perfusion, for reference to allow valid assessment of myocardial viability.

When glucose ^{18}FDG uptake and regional perfusion are considered, three fundamental image patterns are of importance.

- Normal ^{18}FDG uptake and normal perfusion
- Normal or mildly decreased ^{18}FDG uptake exceeding reduced perfusion (metabolism–perfusion mismatch), which are commonly classified as viable myocardium (Fig. 32-5)
- Decreased ^{18}FDG uptake and concordantly reduced perfusion, which are usually considered nonviable scar tissue[49,85] (Fig. 32-6)

Various criteria have been applied to standardize the evaluation of metabolism–perfusion images. Normal values for the regional accumulation of ^{18}FDG, ^{13}NH$_3$ and the difference between uptake of the two substances have been established, and a divergence of more than 2 standard deviations was considered abnormal.[9,69] Other investigators applied threshold values for regional ^{18}FDG uptake relative to blood flow assessed with thallium-201 (^{201}Tl) (normal, >80% of ^{18}FDG accumulation in regions of normal blood flow; reduced, <80 and ≥50% of reference ^{18}FDG activity; absent, <50% of reference activity) and generated tomographic views based on the ratio of ^{18}FDG uptake to myocardial blood flow to facilitate visual assessment of metabolism–perfusion patterns.[7] However, because no rationale for these limits was provided, the values seem to be arbitrarily selected.

Predictive accuracy of ^{18}FDG imaging

Over the past decade, several studies have investigated the clinical value of ^{18}FDG PET with respect to the assessment of myocardial viability.* Perfusion was measured by using ^{13}N ammonia,[33,85-89,93] ^{82}Rb[50,52] or technetium-99m (^{99m}Tc) sestamibi single-photon emission computed tomography

*References 33, 41, 45, 50, 51, 85, 88, 89, 93.

Fig. 32-5. Coronal, sagittal, and transversal myocardial positron emission tomographic sections obtained after the administration of nitrogen-13 ammonia ($^{13}NH_4^+$) at rest *(perfusion)* and 2-[^{18}F]fluoro-2-deoxy-D-glucose *(metabolism)* in a 65-year-old man. The patient had occluded coronary bypass grafts and congestive heart failure and was referred as a potential candidate for heart transplantation versus coronary angioplasty. Concordantly diminished diaphragmatic and posterolateral tracer accumulation was seen on the perfusion and metabolism images, suggesting scar tissue. However, metabolic activity is preserved in the anterolateral and apical perfusion defects *(metabolism–perfusion mismatch)*, indicating viable myocardium *(arrow)*.

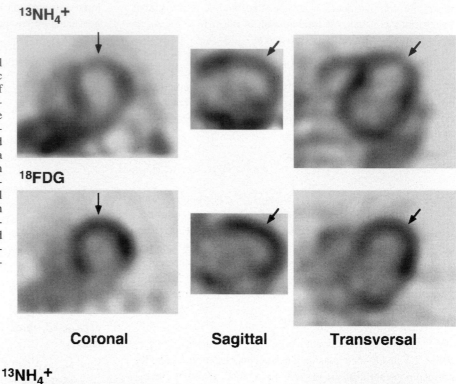

$^{13}NH_4^+$

^{18}FDG

Coronal   Sagittal   Transversal

Fig. 32-6. Coronal, sagittal, and transversal positron emission tomographic sections showing the myocardial distribution of nitrogen-13 ammonia ($^{13}NH_4^+$) at rest *(perfusion)* and 2-[^{18}F]fluoro-2-deoxy-D-glucose *(metabolism)* in an 80-year-old woman with a history of anterior myocardial infarction. Both perfusion and metabolism images show matched anterolateral, apical, and anteroseptal tracer accumulation defects compatible with scar tissue.

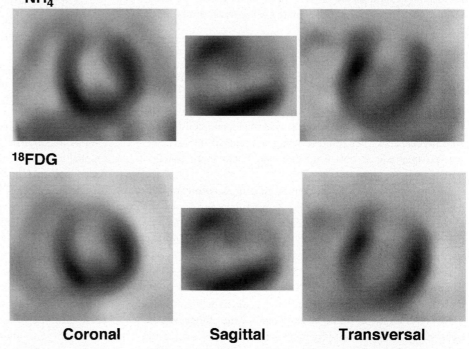

$^{13}NH_4^+$

^{18}FDG

Coronal   Sagittal   Transversal

(SPECT).[41,45] Applying the diagnostic criteria outlined above, these investigations found that ^{18}FDG PET predicted regional systolic functional recovery after coronary bypass surgery with a sensitivity of 73% to 95% and a specificity of 74% to 92%.*

Despite these convincing data, the results of ^{18}FDG PET must be interpreted carefully. Accumulation of ^{18}FDG was found to be linearly related to glucose utilization only under steady-state conditions.[36] Uptake of ^{18}FDG is lower in reversibly injured myocardium following experimental coronary occlusion has been shown to be lower than in remote myocardium and is lower in the early than in the late phase of reperfusion in canine[11] and porcine myocardium.[56] These findings suggest that clinical ^{18}FDG PET is best performed during the subacute phase of myocardial infarction under standardized metabolic conditions.

*References 33, 41, 45, 50, 51, 85, 86, 87, 88, 89, 93.

Prognostic value of [18]FDG imaging

It is of crucial interest to the clinician whether the detection of regional myocardial viability with [18]FDG PET has an impact on overall functional outcome or patient survival. Several studies have addressed this issue. In patients with coronary artery disease and depressed left ventricular function with a mean ejection fraction of 28% ± 6%, the total extent of the metabolism–perfusion mismatch on [18]FDG/^{13}N-ammonia PET correlated linearly with the percentage of improvement in functional status after coronary artery bypass graft surgery ($r = 0.87$; $p < 0.0001$).[20] In another analysis, patients with a mismatch pattern who underwent revascularization had a significantly higher survival rate than those who received medication only (80% compared with 50%; $p = 0.03$) during an average follow-up of 13.6 months.[19] A 12-month follow-up in patients with coronary artery disease and impaired left ventricular function showed a significantly lower rate of adverse cardiac events (death, myocardial infarction, cardiac arrest, or late revascularization) in the presence of a metabolism–perfusion mismatch after successful revascularization compared with medical treatment.[23] A lower rate of adverse cardiac events (unstable angina, myocardial infarction, or cardiac death) during 17 ± 9 months was also observed in postinfarction patients with left ventricular dysfunction and resting [82]Rb perfusion defects that accumulated [18]FDG after revascularization compared with patients who received medical treatment (8% compared with 48%; $p < 0.001$).[43] A recent prospective study with a 2-year follow-up showed that patients with regional wall-motion abnormalities and metabolism–perfusion mismatch on [18]FDG PET and ^{99m}Tc-sestamibi SPECT experienced no adverse cardiac events when they underwent revascularization compared with a 22% event rate among patients who were treated medically ($p < 0.01$).[94] Taken together, these data clearly demonstrate that [18]FDG PET combined with perfusion assessment is a powerful clinical tool for risk stratification in patients with known coronary artery disease and impaired left ventricular function.

COMPARISON WITH OTHER IMAGING METHODS

Various other imaging approaches have been proposed for the assessment of myocardial viability: radioimaging using ^{201}Tl, ^{99m}Tc sestamibi, [82]Rb, or carbon-11 (^{11}C) acetate; stress echocardiography; and magnetic resonance imaging. Of these alternatives, ^{201}Tl imaging using quantitative planar or SPECT techniques and echocardiography under low-dose catecholamine (dobutamine or arbutamine) stress compete in everyday clinical practice with [18]FDG PET. Although several studies have been undertaken that involve one or two of these imaging methods plus [18]FDG PET, few reported investigations have directly compared them with [18]FDG using regional systolic functional improvement after revascularization as an independent gold standard for myocardial viability.

Such a comparative study has recently been published. The investigators evaluated PET using both ^{11}C acetate and [18]FDG for the preoperative assessment of myocardial viability in 34 patients with chronic left ventricular dysfunction and coronary artery disease.[33] Carbon-11 acetate as an indicator of oxidative metabolism[2] was found to provide an estimate of viability compared with [18]FDG (positive predictive value, 67% and 52%; negative predictive value, 89% and 81%, respectively; $p < 0.01$ for each). However, these investigators determined myocardial perfusion from the early myocardial uptake of ^{11}C-acetate and did not combine the perfusion patterns with the data on [18]FDG uptake.[33] This certainly introduced a bias in favor of ^{11}C acetate and may explain the superiority of ^{11}C acetate over [18]FDG, as well as the somewhat low predictive accuracy of [18]FDG, in this investigation.

Several studies found metabolic activity with [18]FDG PET in persistent defects on ^{201}Tl SPECT.[7,8,19,21] However, ^{201}Tl SPECT with reinjection was found to be equivalent to [18]FDG PET.[64] In a meta-analysis evaluating six ^{201}Tl and six [18]FDG studies on the basis of functional improvement after surgery as a gold standard for myocardial viability, an overall trend was seen for better performance with [18]FDG; this trend became significant when only the clinically most relevant group of patients with severely depressed left ventricular function was considered.[76]

As for ^{99m}Tc sestamibi, experimental data indicate that uptake of this tracer requires myocellular viability.[6,27,52,66-68] These findings are in keeping with some clinical observations,[53-55] whereas other results suggested that ^{99m}Tc sestamibi underestimates viability compared with [18]FDG PET[22] or functional recovery after revascularization.[74] Even though the question of whether ^{99m}Tc sestamibi is predominantly a marker of viability or a flow tracer has not been decided, most investigators seem to support the latter view.

A comparative clinical analysis of PET using [82]Rb and [18]FDG (without separate perfusion data) found both approaches to be approximately equivalent for the quantitative assessment of myocardial necrosis and viability.[31]

In a clinical study comparing dobutamine echocardiography with a combination of [18]FDG PET and SPECT as a reference standard for viability, the sensitivity of the sonographic approach was 60% and the specificity 97%.[48] Other investigators comparing ^{99m}Tc sestamibi and dobutamine echocardiography with [18]FDG PET found more myocardial segments, especially severely hypoperfused and akinetic or dyskinetic ones, to be viable with [18]FDG than with the other approaches.[46] This result also suggests a higher sensitivity of metabolic PET. Uptake of [18]FDG was also seen in many segments that were thought to be nonviable with respect to end-diastolic wall thickness and systolic wall thickening on spin-echo magnetic resonance imaging.[63,64]

CONCLUSIONS

Imaging with [18]FDG PET for the assessment of myocardial viability has been validated extensively. Thallium-201 scintigraphy seems to be less sensitive and specific in terms of viability, especially in the clinically most relevant group of patients with severely depressed left ventricular function. Stress echocardiography is a promising alternative for the assessment of myocardial viability; however, it seems to have a lower sensitivity when directly compared with [18]FDG PET. The diagnostic tool of [18]FDG imaging may become more widely available in the near future with the use of SPECT systems for data acquisition. In this regard, both high-energy collimation[3-5,10] and coincidence detection[30,57] have been promising techniques. Patients expected to profit from the assessment of myocardial viability include postinfarction patients with residual ischemia and younger patients with severe coronary heart disease in whom the therapeutic decision between revascularization and cardiac transplantation must be made.

ACKNOWLEDGMENT

The authors thank Diane Martin for preparing the illustrations for this chapter.

REFERENCES

1. Almira EC, Garcia AR, Boshell BR: Insulin binding and glucose transport in cardiomyocytes of a diabetic rat, *Am J Physiol* 250 (4 Pt 1): E402–E406, 1986.
2. Armbrecht JJ, Buxton DB, Schelbert HR: Validation of [1-^{11}C]acetate as a tracer for noninvasive assessment of oxidative metabolism with positron emission tomography in normal, ischemic, postischemic, and hyperemic canine myocardium, *Circulation* 81:1594–1604, 1990.
3. Bax JJ, Visser FC, van Lingen A, et al: Feasibility of assessing regional myocardial uptake of ^{18}F-fluorodeoxyglucose using single photon emission computed tomography, *Eur Heart J* 14:1675–1682, 1993.
4. Bax JJ, Visser FC, van Lingen A, et al: Myocardial F-18 fluorodeoxyglucose imaging by SPECT, *Clin Nucl Med* 20:486–490, 1995.
5. Bax JJ, Visser FC, Blanksma PA, et al: Comparison of myocardial uptake of fluorine-18-fluorodeoxyglucose imaged with PET and SPECT in dyssynergic myocardium, *J Nucl Med* 37:1631–1636, 1996.
6. Beanlands RSB, Dawood F, Wen WH, et al: Are the kinetics of technetium-99m methoxyisobutyl isonitrile affected by cell metabolism and viability? *Circulation* 82:1802–1814, 1990.
7. Bonow RO, Dilsizian V, Cuocolo A, et al: Identification of viable myocardium in patients with chronic coronary artery disease and left ventricular dysfunction. Comparison of thallium scintigraphy with reinjection and PET imaging with ^{18}F-fluorodeoxyglucose, *Circulation* 83:26–37, 1991.
8. Brunken RC, Kotton S, Nienaber CA, et al: PET detection of viable tissue in myocardial segments with persistent defects at Tl-201 SPECT, *Radiology* 172:65–73, 1989.
9. Brunken RC, Mody FV, Hawkins RA, et al: Positron emission tomography detects metabolic viability in myocardium with persistent 24-hour single-photon emission computed tomography ^{201}Tl defects, *Circulation* 86:1357–1369, 1992.
10. Burt RW, Perkins OW, Oppenheim BE, et al: Direct comparison of fluorine-18-FDG SPECT, fluorine-18-FDG PET and rest thallium-201 SPECT for detection of myocardial viability, *J Nucl Med* 36:176–179, 1995.
11. Buxton DB, Schelbert HR: Measurement of regional glucose metabolic rates in reperfused myocardium, *Am J Physiol* 261 (6 Pt 2): H2058–H2068, 1991.
12. Cabin HS, Clubb KS, Vita N, et al: Regional dysfunction by equilibrium radionuclide angiography: a clinicopathologic study evaluating the relation of degree of dysfunction to the presence and extent of myocardial infarction, *J Am Coll Cardiol* 10:743–747, 1987.
13. Camici P, Araujo LI, Spinks T, et al: Increased uptake of ^{18}F-fluorodeoxyglucose in postischemic myocardium of patients with exercise-induced angina, *Circulation* 74:81–88, 1986.
14. Camici P, Bailey IA: Time course of myocardial glycogen repletion following acute transient ischemia, *Circulation* 70:II-85, 1984 (abstract).
15. Camici P, Ferrannini E, Opie LH: Myocardial metabolism in ischemic heart disease: basic principles and application to imaging by positron emission tomography, *Prog Cardiovasc Dis* 32:217–238, 1989.
16. Chen C, Chen I, Fallon JT, et al: Functional and structural alterations with 24-hour myocardial hibernation and recovery after reperfusion. A pig model of myocardial hibernation, *Circulation* 94:507–516, 1996.
17. DeFronzo RA, Tobin JD, Andres R: Glucose clamp technique: a method for quantifying insulin secretion and resistance, *Am J Physiol* 237:E214–E223, 1979.
18. Depre C, Vanoverschelde JL, Melin JA, et al: Structural and metabolic correlates of the reversibility of chronic left ventricular ischemic dysfunction in humans, *Am J Physiol* 268 (3 Pt 2):H1265–H1275, 1995.
19. Di Carli MF, Davidson M, Little R, et al: Value of metabolic imaging with positron emission tomography for evaluating prognosis in patients with coronary artery disease and left ventricular dysfunction, *Am J Cardiol* 73:527–533, 1994.
20. Di Carli MF, Asgarzadie F, Schelbert HR, et al: Quantitative relation between myocardial viability and improvement in heart failure symptoms after revascularization in patients with ischemic cardiomyopathy, *Circulation* 92:3436–3444, 1995.
21. Dilsizian V, Freedman NM, Bacharach SL, et al: Regional thallium uptake in irreversible defects. Magnitude of change in thallium activity after reinjection distinguishes viable from nonviable myocardium, *Circulation* 85:627–634, 1992.
22. Dilsizian V, Arrishi JA, Diodati JG, et al: Myocardial viability in patients with chronic coronary artery disease. Comparison of ^{99m}Tc-sestamibi with thallium reinjection and [^{18}F]fluorodeoxyglucose, *Circulation* 89:578–587, 1994.
23. Eitzman D, al-Aouar Z, Kanter HL, et al: Clinical outcome of patients with advanced coronary artery disease after viability studies with positron emission tomography, *J Am Coll Cardiol* 20:559–565, 1992.
24. Fallavollita JA, Canty JM: ^{18}F-2-deoxyglucose utilization is regionally increased in fasting pigs with hibernating myocardium, *J Am Coll Cardiol* 29:130A, 1997 (abstract).
25. Fedele FA, Gewirtz H, Capone RJ, et al: Metabolic response to prolonged reduction of myocardial blood flow distal to a severe coronary artery stenosis, *Circulation* 78:729–735, 1988.
26. Flameng W, Suy R, Schwarz F, et al: Ultrastructural correlates of left ventricular contraction abnormalities in patients with chronic ischemic heart disease: determinants of reversible segmental asynergy post-revascularization surgery, *Am Heart J* 102:846–857, 1981.
27. Freeman I, Grunwald AM, Hoory S, et al: Effect of coronary occlusion and myocardial viability on myocardial activity of technetium-99m-sestamibi, *J Nucl Med* 32:292–298, 1991.
28. Gambhir SS, Schwaiger M, Huang SC, et al: Simple noninvasive quantification method for measuring myocardial glucose utilization in humans employing positron emission tomography and fluorine-18 deoxyglucose, *J Nucl Med* 39:359–366, 1989.
29. Gjedde A, Wienhard K, Heiss WD, et al: Comparative regional analysis of 2-fluorodeoxyglucose and methylglucose uptake in brain of four stroke patients. With special reference to the regional estimation of the lumped constant, *J Cereb Blood Flow Metab* 5:163–178, 1985.
30. Glass EC, Nelleman P, Hines H, et al: Initial coincidence imaging experience with a SPECT/PET dual head camera. *J Nucl Med* 37:53P, 1996.
31. Gould KL, Yoshida K, Hess MJ, et al: Myocardial metabolism of fluorodeoxyglucose compared to cell membrane integrity for the potassium analogue rubidium-82 for assessing infarct size in man by PET, *J Nucl Med* 32:1–9, 1991.
32. Gropler RJ, Siegel BA, Lee KJ, et al: Nonuniformity in myocardial accumulation of fluorine-18-fluorodeoxyglucose in normal fasted humans, *J Nucl Med* 31:1749–1756, 1990.
33. Gropler RJ, Geltman EM, Sampathkumaran K, et al: Comparison of carbon-11-acetate with fluorine-18-fluorodeoxyglucose for delineating

viable myocardium by positron emission tomography, *J Am Coll Cardiol* 22:1587–1597, 1993.

34. Gropler RJ: Methodology governing the assessment of myocardial glucose metabolism by positron emission tomography and fluorine 18-labeled fluorodeoxyglucose, *J Nucl Cardiol* 1 (2 Pt 2):S4–S14, 1994.

35. Hamacher K, Coenen HH, Stöcklin G: Efficient stereospecific synthesis of no-carrier-added 2-[18F]fluoro-2-deoxy-D-glucose using aminopolyether supported nucleophilic substitution, *J Nucl Med* 27:235–238, 1986.

36. Hariharan R, Bray M, Ganim R, et al: Fundamental limitations of [18F]2-deoxy-2-fluoro-D-glucose for assessing myocardial glucose uptake, *Circulation* 91:2435–2444, 1995.

37. Huang SC, Phelps ME, Hoffman EJ, et al: Noninvasive determination of local cerebral metabolic rate of glucose in man, *Am J Physiol* 238:E69–E82, 1980.

38. Huang SC, Williams BA, Barrio JR, et al: Measurement of glucose and 2-deoxy-2-[18F]fluoro-D-glucose transport and phosphorylation using dual-tracer kinetic experiments, *FEBS Lett* 216:128–132, 1987.

39. Knuuti MJ, Nuutila P, Ruotsalainen U, et al: Euglycemic hyperinsulinemic clamp and oral glucose load in stimulating myocardial glucose utilization during positron emission tomography, *J Nucl Med* 33:1255–1262, 1992.

40. Knuuti MJ, Nuutila P, Ruotsalainen U, et al: The value of quantitative analysis of glucose utilization in detection of myocardial viability by PET, *J Nucl Med* 34:2068–2075, 1993.

41. Knuuti MJ, Saraste M, Nuutila P, et al: Myocardial viability: fluorine-18-deoxyglucose positron emission tomography in prediction of wall motion recovery after revascularization, *Am Heart J* 127(4 Pt 1):785–796, 1994.

42. Krivokapich J, Huang SC, Phelps ME, et al: Estimation of rabbit myocardial metabolic rate for glucose using fluorodeoxyglucose, *Am J Physiol* 243:H884–H895, 1982.

43. Lee KS, Marwick TH, Cook SA, et al: Prognosis of patients with left ventricular dysfunction, with and without viable myocardium after myocardial infarction. Relative efficacy of medical therapy and revascularization, *Circulation* 90:2687–2694, 1994.

44. Liedtke AJ: Alterations of carbohydrate and lipid metabolism in the acutely ischemic heart, *Prog Cardiovasc Dis* 23:321–336, 1981.

45. Lucignani G, Paolini G, Landoni C, et al: Presurgical identification of hibernating myocardium by combined use of technetium-99m-hexakis 2-methoxyisobutylisonitrile single photon emission tomography and fluorine-18 fluoro-2-deoxy-D-glucose positron emission tomography in patients with coronary artery disease. *Eur J Nucl Med* 19:874–881, 1992.

46. Lucignani G, Landoni C, Mengozzi G, et al: Relation between dobutamine trans-thoracic echocardiography, 99mTc-MIBI and 18FDG uptake in chronic coronary artery disease, *Nucl Med Comm* 16:548–557, 1995.

47. Maes A, Flameng W, Nuyts J, et al: Histological alterations in chronically hypoperfused myocardium. Correlation with PET findings, *Circulation* 90:735–745, 1994.

48. Mariani MA, Palagi C, Donatelli F, et al: Identification of hibernating myocardium: a comparison between dobutamine echocardiography and study of perfusion and metabolism in patients with severe left ventricular dysfunction, *Am J Card Imaging* 9:1–8, 1995.

49. Marshall RC, Tillisch JH, Phelps ME, et al: Identification and differentiation of resting myocardial ischemia and infarction in man with positron emission computed tomography, 18F-labeled fluorodeoxyglucose and N-13 ammonia, *Circulation* 67:766–778, 1983.

50. Marwick TH, MacIntyre WJ, Lafont A, et al: Metabolic responses of hibernating and infarcted myocardium to revascularization. A follow-up study of regional perfusion, function, and metabolism, *Circulation* 85:1347–1353, 1992.

51. Marwick TH, Nemec JJ, Lafont A, et al: Prediction by postexercise fluoro-18 deoxyglucose positron emission tomography of improvement in exercise capacity after revascularization, *Am J Cardiol* 69:854–859, 1992.

52. Maublant JC, Gachon P, Moins N: Hexakis (2-methoxy isobutylisonitrile) technetium-99m and thallium-201 chloride: uptake and release in cultured myocardial cells, *J Nucl Med* 29:48–54, 1988.

53. Maublant JC, Citron B, Lipiecki J, et al: Rest technetium-99m-sestamibi tomoscintigraphy in hibernating myocardium, *Am Heart J* 129:306–314, 1995.

54. Maurea S, Cuocolo A, Soricelli A, et al: Enhanced detection of viable myocardium by technetium-99m-MIBI imaging after nitrate administration in chronic coronary artery disease, *J Nucl Med* 36:1945–1952, 1995.

55. Maurea S, Cuocolo A, Soricelli A, et al: Myocardial viability index in chronic coronary artery disease: technetium-99m-methoxy isobutyl isonitrile redistribution, *J Nucl Med* 36:1953–1960, 1995.

56. McFalls EO, Ward H, Fashingbauer P, et al: Myocardial flow and FDG retention in acutely stunned porcine myocardium, *J Nucl Med* 36:637–643, 1995.

57. Miyaoka R et al: Coincidence mode imaging using a standard dual-headed gamma camera, *J Nucl Med* 37:223P, 1996.

58. Opie LH: Myocardial ischemia—metabolic pathways and implications of increased glycolysis, *Cardiovasc Drugs Ther* 4Suppl 4:777–790, 1990.

59. Opie LH: *The heart—physiology and metabolism,* ed 2, New York, 1991, Raven Press.

60. Opie LH, Owen P, Riemersma RA: Relative rates of oxidation of glucose and free fatty acids by ischaemic and non-ischaemic myocardium after coronary artery ligation in the dog, *Eur J Clin Invest* 3:419–435, 1973.

61. Patlak CS, Blasberg RG: Graphical evaluation of blood-to-brain transfer constants from multiple-time uptake data. Generalizations, *J Cereb Blood Flow Metab* 5:584–590, 1985.

62. Patlak CS, Blasberg RG, Fenstermacher JD: Graphical evaluation of blood-to-brain transfer constants from multiple-time uptake data, *J Cereb Blood Flow Metab* 3:1–1, 1983.

63. Perrone-Filardi P, Bacharach SL, Dilsizian V, et al: Metabolic evidence of viable myocardium in regions with reduced wall thickness and absent wall thickening in patients with chronic ischemic left ventricular dysfunction, *J Am Coll Cardiol* 20:161–168, 1992.

64. Perrone-Filardi P, Bacharach SL, Dilsizian V, et al: Regional left ventricular wall thickening. Relation to regional uptake of 18fluorodeoxyglucose and 201Tl in patients with chronic artery disease and left ventricular dysfunction, *Circulation* 86:1125–1137, 1992.

65. Phelps M, Huang SC, Hoffman EJ, et al: Tomographic measurement of local cerebral glucose metabolic rate in humans with (F-18)2-fluoro-2-deoxy-D-glucose: validation of method, *Ann Neurol* 6:371–388, 1979.

66. Piwnica-Worms D, Kronauge JF, Delmon L, et al: Effect of metabolic inhibition on technetium 99m MIBI kinetics in cultured chick myocardial cells, *J Nucl Med* 31:464–472, 1990.

67. Piwnica-Worms D, Kronauge JF, Chiu ML: Uptake and retention of hexakis (2-methoxyisobutyl isonitrile) technetium(I) in cultured chick myocardial cells. Mitochondrial and plasma membrane potential dependence, *Circulation* 82:1826–1838, 1990.

68. Piwnica-Worms D, Chiu ML, Kronauge JF, et al: Divergent kinetics of 201Tl and 99mTc-sestamibi in cultured chick ventricular myocytes during ATP depletion, *Circulation* 85:1531–1541, 1992.

69. Porenta G, Kuhle W, Czernin J, et al: Semiquantitative assessment of myocardial blood flow and viability using polar map displays of cardiac PET images, *J Nucl Med* 33:1628–1636, 1992.

70. Rahimtoola SH: A perspective on the three large multicenter randomized clinical trials of coronary bypass surgery for chronic stable angina, *Circulation* 72:V-123–135, 1987.

71. Rahimtoola SH: The hibernating myocardium, *Am Heart J* 117:211–221, 1989.

72. Ratib O, Phelps ME, Huang SC, et al: Positron tomography with deoxyglucose for estimating local myocardial glucose metabolism, *J Nucl Med* 23:577–586, 1982.

73. Reivich M, Alavi A, Wolf A, et al: Glucose metabolic rate kinetic model parameter determination in humans: the lumped constants and rate constants for [^{18}F]fluorodeoxyglucose and [^{11}C]deoxyglucose, *J Cereb Blood Flow Metab* 5:179–192, 1985.

74. Rocco TP, Dilsizian V, Strauss HW, et al: Technetium-99m isonitrile myocardial uptake at rest. II. Relation to clinical markers of potential viability, *J Am Coll Cardiol* 14:1678–1684, 1989.

75. Ruth TJ, Wolf AP: Absolute cross sections for the production of ^{18}F via the ^{18}O(p,n) ^{18}F reaction, *Radiochim Acta* 26:21–24, 1979.

76. Schelbert HR: Merits and limitations of radionuclide approaches to viability and future developments, *J Nucl Cardiol* 1(2 Pt 2):S86–S96, 1994.

77. Schöder H, Campisi R, Ohtake T, et al: Predictive value of PET blood flow/metabolism mismatch in patients with type II diabetes mellitus, *J Am Coll Cardiol* 29:435A, 1997.

78. Schulz R, Rose J, Martin C, et al: Development of short-term myocardial hibernation. Its limitation by the severity of ischemia and inotropic stimulation, *Circulation* 88:684–695, 1993.

79. Schwaiger M, Schelbert HR, Ellison D, et al: Sustained regional abnormalities in cardiac metabolism after transient ischemia in the chronic dog model, *J Am Coll Cardiol* 6:336–347, 1985.

80. Schwaiger M, Neese RA, Araujo L, et al: Sustained nonoxidative glucose utilization and depletion of glycogen in reperfused canine myocardium, *J Am Coll Cardiol* 13:745–754, 1989.

81. Schwarz ER, Schaper J, vom Dahl J, et al: Myocyte degeneration and cell death in hibernating human myocardium, *J Am Coll Cardiol* 27:1577–1585, 1996.

82. Sivitz WI, Lund DD, Yorek B, et al: Pretranslational regulation of two cardiac glucose transporters in rats exposed to hypobaric hypoxia, *Am J Physiol* 263(3 Pt 2):E562–E569, 1992.

83. Sokoloff L, Reivich M, Kennedy C, et al: The [^{14}C]deoxyglucose method for the measurement of local cerebral glucose utilization: theory, procedure, and normal values in the conscious and anesthetized albino rat, *J Neurochem* 28:897–916, 1977.

84. Stinson EB, Billingham ME: Correlative study of regional left ventricular histology and contractile function, *Am J Cardiol* 39:378–383, 1977.

85. Sun D, Nguyen N, DeGrado TR, et al: Ischemia induces translocation of the insulin-responsive glucose transporter GLUT4 to the plasma membrane of cardiac myocytes, *Circulation* 89:793–798, 1994.

86. Tamaki N, Yonekura Y, Yamashita K, et al: Positron emission tomography using fluorine-18 deoxyglucose in evaluation of coronary artery bypass grafting, *Am J Cardiol* 64:860–865, 1989.

87. Tamaki N, Yonekura Y, Yamashita K, et al: Prediction of reversible ischemia after coronary artery bypass grafting by positron emission tomography, *J Cardiol* 21:193–201, 1991.

88. Tamaki N, Kawamoto M, Takahashi N, et al: Prognostic value of an increase in fluorine-18 deoxyglucose uptake in patients with myocardial infarction: comparison with stress thallium imaging, *J Am Coll Cardiol* 22:1621–1627, 1993.

89. Tillisch J, et al: Reversibility of cardiac wall-motion abnormalities predicted by positron emission tomography. *N Engl J Med* 314:884, 1986.

90. Vanoverschelde JLJ, Wijns W, Depre C, et al: Mechanisms of chronic regional postischemic dysfunction in humans. New insights from the study of noninfarcted collateral-dependent myocardium, *Circulation* 87:1513–1523, 1993.

91. Vanoverschelde JLJ, Wijns W, Borgers M, et al: Chronic myocardial hibernation in humans. From bedside to bench, *Circulation* 95:1961–1971, 1997.

92. vom Dahl J, Herman WH, Hicks RJ, et al: Myocardial glucose uptake in patients with insulin-dependent diabetes mellitus assessed quantitatively by dynamic positron emission tomography, *Circulation* 88:395–404, 1988.

93. vom Dahl J, Eitzman DT, al-Aouar ZR, et al: Relation of regional function, perfusion, and metabolism in patients with advanced coronary artery disease undergoing surgical revascularization, *Circulation* 90:2356–2366, 1994.

94. vom Dahl J, Altehoefer C, Sheehan FH, et al: Effect of myocardial viability assessed by technetium-99m-sestamibi SPECT and fluorine-18-FDG PET on clinical outcome in coronary artery disease, *J Nucl Med* 38:742–748, 1997.

95. Young LH, Renfu Y, Russell R, et al: Low-flow ischemia leads to translocation of canine heart GLUT-4 and GLUT-1 glucose transporters to the sarcolemma in vivo, *Circulation* 95:415–422, 1997.

96. Zaninetti D, Greco-Perotto R, Jeanrenaud B: Heart glucose transport and transporters in rat heart: regulation by insulin, workload and glucose, *Diabetologia* 31:108–113, 1988.

Chapter 33

Detection of viable myocardium by PET and carbon-11 acetate

Robert J. Gropler

Coronary revascularization is the preferred therapy for most patients with advanced coronary artery disease. In patients with chronic coronary artery disease, coronary artery bypass graft surgery will reduce angina, improve functional capacity, and increase survival when applied to appropriate patient subsets. Likewise, percutaneous approaches for revascularizing coronary arteries can result in dramatic improvement of symptoms. In patients with acute myocardial infarction, emergent recanalization of the infarct-related artery by intravenous thrombolytic agents or by primary coronary angioplasty will decrease infarct size, preserve left ventricular function, and improve survival.

With the growth of these coronary revascularization procedures it has been recognized that resting left ventricular dysfunction does not necessarily reflect myocardial scar. For example, in many patients who undergo coronary revascularization, regional or global left ventricular function improves and angina decreases; as a consequence, functional class and survival improve. The recognition of the reversible nature of resting left ventricular dysfunction has led to the concept of myocardial viability: that is, myocardium that will exhibit improved systolic function after coronary revascularization. In contrast, nonviable myocardium is irreversibly damaged and does not exhibit improvement in systolic function. Differentiation of viable from nonviable myocardium is of critical importance for various reasons. It is necessary for identifying which patients with left ventricular dysfunction will benefit from coronary revascularization and, thus, should be subjected to the increased morbidity and mortality associated with these procedures. This delineation is of particular importance in determining whether patients should undergo coronary bypass surgery or be listed for cardiac transplantation. Furthermore, accurate identification of viable myocardium is necessary for facilitating the development and evaluation of the efficacy of novel methods to restore myocardial perfusion, such as transmyocardial revascularization, or to reshape left ventricular geometry, such as cardiac myoplasty.

At present, several methods for detecting viable myocardium exist, including:

1. Measurements of myocardial perfusion
2. Assessment of membrane integrity
3. Measurement of myocardial fatty acid, glucose, and oxidative metabolism
4. The demonstration of improvement in function in response to inotropic stimulation (the contractile reserve phenomenon)

In general, measurements of myocardial perfusion, membrane integrity, and metabolism can be performed with single-photon emission computed tomography (SPECT) or positron emission tomography (PET). In contrast, the demonstration of the contractile reserve phenomenon is typically performed with dobutamine echocardiography. Both the large number of methods currently available and the diversity of the biologic processes that are being measured demonstrate that the need to differentiate viable from nonviable myocardium has not been met optimally. Because of the primacy of myocardial oxygen consumption (MVO$_2$) in the performance of left ventricular function, measurement of MVO$_2$ by PET with carbon-11 acetate is an attractive method for the detection of viable myocardium. In this chapter, the contributions of PET using ^{11}C acetate to further our understanding of myocardial viability and its usefulness in detecting viable myocardium will be discussed.

MYOCARDIAL VIABILITY AND RECOVERY OF MECHANICAL FUNCTION

The exact definition of viable myocardium has been controversial. Because the primary clinical goal of coronary revascularization in patients with resting left ventricular dysfunction is improvement in mechanical function, the recovery of function that results from coronary revascularization is considered indicative of myocardial viability by many investigators.[21] However, as mentioned, coronary revascularization has other benefits including a reduction in angina; improvement in functional class; stabilization of myocardial electrical activity; and, perhaps, prevention or improvement in left ventricular remodeling. Consequently, the presence of any of these end points has been proposed as a marker of viable myocardium.[34] However, unequivocal documentation of these markers of viability is frequently difficult to obtain either because procedures to measure their presence objectively are suboptimal (for example, angina reduction or stabilization of electrical activity) or because their occurrence may be confounded by the extent and location of viable myocardium as well as the presence of concomitant mitral valve regurgitation (that is, improvement in functional class or prevention or improvement in left ventricular remodeling). It should be noted that any of these end points will be somewhat dependent on the admixture of viable, nonviable, and normal tissue present within a region of myocardium subtended by a coronary artery that has been revascularized. The recovery of regional mechanical function is probably the most sensitive of the end points to this situation. However, it is still the most useful reference standard for tissue viability because it is readily measurable; is less likely to be affected by the extent and location of viable myocardium; and, when present, is likely to reflect the presence of other potential end points listed above. Thus, when comparisons are made among different methods for detecting viable myocardium, the recovery of regional mechanical function after successful coronary revascularization is the most logical reference standard to use.

MYOCARDIAL OXYGEN CONSUMPTION: EFFECTS OF ISCHEMIA AND REPERFUSION

The heart is an aerobic organ in that the consumption of oxygen by the myocardium is required for the continued generation of adenosine triphosphate by the electron transport chain, the major source of energy for myocardial cellular processes.[14,40] The heart uses various substrates, particularly fatty acids and glucose, to support overall oxidative metabolism. Under normal conditions, fatty acid oxidation usually predominates. With the onset of moderate-to-marked myocardial is-

chemia, inhibition of fatty acid oxidation occurs and anaerobic metabolism supervenes. Glucose becomes the primary substrate for both the increased anaerobic glycolysis and for continued, albeit diminished, oxidative metabolism.[40,42] With more marked reduction in myocardial blood flow, severe ischemic changes occur. Myocardial consumption of oxygen ceases and, because of accumulation of intracellular lactate and hydrogen ion, anaerobic glycolysis diminishes because of end-product inhibition. Myocardial necrosis ensues. With successful reperfusion, oxidative metabolism is restored, frequently returning to levels similar to those observed before the onset of ischemia.[4,38,49] Fatty acid utilization increases and, with time, overall glucose use decreases.[11,42] Of note, the chronology of normalization of MVO$_2$ seems to depend on the pattern and duration of the initial perfusion abnormality. For example, short repetitive episodes of ischemia interspersed with complete reperfusion result in rapid normalization of MVO$_2$.[38,55] In contrast, in more prolonged ischemia, MVO$_2$ will remain reduced despite successful reperfusion and may not normalize for hours or days.[11,31,51,55]

ADVANTAGES OF CARBON-11 ACETATE FOR MEASUREMENT OF MYOCARDIAL OXYGEN CONSUMPTION

Under most conditions, myocardial blood flow and MVO$_2$ are closely coupled. Because of the unique myocardial kinetics of ^{11}C acetate, it is an excellent tracer for assessing overall myocardial oxidative metabolism.

Myocardial blood flow

Under resting conditions, the first-pass extraction of acetate is approximately 50%.[7] Furthermore, significant egress of ^{11}C activity (in the form of ^{11}carbon dioxide [^{11}CO$_2$]) does not occur for 4 to 5 minutes after tracer delivery, except under conditions of very high MVO$_2$ demand.[7,8] Consequently, under most conditions, the behavior of ^{11}C acetate in myocardium early after the administration of tracer will reflect myocardial blood flow. In humans with coronary artery disease, estimates of relative perfusion from myocardial images obtained 1 to 4 minutes after the administration of ^{11}C acetate correlated closely with estimates of flow obtained with well-established flow tracers, such as oxygen-15 water and nitrogen-13 ammonia.[15,24] More recently, compartmental modeling approaches have been developed that permit quantification of myocardial blood flow in milliliters per gram per minute by PET and ^{11}C acetate.[30,32,37,56]

Oxidative metabolism

Because estimates of myocardial substrate use by PET with ^{11}C palmitate or fluorine-18 fluorodeoxyglucose reflect only a portion of overall oxidative metabolism, an alternative approach using ^{11}C acetate for measuring overall oxidative metabolism was developed. All major substrates that support oxidative metabolism ultimately enter the tricarboxylic acid (TCA) cycle through acetyl-coenzyme A (CoA). Acetate is a short-chained fatty acid that, as mentioned, is extracted readily by human myocardium. Acetate is then converted directly to acetyl-CoA within the mitochondria by acetyl-CoA synthase. Because the primary metabolic fate of acetyl-CoA takes place in the TCA cycle, acetate labeled by ^{11}C can be used to measure the flux of the cycle. Moreover, because of the close coupling of the TCA cycle and oxidative phosphorylation, the oxidation of acetate (reflected in the myocardial turnover of ^{11}C acetate) reflects overall regional myocardial oxidative metabolism. However, certain assumptions must be met in order for this relation to hold. First, acetate cannot be a major energy fuel for the heart. Although acetate can be oxidized by myocardium, the blood concentration of acetate under normal physiologic conditions is so low that the overall contribution to energy production by acid oxidation is negligible. Second, the ratio of TCA flux to overall oxygen consumption must be fairly constant, despite changes in the pattern of substrate utilization. Changes in substrate utilization have minimal effects on this ratio. Exclusive use by the heart of palmitate, glucose, or lactate as the sole substrate to support oxidative metabolism consumes 2.9, 3.0, and 3.0 moles of oxygen per mole of acetyl-CoA consumed, respectively. Consequently, an error of approximately 4% in the measurement of MVO_2 based on the assessment of TCA flux would be induced if overall oxidative metabolism were based solely on the oxidation of palmitate, which shifted to solely the oxidation of glucose. Because oxidative metabolism reflects the various admixtures of oxidation of multiple substrates under most conditions, this error would be even smaller. Finally, the relation between the rate of myocardial turnover of ^{11}C acetate and MVO_2 should not be altered appreciably by other nonoxidative metabolic fates of acetyl-CoA. Acetyl-CoA can be incorporated into fatty acid or into TCA cycle intermediates (in the form of amino acids), as well as into ketones. However, it seems that the flux of acetate through these other pathways is fairly small under various conditions so that the relation between myocardial turnover of ^{11}C acetate and MVO_2 is not altered.

VALIDATION OF MYOCARDIAL CARBON-11 ACETATE KINETICS AS A MEASUREMENT OF MYOCARDIAL OXYGEN CONSUMPTION

Studies in isolated perfused rabbit hearts and the hearts of intact dogs have characterized the myocardial kinetics of ^{11}C acetate. The clearance of ^{11}C activity from the myocardium after administration of ^{11}C acetate reflected almost exclusively the myocardial production of $^{11}CO_2$, which in turn was proportional to the rate of myocardial oxidative metabolism. The clearance of ^{11}C activity was biexponential, with a rapid phase of clearance (k_1) representing the oxidation of ^{11}C acetate to $^{11}CO_2$ and a slower phase (k_2) representing the incorporation of the tracer into amino acids via transamination and subsequent metabolism of TCA intermediates.[7,8,12,13] Studies in isolated perfused rabbit hearts demonstrated that the oxidation of acetate, labeled with either ^{11}C or ^{14}C and measured as the rate of efflux of radiolabeled CO_2, correlated closely with MVO_2 over

a wide range of tissue oxygenation and perfusion.[7,13] Although back-diffusion of radiolabeled acetate and a slight increase in radiolabeled ketones occurred under conditions of ischemia, more than 80% of the total activity was still attributable to radiolabeled CO_2. The relation between k_1 and MVO_2 was not altered by these effects. Similar observations were obtained in intact dog experiments.[8,12] Myocardial uptake of ^{11}C acetate was avid. Myocardial clearance of ^{11}C activity was biexponential, with a rapid phase of clearance correlating closely and directly with oxidation of ^{11}C acetate to CO_2 and MVO_2 over a wide range of conditions in levels of cardiac work and diverse flow conditions. Furthermore, changes in the pattern of substrate utilization by infusions of glucose and insulin or fatty acids did not alter appreciably the relation between myocardial clearance of ^{11}C acetate and MVO_2.[9] In human studies, indirect measurements of oxygen consumption had been directly correlated with ^{11}C acetate turnover kinetics. Excellent correlation was seen between clearance of myocardial ^{11}C activity and the rate-pressure product at rest and during exercise in healthy volunteers.[10]

Recently, approaches have been developed that apply compartmental models of the myocardial kinetics of ^{11}C acetate to the measurement of MVO_2.[2,10,29,43] These methods account for the variability in the input function and contamination of this function by radiolabeled metabolites of ^{11}C acetate, particularly $^{11}CO_2$. Results of studies in experimental animals have demonstrated that values for MVO_2 estimated by modeling correlate closely with directly measured values.[43] Furthermore, the correlation may be higher than that obtained from exponential curve fitting. In addition, myocardial ^{11}C acetate kinetics measured by PET were shown to compare favorably with MVO_2 measured by direct arterial-coronary sinus sampling in patients with normal epicardial vessels and normal left ventricular function and in patients with heart failure due to dilated cardiomyopathy.[2,29] However, it is not known whether compartmental modeling provides more accurate measurements of MVO_2 than exponential curve fitting, particularly in patients with severe left ventricular dysfunction, in which marked widening of the input function can occur.

ANIMAL MODELS OF ISCHEMIA AND REPERFUSION

Studies in isolated heart preparations and in dog hearts showed the utility of PET using acetate labeled with ^{14}C or ^{11}C in delineating the changes in MVO_2 during ischemia and reperfusion.* This technique confirmed previous observations that the rate of restoration of MVO_2 with reperfusion was related to the type, severity, and duration of the ischemic insult. Furthermore, these studies defined the chronology of restoration of MVO_2 after reperfusion, particularly in relation to changes in the pattern of substrate utilization and the recovery of systolic function. For example, with brief episodes of ischemia (typically < 15 minutes) followed by reperfusion, myocardial blood flow and MVO_2 were slightly diminished (Fig.

*References 4, 7, 11, 13, 26, 55

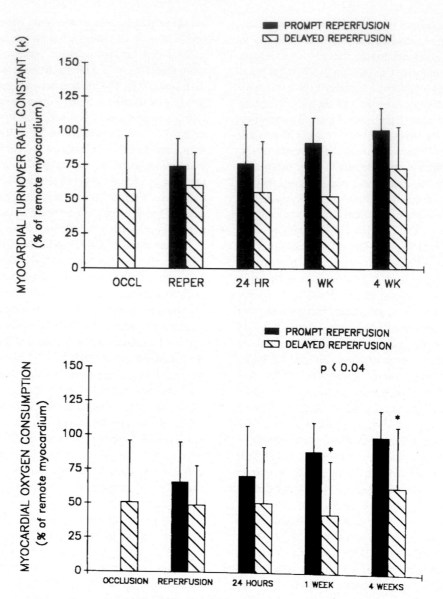

Fig. 33-1. Time course and restoration of myocardial oxygen consumption (MVO$_2$) in dogs as measured by PET and carbon-11 acetate after either prompt reperfusion (following 1 hour of ischemia) or delayed reperfusion (after 4 hours of ischemia). Following prompt reperfusion, MVO$_2$ returned quickly to normal. In contrast, following delayed reperfusion, MVO$_2$ remained depressed for up to 4 weeks after ischemia. (Reproduced with permission of Weinheimer CJ, Brown MA, Nohara R, et al: Functional recovery after reperfusion is predicated on recovery of myocardial oxidative metabolism, *Am Heart J* 125:939-949, 1993.)

33-1) and systolic function was markedly impaired. However, both MVO$_2$ and systolic function increased in response to inotropic stimulation by paired pacing (Fig. 33-2).[4,26,55] These findings confirmed the results of other studies using more invasive approaches that showed that stunned myocardium exhibited both oxidative and functional reserve. Furthermore, these studies demonstrated that the impairment in MVO$_2$ and systolic function present initially did not reflect only abnormalities in the biochemical processes underlying MVO$_2$ or the contractile apparatus. It is more likely that other mechanisms,

such as abnormal excitation contraction coupling due to perturbations and intracellular calcium ion fluxes, were responsible for the abnormalities in systolic function that typify stunned myocardium.

When reperfusion occurs after more-than-prolonged episodes of ischemia (typically 1 to 3 hours), MVO$_2$ does not return to baseline levels for at least 2 to 6 weeks following the initial ischemic insult (Fig. 33-1).[11,55] In addition, recovery of MVO$_2$ is paralleled by the recovery of systolic function. Furthermore, when measurements of MVO$_2$ by PET with ^{11}C ac-

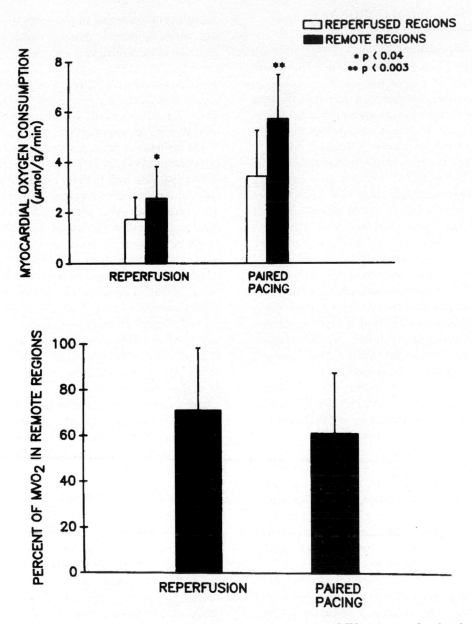

Fig. 33-2. Histograms of regional myocardial oxygen consumption (MVO$_2$) in reperfused and remote myocardium presented in absolute values (μmol/g/min) *(top)* and as a ratio of reperfused to remote myocardium. At rest, reperfused myocardium shows a high MVO$_2$ despite severe dyskinesis. With paired pacing, MVO$_2$ in reperfused myocardium almost doubles, demonstrating the presence of reserved capacity of oxidative metabolism in stunned myocardium. Under resting conditions and in paired pacing, MVO$_2$ was still slightly lower in reperfused myocardium than in remote normal tissue. (Reproduced with permission from Bergmann SR, Weinheimer CJ, Brown MA, et al: Enhancement of regional myocardial efficiency and persistence of perfusion, oxidative, and functional reserve with paired pacing of stunned myocardium, *Circulation* 89:2290-2296, 1994.)

etate are performed in conjunction with measurements of myocardial glucose utilization by FDG and fatty acid metabolism (by ^{11}C palmitate), it becomes clear that the pattern of substrate utilization varies greatly according to whether the myocardium is subjected to ischemia or reperfusion. For example, during ischemia, glucose use predominates, and fatty acid oxidation is markedly impaired.[11] In contrast, after reperfusion, oxidation of

fatty acids become the primary energy source. The results of these studies emphasize the importance of the recovery of MVO$_2$ in presaging the recovery of mechanical function after the termination of reversible ischemia and that measurements of myocardial substrate use will only provide partial information about total MVO$_2$ and, ultimately, the likelihood of recovery of mechanical function.

STUDIES IN HUMANS WITH CORONARY ARTERY DISEASE

Acute coronary syndromes

By using PET with ^{11}C acetate, it is possible to extend the observations of the effects of acute ischemia and reperfusion on MVO_2 obtained in experimental animals to humans with acute myocardial infarction. In patients with acute myocardial infarction treated conservatively (no thrombolytic agents were administered or revascularization procedures performed), MVO_2 in the center of the infarct zone was markedly depressed and did not change appreciably over time.[54] In patients treated with thrombolytic agents or primary angioplasty, MVO_2 was reduced in myocardium subtended by infarct-related arteries compared with normal myocardium remote from the site of infarction.[33] However, the individual values for MVO_2 varied markedly, and many of the segments in the infarct zone demonstrated levels of MVO_2 comparable to that in normal remote myocardium, suggesting that myocardial salvage had occurred. Thus, the potential salutary effects of acute recanalization strategies on MVO_2 were shown.[33] However, as was observed in experimental animals, resting levels of myocardial perfusion normalized rapidly with successful reperfusion; whereas MVO_2 did not reach normal values until 7 to 10 days after the index event.[28]

In addition to demonstrating the effects of ischemia and reperfusion on MVO_2 alone, studies with PET with ^{11}C acetate delineated the relation between alterations in MVO_2 and patterns of substrate utilization in patients with recent infarction. For example, MVO_2 in myocardial segments exhibiting increased glucose metabolism relative to blood flow (a marker of viable myocardium) as measured by PET with FDG was higher than that in myocardial segments exhibiting concordant reductions in flow and glucose metabolism (a marker of viable tissue).[17,52] Thus, with successful reperfusion, preservation of MVO_2 is paralleled by preserved substrate utilization necessary to support overall oxidative metabolism.

Measurements of MVO_2 by PET, referenced to changes in mechanical function in response to coronary bypass surgery or angioplasty, demonstrated the importance of preserved MVO_2 as a determinant of the potential for recovery of mechanical function among patients with recent myocardial infarction (studied within 10 days after the index event) undergoing coronary revascularization.[25] Only measurements of MVO_2 differentiated reversibly dysfunctional or viable segments from irreversibly dysfunctional (nonviable) segments when compared with measurements of regional myocardial perfusion (using ^{15}O water) or overall glucose metabolism (using FDG). Almost one third of nonviable segments showed preserved glucose metabolism with low MVO_2 (suggesting the presence of anaerobic glycolysis), a condition that alone is not capable of maintaining tissue viability in the face of a prolonged ischemic insult.[36] Moreover, about one fifth of viable segments showed marked reductions in glucose metabolism but preserved MVO_2. This pattern suggested that other substrates, most likely free fatty acids, were being used to support oxidative metabolism; this idea is in keeping with results in experimental animals. In ad-

dition, MVO_2 increased in reversibly dysfunctional segments after revascularization, showing that restoration of nutritive perfusion to jeopardized but still viable myocardium had salutary effects on MVO_2 as well as function. These results confirmed in humans the observations from the study of experimental animals that preservation of MVO_2 is a necessary condition for recovery of function consequent to coronary recanalization after myocardial infarction.

On the basis of these findings, it seemed likely that measurements of MVO_2 by PET with ^{11}C acetate would be more effective than PET with FDG for predicting improvement in mechanical function after coronary revascularization in patients with recent myocardial infarction. In a comparison of 19 patients studied within 10 days of infarction, measurements of MVO_2 by PET with ^{11}C acetate were superior to measurements of glucose metabolism by PET with FDG in predicting functional recovery after coronary revascularization (Figs. 33-3 and 33-4).[45] Positron emission tomography with ^{11}C acetate correctly identified reversibly and irreversibly dysfunctional segments 89% and 73% of the time, respectively. In contrast, PET with FDG correctly identified these segments only 65% and 57% of the time. In addition, the magnitude of functional recovery after revascularization correlated with the initial severity of the metabolic abnormality. In patients with recent myocardial infarction, the extent of expected functional recovery can be delineated accurately by measurement of regional oxidative metabolism by PET with ^{11}C acetate. Estimates derived with this method are superior to those obtained with PET using FDG.

Chronic coronary syndromes

Measurements of MVO_2 by PET with ^{11}C acetate have furthered our understanding of the mechanisms responsible for reversible resting systolic dysfunction in patients with coronary artery disease. It has been proposed that viable or reversibly dysfunctional myocardium represents myocardial hibernation.[6,44] This process represents the down regulation of myocardial oxygen demand (represented by a decrease in systolic function) in response to a chronic reduction in blood flow to achieve a better balance in myocardial oxygen supply and demand. Furthermore, it is believed that this new steady state can exist indefinitely and that once blood flow is restored, systolic function will improve or normalize. However, unequivocal evidence to support the existence of this condition is lacking. For example, in isolated perfused rat hearts, moderate reductions in flow were associated with concomitant reductions in MVO_2 without a significant increase in lactate production; these conditions were readily reversible when flow was restored. When reductions of flow became more pronounced, MVO_2 was reduced further, and metabolic patterns consistent with ischemia, such as lactate production, occurred.[35] In dogs, reductions in flow by approximately 50% over a few hours were associated with concomitant reductions in MVO_2 and systolic function. Moreover, lactate production, which initially increased gradually, returned to lactate consumption over the ensuing time in-

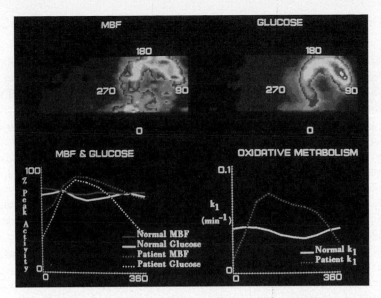

Fig. 33-3. Flow and metabolism in irreversibly dysfunctional myocardium (no change in mechanical dysfunction on serial wall-motion studies) in the inferolateral wall. The midventricular images of flow *(upper left)* and glucose metabolism *(upper right)* are displayed in true short-axis orientation. The lateral wall is at 90° and the anterior wall is at 180°. At the lower left are circumferential profiles of the relative values for regional perfusion *(dark interrupted curve)* and glucose metabolism *(light interrupted curve)*. Profiles representing the lower limits of normal (derived from 10 normal controls) for regional flow and glucose utilization are depicted by the solid dark and light curves, respectively. At the lower right is the profile representing regional values for the myocardial turnover rate constant of acetate (k_1) for this patient *(interrupted curve)* superimposed on the profile depicting the lower limits of normal *(solid curve)*. Myocardial blood flow *(MBF)* and glucose metabolism are reduced concordantly in the inferolateral wall; the values are decreased to less than the lower limits of normal, a pattern consistent with irreversibly damaged tissue. Myocardial oxidative metabolism in the inferolateral wall is also decreased to less than the lower limits of normal for this region, consistent with irreversibly dysfunctional myocardium (From Gropler RJ, Geltman EM, Sampathkumaran K, et al: Comparison of carbon-11-acetate with fluorine-18-fluorodeoxyglucose for delineating viable myocardium by PET, *J Am Coll Cardiol* 22:1587-1597, 1993.)

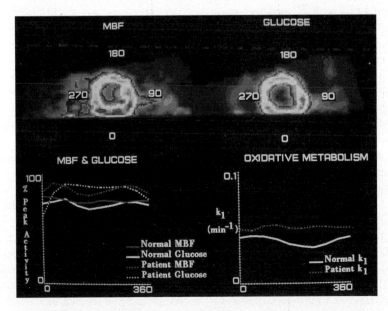

Fig. 33-4. Flow and metabolism in the anterior wall with reversibly dysfunctional myocardium (akinesia present initially, with normal function on follow-up). In the anterior wall, both flow and glucose metabolism are within the normal range predictive of functional recovery. Myocardial oxidative metabolism in the anterior wall is within the normal range as well. Abbreviations as in Figure 33-1 (From Gropler RJ, Geltman EM, Sampathkumaran K, et al: Comparison of carbon-11-acetate with fluorine-18-fluorodeoxyglucose for delineating viable myocardium by PET, *J Am Coll Cardiol* 22:1587-1597, 1993.)

terval. These data suggest that for at least a few hours, there may be a moderate level of hypoperfusion for which the myocardium can compensate with respect to substrate utilization, oxygen consumption, and systolic function. However, the stability of this state is markedly tenuous: Minor changes in heart rate or inotropy lead to subsequent ischemia and infarction.[19] Moreover, maintaining chronic hypoperfusion over a period of weeks has proven to be difficult, because levels of resting perfusion become markedly variable.[48] In humans, the primary line of evidence supporting this concept is the presence of an initial resting perfusion abnormality that redistributes during thallium-201 (^{201}Tl) myocardial scintigraphy in a myocardial segment that shows systolic function after coronary revascularization. However, because the initial ^{201}Tl images are acquired at one point in time, it is unclear if this pattern represents chronic hypoperfusion and, thus, myocardial hibernation or represents intermittent ischemia that was caught at the time of imaging.

In contrast to the situation with myocardial hibernation, a wealth of experimental and clinical evidence supports the concept of myocardial stunning: that is, prolonged but reversible systolic function that persists after successful reperfusion.[3,5,18,49,51] As mentioned previously, MVO_2 in stunned myo-cardium can be reduced to normal depending on the duration, pattern, and severity of the ischemic insult as well as the time interval after the onset of reperfusion. In humans, this concept has been used to explain the persistent systolic dysfunction frequently seen in patients with acute myocardial infarction after successful coronary artery recanalization by either thrombolytic therapy or primary coronary angioplasty.

Results of recent studies using PET with ^{11}C acetate suggest that the attribution of myocardial hibernation and stunning to patients with primarily chronic or acute coronary syndromes, respectively, may not be appropriate. For example, in patients with chronic coronary artery disease, MVO_2, as measured by PET with ^{11}C acetate, in reversible dysfunctional or viable myocardium was, on average, comparable to that found in myocardium with normal function. Given the close coupling of myocardial blood flow and oxygen consumption, this finding suggested that perfusion was within normal limits for many of these patients, a pattern suggestive of intermittent myocardial stunning.[22] Numerous subsequent studies have confirmed this hypothesis by demonstrating that in reversibly dysfunctional or viable myocardium, resting myocardial blood flow (quantified by PET) was comparable to that in normal tissue.[16,41,50,53] In addition, more than half of all viable segments showed normal myocardial blood flow and MVO_2, a state suggestive of myocardial stunning (Fig. 33-5). The rest of the segments exhibited reduced flow and MVO_2 and enhanced glucose metabolism, suggesting myocardial ischemia or hibernation.[16] Moreover, preservation of MVO_2 was a marker of the physiologic response of dysfunctional myocardium to inotropic stimulation.[39] In dysfunctional segments in which MVO_2 was preserved, augmentation in MVO_2, flow, and systolic function were significantly higher than in dysfunctional segments in which MVO_2

was not preserved. These findings are consistent with the presence of stunned myocardium and further substantiate the concept that intermittent episodes of ischemia and reperfusion are a frequent cause of resting reversible left ventricular dysfunction in patients with chronic coronary artery disease. Of note, histologic analysis of direct tissue samples taken at the time of bypass surgery demonstrated profound structural abnormalities in these reversible dysfunctional segments, including cellular swelling, loss of myofibrillar content, and accumulation of glycogen. These histologic findings are consistent with a chronic process and give further credence to the possibility that intermittent myocardial stunning is responsible for the resting systolic function found in patients with chronic coronary artery disease.

The implication of these results is manifold. First, it seems that the flow and metabolic perturbations underlying reversibly dysfunctional or viable myocardium in patients with chronic coronary artery disease are complex. Second, a pattern suggestive of intermittent stunning implies a dynamic process, because intermittent ischemia must occur. Potential mechanisms for dynamic changes in resting myocardial blood flow include repetitive, transitory occlusion and spontaneous reperfusion due to enhanced procoagulant activity or impaired fibrinolysis. Other possibilities include impaired vasomotor tone due to altered production or sensitivity to various vasoactive agents such as nitric oxide, endothelin, or acetylcholine. Delineating the responsible mechanisms will be important because of the likely targets for novel therapeutic agents, particularly in patients in whom the coronary anatomy is not amenable to mechanical revascularization. Finally, it seems that the presence of intermittent ischemia and reperfusion probably represents an unstable process that requires aggressive intervention.

As in patients with recent myocardial infarction, similar observations about the importance of preservation of MVO_2 as a determinant of recovery of mechanical function have been made in patients with left ventricular dysfunction predominantly attributable to chronic coronary artery disease.[22,23] Reversibly dysfunctional or viable myocardium demonstrated significantly higher MVO_2 values than did irreversibly dysfunctional tissue.[23] In contrast, amounts of relative perfusion (measured by using ^{15}O water) or levels of glucose metabolism (measured by using FDG) did not reliably differentiate reversibly dysfunctional from persistently dysfunctional myocardium. Consistent with results in patients with recent myocardial infarction, it seemed that preservation of myocardial glucose use (particularly in the presence of hypoperfusion) predicted functional recovery only when the metabolic pattern in the tissue reflected primarily oxidative metabolism of glucose. Accordingly, it seemed likely that ^{11}C acetate would more effectively predict improvement in mechanical function after coronary revascularization than PET with FDG. In a comparison of 35 patients undergoing coronary revascularization, measurements of MVO_2 by PET with ^{11}C acetate were superior to measurements of glucose metabolism by PET using FDG in predicting functional recovery after coronary revascularization,

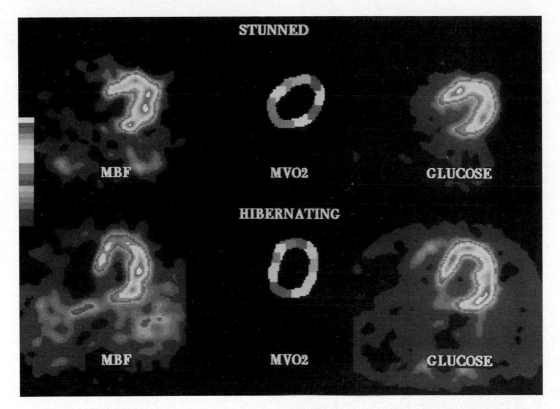

Fig. 33-5. Images of myocardial perfusion and metabolism in patients with diverse perfusion and reversibly dysfunctional segments. The images to the left show relative perfusion with oxygen-15 water; the images in the middle are parametric displays of regional values of myocardial clearance of carbon-11 activity after the administration of ^{11}C acetate and reflect regional oxidative metabolism; images on the right depict regional glucose metabolism with fluorine-18 fluorodeoxyglucose. The septum is to the left and the anterior wall is on top. In the upper example, reversible dysfunction was present in the anterior wall, but myocardial blood flow was normal at 1.2 ml/g/min. Both oxidative metabolism and glucose metabolism were comparable to values in the normally functioning lateral wall. These findings are consistent with stunned myocardium. In the lower panel, reversible dysfunction is present in the anteroapical wall. Perfusion was reduced at 0.50 ml/g/min. Oxidative metabolism was reduced relative to that in the normally functioning posterolateral wall. Glucose metabolism was increased relative to flow. These findings probably reflect myocardial hibernation. (Reproduced with permission: Conversano A, Walsh JF, Geltman FM, et al: Delineation of myocardial stunning and hibernation by positron emission tomography in advanced coronary artery disease, *Am Heart J* 131:440-450,1996.)

regardless of whether receiver-operating characteristic curve analyses or discrete criteria were used.[22] Positron emission tomography with ^{11}C acetate correctly identified reversibly and irreversibly dysfunctional segments 67% and 89% of the time, respectively. In contrast, PET with FDG was correct only 52% and 81% of the time. Both approaches showed better accuracy in segments exhibiting akinetic to aneurysmal changes initially. However, PET with ^{11}C acetate still tended to be more accurate; this method correctly identified reversibly and irreversibly dysfunctional segments 85% and 87% of the time, respectively, whereas PET with FDG was correct in 75% and 82% of cases, respectively. Thus, it seems that the criteria for differentiating viable from nonviable myocardium on the basis of measurements of myocardial metabolism are most accurate when applied to severely dysfunctional myocardium—regions for

which the distinction between viability and nonviability is of most clinical importance.

Recently, it was shown that the response of MVO_2 to intravenous dobutamine may be a more accurate predictor of functional recovery after revascularization than PET measurements of MVO_2 performed at rest.[27] In segments that would recover function after revascularization, a marked increase in MVO_2 was seen during dobutamine infusion. In contrast, in segments that would not recover function, MVO_2 decreased during dobutamine infusion. Unlike in rest conditions, there was no overlap in estimates of MVO_2 by PET with ^{11}C acetate between the two types of segments. Furthermore, the magnitude in increase in MVO_2 during dobutamine infusion correlated directly with the extent of improvement in mechanical function after revascularization.

In addition to predicting improvement in regional systolic function, measurements of MVO_2 can be used to predict improvement in global left ventricular function after coronary revascularization.[46] In patients with ischemic cardiomyopathy (average left ventricular ejection fraction, 24% ± 5%), the presence of at least 6 viable segments (out of 12 potential segments) based on measurements of MVO_2 by PET with ^{11}C acetate resulted in a significant increase in ejection fraction to 32% ± 8% after revascularization. Of note, a direct but weak correlation was seen between the extent of viable myocardium present initially and the magnitude of improvement in ejection fraction after revascularization. The correlation was particularly weak in patients with moderate-to-severe mitral regurgitation or prolonged (> 6 months) symptoms of heart failure before revascularization, suggesting that processes that are likely to distort or remodel left ventricular geometry will confound the interpretation of relation between preservation of metabolic activity and recovery of global left ventricular function.

Because of the close coupling of MVO_2 and perfusion, it has been theorized that estimates of MVO_2 by PET with ^{11}C acetate would not be better discriminators of myocardial viability than estimates of flow. However, results of studies in experimental animals have demonstrated that although a parallelism exists between blood flow and oxygen consumption in ischemic myocardium, the actual correlation differs from that observed in normal myocardium because of altered extraction of oxygen by ischemic myocardium.[20] Similar results are likely to be found in humans. In patients with coronary artery disease localized to the left anterior descending artery and normal left ventricular function, MVO_2 increased to a greater extent than myocardial blood flow (both quantified by PET with ^{11}C acetate) during dobutamine infusion. In contrast, the relation between MVO_2 and myocardial blood flow did not change during the infusion of dobutamine in normal volunteers. These data suggest that in patients with coronary artery disease, oxygen extraction increases when cardiac work is increased. In patients with left ventricular dysfunction undergoing coronary revascularization, logistic regression analysis demonstrated that both MVO_2 (based on exponential curve-fitting of myocardial ^{11}C acetate kinetics) and myocardial blood flow (measured in ml/g/min by PET with [15]O water) were independent predictors of functional recovery after coronary revascularization. However, MVO_2 was the more powerful predictor of functional recovery.[47] Of note, in a similar patient population, when MVO_2 and myocardial blood flow were quantified by compartmental modeling of myocardial ^{11}C acetate kinetics, MVO_2 did not provide unique information about recovery of mechanical function when the level of myocardial blood flow was known.[56] However, it is unclear whether the lack of independence between myocardial blood flow and MVO_2 reflects a true biologic phenomenon or is related to the compartmental model used in this study. Finally, it seems that the relation between MVO_2 and myocardial blood flow changes with the level of blood flow. A flatter relation is seen at moderate-to-high resting flow rates, and a steeper relation occurs at low flow rates (Fig. 33-6).[17] This relation delineated by PET with ^{11}C acetate in humans with recent myocardial infarction is consistent with a theoretical model developed from data obtained in experimental animals.[20]

MYOCARDIAL IMAGING WITH CARBON-11 ACETATE: TECHNICAL CONSIDERATIONS

For performing myocardial viability studies, PET with ^{11}C acetate has numerous advantages over PET with FDG. As mentioned previously, standardization of the substrate environment is not necessary when using ^{11}C acetate whereas the substrate environment must be standardized when using FDG. Moreover, imaging in patients with diabetes mellitus is not problematic with ^{11}C acetate. In addition, estimates of regional myocardial

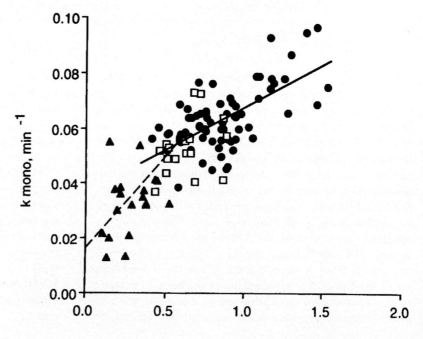

Fig. 33-6. Scatter plot showing the relation between oxidative metabolism *(k mono)* and myocardial blood flow for normal *(closed circles)*, flow-metabolism mismatch *(open squares)*, and flow-metabolism matched defects *(closed triangles)*. The data are fitted as a piecewise linear relation for myocardial blood flows less than 0.56 ml/g/min and greater than 0.56 ml/g/min. The piecewise relation demonstrates the dependency of oxygen extraction on the level of myocardial blood flow. (Reproduced with permission of Czernin J, Porenta G, Brunken R, et al: Regional blood flow, oxidative metabolism, and glucose utilization in patients with recent myocardial infarction, *Circulation* 88:884-895, 1993.)

perfusion in relative or absolute terms can be obtained with this tracer. In contrast, separate administration of a perfusion tracer is necessary when viability studies are performed using PET with FDG. However, ^{11}C acetate has some disadvantages compared with FDG. Because the half-life of ^{11}C is 20.2 minutes, whereas the half-life of ^{18}F is 109.9 minutes, numerous radiopharmaceutical syntheses are necessary when using ^{11}C acetate. Moreover, when imaging analysis is performed, measurement of washout rates is necessary to estimate MVO_2, whereas static imaging can be performed with FDG to obtain a relative estimate of regional myocardial glucose metabolism.

CONCLUSION

Measurement of MVO_2 by PET with ^{11}C acetate has made a remarkable contribution to our understanding of myocardial viability. The effects of myocardial ischemia and reperfusion on MVO_2, particularly with respect to preserving the capacity of jeopardized myocardium to recover systolic function, have been delineated in studies of experimental animals. Exportation of this approach to the study of humans has confirmed these observations in patients with recent myocardial infarction treated with acute coronary recanalization strategies. Measurements of MVO_2 performed in conjunction with measurements of myocardial blood flow have shown that viable myocardium in patients with chronic coronary artery disease is likely caused by intermittent myocardial ischemia and stunning as opposed to a chronic resting hypoperfusion or hibernation. Elucidating the mechanisms responsible for these perfusion abnormalities will facilitate the development of novel therapies and interventions designed to restore perfusion, metabolism, and systolic function in these patients. Another potential research application of PET and ^{11}C acetate will be combining the measurement of MVO_2 with measurement of mechanical work to quantitate energy transduction in ischemic or postischemic myocardium. Such an approach would be valuable in assessing the efficacy of therapies designed to improve systolic function in ischemic or postischemic myocardium in which flow abnormalities still persist but the area is not amenable to mechanical revascularization. In the clinical setting, preservation of MVO_2 has been shown to be an accurate marker of viable myocardium and its ability to recover function after coronary revascularization in patients with acute or chronic coronary syndromes. Thus, PET and ^{11}C acetate will continue to play an important role in both the investigation of the mechanisms responsible for viable myocardium and the detection of this phenomenon in patients with coronary artery disease.

REFERENCES

1. Armbrecht JJ, Buxton DB, Schelbert HR: Validation of [1-^{11}C] acetate as a tracer for noninvasive assessment of oxidative metabolism with positron emission tomography in normal, ischemic, postischemic, and hyperemic canine myocardium, *Circulation* 81:1594–1605, 1990.
2. Beanlands RS, Bach DS, Raylman R, et al: Acute effects of dobutamine on myocardial oxygen consumption and cardiac efficiency determined using Carbon-11 acetate kinetics in patients with dilated cardiomyopathy, *J Am Coll Cardiol* 22:1389–1398, 1993.
3. Becker LC, Levine JH, DiPaula AF, et al: Reversal of dysfunction in postischemic stunned myocardium by epinephrine and postextrasystolic potentiation, *J Am Coll Cardiol* 7:580–589, 1986.
4. Bergmann SR, Weinheimer CJ, Brown MA, et al: Enhancement of regional myocardial efficiency and persistence of perfusion, oxidative, and functional reserve with paired pacing of stunned myocardium, *Circulation* 89:2290–2296, 1993.
5. Bolli R, Zhu WX, Myers ML, et al: Beta-adrenergic stimulation reverses postischemic myocardial dysfunction without producing subsequent functional deterioration, *Am J Cardiol* 56:964–968, 1985.
6. Braunwald E, Rutherford JD: Reversible ischemic left ventricular dysfunction: evidence for the "hibernating myocardium," *J Am Coll Cardiol* 6:1467–1470, 1986.
7. Brown M, Marshall DR, Sobel BE, et al: Delineation of myocardial oxygen utilization with carbon-11-labeled acetate, *Circulation* 76:687–696, 1987.
8. Brown MA, Myears DW, Bergmann SR: Noninvasive assessment of canine myocardial oxidative metabolism with carbon-11 acetate and positron emission tomography, *J Am Coll Cardiol* 12:1054–1063, 1988.
9. Brown MA, Myears DW, Bergmann SR: Validity of estimates of myocardial oxidative metabolism with carbon-11 acetate and positron emission tomography despite altered patterns of substrate utilization, *J Nucl Med* 30:187–193, 1989.
10. Buck A, Wolpers HG, Hutchins GD, et al: Effect of carbon 11-acetate recirculation on estimates of myocardial oxygen consumption by PET, *J Nucl Med* 32:1950–1957, 1991.
11. Buxton DB, Mody FV, Krivokapich J, et al: Quantitative assessment of prolonged metabolic abnormalities in reperfused canine myocardium, *Circulation* 85:1842–1856, 1992.
12. Buxton DB, Nienaber CA, Luxen A, et al: Noninvasive quantitation of regional myocardial oxygen consumption in vivo with [1-^{11}C] acetate and dynamic positron emission tomography, *Circulation* 79:134–142, 1989.
13. Buxton DB, Schwaiger M, Nguyen A, et al: Radiolabeled acetate as a tracer of myocardial tricarboxylic acid cycle flux, *Circ Res* 63:628–634, 1988.
14. Camici P, Ferrannini E, Opie LH: Myocardial metabolism in ischemic heart disease: basic principles and application to imaging by positron emission tomography, *Prog Cardiovasc Dis* 32:217–238, 1989.
15. Chan SY, Brunken RC, Phelps ME, et al: Use of the metabolic tracer carbon-11-acetate for evaluation of regional myocardial perfusion, *J Nucl Med* 32:665–672, 1991.
16. Conversano A, Walsh JF, Geltman EM, et al: Delineation of myocardial stunning and hibernation by positron emission tomography in advanced coronary artery disease, *Am Heart J* 131:440–450, 1996.
17. Czernin J, Porenta G, Brunken R, et al: Regional blood flow, oxidative metabolism, and glucose utilization in patients with recent myocardial infarction, *Circulation* 88:884–895, 1993.
18. Ellis SG, Wynne J, Braunwald E, et al: Response of reperfusion-salvaged, stunned myocardium to inotropic stimulation, *Am Heart J* 107:13–19, 1984.
19. Fedele FA, Gewirtz H, Capone RJ, et al: Metabolic response to prolonged reduction of myocardial blood flow distal to a severe coronary artery stenosis, *Circulation* 78:729–735, 1988.
20. Feigl EO, Neat GW, Huang AH: Interrelations between coronary artery pressure, myocardial metabolism and coronary blood flow, *J Mol Cell Cardiol* 22:375–390, 1990.
21. Gropler RJ, Bergmann SR: Myocardial viability—What is the definition? *J Nucl Med* 32:10–12, 1991.
22. Gropler RJ, Geltman EM, Sampathkumaran K, et al: Comparison of C-11 acetate with fluorine-18-fluorodeoxyglucose for delineating viable myocardium by positron emission tomography, *J Am Coll Cardiol* 22:1587–1597, 1993.
23. Gropler RJ, Geltman EM, Sampathkumaran K, et al: Functional re-

covery after coronary revascularization for chronic coronary artery disease is dependent on maintenance of oxidative metabolism, *J Am Coll Cardiol* 20:569–577, 1992.

24. Gropler RJ, Siegel BA, Geltman EM: Myocardial uptake of carbon-11-acetate as an indirect estimate of regional myocardial blood flow, *J Nucl Med* 32:245–251, 1991.

25. Gropler RJ, Siegel BA, Sampathkumaran K, et al: Dependence of recovery of contractile function on maintenance of oxidative metabolism after myocardial infarction, *J Am Coll Cardiol* 19:989–997, 1992.

26. Hashimoto T, Buxton DB, Krivokapich J, et al: Responses of blood flow, oxygen consumption, and contractile function to inotropic stimulation in stunned canine myocardium, *Am Heart J* 127:1250–1262, 1994.

27. Hata T, Nohara R, Fujita M, et al: Noninvasive assessment of myocardial viability by positron emission tomography with ^{11}C acetate in patients with old myocardial infarction. Usefulness of low-dose dobutamine infusion, *Circulation* 94:1834–1841, 1996.

28. Henes CG, Bergmann SR, Perez JE, et al: The time course of restoration of nutritive perfusion, myocardial oxygen consumption, and regional function after coronary thrombolysis, *Coron Artery Dis* 1: 687–696, 1990.

29. Herrero P, Gropler RJ, Shelton ME, et al: Use of compartmental models of carbon-11 acetate to measure myocardial oxygen consumption: validation in human subjects, *J Nucl Med* 37:161P, 1996.

30. Herrero P, Hartmann JJ, Gropler RJ, et al. Quantification of myocardial perfusion with PET using C-11 acetate and a compartmental model in human subjects, *J Nucl Med* 37:83P, 1996.

31. Heyndrickx GR, Wijns W, Vogelaers D: Recovery of regional contractile function and oxidative metabolism in stunned myocardium induced by 1-hour circumflex coronary artery stenosis in chronically instrumented dogs, *Circ Res* 72:901–913, 1993.

32. Janier MF, André-Fouet X, Landais P, et al: Perfusion-MVO_2 mismatch during inotropic stress in CAD patients with normal contractile function, *Am J Physiol* 271:H59–H67, 1996.

33. Kalff V, Hicks RJ, Hutchins G, et al: Use of carbon-11 acetate and dynamic positron emission tomography to assess regional myocardial oxygen consumption in patients with acute myocardial infarction receiving thrombolysis or coronary angioplasty, *Am J Cardiol* 71: 529–535, 1993.

34. Kaul S: There may be more to myocardial viability than meets the eye, *Circulation* 92:2790–2793, 1995 (editorial).

35. Keller AM, Cannon PJ: Effect of graded reductions of coronary pressure and flow on myocardial metabolism and performance: a model of "hibernating" myocardium, *J Am Coll Cardiol* 17:1661–1670, 1991.

36. Kobayashi K, Neely JR: Control of maximum rates of glycolysis in rat cardiac muscle, *Circ Res* 44:166–175, 1979.

37. Krivokapich J, Huang SC, Schelbert HR: Assessment of the effects of dobutamine on myocardial blood flow and oxidative metabolism in normal human subjects using nitrogen-13 ammonia and carbon-11 acetate, *Am J Cardiol* 71:1351–1356, 1993.

38. Laster SB, Becker LC, Ambrosio G, et al: Reduced aerobic metabolic efficiency in globally "stunned" myocardium, *J Mol Cell Cardiol* 21:419–426, 1989.

39. Lee HH, Davila-Roman VG, Ludbrook PA, et al: Dependency of contractile reserve on myocardial blood flow: implications for the assessment of myocardial viability with dobutamine stress echocardiography, *Circulation* 96:2884–2891, 1997.

40. Liedtke AJ: Alterations of carbohydrate and lipid metabolism in the acutely ischemic heart, *Prog Cardiovasc Dis* 23:321–336, 1981.

41. Marinho NV, Keogh BE, Costa DC, et al: Pathophysiology of chronic left ventricular dysfunction. New insights from the measurement of absolute myocardial blood flow and glucose utilization, *Circulation* 93:737–744, 1996.

42. Myears DW, Sobel BE, Bergmann SR: Substrate use in ischemic and reperfused canine myocardium: quantitative considerations, *Am J Physiol* 253:H107–H114, 1987.

43. Ng CK, Huang SC, Schelbert HR, et al: Validation of a model for [1-^{11}C]acetate as a tracer of cardiac oxidative metabolism, *Am J Physiol* 266 (4 Pt 2):H1304–H1315, 1994.

44. Rahimtoola SH: The hibernating myocardium, *Am Heart J* 117: 211–221, 1989.

45. Rubin PJ, Lee DS, Dávila-Román VG, et al: Superiority of C-11 acetate compared with F-18 fluorodeoxyglucose in predicting myocardial functional recovery by positron emission tomography in patients with acute myocardial infarction, *Am J Cardiol* 78:1230–1235, 1996.

46. Rubin PJ, Miller T, Schechtman KB, et al: Prediction of improvement in left ventricular function after coronary revascularization by measurements of myocardial oxidative metabolism in patients with severe ischemic cardiomyopathy, *Circulation* 92:I550, 1995.

47. Rubin PJ, Schechtman KB, Geltman EM, et al: Preservation of myocardial oxygen consumption identifies viable myocardium independently of measurements of flow or glucose metabolism, *J Nucl Med* 36:68P, 1995.

48. Sherman AJ, Harris KR, Hedjbeli S, et al: Proportionate reversible decreases in systolic function and myocardial oxygen consumption after modest reductions in coronary flow: hibernation versus stunning, *J Am Coll Cardiol* 29:1623–1631, 1997.

49. Stahl LD, Weiss HR, Becker LC: Myocardial oxygen consumption, oxygen supply/demand heterogeneity, and microvascular patency in regionally stunned myocardium, *Circulation* 77:865–872, 1988.

50. Sun KT, Czernin J, Krivokapich J, et al: Effects of dobutamine stimulation on myocardial blood flow, glucose metabolism, and wall motion in normal and dysfunctional myocardium, *Circulation* 94:3146–3154, 1996.

51. Taegtmeyer H, Roberts AF, Raine AE: Energy metabolism in reperfused heart muscle: metabolic correlates to return of function, *J Am Coll Cardiol* 6:864–870, 1985.

52. Vanoverschelde JL, Melin JA, Bol A, et al: Regional oxidative metabolism in patients after recovery from reperfused anterior myocardial infarction. Relation to regional blood flow and glucose uptake, *Circulation* 85:9–21, 1992.

53. Vanoverschelde JL, Wijns W, Depre C, et al: Mechanisms of chronic regional postischemic dysfunction in humans. New insights from the study of noninfarcted collateral-dependent myocardium, *Circulation* 87:1513–1523, 1993.

54. Walsh MN, Geltman EM, Brown MA, et al: Noninvasive estimation of regional myocardial oxygen consumption by positron emission tomography with carbon-11 acetate in patients with myocardial infarction, *J Nucl Med* 30:1798–1808, 1989.

55. Weinheimer CJ, Brown MA, Nohara R, et al: Functional recovery after reperfusion is predicated on recovery of myocardial oxidative metabolism, *Am Heart J* 125:939–949, 1993.

56. Wolpers HG, Burchert W, van den Hoff J, et al: Assessment of myocardial viability by use of ^{11}C-acetate and positron emission tomography. Threshold criteria of reversible dysfunction, *Circulation* 95: 1417–1424, 1997.

Chapter 34

Fatty acid imaging

Nagara Tamaki, Takashi Kudoh, and Eiji Tadamura

Long-chain fatty acids are the principal energy source for the normoxic myocardium and are rapidly metabolized by β-oxidation. Therefore, radiolabeled agents represent potential probes to evaluate the differences in oxidative metabolism that occur in a various cardiac disorders. Approximately 60% to 80% of the adenosine triphosphate (ATP) produced in aerobic myocardium is derived from fatty acid oxidation; the remaining ATP is obtained from glucose and lactate metabolism. In ischemia, glucose metabolism plays a major role in residual oxidative metabolism, whereas oxidation of long-chain fatty acid is greatly suppressed.[37,47] Thus, alteration of fatty acid oxidation is considered to be a sensitive marker of ischemia and myocardial damage.

POSITRON EMISSION TOMOGRAPHY

Several studies have focused on evaluating fatty acid metabolism by using carbon-11 (^{11}C) palmitate and positron emission tomography (PET). After ^{11}C palmitate bound to albumin is administered intravenously, it rapidly clears from the blood. Initial uptake of ^{11}C palmitate correlated well with regional myocardial blood flow.[60] However, the single-pass extraction fraction is not constant; it is influenced by both residence time in the capillary bed and the rate of metabolism extracted into myocytes.[17] During prolonged ischemia, single-pass extraction fraction of the tracer decreases, probably because of the increase in the shunt into the triglyceride pool, and it diffuses back into coronary venous circulation.[81] Thus, regional uptake

of ^{11}C palmitate is reduced in the severely ischemic myocardium. In the clinical setting, quantitative estimation and characterization of myocardial infarction have been evaluated from the defect size on the early ^{11}C palmitate images.[15,36,63]

The clearance of radioactivity from the myocardium has been well documented. The clearance of ^{11}C palmitate showed two components consistent with incorporation of the tracer into at least two pools with different turnover rates. Because the clearance rate of the fast component is closely correlated with ^{11}C carbon dioxide (CO_2) clearance, this is considered to represent β-oxidation of ^{11}C palmitate.[62] On the other hand, the slow component of the tracer washout may reflect slow turnover of triglycerides and phospholipids. During ischemia, the size and the rate of the fast clearance component of the activity are significantly reduced, indicating reduced β-oxidation.[61] The tracer kinetic study, both at rest and during an intervention (such as atrial pacing or dobutamine infusion), may enhance separation of ischemic from normal myocardium on the basis of the differences of the clearance response during the intervention[17,71] (Fig. 34-1). The metabolic response under various types of stress plays a key role in differentiating reversible ischemia from irreversible scar tissue.

Another important aspect of metabolic analysis is the ability to characterize idiopathic myocardial diseases. Heterogeneity of initial ^{11}C palmitate is documented in patients with dilated cardiomyopathy, in contrast to the homogeneous tracer deficit seen in patients with ischemic cardiomyopathy.[8] Recently, myocardial abnormalities in patients with long-chain acyl-coenzyme A (CoA) dehydrogenase deficiency have been characterized by PET with ^{11}C palmitate.[27] Similarly, alteration of fatty acid metabolism is seen in patients with hypertrophic cardiomyopathy.[18] Figure 34-2 shows serial dynamic PET images obtained after ^{11}C palmitate injection in a patient with apical hypertrophic cardiomyopathy. Reduced uptake and washout of the tracer are noted in the apical region compared with the other region, indicating decreased fatty acid uptake and utilization in the abnormally thickened myocardium.

Carbon-11 acetate has been used to assess pathophysiologic conditions in patients with coronary artery disease and car-

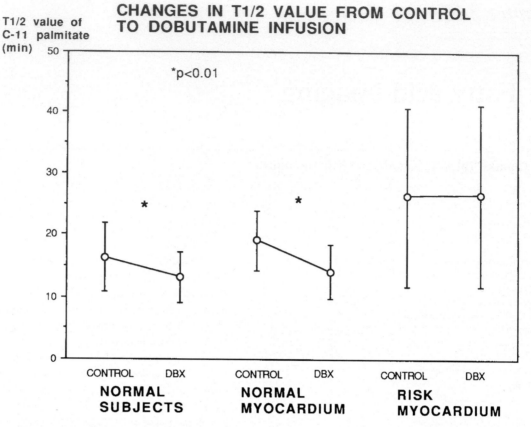

Fig. 34-1. The clearance rate $(T_{1/2})$ of carbon-11 palmitate at rest *(control)* and during dobutamine infusion *(DBX)* in normal patients *(left)*, the normal myocardium *(middle)*, and myocardium at risk *(right)* in patients with coronary artery disease. The $T_{1/2}$ value was reduced during dobutamine infusion, indicating enhanced β-oxidation in the normal myocardium, but this value was scattered in the myocardium at risk, indicating abnormal fatty acid oxidation in many of these segments.

diomyopathy. After administration of ^{11}C acetate, this substance is activated to acetyl-CoA, oxidized in mitochondria by the tricarboxylic acid (TCA) cycle, and washed out from the myocardium as $^{11}CO_2$ and H_2O. The early clearance rate in the myocardium measured by PET corresponds closely to release of $^{11}CO_2$, indicating that oxidative metabolism has occurred.[3] The major advantage of this study is that, unlike glucose or fatty acid metabolism, the oxidative metabolism is not influenced by plasma substrate levels. Gropler et al[16] showed that dysfunctional areas with preserved oxidative metabolism were reversibly ischemic myocardium that had improved regional function after revascularization. The predictive value of ^{11}C acetate was slightly better than that of fluorine-18 fluorodeoxyglucose (FDG). The experimental study also supports the idea that functional recovery after reperfusion was associated with recovery of oxidative metabolism.[80] Hata et al[22] recently showed that oxidative metabolic reserve after low-dose dobutamine infusion was a better marker of recovery of regional function than was resting metabolism alone.

As in the ^{11}C palmitate study, abnormal oxidative metabolism is seen in patients with hypertrophic cardiomyopathy by PET with ^{11}C acetate.[64] However, the chronological changes of metabolic alterations to free fatty acid, oxidation, and glucose

utilization and their relations to prognosis in these patients remain to be clarified.

Because of limited availability of PET, only a few institutes that have a PET camera and a cyclotron can study myocardial energy metabolism in vivo. On the other hand, various iodine-123-(^{123}I)–labeled fatty acid compounds have been introduced to probe myocardial energy metabolism in vivo in routine clinical nuclear medicine facilities.

IODINE-123–LABELED STRAIGHT-CHAIN FATTY ACIDS

Compounds

Radionuclide ^{123}I seems to be the preferred agent for labeling metabolic substrates because it has the chemical property of synthesis by halogen exchange reaction in replacing a molecular methyl group and because it has wide application in clinical practice. Thus, ^{123}I-labeled fatty acids have received great attention for assessing myocardial metabolism.[30,69,70]

There are two groups of iodinated fatty acid compounds: straight-chain fatty acids and modified branched fatty acids. The former compounds are generally metabolized through β-oxidation and released from the myocardium. Therefore, fatty acid utilization can be directly assessed by the washout kinetics

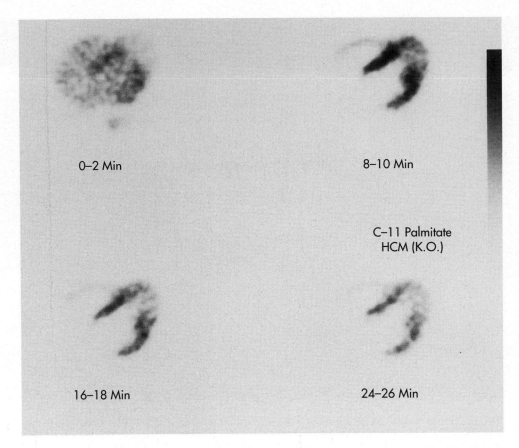

Fig. 34-2. Serial dynamic positron emission tomographic images obtained after carbon-11 palmitate administration in a patient with apical hypertrophic cardiomyopathy. Reduced uptake with washout of the tracer indicates decreased fatty acid uptake and utilization in the apical myocardium.

of the tracer, as with ^{11}C palmitate. However, rapid dynamic acquisition is required. This may become a critical problem when performing tomography with a rotating gamma camera. In addition, back-diffusion and metabolites should be considered in the kinetic model for quantitative analysis of fatty acid metabolism.

The modified fatty acid compounds are used on the basis of the concept of myocardial retention due to metabolic trapping. Therefore, excellent myocardial images are obtained with long acquisition time. On the other hand, their uptake may not directly reflect fatty acid oxidation. Instead, their uptake is based on the fatty acid uptake and turnover rate of the lipid pool. Therefore, the combined imaging of the iodinated fatty acid and thallium perfusion is required to demonstrate perfusion–metabolism mismatch and, thus, to characterize fatty acid utilization.

An early example of a iodinated fatty acid in the iodoalkyl substituted series is 17-iodohexadecanoic acid (HDA).[53] Although the tissue clearance of this tracer was prolonged in ischemic myocardium, suggesting ischemia-induced impairment of fatty acid oxidation,[78] experimental studies indicated that transmembranous exchange of iodine rather than oxidation determined the rate of radioiodine clearance from myocardium.[5,79] In addition, the inability to perform tomography may limit the clinical use of HDA.[7,54]

To eliminate rapid deiodination, Machulla et al[39] introduced the terminally phenylated iodinated straight-chain fatty acid 15(p-(^{123}I)-iodophenyl) pentadecanoic acid (IPPA) (Fig. 34-3). Reske et al[55-58] demonstrated rapid accumulation of this tracer in the heart; it subsequently cleared from the myocardium in the biexponential fashion characteristic of ^{11}C palmitate. Preliminary imaging studies showed a high myocardial uptake with decreased distribution in the areas supplied by the occluded coronary artery.[58] In addition, uptake was linearly correlated to myocardial blood flow during exercise.[4]

Clinical applications

In the clinical studies, segmental reduction of IPPA correlated well with the regional perfusion defect seen on thallium images in patients with coronary artery disease.[19,28] However, IPPA defects were generally more prominent than thallium defects,[55] probably because IPPA has a lower extraction fraction in ischemic areas. An IPPA rest study has been reported as being useful for the detection of coronary artery disease.[82,83] For viability assessment, IPPA uptake was identified in 39% of the segments with a persistent sestamibi defect and normalized in 25% of these segments, indicating the value of IPPA over the sestamibi perfusion study.[33] When dynamic IPPA study data were comparable to those of transmural biopsies and thallium

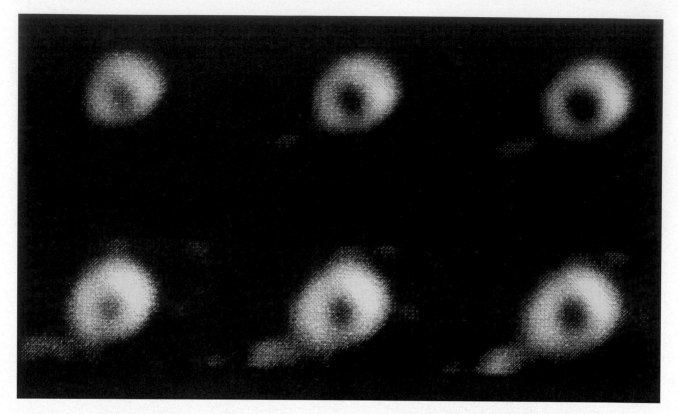

Fig. 34-3. Early *(top)* and late *(bottom)* scans after administration of iodine-123 IPPA in a patient with coronary artery disease. The initial decrease in tracer uptake with partial fill-in in inferoseptal regions indicates decreased fatty acid uptake and oxidation. (Courtesy of Dr. Iskandrian with permission.)

scan, viability assessed by IPPA imaging was similar to that seen with the biopsy findings and, more often, to that seen with the thallium scans.[44,45] A recent study showed the clinical value of IPPA rest imaging for viability assessment based on the prediction of functional recovery after revascularization.[20] Semiquantitative analysis of IPPA kinetics was suggested to have advantages over rest-redistribution thallium imaging.[24]

Thus, because of the unique property of ^{123}I IPPA for tracing perfusion and fatty acid turnover, many clinical data have been reported for its use in the detection of coronary lesions and viability assessment. Its rapid washout from the myocardium, however, may result in difficulties with high-quality SPECT imaging because of low count statistics. Nonetheless, IPPA will play an important role in the precise evaluation of fatty acid turnover in the assessment of pathophysiology in various myocardial diseases.

IODINE-123–LABELED MODIFIED FATTY ACIDS
Compounds

To minimize the limitations of straight-chain fatty acids, many attempts have been made to decrease the washout rate of the tracer from the myocardium for better imaging. Ortho-IPPA (*o*-IPPA) is a product of the synthesis of para-IPPA (*p*-IPPA) with a different isomer.[2] Its unique character relates to its long retention in the myocardium. A similarly high retention in the ischemic myocardium is seen with FDG.[23]

Methyl branching of the fatty acid chain is thought to protect these compounds against metabolism by β-oxidation[52] while allowing them to retain some physiologic properties, such as fatty acid uptake and turnover rate of the triglyceride pool. The degree of branching and the chain length determine the myocardial uptake of these tracers. S-methyl heptadecanoic acid was used in the isolated perfused heart,[38] and several experimental studies were performed to delineate regional differences of myocardial fatty acid uptake.[84,85]

Iodinated branch-chain fatty acids have been introduced to probe fatty acid utilization. 16-[^{123}I]-iodo-3-methylhexadecanoic acid (IMHA) is an example of a methyl-branched analogue. A recent study showed that a reversible IMHA defect was observed more often than reversibility on rest-reinjection thallium scanning.[40]

The use of methyl-branched fatty acid is based on the expected inhibition of β-oxidation by the presence of a methyl group in the β-position. Knapp et al first introduced 15-(*p*-iodophenyl)-3R,S-methyl pentadecanoic acid (BMIPP) and 15-(*p*-iodophenyl)-3,3-dimethyl pentadecanoic acid (DMIPP).[1,29] Animal experiments showed slow clearance of BMIPP, approximately 25% in 2 hours, whereas DMIPP showed no clearance. The fractional distribution of these compounds at 30 minutes after tracer injection in rats indicated that 65% to 80% of the total activity resided in the triglyceride pool. Of the two

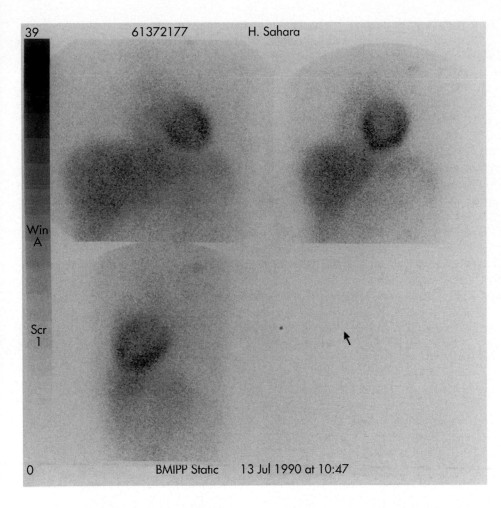

Fig. 34-4. Planar images in the anterior *(left)* and left anterior oblique *(right)* views of a normal patient at 60 minutes after BMIPP injection. A high myocardial uptake of the tracer is seen.

agents, BMIPP has been most widely used, particularly in Japan and Europe.

Basic analysis

Fujibayashi et al indicated that BMIPP uptake correlated with ATP concentration in acutely damaged myocardium treated with dinitrophenol[13] or tetradecylglycidic acid (TDGA), an inhibitor of mitochondrial carnitine acyltransferase I.[14] In an open-chest dog model, they also showed a high retention in and slow washout from the myocardium because of α- and β-oxidation.[11] Likewise, in an ischemic canine model, Nohara et al[50] also showed that BMIPP uptake correlated with ATP levels and may be useful to differentiate ischemic from infarcted myocardium. These results support the importance of ATP levels for the retention of BMIPP, probably because of cytosolic activation of BMIPP into BMIPP-CoA. On the other hand, an inverse correlation was observed between ATP levels and BMIPP uptake in hypertrophied myocardium in Dahl rats.[12] These conflicting results may be explained by differences in separate ATP pools available in mitochondria and the cytosol.[30]

In the ischemic canine model, BMIPP uptake and clearance have been studied with planar imaging, which showed higher uptake of BMIPP than thallium.[43] Similar findings were observed in an ex vivo study in an occlusion–reperfusion model.[48]

These data indicate that BMIPP may provide some measurement of metabolic function independent of myocardial perfusion. However, a BMIPP–perfusion mismatch conflicts with clinical data, in which less BMIPP uptake than perfusion is often observed (as is shown in the following section). Such conflicting results may be explained in part by fatty acid uptake, which is influenced by both residence time in the capillary bed and the rate of metabolism extracted into myocytes. In acute ischemia, prolonged residence time may cause higher retention of fatty acid analogue in the myocardium, with a washout similar to that in normal myocardium. During prolonged ischemia, on the other hand, the single-pass extraction fraction of the tracer decreases, probably because of the increase in the shunt into the triglyceride pool and diffusion back into the coronary venous circulation.[81] Thus, regional uptake of fatty acid analogue may be reduced in the severely ischemic myocardium.

Clinical applications

In clinical studies of BMIPP, rapid myocardial uptake with long retention was observed after BMIPP administration. High myocardial uptake was observed with low background and low uptake in the liver and lung at 60 minutes after BMIPP injection (Fig. 34-4). High-quality SPECT images can be obtained by collecting myocardial images for approximately 20 minutes.

In general, uptake of BMIPP was similar to thallium perfusion (Fig. 34-5).

In a study of myocardial infarction, we initially reported less BMIPP uptake than thallium perfusion in areas of myocardial infarction[72] (Fig. 34-6). Such discordant BMIPP uptake was often seen in recent-onset infarction, areas with recanalized arteries, and regions with severe wall-motion abnormalities in comparison with thallium perfusion abnormalities. Saito et al[59] also showed that iodinated branch-chain fatty acid uptake differed from thallium perfusion in patients with unstable angina and those in whom revascularization was performed. Many other published studies show less BMIPP uptake than perfusion in patients with ischemic heart disease, which correlated well with regional wall-motion abnormalities.* This result indicates that abnormal fatty-acid uptake and retention in ischemic myocardium relative to myocardial perfusion occur. This metabolic abnormality may be reversible long after revascularization therapy in conjunction with improvement in regional wall-motion abnormality.[42,49]

*References 6, 9, 26, 41, 42, 46, 49, 68, 75, 77.

In a study of patients with angina without previous myocardial infarction, a decrease in BMIPP uptake was often seen at rest despite normal perfusion, particularly in persons with unstable and vasospastic angina associated with regional wall-motion abnormality, indicating the presence of metabolic impairment in stunned or hibernating myocardium.[66,76,77] Tateno et al[76] showed a decrease of BMIPP in relation to severity of coronary stenosis and regional asynergy. In addition, such an abnormality was seen more often in patients with unstable angina than those with stable angina.

It is important to know whether BMIPP uptake that is less than thallium perfusion may represent reversible ischemic myocardium. Recent preliminary results showed that discordant BMIPP uptake was observed in areas associated with redistribution on stress thallium scanning (Fig. 34-7) and those with an increase in FDG uptake as a marker of exogenous glucose utilization.[26,73]

In ischemic myocardium, fatty acid oxidation is easily suppressed, and glucose metabolism acts as a major energy source. The study discussed above showed that areas with discordant BMIPP uptake were most likely to show an increase in FDG

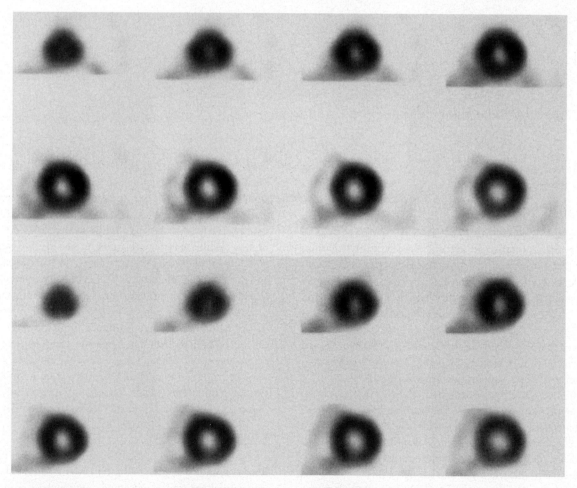

Fig. 34-5. A series of short-axis images of thallium *(top)* and BMIPP *(bottom)* administration in a normal subject. Distribution of BMIPP is homogeneous and similar to that of thallium in the left ventricular myocardium.

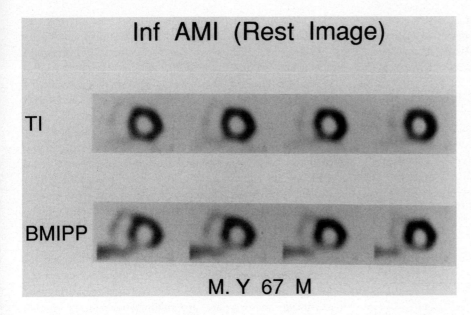

Fig. 34-6. Resting thallium *(top)* and BMIPP *(bottom)* images in a patient with inferior-wall myocardial infarction after successful revascularization of the right coronary artery in the acute stage of infarction. These short-axis images show a significant decrease in BMIPP uptake in the inferior region despite a minimal decrease in thallium uptake.

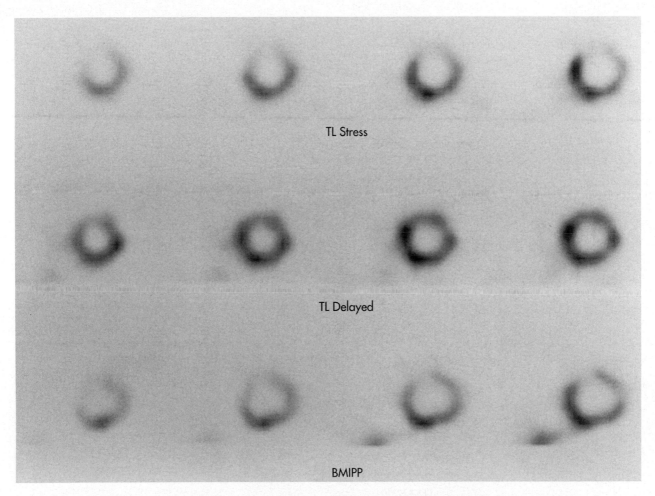

Fig. 34-7. A series of short-axis slices of stress *(top)* and delayed *(middle)* thallium scans and a resting BMIPP scan *(bottom)* in a patient with unstable angina. Decreased BMIPP uptake is observed in the anteroseptal region, where stress-induced hypoperfusion with redistribution is seen on the thallium study.

uptake (PET ischemia) (Table 34-1). In contrast, a concordant decrease in both BMIPP uptake and thallium perfusion may reflect no increase in FDG uptake (PET scar). These data indicate that BMIPP uptake that is less than thallium perfusion may represent ischemic myocardium.

A few reports indicate that discordant BMIPP uptake is a

Table 34-1. Comparison of BMIPP and thallium findings with fluorine-18 fluorodeoxyglucose positron emission tomographic findings in areas at risk in 12 patients with previous myocardial infarction*

	FDG PET Findings		
	PET ischemia	PET scar	Total
BMIPP/thallium findings		*n*	
BMIPP uptake less than thallium perfusion	12	1	13
BMIPP uptake equal to thallium perfusion	6	20	26
Total	18	21	39

*BMIPP = 15-(*p*-iodophenyl)-3R,S-methyl pentadecanoic acid; FDG = fluorine-18 fluorodeoxyglucose; PET = positron emission tomography.

marker of reversible ischemia with regional function may improve after revascularization. Franken et al[10] found that the areas with less BMIPP uptake than technetium-99m sestamibi perfusion showed improved cardiac function shortly after myocardial infarction. Recently, Ito et al[25] also showed recovery of regional dysfunction after myocardial infarction in areas with discordant defect size by BMIPP and thallium imaging (Fig. 34-8). Furthermore, the degree of perfusion–metabolism mismatch may reflect subsequent improvement in postischemic dysfunction.[21] These preliminary data indicate that discordant BMIPP uptake shows an area of reversible ischemic myocardium that is expected to improve dysfunction.

On the basis of the concept that discordant BMIPP uptake may represent ischemic myocardium, combined BMIPP and thallium imaging has been tested for prognostic value. We recently surveyed 50 consecutive patients with myocardial infarction who underwent BMIPP and thallium scanning for the follow-up study with a mean interval of 23 months. Among various clinical, angiographic, and radionuclide indices, discordant BMIPP uptake was the best predictor of future cardiac events, followed by the number of coronary stenoses.[74] Although these data remain preliminary, BMIPP and thallium imaging may have prognostic value for identifying high-risk subgroups among patients with coronary artery disease.

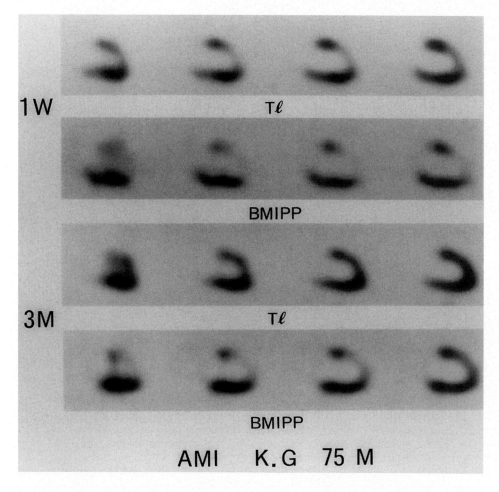

Fig. 34-8. A series of vertical long-axis slices of thallium and BMIPP images obtained 1 week *(top)* and 3 months *(bottom)* after anterior wall myocardial infarction. In the acute stage, a large BMIPP defect, larger than the thallium defect, is noted in the anterior region, which improved slightly in the chronic stage. The improvement in thallium uptake is more prominent than that of BMIPP uptake, indicating that improvement in fatty acid metabolism may be delayed compared with the improvement in perfusion.

Assessment of cardiomyopathy

Cardiac metabolism may play an important role in the assessment of pathophysiology in patients with cardiomyopathy. Alterations of fatty acid metabolism are frequently seen in patients with hypertrophic cardiomyopathy assessed by PET and with ^{11}C palmitate.[18] In Japanese patients with hypertrophic cardiomyopathy, BMIPP has been extensively studied; results indicate that BMIPP is distributed heterogeneously in hypertrophied myocardium independent of thallium perfu-

sion.[34,49,51,65,67] Figure 34-9 show a series of short-axis and horizontal long-axis slices of thallium and BMIPP imaging in a patient with hypertrophic cardiomyopathy. Although thallium uptake is heterogeneous in hypertrophied septal region, BMIPP uptake is strikingly decreased, indicating perfusion–metabolism mismatch. Figure 34-10 shows a series of short-axis and vertical long-axis slices of thallium and BMIPP imaging in the same patient described in Fig. 34-2. Uptake of BMIPP is decreased compared with thallium perfusion in the apex. This

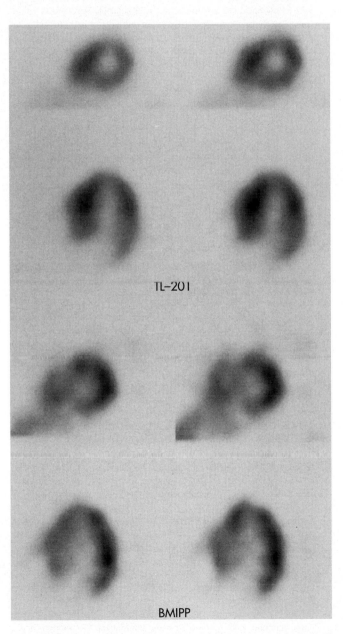

Fig. 34-9. Two representative slices of short-axis and horizontal long-axis thallium images *(top)* and BMIPP images *(bottom)* of a patient with hypertrophic cardiomyopathy. Decrease in BMIPP uptake is observed in septal region where thallium uptake seem to be homogeneous. (From Tanaki et al: *J Nucl Cardiol* 2:256, 1995, with permission.)

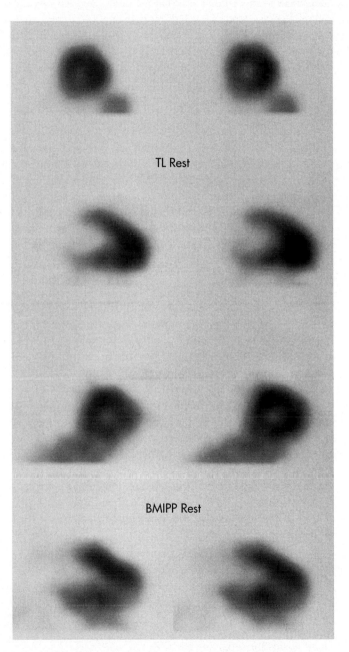

Fig. 34-10. Two representative slices of short-axis and vertical long-axis thallium images *(top)* and BMIPP images *(bottom)* in a patient with hypertrophic cardiomyopathy (the same patient as in Fig. 34-2). Uptake of BMIPP in the apical region is reduced compared with thallium perfusion in this region, whereas decreased fatty acid uptake and utilization is suggested in Fig. 34-2.

finding is similar to those obtained by using PET with ^{11}C palmitate. These data indicate that BMIPP may allow detection of alteration of fatty acid metabolism independent of thallium perfusion. This finding seems to be an early sign in patients with cardiomyopathy. However, more clinical experience is needed to confirm these preliminary results.

A study of congenital heart disease with BMIPP by Kondo et al[31] indicated that contractile dysfunction in cyanotic heart disease was primarily linked to impaired fatty acid metabolism rather than to myocardial scar. On the other hand, no myocardial uptake was seen in 0.9% of more than 1000 patients studied with BMIPP.[32,35] Such patients showed decreased ^{11}C palmitate uptake and increased FDG uptake on PET studies, indicating a metabolic shift from free fatty acid to exogenous glucose in the fasting state.[32]

CONCLUSIONS

Fatty acid is a major energy source in the normal myocardium. In various types of abnormal myocardium, fatty acid oxidation is easily suppressed; thus, assessment of fatty acid metabolism can play an important role in the early detection of myocardial abnormalities and provides insights into pathologic states in the heart. Although ^{11}C palmitate is a well-established tracer used to probe myocardial fatty acid metabolism, several iodinated fatty acid compounds have been introduced for the assessment of fatty acid metabolism, including straight-chain and branch-chain fatty acid compounds. Straight-chain fatty acid has advantages for measuring fatty acid oxidation on the basis of clearance of the tracer from the myocardium. Modified fatty acid can be trapped in the myocardium without further washout. Among these substances, the branch-chain fatty acid compound BMIPP provides excellent images of the left ventricular myocardium and may be used to probe myocardial energy metabolism in vivo. Segments with discordant BMIPP uptake (that is, uptake less than thallium perfusion), which are often seen in patients with coronary artery disease, may represent ischemic but viable myocardium in which an increase in glucose metabolism is also observed. Therefore, combined imaging with BMIPP and thallium permits detection of ischemic but viable myocardium on the basis of alteration of myocardial energy metabolism. In addition, BMIPP holds promise for the demonstration of early alteration of energy metabolism in various myocardial disorders.

ACKNOWLEDGMENT

The authors thank Drs. Naoya Hattori, Yasuhiro Magata, Yasuhisa Fujibayashi, Yoshiharu Yonekura, and Junji Konishi for valuable comments, and Drs. Ryuuji Nohara and Shigetake Sasayama for clinical support. We also acknowledge Nihon MediPhysics for supplying BMIPP.

REFERENCES

1. Ambrose KR, Owen BA, Goodman MM, et al: Evaluation of the metabolism in rat hearts of two new radioiodinated 3-methyl-branched fatty acid myocardial imaging agents, *Eur J Nucl Med* 12:486–491, 1987.

2. Antar MA, Spohr G, Herzog HH, et al: 15-(ortho-^{123}I-phenyl)-pentadecanoic acid, a new myocardial imaging agent for clinical use, *Nucl Med Commun* 7:683–696, 1986.

3. Brown M, Marshall DR, Sobel BE: Delineation of myocardial oxygen utilization with carbon-11-labeled acetate, *Circulation* 76:687–696, 1987.

4. Caldwell JH, Martin GV, Link JM, et al: Iodophenylpentadecanoic acid-myocardial blood flow relationship during maximal exercise with coronary occlusion, *J Nucl Med* 31:99–105, 1990.

5. Cuchet P, Demaison L, Bontemps L, et al: Do iodated fatty acids undergo a nonspecific deiodination in the myocardium? *Eur J Nucl Med* 10:505–510, 1985.

6. De Geeter F, Franken PR, Knapp FF Jr, et al: Relationship between blood flow and fatty acid metabolism in subacute myocardial infarction: a study by means of ^{99m}Tc-sestamibi and ^{123}I-beta-methyl-iodophenyl pentadecanoic acid, *Eur J Nucl Med* 21:283–291, 1994.

7. Dudczak R, Kletter K, Frischauf H, et al: The use of ^{123}I-labeled heptadecanoic acid (HDA) as metabolic tracer: preliminary reports, *Eur J Nucl Med* 9:81–85, 1984.

8. Eisenberg JD, Sobel BE, Geltman EM: Differentiation of ischemic from nonischemic cardiomyopathy with positron emission tomography, *Am J Cardiol* 59:1410–1414, 1987.

9. Franken PR, De Geeter F, Dendale P, et al: Abnormal free fatty acid uptake in subacute myocardial infarction after coronary thrombolysis: correlation with wall motion and inotropic reserve, *J Nucl Med* 35:1758–1765, 1994.

10. Franken PR, Dendale P, De Geeter F, et al: Prediction of functional outcome after myocardial infarction using BMIPP and sestamibi scintigraphy, *J Nucl Med* 37:718–722, 1996.

11. Fujibayashi Y, Nohara R, Hosokawa R, et al: Metabolism and kinetics of iodine-123-BMIPP in canine myocardium, *J Nucl Med* 37:757–761, 1996.

12. Fujibayashi Y, Som P, Yonekura Y, et al: Myocardial accumulation of iodinated beta-methyl-branched fatty acid analog, [^{125}I] (p-iodophenyl)-3-(R,S)-methylpentadecanoic acid (BMIPP), and correlation to ATP concentration—II. Studies in salt-induced hypertensive rats, *Nucl Med Biol* 20:163–166, 1993.

13. Fujibayashi Y, Yonekura Y, Takemura Y, et al: Myocardial accumulation of iodinated beta-methyl-branched fatty acid analogue, iodine-125-15-(p-iodophenyl)-3-(R,S)methylpentadecanoic acid (BMIPP), in relation to ATP concentration, *J Nucl Med* 31:1818–1822, 1990.

14. Fujibayashi Y, Yonekura Y, Tamaki N, et al: Myocardial accumulation of BMIPP in relation to ATP concentration, *Ann Nucl Med* 7:15–18, 1993.

15. Geltman EM, Biello D, Welch MJ: Characterization of nontransmural myocardial infarction by positron-emission tomography, *Circulation* 65:747–755, 1982.

16. Gropler RJ, Geltman EM, Sampathkumaran K, et al: Functional recovery after coronary revascularization for chronic coronary artery disease is dependent on maintenance of oxidative metabolism, *J Am Coll Cardiol* 20:569–577, 1992.

17. Grover-McKay M, Schelbert HR, Schwaiger M, et al: Identification of impaired metabolic reserve by atrial pacing in patients with significant coronary artery stenosis, *Circulation* 74:281–292, 1986.

18. Grover-McKay M, Schwaiger M, Krivokapitch J, et al: Regional myocardial blood flow and metabolism at rest in mildly symptomatic patients with hypertrophic cardiomyopathy, *J Am Coll Cardiol* 13:317–324, 1989.

19. Hansen CL, Corbett JR, Pippin JJ, et al: Iodine-123 phenylpentadecanoic acid and single photon emission computed tomography in identifying left ventricular regional metabolic abnormalities in patients with coronary heart disease: comparison with thallium-201 myocardial tomography, *J Am Coll Cardiol* 12:78–87, 1988.

20. Hansen CL, Heo J, Oliner C, et al: Prediction of improvement in left ventricular function with iodine-123-IPPA after coronary revascularization, *J Nucl Med* 36:1987–1993, 1995.

21. Hashimoto A, Nakata T, Tsuchihashi K, et al: Postischemic functional recovery and BMIPP uptake after primary percutaneous transluminal coronary angioplasty in acute myocardial infarction, *Am J Cardiol* 77:25–30, 1996.

22. Hata T, Nohara R, Fujita M, et al: Noninvasive assessment of myocardial viability by positron emission tomography with ^{11}C acetate in patients with old myocardial infarction. Usefulness of low-dose dobutamine infusion, *Circulation* 94:1834–1841, 1996.

23. Henrich MM, Vester E, von der Lohe E, et al: The comparison of 2-^{18}F-2-deoxyglucose and 15-(ortho-^{123}I-phenyl)-pentadecanoic acid uptake in persisting defects on thallium-201 tomography in myocardial infarction, *J Nucl Med* 32:1353–1357, 1991.

24. Iskandrian AS, Powers J, Cave V, et al: Assessment of myocardial viability by dynamic tomographic iodine-123-iodophenylpentadecanoic acid imaging: comparison with rest-redistribution thallium-201 imaging, *J Nucl Cardiol* 2:101–109, 1995.

25. Ito T, Tanouchi J, Kato J, et al: Recovery of impaired left ventricular function in patients with acute myocardial infarction is predicted by the discordance in defect size on ^{123}I-BMIPP and ^{201}Tl SPECT images, *Eur J Nucl Med* 23:917–923, 1996.

26. Kawamoto M, Tamaki N, Yonekura Y, et al: Combined study with I-123 fatty acid and thallium-201 to assess ischemic myocardium: Comparison with thallium redistribution and glucose metabolism, *Ann Nucl Med* 8:47–54, 1994.

27. Kelly DP, Hartman JJ, Herrero P, et al: Detection of the specific impairment of cardiac fatty acid oxidation in patients with long chain acyl-CoA dehydrogenase deficiency by positron emission tomography, *Circulation* 84 Suppl: ll-630, 1991 (abstract).

28. Kennedy PL, Corbett JR, Kulkarni PV, et al: Iodine 123-phenylpentadecanoic acid myocardial scintigraphy: usefulness in the identification of myocardial ischemia, *Circulation* 74:1007–1015, 1986.

29. Knapp FF Jr, Goodman MM, Callahan AP, et al: Radioiodinated 15-(p-iodophenyl)-3,3-dimethylpentadecanoic acid: a useful new agent to evaluate myocardial fatty acid uptake, *J Nucl Med* 27:521–531, 1986.

30. Knapp FF Jr, Kropp J: Iodine-123-labelled fatty acids for myocardial single-photon emission tomography: current status and future perspectives, *Eur J Nucl Med* 22:361–381, 1995.

31. Kondo C, Nakazawa M, Kusakabe K, et al: Myocardial dysfunction and depressed fatty acid metabolism in patients with cyanotic congenital heart disease, *J Nucl Cardiol* 3:30–36, 1996.

32. Kudoh T, Tamaki N, Magata Y, et al: Metabolism substrate with negative myocardial uptake of iodine-123-BMIPP, *J Nucl Med* 38:548–553, 1997.

33. Kuikka JT, Mussalo H, Hietakorpi S, et al: Evaluation of myocardial viability with technetium-99m hexakis-2-methoxyisobutyl isonitrile and iodine-123 phenyl pentadecanoic acid and single photon emission tomography, *Eur J Nucl Med* 19:882–889, 1992.

34. Kurata C, Tawarahara K, Taniguchi T, et al: Myocardial emission computed tomography with iodine-123-labeled beta-methyl-branched fatty acid in patients with hypertrophic cardiomyopathy, *J Nucl Med* 33:6–13, 1992.

35. Kurata C, Wakabayashi Y, Shouda S, et al: Influence of blood substrate levels on myocardial kinetics of iodine-123-BMIPP, *J Nucl Med* 38:1079–1084, 1997.

36. Lerch RA, Ambos HD, Bergmann SR, et al: Localization of viable, ischemic myocardium by positron-emission tomography with ^{11}C palmitate, *Circulation* 64:689–699, 1981.

37. Liedtke AJ: Alterations of carbohydrate and lipid metabolism in the acutely ischemic heart, *Prog Cardiovasc Dis* 23:321–336, 1981.

38. Livni E, Elmaleh DR, Levy S, et al: Beta-methyl [1-^{11}C] heptadecanoic acid: a new myocardial metabolic tracer for positron emission tomography, *J Nucl Med* 23:169–175, 1982.

39. Machulla HJ, Marsmann M, Dutschka K: Biochemical concept and synthesis of a radioiodinated phenylfatty acid for in vivo metabolic studies of the myocardium, *Eur J Nucl Med* 5:171–173, 1980.

40. Marie PY, Karcher G, Danchin N, et al: Thallium-201 rest-reinjection and iodine-123-MIHA imaging of myocardial infarction: analysis of defect reversibility, *J Nucl Med* 36:1561–1568, 1995.

41. Matsunari I, Saga T, Taki J, et al: Kinetics of iodine-123-BMIPP in patients with prior myocardial infarction: assessment with dynamic rest and stress images compared with stress thallium-201 SPECT, *J Nucl Med* 35:1279–1285, 1994.

42. Matsunari I, Saga T, Taki J, et al: Improved myocardial fatty acid utilization after percutaneous transluminal coronary angioplasty, *J Nucl Med* 36:1605–1607, 1995.

43. Miller DD, Gill JB, Livni E, et al: Fatty acid analogue accumulation: a marker of myocyte viability in ischemic-reperfused myocardium, *Circ Res* 63:681–692, 1988.

44. Murray G, Schad N, Ladd W, et al: Metabolic cardiac imaging in severe coronary disease: assessment of viability with iodine-123-iodophenyl pentadecanoic acid and multicrystal gamma camera, and correlation with biopsy, *J Nucl Med* 33:1269–1277, 1992.

45. Murray G, Schad N, Magill HL, et al: Dynamic low dose I-123 iodophenyl-pentadecanoic acid metabolic cardiac imaging: comparison to myocardial biopsy and reinjection SPECT thallium in ischemic cardiomyopathy and cardiac transplantation, *Ann Nucl Med* 7: SII79–SII85, 1993.

46. Nakajima K, Schimizu K, Taki J, et al: Utility of iodine-123-BMIPP in the diagnosis and follow-up of vasospastic angina, *J Nucl Med* 36:1934–1940, 1995.

47. Neely JR, Rovetto MJ, Oram JF: Myocardial utilization of carbohydrate and lipids, *Prog Cardiovasc Dis* 15:289–329, 1972.

48. Nishimura T, Sago M, Kihara K, et al: Fatty acid myocardial imaging using ^{123}I-β-methyl-iodophenyl pentadecanoic acid (BMIPP): comparison of myocardial perfusion and fatty acid utilization in canine myocardial infarction (occlusion and reperfusion model), *Eur J Nucl Med* 15:341–345, 1989.

49. Nishimura T, Uehara T, Shimonagata T, et al: Clinical experience of ^{123}I-BMIPP myocardial imaging for myocardial infarction and hypertrophic cardiomyopathy, *Ann Nucl Med* 7:SII35–SII39, 1993.

50. Nohara R, Okuda K, Ogino M, et al: Evaluation of myocardial viability with iodine-123-BMIPP in a canine model, *J Nucl Med* 37: 1403–1407, 1996.

51. Ohtsuki K, Sugihara H, Umamoto I, et al: Clinical evaluation of hypertrophic cardiomyopathy by myocardial scintigraphy using ^{123}I-labelled 15-(p-iodophenyl)-3-R,S-methylpentadecanoic acid (^{123}I-BMIPP), *Nucl Med Commun* 14:441–447, 1994.

52. Otto CA, Brown LE, Scott AM: Radioiodinated branched-chain fatty acids: substrates for beta oxidation? *J Nucl Med* 25:75–80, 1984.

53. Poe ND, Robinson GD Jr, Graham LS, et al: Experimental basis for myocardial imaging with ^{123}I-labeled hexadecanoic acid, *J Nucl Med* 17:1077–1082, 1976.

54. Railton R, Rodger JC, Small DR, et al: Myocardial scintigraphy with I-123 heptadecanoic acid as a test for coronary heart disease, *Eur J Nucl Med* 13:63–66, 1987.

55. Reske SN, Biersack HJ, Lackner K, et al: Assessment of regional myocardial uptake and metabolism of ω-(p-^{123}I-phenyl) pentadecanoic acid with serial single-photon emission tomography, *Nuklearmedizin* 21:249–253, 1982.

56. Reske SN, Machulla HJ, Winkler C: Metabolism of 15-p-(I-123-phenyl)-pentadecanoic acid in hearts of rats, *J Nucl Med* 23:10–18, 1982.

57. Reske SN, Sauer W, Machulla HJ, et al. 15(p-[^{123}I]Iodophenyl)pentadecanoic acid as a tracer of lipid metabolism: comparison with [1-^{14}C] palmitic acid in murine tissues, *J Nucl Med* 25:1335–1342, 1984.

58. Reske SN, Sauer W, Machulla HJ, et al: Metabolism of 15(p[123]I-iodophenyl-)pentadecanoic acid in heart muscle and noncardiac tissues, *Eur J Nucl Med* 10:228–234, 1985.

59. Saito T, Yasuda T, Gold HK et al: Differentiation of regional perfusion and fatty acid uptake in zones of myocardial injury, *Nucl Med Commun* 12:663–675, 1991.

60. Schelbert HR, Henze E, Keen R, et al: C-11 palmitate for the noninvasive evaluation of regional myocardial fatty acid metabolism with positron-computed tomography. IV. In vivo evaluation of acute demand-induced ischemia in dogs, *Am Heart J* 106:736–750, 1983.

61. Schon HR, Schelbert HR, Najafi A, et al: C-11 labeled palmitic acid for the noninvasive evaluation of regional myocardial fatty acid metabolism with positron-computed tomography. II. Kinetics of C-11 palmitic acid in acutely ischemic myocardium, *Am Heart J* 103:548–561, 1982.

62. Schon HR, Schelbert HR, Robinson G, et al: C-11 labeled palmitic acid for the noninvasive evaluation of regional myocardial fatty acid metabolism with positron-computed tomography. I. Kinetics of C-11 palmitic acid in normal myocardium, *Am Heart J* 103:532–547, 1982.

63. Sobel BE, Weiss ES, Welch MJ, et al: Detection of remote myocardial infarction in patients with positron emission transaxial tomography and intravenous ^{11}C palmitate, *Circulation* 55:853–857, 1977.

64. Tadamura E, Tamaki N, Matsumori A, et al: Myocardial metabolic changes in hypertrophic cardiomyopathy, *J Nucl Med* 37:572–577, 1996.

65. Takeishi Y, Chiba J, Abe S, et al: Heterogeneous myocardial distribution of iodine-123 15-(p-iodophenyl)-3-R,S-methylpentadecanoic acid (BMIPP) in patients with hypertrophic cardiomyopathy, *Eur J Nucl Med* 19:775–782, 1992.

66. Takeishi Y, Sukekawa H, Saito H, et al: Impaired myocardial fatty acid metabolism detected by ^{123}I-BMIPP in patients with unstable angina pectoris: comparison with perfusion imaging by ^{99m}Tc-sestamibi, *Ann Nucl Med* 9:125–130, 1995.

67. Taki J, Nakajima K, Bunko H, et al: ^{123}I-labelled BMIPP fatty acid myocardial scintigraphy in patients with hypertrophic cardiomyopathy: SPECT comparison with stress ^{201}Tl, *Nucl Med Commun* 14:181–188, 1993.

68. Taki J, Nakajima K, Matsunari I, et al: Impairment of regional fatty acid uptake in relation to wall motion and thallium-201 uptake in ischaemic but viable myocardium: assessment with iodine-123-labelled beta-methyl-branched fatty acid, *Eur J Nucl Med* 22:1385–1392, 1995.

69. Tamaki N, Fujibayashi Y, Magata Y, et al: Radionuclide assessment of myocardial fatty acid metabolism by PET and SPECT, *J Nucl Cardiol* 2:256–266, 1995.

70. Tamaki N, Kawamoto M: The use of iodinated free fatty acids for assessing fatty acid metabolism, *J Nucl Cardiol* 1:S72–S78, 1994.

71. Tamaki N, Kawamoto M, Takahashi N, et al: Assessment of myocardial fatty acid metabolism with positron emission tomography at rest and during dobutamine infusion in patients with coronary artery disease, *Am Heart J* 125:702–710, 1993.

72. Tamaki N, Kawamoto M, Yonekura Y, et al: Regional metabolic abnormality in relation to perfusion and wall motion in patients with myocardial infarction: assessment with emission tomography using an iodinated branched fatty acid analog, *J Nucl Med* 33:659–667, 1992.

73. Tamaki N, Tadamura E, Kawamoto M, et al: Decreased uptake of iodinated branched fatty acid analog indicates metabolic alterations in ischemic myocardium, *J Nucl Med* 36:1974–1980, 1995.

74. Tamaki N, Tadamura E, Kudoh T, et al: Prognostic value of iodine-123 labelled BMIPP fatty acid analogue imaging in patients with myocardial infarction, *Eur J Nucl Med* 23:272–279, 1996.

75. Tamaki N, Tadamura E, Kudoh T, et al: Recent advances in nuclear cardiology in the study of coronary artery disease, *Ann Nucl Med* 11:55–66, 1997.

76. Tateno M, Tamaki N, Yukihiro M, et al: Assessment of fatty acid uptake in ischemic heart disease without myocardial infarction, *J Nucl Med* 37:1981–1985, 1996.

77. Tomiguchi S, Oyama Y, Nabeshima M, et al: Quantitative evaluation of BMIPP in patients with ischemic heart disease, *Ann Nucl Med* 7:SII107–SII112, 1993.

78. van der Wall EE, Heidendal GAK, den Hollander W, et al: Metabolic myocardial imaging with ^{123}I-labeled heptadecanoic acid in patients with angina pectoris, *Eur J Nucl Med* 6:391–396, 1981.

79. Visser FC, van Eenige MJ, Westera G, et al: Metabolic fate of radioiodinated heptadecanoic acid in the normal canine heart, *Circulation* 72:565–571, 1985.

80. Weinheimer CJ, Brown MA, Nohara R, et al: Functional recovery after reperfusion is predicated on recovery of myocardial oxidative metabolism, *Am Heart J* 125:939–949, 1993.

81. Weiss ES, Hoffman EJ, Phelps ME, et al: External detection and visualization of myocardial ischemia with ^{11}C substrates in vitro and in vivo, *Circ Res* 39:24–32, 1976.

82. Wieler H, Kaiser KP, Frank J, et al: Standardized non-invasive assessment of myocardial free fatty acid kinetics by means of 15-(para-iodophenyl) pentadecanoic acid (^{123}I-pPPA)scintigraphy: I. Method, *Nucl Med Commun* 11:865–878, 1990.

83. Wieler H, Kaiser KP, Kuikka JT, et al: Standardized noninvasive assessment of myocardial free fatty acid kinetics by means of 15-(p-iodophenyl) pentadecanoic acid (^{123}I-pPPA) scintigraphy: II. Clinical results, *Nucl Med Commun* 13:168–185, 1992.

84. Yamamoto K, Som P, Brill AB, et al: Dual tracer autoradiographic study of β-methyl-(1-^{14}C) heptadecanoic acid and 15-p-(^{131}I)-iodophenyl-β-methylpentadecanoic acid in normotensive and hypertensive rats, *J Nucl Med* 27:1178–1183, 1986.

85. Yonekura Y, Brill AB, Som P, et al: Regional myocardial substrate uptake in hypertensive rats: a quantitative autoradiographic measurement, *Science* 227:1494–1496, 1985.

NEW APPROACHES

Chapter 35

Neurotransmitter imaging

Ichiro Matsunari, Donald M. Wieland, and **Markus Schwaiger**

The importance of the autonomic nervous system in the pathophysiology of various heart diseases, such as congestive heart failure[17] and arrhythmias,[8] has been increasingly recognized. In the past, evaluation of the autonomic nervous system in vivo was limited to invasive procedures. With the introduction of tracer approaches, noninvasive functional assessment of the cardiac autonomic nervous system by scintigraphic techniques has become possible and may provide important pathophysiologic information in many cardiac disease states. By using catecholamine analogues, such as iodine-123 (^{123}I) metaiodobenzylguanidine (MIBG),[62,130] noninvasive assessment of presynaptic neuronal function has become a reality in the clinical setting. More sophisticated imaging techniques, such as positron emission tomography (PET), have also been developed to assess the sympathetic nervous system by using tracers such as carbon-11 (^{11}C) hydroxyephedrine (HED),[97,103] fluo-

rine-18 (^{18}F) fluorodopamine,[44,45] and CGP 12177,[75] permitting regional quantification of tracer concentration in presynaptic and postsynaptic sites with high spatial resolution.

This chapter describes the basic physiology of the autonomic nervous system, followed by the principles of scintigraphic techniques for neurotransmitter imaging. Current applications of scintigraphic approaches for the noninvasive characterization of the presynaptic nervous system are discussed. Scintigraphic evaluation of the postsynaptic nervous system will be described in Chapter 36.

DESCRIPTION OF THE AUTONOMIC NERVOUS SYSTEM IN THE HEART

The autonomic nervous system, referred to as the visceral nervous system, consists of two main divisions: sympathetic and parasympathetic innervation. The two systems differ in their major neurotransmitters, norepinephrine and acetylcholine, which define the stimulatory and inhibitory physiologic effects of each system.[95] Sympathetic and parasympathetic innervation of the heart facilitates its electrophysiologic and hemodynamic adaptation to changing cardiovascular demands. Both sympathetic and parasympathetic tone control the rate of electrophysiologic stimulation and conduction, whereas contractile performance is primarily modulated by sympathetic neurotransmission. This functional characterization is reflected by the anatomic distribution of sympathetic and parasympathetic nerve fibers and nerve terminals. Sympathetic nerve fibers are characterized by multiple nerve endings that are filled with vesicles containing norepinephrine. Sympathetic nerve fibers travel parallel to the vascular structures on the surface of the heart and penetrate the underlying myocardium in much the same manner as the coronary vessels. On the basis of tissue norepinephrine concentration, the mammalian heart is characterized by dense adrenergic innervation, with a norepinephrine concentration gradient from the atria to the base of the heart and from the base to the apex of the ventricles.[93]

In contrast to sympathetic nerve fibers, parasympathetic innervation is most prevalent in the atria of the heart; the atrioventricular node; and, to a lesser degree, the ventricular myocardium. Parasympathetic fibers in the ventricles seem to travel close to the endocardial surface, unlike the sympathetic innervation. The enzyme choline acetyltransferase (ChAT) has been used as a reliable marker of cholinergic innervation.[101] Choline acetyltransferase concentration is highest in the atria and decreases sharply in the right and left ventricular myocardium. Figure 35-1 shows norepinephrine and acetylcholine synthesis in the sympathetic and parasympathetic nerve terminals, respectively.

Sympathetic nerve terminal

Norepinephrine, the dominant transmitter in the sympathetic nerve system, is synthesized from the amino acid tyrosine by several enzymatic steps.[44] The generation of dopa from tyrosine is the rate-limiting step in the biosynthesis of catecholamines. After conversion of dopa to dopamine by dopa decarboxylase, dopamine is transported into storage vesicles by an energy-requiring mechanism. Norepinephrine is synthesized by the action of dopamine β-hydroxylase on dopamine within the storage vesicles. Nerve stimulation leads to norepinephrine release, which occurs as the vesicles fuse with the neuronal membrane and expel their contents by exocytosis. Single-nerve stimulation, however, leads to exocytosis of only a small fraction of the many thousands of storage vesicles in the sympa-

thetic nerve terminal. The average adrenergic neuron has approximately 25,000 vesicles, and each vesicle contains approximately 250 pg of norepinephrine.[21] Thus, although most norepinephrine is thought to be released by exocytosis, nonvesicular release also occurs.

Apart from neuronal stimulation, norepinephrine release is also regulated by a number of receptor systems. α-2 Receptors on the membrane surface are thought to provide negative feedback of the exocytotic process, and the exocytotic release can thus be inhibited by presynaptic α-2-receptor agonists, such as clonidine, guanabenz, and guanfacin.[38] Muscarinic and adenosine receptors have an antiadrenergic effect in the heart. Neuropeptide Y is stored and released together with norepinephrine from the nerve terminal. Neuropeptide Y is thought to inhibit norepinephrine release by the nerve terminal.[61] Presynaptic angiotensin II receptors and β-receptors, on the other hand, mediate facilitation of norepinephrine release from sympathetic nerve endings. Therefore, some antihypertensive pharmaceuticals, such as angiotensin-converting enzyme inhibitors and nonselective β-blocking agents, can inhibit excessive norepinephrine release.

The complex modulation of sympathetic neurotransmission clearly involves many systems, including dopamine, prostaglandin, and histamine. Only a small amount of the norepi-

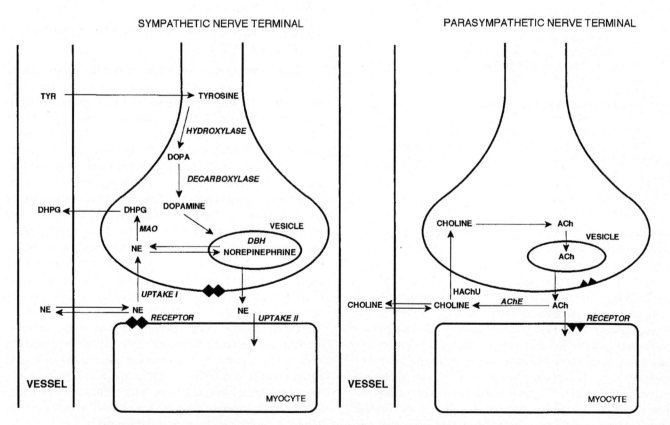

Fig. 35-1. Schematic representation of sympathetic *(left)* and parasympathetic *(right)* nerve endings. ACh = acetylcholine; AChE = acetylcholine esterase; DBH = dopamine β-hydroxylase; DHPG = dihydroxyphenylglycol; HAChu = high-affinity choline uptake; MAO = monoamine oxidase; NE = norepinephrine.

nephrine released by the nerve terminal is actually available to activate receptors on the myocyte surface. Most of the norepinephrine released undergoes reuptake in the nerve terminal (uptake-1 mechanism) and recycles into the vesicles or is metabolized in the cytosol of the nerve terminal. The uptake-1 system is characterized as saturable and sodium, temperature, and energy dependent.[56] It can be inhibited by cocaine and desipramine.[102] Structurally related amines, such as epinephrine, guanitidine, and metaraminol, are also transported by this system. In addition to neuronal uptake through uptake-1, the uptake-2 system removes norepinephrine into nonneuronal tissue.[98] Uptake-2 is characterized as nonsaturable and not sodium, temperature, or energy dependent. It can be inhibited by steroids and clonidine.[100] Free cytosolic norepinephrine is degraded rapidly to dihydroxyphenylglycol by monoamine oxidase. Only a small fraction of the released norepinephrine diffuses into the vascular space, where it can be measured as norepinephrine spillover in the coronary sinus venous blood.

Parasympathetic nerve terminal

Acetylcholine is synthesized within the parasympathetic nerve terminal. Choline is transported into the cytosol of the nerve ending through a high-affinity choline uptake system.[30] In the nerve terminal, choline is rapidly acetylated by ChAT and is subsequently shuttled into storage vesicles. In contrast to amine uptake in the sympathetic nerve terminals, the choline uptake system is restrictive. Even close structural choline analogues are poor substrates for this uptake mechanism. Upon nerve stimulation, acetylcholine is released into the synaptic cleft, where it interacts with muscarinic receptors. Free acetylcholine is rapidly metabolized by acetylcholine esterase.

RADIOPHARMACEUTICALS FOR NEUROTRANSMITTER IMAGING

Metaiodobenzylguanidine

Tracers for neurotransmitter imaging have been developed by either direct labeling of the physiologic neurotransmitter or labeling of their structural analogues (Fig. 35-2). Table 35-1 summarizes the radiopharmaceuticals currently available for the scintigraphic evaluation of the presynaptic nervous function. Iodine-123 MIBG was developed as a norepinephrine ana-

logue by Wieland et al[130] and was first used in the human heart by Kline et al[62] in the early 1980s. This compound is an analogue of guanethidine and has a cellular uptake mechanism similar to that of norepinephrine at the sympathetic nerve terminals. It is transported into cells by uptake-1 and is stored in the vesicles but is not catabolized by monoamine oxidase or COMT. This compound has a low affinity for postsynaptic adrenergic receptors and thus has little pharmacologic action. It has been shown that tissue norepinephrine concentration correlates with MIBG uptake.[22,110]

A potential disadvantage of MIBG is the presence of uptake-2 by nonneuronal tissues, as shown in studies in animal models.[87] However, it is important to consider both the specific activity of MIBG used in previous animal studies, which was considerably lower than that of currently available MIBG, and interspecies variability of MIBG uptake mechanisms in the heart. Because the amount of MIBG that can be transported into neuronal terminals through uptake-1 is limited, a high loading dose of MIBG with low specific activity would cause saturation of the uptake-1 system and, thus, dominance of uptake-2 for MIBG uptake. Mock and Tuli[79] demonstrated that the cardiac uptake of MIBG in rats is dependent on the specific activity, emphasizing the importance of the use of MIBG with high specific activity for better assessment of sympathetic innervation with this tracer. Vaidyanathan and Zalutsky[123] reported that the heart uptake of no-carrier-added MIBG was 1.5 to 3.0 times higher than that of low specific activity. Furthermore, Takatsu, Scheffel, and Fujiwara[116] studied the effect of desipramine on the uptake of MIBG with low (4.1 mCi/mg) and high (200 mCi/mg) specific activity in the mouse heart and observed that the desipramine-inhibitable fraction of MIBG uptake was significantly lower with MIBG of low specific activity (54%) than with MIBG of high specific activity (70%) at 4 hours after injection. Using MIBG of high specific activity (150 mCi/mg) and reserpine as a pharmacologic tool to suppress intravesicular MIBG uptake, the intravesicular fraction of MIBG activity 6 hours after injection reached 63% in the rat heart.[70] Therefore, it is important to pay attention to the specific activity and, thereby, the loading dose of MIBG being used, which varies considerably among the commercially available radiopharmaceuticals.

Table 35-1. Radiopharmaceuticals used for neurotransmitter imaging*

Type of innervation	SPECT	PET
Sympathetic	Iodine-123 metaiodobenzylguanidine	Fluorine-18 fluorometaraminol
		Carbon-11 hydroxyephedrine
		Carbon-11 epinephrine
		Carbon-11 phenylephrine
		Fluorine-18 fluorobenzylguanidine
		Fluorine-18 fluorodopamine
		Fluorine-18 fluoronorepinephrine
Parasympathetic		Fluorine-18 fluoroethoxybenzovesamicol

*PET = positron emission tomography; SPECT = single-photon emission computed tomography.

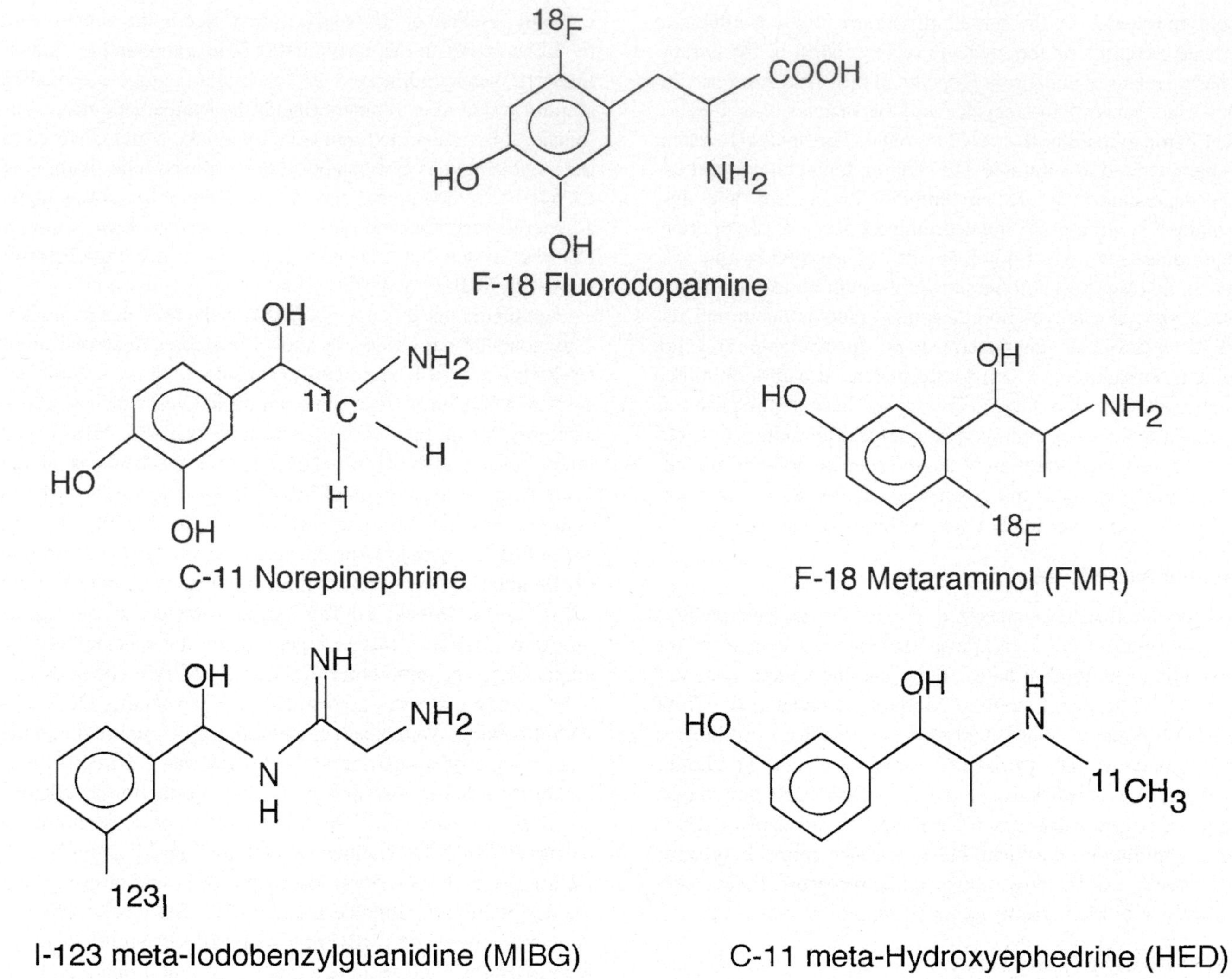

Fig. 35-2. Chemical structure of radiopharmaceuticals for neurotransmitter imaging.

Recent studies in patients who underwent cardiac transplantation[23] suggest that, unlike the results of animal studies, the nonneuronal component of MIBG uptake may be low in human hearts. However, these results should be interpreted with caution, because the transplanted patients were taking steroid-containing medications, which can inhibit the uptake-2 system. In addition, there may be interspecies variability of MIBG uptake mechanisms, which is critically important to the interpretation of the data. Finally, the lipophilicity of the tracer should also be considered a potential mechanism for passive diffusion into the intracellular space, although this may not be significant unless both uptake-1 and uptake-2 are largely inhibited.[26]

MIBG clearance

Uncertainty remains about the interpretation of MIBG clearance from the heart. Several potential mechanisms account for MIBG clearance from the heart, including washout from the extraneuronal space, exocytotic release from storage vesicles, nonexocytotic release through an outward uptake-1 mechanism, and diffusion from the nerve terminal. Clearance of MIBG from the normal human heart seems to be slow (5% to 12% in 3 to 4 hours)[64,121]; this rate is consistent with norepinephrine turnover (half-life, 9.7 hours) measured invasively.[31] Several experimental and clinical studies have suggested that MIBG clearance may correlate with norepinephrine exocytosis and, hence, sympathetic nerve activity in congestive heart failure.[53,117,126] Wakasugi et al,[126] however, suggested that nonexocytotic MIBG release may occur in a rat heart-failure model at advanced stages. Furthermore, Arbab et al[5] demonstrated slower MIBG clearance from the heart in rats with renal failure, probably because of high blood MIBG concentration. In addition, the uptake-2 mechanism and, thereby, MIBG washout from the nonneuronal tissue (which is significantly faster than washout from neuronal tissue) may play a significant role in abnormal states in which the ratio of uptake-1 and uptake-2 activities is altered.[26] The clearance of MIBG from the heart most likely represents several mechanisms and is not specific for sympathetic nerve activity.

Positron-emitting tracers

Because PET has several advantages over SPECT (such as quantification of regional tracer uptake with the use of accurate attenuation correction and higher spatial resolution), efforts have been made to develop positron-emitting tracers for neurotransmitter imaging. ^{18}F-labeled metaraminol is taken up by the sympathetic nerve terminal in a manner similar to that of norepinephrine but is not catabolized by monoamine oxidase.[132] Transient myocardial ischemia resulted in reduced[18] retention of ^{18}F metaraminol in tissue consistent with neuronal dysfunction in reversibly damaged myocardium.[104] Radiopharmaceutical problems associated with low specific activity, however, limited its further clinical application.

Carbon-11 hydroxyephedrine seems to be a more promising tracer because it can be synthesized with high specific activity.[97,131] Experimental studies have indicated a highly specific uptake into sympathetic nerve terminals occurs with little non-neuronal binding.[24] Carbon-11 hydroxyephedrine is currently the most successfully used positron-emitting tracer for neurotransmitter imaging in humans.* More recently, ^{11}C epinephrine has been proposed as a truly physiologic tracer.[14,107] It has been demonstrated that, similar to norepinephrine, accumulation of ^{11}C epinephrine by the heart reflects mainly vesicular storage in the sympathetic neuron. Therefore, ^{11}C epinephrine may be a suitable tracer for the evaluation of sympathetic vesicular function of the heart.[89] Because ^{11}C epinephrine is metabolized by monoamine oxidase (MAO) and catechol-O-methyltransferase (COMT), careful consideration should be given to the influence of metabolic pathways on measurements of ^{11}C retention attributed to vesicular storage functions. Another analogue of epinephrine is ^{11}C phenylephrine, which has been synthesized by Wieland et al[19] at the University of Michigan. This tracer enters the nerve terminal through uptake-1 but is primarily metabolized by the monoamine oxidase enzyme system. Carbon-11 phenylephrine, therefore, allows the evaluation of the enzymatic integrity of the nerve terminal. Other potential tracers include ^{18}F fluorodopamine[16,45] and ^{18}F fluoronorepinephrine.[29] Although the available clinical and experimental data for these tracers are limited, the longer physical half-life of ^{18}F may allow washout analysis to assess sympathetic nerve tone.

Other PET tracers for assessing sympathetic nerve function such as bromine- or ^{18}F-labeled benzylguanidine[9] (an analogue of MIBG) have also been proposed and await further experimental and clinical investigations.

To date, only a few studies have addressed myocardial parasympathetic neuronal imaging, probably because of a low specificity for neuronal uptake and storage. However, recent studies in the brain in mice[96] and rats[58] have shown that ^{125}I-labeled iodobenzovesamicol allowed scintigraphic assessment of cholinergic nerve terminals. Fluorine-18 fluoroethoxybenzovesamicol was developed for parasympathetic neurotransmitter imaging using PET.[25] However, myocardial retention of the tracer was low because of the low cholinergic neuron density, limiting its potential as an imaging agent. Further efforts in developing tracers for the parasympathetic nervous system are required.

IMAGING PROTOCOLS
Metaiodobenzylguanidine

Accelerated washout of MIBG has been reported in various disease conditions, such as congestive heart failure,[52,53] hypertrophic cardiomyopathy,[84] and ischemic heart disease,[85] although the mechanisms remain to be elucidated. Therefore, it is recommended that image sets be obtained at multiple time points after injection, typically early (15 to 30 minutes) and late (3 to 5 hours) after the injection of 3 to 5 mCi (111 to 185 MBq) of MIBG to allow the assessment of MIBG washout from the heart. Each of the early and late image sets includes SPECT as well as planar imaging to measure heart-to-mediastinal uptake ratios and the washout rate of tracer from the heart. Planar imaging is particularly important when myocardial MIBG uptake is too poor to generate SPECT images, as is the case with such disease states as heart failure[74] and diabetes mellitus.[68] Furthermore, myocardial MIBG uptake may be altered by such drugs as labetalol,[60] digoxin, and angiotensin-converting enzyme inhibitors.[37-39] Withdrawal of all cardiac medications may not be practical in the clinical setting. However, one should at least be aware of these drug effects on myocardial MIBG uptake in the interpretation of subsequently obtained images. From a technical viewpoint, one should keep in mind that the performance of certain low-energy collimators may suffer from considerable septal penetration of photons when ^{123}I tracers are imaged, which may limit the accurate measurement of tracer uptake.[27] In addition, simultaneous dual-isotope MIBG imaging with a perfusion tracer, such as ^{201}Tl, may not be optimal because of cross-talk problems.[83]

Hydroxyephedrine and other position emission tomographic tracers

An ^{11}C HED PET protocol typically includes dynamic PET acquisition for 40 to 60 minutes after injection and blood flow imaging using flow tracers, such as nitrogen-13 ammonia or rubidium-82.* For ^{11}C epinephrine PET, in which high levels of ^{11}C metabolites are detected in the blood, correction for metabolite radioactivity in the arterial input function is required for the calculation of tracer retention in the tissue.[82] The use of ^{18}F-labeled tracers allows a longer imaging time period because of their longer physical half-life (110 minutes) compared with [11]C (20 minutes). The longer half-life of ^{18}F may obviate the necessity of an on-site cyclotron and, therefore, may potentially have wide clinical use.

*References 2, 3, 11, 12, 103, 106.

*References 2, 3, 11, 12, 103, 106.

EXPERIMENTAL AND CLINICAL RESULTS
Normal heart

To interpret MIBG images, it is important to know the normal distribution of MIBG in the heart. It has been demonstrated that myocardial MIBG distribution in normal persons is heterogeneous.[41,112] A preliminary study by Sisson et al[94] suggested reduced MIBG uptake at the apex. Gill et al[41] studied the heterogeneity of human myocardial sympathetic innervation with MIBG SPECT. They observed decreased myocardial MIBG uptake in 8 patients older than 40 years of age compared with 7 patients with supraventricular tachycardias younger than 40 years of age. They also noted that the inferior and septal uptake of MIBG was decreased compared with the anterior and lateral walls. This finding was confirmed by Tsuchimochi et al,[121] who found a regional decrease in MIBG uptake in the inferior wall in older patients. They also found that decreased inferior MIBG uptake was more prominent in men than in women, suggesting that age and sex differences may affect the heterogeneity of myocardial MIBG uptake and that the inferior wall of the heart should be interpreted with caution in MIBG images. Estorch et al,[32] on the other hand, performed planar MIBG imaging and observed lower MIBG uptake in terms of the heart-to-mediastinal uptake ratio in older patients, whereas Tsuchimochi et al[121] did not observe such age-related changes in the heart-to-mediastinal uptake ratio. It may also be noteworthy to point out that, unlike Tsuchimochi et al,[121] Estorch et al[32] did not observe regional abnormalities on planar images, although actual data were not provided. Thus, the normal pattern of myocardial MIBG uptake remains to be established.

It is important that potential artifacts associated with conventional SPECT imaging be considered. First, diaphragmatic attenuation may cause a regional decrease in the inferior wall. However, this does not explain why ^{201}Tl, which has a lower photon energy than ^{123}I, did not show decreased activity in the inferior wall, as reported by Gill et al.[41] Second, recent studies have suggested that liver uptake may cause an artifactual inferior defect, especially when 180° data rather than 360° data are used for reconstruction.[71,91] This may at least partially explain the decreased inferior activity; MIBG images usually show high hepatic uptake, and most of the published MIBG SPECT studies utilized 180° acquisition. However, it still may not provide a clear explanation for age- and sex-related differences in regional MIBG uptake.

From a physiologic viewpoint, several potential factors must be considered. It has been reported that plasma catecholamine levels increase with age,[127] suggesting an alteration in the sympathetic nervous system activity with age. High plasma and endogenous catecholamine levels can cause inhibition of MIBG uptake by competition.[86] In addition, previous animal studies have shown that the anterior wall has a predominantly sympathetic afferent innervation, whereas the inferior wall has a predominantly parasympathetic innervation, which may result in reduction of MIBG uptake in the inferior wall.[118]

In contrast to MIBG SPECT studies, HED studies using hydroxyephedrine PET have shown homogeneous myocardial distribution of tracer.[103] This may be explained by the use of attenuation correction, difference in study subjects, or different tracer characteristics between HED and MIBG. It should also be noted that HED distribution may be dependent on myocardial flow, especially when specific activity is high.[2] Another PET study using ^{18}F fluorodopamine also reported homogeneous myocardial tracer uptake.[16] Because no direct comparison of the two tracers has been made, further studies are warranted to address this difference between MIBG SPECT and HED PET.

Myocardial infarction

Myocardial infarction has been shown to induce cardiac denervation exceeding the area of necrosis or scar* (Fig. 35-3). Minardo et al[76] found that MIBG images in dogs after trans-

*References 6, 22, 36, 48, 73, 76, 114.

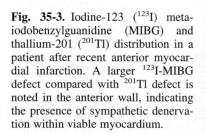

Fig. 35-3. Iodine-123 (^{123}I) meta-iodobenzylguanidine (MIBG) and thallium-201 (^{201}Tl) distribution in a patient after recent anterior myocardial infarction. A larger ^{123}I-MIBG defect compared with ^{201}Tl defect is noted in the anterior wall, indicating the presence of sympathetic denervation within viable myocardium.

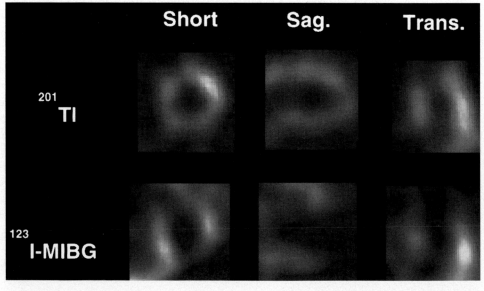

mural myocardial infarction showed perfused but denervated myocardial areas apical to the infarct. Their observation was confirmed by the study by Dae et al,[22] who showed that non-transmural infarction also leads to regional ischemic damage of sympathetic nerves but with minimal extension of denervation beyond the infarct.

Stanton et al[114] studied 19 patients after myocardial infarction with and without ventricular arrhythmia using MIBG and ^{201}Tl imaging. They observed reduced MIBG uptake compared with ^{201}Tl, indicating the presence of denervated but viable myocardium in patients with infarction, particularly those with ventricular tachycardias. However, they failed to show a relation between scintigraphic evidence of denervation and sustained ventricular tachycardias induced during electrophysiologic studies. In the report by McGhie et al,[73] higher MIBG defect scores were observed in patients with ventricular arrhythmias than in those without significant arrhythmias. They also observed that anterior wall infarction was associated with a greater degree of mismatch between perfusion and MIBG uptake than inferior wall infarction. It should be noted, however, that the relatively small number of patients in these studies may have somewhat limited the ability to draw definitive conclusions.

Heart rate variability is considered a powerful predictor of sudden cardiac death after myocardial infarction.[8] Spinnler et al[113] studied 10 patients after myocardial infarction by using serial assessment with MIBG imaging and spectral analysis of heart rate variability. They observed a progressive normalization of electrophysiologic variables, while scintigraphic findings did not change. They concluded that sympathetic denervation as assessed by MIBG imaging may not play a major role in determining the changes in sympathetic and vagal neuronal activities. Mantysaari et al,[69] on the other hand, investigated the association between myocardial sympathetic innervation and heart rate variability in 12 patients after myocardial infarction and observed a larger area of denervated but viable myocardium in patients with low heart-rate variability compared with those with normal heart rate variability.

Thus, although MIBG defects extending beyond necrotic regions are commonly observed in patients after myocardial infarction, the clinical significance of MIBG imaging remains to be elucidated. Published studies were based on relatively small patient populations, which may limit the ability to draw conclusions. Further prospective studies involving a larger patient population are necessary to evaluate the clinical efficacy of MIBG imaging in patients after myocardial infarction.

Reinnervation after myocardial infarction

Although inhomogeneity of cardiac sympathetic reinnervation may play an important role in the risk for arrhythmias early after myocardial infarction, whether reinnervation after myocardial infarction occurs in humans remains controversial. Cardiac sympathetic reinnervation after myocardial infarction has been reported in experimental canine studies.[76,90] Minardo et al[76] observed reinnervation within 14 weeks after infarction in the dog heart. Their results were confirmed by Nishimura et al,[90] who observed recovery in MIBG uptake as well as norepinephrine content during the first 6 weeks after infarction.

In humans, Mitrani et al[77] reported partial sympathetic reinnervation 1 to 8 months after myocardial infarction. This was confirmed by Hartikainen et al,[49] who showed partial reinnervation in the periinfarct zone 3 to 12 months after infarction. Conversely, McGhie et al[73] and Spinnler et al[113] did not detect significant change in MIBG uptake up to 30 months after infarction. Their observations were based on delayed MIBG imaging 4 to 5 hours after injection. Ishida et al,[55] on the other hand, performed early (15 minutes) and delayed (4 hours) MIBG imaging in patients after myocardial infarction and observed improved MIBG uptake on early images but not on delayed images. Considering the growing body of evidence that early MIBG uptake in the human heart may represent neuronal uptake rather than nonneuronal uptake, these observations suggest that recovery of MIBG uptake after myocardial infarction may be a more complex phenomenon than was previously thought.

Using serial HED PET, Allman et al[2] studied the extent and reversibility of neuronal abnormalities in patients with acute myocardial infarction. They observed more extensive HED abnormalities than blood flow abnormalities, particularly in patients with non–Q wave infarction, and saw no change in both extent of abnormality and tracer retention 8 ± 3 months later, suggesting persistent neuronal damage without evidence of reinnervation.

Other forms of ischemic heart disease

In patients with unstable angina, MIBG imaging was successfully used to identify angina-provoking coronary stenoses that could not be determined by perfusion imaging alone,[120,122] indicating the utility of MIBG imaging in this setting. Imaging with MIBG may also be used to detect vasospastic angina, a condition in which perfusion imaging often fails to detect abnormalities.[115] Takano et al[115] reported that uptake mismatch between MIBG and ^{201}Tl imaging was a specific finding in vasospastic angina. However, Sakata et al[99] did not observe reduced MIBG uptake in patients with vasospastic angina, even during the active phase. Of interest, they found reduced myocardial MIBG washout, which may be inhibited by atropine pretreatment in patients in the active phase, suggesting that cardiac sympathetic–parasympathetic interactions may play a role in such patients according to the degree of disease activity. In a recent study by Nakata et al,[88] who performed MIBG imaging in 28 patients with stable coronary artery disease, the diagnostic accuracy of MIBG scintigraphy for detecting coronary artery stenosis was limited, probably because of frequent reductions in MIBG uptake in the inferior wall regardless of the presence or absence of coronary artery disease.

Arrhythmogenic heart disease

A role for the sympathetic nervous system in the generation of arrhythmias has been suggested.[20,54,109,110,133] Different theories have been proposed for the induction of arrhythmias, but in vivo data are limited. Therefore, scintigraphic techniques using MIBG or HED may provide unique information on the pathophysiology of arrhythmogenic heart disease.

Mitrani et al[78] reported that abnormal MIBG uptake occurred in patients with ventricular tachycardia, even in the absence of coronary artery disease. Gill et al[40] observed reduced MIBG uptake in the septal region in patients with ventricular tachycardia. Using HED PET, Calkins et al[11] observed a correlation between reduced HED retention and ventricular refractoriness in patients with a history of sustained ventricular tachycardia. Thus, the presence of denervated but viable myocardium as assessed by scintigraphic techniques may have important implications for the pathogenesis of ventricular arrhythmias.

Wichter et al[129] studied 48 patients with arrhythmogenic right ventricular cardiomyopathy by using MIBG scintigraphy and observed that most patients with this condition (83%) showed reduced MIBG uptake despite normal ^{201}Tl studies. The location of defects on the MIBG scan correlated with the site of origin of ventricular tachycardia determined by invasive electrophysiologic study, suggesting the potential utility of MIBG imaging for noninvasive detection of localized sympathetic denervation.

Sympathetic imbalance with decreased right cardiac sympathetic activity has been attributed to the induction of ventricular arrhythmias in the long Q-T syndrome.[110] Decreased MIBG uptake in the inferior and inferoseptal walls was reported in patients with the long Q-T syndrome,[43] supporting the "sympathetic imbalance" hypothesis. Abnormalities of hydroxyephedrine uptake, however, were not observed in the study by Calkins et al.[12] A prospective study directly comparing MIBG SPECT and HED PET in the same patient population may be necessary to resolve this discrepancy.

Diabetes mellitus

Diabetic patients often develop autonomic neuropathy, and autonomic dysfunction may be associated with increased morbidity in these patients.[34] Therefore, scintigraphic techniques may allow for the objective assessment of sympathetic nervous system function in diabetic patients. Mantysaari et al[68] reported for the first time the relation between clinical autonomic dysfunction and myocardial MIBG uptake. They observed reduced myocardial MIBG uptake in diabetic patients, especially those with autonomic neuropathy. Their findings were confirmed by subsequent studies.[128] In patients with insulin-dependent diabetes mellitus, Kreiner et al[63] observed more frequent abnormalities in MIBG uptake than were expected by a cardiovascular reflex test.

Using HED PET, Allman et al[3] studied diabetic patients with and without autonomic neuropathy and observed regional reduction in cardiac HED retention, predominantly in the apical, inferior, and lateral regions, in patients with autonomic neuropathy compared with normal patients. These findings did not occur in diabetic patients without evident neuropathy. They also observed a correlation between the extent of the scintigraphic abnormality and the severity of autonomic dysfunction.

Because silent myocardial ischemia is known to occur in diabetic patients and because the absence of angina does not necessarily indicate a benign prognosis, several studies have focused on characterizing silent myocardial ischemia in diabetic patients by using MIBG. Langer et al[65] reported that patients with silent myocardial ischemia had more diffuse abnormalities in MIBG uptake than those without silent ischemia. Matsuno et al[72] observed frequent inferior MIBG defects in patients with silent ischemia. These results suggest that sympathetic nervous system function may play an important role in asymptomatic ischemia in diabetic patients. To date, no data are available on hydroxyephedrine PET in diabetic patients with silent myocardial ischemia.

Reinnervation after heart transplantation

In 1990, Schwaiger et al[106] described scintigraphic evidence of reinnervation in patients after heart transplantation by using HED PET. In that study, patients who had undergone transplantation more than 2 years before PET showed partial sympathetic reinnervation in the proximal anterior and septal walls, whereas patients who had recently undergone transplantation (<1 year) did not show evidence of reinnervation. Figure 35-4 displays a representative case 8 years after heart transplantation compared with a normal patient. These observations were confirmed in a subsequent study by De Marco et al,[28] who used serial MIBG imaging to investigate development of sympathetic reinnervation after heart transplantation. Sympathetic reinnervation 1 to 3 years after transplantation was suggested in approximately half of patients who had not shown any signs of sympathetic reinnervation at 1 year after transplantation. This is consistent with the results of a study that suggested that functional autonomic reinnervation of transplanted hearts may occur more than 1 year after transplantation.[59] Of note, they also reported that reinnervation after transplantation was less likely to occur in patients with a preoperative diagnosis of idiopathic cardiomyopathy than in patients with a pretransplantation diagnosis of ischemic or rheumatic heart disease, suggesting that systemic abnormalities in sympathetic nervous function may play a role in the incidence and time course of reinnervation in such patients. Recently, Ziegler et al[134] performed HED PET in 48 patients at various times after heart transplantation and reported that sympathetic reinnervation was a time-dependent phenomenon that paralleled electrophysiologic evidence of functional reinnervation, such as an increase in heart rate variability. The clinical significance of reinnervation in patients who undergo transplantation, however, remains to be determined.

Congestive heart failure

There is general agreement that increased adrenergic nervous system activity plays an important role in the pathophysiology of congestive heart failure.[119] Increased plasma norepinephrine levels,[119] increased spillover of norepinephrine,[51] re-

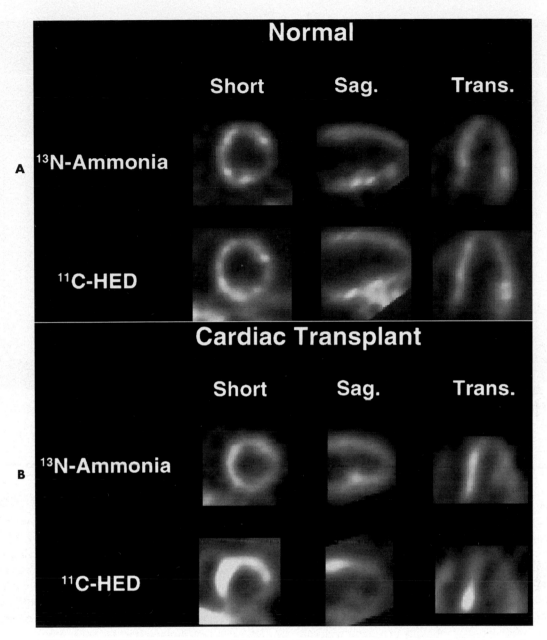

Fig. 35-4. Distribution of carbon-11 (^{11}C) hydroxyephedrine and myocardial blood flow (assessed by nitrogen-13 ammonia) in a normal patient (**A**) and a patient 8 years after heart transplantation (**B**). Severely decreased hydroxyephedrine uptake compared with blood flow is observed in the heart transplant patient, indicating denervation after transplantation. Uptake of hydroxy-ephedrine ^{11}C in the basal anterior and septal walls, however, suggests partial reinnervation in these areas.

duced cardiac stores of norepinephrine,[15] and desensitization of β-adrenoreceptors[10] have been reported in patients with heart failure. This increased sympathetic nervous system activity is perhaps attributable to increased norepinephrine turnover and reduced efficiency of norepinephrine reuptake and storage.[31] It has been also suggested that heart failure patients with high plasma norepinephrine levels have an unfavorable prognosis.[17] Plasma norepinephrine, however, is derived from sympathetic activity throughout the body and, thus, does not necessarily reflect cardiac sympathetic activity. Therefore, noninvasive

scintigraphic techniques may provide important knowledge of cardiac sympathetic nervous system activity, which may be of value in understanding the pathogenesis and prognosis of heart failure.

Numerous studies have shown that abnormal MIBG findings in the setting of heart failure typically include a reduced heart to mediastinal uptake ratio, heterogeneous distribution of MIBG within the myocardium, and increased MIBG washout from the heart.[33,42,52,57,111] A reduced heart to mediastinal uptake ratio (<120%) is reported to be a powerful predictor of

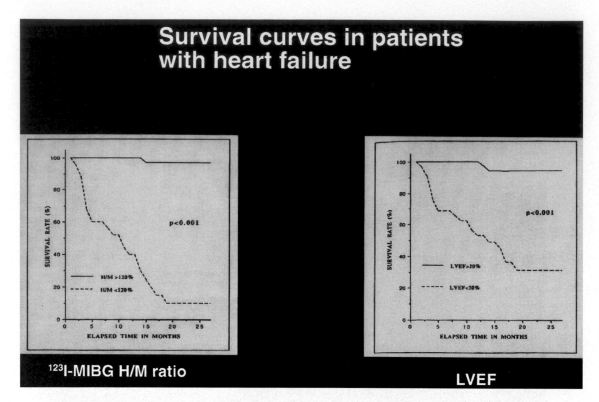

Fig. 35-5. Survival curves with a threshold value of 120% for the heart-to-mediastinal MIBG up-take ratio *(H/M ratio) (left)* and 20% left ventricular ejection fraction *(LVEF) (right),* indicating that an H/M ratio less than 120% is a stronger predictor of poor prognosis than a LVEF less than 20%. (From Merlet P, Valette H, Dubois-Rande JL, et al: Prognostic value of cardiac metaiodobenzyl-guanidine imaging in patients with heart failure, *J Nucl Med* 33:471–477, 1992. With permission.)

poor prognosis in patients with congestive heart failure (Fig. 35-5).[74] It seems that these scintigraphic findings are independent of the underlying cause.[53,85] These abnormal MIBG patterns may reflect accelerated exocytotic or nonexocytotic norepinephrine release with or without reduced norepinephrine uptake, depending on the severity of heart failure.[126]

It has been suggested that such medications as β-blockers[92] and angiotensin-converting enzyme (ACE) inhibitors[18] can improve symptoms, morbidity, and mortality in patients with congestive heart failure. Experimental data using MIBG showed a reduction of sympathetic nerve dysfunction in heart failure after long-term therapy with ACE inhibitors,[117] suggesting a potential role of MIBG imaging in monitoring the effect of pharmacologic therapy. A more recent clinical study also showed improved MIBG uptake after spironolactone therapy in patients with congestive heart failure secondary to coronary artery disease.[7] More clinical and experimental studies focusing on prognosis as well as monitoring the effect of medications are required to determine the role of MIBG imaging in patients with heart failure.

Reduced HED retention has been reported in patients with idiopathic dilated cardiomyopathy.[108] Using quantitative analysis, the reduction of HED retention correlated with the severity of heart failure as expressed by New York Heart Association functional class.[50]

Monitoring patients receiving anticancer drugs

Anthracycline chemotherapeutic agents, such as doxorubicin, are known to cause cardiotoxicity in a dose-dependent fashion. This often limits the use of such chemotherapeutic agents.[1] Recent experimental studies by Wakasugi et al[124,125] have demonstrated that abnormal cardiac adrenergic neuronal activity, as expressed by a reduction of MIBG uptake in the heart, showed a more linear dose-dependent deterioration than left ventricular ejection fraction, suggesting the potential utility of MIBG as a sensitive marker of cardiac damage. In human studies by Lekakis et al[67] and Carrió et al,[13] myocardial MIBG uptake, as expressed by the heart to mediastinum uptake ratio, was decreased after chemotherapy. The clinical impact of MIBG imaging as a tool for monitoring cardiotoxicity induced by anticancer drugs, however, remains to be determined by further studies.

Myocardial hypertrophy and hypertrophic cardiomyopathy

It has been shown that myocardial hypertrophy secondary to mechanical overload, such as valvular aortic stenosis,[35,94] essential hypertension,[81] and pulmonary arterial hypertension,[80] causes reduced MIBG uptake and increased washout. Of interest, the abnormalities seen with MIBG imaging improved after medical treatment and regression of hypertensive cardiac hypertrophy,[81] indicating that such abnormal MIBG findings may be reversible. Rapid clearance of MIBG has also been reported in patients with chronic renal failure receiving dialysis, particularly those with left ventricular hypertrophy and dysfunction,[64] although these findings are opposed by those of other investigators who observed slower MIBG clearance in patients with renal failure.[4] In patients with idiopathic hypertrophic cardiomyopathy, a significant positive correlation between MIBG clearance and septal thickness has been reported.[84]

Using HED PET and compartmental analysis, a significantly reduced distribution volume of HED was reported in patients with hypertrophic cardiomyopathy.[105] Thus, presynaptic imaging using MIBG or hydroxyephedrine may provide new insights into the pathogenesis of myocardial hypertrophy, although the clinical significance of MIBG imaging in these disease conditions remains largely unknown.

CONCLUSIONS AND FUTURE PERSPECTIVES

Myocardial neurotransmitter imaging using MIBG or HED has been successfully performed to assess cardiac autonomic innervation in humans under various clinical conditions. Early detection of abnormalities before the evidence of structural changes is an important goal of these scintigraphic approaches. Monitoring of therapeutic procedures also seems to be a promising application of neurotransmitter imaging.

Several issues remain to be addressed in future studies. First, controversial results of MIBG and hydroxyephedrine imaging have been published for normal persons as well for various disease conditions. It is also noteworthy that several MIBG studies describe regional abnormalities involving the inferior wall. These differences may be attributed to technical differences between SPECT and PET (that is, the attenuation correction and higher spatial resolution of PET compared with SPECT), as well as differences in tracer kinetics and characteristics between MIBG and HED, including differences in specific activity and uptake of the tracer in nerve terminals. Further prospective studies directly comparing SPECT and PET in the same patient population are required to address this issue. Second, the clinical significance and prognostic value of scintigraphic techniques have not yet been fully established. More convincing data involving a large patient population are required to draw significant conclusions about the utility of these scintigraphic techniques in the clinical setting. Finally, future developments aimed at synthesizing new radiopharmaceuticals to discriminate different aspects of autonomic nerve function will further widen the experimental and clinical applications of imaging approaches.

ACKNOWLEDGMENTS

The authors thank Ms. Ngoc Nguyen for the artistic preparation of the illustrations and Drs. Claire S. Duvernoy and Sibylle I. Ziegler for their comments during manuscript preparation.

REFERENCES

1. Alexander J, Dainiak N, Berger HJ, et al: Serial assessment of doxorubicin cardiotoxicity with quantitative radionuclide angiography, N Engl J Med 300:278–283, 1979.
2. Allman KC, Wieland DM, Muzik O, et al: Carbon-11 hydroxyephedrine with positron emission tomography for serial assessment of cardiac adrenergic neuronal function after acute myocardial function in humans, J Am Coll Cardiol 22:368–375, 1993.
3. Allman KC, Stevens MJ, Wieland DM, et al: Noninvasive assessment of cardiac diabetic neuropathy by carbon-11 hydroxyephedrine and positron emission tomography, J Am Coll Cardiol 22:1425–1432, 1993.
4. Arbab AS, Koizumi K, Tateano H, et al: Parameters of dynamic and static iodine-123-MIBG cardiac imaging, J Nucl Med 36:962–968, 1995.
5. Arbab AS, Koizumi K, Araki T: Uptake and washout of I-123-MIBG in neuronal and non-neuronal sites in rat hearts: relationship to renal clearance, Ann Nucl Med 10:211–217, 1996.
6. Barber MJ, Mueller TM, Henry DP, et al: Transmural myocardial infarction in the dog produces sympathectomy in noninfarcted myocardium, Circulation 67:787–796, 1983.
7. Barr CS, Lang CC, Hanson J, et al: Effects of adding spironolactone to an angiotensin-converting enzyme inhibitor in chronic congestive heart failure secondary to coronary artery disease, Am J Cardiol 76:1259–1265, 1995.
8. Barron HV, Lesh MD: Autonomic nervous system and sudden cardiac death, J Am Coll Cardiol 27:1053–1060, 1996.
9. Berry CR, Garg PK, DeGrado TR, et al: Para-[18F]fluorobenzyl-guanidine kinetics in a canine coronary artery occlusion model, J Nucl Cardiol 3:119–129, 1996.
10. Bristow MR, Ginsburg R, Minobe W, et al: Decreased catecholamine sensitivity and β-adrenergic receptor density in failing human hearts, N Engl J Med 307:205–211, 1982.
11. Calkins H, Allman K, Bellins S, et al: Correlation between scintigraphic evidence of regional sympathetic neuronal dysfunction and ventricular refractoriness in the human heart, Circulation 88:172–179, 1993.
12. Calkins H, Lehmann MH, Allman K, et al: Scintigraphic pattern of regional cardiac sympathetic innervation in patients with familial long QT syndrome using positron emission tomography, Circulation 87:1616–1621, 1993.
13. Carrió I, Estorch M, Berna L, et al: Indium-111-antimyosin and iodine-123-MIBG studies in early assessment of doxorubicin cardiomyopathy, J Nucl Med 36:2044–2049, 1995.
14. Chakrabordy PK, Gildersleeve DL, Tocrougian SA, et al: Synthesis of (11C) epinephrine and other biogenic amines by direct methylation of normethyl precursors, J Label Compounds Radiopharm 32:172–173, 1992.
15. Chidsey CA, Braunwald E, Morrow AG, et al: Myocardial norepinephrine concentrations in man: effects of reserpine and of congestive heart failure, N Engl J Med 269:653–658, 1963.
16. Coates G, Chirakal R, Fallen EL, et al: Regional distribution and kinetics of [18F]6-fluorodopamine as a measure of cardiac sympathetic activity in humans, Heart 75:29–34, 1996.
17. Cohn JN, Levine TB, Olivari MT, et al: Plasma norepinephrine as a guide to prognosis in patients with chronic congestive heart failure, N Engl J Med 311:819–823, 1984.
18. Cohn JN, Johnson G, Ziesche S, et al: A comparison of enalapril with hydralazine-isosorbide dinitrate in the treatment of chronic congestive heart failure, N Engl J Med 325:303–310, 1991.
19. Corbett JR, Chiao P-C, del Rosario R, et al: Mapping neuronal enzyme function of the human heart with C-11 phenylephrine, J Nucl Med 35:109P, 1994 (abstract).
20. Corr PB, Gillis RA: Autonomic neural influences on the dysrhythmias resulting from myocardial infarction, Circ Res 43:1–9, 1978.

21. Crout J: The uptake and release of 3H-epinephrine by the guinea pig heart in vivo, *Naunyn Schmiedebergs Arch Pharmacol* 248:85, 1964.

22. Dae MW, Herre JM, O'Connell JW, et al: Scintigraphic assessment of sympathetic innervation after transmural versus nontransmural myocardial infarction, *J Am Coll Cardiol* 17:1416–1423, 1991.

23. Dae MW, DeMarco T, Botvinick EH, et al: Scintigraphic assessment of MIBG uptake in globally denervated and human hearts—implication for clinical studies, *J Nucl Med* 33:1444–1450, 1992.

24. DeGrado TR, Hutchins GD, Tooronsian SA, et al: Myocardial kinetics of carbon-11-meta-hydroxyephedrine: retention mechanisms and effects of norepinephrine, *J Nucl Med* 34:1287–1293, 1993.

25. DeGrado TR, Mulholland GK, Wieland DM, et al: Evaluation of (–)[^{18}F]fluoroethoxybenzovesamicol as a new PET tracer of cholinergic neurons on the heart, *Nucl Med Biol* 21:189–195, 1994.

26. DeGrado TR, Zalutsky MR, et al: Uptake mechanisms of meta-[^{123}I]iodobenzylguanidine in isolated rat heart, *Nucl Med Biol* 22:1–12, 1995.

27. Geeter FD, Franken PR, Defrise M, et al: Optimal collimator choice for sequential iodine-123 and technetium-99m imaging, *Eur J Nucl Med* 23:768–744, 1996.

28. De Marco T, Dae M, Yuen-Green MS, et al: Iodine-123 metaiodobenzylguanidine scintigraphic assessment of the transplanted human heart: evidence for late reinnervation, *J Am Coll Cardiol* 25:927–931, 1995.

29. Ding YS, Fowler JS, Dewey SL, et al: Comparison of high specific activity (–) and (+)-6-[^{18}F]fluoronorepinephrine and 6-[^{18}F]fluorodopamine in baboons: heart uptake, metabolism and the effect of desipramine, *J Nucl Med* 34:619–629, 1993.

30. Ducis I: *The high affinity choline uptake system.* In Whittaker V, ed: *The cholinergic synapse,* New York, 1988, Springer-Verlag.

31. Eisenhofer G, Friberg P, Rundquist B, et al: Cardiac sympathetic nerve function in congestive heart failure, *Circulation* 93:1667–1676, 1996.

32. Estorch M, Carrió I, Berna L, et al: Myocardial iodine-labeled metaiodobenzylguanidine 123 uptake relates to age, *J Nucl Cardiol* 2(2 Pt 1):126–132, 1995.

33. Henderson EB, Kahn JK, Corbett JR, et al: Abnormal I-123 metaiodobenzylguanidine myocardial washout and distribution may reflect myocardial adrenergic derangement in patients with congestive cardiomyopathy, *Circulation* 78(5 Pt 1):1192–1199, 1988.

34. Ewing DJ, Campbell JW, Clarke BF: The natural history of diabetic autonomic neuropathy, *Q J Med* 49:95–108, 1980.

35. Fagret D, Wolf JE, Vanzetto G, et al: Myocardial uptake of metaiodobenzylguanidine in patients with left ventricular hypertrophy secondary to valvular aortic stenosis, *J Nucl Med* 34:57–60, 1993.

36. Fagret D, Wolf JE, Comet M: Myocardial uptake of meta-[^{123}I]-iodobenzylguanidine ([^{123}I]-MIBG) in patients with myocardial infarct, *Eur J Nucl Med* 15:624–628, 1989.

37. Ferguson DW, et al: Sympathoinhibitory responses to digitalis glycosides in heart failure patients: direct evidence from sympathetic neural recordings, *Circulation* 80:65, 1989.

38. Francis GS: Modulation of peripheral sympathetic nerve transmission, *J Am Coll Cardiol* 12:250–254, 1988.

39. Gilbert EM, Sandoval A, Larrabee P, et al: Lisinopril lowers cardiac adrenergic drive and increases β-receptor density in the failing human heart, *Circulation* 88:472–480, 1993.

40. Gill JS, Hunter GJ, Gane G, et al: Asymmetry of cardiac [^{123}I]metaiodobenzyl-guanidine scans in patients with ventricular tachycardia and a "clinically normal" heart, *Br Heart J* 69:6–13, 1993.

41. Gill JS, Hunter GJ, Gane G, et al: Heterogeneity of the human myocardial sympathetic innervation: in vivo demonstration by iodine-123-labeled meta-iodobenzylguanidine scintigraphy, *Am Heart J* 126:390–398, 1993.

42. Glowniak JV, Turner FE, Gray LL, et al: Iodine-123 metaiodobenzylguanidine imaging of the heart in idiopathic congestive cardiomyopathy and cardiac transplants, *J Nucl Med* 30:1182–1191, 1989.

43. Gohl K, Feistel H, Weilel A, et al: Congenital myocardial sympathetic dysinnervation (CMSD)—a structural defect of idiopathic long QT syndrome, *Pacing Clin Electrophysiol* 14:1544–1553, 1991.

44. Goldstein DS, Chang PC, Eisenhofer G, et al: Positron emission tomographic imaging of cardiac sympathetic innervation and function, *Circulation* 81:1606–1621, 1990.

45. Goldstein DS, Eisenhofer G, Dunn BB, et al: Positron emission tomographic imaging of cardiac sympathetic innervation using [^{18}F]6-fluorodopamine: initial findings in humans, *J Am Coll Cardiol* 22:1961–1971, 1993.

46. Hammer R, Berrie C, Birdsall N, et al: Pirenzepine distinguishes between different subclasses of muscarinic receptors, *Nature* 283:90–92, 1980.

47. Hammer R, Giraldo E, Schiavi G, et al: Binding profile of a novel cardioselective muscarinic antagonist, AF-DX 116, to membranes of peripheral tissues and brain in the rat, *Life Sci* 38:1653–1662, 1986.

48. Hartikainen J, Mantysaari M, Kuikka J, et al: Extent of cardiac autonomic denervation in relation to angina on exercise test in patients with recent acute myocardial infarction, *Am J Cardiol* 74:760–763, 1994.

49. Hartikainen J, Kuikka J, Mantysaari M, et al: Sympathetic reinnervation after acute myocardial infarction, *Am J Cardiol* 77:5–9, 1996.

50. Hartman F, Ziegler S, Nekolla S, et al: Regional patterns of myocardial sympathetic observation in dilated cardiomyopathy: An analysis using carbon-II hydroxyephedrine (HED) and position emission tomography, (in press).

51. Hasking GJ, Esler MD, Jennings GL, et al: Norepinephrine spillover to plasma in congestive heart failure: evidence of increased overall and cardiorenal sympathetic nerve activity, *Circulation* 73:615–621, 1986.

52. Henderson EB, Kahn JK, Corbett JR, et al: Abnormal I-123 metaiodobenzylguanidine myocardial washout and distribution may reflect myocardial adrenergic derangement in patients with congestive cardiomyopathy, *Circulation* 78(5 Pt 1):1192–1199, 1988.

53. Imamura Y, Ando H, Mitsuoka W, et al: Iodine-123 metaiodobenzylguanidine images reflect intense myocardial adrenergic nervous activity in congestive heart failure independent of underlying cause, *J Am Coll Cardiol* 26:1594–1599, 1995.

54. Inoue H, Zipes DP: Results of sympathetic denervation in the canine heart: supersensitivity that may be arrhythmogenic, *Circulation* 75:877–887, 1987.

55. Ishida Y, Maeno M, Hirose Y, et al: [Characteristics of regional sympathetic dysfunction in acutely ischemic myocardium assessed by ^{123}I-metaiodobenzylguanidine imaging: impairment of myocardial norepinephrine uptake or retention], *Kaku Igaku* 32:631–642, 1995.

56. Jaques S Jr, Tobes MC, Sisson JC: Sodium dependency of uptake of norepinephrine and m-iodobenzylguanidine into cultured human pheochromocytoma cells: evidence for uptake-one, *Cancer Res* 47:3920–3928, 1987.

57. Schofer J, Spielmann R, Schuchert A, et al: Iodine-123 meta-iodobenzylguanidine scintigraphy: a noninvasive method to demonstrate myocardial adrenergic nervous system disintegrity in patients with idiopathic dilated cardiomyopathy, *J Am Coll Cardiol* 12:1252–1258, 1988.

58. Jung YW, Van Dort ME, Gildersleeve DL, et al: A radiotracer for mapping cholinergic neurons of the brain, *J Med Chem* 33:2065–2068, 1990.

59. Kaye DM, Ester M, Kingwell B, et al: Functional and neurochemical evidence for partial cardiac sympathetic reinnervation after cardiac transplantation in humans, *Circulation* 88:1110–1118, 1993.

60. Khafagi FA, Jhapiro B, Fig LM, et al: Labetalol reduces iodine-131 MIBG uptake by pheochromocytoma and normal tissues, *J Nucl Med* 30:481–489, 1989.

61. Kilborn MJ, Potter EK, McCloskey DI: Neuromodulation of the cardiac vagus: comparison of neuropeptide Y and related peptides, *Regul Pept* 12:155–161, 1985.

62. Kline RC, Swanson DP, Wieland DM: Myocardial imaging in man with I-123 metaiodobenzylguanidine, *J Nucl Med* 22:129–132, 1981.

63. Kreiner G, Wolzt M, Fasching P, et al: Myocardial m-[123I]iodobenzylguanidine scintigraphy for the assessment of adrenergic cardiac innervation in patients with IDDM. Comparison with cardiovascular reflex tests, and relationship to left ventricular function, *Diabetes* 44:543–549, 1995.

64. Kurata C, Wakabayashi Y, Shouda S, et al: Enhanced cardiac clearance of iodine-123-MIBG in chronic renal failure, *J Nucl Med* 36:2037–2043, 1995.

65. Langer A, Freeman MR, Josse RG, et al: Metaiodobenzylguanidine imaging in diabetes mellitus: assessment of cardiac sympathetic denervation and its relation to autonomic dysfunction and silent myocardial ischemia, *J Am Coll Cardiol* 25:610–618, 1995.

66. Lefkowitz RJ, Caron MG: Adrenergic receptors. Models for the study of receptors coupled to guanine nucleotide regulatory proteins, *J Biol Chem* 263:4993–4996, 1988.

67. Lekakis J, Prassopoulos V, Athanassiadis P, et al: Doxorubicin-induced cardiac neurotoxicity: study with iodine-123-labeled meta-iodobenzylguanidine scintigraphy, *J Nucl Cardiol* 3:37–41, 1996.

68. Mantysaari M, Kuikka J, Mustonen J, et al: Noninvasive detection of cardiac sympathetic nervous dysfunction in diabetic patients using [123I]metaiodobenzylguanidine, *Diabetes* 41:1069–1075, 1992.

69. Mantysaari M, Kuikka J, Hartikainen J, et al: Myocardial sympathetic nervous dysfunction detected with iodine-123-MIBG is associated with low heart rate variability after myocardial infarction, *J Nucl Med* 36:956–961, 1995.

70. Matsunari I, Bunko H, Taki J, et al: Regional uptake of iodine-125-metaiodobenzylguanidine in the rat heart, *Eur J Nucl Med* 20:1104–1107, 1993.

71. Matsunari I, Tanishima Y, Taki J, et al: Early and delayed technetium-99m-tetrofosmin myocardial SPECT compared in normal volunteers, *J Nucl Med* 37:1622–1626, 1996.

72. Matsuo S, Takahashi M, Nakamura Y, et al: Evaluation of cardiac sympathetic innervation with iodine-123-metaiodobenzylguanidine imaging in silent myocardial ischemia, *J Nucl Med* 37:712–717, 1996.

73. McGhie AI, Corbett JR, Akers MS, et al: Regional cardiac adrenergic function using I-123 metaiodobenzylguanidine tomographic imaging after acute myocardial infarction, *Am J Cardiol* 67:236–242, 1991.

74. Merlet P, Valette H, Dubois-Rande JL, et al: Prognostic value of cardiac metaiodobenzylguanidine imaging in patients with heart failure, *J Nucl Med* 33:471–477, 1992.

75. Merlet P, Delforge J, Syrota A, et al: Positron emission tomography with 11C CGP-12177 to assess β-adrenergic receptor concentration in idiopathic dilated cardiomyopathy, *Circulation* 87:1169–1178, 1993.

76. Minardo JD, Tuli MM, Mode BH, et al: Scintigraphic and electrophysiological evidence of canine myocardial sympathetic denervation and reinnervation produced by myocardial infarction or phenol application, *Circulation* 78:1008–1019, 1988.

77. Mitrani RD, et al: Regional cardiac sympathetic reinnervation following myocardial infarction in humans, *Circulation* 86 (Suppl 1): I247, 1992 (abstract).

78. Mitrani RD, Klein LS, Miles WM, et al: Regional cardiac sympathetic denervation in patients with ventricular tachycardia in the absence of coronary artery disease, *J Am Coll Cardiol* 22:1344–1353, 1993.

79. Mock BH, Tuli MM: Influence of specific activity on myocardial uptake of [123I]MIBG in rats, *Nucl Med Commun* 9:663–667, 1988.

80. Morimitsu T, Miyahara Y, Sinboku H, et al: Iodine-123-metaiodobenzylguanidine myocardial imaging in patients with right ventricular pressure overload, *J Nucl Med* 37:1343–1346, 1996.

81. Morimoto S, Terada K, Keira N, et al: Investigation of the relationship between regression of hypertensive cardiac hypertrophy and improvement of cardiac sympathetic nervous dysfunction using iodine-123 metaiodobenzylguanidine myocardial imaging, *Eur J Nucl Med* 23:756–761, 1996.

83. Nakajima K, Taki J, Bunko H, et al: Error of uptake in dual energy acquisition with 201Tl and 123I labeled radiopharmaceuticals, *Eur J Nucl Med* 16:595–599, 1990.

84. Nakajima K, Bunko H, Taki J, et al: Quantitative analysis of 123I-meta-iodobenzylguanidine (MIBG) uptake in hypertrophic cardiomyopathy, *Am Heart J* 119:1329–1337, 1990.

85. Nakajima K, Taki J, Tonami N, et al: Decreased 123I-MIBG uptake and increased clearance in various cardiac diseases, *Nucl Med Commun* 15:317–323, 1994.

86. Nakajo M, Jhapiro B, Glowniak J, et al: Inverse relationship between cardiac accumulation of meta-[131I]iodobenzylguanidine (I-131 MIBG) and circulating catecholamines in suspected pheochromocytoma, *J Nucl Med* 24:1127–1134, 1983.

87. Nakajo M, Jhimabukuro K, Yoshimura H, et al: Iodine-131 metaiodobenzylguanidine intra- and extravesicular accumulation in the rat heart, *J Nucl Med* 27:84–89, 1986.

88. Nakata T, Nagao K, Tsuchihashi K, et al: Regional cardiac sympathetic nerve dysfunction and the diagnostic efficacy of metaiodobenzylguanidine tomography in stable coronary artery disease, *Am J Cardiol* 78:292–297, 1996.

89. Nguyen NTB, DeGrado TR, Chakraborty P, et al: Myocardial kinetics of carbon-11 epinephrine in the isolated working rat heart, *J Nucl Med* 38:780–785, 1997.

90. Nishimura T, Oka H, Sago M, et al: Serial assessment of denervated but viable myocardium following acute myocardial infarction in dogs using iodine-123 metaiodobenzylguanidine and thallium-201 chloride myocardial single photon emission computed tomography, *Eur J Nucl Med* 19:25–29, 1992.

91. Nuyts J, Dupont P, Van den Maeghdenbergh V, et al: A study of the liver-heart artifact in emission tomography, *J Nucl Med* 36:133–139, 1995.

92. Packer M, Bristow MR, Cohn JN, et al: The effect of carvedilol on morbidity and mortality in patients with chronic heart failure, *N Engl J Med* 334:1349–1355, 1996.

93. Pierpont GL, DeMaster EG, Reynolds S, et al: Ventricular myocardial catecholamines in primates, *J Lab Clin Med* 106:205–210, 1985.

94. Rabinovitch MA, Rose CP, Schwab AJ, et al: A method of dynamic analysis of iodine-123-metaiodobenzylguanidine scintigrams in cardiac mechanical overload hypertrophy and failure, *J Nucl Med* 34:589–600, 1993.

95. Randall W, Ardell J: *Functional anatomy of the cardiac efferent innervation.* In Kulbertus H, Frank G, eds: *Neurocardiology,* New York, 1988, Future Publishing.

96. Rogers GA, Parsons SM, Anderson DC, et al: Synthesis, in vitro acetylcholine-storage blocking activities, and biological properties of derivates and analogue of trans-2-(4-phenylpiperidino)cyclohexanol (vesamicol), *J Med Chem* 32:1217–1230, 1989.

97. Rosenspire K, Haka MS, Van Dort ME, et al: Synthesis and preliminary evaluation of carbon-11-meta-hydroxyephedrine: a false transmitter agent for heart neuronal imaging, *J Nucl Med* 31:1328–1334, 1990.

98. Russ H, Gliese M, Jonna J, et al: The experimental transport mechanism for noradrenaline (uptake2) avidly transports 1-methylphenylpyridinium (MPP+), *Naunyn Schmiedebergs Arch Pharmacol* 346:158, 1992.

99. Sakata K, Yoshida H, Hoshino T, et al: Sympathetic nerve activity in the spasm-induced coronary artery region is associated with disease activity of vasospastic angina, *J Am Coll Cardiol* 28:460–464, 1996.

100. Salt PJ: Inhibition of noradrenaline uptake 2 in the isolated rat heart by steroids, clonidine and methoxylated phenylethylamines, *Eur J Pharmacol* 20:329–340, 1972.

101. Schmid PG, Greif BJ, Lund OD, et al: Regional choline acetyltransferase activity in the guinea pig heart, *Circ Res* 42:657–660, 1978.

102. Schömig A: Catecholamines in myocardial ischemia. Systemic and cardiac release, *Circulation* 82 (3 Suppl):II13–II22, 1990.

103. Schwaiger M, Kalff V, Rosenspire K, et al: Non-invasive evaluation of sympathetic nervous system in human heart by positron emission tomography, *Circulation* 82:457–464, 1990.

104. Schwaiger M, Guibourg H, Rosenspire K, et al: Effect of myocardial ischemia on sympathetic nervous system assessed by fluorine-18-metaraminol, *J Nucl Med* 31:1352–1357, 1991.

105. Schwaiger M, Hutchins GD, Das SK, et al: C-11 hydroxy-ephedrine kinetics in patients with hypertrophic cardiomyopathy, *J Am Coll Cardiol* 17:343A, 1991 (abstract).

106. Schwaiger M, Hutchins GD, Kalff V, et al: Evidence for regional catecholamine uptake and storage sites in the transplanted human heart by positron emission tomography, *J Clin Invest* 87:1681–1690, 1991.

107. Schwaiger M, Wieland D, Muzik O, et al: Comparison of C-11 epinephrine and C-11 HED for evaluation of sympathetic neurons of the heart, *J Nucl Med* 34:13P, 1993 (abstract).

108. Schwaiger M, Beanlands R, vom Dahl J: Metabolic tissue characterization in the failing heart by positron emission tomography, *Eur Heart J* 15 Suppl D: 14–19, 1994.

109. Schwartz PJ, Zaza A, Pala M, et al: Baroreflex sensitivity and its evolution during the first year after myocardial infarction, *J Am Coll Cardiol* 12:629–636, 1988.

110. Schwartz PJ, Periti M, Malliani A: The long Q-T syndrome, *Am Heart J* 89:378–390, 1975.

111. Simmons WW, Freeman MR, Grima EA, et al: Abnormalities of cardiac sympathetic function in pacing-induced heart failure as assessed by [123I]metaiodobenzylguanidine scintigraphy, *Circulation* 89: 2843–2851, 1994.

112. Sisson JC, Shapiro B, Meyers L, et al: Metaiodobenzylguanidine to map scintigraphically the adrenergic nervous system in man, *J Nucl Med* 28:1625–1636, 1987.

113. Spinnler MT, Lombardi F, Moretti C, et al: Evidence of functional alterations in sympathetic activity after myocardial infarction, *Eur Heart J* 14:1334–1343, 1993.

114. Stanton MS, Tuli MM, Radthe NL, et al: Regional sympathetic denervation after myocardial infarction in humans detected noninvasively using I-123-metaiodobenzylguanidine, *J Am Coll Cardiol* 14:1519–1526, 1989.

115. Takano H, Nakamura T, Satou T, et al: Regional myocardial sympathetic dysinnervation in patients with coronary vasospasm, *Am J Cardiol* 75:324–329, 1995.

116. Takatsu H, Scheffel U, Fujiwara H: Sympathetic tone assessed by washout of iodine 125-labeled metaiodobenzylguanidine from the murine left ventricle—influence of immobilization stress and inhibition of the renin-angiotensin system, *J Nucl Cardiol* 2:507–512, 1995.

117. Takatsu H, Uno Y, Fujiwara H: Modulation of left ventricular iodine-125-MIBG accumulation in cardiomyopathic Syrian hamsters using the renin-angiotensin system, *J Nucl Med* 36:1055–1061, 1995.

118. Thames MD, Klopfenstein HS, Abboud FM, et al: Preferential distribution of inhibitory cardiac receptors with vagal afferents to inferoposterior wall of the left ventricle activated during coronary occlusion in the dog, *Circ Res* 43:512–519, 1978.

119. Thomas JA, Marks BH: Plasma norepinephrine in congestive heart failure, *Am J Cardiol* 41:233–243, 1978.

120. Tomoda H, Yoshioka K, Shiina Y, et al: Regional sympathetic denervation detected by iodine 123 metaiodobenzylguanidine in non-Q-wave myocardial infarction and unstable angina, *Am Heart J* 128:452–458, 1994.

121. Tsuchimochi S, Tamaki N, Tadamura E, et al: Age and gender differences in normal myocardial adrenergic neuronal function evaluated by iodine-123-MIBG imaging, *J Nucl Med* 36:969–974, 1995.

122. Tsutsui H, Ando S, Fukai T, et al: Detection of angina-provoking coronary stenosis by resting iodine 123 metaiodobenzylguanidine scintigraphy in patients with unstable angina pectoris, *Am Heart J* 129:708–715, 1995.

123. Vaidyanathan G, Zalutsky MR: No-carrier-added meta-[123I]iodobenzylguanidine: synthesis and preliminary evaluation, *Nucl Med Biol* 22:61–64, 1995.

124. Wakasugi S, Wada A, Hasegawa Y, et al: Detection of abnormal cardiac adrenergic neuron activity in adriamycin-induced cardiomyopathy with iodine-125-metaiodobenzylguanidine, *J Nucl Med* 33: 208–214, 1992.

125. Wakasugi S, Fischman AJ, Babich JW, et al: Metaiodobenzylguanidine: evaluation of its potential as a tracer for monitoring doxorubicin cardiomyopathy, *J Nucl Med* 34:1283–1286, 1993.

126. Wakasugi S, Inoue M, Tazawa S: Assessment of adrenergic neuron function altered with progression of heart failure, *J Nucl Med* 36:2069–2074, 1995.

127. Weaver LC, Danos LM, Oehl RS, et al: Contrasting reflex influences of cardiac afferent nerves during coronary occlusion, *Am J Physiol* 240:H620–H629, 1981.

128. Wei K, Dorian P, Newman D, et al: Association between QT dispersion and autonomic dysfunction in patients with diabetes mellitus, *J Am Coll Cardiol* 26:859–863, 1995.

129. Wichter T, Hindricks G, Lerch H, et al: Regional myocardial sympathetic dysinnervation in arrhythmogenic right ventricular cardiomyopathy. An analysis using 123I-meta-iodobenzylguanidine scintigraphy, *Circulation* 89:667–683, 1994.

130. Wieland DM, Brown LE, Rosers WL, et al: Myocardial imaging with a radioiodinated norepinephrine storage analog, *J Nucl Med* 22:22–31, 1981.

131. Wieland DM, Hutchins GD, Rosenspire KC, et al: [C11]hydroxy-ephedrine (HED): a high specific activity alternative to 6-[F18]fluorometaraminol (FMR) for heart neuronal imaging, *J Nucl Med* 30:767–768, 1989.

132. Wieland DM, Rosenspire KC, Hutchins GD, et al: Neuronal mapping of the heart with 6-(18F)fluorometaraminol, *J Med Chem* 33:956–964, 1990.

133. Wilber DJ, Baerman J, Olshansky B, et al: Adenosine-sensitive ventricular tachycardia. Clinical characteristics and response to catheter ablation, *Circulation* 87:126–134, 1993.

134. Ziegler SI, Liberfuhl P, Frey A, et al: Incidence and time course of reinnervation in the orthotopic transplanted human heart, *J Nucl Med* 37:70P, 1996 (abstract).

Chapter 36

Receptor imaging

André Syrota and **Pascal Merlet**

Normal functioning of the heart requires precise timing of atrial and ventricular contractions and a force of contraction appropriate for the energy needs of the body. The action of cardiac autonomic neurons, which locally release neurotransmitters, is the most powerful physiologic mechanism to acutely increase contractility or heart rate. The cardiac receptor pathway, especially the β-adrenergic receptor-G-protein-adenylyl cyclase system, is impaired in heart disease. Many medications that have proven efficient in improving mortality and morbidity in patients with heart disease interact with cardiac receptor function.

Most of the available information on receptor abnormalities in heart disease was provided by in vitro binding analyses of myocardial samples obtained by endomyocardial biopsy during cardiac surgery or autopsy. Positron emission tomography (PET) now allows to perform noninvasive quantitative determi-

nation of regional receptor density and affinity in humans. These measurements are based on the synthesis of a radioligand, usually a selective receptor antagonist labeled with a positron-emitting radioisotope. Mathematical compartmental models are fitted to time–activity curves obtained during saturation or displacement experiments to calculate the rate constants and the receptor density in meaningful regions of interest in the myocardium. Recently, some ligands have been developed for use with single-photon emission computed tomography (SPECT); but the available data have not yet provided quantitative findings. Several receptor classes—adrenergic, muscarinic cholinergic, peripheral-type, and benzodiazepine—have been characterized in humans.

CLASSES AND FUNCTIONS OF CARDIAC RECEPTORS

Specific molecular neurotransmitters interact with myocyte surface membrane receptors, including β-adrenergic, α-adrenergic, muscarinic cholinergic, and peripheral-type benzodiazepine receptors. Receptors are membrane proteins or glycoproteins that display a high molecular affinity and selectivity for specific ligands. The binding of a neurotransmitter or a pharmacologic agent to the specific receptor site results in the opening and closing of ion channels brought about by conformational changes of the membrane proteins.

Adrenergic receptors

Adrenergic receptors are characterized by seven helices in their structure; in this respect, they are similar to muscarinic cholinergic receptors as well as to rhodopsin, the retinal color opsin.[85] The seven-helix receptors are attached to the cell membrane and bind ligands in the extracellular space, transducing signals through the action of one or more cytoplasmic guanosine triphosphate–binding proteins called *G proteins*.

Adrenergic receptors include the β-1, β-2, and β-3 subtypes[46]; a possible fourth β-subtype[60]; and the α-1- and α-2-adrenergic classes. β-1 Receptors have equal affinity for epinephrine and norepinephrine, whereas β-2 receptors have a higher affinity for epinephrine than for norepinephrine. β-2 Receptors are involved in the control of heart rate, whereas β-1 receptors affect both the rate and force of cardiac contraction. The widespread distribution of β-adrenergic receptors in the ventricles reflects the fact that sympathetic nerves affect all regions of the heart. β-1-Adrenergic receptors are the predominant β subtype in the human myocardium (about 80% are β-1 receptors and 20% are β-2 receptors).[48,53] The presence of a β-3 subtype in the myocardium has also been demonstrated.[58] The density of β-adrenoceptors in the heart is greater in the apex of the left ventricle than in the base[65] and greater in the subepicardial layer than in subendocardial layer.[80]

The interaction of norepinephrine or agonist medications with β-receptors results in a cascade of molecular events that increase intracellular cyclic adenosine monophosphate (AMP), the second messenger.[94] Several proteins mediate transduction of the neurotransmitter messages. One of these proteins, G(s), is a member of the family of guanine proteins, consisting of an α, β, and γ subunit. The α subunit contains the guanine triphosphate (GTP) binding site, possesses GTPase activity, is responsible for the specific transduction of the epinephrine signals to the effector enzyme,[47] and plays a central role in the regulation of cardiac function.[52] The enzyme adenylyl cyclase is activated by the G(s)-α-subunit when norepinephrine has been bound by its receptor. Activation of adenylyl cyclase results in the synthesis of cyclic AMP, using adenosine triphosphate as the substrate. Just as there are stimulatory Gs proteins, there are three inhibitory G(i) proteins. The mechanism through which activation of G(i) leads to inhibition of adenylyl cyclase is not fully understood.

α-Adrenergic receptors consist of two subtypes: α-1 and α-2. The α-1 receptors are postsynaptic and mediate smooth muscle contraction. The α-2-receptors are found on presynaptic nerve terminals, where they mediate feedback inhibition of norepinephrine release. The α-1-adrenergic pathway in the human myocardium is much less developed than the β-1-adrenergic pathway, and α-1 receptor density is low.[17]

Muscarinic acetylcholine receptors

Muscarinic cholinergic receptors exist in five subtypes: M1, M2, M3, M4, and M5. The M1 class is defined as receptors that exhibit a high affinity for the antagonist pirenzepine, whereas the M2 subclass is defined as receptors that have a low affinity for pirenzepine. Muscarinic receptors in the heart are mainly of the M2 type. Development of AF-DX 116, an M2-antagonist, has led to the suggestion that M2 receptors may be subdivided further into two subtypes: one with a high affinity for AF-DX 116 and one with low affinity for this substance.[51] Cardiac receptors have a high affinity for AF-DX 116 (M2 subclass). The existence of the different muscarinic receptor subtypes has been confirmed by cloning and sequencing DNA genes that code the receptor proteins.[10]

It is important to distinguish between muscarinic acetylcholine receptors located on blood vessels from those found on myocytes. Endothelial muscarinic receptors have a low affinity for the M1-antagonist pirenzepine[56] as well as for the cardioselective antagonist AF-DX 116. Autoradiographic studies with hydrogen-3 (^{3}H) 3-quinuclidyl benzylate (QNB) and iodine-125 (^{125}I) QNB failed to reveal binding sites on endothelial cells but showed them on the smooth muscle cells. This suggests that like myocardial receptors, muscarinic receptors that are present on the smooth muscles of coronary arteries can be detected with imaging techniques.

The physiologic response after ligand binding to muscarinic receptors is mediated by the G proteins, G(p), G(i), and G(k), which bind guanine nucleotides and transduce signals across the cell membrane.[47] The muscarinic M1, M3, and M5 ligand-receptor complex couples with G(p); the M2 and M5 complexes couple with G(i) and G(k), respectively. Both the G(i) and G(k) protein subtypes inhibit cardiac contraction. Activation of G(i) causes a decrease in levels of cyclic AMP, which reduces the activity of AMP-dependent kinases, phosphorylation of calcium channels, and calcium levels inside the cell. The activation of G(k) increases potassium levels, causing hyperpolarization and inhibition of myocyte contractions.

PRINCIPLES OF CARDIAC RECEPTOR IMAGING

Because PET is a tomographic imaging technique that enables quantitative autoradiography by external detection, it makes possible the in vivo investigation of cardiac receptors.[97,98,100] In contrast to SPECT, PET gives the exact value of the regional radioactive concentration of a tracer. It is then possible to select meaningful regions of interest in the septum or the free wall and to plot time–activity curves. Fitting these kinetic data to a mathematical model allows calculation of receptor density or drug affinity in any region of the myocardium. Furthermore, positron-emitting isotopes of natural elements have short half-lives (20 minutes for ^{11}C) and are produced at a very high specific activity (400 to 1000 Ci/mmol), resulting in three advantages. First, drugs labeled by ^{11}C keep their pharmacologic properties contrary to analogues labeled by ^{123}I (unless they naturally contain iodine). Second, the injected amount of drug usually does not exceed 10 to 50 nmol, so that receptor occupancy by the tracer remains low. Third, the radiation burden is low even though the amount of radioactivity injected is relatively high. Disadvantages are the complexity and the cost of PET. Likewise, it is necessary to have in the same facility a cyclotron to produce ^{11}C, a radiochemistry laboratory to synthesize the ^{11}C-labeled molecule in less than 40 minutes, and a positron camera.

SPECIFICITY OF IN VIVO RECEPTOR STUDIES

In vivo studies must deal with two kinds of problems. First, the radioactive ligand, which is usually injected intravenously, must reach its receptor sites within the studied organ without any modification. Second, the radioligand within the organ must interact with high affinity only with its specific receptor sites and must not bind to other receptors or to nonspecific binding sites.

Access of ligands to myocardium

After intravenous injection, the radiotracer can bind to proteins or penetrate into erythrocytes, thus reducing the amount of free ligand available for binding. Ligands such as peptides can be enzymatically degraded by circulating peptidases. Other molecules can be rapidly metabolized by the liver.

Another complication of in vivo studies is the presence of different serial barriers between the site of injection and the receptor sites, such as the lungs and the capillary membrane. Lipophilic molecules are completely extracted during a single pass through the lung circulation. They can be metabolized by the pulmonary endothelial or epithelial cells before reaching the cardiac receptors.[84] The second barrier is the capillary barrier of the target organ. However, in contrast to the blood-brain barrier, the capillary membrane in the heart is permeable to small hydrophilic molecules. The biodistribution of the radiotracer is also important to consider; it may be extracted, trapped, or metabolized by organs other than the lungs and the heart. Many drugs are transformed into metabolites in the liver. Some of these metabolites will still be labeled by the positron-emitting isotope, but their physical and pharmacologic properties may have changed. Both the lipophilicity and the affinity of the metabolites may have been modified by several orders of magnitude.

Interaction of ligand within the myocardium

Additional complexities are related to the removal process of the radioligand within the myocardium, such as uptake by different cells, enzymatic or chemical degradation, and intracellular trapping. A radioligand can also bind to different receptors or different receptor subtypes. Positron emission tomography detects the total radioactivity in the heart and, unlike the case with in vitro studies, the distinction between specific binding and nonspecific binding is not easy. Because nonspecific binding increases linearly with plasma ligand concentration, whereas specific binding is saturable, the ratio of specific-to-nonspecific binding can be increased by minimizing radiotracer plasma concentrations and maximizing specific radioactivity of the radioligand to detect enough radioactivity in the tissue.

Identification criteria of ligand-receptor interaction

Receptor-mediated localization of a ligand in the myocardium must be validated in vivo by the same criteria as those used for in vitro binding studies: saturability, stereospecificity, and a correlation between the binding and the biological effect.

The saturability of the ligand-receptor complex can be demonstrated by two kinds of experiments. In displacement experiments, an excess of cold agonist or antagonist is intravenously injected sometime after injection of the labeled ligand. The radioactive concentration in myocardium then rapidly decreases with time because of the competitive inhibition between the tracer and the excess of unlabeled ligand. The

receptor sites can also be blocked by an excess of unlabeled ligand injected before the radioligand. In this case, the tracer radioactive concentration in the tissue is lower than that measured in the absence of injection of the cold molecule.

Stereoselectivity is a powerful proof for receptor binding. If two stereoisomers are available, one with and one without pharmacologic activity, the displacement must be obtained only with the active isomer.[73]

A correlation between binding and a biological effect is essential for distinguishing between a displaceable binding site with no signal transmission and a receptor-binding site that is related to physiologic responses. A correlation between receptor binding and biological effect was shown with ^{11}C pindolol, [11]C Ciba Geigy Product (CGP) 12177, and ^{11}C MQNB (N-methylquinuclidinyl benzylate). The percentage of ^{11}C MQNB or ^{11}C CGP 12177 displaced by various amounts of unlabeled atropine or propranolol was proportional to the decrease or increase in heart rate.[73] Moreover, in patients with heart failure due to idiopathic dilated cardiomyopathy, decreased β-receptor sites assessed by PET with ^{11}C-CGP 12177 correlated fairly well with impaired β-contractile responsiveness to intracoronary dobutamine infusion, confirming a direct link between changes in the receptor number and its biological function.[75]

Once all of these criteria have been fulfilled, it becomes possible to develop a mathematical model that transforms values of radioactive concentrations measured in selected regions of interest of PET images into values of affinity constants and receptor density.[33]

The multiinjection modeling approach

The most general method used to estimate receptor concentration consists of the identification of all model variables and may require multiple injections.[34] Therefore, the estimation of receptor concentration implies the use of an experimental protocol including at least two injections, one of which results in a significant percentage of receptor occupancy.[99]

The first example of this multiinjection approach was the study of the binding of ^{11}C MQNB to muscarinic receptors in dog heart.[34] Attempts to identify the model variables from data obtained with a single tracer injection led to disappointing numeric results, because most of the variables had to be considered unidentifiable. The possibility of improving variable estimation by using a new experimental design consisting of a first tracer injection followed 30 minutes later by an injection of the cold ligand (displacement experiment) was then investigated. However, this second protocol led to two different solutions. A biologically valid solution was obtained by using a third protocol including both a displacement and a coinjection. A fourth injection (an injection of a large mass of unlabeled ligand) allowed the estimation of irreversible and nonspecific binding.

Such complex protocols may be unsuitable for clinical studies. Therefore, information obtained from animal experiments is useful to set up and validate simplified protocols applicable to human studies. In the case of the investigation of muscarinic receptors, the best protocol in terms of clinical feasibility consisted of a tracer injection followed 30 minutes later by a coinjection of labeled and unlabeled ligand, inducing partial occupancy of the available receptor sites.[34] It has also been shown that with ^{11}C MQNB, the slope of the Patlak plot is not related to the binding of free ligand (variable k_3) but corresponds to the transfer of the ligand from the blood to the free ligand compartment.[34] In this case, the Patlak method did not provide any information on the receptor density.

In the case of ^{11}C CGP, displacement studies with a large excess of unlabeled β-blocking drug cannot be performed in patients. A graphical method that does not need the input function has been developed. It easily provides measurement of receptor density.[32]

IN VIVO CHARACTERIZATION OF CARDIAC RECEPTORS

β-Adrenergic receptors

Five antagonists—propranolol, practolol, pindolol, carazolol, and CGP 12177—have been labeled with ^{11}C for PET.[3–6,11,12,50,86] They differ in affinity, liposolubility, and subtype-selectivity. Carbon-11 propranolol, a lipophilic nonselective antagonist, cannot be used for studying β-adrenergic receptors with PET because of its high accumulation in the lungs. Carbon-11 practolol is a hydrophilic molecule that binds to β-1 receptors. A few minutes after intravenous injection in humans, the heart is well visualized, but the tracer concentration decreases rapidly with time, even when it is injected at a very high specific activity (Fig. 36-1). The percentage of bound tracer that could be displaced by an excess of unlabeled antagonist (practolol, propranolol, atenolol, or pindolol) 20 minutes later is also low. The results can be explained by the relatively low affinity of practolol. By contrast, ^{11}C pindolol and ^{11}C CGP 12177 have high affinity and low lipophilicity.

Fluorocarazolol has been labeled with [18]F.[41] PET studies using ^{11}C carazolol in pigs have shown that specific receptor binding was 75% of the total uptake in the heart, an effect that was preventable and displaceable with propranolol.[7] Dose-dependent competition showed that carazolol binds in vivo to β-1 and β-2 subtypes. Fluorocarazolol is subject to fast metabolization, implying difficulties in evaluating the input function, and it displays a high lipophilicity, implying a high accumulation in the lungs.[41,109,116] However, this ligand, as well as fluorometoprolol,[29] can be used to visualize pulmonary β-adrenergic receptors with PET.[42]

The antagonist CGP 12177 originally was developed as a hydrophilic antagonist to detect cell surface β-1- and β-2-adrenergic receptors. It is usually considered to have no β-adrenoceptor subtype selectivity, although a low β-1 selectivity has been demonstrated with rat ventricular microsomes.[81] Subsequently, it was found to be a partial agonist for the atypical or β-3-adrenergic receptor.[83] The inotropic effects of CGP 12177 have been investigated on paced preparations of isolated right atrial appendages obtained from patients without advanced heart failure undergoing open-heart surgery.[59] The potent positive inotropic effects of CGP 12177 and their resistance to blockade by propranolol but antagonism by bupranolol are consistent with the existence in human atrial myocardium of a minor third β-adrenoceptor population, possibly related to β-3-adrenoceptors.

Ligand CGP 12177 has low nonspecific binding on membranes and low intracellular uptake.[93] In addition, it does not bind to receptors that are removed from the plasma membrane and internalized during short-term desensitization.[54] It is therefore an ideal probe to specifically measure the cell surface receptors in vivo: that is, the "functionally active" β-receptors.[66] This ligand labeled with ^{11}C has fulfilled all the criteria needed to characterize the β-receptors.[75] A high myocardial uptake was measured with PET after injection of ^{11}C CGP 12177, and a displacement of bound tracer was obtained after injection of an excess of cold ligand. Saturation of the β-adrenergic receptor was demonstrated by preinjection of an unlabeled β-blocker a few minutes before injection of ^{11}C CGP. A correlation was observed between the tracer displacement and the decrease in heart rate induced by the displacing agent. This is a strong indication that receptor sites and not only binding sites are visualized.

The potential of PET with ^{11}C CGP 12177 for clinical investigation has been pointed out.[75] The ability of PET with ^{11}C CGP 12177 to determine myocardial β-receptor changes was evaluated in patients with idiopathic dilated cardiomyopathy and in healthy persons (Fig. 36-2). The β-receptor density obtained from PET correlated well with the β-receptor density determined with endomyocardial biopsy samples by an in vitro binding technique using ^{3}H CGP 12177.[75]

An experimental pharmacologic study in rats failed to demonstrate a potential to reflect binding to adrenoceptor of

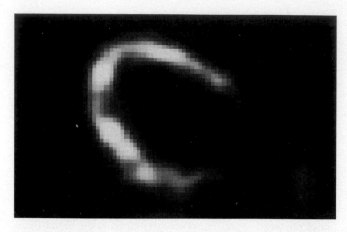

Fig. 36-1. Representative midventricular tomogram acquired with positron emission tomography after intravenous administration of carbon-11 choline glycerophosphatide in a normal patient. This ligand binds with high affinity to the externalized β receptors. The left ventricle is to the left. The lateral left ventricular wall is to the left, the septum is to the right, and the anterior wall is at the top. The regional distribution of the tracer is homogenous, and the heart to lung ratio of activity is high.

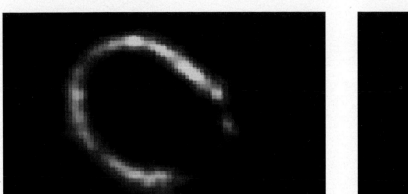

Fig. 36-2. Midventricular tomogram acquired after intravenous administration of carbon-11 choline glycerophosphatide (CGP) in a patient with severe left ventricular dysfunction related to idiopathic dilated cardiomyopathy. Compared with the normal patient, the myocardial uptake of labeled CGP seems to be high. However, decreased concentration of available receptor sites was found when mathematical analysis was done, because the images are normalized.

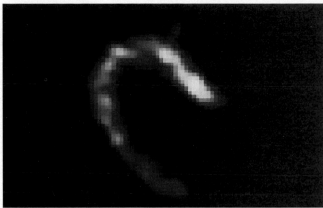

Fig. 36-3. Midventricular tomogram acquired after intravenous administration in a normal subject of carbon-11 N-methyl 3-quinuclidinyl benzilate, an antagonist of the muscarinic acetylcholine receptors. The orientation is the same as that in Fig. 36-1. A high activity is seen in the myocardium. Activity in the right ventricle is lower than that in the left ventricle. Lungs and blood activities are very low.

CGP 26505, a β-1-adrenoceptor antagonist.[107] Thus, ^{11}C CGP 12177 remains the ideal PET ligand for in vivo characterization of β-adrenergic receptors in the human heart.

Some SPECT ligands have been developed. The asymmetric synthesis and structural characterization of different new iodine-containing β-adrenoceptor antagonist derivatives have been reported.[36,108] Thus far, no optimal ligands are available to image cardiac β-adrenoceptors with SPECT. Among them, the iodinated analogue of CGP 12177 and one analogue of the nonselective β-adrenoceptor antagonist penbutolol have been pharmacologically characterized.[36] Although some analogues showed reasonable affinity in vitro for the receptor, their binding in vivo proved to be largely nonspecific, suggesting that these compounds are unsuitable for imaging purposes.

α-Adrenergic Receptors

Prazosin, a selective α-1 adrenergic blocker, was labeled with ^{11}C and injected into dogs.[40] Positron emission tomography showed a high and homogeneous myocardial uptake and a much lower pulmonary uptake. However, the criteria needed for the characterization of receptors could not be fulfilled because of high nonspecific binding.

Muscarinic acetylcholine receptors

The radiolabeled muscarinic antagonists ^{3}H QNB and ^{3}H NMS (N-methylscopolamine) have been widely used in in vitro studies.[39,87] The former agent binds to M1 and M2 receptor subtypes. When ^{3}H QNB was used to label intact cells instead of membrane preparations, some trapping of the ligand occurred within the cells, presumably by the lysosomes. The same phenomenon occurred with ^{3}H dexetimide.[49] Hydrogen-3 QNB labels more sites than ^{3}H-NMS or ^{3}H-MQNB, a quaternary derivative of ^{3}H QNB.[22] It is likely that the subset of receptors de-

tected only by ^{3}H QNB does not participate in physiologic responses, possibly because they are sequestered in a hydrophobic compartment within the cell membrane.[22]

Therefore, the hydrophilic ligand MQNB, the methiodide salt of QNB, was labeled with ^{11}C to study the muscarinic acetylcholine receptors in vivo by PET.[73] This ligand is a potent antagonist that is not extracted by the lungs and displays a high affinity for the cholinergic receptors (Fig. 36-3).[96]

All of the criteria needed to characterize the muscarinic receptor were validated in baboons and humans with ^{11}C MQNB.[96]

After a bolus intravenous injection of ^{11}C MQNB at a high specific activity, the ^{11}C MQNB blood concentration decreased rapidly to a negligible value a few minutes after injection. In contrast, the ^{11}C MQNB concentration increased rapidly in the myocardium to its maximum in 1 to 5 minutes and remained constant for 70 minutes. Rapid intravenous injection of atropine led to a rapid decrease in the septal ^{11}C MQNB concentration. The maximal percentage of ^{11}C MQNB that could be displaced in dogs was 94%. Because atropine did not discriminate between muscarinic receptor subtypes in the heart, one could assume that less than 6% of the ^{11}C MQNB bound in the heart corresponds to nonspecific binding. The specific binding is stereospecific because dexetimide, the pharmacologically active isomer, but not levetimide can displace ^{11}C MQNB from its binding sites.[73]

The ventricles primarily receive postganglionic cholinergic fibers from ganglion cells localized in the atria. The release of acetylcholine at parasympathetic nerve endings in the ventricles would thus depend on the activity of atrial cells mediating both the atrial chronotropic and the ventricular inotropic effects. Reduced frequency is related to a predominant vagal influence. The greater ^{11}C MQNB binding in the septum linked to vagal stimulation could be explained by an increase in the number or the affinity of antagonist binding sites. In the physiologically active state, the agonist is released from the receptor in a low-affinity form, and more sites are available for ^{11}C MQNB binding.[96] The presence of two interconvertible forms of the muscarinic cholinergic receptor, favored by agonists and antagonists and displaying high-agonist-to-low-antagonist and low-agonist-to-high-antagonist affinities, respectively, has been demonstrated.[23] According to this hypothesis, vagal stimulation would be characterized by a conversion to a low-agonist-to-high-antagonist affinity form of the muscarinic receptor. These findings suggest that PET allows identification of the physiologically active form of the muscarinic receptor.[96]

Affinity constant and B_{max} values for ^{11}C-MQNB binding to cardiac muscarinic receptors have been calculated in dogs by using the multiinjection modeling approach described previously, including displacement experiment with an excess of unlabeled MQNB.[30,34] The experimental protocol was recently optimized to make this approach suitable for human studies in six normal persons by the use of a three-injection protocol. This protocol includes a tracer injection, followed 30 minutes later by an injection of an excess of unlabeled MQNB (displacement) and another 30 minutes later by a simultaneous injection of unlabeled and labeled MQNB (coinjection).[31] A simplified two-injection protocol (tracer injection and coinjection) was compared with the three-injection protocol in five other normal persons. The results were similar in terms of B_{max}. In the left ventricle, the mean values of the receptor concentration B_{max} and the equilibrium dissociation constant K_D were 26±7 pmol/ml of tissue and 2.0±0.5 pmol/ml of tissue, respectively. A very low nonspecific binding was found in two persons by using a double-displacement protocol.[31]

The agents 2- and 4-[^{18}F]fluorodexetimide and the racemic E-1-azabicyclo[2.2.2]oct-3-yl α-(1-bromo-1-1-propen-3-yl)-α-hydroxy-α-phenylacetate, as well as AF-DX 116 and AF-DX 384, are potential candidates for imaging muscarinic acetylcholinergic receptors by PET.[55,77,95] The pharmacological characteristics, tissue distribution, and metabolization of these ligands confirm their ability to evaluate M2-muscarinic receptors but they do not seem superior to MQNB.

Peripheral-type benzodiazepine receptor

Specific high-affinity benzodiazepine binding sites have been demonstrated in several peripheral organs, including the heart.[102] New ligands that bind only to peripheral-type sites have been synthesized. The ligands RO 5-4864 and PK 11195 have a very high affinity for peripheral sites.[67,68] In vitro, the PK 11195 binding sites in rat cardiac membranes are specific and saturable with a K_D of 1.41 nM and a B_{max} of 2250 pmol/g of protein. The agent PK 11195 was labeled with ^{11}C at a very high specific activity[24] and was injected intravenously in dogs and humans. An initial uptake of ^{11}C PK-11195 was seen in the lung, followed by a high uptake in the heart. Benzodiazepine binding sites were uniformly distributed.[26] The amount of PK 11195 found in the heart was proportional to the quantity injected at values below 40 nmol/kg, whereas above this value, the curve showed a plateau due to saturation of the benzodiazepine binding sites.

Other criteria needed for identification of a ligand-receptor interaction by PET were validated. Saturability was demonstrated by coinjection or displacement experiments with unlabeled PK 11195 and other ligands that compete for peripheral-type sites, such as RO 5-4864 and diazepam. Ligands that only bind to brain-type sites, such as RO 15-1788 and clonazepam, were ineffective.[26] The physiologic function of these receptors is still largely unknown. Some data have suggested that PK 11195 binds to the mitochondrial outer membrane.[1] In cardiac muscle and vascular smooth muscle, benzodiazepines have been shown to interfere with Ca^{++} movements. The ligand PK 11195 antagonized the effects of several calcium-channel blockers (diltiazem, nitrendipine, verapamil) and a calcium-channel agonist (BAY K 8644) in a guinea pig papillary muscle preparation.[76] It also inhibited arrhythmias induced by ischemia and abnormalities after reperfusion in the dog heart. Chemical sympathectomy increased B_{max} in the left ventricle (34%) 1 week after administration of 6-hydroxydopamine or reserpine. Despite these appealing findings, no clear interest for PET study of these receptors in clinical situations has been reported.

CLINICAL APPLICATIONS

Heart failure

Heart failure is a problem of increasing importance in cardiovascular medicine. Sympathetic stimulation is one of the main compensatory mechanisms for the failing heart. As failure progresses, cardiac stores of norepinephrine are depleted but circulating norepinephrine concentration is elevated. This effect has been directly related to the degree of left ventricle dysfunction and to the risk of death. Even though plasma levels of norepinephrine are elevated in response to heart failure, ino-tropic responsiveness to catecholamines is abnormal.[15]

The failing heart is characterized not only by a decrease in the catecholamine content of myocytes and impairment of norepinephrine release and uptake but also by abnormalities of cardiac nerve terminals. Presynaptic uptake of norepinephrine is reduced in experimental heart models.

In heart failure, α-receptor density is normal or slightly increased, suggesting that the α-1 receptor pathway has no compensatory role in supporting the heart. The uncompromised α-1 receptor pathway in the failing heart plays a role in the stimulation of cardiac hypertrophy.[18] An important characteristic of heart failure is reduced agonist-stimulated adenylyl cyclase activity (receptor desensitization) due to both diminished receptor number (receptor downregulation) and impaired receptor function (receptor uncoupling). These changes in the adrenergic receptor system may account in part for some of the abnormalities of contractile function in this disease. Blunted cardiac responsiveness to β-adrenergic stimulation, associated with substantial reduction of the β-adrenergic receptor density, has been shown in failing human myocardium in in vitro studies.[15] This phenomenon probably also occurs in children with congestive heart failure, because in noncyanotic congenital children, lymphocyte β-adrenergic receptor density was shown to be decreased in relation to the degree of left-to-right shunt and pulmonary pressure.[115]

Autoradiography of ^{125}I iodocyanopindolol–binding sites from failing human heart has shown that the subendocardium contained the greatest reduction in β-adrenergic receptor density.[80] Heart failure produces a loss in β-1-receptors, whereas the density of β-2-receptors remains constant. This relative loss of β-1 receptors leads to a shift in the proportion of β-1 receptors compared with β-2 receptors from approximately 80:20 in nonfailing heart to 60:40 in failing ventricular myocardium.[16] This subtype alteration is heterogeneous in transmural distribution.[2] The density of β receptors and, by inference, the density of β-1 receptors begins to decrease in mild heart failure and becomes more reduced as heart failure progresses.[45] A progressive 60% to 70% loss in β-1 receptor density leads to a marked decrease in selective β-1 agonist–stimulated adenylate cyclase activity.[63,113] Thus, downregulation of β-1 receptors seems to be a main factor in the decreased β-1 agonist sensitivity of the failing heart, especially in idiopathic cardiomyopathy.[14] Although the density of β-2 receptors is preserved, adrenergic receptor occupancy is mildly uncoupled from pharmacologic response in failing myocardium. β-1 Receptors seem to be uncoupled in ischemic cardiomyopathy.[14] The decreased density of β-1 adrenergic receptor density in failing human ventricular myocardium seems to be related to decreased levels of β-1 receptor messenger RNA.[20,43] In end-stage heart failure, the expression of different myocardial regulatory proteins involved in the β-adrenergic cyclic AMP signalling pathway is altered.[91] Uncoupling of β-2 adrenergic receptor in idiopathic cardiomyopathy and of β-1 adrenergic receptor in ischemic cardiomyopathy is related to increased functional activity of G(i), thereby inhibiting cyclic AMP formation and receptor phosphorylation.[14,82,103] The aging human heart shows some similarities with the failing human heart: In both settings, β-adrenergic receptor–mediated effects and all other cyclic AMP–dependent effects are depressed and G(i) protein is increased.[28]

A 50% decrease in left ventricular β receptors was found by using PET and ^{11}C CGP 12177 in patients with idiopathic dilated cardiomyopathy compared with controls, a result that is in agreement with in vitro data.[75] Moreover, a decreased number of β receptors correlated well with impaired contractile responsiveness to intracoronary dobutamine infusion, indicating a direct link between the level of downregulation and the corresponding impaired biological effect. Recently, a relation between the decrease in β receptor density and the neuronal norepinephrine function was found in patients with idiopathic dilated cardiomyopathy by using PET with ^{11}C CGP 12177 and planar scintigraphy with ^{123}I MIBG.[98] However, no correlation was found between plasma norepinephrine concentration and β receptor density. This finding supports the concept of β receptor downregulation as a consequence of presynaptic adrenergic nerve dysfunction. This observation is also concordant with the

predominance of the decrease in specific tritiated norepinephrine accumulation that paralleled a predominant β receptor downregulation in subendocardial regions of failing left ventricles.[2] β-Adrenergic neuroeffector abnormalities in the failing human heart are therefore probably produced by local rather than systemic mechanisms.[19]

Parasympathetic neurotransmission was thought to play a lesser role than that of sympathetic neurotransmission in the diseased myocardium, but muscarinic cholinergic agonists counteract the stimulating effect of adrenergic overactivity in the heart. Several lines of evidence suggest that the parasympathetic receptor–effector system is altered in heart failure. A chronic attenuation of cardiac vagal tone has been inferred from studies of heart rate variability in patients with cardiomyopathy.[8,38,90] This alteration of cardiac vagal tone evolves early in the course of ventricular dysfunction in animal models.[37] Parasympathetic agonists restore tonic and reflex vagal activity.[62]

Increased modulation of β-adrenergic inotropic left stimulation by parasympathetic agonists was recently demonstrated in patients with heart failure.[64] A reduction in GTP-stimulated adenylate cyclase activity and an increased concentration or activity of G(i)-α regulatory protein have been reported in animals and in humans.[9,90,112] In experimental cardiac failure, changes occur in cardiac muscarinic receptors,[112,114] but no significant abnormalities have been found by in vitro binding techniques in the myocardium of patients with end-stage heart failure.[9] However, atrial myocytes isolated from failing human explanted hearts exhibited a lower resting membrane potential and reduced sensitivity to acetylcholine compared with control (donor) atria.[61] Whole-cell and single-channel measurements suggest that these alterations are caused by reduced I-K(acetylcholine) channel density sensitivity to M2 cholinergic receptor–linked G protein G$_i$-mediated channel activation. The first demonstration of changes in muscarinic receptors in failing human left ventricle was by PET with ^{11}C MQNB. In patients with congestive heart failure due to idiopathic cardiomyopathy, the mean value of left ventricular muscarinic receptors was increased compared with normal values (Fig. 36-4).[69]

Ischemia

Major changes in β-adrenoceptor regulation take place in the ischemic myocardium,[72,78,79] some of which are responsible for arrhythmias. These results were not confirmed by others,[57] and the discrepancies were perhaps related to differences in durations of ischemia or reperfusion or in membrane preparation. During myocardial ischemia, a local release of noradrenaline coincides with an increased density of β-adrenergic receptors.[104] Moreover, the increase in the number of β-adrenergic receptors is paralleled by increased membrane activity of the β-adrenergic receptor kinase (β-ARK) that specifically phosphorylates and thereby inactivates β-adrenergic receptors after stimulation by receptor agonists, facilitating the binding of the inhibitor protein β-arrestin to the receptors. Activation of β-ARK involves a translocation of the enzyme to the mem-

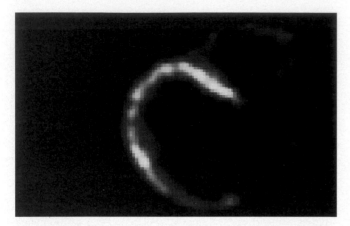

Fig. 36-4. Midventricular tomogram acquired after intravenous administration of carbon-11 N-methyl 3-quinuclidinyl benzilate in a patient with nonischemic dilated cardiomyopathy. In such patients, an increased number of muscarinic acetylcholine receptors was seen by using this positron emission tomographic approach.

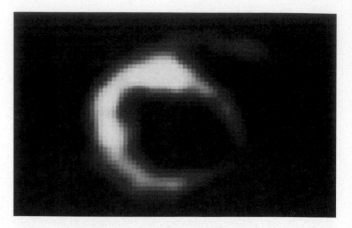

Fig. 36-5. Midventricular tomogram acquired after administration of carbon-11 choline glyceropeptide in a patient with primary hypertrophic cardiomyopathy who had had an episode of decompensed heart failure. A significant decrease in β receptor sites has been found in such patients, similar to that found in patients with idiopathic dilated cardiomyopathy.

brane.[104] Inversely, the induction of ischemia in isolated perfused rat heart produced no change in cardiac Al adenosine receptor density or affinity, whereas a 75% downregulation of M2 muscarinic cholinoceptors was found (but only for sustained ischemic injury).[105] In the same experiment, no change in Al adenosine receptor or in M2 muscarinic cholinoceptor messenger RNA concentrations was found by quantitative polymerase chain reactions. Finally, in the pig model of stunned myocardium, an increased β receptor density was demonstrated by using ^{125}I iodocyanopindolol binding.[89] Neither PET nor SPECT data are available in human myocardial ischemia.

Hypertrophy

In experimental renovascular or spontaneous hypertension, β-adrenergic receptor density is normal, increased,[71] or unchanged.[25] In experimental left ventricular hypertrophy secondary to aortic banding, physiologic responsiveness to catecholamines is normal, with increased β-adrenergic receptor density but decreased antagonist affinity.[110]

Primary hypertrophic cardiomyopathy represents a clinical entity that is totally different from dilated cardiomyopathy. Characteristics include mainly asymmetric hypertrophy associated with hyperdynamic contractility, diastolic filling abnormalities, and propensity for arrhythmias. These characteristics have suggested a potential role of an altered sympathetic system in the evolution of the disease. In patients with primary hypertrophic cardiomyopathy, no change in β-adrenergic receptor density has been found by using in vitro binding techniques.[48] However, by using PET and ^{11}C CGP 12177, a diffuse reduction in myocardial β-receptors has been shown in patients with primary hypertrophic cardiomyopathy without heart failure and increased circulating norepinephrine levels.[27] In hypertrophic patients with heart failure,[27] an even greater decrease in β-AR density was shown with PET; the downregulation of this receptor is related to echographic indices of left ventricular dysfunc-

tion (see Fig. 36-5 for personal data). This discrepancy may be attributable to patient or control selection as well as to methodologic differences.

Denervation

Denervation supersensitivity occurs in patients treated with β-blockers or in naturally occurring neuronal denervation. Chronic denervation results in β-adrenergic receptor upregulation and supersensitivity in the surgically denervated heart.[13,111] Supersensitivity is due to upregulation of β-adrenergic receptors and to the lack of reuptake resulting from the absence of sympathetic nerve endings. In a model of canine denervation obtained by autotransplantation, the density of cardiac β-receptors measured by PET was found to return to a normal level in parallel with that seen in late sympathetic reinnervation.[106]

When cardiac β-receptor sensitivity to isoprenaline in the denervated donor heart in patients who received heart transplants was compared with that of the innervated recipient, β receptor density increased and β receptor affinity did not change in the transplanted heart. However, no change in β-adrenergic receptor density was found in biopsy samples from patients who received heart transplants.[21] Similar results were obtained in vivo with ^{11}C CGP 12177.[74] These findings indicate that the observed supersensitivity of the transplanted heart to extrinsic catecholamines is of presynaptic origin. Decreased myocardial adenylate cyclase activity in response to guanine nucleotide stimulation was recently demonstrated in denervated myocardium of transplant patients, suggesting that changes in left ventricular muscarinic receptors may occur.[35] No difference in the concentration and affinity constant of muscarinic receptors by PET with ^{11}C MQNB was found in transplant patients compared with controls.[70] This suggests abnormalities of the signal-transduction function, such as changes in the guanine nucleotide-binding proteins.

Desensitization

Densensitization is caused by changes in the β-adrenergic receptor-G protein-adenylyl cyclase complex as a result of chronic exposure to high levels of β-adrenergic agonist at the receptor sites.[92] On the functional level, the most important mechanism of desensitization involves the phosphorylation of β-adrenergic and homologous receptors by specific receptor kinases, termed the G protein–coupled receptor kinases. This phosphorylation is followed by binding of arrestins to the receptors, which causes uncoupling of receptors and G proteins and thus results in a loss of receptor function. On the expression level, two major pathways seem to lead to a reduction of the receptor number: degradation of the receptors themselves or reduced receptor synthesis brought about by reduced receptor messenger RNA levels. Heart failure, as described above, is accompanied by a markedly reduced responsiveness of the β-adrenergic receptor system, which in many ways resembles the phenomenon seen in agonist-induced receptor desensitization. Levels of β-1-adrenergic receptors are reduced, and this reduction is paralleled by similar decreases in the levels of the corresponding messenger RNA. At the same time, the activity and the messenger RNA levels of some G protein–coupled receptor kinase isoforms are increased. These alterations may contribute to the loss of β-adrenergic receptor responsiveness in heart failure and may result in further impairment of cardiac function.

Homologous desensitization is characterized by a reduced responsiveness only to the specific desensitizing hormone without affecting the responsiveness of the adenylyl cyclase enzyme to other hormones. Heterologous desensitization is characterized by diminished responsiveness of adenylyl cyclase to a wide spectrum of stimulators, including other hormones, fluoride, and guanine nucleotides.[101]

Human myocardium relies mainly on β receptors to augment contractility and seems to have no or few "spare" receptors. The close correlation found in heart failure patients between the β receptor concentration assessed by PET and the contractile responsiveness to intracoronary infusion of dobutamine[75] suggests that the downregulation of β receptors is the main mechanism of β adrenergic desensitization. This is consistent with other findings that showed reduced basal, Gpp(NH)p-, and isoproterenol-stimulated adenylyl cyclase activity but unchanged forskoline-stimulated adenylyl cyclase, suggesting that reduced isoproterenol-stimulated adenylate cyclase is due to reduced β-adrenergic receptor density rather than to increased inhibitory subunit of G protein.

Asthma

One PET study evaluated the density of β receptor in the heart and the lungs of patients with asthma.[44] No difference in either pulmonary or cardiac β-receptor density was seen between asthmatic patients and controls.

Syndrome X

Recent research has questioned the ischemic hypothesis of etiology of syndrome X (anginal pain and ischemia-like changes on the stress electrocardiogram but a normal coronary arteriogram).[88] Abnormalities of pain perception and abnormal sympathetic nervous system activation with increased myocardial catecholamine concentrations have also been implicated. In patients with syndrome X, β adrenoceptor density assessed by using PET with ^{11}C CGP 12177 was found to be normal.

CONCLUSION

Positron emission tomography only recently emerged as a new tool to study the physiologic regulation of receptors. The binding of a neurotransmitter to its receptor sets in motion a series of molecular events through the second messenger system, culminating in the observed response. This series of molecular interactions has been shown to be altered in several cardiac diseases. Several pathologic and therapeutic concepts in cardiology have been based on sympathetic neuroeffector mechanisms in the heart. A limitation in evaluating these concepts has been the difficulty of measuring cardiac autonomic function in vivo and noninvasively. Positron emission tomography, but not SPECT, offers this opportunity. Although the partial volume effect still precludes evaluation of the transmural distribution of cardiac receptors, one of the main advantages of PET is the possibility of studying their regional distribution. Furthermore, PET may be useful in exploring the receptor alterations in the early stages of different diseases. As a noninvasive test, PET can be repeated, and this may provide information on the effects of pharmacologic agents interacting with myocardial receptors.

REFERENCES

1. Anholt RRH, Pedersen PL, De Souza EB: The peripheral-type benzodiazepine receptor. Localization to the mitochondrial outer membrane, *J Biol Chem* 261:576–583, 1986.
2. Beau SL, Tolley TK, Saffitz JE: Heterogeneous transmural distribution of beta-adrenergic receptor subtypes in failing human hearts, *Circulation* 88:2501–2509, 1993.
3. Berger G, Maziere M, Prenant C, et al: Synthesis of ^{11}C-propranolol, *J Radioanal Chem* 74:301–306, 1982.
4. Berger G, Dormont D, Syrota A, et al: [11]C ligand binding to adrenergic and muscarinic receptors in the human heart studied in vivo by PET, *J Nucl Med* 24:P20, 1983 (abstract).
5. Berger G, Prenant C, Sastre J: Synthesis of a beta-blocker for heart visualization: [^{11}C] practolol, *Int J Appl Radiat Isot* 34:1556–1557, 1983.
6. Berridge MS, Cassidy EH, Terris AH, et al: Preparation and in vivo binding of ^{11}C carazolol, a radiotracer for the beta-adrenergic receptor, *Int J Rad Appl Instrum* 19:563–569, 1992.
7. Berridge MS, Nelson AD, Zheng L: Specific beta-adrenergic receptor binding of carazolol measured with PET, *J Nucl Med* 35:1665–1676, 1994.
8. Binkley PF, Nunziata E, Haas GJ, et al: Parasympathetic withdrawal is an integral component of autonomic imbalance in congestive heart failure: demonstration in human subjects and verification in a paced canine model of ventricular failure, *J Am Coll Cardiol* 18:464–472, 1991.
9. Böhm M, Gierschik P, Jakobs KH, et al: Increase of Gi alpha in human hearts with dilated but not ischemic cardiomyopathy, *Circulation* 82:1249–1265, 1990.
10. Bonner TI, Buckley NJ, Young AC, et al: Identification of a family of muscarinic acetylcholine receptor genes, *Science* 237:527–532, 1987.
11. Boullais C, Crouzel C, Syrota A: Synthesis of 4-(3-t-butylamino-2-hydroxypropoxy)-benzimidazol-2 (^{11}C)-one (CGP 12177), *J Label Compound Radiopharm* 23:565–567, 1986.

12. Brady F, Luthra SK, Tochon-Danguy HJ, et al: Asymmetric synthesis of a precursor for the automated radiosynthesis of S-(3'-t-butylamino-2'-hydroxypropoxy)-benzimidazol-2-[^{11}C] one (S-[^{11}C] CGP 12177) as a preferred radioligand for beta-adrenergic receptors, *Int J Rad Appl Instrum* 42:621–628, 1991.

13. Bristow MR: The surgically denervated, transplanted human heart, *Circulation* 82:658–660, 1990.

14. Bristow MR, Anderson FL, Port JD, et al: Differences in beta-adrenergic neuroeffector mechanisms in ischemic versus idiopathic dilated cardiomyopathy, *Circulation* 84:1024–1039, 1991.

15. Bristow MR, Ginsburg R, Minobe W, et al: Decreased catecholamine sensitivity and beta-adrenergic-receptor density in failing human hearts, *N Engl J Med* 307:205–211, 1982.

16. Bristow MR, Ginsburg R, Umans V, et al: Beta 1- and beta 2-adrenergic-receptor subpopulations in nonfailing and failing human ventricular myocardium: coupling of both receptor subtypes to muscle contraction and selective beta 1-receptor down-regulation in heart failure, *Circ Res* 59:297–309, 1986.

17. Bristow MR, Hershberger RE, Port JD, et al: β-adrenergic pathways in nonfailing and failing human ventricular myocardium, *Circulation* 82:I12–I25, 1990.

18. Bristow MR, Minobe W, Rasmussen R, et al: Alpha-1 adrenergic receptors in the nonfailing and failing human heart, *J Pharmacol Exp Ther* 247:1039–1045, 1988.

19. Bristow MR, Minobe W, Rasmussen R, et al: β-Adrenergic neuroeffector abnormalities in the failing human heart are produced by local rather than systemic mechanisms, *J Clin Invest* 89:803–815, 1992.

20. Bristow MR, Minobe WA, Raynolds MV, et al: Reduced beta 1 receptor messenger RNA abundance in the failing human heart, *J Clin Invest* 92:2737–2745, 1993.

21. Brodde OE, Khamssi M, Zerkowski HR: Beta-adrenoceptors in the transplanted human heart: unaltered beta-adrenoceptor density, but increased proportion of beta 2-adrenoceptors with increasing post-transplant time, *Naunyn Schmiedebergs Arch Pharmacol* 334:430–436, 1991.

22. Brown JH, Goldstein D: Analysis of cardiac muscarinic receptors recognized selectively by nonquaternary but not by quaternary ligands, *J Pharmacol Exp Ther* 238:580–586, 1986.

23. Burgisser E, De Lean A, Lefkowitz RJ: Reciprocal modulation of agonist and antagonist binding to muscarinic cholinergic receptor by guanine nucleotide, *Proc Natl Acad Sci U S A* 79:1732–1736, 1982.

24. Camsonne R, Crouzel C, Comar D, et al: Synthesis of N-(^{11}C) methyl, N-(methyl-1 propyl), (chloro-2 phenyl)-1 isoquinoleine carboxamide receptors, *J Label Compound Radiopharm* 21:985–991, 1984.

25. Cervoni P, Herzlinger H, Lai FM, et al: A comparison of cardiac reactivity and beta-adrenoceptor number and affinity between aorta-coarcted hypertensive and normotensive rats, *Br J Pharmacol* 74:517–523, 1981.

26. Charbonneau P, Syrota A, Crouzel C, et al: Peripheral-type benzodiazepine receptors in the living heart characterized by positron emission tomography, *Circulation* 73:476–483, 1986.

27. Choudhury L, Guzzetti S, Lefroy DC, et al: Myocardial β adrenoceptors and left ventricular function in hypertrophic cardiomyopathy, *Heart* 75:50–54, 1996.

28. Davies CH, Ferrara N, Harding SE: β-adrenoceptor function changes with age of subject in myocytes from non-failing human ventricle, *Cardiovasc Res* 31:152–156, 1996.

29. de Groot TJ, van Waarde A, Elsinga PH, et al: Synthesis and evaluation of 1'-[^{18}F] fluorometoprolol as a potential tracer for the visualization of beta-adrenoceptors with PET, *Nucl Med Biol* 20:637–642, 1993.

30. Delforge J, Janier M, Syrota A, et al: Noninvasive quantification of muscarinic receptors in vivo with positron emission tomography in the dog heart, *Circulation* 82:1494–1504, 1990.

31. Delforge J, Le Guludec D, Syrota A, et al: Quantification of myocardial muscarinic receptors with PET in humans, *J Nucl Med* 34:981–991, 1993.

32. Delforge J, Syrota A, Lancon JP, et al: Cardiac beta-adrenergic receptor density measured in vivo using PET, CGP 12177, and a new graphical method, *J Nucl Med* 32:739–748, 1991.

33. Delforge J, Syrota A, Mazoyer BM: Experimental design optimization: theory and application to estimation of receptor model parameters using dynamic positron emission tomography, *Phys Med Biol* 34:419–435, 1989.

34. Delforge J, Syrota A, Mazoyer BM: Identifiability analysis and parameter identification of an in vivo ligand-receptor model from PET data, *IEEE Trans Biomed Eng* 37:653–661, 1990.

35. Denniss AR, Marsh JD, Quigg RJ, et al: β-adrenergic receptor number and adenylate cyclase function in denervated transplanted and cardiomyopathic human hearts, *Circulation* 79:1028–1034, 1989.

36. Dubois EA, Somsen GA, van den Bos JC, et al: Development of radioligands for the imaging of cardiac beta-adrenoceptors using SPECT. Part II: Pharmacological characterization in vitro and in vivo of new ^{123}I-labeled beta-adrenoceptor antagonists, *Nucl Med Biol* 24:9–13, 1997.

37. Eaton GM, Cody RJ, Nunziata E, et al: Early left ventricular dysfunction elicits activation of sympathetic drive and attenuation of parasympathetic tone in the paced canine model of congestive heart failure, *Circulation* 92:555–561, 1995.

38. Eckberg DL, Drabinsky M, Braunwald E: Defective cardiac parasympathetic control in patients with heart disease, *N Engl J Med* 285:877–883, 1971.

39. Gibson RE, Eckelman WC, Vieras F, Reba RC: The distribution of the muscarinic acetylcholine receptor antagonists, quinuclidinyl benzilate and quinuclidinyl benzilate methiodide (both triated) in rat, guinea pig and rabbit, *J Nucl Med* 20:865–870, 1979.

40. Ehrin E, Luthra SK, Crouzel C, et al: Preparation of carbon-11 labelled prazosin, a potent and selective alpha-ladrenoceptor antagonist, *J Label Compound Radiopharm* 25:177–183, 1988.

41. Elsinga PH, Van Waarde A, Visser GM, et al: Synthesis and preliminary evaluation of (R,S)-1-[2-((carbamoyl-4-hydroxy)phenoxy)ethyl-amino]-3-[4-(1-[^{11}C]-methyl-4-trifluoromethyl-2-imidazolyl) phenoxy]-2-propanol ([^{11}C] CGP 20712A) as a selective beta 1-adrenoceptor ligand for PET, *Nucl Med Biol* 21:211–217, 1994.

42. Elsinga PH, Vos MG, van Waarde AH, et al: (S,S)- and (S,R)-1'-[^{18}F]fluorocarazolol, ligands for the visualization of pulmonary β-adrenergic receptors with PET, *Nucl Med Biol* 23:159–167, 1996.

43. Engelhardt S, Bohm M, Erdmann E, et al: Analysis of beta-adrenergic receptor mRNA levels in human ventricular biopsy specimens by quantitative polymerase chain reactions: progressive reduction of beta$_1$-adrenergic receptor mRNA in heart failure, *J Am Coll Cardiol* 27:146–154, 1996.

44. Quing F, Rahman SU, Rhodes CG, et al: Pulmonary and cardiac β-adrenoceptor density in vivo in asthmatic subjects, *Am J Respir Crit Care Med* 155:1130–1134, 1997.

45. Fowler MB, Laser JA, Hopkins GL, et al: Assessment of the beta-adrenergic receptor pathway in the intact failing human heart: progressive receptor down-regulation and subsensitivity to agonist response, *Circulation* 74:1290–1302, 1986.

46. Gauthier C, Tavernier G, Charpentier F, et al: Functional β$_3$-adrenoceptor in the human heart, *J Clin Invest* 98:556–562, 1996.

47. Gilman AG: G proteins: transducers of receptor-generated signals, *Annu Rev Biochem* 56:615–649, 1987.

48. Golf S, Lovstad R, Hansson V: Beta-adrenoceptor density and relative number of beta-adrenoceptor subtypes in biopsies from human right atrial, left ventricular and right ventricular myocard, *Cardiovasc Res* 19:636–641, 1985.

49. Gossuin A, Maloteaux JM, Trouet A, et al: Differentiation between ligand trapping into intact cells and binding on muscarinic receptors, *Biochem Biophys Acta* 804:100–106, 1984.

50. Hammadi A, Crouzel C: Asymmetric synthesis of (2S) and (2R)-4-(butylamino-2-hydroxypropoxy-benzamidazol-2-^{11}C) one (S) and (R) (^{11}C CGP 12177) from optically active precursors, *J Label Compound Radiopharm* 29:681–690, 1991.

51. Hammer R, Giraldo E, Schiavi GB, et al: Binding profile of a novel cardioselective muscarine receptor antagonist, AF-DX 116, to membranes of peripheral tissues and brain in the rat, *Life Sci* 38:1653–1662, 1986.

52. Hein L, Kobilka BK: Adrenergic receptors—from molecular structure to in vivo function, *Trend Cardiovasc Med* 7:137–145, 1997.

53. Heitz A, Schwartz J, Velly J: Beta-adrenoceptors of the human myocardium: determination of beta 1 and beta 2 subtypes by radioligand binding, *Br J Pharmacol* 80:711–717, 1983.

54. Hertel C, Muller P, Portenier M, et al: Determination of the desensitization of beta-adrenergic receptors by [3H]CGP-12177, *Biochem J* 216:669–674, 1983.

55. Hwang DR, Dence CS, McKinnon ZA, et al: Positron labeled muscarinic acetylcholine receptor antagonist: 2- and 4-[18F]fluorodexetimide. Syntheses and biodistribution, *Int J Rad Appl Instrum [B]* 18:247–252, 1991.

56. Hynes MR, Banner W Jr, Yamamura HI, et al: Characterization of muscarinic receptors of the rabbit ear artery smooth muscle and endothelium, *J Pharmacol Exp Ther* 238:100–105, 1986.

57. Karliner JS, Stevens M, Grattan M, et al: Beta-adrenergic receptor properties of canine myocardium: effects of chronic myocardial infarction, *J Am Coll Cardiol* 8:349–356, 1986.

58. Kaumann AJ: Some aspects of heart beat adrenoreceptor function, *Cardiovasc Drugs Therapy* 5:549–560, 1991.

59. Kaumann AJ: (-)-CGP 12177 induced increase of human atrial contraction through a putative third β-adrenoceptor, *Br J Pharmacol* 117:93–98, 1996.

60. Kaumann AJ: Four β-adrenoceptor subtypes in the mammalian heart, *Trends Pharmacol Sci* 18:70–76, 1997.

61. Koumi S, Arentzen CE, Backer CL, et al: Alterations in muscarinic K+ channel response to acetylcholine and to G protein-mediated activation in atrial myocytes isolated from failing human hearts, *Circulation* 90:2213–2224, 1994.

62. La Rovere MT, Mortara A, Pantaleo P, et al: Scopolamine improves autonomic balance in advanced congestive heart failure, *Circulation* 90:838–843, 1994.

63. Lai LP, Suematsu M, Elam H, et al: Differential changes of myocardial beta-adrenoceptor subtypes and G-proteins in dogs with right-sided congestive heart failure, *Eur J Pharmacol* 309:201–208, 1996.

64. Landzberg JS, Parker JD, Gauthier DF, et al: Effects of intracoronary acetylcholine and atropine on basal and dobutamine-stimulated left ventricular contractility, *Circulation* 89:164–168, 1994.

65. Lathers CM, Levin RM, Spivey WH: Regional distribution of myocardial beta-adrenoceptors in the cat, *Eur J Pharmacol* 130:111–117, 1986.

66. Law MP: Demonstration of the suitability of CGP 12177 for in vivo studies of beta-adrenoceptors, *Br J Pharmacol* 109:1101–1109, 1993.

67. Le Fur G, Guilloux F, Rufat P, et al: Peripheral benzodiazepine binding sites: effect of PK 11195, 1-(2-chorophenyl)-N-methyl-(1-methylpropyl)-3 isoquinolinecarboxamide. II. In vivo studies, *Life Sci* 32:1849–1856, 1983.

68. Le Fur G, Perrier ML, Vaucher N, et al: Peripheral benzodiazepine binding sites: effect of PK 11195, 1-(2-chlorophenyl)-N-methyl-N-(1-methylpropyl)-3-isoquinolinecarboxamide. I. In vivo studies, *Life Sci* 32:1839–1847, 1983.

69. Le Guludec D, Cohen-Solal A, Delforge J, et al: Increased myocardial muscarinic receptor density in idiopathic dilated cardiomyopathy: an in vivo PET study, *Circulation* 96:3416–3422, 1997.

70. Le Guludec D, Delforge J, Syrota A, et al: In vivo quantification of myocardial muscarinic receptors in heart transplant patients, *Circulation* 90:172–178, 1994.

71. Limas CJ: Increased number of beta-adrenergic receptors in the hypertrophied myocardium, *Biochem Biophys Acta* 588:174–178, 1979.

72. Maisel AS, Motulsky HJ, Insel PA: Externalization of beta-adrenergic receptors promoted by myocardial ischemia, *Science* 230:183–186, 1985.

73. Mazière M, Comar D, Godot JM, et al: In vivo characterization of myocardium muscarinic receptors by positron emission tomography, *Life Sci* 29:2391–2397, 1981.

74. Merlet P, Benvenuti C, Valette H, Delforge J: Myocardial β-adrenergic receptors in heart transplanted patients: assessment with ^{11}C-CGP 12177 and positron emission tomography, *Circulation* 86:245–245, 1993 (abstract).

75. Merlet P, Delforge J, Syrota A, et al: Positron emission tomography with ^{11}C CGP-12177 to assess β-adrenergic receptor concentration in idiopathic dilated cardiomyopathy, *Circulation* 87:1169–1178, 1993.

76. Mestre M, Carriot T, Belin C, et al: Electrophysiological and pharmacological evidence that peripheral type benzodiazepine receptors are coupled to calcium channels in the heart, *Life Sci* 36:391–400, 1985.

77. Mickala P, Boutin H, Bellanger C, et al: In vivo binding, pharmacokinetics and metabolism of the selective M2 muscarinic antagonists [3H] AF-DX 116 and [3H] AF-DX 384 in the anesthetized rat, *Nucl Med Biol* 23:173–179, 1996.

78. Mukherjee A, Bush LR, McCoy KE, et al: Relationship between beta-adrenergic receptor numbers and physiological responses during experimental canine myocardial ischemia, *Circ Res* 50:735–741, 1982.

79. Mukherjee A, Wong TM, Buja LM, et al: Beta adrenergic and muscarinic cholinergic receptors in canine myocardium. Effects of ischemia, *J Clin Invest* 64:1423–1428, 1979.

80. Murphree SS, Saffitz JE: Distribution of beta-adrenergic receptors in failing human myocardium. Implications for mechanisms of down-regulation, *Circulation* 79:1214–1225, 1989.

81. Nanoff C, Freissmuth M, Schütz W: The role of a low beta 1-adrenoceptor selectivity of [3H] CGP-12177 for resolving subtype-selectivity of competitive ligands, *Naunyn Schmiedebergs Arch Pharmacol* 336:519–525, 1987.

82. Neumann J, Schmitz W, Scholtz H, et al: Increase in myocardial Gi-proteins in heart failure, *Lancet* 22:936–937, 1988.

83. Pak MD, Fishman PH: Anomalous behavior of CGP 12177A on β1-adrenergic receptors, *J Recept Signal Transduct Res* 16:1–23, 1996.

84. Pascal O, Syrota A, Berger G, et al: *Lung uptake of ^{11}C-imipramine and ^{11}C-propranolol in patients with sarcoidosis evaluated by positron emission tomography.* In Marsac J, Chretien J, eds: *Sarcoidosis and other granulomatous disorders,* Pergamon Press, Paris, 404–408, 1981.

85. Peralta EG, Winslow JW, Peterson GL, et al: Primary structure and biochemical properties of an M2 muscarinic receptor, *Science* 236:600–605, 1987.

86. Prenant C, Sastre J, Crouzel C, et al: Synthesis of ^{11}C-pindolol, *J Label Compound Radiopharm* 24:227–232, 1987.

87. Fields JZ, Roeske WR, Morkin E, et al: Cardiac muscarinic cholinergic receptors. Biochemical identification and characterization, *J Biol Chem* 253:3251–3258, 1978.

88. Rosen SD, Boyd H, Rhodes CG, et al: Myocardial beta-adrenoceptor density and plasma catecholamines in syndrome X, *Am J Cardiol* 78(1):37–42, 1996.

89. Sato S, Sato N, Kudej RK, et al: β-Adrenergic receptor signalling in stunned myocardium of conscious pigs. *J Mol Cell Cardiol* 29(5):1387–1400, 1997.

90. Saul JP, Arai Y, Berger RD, et al: Assessment of autonomic regulation in chronic congestive heart failure by heart rate spectral analysis, *Am J Cardiol* 61:1292–1299, 1988.

91. Schmitz W, Boknik P, Linck B, et al: Adrenergic and muscarinic receptor regulation and therapeutic implications in heart failure, *Mol Cell Biochem* 157:251–258, 1996.

92. Sibley DR, Daniel K, Strader CD, et al: Phosphorylation of the β-

adrenergic receptor in intact cells: relationship to heterologous and homologous mechanisms of adenylate cyclase desensitization, *Arch Biochem Biophys* 258:24–32, 1987.

93. Staehelin M, Simons P, Jaeggi K, et al: CGP-12177. A hydrophilic beta-adrenergic receptor radioligand reveals high affinity binding of agonists to intact cells, *J Biol Chem* 258:3496–3502, 1983.

94. Stiles GL, Lefkowitz RJ: Cardiac adrenergic receptors, *Annu Rev Med* 35:149–164, 1984.

95. Strijckmans V, Luo H, Coulon C, et al: Z-(-,-)-[Br-76] BrQNP: a high affinity PET radiotracer for central and cardiac muscarinic receptors, *J Label Compound Radiopharm* 38:883–895, 1996.

96. Syrota A, Comar D, Paillotin G, et al: Muscarinic cholinergic receptor in the human heart evidenced under physiological conditions by positron emission tomography, *Proc Natl Acad Sci U S A* 82:584–588, 1985.

97. Syrota A, Merlet P: *Positron emission tomography: evaluation of cardiac receptors and neuronal function.* In Skorton DJ, Schelbert HR, Wolf GL, eds: *Marcus Cardiac Imaging,* Orlando, 1995, W.B. Saunders Company.

98. Syrota A, Merlet P, Delforge J: *Cardiac neurotransmission.* In Wagner HN Jr, Szabo Z, Buchanan JW, eds: *Principles of nuclear medicine*, Philadelphia, 1995, W.B. Saunders Company.

99. Syrota A, Paillotin G, Davy JM, et al: Kinetics of in vivo binding of antagonist to muscarinic cholinergic receptor in the human heart studied by positron emission tomography, *Life Sci* 35:937–945, 1984.

100. Syrota A, Valette H, Merlet P: *Cardiac neurotransmission.* In Schwaiger M, ed: *Cardiac positron emission tomography,* Dordrecht, 1995, Kluwer Academic Publishers.

101. Travis MD, Whalen EJ, Lewis SJ: Heterologous desensitization of beta-adrenoceptor signal transduction in vivo, *Eur J Pharmacol* 328:R1–R3, 1997.

102. Trifiletti RR, Lo MMS, Snyder SH: Kinetic differences between type I and type II benzodiazepine receptors, *Mol Pharmacol* 26:228–240, 1984.

103. Ungerer M, Bohm M, Elce JS, et al: Altered expression of beta-adrenergic receptor kinase and beta 1-adrenergic receptors in the failing human heart, *Circulation* 87:454–463, 1993.

104. Ungerer M, Kessebohm K, Kronsbein K, et al: Activation of beta-adrenergic receptor kinase during myocardial ischemia, *Circ Res* 79:455–460, 1996.

105. Ungerer M, Stocker M, Richardt G: A_1 adenosine receptors and muscarinic cholinoceptors in myocardial ischemia, *Naunyn Schmiedebergs Arch Pharmacol* 354:44–52, 1996.

106. Valette H, Syrota A, Deleuze P, et al: Late sympathetic reinnervation and normalization of canine myocardial beta-adrenergic receptor density following denervation, *J Nucl Med* 36:1727, 1995.

107. Van Waarde A, Meeder JG, Blanksma PK, et al: Uptake of radioligands by rat heart and lung in vivo: CGP 12177 does and CGP 26505 does not reflect binding to beta-adrenoceptors, *Eur J Pharmacol* 222:107–112, 1992.

108. van den Bos JC, van Doremalen PA, Dubois EA, et al: Development of radioligands for the imaging of cardiac beta-adrenoceptors using SPECT. Part 1. Asymmetric synthesis and structural characterization of five new iodine-containing beta-adrenoceptor antagonist derivatives, *Nucl Med Biol* 24:1–7, 1997.

109. van Waarde A, Visser TJ, Posthumus H, et al: Quantification of the β-adrenoceptor ligand S-1'-[^{18}F] fluorocarazolol in plasma of humans, rats and sheep, *J Chromatogr B Bio Med Appl* 678:253–260, 1996.

110. Vatner DE, Homcy CJ, Sit SP, et al: Effects of pressure overload, left ventricular hypertrophy on β-adrenergic receptors, and responsiveness to catecholamines, *J Clin Invest* 73:1473–1482, 1984.

111. Vatner DE, Lavallee M, Amano J, et al: Mechanisms of supersensitivity to sympathomimetic amines in the chronically denervated heart of the conscious dog, *Circ Res* 57:55–64, 1985.

112. Vatner DE, Lee DL, Schwarz KR, et al: Impaired cardiac muscarinic receptor function in dogs with heart failure, *J Clin Invest* 81:1836–1842, 1988.

113. Vatner DE, Vatner SF, Fujii AM, et al: Loss of high affinity cardiac beta adrenergic receptors in dogs with heart failure, *J Clin Invest* 76:2259–2264, 1985.

114. Wilkinson M, Horackova M, Giles A: Reduction of ventricular M2 muscarinic receptors in cardiomyopathic hamster (CHF 147) at the necrotic stage of the myopathy, *Pflugers Arch* 426:516–523, 1994.

115. Wu JR, Chang HR, Chen SS, et al: Circulating noradrenaline and β-adrenergic receptors in children with congestive heart failure, *Acta Paediatr* 85:923–927, 1996.

116. Zheng L, Berridge MS, Ernsberger P: Synthesis, binding properties, and ^{18}F labeling of fluorocarazolol, a high-affinity beta-adrenergic receptor antagonist, *J Med Chem* 37:3219–3230, 1994.

Chapter 37

Imaging in ischemic cardiomyopathy: therapeutic considerations

Avijit Lahiri and **Roxy Senior**

The economic and human burden of congestive heart failure is a major hurdle for Western society that is likely to continue into the new century. The cost of management of congestive heart failure has escalated, and management of the condition is far from ideal.[36] In this chapter, we discuss the utility of imaging methods as used to assess congestive heart failure in the context of therapeutic management. To develop adequate imaging techniques, which will provide us with tools for better management of the heart failure patient, it is imperative that we understand the complex pathophysiology of congestive heart failure in patients with ischemic heart disease.

TREATMENT OPTIONS IN CONGESTIVE HEART FAILURE

The history of the pharmacologic management of heart failure is, to a surprisingly large extent, a story of theoretical promise and clinical disappointment. The traditional mechanistic model of cardiac failure, the perpetual cycle of diminished contractility and peripheral vasoconstriction, suggests that dilating the peripheral vessels or augmenting the force of myocardial contraction are the approaches most likely to succeed. The mechanistic model describes a small part of a complex and still ill-defined entity. The central issue is undoubtedly left ventricular dysfunction, but the host of compensatory responses

evoked by dysfunction defies any simple description and makes any prediction of the long-term effect of pharmacologic intervention risky. Left ventricular ejection fraction remains the single most important factor in defining heart failure and in predicting its outcome.[12,31] In the Coronary Artery Surgery Study (CASS), for example, mortality during the first 30 days after myocardial infarction was doubled in patients in whom the left ventricular score (the sum of five segmental ratings of wall motion) was 10 or more; the risk increase was identical in patients treated medically and those who underwent coronary artery bypass graft surgery.[18] The problem is that although left ventricular dysfunction increases the risk for death, it does not necessarily cause symptoms, reduce exercise tolerance, or provide useful information on response to treatment. Thus, radionuclide ventriculography remains a hallmark for assessment of left ventricular ejection fraction. Ischemia must be featured in any comprehensive definition of congestive heart failure because subendocardial ischemia on its own can produce transmural myocardial dysfunction. Another ischemic component of heart failure is the hibernating, metabolically suppressed myocardium often associated with left ventricular wall akinesis and dyskinesis in patients with coronary heart disease.[22,45,51,62] An exhaustive search for myocardial ischemia is an essential part of the investigation of patients with heart failure. Imaging methods used for detection of myocardial ischemia in the context of heart failure will also be discussed.

Vasodilators

Vasodilators, first as intravenous infusions of phentolamine, nitroprusside, or nitroglycerin and later as long-acting nitrates, hydralazine, and angiotensin-converting enzyme (ACE) inhibitors, have long been part of the management of heart failure.[2,30,33,35] Hemodynamic benefit was easy to demonstrate; an effect on mortality proved more elusive. The first Veterans Administration (VHeFT) study showed that the combination of hydralazine and isosorbide dinitrate lowered mortality by one third,[13] and in the second study, enalapril reduced mortality by a further 18%.[14] The Cooperative New Scandinavian Enalapril Survival Study showed that enalapril lowered mortality by as much as 31% in patients with severe heart failure (functional class IV). The value of ACE inhibitors has been amply confirmed in the two Studies of Left Ventricular Dysfunction trials, which showed a risk reduction of 16% and a decrease in the number of patients admitted to the hospital for worsening heart failure.[58,59] The Survival and Ventricular Enlargement study showed that these benefits extended to patients in whom heart failure followed a myocardial infarction and in whom the risk for death was reduced by 21% with captopril.[42] Another major group of vasodilators, the calcium antagonists, produce short-term hemodynamic improvement but no long-term advantage. Good evidence shows that in patients with heart failure, calcium antagonists increase rather than diminish mortality.[25,29] The same seems to be true of a more recent agent, flosequinan, which produced balanced vasodilatation and reduced both preload and afterload. At a dose of 100 mg/d, flosequinan killed more patients than it saved, and the drug was withdrawn from use.[44] The large-scale trial of prostacyclin in patients with severe chronic refractory heart failure was stopped because the mortality in the treatment group exceeded that in the placebo group despite improved hemodynamics.[3,71]

Inotropes

The history of inotropic therapy in the management of heart failure is a chronicle of disappointments. Dobutamine produces impressive short-term clinical and hemodynamic benefit, but attempts to exploit these effects in the management of outpatients led to ventricular arrhythmias and increased mortality.[20] The phosphodiesterase inhibitors followed the same path from short-term benefit to long-term disaster,[40,64] as did the partial β-agonist xamoterol.[68] No exception to this gloomy history is the new drug vesnarinone, a phosphodiesterase inhibitor that prolongs the duration of the action potential by its effect on ion channels.[46] Vesnarinone increased mortality fivefold, an adverse effect more dramatic than that seen with any other inotrope.[27] Recent studies have shown that digoxin does not seem to confer any survival benefit in congestive heart failure.[21] Thus, it seems that enhancing contractility and vasodilatation alone may not necessarily be a good therapeutic end point in congestive heart failure; clearly, short-term success may spell long-term disaster (Table 37-1).

Hemodynamics and mortality in congestive heart failure

The interesting point that emerges from the long-term trials of drugs in congestive heart failure is that reductions in mortality and morbidity bear little relation to changes in hemodynamics. In the first VHeFT trial, prazosin was a more effective vasodilator than the hydralazine–nitrate combination, but it had no significant effect on mortality.[13] In the second VHeFT trial, the hydralazine–nitrate combination increased peak oxygen consumption and ejection fraction to a greater extent than enalapril, but it was enalapril, not hydralazine–nitrate, that reduced mortality.[14] The same discrepancy between hemodynamics and clinical outcome seems to apply to patients receiving cardiac transplants. Stevenson et al[60] compared ejection fraction and exercise capacity in patients who underwent cardiac transplantation with those of transplant candidates who were maintained with ACE inhibitors, digoxin, and diuretic agents. The similarity in exercise performance was unexpected in the two groups, and the results show clearly how poorly hemodynamic changes are reflected in an increase in physical capacity. The results of the ACE inhibitor studies suggest that the drugs might prolong survival because of a nonperipheral vasodilator effect caused by the antagonism of vasoconstrictor neurohormones or by some direct metabolic or cardioprotective effect. Some evidence shows that this is the case. The clinical deterioration associated with the use of calcium antagonists in congestive heart failure seems to be more a consequence of increased plasma levels of renin, vasopressin, and noradrenaline than of negative inotropicity.[4] Digoxin, the original inotrope, reduces the levels of noradrenaline, renin, and aldosterone, and

Table 37-1. Effect of therapy on mortality in congestive heart failure in large controlled studies

Improves mortality in ischemic heart disease and idiopathic dilated cardiomyopathy	Improves mortality in idiopathic dilated cardiomyopathy only	No effect on mortality	Increases mortality
Nitrates and hydralazine	Bisoprolol	Prazosin	Milrinone
Angiotensin-converting enzyme inhibitors	Amiodarone	Digoxin	Amrinone
Carvedilol	Amlodipine		Vesnarinone
Warfarin	Felodipine		Dobutamine
			Enoximone
			Ibupamine
			Prostaglandin derivatives
			Flosequinan
			Xamaterol
			Nifedipine
			Flolan

a decrease in noradrenaline level is correlated with an increase in cardiac index. Despite this fact, digoxin showed no survival benefit.[21,47] Cohn et al[15] have shown that plasma noradrenaline is an entirely independent predictor of mortality in patients with congestive heart failure, and in the VHeFT II trial, it was the only factor that paralleled the increased survival rate.[28] The higher the patient's baseline noradrenaline level, the higher their mortality over the 5 years of the trial (Fig. 37-1). Plasma noradrenaline clearly delineates the risk categories, but the relation between renin and increased mortality is much less clear.

Adrenergic receptor density and mortality in congestive heart failure

Chronic sympathetic activation in congestive heart failure produces receptor downregulation, a decrease in the surface density of cardiac β-1 receptors.[8] The existence of downregulation as a physiologic entity has been accepted for years, but recent evidence suggests that the decrease in adrenergic receptor density in patients with congestive heart failure is an independent predictor of early death.[37] Merlet et al[37] used iodine-123 (^{123}I) metaiodobenzylguanidine (MIBG) as a direct marker of cardiac adrenergic activity in 90 patients with at least one episode of decompensated congestive heart failure related to idiopathic or ischemic cardiomyopathy. They also used radionuclide venticulography to measure left ventricular ejection fraction, M-mode echocardiography to measure end-diastolic and end-systolic diameter, and radiology to measure the cardiothoracic ratio. There were 22 deaths in the course of the study. Multivariate analyses related the baseline measurements to survival (Table 37-2), and life table analysis related them to duration of life (Tables 37-3 and 37-4). The results were analyzed separately for patients with idiopathic or ischemic cardiomy-

Table 37-2. Predictors of survival: multivariate analysis*

Variable	P Value
Reduced cardiac MIBG uptake	<0.0001
Cardiothoracic ratio	0.0017
End-diastolic diameter	0.0264
Left ventricular ejection fraction	0.0301

*MIBG = metaiodobenzylguanidine.

Table 37-3. Predictors of life duration: life table analysis*

Variable	P Value
Reduced cardiac MIBG uptake	<0.0001
Cardiothoracic ratio	0.0013
Left ventricular ejection fraction	0.0098

*MIBG = metaiodobenzylguanidine.

Table 37-4. Predictors of survival: multivariate analysis*

Variable	P value Idiopathic cardiomyopathy	P value Ischemic cardiomyopathy
Reduced cardiac MIBG uptake	<0.0001	0.0004
End-diastolic diameter	n.s.	n.s.
Left ventricular ejection fraction	n.s.	0.02

*MIBG = metaiodobenzylguanidine; n.s. = not significant.

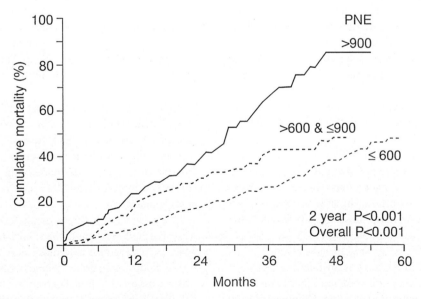

Fig. 37-1. The effect of increasing levels of plasma norepineprine (PNE) on mortality in patients with congestive heart failure. (Adapted from data published in Cohn JH et al: Plasma norepinephrine as a guide to prognosis in patients with chronic congestive heart failure, *N Engl J Med* 311:819-823, 1984.)

opathy (Table 37-4). Cardiac MIBG uptake, and by implication, β-adrenergic receptor density predict outcome more effectively than any of the standard noninvasive measurements of left ventricular function in patients with congestive heart failure. This evidence of cardiac adrenergic dysfunction is much more specific than that derived from measurements of plasma noradrenaline, reflecting the generalized and systemic adrenergic activity. This reduced uptake of an adrenergic marker could be a consequence of receptor internalization rather than reduced receptor density, but Bristow et al[9] recently showed that the ventricles of patients in congestive failure have a lower surface density of β-1-adrenergic receptors and a deficiency in β-1 receptor messenger RNA. This suggests that the fundamental mechanism of adrenergic dysfunction in patients with congestive failure may be an alteration in gene expression. Imaging methods that address this system may provide a powerful tool for monitoring outcome in patients with congestive heart failure.

The antiadrenergic approach: β-blockers in heart failure

When β-blockers were introduced 30 years ago, heart failure was an emphatic contraindication, and using them defied the prevailing orthodoxy that the failing heart was dependent on sympathetic drive. In 1975, when Waagstein et al[66] showed that β-blockers were effective in patients with congestive cardiomyopathy, few were convinced.[66] This skepticism was understandable: The original report was a series of uncontrolled observations, and the follow-up, which showed that β-blockers could prolong survival, used historical rather than concurrent controls.[61] Englemeier et al,[26] in a controlled trial of metoprolol in dilated cardiomyopathy, showed that patients who received β-blockers felt better, could exercise longer, and had improved cardiac function.[26] Results in the patients who developed congestive failure in the postinfarction β-blocker Heart Attack Trial of propranolol showed that the benefits of β-blockade were greater in patients with congestive failure than in those without this condition and pointed to the same conclusion.[10] Basu et al[5] from our group showed similar effects with carvedilol (a new multiple-action vasodilating β-blocker) in acute myocardial infarction with cardiac failure in the thrombolytic era.[5]

Evidence indicates that β-blockers improve systolic function in patients with heart failure and that the improvement in cardiac function is greater than that produced by any other form of treatment.[23,38] Possible reasons for initial worsening of heart failure that sometimes follows after doses of β-blockers is the fact that these drugs increase vascular resistance, cardiac volumes, and thus afterload in the absence of vasodilatation. Furthermore, the acute effect of reducing heart rate in a tachycardia-dependent patient can decrease cardiac output before producing any significant receptor upregulation. Compounds with a vasodilator component that minimize or reduce systemic resistance and leave cardiac output unchanged may be preferred in patients with congestive heart failure. Thus, one may be able to measure myocardial catecholamine turnover by using [123]I-

MIBG imaging and to streamline therapeutic management by selecting patients with the greatest degree of downregulation due to neurohormonal activation. By using this technique, one may be able to dedicate correct imaging methods to guide therapy. However, because ^{123}I MIBG is not taken up by the failing heart muscle, or the infarcted myocardium, imaging may be difficult in ischemic cardiomyopathy. Thus, a combination of a perfusion tracer (such as thallium-201 [^{201}Tl] or technetium-99m [^{99m}Tc] sestamibi) may be used to define viable but downregulated myocardium. This hypothesis requires further evaluation.

Clearly, much has changed in the past few years, with the development of new multiple-action drugs, such as carvedilol.[5,17,32] We believe that understanding the effects of carvedilol in congestive heart failure may be the key to understanding the complexity of end-stage ischemic cardiomyopathy. Carvedilol is a nonselective β-blocker, has α_1 blocking properties (vasodilatation and, probably, free-radical suppression), is a potent antioxidant, reduces endothelial cell proliferation, and suppresses free radical production.[49,50,69,70] Carvedilol has been shown to reduce mortality in congestive heart failure over and above conventional treatment in an unprecedented manner.[7,39] We have previously shown that carvedilol improves both systolic and diastolic left ventricular function,[34] improves hibernating myocardium,[16] and reduces cardiac arrhythmias[57] in patients with ischemic heart disease and left ventricular dysfunction.

ISCHEMIC CARDIOMYOPATHY

Table 37-1 shows a list of drugs that increase mortality in congestive cardiac failure. It is clear from these data that understanding the underlying etiology and pathophysiology of congestive heart failure is of utmost importance, because the choice of therapy and investigations will depend greatly on these issues. Many drugs improve mortality in idiopathic dilated cardiomyopathy, but only a handful favorably alter mortality in ischemic cardiomyopathy. Thus, it seems that ischemia per se may play a major role in the genesis of worsening heart failure in this condition.

Ischemic cardiomyopathy defines patients who are at variable clinical states with compromised cardiac function due to ischemic heart disease and are nonhomogenous. Thus, their management is difficult and cannot be complete without detailed knowledge of their underlying myocardial perfusion or contractile reserve. Only then can relevant therapeutic decisions be made.

The early warning signs of the failure of medical regimens were inherently present in the CASS data. It was surprising that when patients were randomized into surgical (coronary artery bypass graft) and medical therapy cohorts, the overall survival was not different.[18] It became apparent that patients with high-risk disease benefited significantly. What was surprising at the time was that patients with a left ventricular ejection fraction of 26% or less did significantly better with surgery (revascularization) than with medical treatment (Fig. 37-2). This was the first large-scale trial to indicate that silent ischemia or hibernating

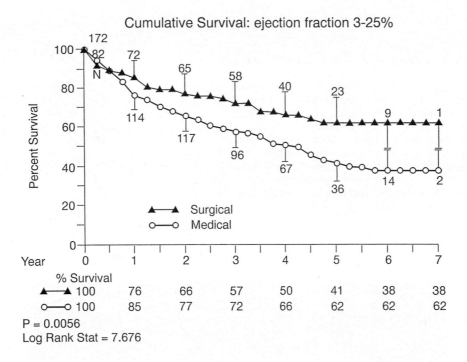

Fig. 37-2. Data from the Coronary Artery Surgery Study show benefit of coronary artery bypass graft surgery on survival in patients with low ejection fraction compared to medical treatment. (From Alderman EL, Fisher LD, Litwin P, et al: Results of coronary artery surgery in patients with poor left ventricular function (CASS), *Circulation* 68:785-795, 1983.)

myocardium may be implicated in the genesis of heart failure and that survival could be prolonged by revascularization.

Myocardial perfusion and metabolism

Recently, many studies have been performed with positron emission tomography (PET), single-photon perfusion imaging agents (^{201}Tl or ^{99m}Tc sestamibi); and dobutamine echocardiography, which clearly groups patients with ischemic cardiomyopathy into those who have hibernating myocardium (viable but dysfunctional myocardium with reduced myocardial blood flow) or those who have left ventricular dysfunction due to nonviable myocardium or scar.[6,11,43,51] In a seminal study with PET, Di Carli et al[19] clearly demonstrated the value of revascularization in patients with congestive cardiac failure secondary to coronary artery disease. Significant improvement in survival and morbidity occurred when myocardial viability was present in severely dysfunctional myocardium. It was clearly demonstrated that the greater the degree of metabolism–flow mismatch (extent of hibernating myocardium), the better the result of revascularization.[19]

Because PET is not freely available to most physicians, others have adapted the metabolic properties of ^{201}Tl[8,57] and ^{99m}Tc sestamibi[63] to detect viable myocardium in patients with left ventricular dysfunction. The aim of this chapter is not to compare the various methods and protocols but to present the theoretical basis for the evaluation of hibernating myocardium and to discuss the direction of future studies.

Because hibernating, stunned, and necrotic myocardium can coexist in the same patient and because demarcation of these

states is not always clear, it may be difficult to understand the consequences of therapy in this complex pathologic state. Hibernating myocardium is often segmental and is associated with coronary artery stenosis. It has been described as a state of "metabolic adaptation" to low flow.[48] Rahimtoola[45] first described the benefit of revascularization and restitution of blood flow and demonstrated significant recovery of contractile function in patients with severe ischemic left ventricular dysfunction. By using a combination of low-dose dobutamine infusion during echocardiography (assessment of contractile reserve) and nitrate-enhanced ^{201}Tl imaging at rest (to assess metabolic state and blood flow), we have shown that patients with severe left ventricular dysfunction and congestive heart failure can be safely selected for revascularization.[51] Revascularization produced excellent survival and significantly improved global left ventricular function in these patients[51] (Figs. 37-3 and 37-4).

Myocardial ischemia and ischemic cardiomyopathy

Ischemic cardiomyopathy is a term used loosely to describe left ventricular dysfunction in the presence of coronary artery disease. However, the term *ischemic* is probably derived from *ischemic heart disease* and does not imply that there is ongoing ischemia, because most therapy (medical) for congestive heart failure was not directed towards ischemia but may have in fact induced ischemia. Clinical trials have shown that many drugs that enhance myocardial oxygen demand are associated with increased mortality; in contrast, β-blockers and ACE inhibitors reduce myocardial demand and also seem to improve survival in congestive heart failure.[32] Approximately 80% of patients in

Fig. 37-3. Left ventricular ejection fraction *(LVEF)* at rest *(basal)* and 3 months after revascularization *(post).* **A,** Patients with improved wall thickening in two or more contiguous segments as demonstrated by dobutamine echocardiography. **B,** Patients with at least grade 3 thallium-201 uptake in two or more contiguous segments before surgery. The solid line indicates patients with greater than or equal to 5% improvement in LVEF after revascularization; the dashed line indicates patients with less than 5% improvement in ejection fraction after revascularization. Error bars show the mean (SD). * = $p<0.001$; ** = $p<0.005$ (patient *t* test). (From Senior R, Glenville B, Basu S, et al: Dobutamine echocardiography and thallium-201 imaging predict functional improvement after revascularization in severe ischaemic left ventricular dysfunction, *Br Heart J* 74:358-364, 1995.)

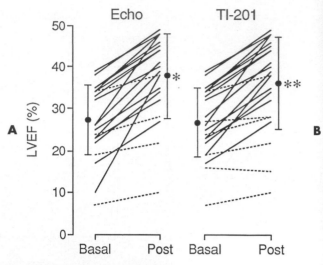

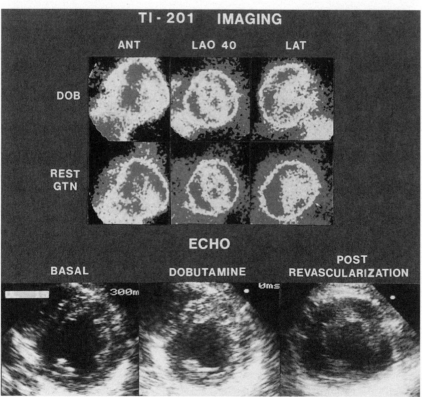

Fig. 37-4. Composite image of a patient with a preoperative left ventricular ejection fraction of 17%, triple-vessel disease, and New York Heart Association class IV congestive heart failure. *Top,* Dobutamine and rest-redistribution thallium-201 (^{201}Tl) imaging at 1 hour after treatment with glyceryl trinitrate *(GTN)* shows retained viability in the anterior, septal, and lateral walls. *Bottom,* Short-axis end-systolic echocardiographic images at rest *(basal) (left)* and low-dose dobutamine *(middle)* before surgery and at rest 3 months after revascularization *(right).* The basal echocardiogram shows discordance caused by severe global hypokinesia (left ventricular ejection fraction, 17%). The dobutamine echocardiogram shows improved wall thickening in the anteroseptal, lateral, and inferior walls (left ventricular ejection fraction 30%) but not in the inferoposterolateral wall, which shows a matching perfusion defect in the same region with ^{201}Tl. Three months after revascularization, improved contractility was seen in the anteroseptal and lateral walls (predicted by ^{201}Tl and dobutamine echocardiography). The postoperative left ventricular ejection fraction improved to 32%. Reduced anterolateral perfusion can be seen on ^{201}Tl imaging during dobutamine infusion despite increased contractility as demonstrated by echocardiography in the same region. (From Senior R, Glenville B, Basu S, et al: Dobutamine echocardiography and thallium-201 imaging predict functional improvement after revascularization in severe ischaemic left ventricular dysfunction, *Br Heart J* 74:358-364, 1995.)

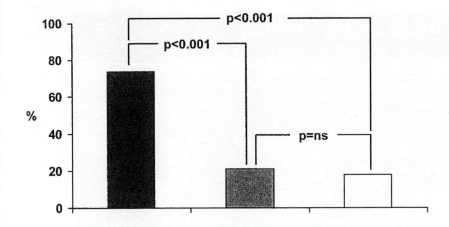

reversible perfusion defect (MIBI) ▨ **exercise ST depression** ☐ **angina**

Fig. 37-5. Painless reversible perfusion defects on technetium-99m sestamibi scans occur more often than ST-segment changes or angina in patients with ischemic cardiomyopathy. (From Senior R, Kaul S, Raval U, et al: Painless myocardial ischaemia is frequently associated with hibernating myocardium in congestive heart failure, *Eur Heart J* 17(Suppl):154, 1996 (abstract). With permission of the publisher WB Saunders Company Limited, London.)

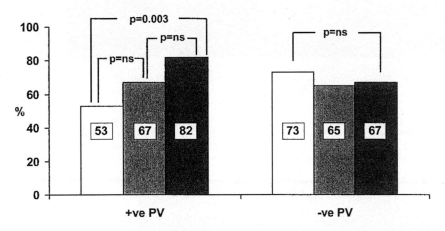

☐ **cellular viability** ▨ **reversible ischaemia** ■ **viability + ischaemia**

Fig. 37-6. The predictive value *(PV)* of combined cellular viability and reversible perfusion defects was significantly better than viability alone for predicting recovery of regional left ventricular function after revascularization. (From Senior R, Kaul S, Raval U, et al: Demonstration of reversible ischaemia is a better predictor of functional recovery after revascularization than presence of cellular variability alone in ischaemic cardiomyopathy, *Eur Heart J* 18(suppl):245, 1997 (abstract). With permission of the publisher WB Saunders Company Limited, London.)

the large trials in congestive heart failure had underlying ischemic heart disease, and myocardial "ischemia" may have played a part in the genesis of worsening heart failure or death.[58] Because hibernating myocardium is not an uncommon finding and because the phenomenon may be associated with severe prolonged and repetitive ischemia, further increases in myocardial demand may induce ischemia. This enhanced oxygen demand can be a catecholamine-induced or effort-induced stress.

In patients with coronary artery disease and left ventricular dysfunction, low-dose and high-dose dobutamine echocardiography may be used to clearly describe a phenomenon termed the *biphasic response*.[56] At lower levels of inotropic stress, viable but hibernating myocardium will often show increased wall thickening (a sign of viability and contractile reserve), but at a higher dose of dobutamine, this is followed by a significant decrease in wall thickening due to myocardial ischemia in the same segment. This ischemia is caused by increased myocardial demand that surpasses the ischemic threshold.[56] This phenomenon was recently used as a prognostic marker by other investigators and implies that ischemia

may be an important underlying determinant of outcome in patients with coronary artery disease and left ventricular dysfunction.[67]

There has been considerable confusion with regard to ischemia in patients with ischemic cardiomyopathy. Senior et al[53] prospectively studied 57 unselected patients with congestive heart failure secondary to coronary artery disease who had a left ventricular ejection fraction less than 35% by stress–rest (nitrate-enhanced) ^{99m}Tc sestamibi single-photon emission computed tomography. The classic hallmarks of ischemia (angina and ST-segment depression) were poor indicators of ischemia, but reversible ischemia was present in 74% of patients (Fig. 37-5).[53] Thus, in the absence of classic hallmarks, painless ischemia was a common finding. In the same study, revascularization was performed in 23 patients, and reversible ischemia was found to be a better predictor of functional recovery than myocardial viability alone (Fig. 37-6).[54] Figure 37-7 shows ^{99m}Tc sestamibi images of a patient who was on a heart transplantation waiting list for end-stage heart failure, in whom revascularization produced considerable improvement in function. Figure 37-8 shows echocardiographic images from the same pa-

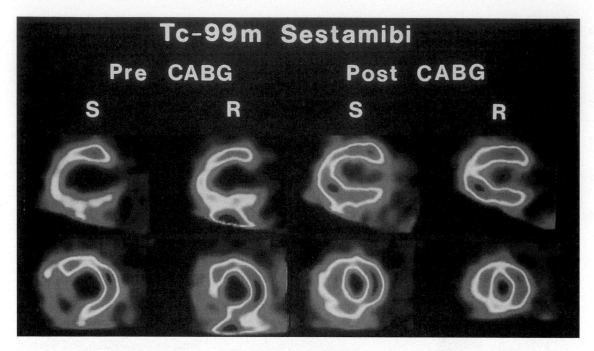

Fig. 37-7. Technetium-99m sestamibi *(MIBI)* single-photon emission computed tomography in a 42-year-old man with New York Heart Association class IV heart failure *(CHF)* who was awaiting heart transplantation. The rest *(R)* nitrate-enhanced MIBI image shows extensive myocardial viability despite left ventricular ejection fraction of 17% (Fig. 37-8). Extensive ischemia was noted by stress *(S)* MIBI after 2 minutes of a modified Bruce protocol. Three months after triple-vessel revascularization, exercise tolerance increased to 10 minutes of Bruce protocol, with a normal MIBI, improvement in left ventricular ejection fraction to 48% (Fig. 37-8), and no evidence of CHF.

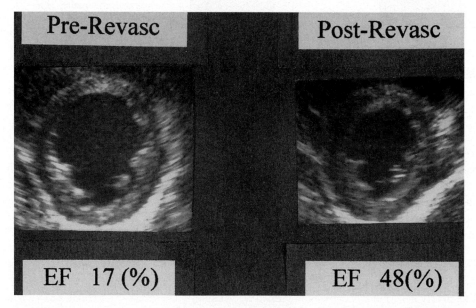

Fig. 37-8. Same patient as in Fig. 36-7. The end-systolic short-axis echocardiographic images show significant improvement in left ventricular function after revascularization (ejection fraction, 17% to 48%).

tient, who had a profound improvement in left ventricular ejection fraction from 17% to 48% 3 months after surgery.

Prognosis

It is clear that revascularization in patients with poor cardiac function improves prognosis. The question is, do we need to as-

sess myocardial viability, hibernating myocardium, or reversible ischemia, or could one revascularize without performing an imaging study? Studies from Yale University have shown improvements in left ventricular ejection fraction function and survival in patients with impaired left ventricular function who were undergoing surgical coronary revasculariza-

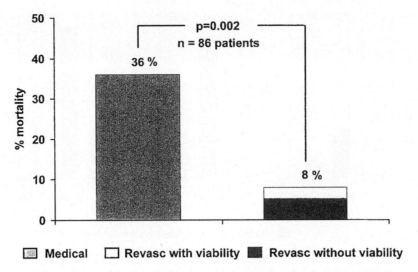

Fig. 37-9. Prognostic value of revascularization in ischemic cardiomyopathy during a 5-year follow-up (86 patients). Of 30 patients who underwent revascularization, only 1 patient with myocardial viability died after surgery. (From Senior R, et al: Personal Communication, 1997.)

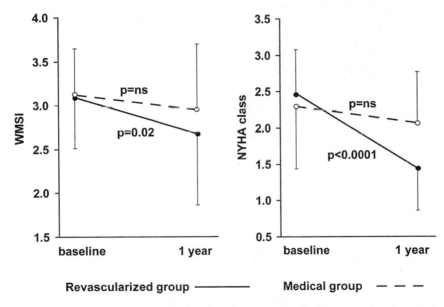

Fig. 37-10. The benefit of revascularization (30 patients) compared with conventional medical treatment (56 patients). NYHA = New York Heart Association class for congestive heart failure; WMSI = wall-motion score index (by echocardiography). (From Senior R, et al: Personal Communication, 1997.)

tion.[24] This result supports the original data from the CASS trial.[1] Thus, the question remains, what is the implication of performing revascularization surgery in patients without myocardial viability?

Recent studies by Pagley et al[41] clearly show that patients without myocardial viability and with left ventricular dysfunction have a poorer outcome after revascularization. Studies from our group support this hypothesis.[52] A 5-year follow-up study of 86 patients (mean left ventricular ejection fraction 25% ± 9%) with congestive cardiac failure due to coronary

artery disease had a better survival outcome compared to those who received conventional medical therapy. However, these patients were not treated with new-generation β-blockers, such as carvedilol. Eighteen patients (36%) died in the medical therapy group compared with 3 (8%) in the revascularization group (Fig. 37-9). Of note, of the three patients who died in the revascularization group, only 1 had residual myocardial viability. Revascularization also produced reductions in regional wall-motion score index and New York Heart Association functional class (Fig. 37-10).[52]

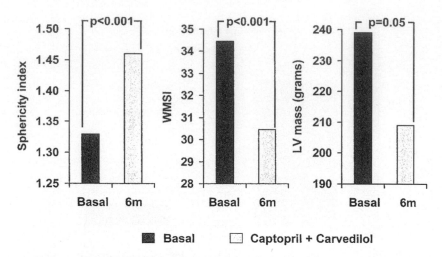

Basal   ☐ Captopril + Carvedilol

Fig. 37-11. Echocardiographic estimation of remodeling in 18 patients with congestive heart failure undergoing treatment with carvedilol and captopril. Note the changes in wall-motion score index *(WMSI)* and left ventricular mass.

Remodeling

One of the most unwanted complications of chronic congestive heart failure is pathologic remodeling. This is the heart's adaptation to mechanical and subsequent neurohormonal stress. Recent studies by Villanueva et al[65] showed that revascularization produces a significant improvement in microvascular function and reverse remodeling. Thus, regression of remodeling will significantly alter regional and global left ventricular function and wall thickening, and the improvement in left ventricular wall motion may be a composite of regression of remodeling and ischemia-induced dyskinesis. This phenomenon is clearly seen in results of an ongoing study of a combination of carvedilol and captopril in 18 patients with congestive heart failure after 6 months of treatment.[55] Regression of remodeling was associated with reduction in left ventricular mass, regional wall-thickening abnormality, and alteration of cardiac geometry (the sphericity index) (Fig. 37-11). These data may partly explain the complex underlying mechanisms at play after revascularization. The improvement in wall motion abnormality may be a result of combination of improvements in regional hypoxia and regression of remodeling. Radionuclide ventriculography may be used to calculate change in cardiac shape as well, but these studies are probably best done with echocardiography and magnetic resonance imaging.

In patients with congestive heart failure, it is important to assess the effects of revascularization in light of newer medical therapies, since much has changed in the last decade. Although "blood is the best medicine for ischemic cardiomyopathy," a substantial group of patients with congestive heart failure and hibernating myocardium remains who will not be able to undergo revascularization because of poor coronary anatomy or limited resources. Nuclear cardiology techniques should be rationally applied to risk stratification and therapeutic selection in patients with ischemic cardiomyopathy.

ACKNOWLEDGMENT

We thank Ms. Usha Raval and Mr. Christopher Kinsey for technical support and Mrs. Minal Shah for preparation of the manuscript.

REFERENCES

1. Alderman EL, Fisher LD, Litwin P, et al: Results of coronary artery surgery in patients with poor left ventricular function (CASS), *Circulation* 68:785–795, 1983.
2. Armstrong PW, Armstrong JA, Marks GS, et al: Pharmacokinetic-hemodynamic studies of intravenous nitroglycerin in congestive cardiac failure, *Circulation* 62:160–166, 1980.
3. Armstrong PW, Moe GW: Medical advances in the treatment of congestive heart failure, *Circulation* 88:2941–2952, 1994.
4. Barjon JN, Rouleau JL, Bichet D, et al: Chronic renal and neurohumoral effects of the calcium entry blocker nisoldipine in patients with congestive heart failure, *J Am Coll Cardiol* 9:622–630, 1987.
5. Basu S, Senior R, Raval U, et al: Beneficial effects of intravenous and oral carvedilol treatment in acute myocardial infarction. A placebo-controlled, randomized trial, *Circulation* 96:183–191, 1997.
6. Bonow RO, Dilsizian V, Cuocolo A, et al: Identification of viable myocardium in patients with chronic coronary artery disease and left ventricular dysfunction. Comparison of thallium scintigraphy with reinjection and PET imaging with ^{18}F-fluorodeoxyglucose, *Circulation* 83:26–37, 1991.
7. Bristow MR, Gilbert EM, Abraham WT, et al: Carvedilol produces dose-related improvements in left ventricular function and survival in subjects with chronic heart failure. MOCHA Investigators, *Circulation* 94:2807–2816, 1996.
8. Bristow MR, Ginsburg R, Minobe W, et al: Decreased catecholamine sensitivity and β-adrenergic-receptor density in failing human hearts, *N Engl J Med* 307:205–211, 1982.
9. Bristow MR, Minobe WA, Raynolds MV, et al: Reduced β 1 receptor messenger RNA abundance in the failing human heart, *J Clin Invest* 92:2737–2745, 1993.
10. Chadda K, Goldstein S, Byington R, et al: Effect of propranolol after acute myocardial infarction in patients with congestive heart failure, *Circulation* 73:503–510, 1986.
11. Cigarroa CG, deFilippi CR, Brickner ME, et al: Dobutamine stress echocardiography identifies hibernating myocardium and predicts re-

covery of left ventricular function after coronary revascularization, *Circulation* 88:430–436, 1993.

12. Cintron G, Johnson G, Francis G, et al: Prognostic significance of serial changes in left ventricular ejection fraction in patients with congestive heart failure. The V-HeFT VA Cooperative Studies Group, *Circulation* 87 (6 Suppl):VI17–VI23, 1993.

13. Cohn JN, Archibald DG, Ziesche S, et al: Effect of vasodilator therapy on mortality in chronic congestive heart failure. Results of a Veterans Administration Cooperative Study, *N Engl J Med* 314:1547–1552, 1986.

14. Cohn JN, Johnson G, Ziesche S, et al: A comparison of enalapril with hydralazine-isosorbide dinitrate in the treatment of chronic congestive heart failure, *N Engl J Med* 325:303–310, 1991.

15. Cohn JN, Levine TB, Olivari MT, et al: Plasma norepinephrine as a guide to prognosis in patients with chronic congestive heart failure, *N Engl J Med* 311:819–823, 1984.

16. Das Gupta P, Broadhurst P, Raftery EB, et al: Value of carvedilol in congestive heart failure secondary to coronary artery disease, *Am J Cardiol* 66:1118–1123, 1990.

17. Das Gupta P, Lahiri A: Can intravenous β-blockade predict long-term hemodynamic benefit in chronic congestive heart failure secondary to ischemic heart disease? *J Cardiovasc Pharmacol* 19 Suppl 1:S62–S67, 1992.

18. Davis KB, Alderman EL, Kosinski AS, et al: Early mortality of acute myocardial infarction in patients with and without prior coronary revascularization surgery. A Coronary Artery Surgery Study Registry Study, *Circulation* 85:2100–2109, 1992.

19. Di Carli MF, Asgarzadie F, Schelbert HR, et al: Quantitative relation between myocardial viability and improvement in heart failure symptoms after revascularization in patients with ischemic cardiomyopathy, *Circulation* 92:3436–3444, 1995.

20. Dies F, Krell MJ, Whitlow CS, et al: Intermittent dobutamine in ambulatory outpatients with chronic cardiac failure, *Circulation* 74(Suppl 2):II-138, 1986.

21. The effect of digoxin on mortality and morbidity in patients with heart failure. The Digitalis Investigation Group, *N Engl J Med* 336:525–533, 1997.

22. Edwards NC, Sinusas AJ, Bergin JD, et al: Influence of subendocardial ischemia on transmural myocardial function, *Am J Physiol* 262:H568–H576, 1992.

23. Eichhorn EJ, Bedotto JB, Malloy CR, et al: Effect of β-adrenergic blockade on myocardial function and energetics in congestive heart failure. Improvements in hemodynamic, contractile, and diastolic performance with bucindolol, *Circulation* 82:473–483, 1990.

24. Elefteriades JA, Morales DLS, Gradel C, et al: Results of coronary artery bypass grafting by a single surgeon in patients with left ventricular ejection fractions ≤30%, *Am J Cardiol* 79:1573–1578, 1997.

25. Elkayam U, Amin J, Mehra A, et al: A prospective, randomized, double-blind, crossover study to compare the efficacy and safety of chronic nifedipine therapy with that of isosorbide dinitrate and their combination in the treatment of chronic congestive heart failure, *Circulation* 82:1954–1961, 1990.

26. Engelmeier RS, O'Connell JB, Walsh R, et al: Improvement in symptoms and exercise tolerance by metoprolol in patients with dilated cardiomyopathy: a double-blind, randomized, placebo-controlled trial, *Circulation* 72:536–546, 1985.

27. Feldman AM, Bristow MR, Parmley WW, et al: Effects of vesnarinone on morbidity and mortality in patients with heart failure, *New Engl J Med* 329:149–155, 1993.

28. Francis GS, Cohn JN, Johnson G, et al: Plasma norepinephrine, plasma renin activity, and congestive heart failure. Relations to survival and the effects of therapy in VHeFT II. The VHeFT VA Cooperative Studies Group, *Circulation* 87(Suppl):VI40–VI48, 1993.

29. Goldstein RE, Boccuzzi SJ, Cruess D, et al: Diltiazem increases late-onset congestive heart failure in postinfarction patients with early reduction in ejection fraction. The Adverse Experience Committee; and

30. the Multicenter Diltiazem Postinfarction Research Group, *Circulation* 83:52–60, 1991.

30. Guiha NH, Cohn JN, Mikulic E, et al: Treatment of refractory heart failure with infusion of nitroprusside, *N Engl J Med* 291:587–592, 1974.

31. Ho KKL, Anderson KM, Kannel WB, et al: Survival after the onset of congestive heart failure in Framingham Heart Study subjects, *Circulation* 88:107–115, 1993.

32. Lahiri A: Neurohumoral mechanisms in congestive heart failure and the role of drugs with multiple actions: a review of carvedilol, *American Journal of Therapeutics* 3:237–247, 1996.

33. Lahiri A, Crawley JCW, Sonecha TN, et al: Acute and chronic effects of sustained action buccal nitroglycerin in severe congestive heart failure, *Int J Cardiol* 5:39–48, 1984.

34. Lahiri A, Rodrigues EA, Al-Khawaja I, et al: Effects of a new vasodilating beta-blocking drug, carvedilol, on left ventricular function in stable angina pectoris, *Am J Cardiol* 59:769–774, 1987.

35. Majid PA, Sharma B, Taylor SH: Phentolamine for vasodilator treatment of severe heart-failure, *Lancet* 2:719–724, 1971.

36. Massie BM, Shah NB: The heart failure epidemic: magnitude of the problem and potential mitigating approaches, *Curr Opin Cardiol* 11:221–226, 1996.

37. Merlet P, Valette H, Dubois-Randé JL, et al: Prognostic value of cardiac metaiodobenzylguanidine imaging in patients with heart failure, *J Nucl Med* 33:471–477, 1992.

38. Olsen SL, Gilbert EM, Renlund DG, et al: Carvedilol improves left ventricular function in idiopathic dilated cardiomyopathy, *Circulation* 84(Suppl II):II564, 1991.

39. Packer M, Bristow MR, Cohn JN, et al: The effect of carvedilol on morbidity and mortality in patients with chronic heart failure, *N Engl J Med* 334:1349–1355, 1996.

40. Packer M, Carver JR, Rodeheffer RJ, et al: Effect of oral milrinone on mortality in severe chronic heart failure. The PROMISE Study Research Group, *N Engl J Med* 325:1468–1475, 1991.

41. Pagley PR, Beller GA, Watson DD, et al: Improved outcome after coronary bypass surgery in patients with ischemic cardiomyopathy and residual myocardial viability, *Circulation* 96:793–800, 1997.

42. Pfeffer MA, Braunwald E, Moyé LA, et al: Effect of captopril on mortality and morbidity in patients with left ventricular dysfunction after myocardial infarction. Results of the survival and ventricular enlargement trial. The SAVE Investigators, *N Engl J Med* 327:669–677, 1992.

43. Pierard LA, De Landsheere CM, Berthe C, et al: Identification of viable myocardium by echocardiography during dobutamine infusion in patients with myocardial infarction after thrombolytic therapy: comparison with positron emission tomography, *J Am Coll Cardiol* 15:1021–1031, 1990.

44. Prospective Randomized Flosequinan Longevity Evaluation (PROFILE), (in press).

45. Rahimtoola SH: The hibernating myocardium, *Am Heart J* 117:211–221, 1989.

46. Rapundalo ST, Lathrop DA, Harrison SA, et al: Cyclic AMP-dependent and cyclic AMP-independent actions of a novel cardiotonic agent, OPC-8212, *Naunyn Schmiedebergs Arch Pharmacol* 338:692–698, 1988.

47. Ribner HSA, Plucinski DA, Hsieh AM, et al: Acute effects of digoxin on total systemic vascular resistance in congestive heart failure due to dilated cardiomyopathy: a hemodynamic-hormonal study, *Am J Cardiol* 56:896–904, 1985.

48. Ross J Jr: Myocardial perfusion-contraction matching. Implications for coronary heart disease and hibernation, *Circulation* 83:1076–1083, 1991.

49. Ruffolo RR, Boyle DA, Brooks DP, et al: Carvedilol: a novel cardiovascular drug with multiple actions, *Cardiovascular Drug Review* 10:127–157, 1992.

50. Ruffolo RR Jr, Gellai M, Hieble JP, et al: The pharmacology of carvedilol, *Eur J Clin Pharmacol* 38:S82–S88, 1990.

51. Senior R, Glenville B, Basu S, et al: Dobutamine echocardiography

and thallium-201 imaging predict functional improvement after revascularization in severe ischaemic left ventricular dysfunction, *Br Heart J* 74:358–364, 1995.

52. Senior R, Kaul S, Lahiri A: Improved survival after revascularization in patients with ischaemic cardiomyopathy, *European Heart Journal* Suppl, in press (abstract).

53. Senior R, Kaul S, Raval U, et al: Painless myocardial ischaemia is frequently associated with hibernating myocardium in congestive heart failure, *Eur Heart J* 17(Suppl):154, 1996 (abstract).

54. Senior R, Kaul S, Raval U, et al: Demonstration of reversible ischaemia is a better predictor of functional recovery after revascularization than presence of cellular variability alone in ischaemic cardiomyopathy, *Eur Heart J* 18(Suppl):245, 1997 (abstract).

55. Lahiri A: The role of neurohormonal antagonists in hibernating myocardium, *Journal of Cardiovascular Pharmacology* Suppl, (in press).

56. Senior R, Lahiri A: Enhanced detection of myocardial ischemia by stress dobutamine echocardiography utilizing the "biphasic" response of wall thickening during low and high dose dobutamine infusion, *J Am Coll Cardiol* 26:26–32, 1995.

57. Senior R, Muller-Beckmann B, DasGupta P, et al: Effects of carvedilol on ventricular arrhythmias, *J Cardiovasc Pharmacol* 19 Suppl 1: S117–S121, 1992.

58. Effect of enalapril on survival in patients with reduced left ventricular ejection fractions and congestive heart failure. The SOLVD Investigators, *N Engl J Med* 325:293–302, 1991.

59. Effect of enalapril on mortality and the development of heart failure in asymptomatic patients with reduced left ventricular ejection fractions. The SOLVD Investigators, *N Engl J Med* 327:685–691, 1992.

60. Stevenson LW, Sietsema K, Tillisch JH, et al: Exercise capacity for survivors of cardiac transplantation or sustained medical therapy for stable heart failure, *Circulation* 81:78–85, 1990.

61. Swedberg K, Hjalmarson A, Waagstein F, et al: Prolongation of survival in congestive cardiomyopathy by β-receptor blockade, *Lancet* 1:1374–1376, 1979.

62. Tillisch J, Brunken R, Marshall R, et al: Reversibility of cardiac wall-motion abnormalities predicted by positron tomography, *N Engl J Med* 314:884–888, 1986.

63. Udelson JE, Coleman PS, Metherall J, et al: Predicting recovery of severe regional ventricular dysfunction. Comparison of resting scintigraphy with ^{201}Tl and ^{99m}Tc-sestamibi, *Circulation* 89:2552–2561, 1994.

64. Uretsky BF, Jessup M, Konstam MA, et al: Multicenter trial of oral enoximone in patients with moderate to moderately severe congestive heart failure. Lack of benefit compared with placebo. Enoximone Multicenter Trial Group, *Circulation* 82:774–780, 1990.

65. Villanueva FS, Glasheen WP, Sklenar J, et al: Characterization of spatial patterns of flow within the reperfused myocardium by myocardial contrast echocardiography. Implications in determining extent of myocardial salvage, *Circulation* 88:2596–2606, 1993.

66. Waagstein F, Hjalmarson A, Varnauscas E, et al: β-Blockers in dilated cardiomyopathy, *Br Heart J* 37:1022–1036, 1975.

67. Williams MJ, Odabashian J, Lauer MS, et al: Prognostic value of dobutamine echocardiography in patients with left ventricular dysfunction, *J Am Coll Cardiol* 27:132–139, 1996.

68. Xamoterol in severe heart failure. The Xamoterol in Severe Heart Failure Study Group, *Lancet* 336:1–6, 1990.

69. Yue T-L, Gu JL, Feurstein G: Carvedilol, a new beta-adrenoceptor antagonist and vasodilator antihypertensive drug, inhibits oxygen radical mediated lipid peroxidation in swine ventricular membranes, *Pharmacol Commun* 1:27–35, 1992.

70. Yue TL, McKenna PJ, Ruffolo RR Jr, et al: Carvedilol, a new beta-adrenoceptor antagonist and vasodilator antihypertensive drug, inhibits superoxide release from human neutrophils, *Eur J Pharmacol* 214:277–280, 1992.

71. Yui Y, Nakajima H, Kawai C, et al: Prostacyclin therapy in patients with congestive heart failure, *Am J Cardiol* 50:320–324, 1982.

Index

Page numbers in *italics* indicate illustrations; "t" indicates tables.

ST-segment depression with, 324
in thallium-201 SPECT, 242, 249, 251-252, 252t
propranolol and, *265*
protocol, 238
Dobutamine atropine stress, technetium-99m imaging with, prognosis and, 335
Dobutamine echocardiography, 326
clinical results, 374
disadvantages, 372, 373
in ischemic cardiomyopathy, *618*
in myocardial viability assessment, 507, 508, *508*, 509, 557
physiology, 369-370
in preoperative risk stratification, 356-357, 357t
in revascularization procedures, 420
Dodge-Sandler analogs, 218, *218*, 221
Dog model of radiotracer evaluation, 38, *60*
Dopamine, 315t
Doppler flow wire measurements, 407
Dripps-ASA index, 347, 347t
Drug abuse, gated SPECT studies in, 225
Drug effects on left ventricular function and volume, radionuclide angiographic assessment of, 210, 211
Dual isotope SPECT; *see* Single-photon emission computed tomography, dual isotope
Duke treadmill scores, dual isotope SPECT and, 292, *293*
Dynamic cardiac SPECT, 137-187
data analysis, 139
effects of physical aspects of image detection, 162
attenuation, 171, 171t
cardiac motion, 165, *166-167*
detector motion, 165-166, *168*
input function shape and acquisition interval, 166, 168-171, *169-170*, 171t
other physical factors in image detection, 171-172
partial volume, 162-165, *163*, 163-164t
estimation of kinetic parameters, 148-149
compensation of inconsistent projection data due to time-varying activity during camera rotation, 155-156, *156*
directly from projections, 156-162, *158-159*, 160t
from dynamic reconstructed images, 149-155, 154t, *154-155*
estimation of model parameters in dogs, 172
animal preparation, 172
data acquisition, 172-173
data analysis, 173, *173*
data visualization, 175, 176t, *177-179*, 178
initial results, 173, 173t, *174*, 175, 175t
objectives, 172
extraction of time-activity curves in, 146-148
future directions and summary, 178-181
imaging characteristics, 139-140
research and applications, 137-138
tracer kinetic modeling principles in, 140-142, *141*
compartment models for measuring cardiac function, 142-146, *143-145*
Dynamic imaging, in biological models of radiotracer evaluation, 39-43
Dysprosium-DTPA-BMA, 380

E

Echocardiography
in acute chest pain, 472
with dobutamine; *see* Dobutamine echocardiography
future of, 376
in ischemic cardiomyopathy, *618, 620, 622*
multimodality registration and, 110
myocardial contrast
microbubbles in, 384-385, *385-388*, 387t
relation between tracer concentration and signal intensity in, 391-393, *392-393*
temporal and spatial resolution, 393-394, *394-395*
stress; *see* Stress echocardiography
two-dimensional

in myocardium at risk estimation, 434-435, *434-435*
pharmacologic stress testing with, 326
Echogen, 398t
Efflux rate, 15
Ejection fraction; *see also* Left ventricular ejection fraction
in aortic regurgitation, 210
defect size and, 435, *436*
in first-pass and equilibrium radionuclide angiography, 206, *209*
global
in final infarct size measurement, 442
in myocardium at risk estimation, 434
late resting, in final infarct size measurement, 439
measured by miniaturized nonimaging detectors, *193-197*
in mitral regurgitation, 210-211, *211*
in myocardial diseases, 211
Electrocardiography
in acute chest pain, 470, *473, 482-483*, 492
technetium-99m imaging vs., *477, 479*
exercise; *see also* Exercise testing
prognostic value of, 338, *338, 339*
in final infarct size quantification, 439, 442
in myocardium at risk estimation, 434
in unstable angina, 492, *493*, 494-495
Emergency imaging studies, in acute chest pain, 480-485, 492-494
Emission imaging, in SPECT, attenuation map estimation and, *130*, 130-132, 132t
Enalapril, 613-614
End-diastolic volumes, measured by miniaturized nonimaging detectors, *196-197*
End-systolic volumes
after acute myocardial infarction, infarct size and, 436t, *437*
measured by miniaturized nonimaging detectors, *196-197*
Energy distribution methods, for scatter compensation in SPECT, 129-130
Energy transfer in heart muscle, 534
Energy-providing substrates for heart, 534-538, *535, 537*
Epinephrine, 315t
Equilibrium, tracer uptake and, 16
Equilibrium methods, in left ventricular function and volume measurement, 203, 204-205, 206-208
Estrogen, cardioprotective role of, 298
Ethiodol, 384, *384*
Exercise testing; *see also* Stress echocardiography
bicycle, 349, 372-373
contraindications, 313
in coronary artery disease, 373, 374
electrocardiography
prognostic value of, 338, *338, 339*
in revascularization procedures, 419-420
pharmacologic stress testing vs., 327
predischarge, in risk stratification after acute myocardial infarction
electrocardiographic stress testing, 454-455
multivessel disease detection, 457-458, *457-458*
myocardial perfusion imaging, 455-456, *457*
perfusion imaging in thrombolytic era, 456
reduction in late heart failure after infarction, *460*, 460-461
separation of high-risk and low-risk subsets, 458-460, 459t, *459-460*
in preoperative risk stratification, 348-350, 349t
radionuclide angiography, 205, 209-210, 368, 400, 418-419, 462-463
recurrent chest pain after angioplasty and, 411, *412*
restenosis and, 414
technetium-99m–labeled agents in, 275-277, *276*
in unstable angina, 495, 496
in women, 301-302, *302*, 302t, 303
Exercise thallium-201 SPECT
antiischemic therapy results assessed with, 261-263, *262-265*
in coronary artery disease detection, 242, *243*, 243t
bypass graft stenosis, 244-245, *246*
effect of stenosis severity on results of scintigraphy, 245-246, *247*, 248
individual coronary artery stenosis, 242, 244, *244*, 245t
influence of exercise performance, 248-249, *248-249*
prognostic value of, 338, 339
protocols, 237-238